Textbook of Interventional Cardiovascular Pharmacology

Textbook of Interventional Cardiovascular Pharmacology

Nicholas N. Kipshidze MD PhD
FACC FESC FSCAI
Professor of Medicine and Surgery
Consultant Cardiologist
Cardiovascular Research Foundation
Director of Research
Lenox Hill Heart and Vascular Institute
New York NY USA
Director and Physician in Chief
Central University Hospital
Tbilisi Georgia

Jawed Fareed PhD FACB
Professor of Pathology and
Pharmacology
Director of Hemostasis and
Thrombosis Research Laboratories
and Department of Pathology
Loyola University, Stritch School
of Medicine
Maywood IL USA

Jeffrey W. Moses MD FACC
Professor of Medicine
Director, Center for Interventional
Vascular Therapy
Director, Cardiac Catheterization
Laboratories
Columbia University Medical Center
New York-Presbyterian Hospital
New York NY USA

Patrick W. Serruys MD PhD
FACC FESC
Professor and Head
Interventional Department
Thoraxcenter
Erasmus University Medical Center
Rotterdam
The Netherlands

Associate Editor:
Cathy Kennedy MLS
Columbia University Medical Center
New York NY
USA

Forewords by Valentin Fuster MD PhD and Richard H. Kennedy PhD

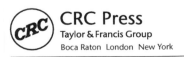
CRC Press
Taylor & Francis Group
Boca Raton London New York

CRC Press is an imprint of the
Taylor & Francis Group, an **informa** business

CRC Press
Taylor & Francis Group
6000 Broken Sound Parkway NW, Suite 300
Boca Raton, FL 33487-2742

First issued in paperback 2019

© 2010 by Taylor & Francis Group, LLC
CRC Press is an imprint of Taylor & Francis Group, an Informa business

No claim to original U.S. Government works

ISBN-13: 978-1-84184-438-1 (hbk)
ISBN-13: 978-0-367-38902-4 (pbk)

A CIP record for this book is available from the British Library.

Library of Congress Cataloging-in-Publication Data available on application

Visit the Taylor & Francis Web site at
http://www.taylorandfrancis.com

and the CRC Press Web site at
http://www.crcpress.com

Contents

Part I Systemic and Endoluminal Therapy

Contributors

Alexandre C. Abizaid MD PhD
Institute Dante Pazzanese of Cardiology
São Paulo
Brazil

Steven J. Adelman PhD
Nano Medical, Inc.
Doylestown PA
USA

Raul Altman MD PhD
Centro de Trombosis de Buenos Aires
Buenos Aires
Argentina

James J. Barry PhD
Boston Scientific Corporation
Corporate Research and Advanced Technology
    Department
Natick MA
USA

Michel E. Bertrand MD FRCP FACC FAHA
Lille Heart Institute
Lille
France

Rodger L. Bick MD PhD FACP
Clinical Professor of Medicine
University of Texas Southwestern Medical Center
Director, Thrombosis Hemostasis and Vascular
    Medicine Clinical Center
Dallas TX
USA

Munir Boodhwani MD
BIDMC/Harvard Medical School
Boston MA
USA

Mehgan Businaro MD
Midwestern University
Downers Grove IL
USA

Valeri S. Chekanov MD PhD
Heart Care Associates
Milwaukee Heart Institute
Milwaukee WI
USA

Derek P. Chew MBBS MPH FCSANZ
Green Lane Cardiovascular Research Unit
Flinders University and Medical Centre
Adelaide
Australia

Antonio Colombo MD
EMO Centro Luore Columbus and San
    Raffaele Hospital
Milan
Italy

Umberto Cornelli MD PhD
President, European Society of Biological Nutrition
Loyola University Medical School
Chicago IL
USA

Erwin Coyne PhD
Hines Veteran Affairs Hospital
Hines IL
USA

George D. Dangas MD PhD
Department of Medicine
Columbia University Medical Center
Program Director, Interventional Cardiology
New York-Presbyterian Hospital
New York NY
USA

Rajesh M. Dave MD
Associate Cardiologists
Harrisburg PA
USA

Raphaelle Dumaine MD
Institut de Cardiologie
Pitié-Salpêtriére University Hospital
Paris
France

Victor J. Dzau MD
Professor of Medicine
Duke University Medical Center
Durham NC
USA

Robert Falotico MD PhD
Cordis Corporation
Warren NJ
USA

Jawed Fareed PhD FACB
Professor of Pathology and Pharmacology
Director of Hemostasis and
    Thrombosis Research Laboratories
    and Department of Pathology
Loyola University, Stritch School of Medicine
Maywood IL USA

Omar Farouque MBBS (Hons) PhD
FRACP FACC
Interventional Cardiologist
Department of Cardiology
Austin Health
Melbourne
Australia

James J. Ferguson MD
Cardiology Research
Bayler College of Medicine
The University of Texas Health Care Center
Houston TX
USA

Anthony Gershlick MBBS MRCS LRCP
Cardiology Clinical Sciences Department
Glenfield Hospital
Leicester
UK

Mihai Gheorghiade MD FACC
Feinberg School of Medicine
Northwestern University
Chicago IL
USA

Clarence E. Grim BS MS MD
Clinical Professor of Medicine and Epidemiology
Shared Care Research, Education and Consulting Inc.
Milwaukee WI
USA

Paul A. Gurbel MD
Director, Sinai Center for Thrombosis Research
Sinai Hospital of Balimore
Associate Professor of Medicine
Department of Medicine
Johns Hopkins University
Baltimore MD
USA

Amir Halkin MD
Lenox Hill Heart and Vascular Institute
New York NY
USA

María de Lourdes Herrera PhD
Centro de Trombosis de Buenos Aires
Buenos Aires
Argentina

Ralph Hein MD
Cardiovascular Center Frankfurt
Frankfurt
Germany

Markus Hinder MD
Sanofi-Aventis, Science & Medical Affairs
Frankfurt
Germany

David R. Holmes, Jr MD
Division of Cardiovascular Diseases and
    Internal Medicine
Mayo Clinic
Rochester MN
USA

Debra A. Hoppensteadt PhD
Department of Pathology
Loyola University, Stritch School of Medicine
Maywood IL
USA

Yanming Huang MD PhD
Departments of Cardiology and Cell Biology
The Cleveland Clinic Foundation
Cleveland OH
USA

Ioannis Iakovou MD
Department of Cardiology
Army Hospital of Thessaloniki and
    Blue Cross Heart Centre
Thessaloniki
Greece

Omer Iqbal MD FACC
Department of Pathology
Loyola University, Stritch School of Medicine
Maywood IL
USA

Patrick Iversen PhD
AVI-BioPharma
Corvallis OR
USA

Sriram S. Iyer MD
Lenox Hill Hospital
New York NY
USA

Graham Jackson FRCP
Guys & St. Thomas Hospital
Cardiology Department
London
UK

Michael R. Jaff DO FACP FACC
Assistant Professor of Medicine
Harvard Medical School
Director, Vascular Medicine
Massachusetts General Hospital
Boston MA
USA

Walter Jeske PhD
Cardiovascular Institute
Loyola University Medical Center
Maywood IL
USA

Torfi F. Jonasson MD PhD
Department of Cardiology
University Hospital of Iceland
Reykjavik
Iceland

Luc J. Jordaens MD PhD
Erasmus University
Thoraxcenter
Rotterdam
The Netherlands

Brigitte Kaiser MD PhD
Friedrich Schiller University Jena
Faculty of Medicine
Institute for Vascular Medicine
Jena
Germany

Kalpana R. Kamath PhD
Boston Scientific Corporation
Corporate Research and Advanced
    Technology Department
Natick MA
USA

Barry T. Katzen MD
Founder and Medical Director
Baptist Cardiac and Vascular Institute
Miami FL
USA

Sanjay Kaul MD
Director, Vascular Physiology and
    Thrombosis Laboratory
Division of Cardiology
Cedars-Sinai Medical Center
Professor, David Geffen School of
    Medicine UCLA
Los Angeles CA
USA

Nicholas N. Kipshidze MD PhD
FACC FESC FSCAI

Professor of Medicine and Surgery

Consultant Cardiologist
Cardiovascular Research Foundation
Director of Research
Lenox Hill Heart and Vascular Institute
New York NY USA
Director and Physician in Chief
    Central University Hospital
Tbilisi Georgia

Roger J. Laham MD
BIDMC/Harvard Medical School
Boston MA
USA

Zoran Lasic MD FACC
Department of Interventional Cardiology
Lenox Hill Hospital
New York NY
USA

Volker Laux PhD
Thrombosis Research Department
Bayer Healthcare AC
Wuppertal
Germany

Edwin Lee MD PhD
Fellow in Cardiology
Albert Einstein College of Medicine
Montefiore Medical Center
Bronx NY
USA

Sam J. Lehman MBBS
Flinders University and Medical Centre
Adelaide
Australia

Martin B. Leon MD FACC
Cardiovascular Research Foundation,
Center for Interventional Vascular Therapy
Columbia University Medical Center
New York NY
USA

Basil S. Lewis MD FRCP FACC
Department of Cardiovascular Medicine
Lady Davis Carmel Medical Center
Haifa
Israel

Bruce E. Lewis MD
Division of Cardiology
Loyola University Medical Center
Maywood IL
USA

Ferdinand Leya MD
Division of Cardiology
Loyola University Medical Center
Maywood IL
USA

Xiaoshun Liu MD PhD
Department of Cardiology
University Hospital
Leuven
Belgium

Alexandra A. MacLean MD
Assistant Professor of Surgery
Department of Surgery
New York Hospital, Queens
Flushing NY
USA

Carlo Di Mario MD PhD FACC, FESC
Department of Cardiology
Royal Brompton Hospital
London
UK

Takefumi Matsuo MD
Hyogo Prefectural Awaji Hospital
Hyogo-ken
Japan

Luis G. Melo PhD
Associate Professor of Physiology
Department of Physiology
College of Medicine
Queen's University
Kingston Ontario
Canada

Harry L. Messmore MD
Cancer Center
Loyola University Medical Center
Maywood IL
USA

Kathleen M. Miller PhD
Boston Scientific Corporation
Corporate Research and Advanced
    Technology Department
Natick MA
USA

Gilles Montalescot MD FESC
Institut de Cardiologie
Pitie-Salpetriere University Hospital
Paris
France

John F. Moran MD
Professor of Medicine
Loyola University, Stritch School
    of Medicine
Maywood IL
USA

Jeffrey W. Moses MD FACC
Professor of Medicine
Director, Center for Interventional
    Vascular Therapy
Director, Cardiac Catheterization
    Laboratories
Columbia University Medical Center
New York-Presbyterian Hospital
New York NY USA

Shaker A. Mousa PhD MBA FACC FACB
Pharmaceutical Research Institute
Albany College of Pharmacy
Albany NY
USA

Hans Ohlin MD PhD
Department of Cardiology
University Hospital Lund
Lund
Sweden

Masanori Osakabe
Metsubishi Pharma Corporation
Tokyo
Japan

Harald Ott MD
Scientific Director
Center for Cardiovascular Repair
University of Minnesota
Minneapolis MN
USA

Alok S. Pachori PhD
Instructor in Medicine
Duke University Medical Center
Durham NC
USA

Ravi K. Ramana DO
Division of Cardiology
Loyola University Medical Center
Maywood IL
USA

Alfredo E. Rodriguez MD PhD FACC FSCAI
Otamendi Hospital - Cardiac Unit
Buenos Aires
Argentina

Gary S. Roubin MD PhD
Lenox Hill Hospital
New York NY
USA

Alejandra Scazziota PhD
Centro de Trombosis de Buenos Aires
Buenos Aires
Argentina

Ivan De Scheerder MD PhD
Global Medical Services
Keeromstraat
Herent
Belgium

M. F. Scholten MD
Erasmus University
Thoraxcenter
Rotterdam
The Netherlands

Patrick W. Serruys MD PhD FACC FESC
Professor and Head
Interventional Department
Thoraxcenter
Erasmus University Medical Center
Rotterdam
The Netherlands

Asad Shaikh MD
Dayton Interventional Radiology
Kettering OH
USA

Rakesh Sharma MRCP PhD
Department of Cardiology
Royal Brompton Hospital
London
UK

Horst Sievert MD
Professor of Medicine
Cardiovascular Center
Frankfurt
Germany

Christodoulos Stefanadis MD PhD
Professor of Cardiology
Athens Medical School
Paleo Psychico
Athens
Greece

Shunji Suzuki MD
HIT Information Center
Hyogo-ken
Japan

Neil Swanson MD
Cardiology Clinical Sciences Department
Glenfield Hospital
Leicester
UK

Mubin Syed MD
Clinical Associate Professor of Radiology
Wright State University School of Medicine
Dayton OH
USA

Jean-François Tanguay MD
Department of Medicine
Montreal Heart Institute
Montreal Quebec
Canada

Udaya S. Tantry PhD
Sinai Center for Thrombosis Research
Sinai Hospital of Baltimore
Baltimore MD
USA

Doris A. Taylor PhD
Scientific Director
Center for Cardiovascular Repair
University of Minnesota
Minneapolis MN
USA

Andrew M. Tonkin MBBS MD FRACP
Head, Cardiovascular Research Unit
Department of Epidemiology and
    Preventive Medicine
Monash University
Central and Eastern Clinical School
Alfred Hospital
Melbourne
Australia

Konstantinos Toutouzas MD PhD
Athens Medical School
Athens
Greece

Waqas Ullah MBBS
Department of Cardiology
Royal Brompton Hospital
London
UK

Yves L. E. Van Belle MD
Erasmus University
Thoraxcenter
Rotterdam
The Netherlands

Freek W. A. Verheugt MD
Professor of Cardiology
University Medical Center St. Radboud
Nijmegen
The Netherlands

Jiri Vitek MD PhD
Lenox Hill Hospital
New York NY
USA

Ron Waksman MD
Washington Hospital Center
Washington DC
USA

Jeanine M. Walenga PhD
Professor, Thoracic and Cardiovascular Surgery
Loyola University, Stritch School of Medicine
Maywood IL
USA

Lan Wang MD
Institute of Pathology
Casewestern Reserve University
Cleveland OH
USA

Hikari Watanabe MD
Mitsubishi Pharma Corporation
Tokyo
Japan

William Wehrmacher MD
Cancer Center
Loyola University Medical Center
Maywood IL
USA

Mitchell D. Weinberg MD
New York-Presbyterian Hospital
Columbia University Medical Center
New York NY
USA

Thomas L. Wenger MD FACC
President
Wenger Consulting
Durham NC
USA

Harvey D. White DSc FCSANZ
Director of Coronary Care Unit
Green Lane Cardiovascular Unit
Auckland City Hospital
Auckland
New Zealand

Neil Wilson MD
Cardiovascular Center
Frankfurt
Germany
Department of Paediatric Cardiology
John Radcliffe Hospital
Oxford
UK

Joanna J. Wykrzykowska MD
BIDMC/Harvard Medical School
Boston MA
USA

Nicholas H. G. Yeo
Chief Executive Officer
Vascular Reconditioning, Inc.
Snoqualmie WA
USA

Jonathon Zhao PhD
Cordis Corporation
Warren NJ
USA

Foreword

I am pleased to write this introduction for the *Textbook of Interventional Cardiovascular Pharmacology*. This definitive international textbook on cardiovascular pharmacology for interventional procedures incorporates contributions from world opinion leaders and a transatlantic perspective. This textbook is a first of its kind for practicing interventional cardiologists, cardiologists, and pharmacologists.

Edited by Nicholas N. Kipshidze, Jawed Fareed, Jeffrey W. Moses, and Patrick W. Serruys, the *Textbook of Interven- tional Cardiovascular Pharmacology* is an outstanding text that focuses primarily on currently used pharmacologic agents, interventional approaches, and the delivery techniques available for treatment of cardiovascular diseases. In looking forward, the book also covers the exciting potential of various experimental drug therapies such as angiogenetic agents to treat the ischemic heart and limb, cardiovascular cell transplantation to treat the underlying injuries associated with cardiac and vascular disease, and the promising results of clinical trials in these rapidly moving fields. To this end the editors have assembled an impressive roster of international contributors who are all active in the field of interventional cardiology and write from a hands-on perspective. They have analyzed an enormous range of various cardiovascular pharmacological therapies in superbly illustrated and clearly focused chapters.

The book is comprised of five sections with part I covering systemic and endoluminal therapy with an incisive overview of hemostasis and thrombosis; part II covers local therapy with several chapters devoted to drug-eluting stents and restenosis therapies; part III covers cell therapy and therapeutic angiogenesis and includes chapters on cell transplantation and clinical trials in cellular therapy; part IV covers adjunctive pharmacotherapy with chapters devoted to various patient populations including those with heart failure, diabetes, atrial fibrillation, peripheral artery disease,

acute coronary syndrome, and chronic total occlusions; and part V covers noncoronary interventions such as carotid artery stenting, repair of abdominal aortic aneurysms, and alcohol septal ablation. The text is written with best clinical practice in mind yet provides much information that is translational in nature. The final chapter is an epilogue that provides an objective opinion on current drug development in vascular medicine and interventions. In addition, there is a handy drug table comparing the pharmacokinetics of the various anticoagulants used in cardiovascular medicine.

Perhaps for the next edition the editors will include a separate section on imaging since it is a very important development in this decade and promises to stimulate the interest of all concerned and interested in cardiovascular disease, from those in basic science, to those in the interventional and pharmacological fields and to those interested in clinical trials and outcomes.

In summary Nicholas N. Kipshidze, Jawed Fareed, Jeffrey W. Moses, and Patrick W. Serruys have put together an outstanding textbook covering a broad range of topics in cardiovascular pharmacology. I would recommend this book to anyone working in the field of cardiovascular disease, clinical research, and pharmacology.

Valentin Fuster MD PhD
Director, Zena and Michael A. Wiener Cardiovascular
Institute and the Marie-Josee and Henry R. Kravis Center
for Cardiovascular Health
The Mount Sinai Medical Center
Professor of Medicine
Mount Sinai School of Medicine
New York NY
USA
Past President, American Heart Association
Immediate Past President, World Heart Federation

Foreword

The *Textbook of Interventional Cardiovascular Pharmacology* is an excellent up-to-date text that focuses on agents, interventional approaches, and delivery techniques that are available for treatment of, and to some extent prevention of, disease states arising from vascular and intravascular pathologies. Part I focuses on hemostasis and thrombosis, including chapters on available anticoagulant, antiplatelet, and fibrinolytic therapies. Also covered in this section are anti-restenotic drugs and approaches at minimizing proliferative and atherosclerotic processes. The second section, on local therapy, includes chapters on drug-eluting stents, antiproliferative and antimigratory drugs, and use of growth factor, gene therapy, antisense, and photodynamic approaches. Part III examines current knowledge regarding cell therapy approaches for cardiovascular repair. Part IV addresses use of adjunctive pharmacotherapy in a number of patient populations, such as those with heart failure, diabetes, peripheral artery disease, and erectile dysfunction, and the final section discusses non-coronary interventions and structural diseases of the heart.

Each chapter in this work provides a thorough evaluation and concise presentation that highlights both recent advances in the field as well as the current overall understanding of the topic. Although written with the best clinical practice in mind, the text provides a wealth of information that is truly translational in nature, bridging pathogenesis and mechanism of action with therapeutic approach. I commend the editors for developing the vision of such a text, and congratulate each of the authors for the depth and clarity of their presentation. I would recommend this text to anyone working in the field of vascular and intravascular disease. Basic, clinical, and translational scientists, practicing clinicians, and clinical and research trainees can all benefit from the information included in individual chapters as well as from the overall scope and breadth of knowledge presented.

Richard H. Kennedy PhD
Senior Associate Dean for Research
Professor of Physiology and Pharmacology
Loyola University
Stritch School of Medicine
Chicago IL
USA

Preface

The last quarter of a century has seen dramatic developments in the management of cardiovascular diseases. Besides the pioneering developments in the medical management of cardiovascular disorders the field of interventional cardiology has also emerged as a major discipline with a huge impact on the clinical management of acute coronary syndrome, chronic coronary artery disease, congestive heart failure, and peripheral vascular and valvular diseases. Percutaneous interventions necessitated the development of newer agents and drugs for the imaging, anticoagulation, vascular tone control, and post-interventional proliferative control processes. Drug coating of mechanical devices posed yet another challenge in addressing the safety issues related to these modified devices.

The last decade has witnessed a major breakthrough in the use of mechanical support devices such as stents and newer drugs, which has revolutionized the field of interventional cardiology. Moreover, novel uses of drugs, such as drug-coated stents and grafts have emerged. While conventional drugs, such as aspirin, heparin, and clopidrogel, are commonly used in the short-and long-term treatment of patients who have undergone interventions, many newer drugs and drug combinations have been developed.

The molecular and cellular understanding of the pathogenesis of cardiovascular diseases, in particular acute coronary syndromes, and the use of interventional procedures in their management has identified several newer targets to optimize clinical management of patients undergoing these procedures. In the area of newer drugs developed in conjunction with interventional procedures, progress has been remarkable and there has been an influx of massive information on their pharmacology and toxicology. Recognizing the importance of this developing area and its impact on interventional cardiology practice, the editors identified the need of a comprehensive reference book covering this topic. Having such information in one volume is projected to meet the need of practicing interventional cardiologists to obtain objective knowledge of the newer drugs used in interventional cardiology. It is hoped that this book will provide a comprehensive coverage of pharmacologic agents which are currently used and for those that are in clinical trials and will soon become available for clinical use. The use of drugs for the acute and extended indications in this area is in transition. The recommendations from peer groups undergo periodic revisions due to the introduction of newer devices and/or newer drugs. Thus, it provides a moving target to develop guidelines. This book is intended to provide some of the fundamental knowledge as a foundation to appreciate the ongoing developments in the area of interventional sciences.

This book is comprised of over fifty chapters, each of which is written by an expert in the assigned topic. Assembling a multi-authored specialized pharmacology book is a major challenge for both the authors and the editors. Because of the influx of newer information, differing opinions, data interpretation and regulatory positions, the authors are challenged to provide the most practical, unbiased and helpful information on specific topics. The editors are grateful to the authors contributing to this book for their excellent and objective manuscripts which are written in an integrated fashion to provide an updated and comprehensive account of different drugs and devices.

This book is divided into five parts comprised of systemic and endoluminal therapy, local therapy, therapeutic angiogenesis, adjunctive pharmacotherapy and noncoronary interventions. The first chapter is on hemostasis and thrombosis and is included since many of the new drugs target the components of the hemostatic system including cellular sites and receptors on platelets, endothelial cells, white cells and blood proteins. The last chapter is written as an epilogue to provide an objective opinion on current drug development in vascular medicine and interventions. It is hoped that the individual chapters included will provide updated references to practicing clinicians and those who are involved in the development of newer drugs.

This book is also intended to serve as a comprehensive reference and a practical guide in the application of drugs and devices used for primary coronary angioplasty, coronary thrombolysis and the correction in ST segment elevation in acute coronary syndrome. Specialized topics such as drug coated stents, molecular therapies, cellular therapies, newer pharmacologic approaches and specific topics on noncoronary interventions are also reported. It is hoped that this book will be periodically updated to reflect the ongoing developments in this fast moving area.

Nicholas N. Kipshidze
Jawed Fareed
Jeffrey W. Moses
Patrick W. Serruys

Acknowledgments

The editors are tremendously grateful to all of the contributing authors, who have voluntarily provided their expert chapters. The editors are also grateful to Ms. Cathy Kennedy, associate editor, who has been extremely helpful throughout this project and without whose help it would have been difficult to publish this book. The publishers, in particular Mr. Oliver Walter, development editor, and Mr. Alan Burgess, commissioning editor, are to be thanked for their commitment and support in publishing this timely book on interventional pharmacology.

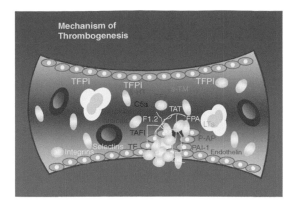

Figure 1.1
The primary hemostatic response. *(See p. 2.)*

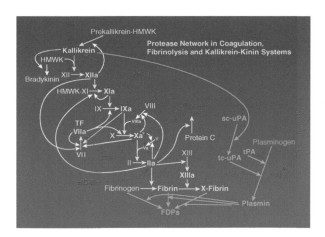

Figure 1.2
The coagulation cascade. *(See p. 2.)*

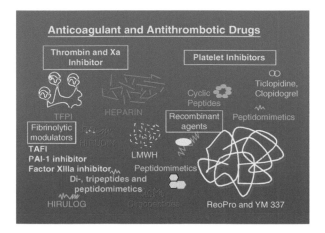

Figure 1.3
Current anticoagulant and anti-thrombotic drugs *(See p. 20.)*

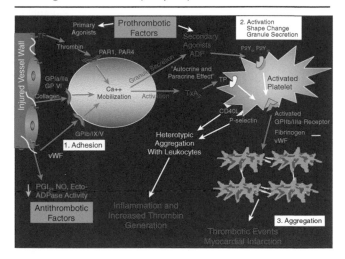

Figure 13.1
Role of platelet activation and aggregation in cardiovascular diseases. *(See p. 140.)*

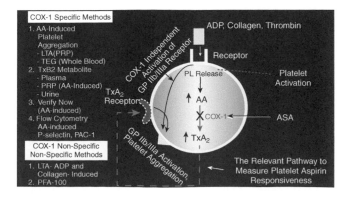

Figure 13.2
Mechanism of action of aspirin and laboratory evaluation of aspirin responsiveness. *(See p. 141.)*

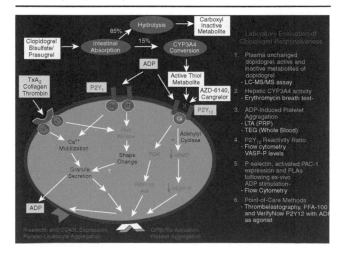

Figure 13.3
Mechanism of action of clopidogrel and laboratory evaluation of clopidogrel nonresponsiveness. *(See p. 145.)*

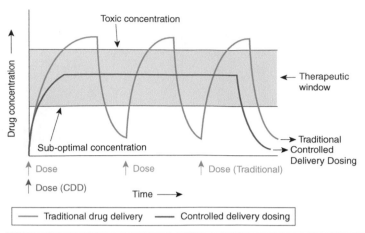

Toxic concentration

Therapeutic window

Sub-optimal concentration

Drug concentration →

↑ Dose   ↑ Dose   ↑ Dose (Traditional)

↑ Dose (CDD)   Time →

Traditional
Controlled
Delivery Dosing

—— Traditional drug delivery   —— Controlled delivery dosing

Figure 22.1

Drug levels in the blood with traditional drug delivery and controlled-delivery dosing. *(See p. 268.)*

Rat subcutaneous implant

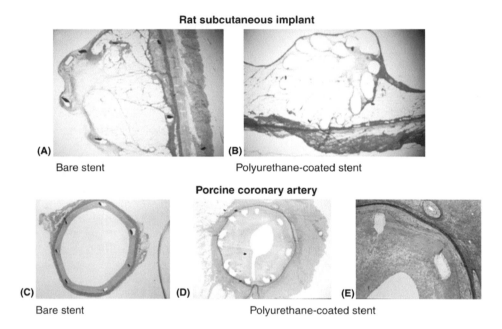

(A) Bare stent

(B) Polyurethane-coated stent

Porcine coronary artery

(C) Bare stent

(D) (E) Polyurethane-coated stent

Figure 22.3

Effect of animal model and implant site on biologic response to polyurethane stents. *(See p. 272.)*

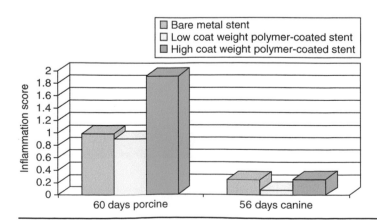

☐ Bare metal stent
☐ Low coat weight polymer-coated stent
☐ High coat weight polymer-coated stent

Inflammation score

60 days porcine   56 days canine

Figure 22.5

Strut-associated inflammation in response to the polyethylene-co-vinyl acetate—poly-*n*-butyl methacrylate polymers in porcine and canine models at two months. *(See p. 273.)*

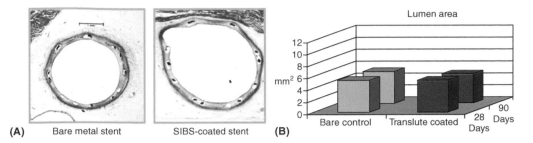

(A) Bare metal stent   SIBS-coated stent   **(B)**

Figure 22.8

Vascular compatibility of poly(styrene-*b*-isobutylene-*b*-styrene) (SIBS) as examined in the porcine coronary model. *(See p. 274.)*

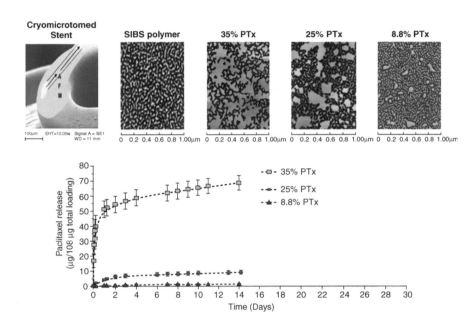

Figure 22.9

Atomic force microscopy images and drug release kinetics of the paclitaxel-poly(styrene-*b*-isobutylene-*b*-styrene) polymer combination. *(See p. 275.)*

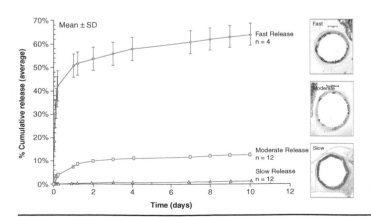

Figure 22.10

Vascular response to slow-, moderate-, and fast-release formulations of paclitaxel in the porcine coronary artery model. *(See p. 275.)*

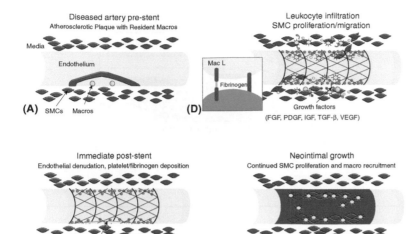

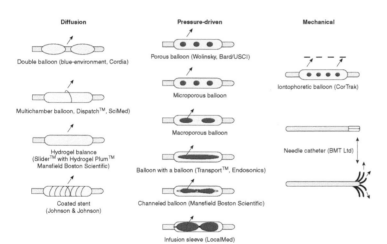

Figure 25.1
Pathophysiology of restenosis *(See p. 300.)*

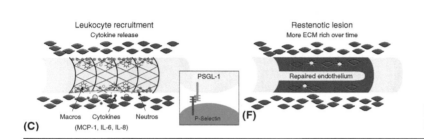

Figure 25.2
Types of catheter-based local delivery devices. *(See p. 302.)*

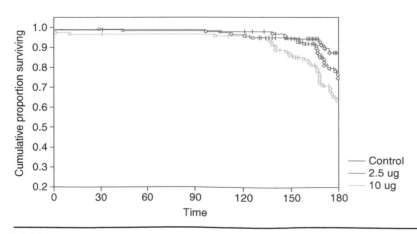

Figure 25.3
Event-free survival at six months in the ACTinomycin-eluting stent improves outcomes by reduction of neointimal hyperplasia trial of the actinomycin-eluting stent. *(See p. 304.)*

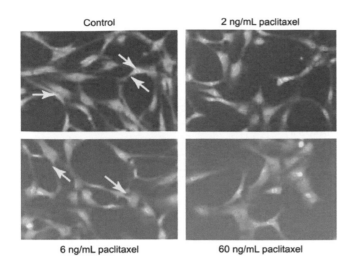

Control · 2 ng/mL paclitaxel

6 ng/mL paclitaxel · 60 ng/mL paclitaxel

Figure 25.5
Effect of paclitaxel on smooth muscle cell morphology.
(See p. 305.)

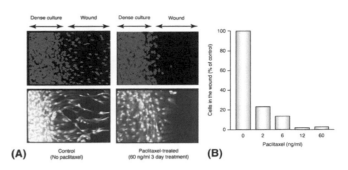

(A) Control (No paclitaxel) · Paclitaxel-treated (60 ng/ml 3 day treatment) **(B)**

Figure 25.6
The effects of paclitaxel on smooth muscle cell migration.
(See p. 306.)

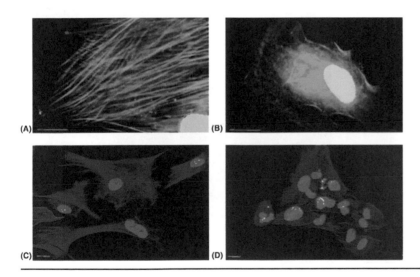

(A) **(B)** **(C)** **(D)**

Figure 25.7
Immunofluorescence micrographs demonstrating the effect of 1.0 μmol/L paclitaxel on the distribution of the contractile filament smooth muscle α-actin and the intermediate filament vimentin in haSMCs.
(See p. 307.)

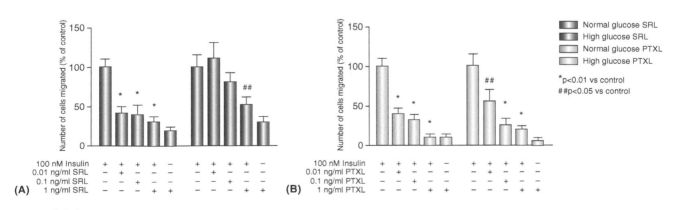

Normal glucose SRL
High glucose SRL
Normal glucose PTXL
High glucose PTXL

*p<0.01 vs control
##p<0.05 vs control

Figure 25.8
The effects of sirolimus and paclitaxel on smooth muscle cell migration under conditions of normal and high glucose. *Source: (See p. 307.)*

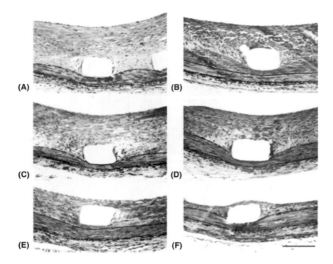

Figure 25.10
Inhibition of restenosis by paclitaxel inhibits in a porcine coronary model. *(See p. 309.)*

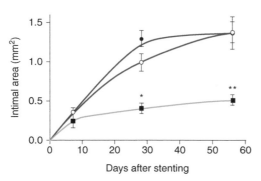

─○─ Uncoated stent
─●─ Poly(lactide-co-Σ-caprolactone)-coated stent
─■─ Poly(lactide-co-Σ-caprolactone)-coated paclitaxel-releasing stent

Figure 25.11
Sustained reduction in neointimal hyperplasia in the rabbit iliac model. *(See p. 309.)*

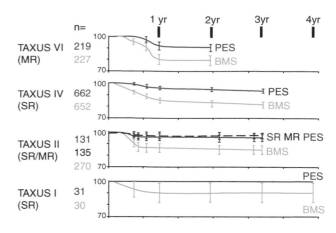

Figure 25.12
Sustained freedom from target lesion revascularization in TAXUS clinical trials.*(See p. 309.)*

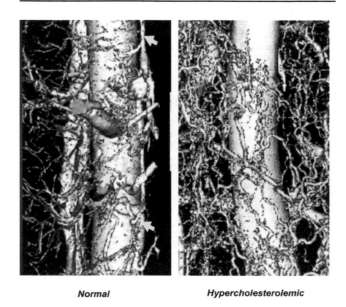

Normal   *Hypercholesterolemic*

Figure 28.1
The development of neovascularization in a hypercholesterolemic model is shown in the right panel. *(See p. 341.)*

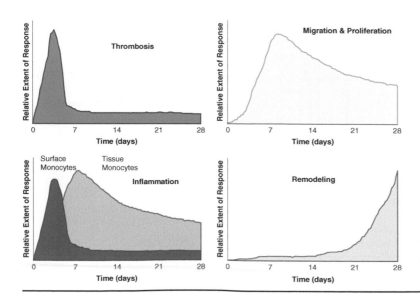

Figure 27.3
The phases and their timing in the restenosis process. *(See p. 329.)*

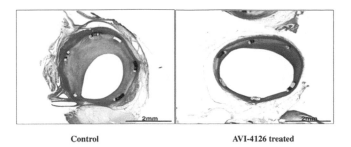

Figure 32.2
Polymer-coated stent delivery of c-myc antisense phosphorodiamidate morpholino oligomers into swine vessels. *(See p. 376.)*

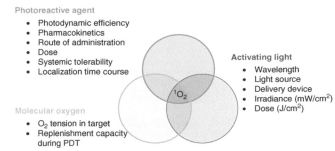

Figure 33.2
Summary of the interaction of the three elements required for photodynamic effect. *(See p. 382.)*

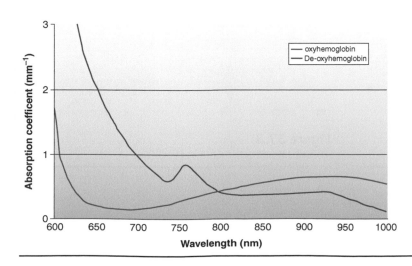

Figure 33.3
Microscopy with 405 nm excitation reveals red fluorescence from talaporfin (LS11/NPe6) *(See p. 384.)*

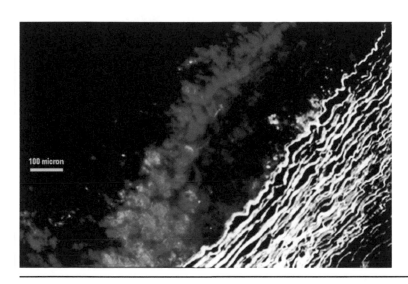

Figure 33.4
Absorption coefficient of oxyhemoglobin and de-oxyhemoglobin as a function of wavelength. *(See p. 386.)*

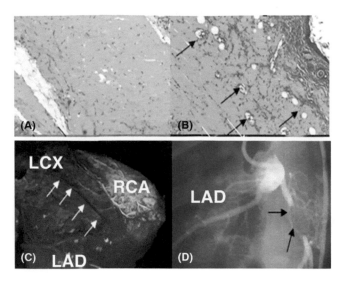

Figure 35.3
Histological analysis in the ameroid constrictor model
(See p. 409.)

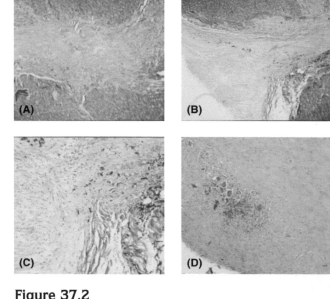

Figure 37.2
Fibrosis and lack of viability of skeletal myoblasts injected into
the myocardium of dogs. *(See p. 441.)*

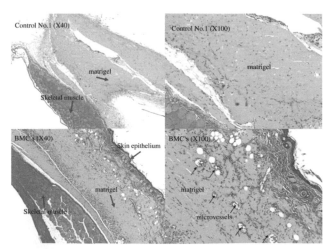

Figure 37.1
Bone marrow cell-induced capillary and neovessel formation.
(See p. 440.)

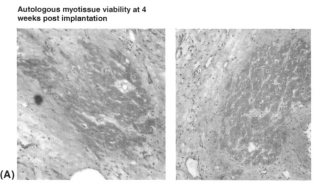

Figure 37.3
(A) Viability of myotissue *(See p. 448.)*

1

An overview of hemostasis and thrombosis

Walter Jeske, Debra A. Hoppensteadt, Asad Shaikh, Jeanine M. Walenga, Mamdouh Bakhos, and Jawed Fareed

Overview

In addition to surgical management of thrombotic disorders, in particular those involving the arterial system including Acute Coronary Syndrome (ACS), atrial fibrillation, thrombotic and ischemic stroke, and other ischemic and occlusive disorders, advanced interventional methods including stenting and molecular/cellular approaches involving genes and stem cell-based approaches are now used. Each year in the United States myocardial infarction contributes to over 600,000 deaths and an additional 800,000 deaths are attributed to this syndrome in hospital discharged patients. Thus, almost 1.5 million deaths are related to myocardial infarction and its manifestations. Percutaneous Interventions (PCI) have significantly contributed to the management of acute coronary syndrome and improved the clinical outcome in this syndrome. Similarly, interventional procedures have also been used in the management of atrial fibrillation and embolic stroke. Although the interventional methods have been extremely valuable, there are several specific pathophysiologic and pharmacologic problems, which require a continual review and assessment to optimize patient care. Coronary Interventions represent a controlled injury to the vessel wall resulting in the generation of tissue factor that initially promotes thrombogenesis at the site of injury. Regardless of the extent of this injury, both the acute and late occlusive process are often associated with PCI, necessitating pharmacological and mechanical measures to avoid occlusive events. Many of the fateful events occur in patients free of coronary artery diseases, with almost an equal number of events occuring in those with known coronary artery diseases already receiving therapy, including PCI and aggressive medical therapy with statins, antiplatelet drugs, and anticoagulants. A great number of these infarctions result from the rupture of high-risk unstable plaque that in most cases did not impede flow before the acute events. Therefore, it is quite clear that newer approaches must be developed to understand the pathogenesis of occlusive coronary events and to develop methods for their optimal management. Risk assessment involving newer approaches based on genetic predisposition, lifestyle, and other contributing factors may be important. Other problems related to the management of vascular injury, the patency of the stents, and the role of different drugs used in the control and mediation of the thrombotic and bleeding complications observed during and after PCI require serious considerations. Interventional approaches have been in an evolutionary phase for the past two decades. Besides the proper understanding of pathogenesis of the lesions requiring interventions, post-interventional monitoring and additional control of the pathogenesis of thrombotic and fibrotic complications is equally important. Excessive bleeding with the use of newer anticoagulants, thrombotic complications with drug-coated stents and molecular and cellular abberations due to gene and stem cell approaches will require further understanding of the mechanisms involved in these processes. A firm understanding of the hemostasis and thrombosis is crucial in the optimal management of patients undergoing interventions.

Introduction to hemostasis and thrombosis

Hemostasis as defined by Virchow in the last century is a fine balance between blood flow, humoral factors, and cellular elements of the vascular system. Today, molecular and cellular biology has advanced our understanding of the thrombotic and hemostatic processes and their regulation. Thrombotic and bleeding disorders are the most frequent causes of death. Heparin and warfarin have remained the sole antithrombotic agents to manage thrombosis. However, specific plasmatic and cellular sites in the thrombotic network can now be targeted and specific drugs based on the inhibition of factors Xa and IIa are being developed. Antibodies against specific platelet receptors as well as specific anti-tissue factor, antithrombin, and anti-Xa agents are being developed. Mutations of endogenous inhibitors have been identified as causes of congenital thrombophilias. The use of heparin has also greatly advanced with the availability of low molecular weight heparins. Several newer approaches to treat bleeding diatheses, including the use of recombinant factor VIII and VIIa, have evolved. Heparin is no longer solely a surgical anticoagulant, but is used to treat a variety of conditions including venous thrombosis, unstable angina, and myocardial infarction and is used in procedures such as angioplasty and stent implantation. The mechanism of heparin's action has become more complex with the discovery of tissue factor pathway inhibitor (TFPI), thrombin activatable fibrinolytic inhibitor, selectins, and other cellular targets where the drug is able to produce its effects.

Blood normally is maintained in the fluid state so that nutrients can be delivered to the various tissues of the body. When the integrity of the vascular system has been compromised, it becomes necessary for the blood to clot. As shown in Figure 1, the initial response to a break in the continuity of the vasculature is the formation of the platelet plug. Platelets in the flowing blood rapidly adhere to the exposed subendothelial vessel wall matrix and become activated. During this activation process, components of the platelet α and β granules (ATP, ADP, factor V, 5-HT) are released, causing further platelet aggregation. Also during these morphologic changes, activated platelets express protein and cell receptors and procoagulant phospholipids are expressed upon their surface. The damaged endothelium is also capable of releasing certain procoagulant substances and downregulates the fibrinolytic process, inflammation, complement activation, and the kallikrein system.

The negatively charged phospholipid phosphatidylserine is asymmetrically distributed in mammalian cell membranes, primarily on the inner leaflet. Upon exposure to collagen or thrombin, the distribution of phospholipids changes with increasing phosphatidylserine in the external membrane leaf (1). The increased expression of phosphatidylserine on the outer leaflet of the membrane creates a procoagulant surface on which several steps of the coagulation cascade take place.

The platelet plug initially arrests the loss of blood. This, however, is not a permanent blockade. The formation of a fibrin-based clot acts to stabilize the initial platelet plug. The coagulation system is a complex network of zymogens, which must be activated to ultimately form the fibrin strands of the blood clot. Upon activation, most of these coagulation proteins are converted into active serine proteases, which are similar to trypsin and chymotrypsin. Traditionally, coagulation has been viewed as having two distinct branches (2,3), the intrinsic and the extrinsic pathways. Today it has been widely accepted that the two pathways are linked prior to the generation of factor Xa (4). A schematic of the coagulation cascade is depicted in Figure 2.

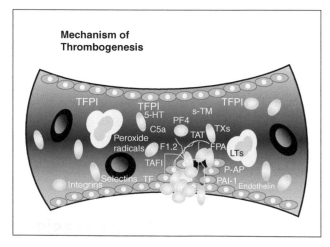

Figure 1
(*See color plate.*) The primary hemostatic response. Following loss of vascular integrity platelets adhere to subendothelial wall matrix, which triggers their activation. *Abbreviations*: HT, hydroxy tryptamine; TFPI, tissue factor pathway inhibitor.

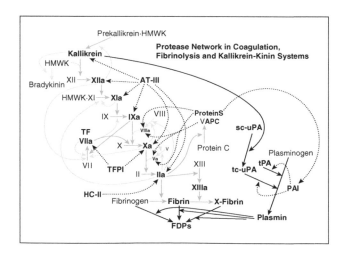

Figure 2
(*See color plate.*) The coagulation cascade. The formation of fibrin strands is the result of a sequential activation of a number of enzymes. The hemostatic balance is maintained by endogenous inhibitors such as AT, HC-II, and TFPI. *Abbreviations*: AT, antithrombin; TFPI, tissue factor pathway inhibitor.

Intrinsic pathway of coagulation

In the intrinsic pathway, factor XII becomes activated in the contact phase of coagulation. This occurs when factor XII, factor XI, prekallikrein, and high molecular weight kininogen come together on a negatively charged surface. While this reaction can take place in the laboratory on a negatively charged surface such as glass or kaolin, the physiologic surface is unknown. It has been proposed that this could be a tissue rich in collagen or sulphatides (5). By binding to the negatively charged surface, factor XII is converted to its active form through an unknown mechanism. The formation of factor XIIa is amplified by a positive feedback loop. Factor XIIa is capable of converting prekallikrein to kallikrein. Likewise, kallikrein converts factor XII to its active form. Factor XIIa also converts factor XI to factor XIa which in turn activates factor IX. Factor IXa, along with its cofactor factor VIII, calcium ions, and phospholipid membranes form the "tenase" complex which converts factor X to factor Xa thereby initiating the common pathway of coagulation. The phospholipid membrane in these complexes serves to lower the Km of the reaction. The phospholipid allows the enzyme to become saturated more easily and serves to localize the coagulation response to where it is most needed. The cofactor, factor V, increases the catalytic efficiency of the enzyme (6). Factor Xa joins with its cofactor factor V, calcium ions and phospholipid membranes to form the prothrombinase complex. The prothrombinase complex then acts to convert prothrombin into the active enzyme thrombin. Factors V and VIII are activated through proteolytic cleavage by factor Xa or thrombin. They are not, however, active proteases. Factor V is believed to have two rate-enhancing effects on the prothrombinase complex. In the prothrombinase complex, factor Xa and factor V are present in stoichiometric amounts resulting in an unknown alteration in the active site of factor Xa which increases its catalytic efficiency (7). Factor V also binds to prothrombin thus sequestering it at the site of assembly of the prothrombinase complex. Overall, these two actions of factor V result in a 300,000-fold increase in the rate of prothrombin conversion.

Thrombin serves many functions in coagulation. First, thrombin cleaves the soluble protein fibrinogen to generate the insoluble fibrin monomer. Fibrinogen circulates as a disulfide-linked dimer containing two A-α chains, two B-β chains, and two gamma chains. Cleavage of fibrinogen by thrombin results in the release of fibrinopeptides A and B and the exposure of charged domains at opposite ends of the molecule (8). Exposure of these charged domains leads to polymerization of the monomers. The release of fibrinopeptides A and B occur at different rates with fibrinopeptide A preferentially removed in mammalian systems (9,10). Removal of fibrinopeptide A leads to end-to-end fibrin polymerization whereas loss of fibrinopeptide B allows side-to-side polymerization of the end-to-end linked monomers (11). It is these monomers which are cross-linked by the transaminase factor XIIIa to form the meshwork of the thrombus. Thrombin also acts to augment its own generation by being a part of several positive feedback loops in the coagulation cascade. In these loops, thrombin activates factors XII, XI, VIII, and V. By activating the precursors to its own generation, thrombin greatly amplifies its own generation. Thrombin also activates platelets (12), activates the inhibitor Protein C through binding with thrombomodulin (13), and stimulates activated endothelial cells to release tissue plasminogen activator (14).

Extrinsic pathway of coagulation

The extrinsic pathway of coagulation is activated when circulating factor VII encounters tissue factor. Tissue factor is a transmembrane glycoprotein, which is normally expressed by subendothelial fibroblast-like cells, which surround the blood vessel. An intact endothelium normally shields the circulating blood from exposure to tissue factor. The tissue factor molecule consists of a 219 amino acid hydrophilic extracellular domain, a 23 amino acid hydrophobic region that spans the membrane, and a 21 amino acid cytoplasmic tail that anchors the molecule to the cell membrane (15,16). Other sites of tissue factor expression include activated monocytes, activated endothelial cells, and atherosclerotic plaques.

Factor VII exhibits a weak procoagulant activity on its own, typically accounting for about 1–2% of the total factor VII/VIIa activity (17). Upon binding to tissue factor, a 10,000,000-fold increase in factor VIIa enzymatic activity is observed (18). Both factor VII and factor VIIa bind to tissue factor with equal affinity (19). How factor VII is initially activated is not known, though it is hypothesized that factor Xa can activate factor VII in a back-activation reaction. The factor VIIa–tissue factor complex can then activate factor X leading to the generation of thrombin and ultimately to the formation of fibrin strands.

It has been shown in 1977 and more recently appreciated that the tissue factor–factor VIIa complex also activates factor IX to factor IXa, thus interacting with "intrinsic" pathway enzymes (4). This is believed to be important for maintaining the clotting process. Direct activation of factor X by factor VIIa–tissue factor can rapidly initiate coagulation, but both of these enzymes are quickly inhibited by the endogenous inhibitor TFPI. By activating factor IX, the tissue factor–VIIa complex initiates two pathways for thrombin generation. The small amounts of factor Xa generated prior to TFPI inhibition are sufficient to cleave prothrombin and generate a small amount of thrombin. This thrombin is then capable of back-activating factors V, VIII, and possibly XI, thereby sustaining clot formation through generation of thrombin via the intrinsic pathway. It has been observed that the activation of factor X by the factor IXa–VIII complex in the presence of calcium and phospholipids is 50 times greater than by the tissue factor–VIIa complex (20). Factor XI activation has been shown to occur in the presence of thrombin and a polyanion cofactor (21,22). Activation without the cofactor has been observed to be poor. A physiologic cofactor has not been elucidated. It has been reasoned that if the direct activation of factor X by VIIa–tissue factor is the sole source of thrombin generation, there would be no manifestation of hemophilia, a genetic deficiency of either factor IX or factor VIII.

Role of platelets in hemostasis and thrombosis

Platelets are disc-shaped, anuclear cells which circulate in a non-adhesive state in the undamaged circulation (23). These cells contain a contractile system and a number of storage granules. The α storage granules contain platelet factor 4 (PF4), ß-thromboglobulin, platelet derived growth factor (PDGF), fibrinogen, factor V, and von Willebrand factor (24). The dense or β-granules contain ATP, ADP, and serotonin (25,26).

The first step toward platelet aggregation is platelet adhesion. Normally, platelets do not adhere to the vessel walls due to the non-thrombogenic properties of the endothelium. Endothelial cells produce heparin sulfate (to activate antithrombin), thrombomodulin (for activation of protein C), plasminogen activators (to induce fibrin degradation), and TFPI (to inhibit tissue factor activity). In addition, these cells also produce prostacyclin (PGI_2) that inhibits platelet activation by raising platelet cAMP levels and endothelial derived relaxing factor (EDRF; NO), which inhibits platelet activation through a cGMP dependent mechanism. When this antithrombotic continuum of cells is interrupted by vascular injury, platelets adhere to the exposed subendothelial tissues.

Following adhesion, platelets become activated. In this activation process, there is a morphologic shape change in the platelet, with pseudopod formation observed. This brings about a change in the conformation of the glycoprotein IIb/IIIa receptor on the platelet surface, which allows for fibrinogen binding (23). Fibrinogen binding serves as a bridge that links individual platelets into larger aggregates. An increase in cytosolic calcium levels leads to activation of internal platelet enzymes with the subsequent release of platelet granule contents. The formation of these platelet aggregates is the process of primary hemostasis, the first step to arrest blood loss.

The release of platelet granule contents leads to further platelet activation and aggregation and an activation of coagulation. Most of the known aggregating agents cause release of the storage granule contents. These agonists include thrombin, ADP, collagen, TXA_2, platelet activating factor, serotonin, epinephrine, immune complexes, and fibrinogen (23). Thrombin is the most potent aggregating agent, capable of causing platelet aggregation without any contribution from thromboxane A_2 or ADP (23). Serotonin and epinephrine do not induce aggregation on their own, but synergistically promote aggregation induced by other agents (27,28,29).

Platelet membranes contain a variety of receptors for the various agonists including the thrombin receptor, the TXA_2 receptor, 5-HT_2 receptors, and α_2-adrenergic receptors. In addition, a number of glycoproteins present on the membrane serve as receptors for collagen (GP Ia/IIa), fibrinogen (GP IIb/IIIa), von Willebrand factor (GP Ib), and fibronectin (GP IIb/IIIa) (27,28,29). A high molecular weight chondroitin sulfate proteoglycan has been shown to be released from the surface of the platelet during the aggregation process (30). This proteoglycan contains homopolymers of 4-O chondroitin sulfate that inhibit ADP induced aggregation of platelets (30).

Activated platelets also provide a procoagulant surface on which several reactions of the coagulation cascade take place. Unstimulated platelets provide only a minimally effective surface on which the "tenase" and prothrombinase complexes can assemble (31,32,33). This is due to the bilayer partitioning of various phospholipids. In unstimulated platelets, the outer leaflet of the membrane consists of mostly phosphatidylcholine while the inner leaf contains most of the phosphatidylserine. Two mechanisms have been proposed for maintaining this distribution (34,35). When platelets are stimulated to release their granular contents, the procoagulant phospholipids are brought to the surface as the granules fuse to the membranes (31). This expression of phosphatidylserine on the outer leaflet along with factor V release from the α-granule greatly accelerates the formation of thrombin (36,37,38).

Platelet activation leads to the formation of platelet-derived microparticles derived from the platelet surface. These microvesicles typically account for 25% to 30% of platelet procoagulant activity and factor V binding sites (34,39).

Role of platelet integrins in the regulation of hemostasis

A number of the glycoproteins on the surface of the platelet belong to the superfamily of adhesive protein receptors known as integrins. Integrins are α/β heterodimer protein complexes which are present on the surface of adherent cells of most species (40,41,42). These integrins mediate cell–cell and cell–matrix interactions involved in a diverse number of biologic functions (43,44). Integrins are divided into subfamilies based on the identity of the β-subunit. The first two subfamilies of integrins, the VLA complexes and the Leu-Cams, are found on white cells and mediate various leukocyte aggregation responses (45,46). Platelets contain two members of the third subfamily of integrins, glycoprotein IIb/IIIa, and the vitronectin receptor (47,48).

Integrins function by interacting with a number of extra-cellular glycoprotein ligands such as fibronectin, laminin, collagen, vitronectin, fibrinogen, and von Willebrand factor (49). Integrins are capable of binding several ligands; the nature of the ligand specificity is not known.

Platelet membranes contain five integrin-like receptors that are involved in the formation of the primary hemostatic plug. These include VLA-2, VLA-5, VLA-6, glycoprotein IIb/IIIa, and the vitronectin receptor. Of these, GP IIb/IIIa is the most abundant (50). VLA-2 (GPIa/IIa) is the binding site for collagen on the platelet surface (51). VLA-5 and VLA-6 are responsible for the binding to vitronectin and laminin, respectively (45). The extent to which these receptors contribute to platelet adhesion in vivo is not known. The physiologic function of the vitronectin receptor is not known.

Platelet aggregation requires that platelets become activated by at least one platelet agonist, the presence of functional GPIIb/IIIa molecules, and the presence of at least one GPIIb/IIIa ligand (52). Lack of GPIIb/IIIa complexes leads to the congenital bleeding disorder known as Glanzmann's thrombasthenia (53). In nonactivated platelets, GPIIb/IIIa is capable of binding only immobilized fibrinogen. Platelet activation allows plasma-borne adhesive proteins to bind to GPIIb/IIIa complexes (54). The activation of the IIb/IIIa complex occurs by an unknown mechanism though the number of receptors on the membrane is not altered by activation (50). Fibrin polymers bind to the activated GPIIb/IIIa complexes and anchor the platelet plug in place.

Recent studies have shown that the binding of ligands to GPIIb/IIIa also activates a number of cellular processes important for platelet stimulation (50) including the synthesis of 3-phosphorylated phosphatidylinositols, the release of arachidonic acid, and the increase in plasma calcium levels. Stimulation of these processes allows for bidirectional signaling between the intracellular and extracellular compartments.

Role of leukocytes in thrombogenesis

Leukocytes typically express minimal amounts of procoagulant activity in the unstimulated state (55). Cytokines such as interleukin-1 (IL-1) and tumor necrosis factor (TNF) can elicit the expression of tissue factor on endothelial and mononuclear cells (56). Monocyte procoagulant activity is also induced by endotoxin, the complement system, phorbol esters, prostaglandins, and a number of other agonists (57). Procoagulant activity associated with leukocytes is not limited

to the expression of tissue factor. Several monocyte/macrophage derived procoagulant activities have been characterized including tissue factor (58,59,60), factor VII (60), and factor XIII (61). In addition, some monocytes and macrophages have been shown to express functional factor V/Va (62) and to possess binding sites for factor X (63). The factor Xa binding site on leukocytes has been shown to be the integrin CD11b/CD18 (63). Not only does this integrin bind factor X, but it also proteolytically activates factor X to Xa, allowing for initiation of coagulation on the surface of the monocytes and neutrophils (63). Monocytes have also been shown to contain a receptor for the factor IXa/VIII complex, which allows the reactions of the intrinsic pathway of coagulation to take place on the surface of the monocyte (64).

Prothrombin has been shown to be efficiently activated on the cell surface of monocytes and lymphocytes (65). As with platelets, the prothrombinase activity on monocytes is increased with activated monocytes as compared to the non-activated cells (66).

It has been stated that when coagulation takes place on the surface of leukocytes, it "... assumes the aspects of a broad inflammatory mechanism, directly influencing cellular motility and adhesion, phagocytosis, cell-cell communication, and normal or deregulated cellular growth" (63). Fibrin formation not only forms the basis for a blood clot, but can also serve to limit the inflammatory response. In addition, products of the coagulation process such as thrombin, fibrinopeptides, and fibrin degradation products have chemotactic and mitogenic properties (67,68).

Studies have indicated that leukocytes play a critical role in the activation of coagulation in patients with septicemia and in animal models of acute lung injury (69). One study has presented direct evidence indicating the role of tissue factor expression on activated endothelial cells on in vivo thrombogenesis (70).

Role of the endothelium

The endothelium plays a relatively important role in the modulation of overall coagulation and fibrinolytic and platelet dependent processes. Endothelial cells are reactive to various physiologic and pathologic states and release various mediators, which modulate plasmatic processes. The role of endothelial function in mediating the overall coagulation process can be summarized by the following:

1. Regulation of thrombin function by binding to thrombomodulin
2. Release of fibrinolytic mediators in the regulation of the fibrinolytic system
3. Release of prostaglandin derivatives in the control of platelet function and vascular hemodynamics

4. Release of nitric oxide, TFPI and other substances to mediate various functions

Under normal conditions, endothelial cells play a regulatory role in balancing cellular and plasmatic reactions. However, in pathologic states, such as ischemia and occlusive states (thrombotic or restenotic), endothelial function changes markedly, with endothelial cells producing various substances that mediate the pathologic changes. Some of these functions are summarized as follows:

1. Release of tissue factor to initiate the clotting process
2. Release of PAI to inhibit the fibrinolytic response
3. Generation of procoagulant proteins and von Willebrand factor to activate thrombogenesis

It is therefore important to consider the endothelium as a major player in the overall regulation of hemostasis.

Endogenous inhibitors of coagulation

Antithrombin

Antithrombin is a single chain glycoprotein with a molecular weight of approximately 58 kDa (71). The primary structure of this serine protease inhibitor (SERPIN) has been determined by protein and cDNA sequencing of clones from several species (72,73). Normal plasma levels of antithrombin are approximately 2 to 3 μM (74). In the beginning of the century, it was suspected that a natural inhibitor of thrombin was present in the plasma (75). The first hints of antithrombin's existence were detected shortly after the discovery of heparin when it was discovered that heparin required a cofactor to exhibit its anticoagulant activity (76,77). At this point, the molecule was termed heparin cofactor (77). It was not until the late 1960s that Abildgaard demonstrated that the proteins antithrombin and heparin cofactor were one in the same (78).

Antithrombin is a member of the SERPIN superfamily of proteins, which includes the inhibitors α_2-antiplasmin, α_1-antichymotrypsin, and α_1-proteinase inhibitor (79). Antithrombin is considered to be the primary inhibitor of coagulation (80) and targets most coagulation proteases as well as the enzymes trypsin, plasmin, and kallikrein (81). Inhibition takes place when a stoichiometric complex between the active site serine of the protease and the ARG393-SER394 bond of antithrombin forms (82,83). The tertiary structure of antithrombin resembles α_1-antitrypsin in that it is folded into N-terminal domain helices and β-sheets. This tertiary structure is maintained by the formation of three disulfide bonds (71). Four glycosylation sites exist on human

antithrombin, two of which are suspected to actually contain carbohydrate chains. The glycosylation of these sites appears to effect heparin binding to the inhibitor (84). The efficient inhibition of proteases by antithrombin requires heparin as a cofactor. Without heparin, the inhibition rate constants for thrombin and factor Xa have been estimated to be 1×10^3 and 3×10^3 L/mol sec^{-1}, respectively. In the presence of heparin, these rates of inhibition are accelerated to 3×10^7 and 4×10^6 L/mol sec^{-1}, respectively, for thrombin and factor Xa (85). The binding site for heparin is located on the N-terminal domain of the molecule.

Two mechanisms have been proposed to account for heparin's ability to catalyze the antiprotease actions of antithrombin. The first suggests that heparin binds to antithrombin and causes a conformational change at the active site (82). The second model, the ternary complex or template model, proposes that heparin acts catalytically by binding both antithrombin and the serine protease, thereby bringing them in close proximity (81). Both models may be operative depending upon the serine protease being inhibited. Conformational changes of antithrombin upon heparin binding have been observed spectroscopically (82). Furthermore, the ability of a pentasaccharide region of heparin to promote the antithrombin mediated inhibition of factor Xa supports this model. The inhibition of thrombin appears to be better explained by the template model. Conformational changes induced by heparin binding do not alter the reactivity of antithrombin towards thrombin (86). In addition, heparin pentasaccharides do not promote thrombin inhibition. Rather, chains of greater than 18 saccharide units are needed for this inhibition. Kinetic studies indicate that heparin must bind both thrombin and antithrombin (87). It is not clear if one binding must precede the other for optimal inhibition to occur (82.84,87).

Deficiency of antithrombin predisposes the patient to thrombotic complications. Antithrombin deficiencies can be the result of low protein levels or due to functionally abnormal molecules. Low protein levels can be brought about by reduced synthesis or an increased turnover of the molecule. Functional deficiencies can be brought about by mutations in either the reactive site or heparin binding sites. A number of such mutations have been documented (81,86,87).

Heparin cofactor II

Heparin cofactor II is a second plasma SERPIN which has resemblance to antithrombin in that it is activatable by glycosaminoglycan binding. This protein has also been called antithrombin BM, dermatan sulfate cofactor, and human leuserpin 2 (88). The existence of this second inhibitor and heparin cofactor was first shown by Briginshaw in 1974 (89). Whereas antithrombin is observed to have progressive antithrombin activity and to also inhibit factor Xa, the second cofactor exhibits only weak progressive activity and does not inhibit factor Xa. Tollefsen observed two different thrombin inhibitor complexes, one of which could not be identified with antisera to known protease inhibitors (90). Several clinical studies observed a discrepancy between heparin cofactor activity levels and plasma antithrombin antigen levels (91). The existence of the inhibitor was confirmed when the protein was isolated from human plasma and from Cohn fraction IV (90). The heparin cofactor II protein has a molecular weight of 62 to 72 kDa, depending upon the methodology used (90).

Like antithrombin, heparin cofactor II inhibits proteases by forming a 1:1 stoichiometric complex with the enzyme. The protease attacks the reactive site of heparin cofactor II located on the C-terminus, resulting in the formation of a covalent bond. Heparin cofactor II has higher protease specificity than antithrombin. Of the coagulation enzymes, heparin cofactor II is known only to inhibit thrombin (92). Additionally, heparin cofactor II has been shown to inhibit chymotrypsin (93) and leukocyte cathepsin G (94). This protease specificity appears to be due to the active site bond present in heparin cofactor II. Whereas antithrombin contains an Arg-Ser bond as its active site, heparin cofactor II is unique in containing a Leu-Ser bond. This suggests than another portion of the heparin cofactor II molecular may be required for protease binding.

As in the case of antithrombin, the inhibition of protease activity by heparin cofactor II is promoted by glycosaminoglycan binding. Whereas the activation of antithrombin is dependent upon the presence of a specific sequence in the heparin chain, heparin cofactor II can be activated by a wide variety of agents. Heparins, heparans, and dermatan sulfate all promote thrombin inhibition via heparin cofactor II. In the absence of glycosaminoglycan, thrombin variants recognize antithrombin and heparin cofactor II to a similar degree, indicating that neither the autolysis loop nor the β-loop of thrombin is required for SERPIN/protease interaction. Upon addition of heparin, the interaction of antithrombin with the thrombin variants is not altered, suggesting the importance of the anion binding exosite II for the heparin bridge between thrombin and antithrombin. These same studies indicate the importance of anion binding exosite I for the inhibition of thrombin by heparin cofactor II as gamma thrombin, lacking this site, is not inhibited. Based on these results, a complex double bridge mechanism for heparin cofactor II mediated thrombin inhibition has been postulated. In this mechanism, heparin or dermatan sulfate binds to the glycosaminoglycan-binding site on heparin cofactor II and anion binding site I on thrombin. Upon heparin binding to heparin cofactor II, the acidic domain is displaced and is free to interact with the β-loop region of the anion binding exosite of thrombin, facilitating its rapid inhibition.

The normal plasma level of heparin cofactor II is approximately $1.2 \pm 0.2\,\mu M$ (90). Two patients to date have been described as having thrombosis related to heparin cofactor II deficiency (95).

Tissue factor pathway inhibitor

TFPI is one of the coagulation protease inhibitors found endogenously within the vasculature. TFPI has alternately been known as lipoprotein associated coagulation inhibitor (LACI) or extrinsic pathway inhibitor (EPI). This 42 kDa inhibitor has been shown to contain three Kunitz domains tandemly linked between a negatively charged amino terminus and a positively charged carboxy terminus (96). The active site of the first Kunitz domain binds to the active site of the VIIa–tissue factor complex while the active site of the second Kunitz domain binds to the active site of factor Xa. Mutation of the active site of the third Kunitz domain has no effect on the inhibition of either factor VIIa or factor Xa. This protein has been produced by recombinant methods and can be used for the study of thrombosis in simulated conditions. Modification of the second Kunitz domain has also been shown to result in a loss of inhibition of tissue factor–VIIa activity. In experiments where the third Kunitz domain has been truncated, TFPI still inhibits factor VIIa–tissue factor complexes on cell surfaces in culture (97). The carboxy terminus of TFPI is required for the optimal inhibition of factor Xa, perhaps affecting the rate at which TFPI can bind to Factor Xa. No difference is observed between the inhibition of factor VIIa–tissue factor by full-length TFPI or by a truncated form of TFPI (98). Two studies have examined the kinetics of TFPI inhibition of factor Xa (99,100). Both studies have indicated that more than just the second Kunitz domain is required for factor Xa binding as the association rate constants for full-length TFPI are higher than for carboxy-terminus or Kunitz 3 truncated TFPI. The third Kunitz domain has recently been shown to contain a second heparin-binding site (101).

In normal tissues of the vasculature, TFPI is produced by megakaryocytes and the endothelium (102). Once produced, this TFPI is stored in three intravascular pools. These pools are located in the plasma, in platelets, and bound to the endothelium (103). The smallest pool of TFPI is found in the platelets, accounting for less than 2.5% of the intravascular total. This small pool of TFPI is released upon platelet activation (104). 10% to 50% of the intravascular TFPI is in the plasma. Most plasma-based TFPI is bound to plasma lipoproteins (104,105). Approximately 5% of the plasma pool of TFPI circulates in the free form (103,104,105). The lipoprotein-bound TFPI is reported to be of relatively low inhibitory activity (104). The largest pool of TFPI is found bound to the endothelial surface (103,104,106). This pool can account for 50% to 90% of the total intravascular TFPI.

The TFPI pool bound to the endothelium has been shown to be heparin releasable in a number of studies (104,106). Venous occlusion and agents such as 1-deamino-8-D-arginine vasopressin (DDAVP) that induce exocytosis of endothelial granular proteins do not cause the release of TFPI (106). Repeated heparin administration is observed to release similar amounts of TFPI with no tachyphylaxis (106). It is believed that the endothelial pool of TFPI is bound to glycosaminoglycans on the surface of the endothelium. Heparin injection, then, is thought to displace TFPI from the endogenous glycosaminoglycans. The amount of TFPI in the plasma following heparin administration is determined by the heparin concentration. TFPI levels 2- to 10-fold baseline have been reported following heparin and low molecular weight heparin (LMWH) administration. The chemical nature of the LMWH also affects the degree of TFPI release. It has been shown that when different LMWHs are administered at the same anti-Xa unit dosage, plasma TFPI levels vary by as much as 30% (107). Neutralization of heparin by protamine sulfate or protamine chloride results in a dramatic decrease in plasma TFPI levels (103,108).

TFPI acts in vitro as an anticoagulant when measured by a number of assays. Both the thromboplastin induced clotting time and the activated partial thromboplastin time are prolonged by TFPI (103). Factor Xa based assays such as the Heptest and the amidolytic anti-Xa assay are also affected by recombinant TFPI (108). Higher amounts of TFPI are required in the prothrombin time and APTT for prolongation of the clotting time than are needed in the Heptest. The prothrombin time is a more sensitive assay for the anticoagulant effects of TFPI than is the APTT, suggesting that the main in vitro inhibitory effect of TFPI is the inhibition of factor VIIa (103). Co-supplementation of heparin and rTFPI to plasma in vitro has differing effects depending upon the assay used. Kristensen (109) observed that heparin and rTFPI additively prolong the Heptest clotting time. It has been shown that the prolongation of the APTT and PT assays by heparin and TFPI is synergistic (103–108). A study by Nordfang et al., however, suggests that the increased effect of TFPI in the presence of heparin is due to heparin antithrombin complexes, as addition of heparin exhibited no effect in antithrombin deficient plasma (98). The rate of Xa inhibition by rTFPI was observed to increase 2.5-fold upon the addition of heparin, though not with full-length TFPI (105).

TFPI, when administered to rabbits, has been shown to have an antithrombotic effect when thromboplastin was used as a thrombogenic challenge (110). TFPI was also shown to be an effective inhibitor when thrombosis was induced in rabbit jugular veins by endothelial destruction and restricted blood flow. The antithrombotic and antiprotease actions of TFPI have been tested in several other animal models. Warn-Cramer et al. investigated the effect of immunodepletion of TFPI in factor VIIa and Xa induced coagulation in rabbits (111). These rabbits were observed to be sensitized to the procoagulant effects of factor VIIa, but not factor Xa in the absence of factor VIIa. Two studies have indicated that TFPI administration reduces the lethal effects of E. coli administration in a septic shock model in baboons (112). These studies also indicated that TFPI may have an anti-inflammatory effect, as an attenuation of the IL-6 response was also observed. Administration of TFPI has been observed to prevent

reocclusion of arteries in dogs following clot lysis with t-PA. Topical administration of TFPI has been shown to prevent thrombosis in a rabbit model of vascular trauma (113).

Protein C

The protein C pathway is one of the natural anticoagulant systems that keeps blood in the fluid state. When thrombin is formed, it stimulates coagulation and its own formation by activating factors V and VIII through proteolytic cleavage (114). Factors VIIIa and Va bind to negatively charged phospholipids on activated platelets and act as binding sites for factors IXa and Xa, respectively, allowing for formation of the "tenase" and prothrombinase complexes (20).

Thrombin can also act to limit its own procoagulant activity. When thrombin is in circulation, it binds a high affinity receptor on the endothelium known as thrombomodulin (33). The k_d for this binding is 0.2 to 0.5×10^{-9} M (115). Thrombomodulin is a membrane spanning protein containing multiple functional domains and a molecular weight of approximately 60 kDa (116). When thrombin binds to thrombomodulin, a change in substrate specificity is noted. While this complex is a potent activator of protein C, the bound thrombin no longer cleaves fibrinogen, is not able to activate other coagulation proteases such as factors V and VIII, and does not activate platelets (33,115). The thrombin–thrombomodulin complex is a 20,000-fold better activator of protein C than is free thrombin (33,116). Thrombomodulin is present on the endothelium in most arteries, veins, and capillaries (117,118).

Protein C is a vitamin K-dependent zymogen identified by Stenflo that has been shown to be identical to autoprothrombin IIa (118,119). Upon activation, protein C exhibits anticoagulant properties (120). Alterations of thrombin's substrate specificity upon binding to thrombomodulin are thought to be due both to steric hinderance of thrombin's active site and to conformational changes in the active site (118,119,120). Protein C is made up of disulfide-linked heavy and light chains and has a molecular weight of approximately 62 kDa (121). Protein C derives its anticoagulant properties from its ability to cleave and inactivate membrane bound forms of factors Va and VIIIa (33). Factors V and VIII as well as non-membrane bound forms of factors Va and VIIIa are not cleaved by protein C.

Protein C requires two cofactors in order to express its anticoagulant activity, protein S and factor V. Protein S is another vitamin K dependent plasma protein whose free form expresses protein C cofactor activity for the degradation of factors Va and VIIIa (116). Protein S is a single chain, 70 kDa glycoprotein, and has the highest affinity for negatively charged phospholipids among vitamin K dependent proteins (116). Protein S forms a 1:1 complex with protein C on the lipid membrane, which may account for its ability to increase the affinity of activated protein C for such membranes (122). Though the mechanism of action of protein S is not completely understood, it may be related to its ability to make factors Va and VIIIa available for proteolytic cleavage by activated protein C (123). Less is known about factor V's role as an activated protein C cofactor, though it is hypothesized that factor V and protein S may synergistically act to localize protein C activity to the surface of membranes (116).

As low levels of protein C activation peptide are found in healthy individuals, it is suggested that protein C is constantly activated to a small degree (124). Protein C administration has been shown to inhibit both arterial and venous thrombosis in animal models (125). Heterozygous protein C deficiency or activated protein C resistance due to factor V mutation is thought to explain 60% to 70% of the cases of familial thrombophilia (116).

Protease nexins

Protease nexins 1 and 2 are endogenous serine protease inhibitors, which have molecular weights of 43 and approximately 100 kDa, respectively (126). Both protease nexin 1 and protease nexin 2 have effects on the coagulation system. Based on cell culture studies, protease nexin 1 appears to be produced by fibroblasts, smooth muscle cells, and epithelial cells (127,128). Protease nexin 1 has a 30% sequence homology with antithrombin and like AT, has a high affinity heparin-binding site. Heparin binding to protease nexin 1 accelerates protease inhibition (127,128). Protease nexin 1 appears to be limited to the extravascular compartment as human plasma contains only small amounts of this inhibitor (20 pM) (126). Protease nexin 1 inhibits several serine proteases including thrombin, urokinase, plasminogen activator, and activated protein C (126,128). Upon formation of a stable complex with the target protease, the complex binds back to the cells where it is internalized and degraded (127). The physiologic role of protease nexin 1 appears to be related to protection of the extracellular matrix from degradation by urokinase and plasminogen activator (129). This is supported by the fact that protease nexin 1 binds tightly to the extracellular matrix, thereby localizing its activity.

Protease nexin 2 is identical to the secreted form of the amyloid precursor protein containing the Kunitz-type serine protease inhibitor domain (128,129). Protease nexin 2 circulates in blood stored as a platelet α-granule protein, which is secreted upon platelet activation (127). Protease nexin 2 inhibits trypsin- and chymotrypsin-like serine proteases and is also a potent inhibitor of factor XIa (126,127,128). Its location in platelets and its ability to inhibit factor XIa suggests a role in regulating blood coagulation for protease nexin 2.

Other inhibitors

A number of other serine protease inhibitors are known to play a role in modulating physiologic functions. Plasminogen activator inhibitors serve to limit the normal activation of the fibrinolytic process. High levels of PAI-1 are associated with an increased risk of thromboembolic disease (129). PAI-1 has also been shown to regulate the degradation of extracellular matrix, which may be important in modulating cancer invasion. α_2-Antiplasmin rapidly inhibits the fibrinolytic activity of plasmin (130). α_2-Macroglobulin has been described as a "panproteinase inhibitor" in light of evidence that it interacts with nearly any proteinase (131). In addition, α_2-macroglobulin may play a role in inflammation and immune reactions through its ability to regulate the distribution and activity of numerous cytokines including transforming growth factor β, tumor necrosis factor α, platelet derived growth factor, and several interleukins (132). The complement and contact systems are regulated by c_1-esterase inhibitor through the inhibition of complement components C1r and C1s (133). Deficiency of c_1-esterase inhibitor is associated with angioedema (134). Histidine-rich glycoprotein has been shown to bind to plasminogen and interfere with its interaction with fibrin (135). Additionally, histidine-rich glycoprotein is known to bind to heparin and related glycosaminoglycans (135). High levels of this protein have not been definitively linked to thrombosis (136).

Thrombin activatable fibrinolytic inhibitor

Thrombin activatable fibrinolytic inhibitor (TAFI) was discovered by two independent groups as a basic carboxypeptidase present in fresh serum obtained from clotted human blood, and was characterized to be distinct from the constitutive basic carboxypeptidase (137). Because of its relative instability, this enzyme was also designated as carboxypeptidase U (unstable). It was also found that arginine residues, from such substrates as fibrin strands, were digested more efficiently than lysine and thus it was also designated as carboxypeptidase R (arginine). Subsequent studies on cDNA encoding revealed TAFI to be a zymogen with a high degree of homology to pancreatic procarboxypeptidase (138). The amino acid sequence of TAFI is also reported to be identical to plasma procarboxypeptidase B, U, and R. Beside thrombin-thrombomodulin, TAFI can be activated by plasmin. Activated TAFI inhibits fibrin clot lysis by removing the carboxyl terminal lysine residues from partially degraded fibrin that mediate positive feedback in the fibrinolytic cascade. TAFI has been shown to remove the carboxyl terminal arginine from thrombin and a variety of polypeptides such as anaphylatoxins and kinins (137,139). More recently, it has been demonstrated that TAFI is an acute phase protein. Injections of bacteria lipopolysaccharide elicit fibrinolytic deficit and increases in hepatic TAFI mRNA (140). Recent data obtained in our laboratories in collaboration with Dr. Ravindranath have also demonstrated that TAFI is upregulated in rats with burn injury and septic shock. A recent publication also reported on the modulation of TAFI gene expression in acute phase and other inflammatory states in HepG2 cells by Northern blot analysis and on TAFI promoter activity by transient transfection into HepG2 cells with luciferase reporter plasmids harboring the TAFI 5'-flanking region (141). These observations may have a direct impact on the pathogenesis of both the acute and chronic events leading to ischemic and occlusive processes, which are involved in the pathogenesis of acute coronary syndromes and ischemic and thrombotic vascular deficit.

Elevated TAFI levels have been found in men with symptomatic coronary artery disease (142). TAFI is also reported to be a risk factor for deep venous thrombosis. A recent report on the high levels of TAFI in the acute phase of ischemic stroke revealed not only elevated levels but also an incremental increase in TAFI with the degree of neurologic deterioration (143). Therefore, the observation by Boffa et al. on the acute phase nature of this protein requires further validation. In addition, Juhan-Vague et al. stated that there is a correlation between TAFI levels and cardiovascular risk factors (144). Animal models may be needed to truly validate studies on TAFI upregulation and its relation to thrombosis.

Abnormal hemostasis leading to thrombosis and bleeding

Thrombotic microangiopathies

As previously discussed, hemostasis results from a dynamic equilibrium between endothelial injury, stasis or turbulance of blood flow, and blood hypercoagulation. Any of the following disorders may cause a disturbance in this delicate balance resulting in either bleeding or thrombosis. There are several quantitative platelet disorders that can lead to a thrombotic state. One such category of disorders is the thrombotic microangiopathies. The thrombotic microangiopathies include the thrombotic thrombocytopenic purpura (TTP) and hemolytic uremic syndrome (HUS).

TTP occurs in approximately 1000 individuals in North America every year. The diagnosis is mainly clinical and suspected when patients present with any combination of renal insufficiency, thrombocytopenia, and central nervous system symptomatology (145,146). Altered mental status,

seizures and strokes, or complications of renal insufficiency are usually seen among patients presenting to the intensive care units. Microangiopathic hemolytic anemia, shistocytes on the peripheral smear, and renal insufficiency are commonly present. Extremely high levels of LDH serve as a prognostic factor. The platelet thrombi in TTP contain von Willebrand factor (vWF) and fibrin. The vWF multimers may be involved in platelet aggregation. Unless treated rapidly with plasma exchange therapy and intravenous glucocorticoids, TTP can be fatal. Daily plasma exchange therapy is continued until the LDH level normalizes. Platelet transfusions are contraindicated. TTP occurring during pregnancy may present difficulty in the diagnosis because of the overlap in symptoms between TTP and hemolysis, elevated liver enzymes, low platelets (HELLP) syndrome (147). vWF-cleaving metalloprotease, ADAMTS-13, produced predominantly by liver cells, has been recently characterized.

Hemolytic uremic syndrome

HUS has also been associated with thrombosis. First identified in children, HUS is also seen in adults in association with pregnancy, chemotherapy, immune suppression, transplantation, or exposure to drugs (148,149). A majority of childhood HUS results after a bloody diarrhea caused by verotoxin producing E. coli serotype O157:H7 (150). The non diarrhea-associated HUS is due to mitomycin C, cyclosporin, FK506 (tacrolimus), drug combination therapy, and total body irradiation. The familial (congenital) HUS accounting for 5–10% of all cases of HUS has a mortality rate of 54%, much higher than that of typical childhood HUS (3–5%). Histopathological exam of the renal biopsies reveal intraglomerular thrombi causing severe ischemic injury to the renal cortex. The renal dysfunction is severe in HUS, requiring dialysis.

Alloimmune thrombocytopenia

Alloimmune thrombocytopenia is one of the complications that can occur 5–10 days after a blood transfusion. The alloantibodies developed react with the platelet membrane glycoproteins PLA1 and PLA2 epitopes on GPIIIa, the BAKa and BAKb epitopes on GPIIb, the Pena epitope on GPIIIa, and the Bra on GPIa (151). Shulman demonstrated that membrane-associated GPIIIa bearing the PLA1 epitope exists in normal plasma. About 1% of the total PLA1 antigen present in the circulation exists in this form and is sufficient to transfer the PLA1 antigen site to platelets of a PLA1 negative recipient (152). Acute destruction of autologous platelets after blood tranfusion in these patients occurs due to this mechanism (152). The alloantigens transfused or released from platelets after transfusion attach to the autologous platelets thereby becoming sensitized to the later formed alloantibodies. Autoantibodies that react with a patient's platelets may be produced along with the alloantibody. About 2% of transfusions are mismatched for PLAI. The PLAI-reactive alloantibodies characteristic of PTP are complement fixing, in contrast to the alloantibodies that cause neonatal alloimmune thrombocytopenia (NATP). Patients with PTP are treated with prednisone or other corticosteroids. While untreated patients recover spontaneously within a month, about 10% of the patients develop intracranial hemorrhage and succumb to it (153).

Drug induced thrombocytopenia

With the introduction of newer agents for the treatment of thrombosis, the true incidence of drug-induced thrombocytopenia may be higher (154) than the original estimation of approximately 1 per 100,000 population in developed countries (155,156,157). The following criteria are generally used in the diagnosis of drug-induced thrombocytopenia (159):

1. There should be a proper temporal relationship between the onset of thrombocytopenia and the initiation of therapy.
2. No reasonable alternative explanation exists for the thrombocytopenia other than the drug therapy initiated.
3. The platelet count should revert to normal after discontinuation of the drug therapy.
4. Diagnosis is confirmed by in vitro testing or rechallenging with the suspected drug when indicated.

Several drugs from acetaminophen to valproic acid cause drug-induced antibody-mediated thrombocytopenia. While mitomycin C, cyclosporin, FK506 (tacrolimus), combination chemotherapeutic agents, and total body irradiation can cause drug-induced thrombocytopenia with thrombotic microangiopathy, drugs that cause immune platelet destruction include heparin, GPIIb/IIIa antagonists, quinidine, quinine, sulfa containing drugs, penicillins, gold, cocaine, and valproic acid.

Heparin-induced thrombocytopenia

HIT occurs in approximately 5% of patients receiving heparin for at least 5 days. The diagnosis of this condition is clinical. Platelet counts drop below 100,000/μl or there is more than a 50% drop of the baseline platelet count, following administration of heparin. This occurs independently of the route of administration and is not associated with any other explanation for the thrombocytopenia. Some of the patients developing HIT go on to develop heparin-induced thrombocytopenia/thrombosis syndrome (HITTS). While the incidence of HIT or HITTS may be lower with LMWHs, the cross reactivity of the LMWHs can cause HIT. Although the incidence of HIT is approximately 5%, the morbidity and mortality rates are so high that failure to diagnose early can result in catastrophic complications (159,160). The terminology HIT type I is used to indicate heparin-induced thrombocytopenia occurring via a non-immune platelet activating mechanism. HIT type II refers to the immune-mediated syndrome. The pathophysiology of HIT is still not completely understood. It is hypothesized that binding of heparin complexes to platelets triggers the platelet activation. The IgG antibodies react with a complex of heparin and platelet factor 4 forming an immune complex, which binds to an unknown site on the platelet surface. Platelet activation is triggered when the Fc portion of the IgG antibody bound to the heparin-PF4 complex reacts with the Fc receptor on adjacent platelets (161). The laboratory testing for confirmation of HIT diagnosis can be performed by platelet aggregation, serotonin release, ELISA (platelet IgG), ELISA (platelet factor 4-heparin), platelet activation, and lumi-aggregometry. Once the diagnosis is confirmed, heparin administration in any form should be completely stopped.

The United States Food and Drug Administration (US FDA) has approved argatroban and recombinant hirudin to be used as alternate anticoagulants in patients with HIT. While anti-hirudin antibodies may form, which can neutralize hirudin and jeopardize the anticoagulant management, no such antibodies have been detected with the use of argatroban in HIT patients. Overlap of parenteral and oral anticoagulation may be required to avoid paradoxical hypercoagulable complications of warfarin. Antithrombin drugs are known to prolong the INR. In patients with HIT, warfarin should not be started until the patient is adequately anticoagulated and the platelet count has risen above 100,000/μl, with a parenteral anticoagulant such as danaparoid, argatroban, or recombinant hirudin. An increase in the platelet count to at least 100,000/μl indicates that the patient is responding to the alternate anticoagulant. For patients in whom HIT has not been diagnosed until treatment with warfarin has commenced, it is advised to stop the warfarin, since it prolongs both the INR and APTT. In this case, suboptimal anticoagulation with antithrombin drugs may result due to APTT-based monitoring. Furthermore, APTT is not a specific test for the monitoring of direct thrombin inhibitors. Instead, ecarin clotting time (ECT) should be used for the monitoring of antithrombin drugs. In patients treated with danaparoid, there is no need to stop warfarin since danaparoid does not interfere with INR. For patients who are on recombinant hirudin in whom initiation of warfarin is required, it is recommended to reduce the dose of hirudin until the APTT is at the lower end of the therapeutic range before starting warfarin (162).

Immune thrombocytopenic purpura

Though most commonly found in children, (ITP) is being recognized with increasing frequency among older patients. Its annual incidence is about 27 cases per every million population (163). Antiplatelet antibodies cause increased platelet destruction. It may be associated with decreased marrow production of platelets. The peripheral blood smear characteristically shows thrombocytopenia with either normal sized or slightly larger platelets, with normal red cell and white cell number and structure. Splenomegaly is rarely present. For evaluation of ITP, bone marrow aspiration may be appropriate in patients over the age of 60 years to rule out myelopdysplasia and in patients in whom splenectomy is being considered (164). Treatment of bleeding patients include platelet transfusion, high dose parenteral glucocorticoids, and intravenous immunoglobulins (IVIg) (164). Differential diagnoses of ITP include pseudothrombocytopenia (autoantibody against a neo-epitope on GPIIb/IIa, exposed by ethylene diaminotetraacetic acid), drug-induced thrombocytopenia, pregnancy, hypersplenism due to chronic liver disease, infections, congenital thrombocytopenia, myelopdysplasia, disseminated intravascular coagulation (DIC), TTP/HUS, acquired pure megakaryocytic aplasia, and thrombocytopenia associated with other autoimmune disorders. Since prevention of bleeding is the only goal of management, platelet counts should be maintained. The risk of bleeding may be more in adults because of the associated hypertension (165,166). The major concern for pregnant women with ITP is the development of thrombocytopenia in the newborn from the passive transfer of maternal antiplatelet antibodies. The platelet count characteristically falls during the first week and most intracranial hemorrhages may occur during this period. Careful monitoring of the infant's platelet count is essential in order to prevent neonatal bleeding complications.

Thrombocytosis

Platelet counts above 400,000/μl are referred to as thrombocytosis. Thrombocytosis is classified as being either primary or secondary. Primary thrombocytosis or essential thrombocythemia is associated with chronic myeloproliferative disorders such as chronic myeloid leukemia, polycythemia vera, and agnogenic myeloid metaplasia. Exclusion-based diagnosis of essential thrombocythemia is made when patients present with characteristic findings of autonomous proliferation of platelets by megakaryocytes or by presence of megakaryocytes that are hypersensitive to thrombopoietin (167). Thrombopoietin binds to the c-Mpl receptors on the surface of platelet membranes, which are first internalized and then degraded (168). The salient features of essential thrombocythemia include platelet count of >600,000/μl, hemoglobin level of 13 g/dl, failure of iron supplementation to normalize the platelet count, absence of Philadelphia chromosome, collagen fibrosis without splenomegaly, and leukoerythroblastosis and no known cause for reactive thrombocytosis (169). Cytoreductive therapy with hydroxyurea, anagrelide, interferon–alpha, alkylating agents such as busulfan, chlorambucil, pipabroman and thiotepa, radioactive phosphorus, or plateletpheresis is indicated for patients who are likely to develop thrombosis or bleeding. Smoking cessation and proper management of diabetes and hypertension is important in the management of hypercoagulability. Secondary or reactive thrombocytosis due to increased megakaryocyte production of platelets is stimulated by various cytokines, including interleukin (IL)-1, IL-3, IL-6, and IL-11, and is more commonly seen than the primary. Although increased levels of IL-1, IL-4, IL-6, and C-reactive protein (CRP) are found in secondary thrombocytosis, normal levels are found in primary thrombocytosis (170,172).

Qualitative platelet disorders are defined as both the congenital and acquired disorders of platelet function. Congenital disorders of platelet function include defects in platelet-vessel wall interaction (von Willebrand disease with deficiency of vWF) and Bernard-Soulier syndrome (defect in GPIb), disorders of aggregation, disorders of platelet secretion and signal transduction, abnormalities in arachidonic acid pathways, and disorders of platelet coagulant protein interaction. Bernard-Soulier syndrome is an autosomal recessive disorder due to abnormality in platelet GPIb-IX-V complex that mediates the binding of vWF to platelets during adhesion. Glanzmann's thrombasthenia is an autosomal recessive disorder characterized by impaired platelet aggregation, a prolonged bleeding time, and mucocutaneous bleeding.

The acquired disorders of platelet function arise by different mechanisms. In most of the conditions the mechanisms of platelet dysfunction are not understood. Several disorders may result from defects in platelet adhesion, aggregation, secretion, or platelet coagulant activities. In myeloproliferative disorders including essential thrombocythemia, polycythemia vera, chronic myelogenous leukemia, and agnogenic myeloid dysplasia, the platelet abnormalities result from their generation from an abnormal clone of stem cells, or secondary to enhanced platelet activation resulting in qualitative platelet defects leading to bleeding and thromboembolic complications. Conditions in which acquired disorders of platelet function are recognized include uremia, acute leukemia and myelodysplastic syndrome, dysproteinemias, cardiopulmonary bypass, acquired von Willebrand disease, acquired storage pool disease, liver disease, antiplatelet antibodies, and with certain drug treatments.

Several disorders of coagulation and fibrinolysis have been identified that lead to thrombosis or bleeding. These include von Willebrand disease (vWD), hemophilia, coagulation factor deficiencies, acquired/congenital inhibitors of coagulation, and antiphospolipid syndrome.

Von Willebrand's disease

vWD is an autosomal dominant bleeding disorder with an estimated incidence of 1% of the population (26). Functions of vWF include platelet–subendothelial binding, binding to platelet receptor GPIb and to subendothelial collagen; platelet–platelet binding, its binding to platelet receptor GPIb in areas of shear stress, causing platelet aggregation; carrier for factor VIII in plasma, binding to factor VII and protecting it from proteolysis and prolonging its half-life. Bleeding at any age can manifest as bruising and mucous membrane bleeding such as epistaxis, oral bleeding, menorrhagia, and gastrointestinal bleeding (169). Normal variations in collagen receptor may affect the degree of bleeding in patients with mild vWD (170). Laboratory diagnostic assays for vWF include vWF antigen, vWF activity (ristocetin cofactor activity), factor VIII activity, and bleeding time. Useful assays for the classification of vWD include ristocetin-induced platelet aggregation (RIPA) and vWF multimer analysis. VWD is classified into types 1, 2, and 3. VWD type 1 is a quantitative decrease in circulating vWF seen in 70% to 75% of vWD patients. Type 2 comprises of 20% to 25% of vWD patients and type 3 occurs in rare homozygous or heterozygous groups of patients. Different treatment approaches for vWD include (DDAVP, desmopressin), vWF-containing plasma replacement, antifibrinolytic therapy such as ϵ-amino caproic acid (EACA) or tranexemic acid, topical agents such as micronized collagen (Avitene), and fibrin glue. Estrogens increase the synthesis of vWF and are quite helpful in women with vWD. Patients presenting to emergency rooms with bleeding may be treated with DDAVP. In severe cases of bleeding, replacement therapy with "intermediate purity" factor VIII concentrates that contain vWF or more highly purified vWF concentrates may be given to keep the vWF between 50% and 100%.

Hemophilia A and hemophilia B

There are two types of hemophilias that have been identified, hemophilia A (factor VIII deficiency) and hemophilia B (factor IX deficiency). The incidence of hemophilia A is 1 in every 5000 live male births and for hemophilia B the incidence is 1 in every 30,000 live male births. Both types of hemophilia are transmitted genetically as X-linked recessive disorder with criss-cross inheritance where males are affected and their daughters and mothers are carriers. The inversion of intron 22 is the most common mutation in hemophilia A and accounts for nearly 45% of cases. Large gene deletions may also be involved less commonly in hemophilia A. Several point mutations and deletions resulting in nonfunctioning and defective Factor IX protein (cross-reacting material or CRM +) are responsible for Hemophilia B. Large gene deletions and nonsense mutations that are CRM negative lead to factor IX alloantibodies (171). Clinically, hemophilias A and B manifest as intra-articular (hemearthroses and hemophilic arthropathy) and intramuscular bleeding. The typical joints involved are knees (>50% of all events), elbows, ankles, shoulders, and wrists (172). Intramuscular hemorrhage accounting for 30% of bleeding events occurring in large muscles resolve without complications. However, bleeding into closed fascial compartments may cause severe compression of vital structures resulting in ischemia, gangrene, flexion contractures, and neuropathy (compartment syndrome). Bleeding into the psoas muscle or retroperitoneal hemorrhage can cause sudden inguinal pain, decreased range of motion of the ipsilateral hip, and marked flexion and lateral rotation. While spontaneous hematuria occurs frequently, the cause of death in hemophilias is intracranial hemorrhage. Other bleeding complications seen are gastrointestinal and oropharyngeal bleeding and 1% to 2% of patients with recurrent bleeding may develop pseudotumor formation composed of old clots and necrotic tissue.

Male patients with easy bruisability or bleeding with an isolated prolongation of the APTT are suspected of having hemophilia A and B. The PT, platelet counts, and platelet function studies in these patients are normal. Mixing studies with patient's plasma and normal pooled plasma at 37°C promptly corrects the prolonged APTT. Correction of the prolonged APTT in the mixture at both 0 and 120 minutes of incubation excludes the presence of alloantibody inhibitors directed against a specific clotting factor, the presence of lupus-like anticoagulants directed against the phospholipid in the APTT assay, or any weak neutralizing inhibitors.

The presence of lupus anticoagulant may be confirmed by a diluted phospholipid-based assay like the dilute Russell's viper venom time, the tissue thromboplastin inhibition time, or the platelet neutralizing procedure, which utilizes platelets as a source of phospholipids. If mixing studies indicate a clotting factor deficiency, activity levels of specific clotting factors in the intrinsic pathway including factors XII, XI, IX, and VIII should be performed. The factor VIII:C chromogenic assays based on the quantity of factor Xa generated in the presence of factor VIII:C, factor IXa, IIa, calcium, and phospholipid is routinely being performed in laboratories across Europe. The APTT-based one-stage clotting times are performed in the United States. In patients, especially females, with low levels of factor VIII activity, a diagnosis of von Willebrand disease type 2 should be considered. These phenotypic hemophiliacs with normal vWF protein on RIPA have abnormal factor VIII binding assays due to point mutations at the binding site for factor VIII on the vWF protein. About 50% of the severe hemophilia A and 5% of hemophilia B patients develop neutralizing alloantibody inhibitors. These may be suspected in hemophiliacs whose incremental response to clotting factor concentrate therapy is less than 60% of the expected increase over the baseline value. The alloantibody inhibitor can be quantitated using the Bethesda assay (175), where one Bethesda Unit is defined as the amount of antibody in a patient's plasma that causes a 50% decrease in factor VIII activity in pooled normal plasma (PNP) after incubation at 37°C for 2 hours. Infusions of FEIBA offer a therapeutic strategy in the management of bleeding associated with allo- and auto-factor VIII antibodies. Gene therapy in the treatments of hemophilia A and B, although still in early stages of development, may offer new hope in the effective management.

Coagulation factor deficiencies

Factor deficiencies include disorders of fibrinogen such as afibrinogenemia and dysfibrinogenemias, prothrombin deficiency, factor V, VII, X, XI, XII, and XIII deficiency, prekallikrein and high-molecular-weight kininogen deficiency, combined factor deficiencies, α_2 anti-plasmin deficiency, α_1 antitrypsin Pittsburgh, and protein Z deficiency.

The acquired inhibitors of coagulation are usually IgG circulating immunoglobulins that neutralize the activity of a specific coagulation protein or accelerate its clearance from the plasma. They are referred to as alloantibodies when they are developed following the administration of blood products to individuals with congenital factor deficiencies. They are called autoantibodies when they occur among patients who have no pre-existing coagulation defect. Autoantibodies against factor VIII are found in about 1 in every one million individuals; this is referred to as acquired hemophilia. Bleeding is severe occurring spontaneously or following minor trauma. Conditions that are associated with the development of factor VIII inhibitors are systemic lupus erythematosus, inflammatory bowel disease (IBD), post-partum, malignancy, and skin disorders (176,177). Immunosuppression with corticosteroids alone or in combination with azathioprine or cyclophosphamides is needed for rapid clearance of factor VIII inhibitors (178,179). DDAVP therapy causes rapid elevation of factor VIII levels in normal individuals and in patients with acquired hemophilia. When the factor VIII inhibitor levels are very high, bypassing agents (FIX complex concentrates, Factor Eight Inhibitor Bypass Activator-FEIBA) that activate the intrinsic and extrinsic pathways of coagulation to generate thrombin in the absence of Factor VIII may be used (180).

Antiphospholipid syndrome

Antiphospholipid antibodies (APA), first described as circulating anticoagulants because of their interference in phospholipid-dependent assays such as the APTT and often detected in patients with systemic lupus erythematosus (SLE), were referred to as lupus anticoagulants. They were later reported to cause thrombosis in patients with SLE. The association of APA with thrombosis, fetal loss, and thrombocytopenia was termed antiphospholipid syndrome (179). IgG, IgM, and even IgA antibodies directed against prothrombin or β-2 glycoprotein 1 may be involved in APA syndrome. The majority of patients testing positive for lupus anticoagulants also have anticardiolipin antibody (ACA). APA syndrome is usually suspected when younger patients present with recurrent pregnancy loss or arterial and/or venous thrombosis manifested as stroke or myocardial infarction (182,183). Other associated conditions include thrombocytopenia, arthralgia, rash, livedo reticularis, digital dermal necrosis, and pulmonary hypertension (184). Both immunologic and clot-based assays have to be performed and more than two tests for lupus anticoagulants need to be positive in order to make a confirmatory diagnosis of APA syndrome. Moderate to high levels of IgG and IgM need to be detected on two occasions six weeks apart to make the diagnosis (183). Primary APA syndrome occurs with a male to female ratio of 1:2, in the absence of SLE or other autoimmune disorders. However, secondary APA syndrome occurs among patients who have other autoimmune disorders with a male to female ratio of 1:9. Neurologic manifestations of APA syndrome include vascular dementia, cerebral infarction, transient ischemic attack, amaurosis fugax, retinal infarction, acute ischemic encephalopathy, and myelopathy. The treatment of choice in women with previous fetal loss and ACA is unfractionated heparin given at a dose of 5,000 units SC twice daily. Although LMWHs have not been tried in large-scale clinical trials, based on the results of meta-analyses, LMWH at a dose of 75 to 150 units/kg with frequent monitoring of anti-Xa levels may be an alternate regimen. Since the pharmacokinetics of heparin and LMWHs may be altered in APA syndrome, the dosages should be carefully calibrated.

Thrombotic disorders

The thrombotic disorders include atherothrombosis, endothelial dysfunction, hypercoagulable states, and the thrombophilias. Atherothrombosis or atherosclerosis is a systemic disease of the vessel wall occuring in the aorta, carotid, coronary, and peripheral arteries. The associated inflammatory response is mediated by macrophages and T-lymphocytes with continued smooth muscle cell proliferation. The levels of endothelin-1 (ET-1), an extremely potent smooth muscle cell mitogen acting through G_i-protein-coupled ET(A) and ET(B) receptors, are increased in atherosclerosis (185). Endothelin blockade inhibits fatty streak formation and restores nitric oxide-mediated endothelial function. Nitric oxide may promote smooth muscle cell apoptosis. Recently, it was shown that the plasma levels of inflammatory markers were higher in patients with coronary artery disease and peripheral arterial disease than in patients with coronary artery disease alone (186). Although increased levels of C-reactive protein are linked to increased cardiovascular risk, the coexistence of peripheral arterial disease adds additional risk of mortality in coronary artery disease patients. Besides CRP, other markers of inflammation include cell adhesion molecules, cytokines, and proatherogenic enzymes. The T-786 endothelial nitric oxide synthase genotype has recently been reported in the Genetic and ENvironmental factors In Coronary Atherosclerosis (GENICA) study as a novel risk factor for coronary artery disease in Caucasian patients (187). Nitric oxide, a major mediator of endothelium-dependent vasodilation, made by endothelial nitric oxide synthase (eNOS), not only plays a key role in the regulation of vascular tone and blood pressure but is also involved in atherogenesis. The stable plaque becomes vulnerable to rupture when the fibrous cap is thin. Once ruptured, the procoagulant material released causes thrombosis.

The endothelium is the largest endocrine, paracrine, and autocrine gland known. The endothelium plays a key role in vascular homeostasis. Endothelial activation or endothelial dysfunction results in increased expression of adhesion molecules such as E-selectin, intercellular adhesion molecule-1 (ICAM-1), and vascular cell adhesion molecule (VCAM-1). Endothelial dysfunction also leads to increased production of monocyte chemotactic protein-1 (MCP-1), interleukin-8, platelet-derived growth factor, and mononuclear cell-stimulating factor. Endothelial cells serve regulatory functions in maintaining vascular integrity. Therefore, with endothelial dysfunction there is a disturbance in these regulatory functions leading to vasospasm, thrombosis, inflammation, intimal growth, plaque activation, and plaque rupture resulting in atherothrombosis, ischemia, and infarction. Endothelial dysfunction is associated with aging, atherosclerosis, and associated conditions such as hyperhomocysteinemia, infectious diseases, inflammatory cytokines, vascular injury, ischemia, and reperfusion. Endothelial dysfunction causes downregulation of nitric oxide leading to vasoconstriction, platelet adhesion, vascular smooth muscle cell proliferation, leukocyte adhesion, expression of adhesion molecules resulting in monocyte adhesion, foam cell formation, and plaque inflammation. Endothelial dysfunction also leads to decreased prostacyclin production and increased production of endothelin. Furthermore, endothelial dysfunction also causes decreased tPA and PAI-1 leading to impaired fibrinolysis. Understanding the earliest changes in endothelial dysfunction may identify strategies to modulate them in a timely fashion. Reversing endothelial dysfunction will reduce the risk of

cardiovascular disease. Newer therapies known to improve endothelial function have been advocated. These include lipid-lowering therapy, smoking cessation, exercise, ACE inhibitors, hormone replacement therapy, angiotensin receptor blockers, control of blood glucose in diabetics, and combination antioxidants (188). The recently commenced Multi-Ethnic Study of Atherosclerosis (MESA) will evaluate the predictive value of several measures of endothelial dysfunction and other markers of atherosclerosis (189). The precise mechanism of endothelial dysfunction remains to be elucidated.

The hypercoagulable states can be inherited or acquired. One inherited hypercoagulable state is antithrombin (AT) deficiency. AT deficiency is an autosomal dominant condition. The type I antithrombin deficiency is characterized by reduced synthesis of normal protease inhibitor molecules. The antigenic and functional activities of antithrombin are reduced due to small deletions or insertions or single base substitutions. Type II antithrombin deficiency is due to defects within the protease inhibitor. While the immunologic activity levels are normal, the plasma levels of antithrombin are reduced. About 42% of afflicted individuals develop clinical manifestations spontaneously. Manifestations related to pregnancy, parturition, oral contraceptives, or trauma occur in 58% of AT deficient individuals (190).

The inherited (primary) hypercoagulable states include activated protein C resistance due to the factor V Leiden mutation, prothrombin gene mutation, antithrombin deficiency, protein C or protein S deficiency, and dysfibrinogenemia. The most important cause of activated Protein C resistance is the defect in factor V involving the mutation of Arg506 to Gln506 (191).

The acquired (secondary) hypercoagulable states include prolonged air travel, postoperative state, advanced age, estrogen use (oral contraceptives), pregnancy, and postpartum period. Long distance air travel is increasing and cases of venous thromboembolism (VTE) following air travel have attracted both considerable public attention and legal claims against airlines (193). The World Health Organization in collaboration with several international aviation authorities are planning large prospective studies to further establish the importance of travel and travel-related conditions to the development of venous thromboembolic complications. Public and professional understanding of travel-related venous thromboembolic complications and close interactions between physicians, health care authorities and national and international aviation authorities would help to provide safer long distance air travel.

Oral contraceptives have been linked to an increased incidence of thromboembolic complications. Oral contraceptive usage with smoking causes increased risk of thrombosis. Since estrogen was suspected of causing the complications, formulations with less than 50 µg of estrogen and a newer progesterone with lower androgenic effects, levonorgestrel, were introduced. Selective estrogen receptor modulators

(SERMS), nonsteroidal antiestrogens, have a combination of estrogenic and antiestrogenic activity and provide antitumor activity in the breast without antiestrogenic effects such as decreased bone density and increased cardiovascular risk. Besides tamoxifen and raloxifene, nonsteroidal agents related to tamoxifene (toremifene, idoxifene, droloxifene, and TAT-59), other novel nonsteroidal agents including raloxifene and LY-353381, and pure steroidal antiestrogenic agents like ICI 182,780 and EM 800 have been developed.

A malignancy-associated hypercoagulable state occurs in about 11% patients with various cancers (194). However, autopsy studies have shown higher figures with some cancers (30% in pancreatic cancers and more than 50% with cancer of the body or tail of pancreas) (195). Carcinomas of the gastrointestinal tract, ovary, prostate, and lung are also associated with thromboembolic complications. Patients with malignancy have increased rates of postoperative venous thrombotic complication (196). Nonbacterial thrombotic endocarditis (NBTE), characterized by sterile vegetations composed of platelets and fibrin on heart valves, is found most commonly in adenocarcinomas and in 7% of lung cancer patients. In autopsy studies, cancer was found in nearly 75% of cases with NBTE (197).

Disseminated intravascular coagulation (DIC) in malignancy results from activation of the coagulation system. After infection and trauma, malignancy is the third most common condition to cause DIC. DIC occurs in 15% of the patients with malignancy. DIC is reported in nearly all patients with acute promyelocytic leukemia. Malignancy-associated hypercoagulation is invariably associated with inflammation. Inflammatory markers such as C-reactive protein (CRP), monocyte chemotactic protein-1 (MCP-1), and soluble CD40 ligand (sCD40L) are markedly elevated in plasma samples obtained from cancer patients (196). Similarly other elevated levels of markers such as nitric oxide and TNFα have also been reported (199,200).

Recombinant human erythropoietin (rHuEpo) may increase the risk of thrombosis (201). It has been reported that patients with carcinoma of the cervix who received chemotherapy and rHuEpo have an increased risk of symptomatic venous thrombosis (201). In clinical trials where the maintenance hematocrit was 3% on PROCRIT, clotting of the arteriovenous shunts occurred at an annual rate of about 0.25 events per patient per year. However, other thrombotic conditions such as cerebrovascular events, transient ischemic attacks, myocardial infarction, or pulmonary embolism occurred at a rate of 0.04 events per patient per year (202). In a separate study of 1,111 untreated patients on hemodialysis, clotting of arteriovenous shunts occurred at a rate of 0.5 events per patient per year. In patients with chronic renal failure on hemodialysis who also had congestive heart failure, ischemic heart disease and venous thrombosis were increased in patients who were treated with PROCRIT targeted to a hematocrit level of $42 \pm 3\%$ compared to those targeted to $30 \pm 3\%$ (202). It has also been reported

that erythropoietin triggers a signaling pathway in endothelial cells and increases thrombogenicity of their extracellular matrices in vitro (203).

Other coagulation disorders
Disseminated intravascular coagulation

DIC is also known as defibrination syndrome, acquired afibrinogenemia, consumptive coagulopathy, and consumptive thrombohemorrhagic disorder. DIC may be initiated with tissue damage, infections, neoplasia, and obstetric conditions. Tissue damage, endothelial injury, and the exposure of blood to bacterial products, necrotic cells, and subendothelial tissue activate both the intrinsic and extrinsic pathways of coagulation. Extrinsic pathway activation is more important in initiating DIC (204). The bacterial products and endotoxin can activate the contact system. The activation of these pathways of coagulation eventually generates thrombin. Thrombin activates platelets and fibrinogen and activates factors V, VIII, and XIII, resulting in a prothrombotic state. Thrombin first binds with thrombomodulin to form a thrombin:thrombomodulin complex that activates proteins C and S which in turn neutralizes PAI-1 and enhances the fibrinolytic system. Thus in this pathway, thrombin which is normally a powerful procoagulant becomes a powerful anticoagulant. Endotoxin, interleukin-1 (IL-1), IL-6, and TNF release tPA and uPA from the endothelium which activates plasminogen to plasmin. Plasmin in turn degrades fibrin, fibrinogen forming fibrinogen (FgDP) and fibrin degradation products (FDP) and D-dimers. The increased levels of PAI-1 inhibit plasminogen activation. If the levels of PAI-1 are greatly increased, the fibrinolytic system completely shuts down resulting in catastrophic thrombotic complications. Although α_2-antiplasmin can inhibit the activity of plasmin, this is also greatly overwhelmed in DIC. Thus, in a runaway hemostatic situation, the key hemostatic forces such as TF, activated factors V and VIII, other activated coagulation factors and thrombin, and other fibrinolytic forces such as tPA and plasmin fight against their corresponding inhibitors—namely TFPI, protein C and protein S, antithrombin, PAI-1, and α_2-antiplasmin. As a result there is enhanced thrombin generation, enhanced fibrin formation and platelet activation, enhanced fibrinolytic activation (decreased PAI-1) or enhanced thrombosis (increased PAI-1), and unopposed fibrinolysis. Thus, bleeding and thrombosis can occur together in the patient having multiple organ failure due to fibrin deposition. The diagnosis of DIC is indeed clinical and laboratory tests such as PT, APTT, thrombin time (TT), platelet count, FDP, and blood smears are done to confirm the diagnosis. The best treatment is to determine the cause of

DIC and treat it first, after which symptomatic treatment may be provided.

Hemostatic problems during and after pregnancy

The inherited bleeding disorders include von Willebrand and less commonly, factor deficiencies and inherited platelet disorders. The acquired disorders that manifest before pregnancy include ITP and clotting factor inhibitors. The conditions that are associated with pregnancy are disseminated intravascular coagulation and hemolysis with elevated liver functions and low platelets (HELLP) syndrome. Obstetrical complications include placenta previa, abruptio placenta, ectopic pregnancy, abortion, miscarriage, and retained products of conception. Normal pregnancy is a procoagulant state with altered coagulation and fibrinolysis; the concentrations of some coagulation factors and PAI-1 are known to increase. Factor VIII and von Willebrand factor levels increase steadily during the pregnancy (263). Since HELLP invariably leads to postpartum complications and thrombosis, heparin administration postpartum is considered reasonable. The risk of VTE in pregnancy is approximately six times greater than in non-pregnant women amounting to greater morbidity and mortality during pregnancy and puerperium. Untreated DVT resulting in pulmonary embolism is the most common cause of maternal mortality (264).

Thrombotic and embolic disorders

Twenty-five percent of thrombophilic patients develop thrombosis at unusual sites resulting in cerebral venous thrombosis, mesenteric vein thrombosis, hepatic venous thrombosis, retinal vein thrombosis, purpura fulminans, splenic vein thrombosis, portal vein thrombosis, renal vein thrombosis, or axillary vein thrombosis. The thrombotic disorders may involve inflammatory factors that contribute to the vascular deficit. In addition, embolic events also play a role in the development of these thrombotic complications.

Cerebral venous thrombosis

Thrombosis of superficial and deep cerebral veins as well as the venous sinuses is referred to as cerebral venous thrombosis. Advances in imaging techniques are making it possible to diagnose these conditions more frequently. The clinical features of cerebral vein thrombosis include headache, papilledema, fever, seizures, and altered mental status. Deep cerebral venous thrombosis includes thrombosis of the internal cerebral vein and the great vein of Galen. Heparin treatment results in almost full recovery. Cerebral venous thrombosis often terminates in intracerebral hemorrhage due to infarctive ischemia.

Retinal vein thrombosis

Common risk factors for developing branch retinal vein thrombosis (BRVT) and central retinal vein thrombosis (CRVT) include increased plasma fibrinogen, diabetes, decreased exercise, hypertension, and hyperviscosity (205). Sickle cell anemia, polycythemia vera, and other proliferative disorders may also lead to this syndrome.

Veno-occlusive disease

Hepatic veno-occlusive disease (VOD) is the most common and severe complication of chemotherapy and radiation regimens used to prepare patients for autologous or allogenic stem cell transplantation (206). Chemicals such as arsenic and pyrrolidine alkaloids are known to be associated with VOD of the liver. Signs and symptoms of liver toxicity such as sudden weight gain, hepatomegaly, liver tenderness, hyperbilirubinemia (>2 mg/dL), and peripheral edema appearing one week after bone marrow transplantation are characteristic. PAI-1 levels are increased, differentiating this from graft versus host disease. Although several agents have been used in the treatment of hepatic VOD, defibrotide, a polydeoxyribonucleotide derivative used on a compassionate basis was found to be effective without inducing significant bleeding complications (207,208).

Budd-Chiari syndrome

Hepatic venous thrombosis, also known as Budd-Chiari syndrome, is caused by hypercoagulable disorders precipitated by pregnancy, infection, and birth control medication. An acute painful abdomen, sudden enlargement of the liver, and the presence of ascites make up a triad of clinical symptoms that are important in the diagnosis of this syndrome. Myeloproliferative disorders such as polycythemia vera and paroxysmal nocturnal dyspnea were previously thought to be responsible. Factor V Leiden and prothrombin 20210 mutations are also known to be responsible. Other intra-abdominal thromboses include portal vein thrombosis, mesenteric vein thrombosis and renal vein thrombosis.

Sepsis

Sepsis is a systemic inflammatory response to infection. When the inflammatory response extends to multiple organ dysfunction, the condition is termed severe sepsis. Sepsis remains a leading cause of mortality in the critically ill. The response to invading microorganisms may be considered as a balance between a pro-inflammatory and anti-inflammatory reaction. While an inadequate pro-inflammatory reaction and a strong anti-inflammatory response could lead to over-whelming infection and the death of the patient, a strong and uncontrolled pro-inflammatory response, manifested by the release of pro-inflammatory mediators, may lead to microvascular thrombosis and multiple organ failure. Endotoxin triggers sepsis via the release of various mediators such as TNFα and IL-1. These cytokines activate the complement and coagulation systems and release adhesion molecules, prostaglandins, leukotrienes, reactive oxygen species, and nitric oxide. Other mediators involved in sepsis syndrome include IL-6 and IL-8, arachidonic acid metabolites, platelet activating factor, histamine, bradykinin, angiotensin, and vasoactive intestinal peptide. These inflammatory responses are counteracted by IL-10. Most clinical trials targeting various mediators of the pro-inflammatory response have failed due to a lack of a correct definition of sepsis. Targeting the coagulation system with various anticoagulant agents including activated protein C and TFPI is a rational approach. Many clinical trials have been conducted to evaluate these agents in severe sepsis. While trials on antithrombin and TFPI were not very successful, the double-blind, placebo-controlled, phase III trial of recombinant human activated protein C, Worldwide Evaluation in Severe Sepsis (PROWESS) was successful, demonstrating a significant decrease in mortality when compared to the placebo group. A better understanding of the pathophysiologic mechanism of severe sepsis will provide better treatment options, and combination antithrombotic treatment may provide a multi-pronged approach for the treatment of severe sepsis.

HIV/AIDS-associated thrombocytopenia and thrombosis

A serious complication of HIV infection is HIV-associated thrombocytopenia. This results from immune-mediated platelet destruction and decreased or defective platelet production due to infection of megakaryocytes with HIV-1 (211). HIV-related thrombocytopenia may be associated with an accelerated progression to AIDS and decreased survival rates. Hence management of thrombocytopenia in AIDS patient is crucial to prevent severe complications. Severe bleeding complications in HIV-infected hemophilia patients treated with protease inhibitors

such as ritonavir, indinavir, and sequinavir are quite frequent. This increased bleeding is due to inhibition of cytochrome P450, which plays an important role in arachidonic acid metabolism and thus interferes with platelet function. The frequency of thrombosis in HIV patients is 2.6/1000 patient-years. Leg swellings or tenderness should be evaluated by Doppler ultrasound to confirm the presence of thrombosis. Anticoagulants are generally well tolerated by HIV patients. Prophylactic anticoagulants may be used at the discretion of the clinician. AIDS-associated thrombotic microangiopathy may be managed by reducing the amounts of circulating VWF. Plasma infusion or exchange using fresh frozen plasma, cryoprecipitate-depleted fraction of plasma (cryosupernatant), or solvent/detergent-treated plasma for replacement may be considered as treatment of choice for thrombotic thrombocytogenic purpura (TTP) (212).

Postphlebitic syndrome

Post-phlebitic syndrome, a complication of acute DVT, is estimated to occur in approximately 4% of the population (213). This syndrome is characterized by persistent pain, edema, hyperpigmentation, induration of the skin, and stasis ulceration (214). The post-phlebitic syndrome may be due to venous hypertension as a result of outflow obstruction or damage to the valves and in the cutaneous microcirculation may manifest as tissue hypoxia and lymphatic obstruction. Chronic venous insufficiency may lead to post-phlebetic syndrome. The syndrome may be the result of abnormalities in the superficial, the perforator, or the deep venous system. The diagnosis is purely clinical. The pharmacologic treament of post-phlebetic syndrome is rather limited, with pentoxifylline reported to improve the healing rate of skin ulcers.

Less common congenital disorders of hemostasis

In children the majority of cases of cerebral venous thrombosis occur under the age of 1 year. The optimal diagnostic test is MRI with MRV. CT is less sensitive than MRI. The treatment of cerebral venous thrombosis in children is controversial. While some clinicians use anticoagulants, others prefer to treat conservatively.

Neuraxial anesthesia and anticoagulation

The most serious complication of neuraxial block (epidural or spinal anesthesia) is spinal hematoma with resulting paraplegia. Based on the pharmacokinetic and pharmacodynamic profile of a particular antithrombotic drug, the hematologist can formulate a dosage strategy that minimizes the risk of thrombosis and bleeding and at the same time provides the most appropriate anesthesia and analgesia. The LMWH enoxaparin is approved in the United States for the prophylaxis of venous thromboembolism following total hip replacement surgery. Several cases of spinal hematoma were reported in enoxaparin-treated patients receiving neuraxial anesthesia (215). The incidence of spinal hematoma due to enoxaparin treatment is estimated to be 1 in 3,100 continuous epidural anesthesias and 1 in 4,100 spinal anesthesias (216). In this study, the median age of the patients was 78 years and 78% were women. Some patients had pre-existing spinal abnormalities and one-third of the patients were using non-steroidal anti-inflammatory agents (NSAIDs). It is well known that NSAIDS impair hemostasis. Despite the frequent use of neuraxial anesthesia in Germany, the reported incidence of spinal hematoma is low (217,218). LMWH is increasingly being used as "bridging" therapy for chronically anticoagulated patients who need anticoagulation reversal for an operative procedure. Neuraxial anesthesia should be well timed and delayed for at least 24 hours after the last subcutaneous administration of LMWH. For patients exhibiting renal dysfunction with a serum creatinine level >2.0, the clearance of LMWH is delayed. In such patients, neuraxial anesthesia should be delayed until the anti-Xa level is not higher than 0.1 IU/ml.

Inferior vena caval interventions in thromboembolic disease

Pulmonary embolism is the third leading cause of death in United States. Vena caval filters were designed to prevent a thrombus from embolizing from the deep veins of the legs to the pulmonary vessels causing pulmonary embolism. The filters are placed in the inferior or superior vena cava. Anticoagulation is used to treat the underlying DVT, to control the hypercoagulable state, and to prevent the development of clots in the filter. Temporary filters are being evaluated for their safety. There are some patients who cannot receive anticoagulation for various reasons. In these patients, temporary filters may be placed until anticoagulation can be safely used. Tethered filters and retrievable filters are the two main types of temporary filters available. Temporary filters with trapped emboli may pose a problem. In such cases, lysis of the thrombus before removal of the filter or placement of a permanent filter above the temporary one may be useful.

Surgery and thrombosis

Surgery and trauma increase the risk of thrombosis up to 100-fold. Patients with thrombophilic conditions are more prone to develop postsurgical thrombosis, while hemophiliac patients may bleed profusely from surgical interventions. Tables 1–4 provide data from the International Consensus Statement on the relative risk of thromboembolic complications in patients who undergo surgical interventions (219,220,221,222). Factors such as age, obesity, malignancy, thrombophilic states, varicose veins, and previous history of thrombosis increase this risk. This risk is also increased by the duration of surgery, type of anesthetic used, presurgical and postsurgical immobility, level of hydration, and presence of sepsis and inflammation (223). Results from studies carried out on patients who have undergone general surgery and arthroplasty indicate that the thrombotic risk remains even after hospital discharge. Thus, prolonged thromboprophylaxis with anticoagulants may decrease the incidence of venographically detected DVT.

Vascular interventions and hemostatic balance

Vascular intervention results in cellular injury and the release of several mediators of thrombotic and inflammatory processes. Endothelial cell injury results in luminal thrombosis, inflammatory cell infiltration, cellular proliferation, and

Table 1	Incidence of DVT in various patient groups	
Patient group	*DVT incidence (%)*
Stroke	56
Elective hip replacement	51
Multiple trauma	50
Total knee replacement	47
Hip fracture	45
Retropubic prostatectomy	32
General surgery	25
Spinal cord injury	35
Neurosurgery	22
Gynaecologic surgery, malignancy	22
Myocardial infarction	22
General medical	17
Gynaecologic surgery	14
Geriatric	9
Transurethral prostatectomy	9
Source: From Ref. 219.	

Table 2   Frequency of proximal DVT in the absence of prophylaxis diagnosed by surveillance with objective methods[a]

Patient group	Incidence of DVT (%)
General surgery	6.9
Elective hip replacement	23
Total knee replacement	7.6

[a]Fibrinogen uptake test or phlebography.
Source: From Ref. 220.

Table 4   Frequency of fatal pulmonary embolism without prophylaxis

Patient group	Incidence of DVT (%)
General surgery	0.87
Elective hip replacement	1.65
Fractured neck of femur	4.0

Source: From Refs. 221, 222, 227.

vascular spasm. Interventional injury to smooth muscle cells and adventitial cells leads to the cell proliferation and migration, which are responsible late occlusive processes. Progressively, this lesion remodels and may either result in increased or decreased luminal diameter. In the pre-stenting era, restenosis occurred in a significant number of lesions after interventions. With the use of stents and other vascular stabilitzing devices, the restenosis rate is markedly decreased; however, significant thrombotic complications are reported with the drug-eluting stents.

Repeated administration of contrast media and other agents also contribute to vascular injury and or endothelial dysfunctions. Since most vascular interventional procedures result in an injury at the culprit site or other sites, thrombogeneic material such as tissue factor is generated. This necessitates proper anticoagulation. The lesion remains thrombogenic for the intial phase requiring a careful anticoagulant/antithrombotic approach. Thus during the procedure, heparin and related anticoagulant and antiplatelet drugs are used. In certain cases, thrombolytic agents are also used. Bleeding complications can be observed, requiring proper hemostatic measures. The intial management of the thrombogenic site can be managed by using pharmacologic processes. However with the use of drug-coated stents, additional approaches are needed to prevent thrombotic complications. Longer-term usage of antiplatelet drugs may be helpful in further reducing these complications. The interventional approaches will undergo additional advancement

due to the expansion of pathophysiologic and pharmacologic developments. Therfore, it would be important to take into account the periodic recommendations for the control of bleeding, thrombotic, and other occlusive complications associated with these approaches.

Pharmacologic management of thrombosis

Over the past decade, interest in anticoagulant and thrombolytic drugs has grown dramatically, as evidenced by a continual increase in the number of drugs introduced for both pre-clinical and clinical development (224,225). These drugs include new heparins, synthetic heparinomimetic agents, antithrombin agents, anti-Xa agents, biotechnology-derived antithrombotic proteins, antiplatelet drugs, and novel thrombolytic agents. The newer drugs represent a wide array of chemically and biologically derived substances as shown in Figure 3. The outstanding scientific research and development

Table 3   Frequency of clinical pulmonary embolism in the absence of prophylaxis

Patient group	Incidence of DVT (%)
General surgery	1.6
Elective hip replacement	4
Traumatic orthopedic surgery	6.9

Source: From Refs. 221, 222, 227.

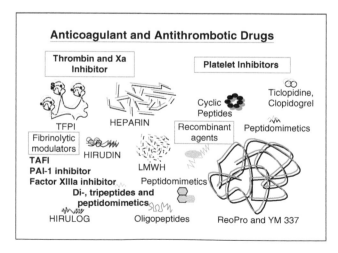

Figure 3
(See color plate.) Current anticoagulant and antithrombotic drugs encompass a wide variety of chemically and biologically-derived substances.

Table 5 Aspirin vs. ADP receptor inhibitors	
Aspirin	*ADP receptor inhibitor*
Polypharmacologic effects	Single receptor targeting agent
Produces both platelet and vascular effects	Only produces platelet mediated responses
Multiple actions (analgesic, anti-inflammatory)	Only produces inhibition of platelets

activities in academic centers and pharmaceutical industry have resulted in a steady flow of new products.

Third party validation of developed products and numerous clinical trials have been carried out globally to validate the claims of safety and efficacy of the newer drugs. The results of these studies constitute a significant portion of the progress reported at various scientific forums. Through their fast track and revised policies, regulatory bodies such as the EMEA (European Medicine Evaluation Agency), US FDA and other regional agencies have continually contributed to the timely evaluation and approval of new drugs by providing input at various stages of drug development. Such close interactions have clarified various issues related to drug development and in fact have accelerated the approval process of many new drugs such as low molecular weight heparins (LMWHs), synthetic heparin pentasaccharide (Arixtra), newer antithrombin agents, and activated protein C (Xigris). Many of the new antiplatelet drugs and thrombolytic agents have also gained approval for multiple indications. The concept of polytherapy including combination of different drugs has been introduced.

Owing to the dramatic development and the relatively defined chemical and biologic profile of the newer drugs such as the anti-Xa/anti-IIa agents and newer antiplatelet drugs, it is now widely believed that conventional anticoagulants such as the heparins, warfarin, and aspirin will eventually be replaced by newer drugs. This is mainly attributed due to adverse reactions associated with their use. The safety of newer drugs is not totally clear at this time. Besides being monotherapeutic, these drugs exhibit several side effects such as the increase in liver enzymes, thrombocytopenia, and that their prolonged use may result in additional vascular and target organ complications. Unfractionated heparin has been in use for nearly 50 years. It is the only anticoagulant drug with an antidote. In many countries this anticoagulant is still the main drug for the management of thrombotic and cardiovascular indications.

The use of unfractionated heparin has been optimized by the development of the LMWHs. This is primarily due to our current understanding of the chemistry and biology of heparin. Antithrombin drugs such as hirudin, argatroban, and bivalirudin have been in development for many years. These drugs are useful as substitutes for heparin in such conditions as heparin-induced thrombocytopenia; however, these drugs do not have an antidote and cannot be used for surgical indications at

this time. The direct factor Xa inhibitors and the heparinomimetics do not have a direct effect on thrombin and produce minimal anticoagulant effects. As such, these drugs may not be useful in the management of patients who have heparin compromise. However, the long-term use of these agents requires further clinical validation. The indications for the newer drugs may be somewhat limited as these drugs are usually monotherapeutic, in contrast to heparin, which exhibits multiple actions.

It has been more than forty years since the oral anticoagulant drugs such as warfarin were introduced for the management of thrombotic and cardiovascular disorders. Variations in response, the need for monitoring, and delayed onset/cessation are some of the problems associated with their use. More recently, the oral antithrombin drugs such as ximelagatran have been developed as potential substitutes for warfarin. While this agent was shown to be effective, or in some cases non-inferior, to warfarin, its use has been associated with an increase in liver enzyme levels and this agent has been shown to pass the placental and blood brain barriers. Furthermore, the thrombin inhibitors may compromise the regulatory function of this enzyme.

Aspirin has been in clinical use for more than one hundred years. The antiplatelet effect of this agent was recognized some forty years ago. Since then aspirin has been a life-saving drug for several types of thrombotic indications. Several

Table 6 Key questions on the fate of conventional anticoagulants and antithrombotics
1. Will aspirin be replaced by newer antiplatelet drugs or drug combinations? No. Aspirin will remain the #1 antiplatelet drug for some time
2. Will Warfarin be replaced by oral antithrombin and anti-Xa agents? Only in some qualified indications
3. Will unfractionated heparin use be obsolete in the near future? Unlikely. It will remain an anticoagulant of choice for surgical and interventional use

newer formulations of aspirin have been developed. It now represents a universal antithrombotic drug in both thrombotic and cardiovascular indications. The newly developed COX inhibitors produce some specific effects of aspirin and may or may not exhibit the same therapeutic effects in thrombosis. Moreover, COX-2 inhibitors have been reported to be associated with adverse thrombotic complications. In comparison with aspirin, the ADP receptor inhibitors are single target drugs (Table 5). The selective ADP receptors when combined with aspirin exhibit superior efficacy compared to monotherapy. However, their clinical spectrum without aspirin will be limited. The same is true for the phosphodiesterase inhibitors.

The coming years will witness dramatic developments in the management of thrombotic and cardiovascular disorders. Synthetic and recombinant approaches will provide cost-effective and clinically useful drugs. LMWHs and synthetic heparin analogs are expected to have significant effects on the overall management of thrombotic and cardiovascular disorders. Factors such as managed care, regulatory issues, polytherapy, and combined pharmacologic and mechanical approaches will redirect the focus of the management of DVT, myocardial infarction, and thrombotic and ischemic stroke. The direct antithrombin agents such as hirudin and bivalirudin will be of great value for surgical and interventional anticoagulation and various acute indications. Postsurgical and interventional control of thrombotic processes may require combination therapy and heparin derived agents such as fondaparinux and non-heparin glycosaminoglycans such as dermatan sulfate. Biotechnology-derived heparin analogues will also be developed as potential replacements for heparins.

It is now widely believed that the days for the classical anticoagulants are numbered and in the foreseeable future these drugs may not exist. However, this is not the case when one reads the recommendations of the American College of Chest Physicians and the approval labels for the drugs (226). Considering the results of several new clinical trials, the ACCP and the International Union of Angiology Consensus Conferences on Antithrombotic Therapy have included definitive recommendations on the clinical effectiveness of the classical drugs for both arterial and venous thrombotic diseases. In addition, these recommendations include specific guidelines on additional indications where these drugs will likely be useful. Thus, it is very likely that heparin, warfarin, and aspirin will continue to be important drugs in hematologic and oncologic disorders for some time.

When the classic anticoagulants are described in some recent publications, they are often labeled as "bad" drugs with many adverse effects. In fact, the classical anticoagulants may not have any more adverse effects than the newer drugs. Needless to say, all pharmacologic agents have their limitations. Heparin, aspirin, and warfarin certainly have drawbacks, some of which have already been addressed, although improvements have been made.

The development of LMWHs is an example of the optimized use of a pharmacologic agent. Their use has nearly eliminated the risk of heparin-induced thrombocytopenia, and these drugs have achieved standard-of-care status for many venous and arterial thrombosis indications. LMWHs are currently being examined for their effectiveness as surgical and interventional anticoagulation. Improved monitoring and dosage optimization are currently being pursued. Another example is the SPORTIF trial in which the oral anticoagulant, warfarin, was found to be essentially equivalent to the new oral anti-thrombin agent, ximelagatran, without risk of significant bleeding. Moreover, warfarin use was not associated with an elevation of liver enzymes.

Despite the problem of heparin-induced thrombocytopenia, heparin has remained the drug of choice for surgical anticoagulation. This is due to the high bleeding risk associated with the new antithrombin agents when used at higher doses coupled with the lack of an antagonist. The heparin-protamine combination has been used with much success for many years, making unfractionated heparin the only reliable anticoagulant that can be used in surgical and interventional indications.

It is noteworthy to state that thrombosis is a polycomponent syndrome that optimally requires a multitargeted therapeutic approach. Despite an advanced understanding of the molecular mechanisms of thrombotic disorders, only mono-therapeutic drugs that have a single target of action have been developed. These mono-therapeutic agents like fondaparinux, ximelagatran, and clopidogrel are molecularly and functionally defined. Their applications have been validated in well designed, sponsored clinical trials for specific indications. But, like the classical drugs, these new drugs were also found to have adverse effects. Bleeding, a lack of dose response, questions on how to appropriately monitor biologic effects, and a lack of antidotes remain problematic issues.

Some of the key questions on the fate of the conventional drugs such as heparin, oral anticoagulants, and aspirin are mostly related to their safety, as their efficacy is not in question (Table 6). These drugs will remain the gold standards despite their known drawbacks. They require further optimization and can be used for various indications in a cost-effective manner. The newer drugs, however, provide alternatives that in the next few years may lead to improved, cost-effective treatments. The actions of non-anticoagulant drugs such as the cholesterol lowering agents (statins), specific inhibitors of cyclooxygenase, nitric oxide donors, and drugs modulating endothelial function will also impact the combination therapy of thrombotic and cardiovascular diseases.

Synopsis

The process of blood coagulation is no longer considered to be a simple transformation of fibrinogen to fibrin by the action of thrombin. Rather, this remarkably complex process is a result of several transformations, which are mediated by enzymes, activators, inhibitors, and cellular contributors. The process of coagulation contributes significantly to thrombogenesis; however, it is no longer considered to be the sole event. The role of platelets, leukocytes, and endothelial cells has gradually been accepted to be crucial in the overall regulation of thrombogenesis.

Surgical interventions produce a major stimulus for coagulation through the release of large amounts of tissue factor, enzymes, platelet activation from the extracorporeal circulation, and endothelial distress. This necessitates the use of anticoagulant and antithrombotic agents to keep blood coagulation under control. The understanding of the activation processes has led to the development of newer approaches to inhibit the coagulation process. Furthermore, physiologic means such as hypothermia and blood salvage techniques have added to the restoration approaches during cardiovascular surgical procedures. Endogenous inhibitors such as antithrombin, protein C, and TFPI play a major role in the control of thrombogenesis. Heparin and warfarin have been crucial in controlling the thrombotic process both during and after surgical procedures. Alternate anticoagulant drug development will continue to provide us new drugs to control the coagulation process. However, clinical studies on long-term safety and efficacy will be needed prior to replacing the conventional anticoagulants such as heparin and oral anticoagulant drugs.

Bleeding risk is also a major factor contributing to the mortality and morbidity in patients undergoing surgical procedures. Appropriate hemostatic measures, the optimized use of anticoagulants, and the identification of predisposing factors in a given patient may be helpful in minimizing surgical bleeding. The available plasma-derived hemostatic factors, recombinant factor VIII and VIIa, and antifibrinolytic agents such as aprotinin and lysine analogs (epsilon aminocaproic and transexamic acid) are useful in the control of surgical bleeding.

Advances in the molecular understanding of the hemostatic process and pathogenesis of hemostatic disorders and the application of genomic and proteomic techniques will have a major impact in the risk stratification of surgical patients. The application of such technology will also be helpful in tailoring the use of anticoagulant and prohemostatic agents to facilitate improved clinical outcome.

References

1   Bevers EM, Rosing J, Zwaal RFA. Development of procoagulant binding sites on the platelet surface. In: Westweek J, Scully MF, McIntyre DE, Kakkar W, eds. Mechanisms of Stimulus Response Coupling in Platelets. New York: Plenum Press, 1985:359–372.

2   Davie EW, Ratnoff OD. Waterfall sequence for intrinsic blood clotting. Science 1964; 145:1310–1312.

3   MacFarlane RG. An enzyme cascade in the blood clotting mechanism and its function as a biochemical amplifier. Nature 1964; 202:498–499.

4   Osterud B, Rapaport SI. Activation of factor IX by the reaction product of tissue factor and factor VII: additional pathway for initiating blood coagulation. Proc Natl Acad Sci USA 1977; 74:5260–5264.

5   Scully MF. The biochemistry of blood clotting: The digestion of a liquid to form a solid. Essays in Biochem 1992; 27:17–36.

6   Hemker HC, Kessels H. Feedback mechanisms in coagulation. Haemostasis 1991; 21:189–196.

7   Mann KG, Jerry RJ, Krishnaswamy S. Cofactor proteins in the assembly of blood clotting enzyme complexes. Annu Rev Biochem 1988; 57:915–956.

8   Hettasch JM, Greenberg CS. Fibrin formation and stabilization. In: Loscalzo J, Schafer AI, eds. Thrombosis and Hemorrhage, 2nd ed. Baltimore, MD: Williams & Wilkins, 1998:129–154.

9   Blomback B, Vestermark A. Isolation of fibrinopeptides by chromatography. Arkiv Kemi 1958; 12:173–182.

10 Shainoff JR, Dardik BN. Fibrinopeptide B and aggregation of fibrinogen. Science 1979; 204(4389):200–202.

11 Laurent TC, Blomback B. On the significance of the release of two different peptides from fibrinogen during clotting. Acta Chem Scand 1958; 12:1875–1877.

12 Coughlin SR, Vu TKH, Hung DT, Wheaton VI. Characterization of a functional thrombin receptor. Issues and opportunities. Clin Invest 1992; 89:351–353.

13 Esmon CT. The roles of protein C and thrombomodulin in the regulation of blood coagulation. J Biol Chem 1989; 264:4743–4761.

14 Olson ST, Bjork I. Regulation of thrombin by antithrombin and heparin cofactor II. In: Berliner LJ, ed. Thrombin: Structure and Function. New York: Plenum Press, 1992:159–217.

15 Bach R, Konigsberg W, Nemerson Y. Human tissue factor contains thioester linked palmitate and stearate on the cytoplasmic half cystine. Biochemistry 1988; 27:4227–4231.

16 McVey JH. Tissue factor pathway. Bailliere's Clin Haemat 1994; 7(3):469–484.

17 Morrissey JH, Mack BG, Neuenschwander PF, Comp PC. Quantitation of activated factor VII levels in plasma using a tissue factor mutant selectively deficient in promoting factor VII activation. Blood 1993; 81:734–744.

18 Edgington TS, Mackman N, Brand K, Ruf W. The structural biology of the expression and function of tissue factor. Thromb Haemost 1991; 66:67–77.

19 Nemerson Y. Tissue factor and haemostasis. Blood 1988; 71:1–8.

20 Mann KG, Nesheim ME, Church WR, Haley P, Krishnaswamy S. Surface-dependent reactions of the vitamin K-dependent enzyme complexes. Blood 1990; 76:1–16.

21 Naito K, Fujikawa K. Activation of human blood coagulation factor XI independent of factor XII: factor XI is activated by thrombin and factor Xia in the presence of negatively charged surfaces. J Biol Chem 1991; 66:7353–7358.

22 Gailani D, Broze GJ. Factor XI activation in a revised model of blood coagulation. Science 1991; 253:909–912.

23 Packham MA. Role of platelets in thrombosis and hemostasis. Can J Physiol Pharmacol 1994; 72:278–284.

24 Kaplan KL. Platelet granule proteins: localization and secretion. In: Gordon AS, ed. Platelet in Biology and Pathology. Vol. 5. Amsterdam: Elsevier, 1981:77.

25 Holmsen H. Platelet secretion. In: Colman RW, Hirsh J, Marder VJ, Salzman EW, eds. Hemostasis and Thrombosis. Philadelphia: Lippincott, 1987:606.

26 Niewiarowski S, Holt JC. Biochemistry and physiology of secreted platelet proteins. In: Colman RW, Hirsh J, Marder VJ, Salzman EW, eds. Hemostasis and Thrombosis. Basic Principles and Clinical Practice. 2nd ed. Philadelphia: Lippincott, 1987:618–630.

27 Coller B. Platelets in cardiovascular thrombosis and thrombolysis. In: Fozzard UA, Haber E, Jennings RB, Katz AM, Morgan HE, eds. The Heart and Cardiovascular System. 2nd ed. New York: Raven Press, 1992:219–273.

28 Hourani SMO, Cusack NJ. Pharmacological receptors on blood platelets. Pharmacol Rev 1991; 43:243–298.

29 Siess W. Molecular mechanisms of platelet activation. Physiol Rev 1989; 69:58–78.

30 Nader HB. Characterization of heparan sulfate and a particular chondroitin 4-sulfate proteoglycan from platelets. Inhibition of the aggregation process by platelet chondroitin sulfate proteoglycan. J Biol Chem 1991; 266(16):10518–10523.

31 Zwaal RFA, Bevers EM, Comfurius P, Rosing J, Tilly RHJ, Verhallen PFJ. Loss of membrane phospholipid asymmetry during activation of blood platelets and sickled red cells; mechanisms and physiological significance. Mol Cell Biochem 1989; 91:23–31.

32 Wiedmer T, Esmon CT, Sims PJ. Complement proteins C5b-9 stimulate procoagulant activity through platelet prothrombinase. Blood 1986; 68:875–880.

33 Esmon CT. Molecular events that control the protein C anticoagulant pathway. Thromb Haemost 1993; 70:29–35.

34 Sandberg H, Bode AP, Dombrose FA, Hoechli M, Lentz BR. Expression of coagulant activity in human platelets: release of membranous vesicles providing platelet factor 1 and platelet factor 3. Thromb Res 1985; 39:63–79.

35 Tilly RHJ, Senden JMG, Comfurius P, Bevers EM, Zwaal RFA. Increased aminophospholipid translocase activity in human platelets during secretion. Biochem Biophys Acta 1990; 1029:188–190.

36 Tracy PB, Nesheim ME, Mann KG. Platelet factor Xa receptor. Meth Enzymol 1992; 215:329–360.

37 Miletich JP, Jackson CM, Majerus PW. Interaction of coagulation factor Xa with human platelets. Proc Natl Acad Sci USA 1977; 74:4033–4036.

38 Ittyerah TR, Rawala R, Colman RW. Immunochemical studies of factor V of bovine platelets. Eur J Biochem 1981; 120:235–241.

39 Sims PJ, Wiedmer T, Esmon CT, Weiss HJ, Shattil SJ. Assembly of the platelet prothrombinase complex is linked to vesiculation of the platelet plasma membrane. J Biol Chem 1989; 264:17,049–17,057.

40 Bogaert TN, Brown N, Wilcox M. The Drosophila PS2 antigen is an invertebrate integrin that, like the fibronectin receptor, becomes localized to muscle attachments. Cell 1987; 51:929–940.

41 DeSimone DW, Hynes RO. Xenopus laevie integrins. Structural conservation and evolutionary divergence of integrin beta. J Biol Chem 1988; 263(11):5333–5340.

42 Marcantonio EE, Hynes RO. Antibodies to the conserved cytoplasmic domain of the integrin beta 1 subunit react with proteins in vertebrates, invertebrates and fungi. J Cell Biol 1988; 106(5):1765–1772.

43 Hynes RO. Integrins: a family of cell surface receptors. Cell 1987; 48:549–554.

44 Takada Y, Strominger JL, Hemler ME. The very late antigen family of heterodimers is part of a superfamily of molecules in adhesion and embryogenesis. Proc Natl Acad Sci USA 1987; 84(10):3239–3243.

45 Hemler ME, Crouse C, Takada Y, Sonnenberg A. Multiple very late antigen (VLA) heterodimers on platelets. Evidence for distinct VLA-2, VLA-5 (fibrinogen receptor) and VLA-6 structures. J Biol Chem 1988; 263(16):7660–7665.

46 Anderson DC, Springer TA. Leukocyte adhesion deficiency: an inherited defect in the Mac-1, LFA-1, and P150 glycoproteins. Annu Rev Med 1987; 38:175–194.

47 Cheresh DA, Spiro RC. Biosynthetic and functional properties of an Arg-Gly-Asp directed receptor involved in human melanoma cell attachment to vitronectin, fibrinogen, and von Willebrand factor. J Biol Chem 1987; 262(36):17,703–17,711.

48 Lam SC, Plow EW, D'Souza SE, Cheres DA, Frelinger AL, Ginsberg MH. Isolation and characterization of a platelet membrane protein related to the vitronectin receptor. J Biol Chem 1989; 264:3742–3749.

49 Humphries JD, Byron A, Humphries MJ. Integrin ligands at a glance. Journal of Cell Science 2006; 119:3901–3903.

50 Phillips DR, Chaio IF, Scarborough RM. GPIIB/IIIa: the responsive integrin. Cell 1991; 65:359–362.

51 Perrschke EB, López JA. Platelet membranes and receptors. In: Loscalzo J, Schafer AI, eds. Thrombosis and Hemorrhage, 2nd ed. Baltimore, MD: Williams & Wilkins, 1998.

52 Shattil SJ, Bennett JS. Platelets and their membranes in hemostasis: physiology and pathophysiology. Ann Intern Med 1981; 94(1):108–118.

53 Bennet JS, Vilaire G. Exposure of platelet fibrinogen receptors by ADP and epinephrine. J Clin Invest 1979; 64(5):1393–1401.

54 Jackson SP, Yuan Y, Schoenwaelder SM, Mitchell CA. Role of the platelet integrin glycoprotein IIb-IIIa in intracellular signalling. Thromb Res 1993; 71:159–168.

55 Drake TA, Morissey JH, Edgington TS. Selective expression of tissue factor in human tissues. Am J Pathol 1989; 134:1087–1097.

56 Carlsen E, Flatmark A, Prydz H. Cytokine-induced procoagulant activity in monocytes and endothelial cells. Further enhancement by cyclosporine. Transplantation 1988; 46:575–580.

57 Edwards RL, Rickles FR. The role of leukocytes in the activation of blood coagulation. Semin Hematol 1992; 29(3):202–212.

58 Gregory SA, Morissey JH, Edgington TS. Regulation of tissue factor gene expression in the monocyte procoagulant response to endotoxin. Mol Cell Biol 1989; 9:2752–2755.

59 McGee MP, Devlin R, Saluta G, Koren H. Tissue factor and factor VII messenger RNAs in human alveolar macrophages: effects of breathing ozone. Blood 1990; 75:122–127.

60 McGee MP, Wallin R, Devlin R, Rothberger H. Identification of mRNA coding for factor VII protein in human alveolar macrophages. Coagulant expression may be limited due to postribosomal processing. Thromb Haemost 1989; 61:170–174.

61 Weisberg LJ, Shin DT, Conkling PR. Identification of normal human peripheral blood monocytes and liver as sites of

synthesis of coagulation factor XIII alpha chain. Blood 1987; 70:579–582.

62 Rothberger H, McGee MP. Generation of coagulation factor V activity by cultured rabbit alveolar macrophages. J Exp Med 1984; 160:1880–1890.

63 Altieri DA. Coagulation assembly on leukocytes in transmembrane signaling and cell adhesion. Blood 1993; 81(3):569–579.

64 McGee MP, Li LC. Functional difference between intrinsic and extrinsic coagulation pathways. Kinetics of factor X activation on human monocytes and alveolar macrophages. J Biol Chem 1991; 266:8079–8085.

65 Tracy PB, Eide LL, Mann KG. Human prothrombinase complex assembly and function on isolated peripheral blood cell populations. J Biol Chem 1985; 260:2119–2124.

66 Robinson RA, Worfolk L, Tracy PB. Endotoxin enhances expression of monocyte prothrombinase activity. Blood 1992; 79:406–416.

67 Perdue JF, Lubenskyi W, Kivity E, Sonder SA, Fenton JW. Protease mitogenic response of chick embryo fibroblasts and receptor binding/processing of human α-thrombin. J Biol Chem 1981; 256:2767–2776.

68 Senior RM, Skogen WF, Griffin GL, Wilner GD. Effects of fibrinogen derivatives upon the inflammatory response. J Clin Invest 1986; 77:1014–1021.

69 Car BD, Suyemoto M, Neilsen NR, Slauson DO. The role of leukocytes in the pathogenesis of fibrin deposition in bovine acute lung injury. Am J Pathol 1991; 138(5):1191–1198.

70 Nawroth P, Handley D, Esmon C, Stern DM. Interleukin 1 induces endothelial cell procoagulant while suppressing cell surface anticoagulant activity. Proc Natl Acad Sci USA 1986; 83:3460–3464.

71 Mourey L, Samama JP, Delarue M, Choay J, Lormeau JC, Petitou M, et al. Antithrombin III: structural and functional aspects. Biochemie 1990; 72:599–608.

72 Chandra T, Stackhouse R, Kidd VJ, Woo SLC. Isolation and sequence characterization of a cDNA clone of human antithrombin III. Proc Natl Acad Sci USA 1978; 80:1845–1848.

73 Sheffield WP, Brothers AB, Wells MJ, Haiton MWC, Clarke BJ, Blajchman MA. Molecular cloning and expression of rabbit antithrombin III. Blood 1992; 79(9):2330–2339.

74 Conrad J, Brosstad F, Larsen ML, Samama M, Abildgaard U. Molar antithrombin concentration in normal human plasma. Haemostasis 1983; 13:363–368.

75 Howell WH. The coagulation of blood. In: The Harvey Lectures. Vol 12. Philadelphia: Lippincott, 1918:272–323.

76 Howell WH. The purification of heparin and its presence in blood. Am J Physiol 1925; 71:553–562.

77 Brinkhous KM, Smith HP, Warmer ED, Seegers WH. The inhibition of blood clotting: an unidentified substance which acts in conjunction with heparin to prevent the conversion of prothrombin into thrombin. Am J Physiol 1939; 125:683–687.

78 Abildgaard U. Highly purified antithrombin III with heparin cofactor activity prepared by disc electrophoresis. Scand J Clin Lab Invest 1968; 21:89–91.

79 Pizzo SV. The physiologic role of antithrombin III as an anticoagulant. Semin Hematol 1994; 31(2):4–7.

80 Pratt CW, Church FC. Antithrombin: structure and function. Semin Hematol 1991; 28(1):3–9.

81 Bjork I, Danielsson A. Antithrombin and related inhibitors of coagulation proteinases. In: Barrett AJ, Salvesen GS, eds. Proteinase Inhibitors. Amsterdam, The Netherlands: Elsevier, 1986:489–513.

82 Rosenberg RD, Damus PS. The purification and mechanism of action of human antithrombin-heparin cofactor. J Biol Chem 1973; 248:6490–6505.

83 Damus PS, Hicks M, Rosenberg RD. Anticoagulant action of heparin. Nature 1973; 246:355–357.

84 Brennan SO, George PM, Jordan RE. Physiological variant of antithrombin III acks carbohydrate side chain at ASN 135. FEBS Letters 1987; 219:431–436.

85 Jordan RE, Oosta GM, Gardner WT, Rosenberg RD. The kinetics of hemostatic enzyme–antithrombin interactions in the presence of low molecular weight heparins. J Biol Chem 1980; 255:10,081–10,090.

86 Peterson CB, Morgan WT, Blackburn MN. Histidine-rich glycoprotein modulation of the anticoagulant activity of heparin. J Biol Chem 1987; 262:7567–7574.

87 Nesheim M, Blackburn MN, Lawler CM, Mann KG. Dependence of antithrombin III and thrombin binding stoichiometries and catalytic activity on the molecular weight of affinity purified heparin. J Biol Chem 1986; 261:3214–3221.

88 Abildgaard U, Larsen ML. Assay of dermatan sulfate cofactor (heparin cofactor II) activity in human plasma. Thromb Res 1984; 35:257–266.

89 Briginshaw GF, Shanberge JN. Identification of two distinct heparin cofactors in human plasma. Inhibition of thrombin and activated factor X. Thromb Res 1974; 4:463–477.

90 Tollefsen DM, Blank MK. Detection of a new heparin dependent inhibitor of thrombin in human plasma. J Clin Invest 1981; 68:589–596.

91 Bauer KA. Inherited and acquired hypercoagulable states. In: Loscalzo J, Schafer AI, eds. Thrombosis and Hemorrhage, 2nd ed. Baltimore, MD: Williams & Wilkins, 1998.

92 Travis J, Salvesen GS. Human plasma proteinase inhibitors. Ann Rev Biochem 1983; 52:655–709.

93 Church FC, Noyes CM, Griffith MJ. Inhibition of chymotrypsin by heparin cofactor II. Proc Natl Acad Sci USA 1985; 82:6431–6434.

94 Parker KA, Tollefsen DM. The protease specificity of heparin cofactor II. Inhibition of thrombin generated during coagulation. J Biol Chem 1987; 260:3501–3503.

95 Sie P, DuPouy D, Pichon J, Boneu B. Constitutional heparin cofactor II deficiency associated with recurrent thrombosis. Lancet 1985; 2:414–416.

96 Girard TJ, Warren LA, Novotny WF, Likert KM, Brown SG, Miletich JP, et al. Functional significance of the Kunitz-type inhibitory domains of lipoprotein-associated coagulation inhibitor. Nature 1989; 338:518–520.

97 Hamamoto T, Yamamoto M, Nordfang O, Petersen JGL, Foster DC, Kisiel W. Inhibitory properties of full-length and truncated tissue factor pathway inhibitor (TFPI). J Biol Chem 1993; 268(12):8704–8710.

98 Nordfang O, Kristensen HI, Valentin S, Ostergaard P, Wadt J. The significance of TFPI in clotting assays—comparison and combination with other anticoagulants. Thromb Haemost 1993; 70(3):448–453.

99 Lindhout T, Willems G, Blezer R, Hemker H. Kinetics of the inhibition of human factor Xa by full-length and truncated

recombinant tissue factor pathway inhibitor. Biochem Jour 1994; 297(Pt 1):131–136.

100 Huang ZF, Wun TC, Broze GJ. Kinetics of factor Xa inhibition by tissue factor pathway inhibitor. J Biol Chem 1993; 268(36):26,950–26,955.

101 Enjyoji K, Miyaya T, Kamikubo Y, Kato H. Effect of heparin on the inhibition of factor Xa by tissue factor pathway inhibitor: a segment, Gly 212–Phe 243, of the third Kunitz domain is a heparin binding site. Biochemistry 1995; 34:5725–5735.

102 Lindahl AK, Abildgaard U, Larsen ML, Aamodt LM, Nordfang O, Beck TC. Extrinsic pathway inhibitor (EPI) and the post-heparin anticoagulant effect in tissue thromboplastin induced coagulation. Thromb Res 1991; (suppl 14):39–48.

103 Lindahl AK, Sandset PM, Abildgaard U. The present status of tissue factor pathway inhibitor. Blood Coag Fibrinol 1992; 3:439–449.

104 Novotny WF, Palmier MO, Wun TC, Broze GJ, Miletich JP. Purification and properties of heparin releasable lipoprotein-associated inhibitor. Blood 1991; 78:394–400.

105 Broze GJ, Miletich JP. Isolation of tissue factor inhibitor produced by HEPG2 hepatoma cells. Proc Natl Acad Sci USA 1987; 84:1886–1890.

106 Sandset PM, Abildgaard U, Larsen ML. Heparin induces release of extrinsic pathway inhibitor (EPI). Thromb Res 1988; 50:803–813.

107 Alban S, Gastpar R. Plasma levels of total and free tissue factor pathway inhibitor as individual pharmacological parameters of various heparins. Thromb Haemost 2001; 85(5):824–829.

108 Hoppensteadt DA, Fasanella A, Fareed J. Effect of protamine on heparin releasable TFPI antigen levels in normal volunteers. Thromb Res 1995; 79(3):325–330.

109 Kristensen HI, Ostergaard P, Nordfang O, Abilolgaard U. Effect of tissue factor pathway inhibitor (TFPI) in the HEPTEST assay and in an amidolytic anti factor Xa assay for LMW heparin. Thromb Haemost 1992; 68(3):310–314.

110 Day KC, Hoffman LC, Palmier MO, et al. Recombinant lipoprotein-associated coagulation inhibitor inhibits tissue thromboplastin-induced intravascular coagulation in the rabbit. Blood 1990; 76:1538–1545.

111 Warn-Cramer BJ, Rapaport SI. Studies of factor Xa/phospho-lipid induced intravascular coagulation on rabbits. Effects of immunodepletion of tissue factor pathway inhibitor. Arteriosclerosis Thrombosis 1993; 13(11):1551–1557.

112 Creasey AA, Chang ACK, Feigen L, Wun TC, Taylor FB, Hinshaw LB. Tissue factor pathway inhibitor reduces mortality from *Escherichia coli* septic shock. J Clin Invest 1993; 91:2850–2860.

113 Khouri RK, Koudsi D, Fu K, Ornberg RL, Wun TC. Prevention of thrombosis by topical application of tissue factor pathway inhibitor in a rabbit model of vascular trauma. Ann Plast Surg 1993; 30(5):398–404.

114 Kane WH, Davie EW. Blood coagulation factors V and VIII: structural and functional similarities and their relationship to hemorrhagic and thrombotic disorders. Blood 1988; 71: 539–555.

115 Owen WG, Esmon CT. Functional properties of an endothelial cell cofactor for thrombin catalyzed activation of protein C. J Biol Chem 1981; 256:5532–5535.

116 Dahlback B. The protein C anticoagulant system: inherited defects as basis for venous thrombosis. Thromb Res 1995; 77(1):1–43.

117 Maruyama I, Bell CE, Majerus PW. Thrombomodulin is found on endothelium of arteries, veins, capillaries, lymphatics, and syncytioblasts of human placenta. J Cell Biol 1985; 101:363–371.

118 Stenflo J. A new vitamin K-dependent protein. J Biol Chem 1976; 251:355–363.

119 Seegers WH, Novoa E, Henry RL, Hassouna HI. Relationship of "new" vitamin K-dependent protein C and "old" autopro-thrombin II-A. Thromb Res 1976; 8:543–552.

120 Kisiel W, Canfield WM, Ericsson LN, Davie EW. Anticoagulant properties of bovine plasma protein C following activation by thrombin. J Biol Chem 1977; 16:5824–5831.

121 Beckman RJ, Schmidt RJ, Santerre PF, Plutzky J, Crabtree GR, Long GL. The structure and evolution of a 461 amino acid human protein C precursor and its messenger Rna, based upon the DNA sequence of cloned human liver cDNAs. Acids Res 1985; 13:5233–5247.

122 Walker FJ, Fay PJ. Regulation of blood coagulation by the protein C system. FASEB J 1992; 6(8):2561–2567.

123 Solymoss S, Tucker MM, Tracy PB. Kinetics of inactivation of membrane-bound factor V by activated protein C. J Biol Chem 1988; 263:14,884–14,890.

124 Bauer KA, Kass BL, Beeler DL, Rosenberg RD. The detection of protein C activation in humans. J Clin Invest 1994; 74:2033–2041.

125 Gruber A, Hanson SR, Kelly AB, et al. Inhibition of thrombus formation by activated recombinant protein C in a primate model of arterial thrombosis. Circulation 1990; 82:578–585.

126 Preissner KT. Anticoagulant potential of endothelial cell membrane components. Haemostasis 1988; 18:271–273.

127 Baker JB, Low DA, Simmer RL, Cunningham DD. Protease nexin: a cellular component that links thrombin and plasminogen activator and mediates their binding to cells. Cell 1980; 21:37–45.

128 Eaton DL, Baker JB. Evidence that a variety of cultured cells secrete protease nexin and produce a distinct cytoplasmic serine protease-binding factor. J Cell Physiol 1983; 117:175–182.

129 Reilly TM, Mousa SA, Seetharam R, Racanelli AL. Recombinant plasminogen activator inhibitor type 1: a review of structural, functional, and biological aspects. Blood Coag Fibrinol 1994; 5(1):78–83.

130 Edelberg J, Pizzo SV. Lipoprotein (a) regulates plasmin generation and inhibition. Chem Phys Lipids 1994; 67:63–68.

131 Borth W. Alpha 2-macroglobulin, a multifunctional binding protein with targeting characteristics. FASEB J 1992; 6(15):3345–3353.

132 LaMarre J, Wollenberg GK, Gonias SL, Hayes MA. Cytokine binding and clearance properties of proteinase-activated alpha 2-macroglobulins. Lab Invest 1991; 65(1):3–14.

133 Hack CE, Oglivie AC, Eisele B, Jansen PM, Wagstaff J, Thijs LG. Initial studies on the administration of C1-esterase inhibitor to patients with septic shock or with a vascular leak syndrome induced by interleukin-2 therapy. Prog Clin Biol Res 1994; 388:335–357.

134 Carreer FM. The C1 inhibitor deficiency. Eur J Clin Chem Clin Biochem 1992; 30(12):793–807.

135 Lijnen HR, Hoylaerts M, Collen D. Isolation and characterization of human plasma protein with high affinity for lysine binding sites in plasminogen. J Biol Chem 1980; 225:10,214–10,222.

136 Engesser L, Kluft C, Briet E, Brommer E. Familial elevation of plasma histidine-rich glycoprotein in a family with thrombophilia. Br J Haematol 1987; 67:355–358.

137 Campbell W, Okada N, Okads H. Carboxypeptidase R is an inactivator of complement-derived inflammatory peptides and an inhibitor of fibrinolysis. Immuno Rev 2001; 180:162–167.

138 Bajzar L. Thrombin activatable fibrinolysis inhibitor and an antifibrinolytic pathway. Thrombosis Vascular Biol 2000; 20(12):2511–2518.

139 Tan AK, Eaton DL. Activation and characterization of procarboxypeptidase B from human plasma. Biochemistry 1995; 34:5811–5816.

140 Sato T, Miwa T, Asatsu H, et al. Pro-carboxypeptidase R is an acute phase protein in the mouse, whereas carboxypeptidase N is not. J Immunol 2000; 165:1053–1058.

141 Boffa MB, Hamill JD, Maret D, et al. Acute phase mediators modulate thrombin-activable fibrinolysis inhibitor (TAFI) gene expression in HepG2 cells. J Biol Chem 2003; 278(11):9250–9257.

142 Bajzar L. Thrombin activatable fibrinolysis inhibitor and an antifibrinolytic pathway. Arterioscler Thromb Vasc Biol 2000; 20(12):2511–2518.

143 Kakkar VV, Hoppensteadt DA, Fareed J, et al. Randomized trial of different regimens of heparins and in vivo thrombin generation in acute deep vein thrombosis. Blood 2002; 99(6):1965–1970.

144 Lau HK, Segev A, Hegele RA, et al. Thrombin-activatable fibrinolysis inhibitor (TAFI): a novel predictor of angiographic coronary restenosis. Thromb Haemost 2003; 90(6): 1187–1191.

145 Medina PJ, Sipols JM, George JN. Drug-associated thrombotic thrombocytopenic purpura-hemolytic uremic syndrome. Curr opin Hematol 2001; 8:286–293.

146 George JN. How I treat patients with thrombotic thrombocytopenic purpura- hemolytic uremic syndrome. Blood 2000; 96:1223–1229.

147 Egerman RS, Sibai BM. HELLP syndrome. Clin Obstet Gynecol 1999; 42:381–389.

148 Byrnes JJ, Moake JL. Thrombotic thrombocytopenic pupura and the hemolytic uremic syndrome: evolving concepts of pathogenesis and therapy. Clin Hematol 1986; 15:413–442.

149 Moake JL, Bynes JJ. Thrombotic microangiopathies associated with drugs and bone marrow transplantation. Hematol Oncol Clin North Am 1996; 10:485–497.

150 Karmali MA, Petric M, Lim C, et al. The association between idiopathic heolytic uremic syndrome and infection by verotoxin-producing Escherichia coli. J infec Dis 1985; 151:775–782.

151 Christie DJ, Pulkrabek S, Putnam JL, et al. Posttransfusion purpura due to an alloantibody reactive with glycoprotein Ia/IIa (anti-HPA-5b). Blood 1991; 77:2785–2789.

152 Shulman NR. Post-transfusion pupura. In: Nance ST, ed. Clinical and Basic Science Aspects if Immunohematology. Arlington, VA: American Association of Blood Banks, 1991:137–154.

153 Shulman NR, Jordan JV. Platelet immunology. In: Coleman RW, Hirsh J, Marder VJ, Salzman EW, eds. Hemostasis and Thrombosis. Philadelphia: JB Lippincott, 1987:452–529.

154 Classen DC, Pestonik SL, Evans RS, et al. Computerized surveillance of adverse drug events in hospital patients. JAMA 1991; 266:2847–2851.

155 Bottiger LE, Bottiger B. Incidence and cause of aplastic anemia, hemolytic anemia, agranulocytosis and thrombocytopenia. Acta Med Scand 1981; 210:475–479.

156 Bottiger L, Westerholm B. Thrombocytopenia. II. Drug-induced thrombocytopenia. Acta Med Scand 1973; 191:541–548.

157 Pedersen-Bjergaard U, Andersen M, Hansen PB. Thrombocytopenia induced by noncytotoxic drugs in Denmark 1968–1991. J Intern Med 1996; 239:509–515.

158 George JN, Raskob GE, Haha SR, et al. Drug-induced thrombocytopenia: a systematic review of published cases. Ann Intern Med 1998; 129:886–890.

159 Demasi R, Bode AP, Knupp C, et al. Heparin-induced thrombocytopenia. Am Surg 1994; 60:26–29.

160 Weisman RE, Tobin RW. Arterial embolism occurring systemic heparin therapy. AMA Arch Surg 1958; 76:219–226.

161 Aster RH. Heparin-induced thrombocytopenia and thrombosis. N Engl J Med 1995; 332:1374–1376.

162 Hoechst Marion Roussel, prescribing information (as of March 1998) for Refludan. HMR. The pharmaceutical Company of Hoechst, Kansas City, MO.

163 Frederiksen H, Schmidt K. The incidence of ITP in adults increases with age. Blood 1999; 94:909–913.

164 George JN, Woolf SH, Raskob GE, et al. Idiopathic thrombocytopenic purpura: a practice guideline developed by explicit methods for the American Society of Hematology. Blood 1996; 88:3–40.

165 Guthrie TH, Brannan DP, Prisant LM. Idiopathic thrombocytopenic purpura in the older adult patient. Am J Med Sci 1988; 296:17–21.

166 Cortellazo S, Finazzi G, Buelli M, et al. High risk of severe bleeding in aged patients with chronic idiopathic thrombocytopenic purpura. Blood 1991; 77:31–33.

167 Axelrad AA, Fskinazi D, Amato D. Hypersensitivity of circulating progenitor cells to megakaryocyte growth and development of factor (PEG-rHu MGDF) in essential thrombocythemia. Blood 1998; 92(suppl 1):488a.

168 Kaushansky K. Thrombopoietin. N Engl J Med 1998; 339:746–753.

169 Murphy S, Iland H, Rosnethal D, et al. Essential thrombocythemia: an interim report from the polycythemia vera study group. Semin Hematol 1986; 23:177–182.

170 Rodeghiero F, Castaman G, Dini E. Epidemiological investigation of the prevalence of von Willebrand's disease. Blood 1987; 69:454–459.

171 Miller CH, Graham JB, Goldin LR, Elston RC. Genetics of classic von Willebrand's disease. I. Phenotype variation within families. Blood 1979; 54:117–136.

172 Di Paola J, Frederici AB, Mannucci PM, et al. Low platelet alpha2 beta1 levels in type I von Willebrand disease correlate with impaired platelet function in a high shear stress system. Blood 1999; 93:3578–3582.

173 White GC, Beebe A, Nielsen B. Recombinant factor IX. Thromb Haemost 1997; 77:261–265.

174 Arnold WD, Hilgartner MW. Hemophilic arthropathy. Current concepts of pathogenesis and management. J Bone Joint Surg [AM] 1997; 59(3):287–305.

175 Kasper CK, Aledort LM, Counts RB, et al. A more uniform measurement of factor VIII inhibitors. Thromb Diath Haemorrhag 1975; 34:869–872.

176 Green D, Lechner K. A survey of 215 non-hemophilic patients with inhibitors to factor VIII. Thromb Haemost 1981; 45:200–203.

177 Morrison AE, Ludlam CA, Kessler C. Use of porcine factor VIII in the treatment of patients with acquired hemophilia. Blood 1993; 81:1513–1520.

178 Spero JA, Lewis JH, Hasiba U. Corticosteroid therapy for acquired FVIII:c inhibitors. Br J Haematol 1981; 48:635–642.

179 Green D. Suppression of an antibody to factor VIII by a combination of factor VIII and cyclophosphamide. Blood 1971; 37:381–387.

180 Sultan Y, Loyer F. In vitro evaluation of factor VIII-bypassing activity of activated prothrombin complex concentrates and factor VIIa in the plasma of patients with factor VIII inhibitors: thrombin generation test in the presence of collagen-activated platelets. J Lab Clin Med 1993; 121:444–452.

181 Hughes GRV. The antiphospholipid syndrome. Lupus 1996; 5:345–346.

182 Greaves M. Antiphospholipid antibodies and thrombosis. Lancet 1999; 353:1348–1353.

183 Wilson W, Gharavi AE, Koike T, et al. International consensus statement on preliminary classification criteria for definite antiphospholipid syndrome. Arthritis Rheum 1999; 42:1309–1311.

184 Asherson RA. Antiphospholipid antibodies. Clinical complications reported in medical literature. In: Harris EN, Exner T, Hughes GRV, Asherson RA, eds. Phospholipid-Binding Antibodies. Boston: CRC Press, Inc., 1991:388–402.

185 Barton M. Endothelial dysfunction and atherosclerosis: endothelin receptor antagonists as novel thaerapeutics. Curr Hypertens Rep 2000; 2:84–91.

186 Brevetti G, Piscione F, Silvestro A, et al. Increased inflammatory status and higher prevalence of three-vessel coronary artery disease in patients with concomitant coronary and peripheral atherosclerosis. Thromb Haemost 2003; 89:1058–1063.

187 Rossi GP, Cesari M, Zanchetta M, et al. The T-786 endothelial nitric oxide synthase genotype is a novel risk factor for coronary artery disease in caucasian patients for the GENICA study. J Am Coll Cardiol 2003; 41:930–937.

188 Widlansky ME, Gokce N, Keaney JF, Jr. et al. The clinical implications of endothelial dysfunction. JACC 2003; 42(7):1149–60.

189 Bild DE, Bluemke DA, Burke GL, et al. Multi-ethnic study of atherosclerosis: objectives and design. Am J Epidemiol 2002; 156:871–881.

190 Thaler E, Lechner K. Antithrombin III deficiency and thromboembolism. In: Prentice CRM, ed. Clinics in Hematology. London: WB Saunders, 1981:369–380.

191 Bertina RM, Koelman BPC, Koster T, et al. Mutation in blood coagulation factor V associated with resistance to activated protein C. Nature 1994; 369:64–67.

192 Dahlback B, Carlsson M, Svensson PJ. Familial thrombophilia due to a previously unrecognized mechanism characterized by poor anticoagulant response to activated protein C: prediction of a cofactor to activated protein C. Proc Natl Acad Sci USA 1993; 90:1004–1008.

193 Iqbal O, Eklof B, Tobu, Fareed J. Air travel-associated venous thromboembolism. Med Princ Pract 2003; 12:73–80.

194 Sack GH, Jr, Levin J, Bell WR. Trousseau's syndrome and other manifestations of chronic disseminated coagulopathy in patients with neoplasms: clinical and pathophysiologic and therapeutic features. Medicine (Baltimore) 1977; 56:1–37.

195 Sproul EE. Carcinoma and venous thrombosis: the frequency of association of carcinoma in the body or tail of the pancreas with multiple venous thrombosis. Am J Cancer 1938; 34:566–585.

196 Kakkar VV, Howe CT, Nicolaides AN, et al. Deep vein thrombosis of the leg. Is there a high risk group? Am J Surg 1970; 120:527–530.

197 Deppisch LM, Fayemi AO. Nonbacterial thrombotic endocarditis: clinicopathologic correlations. Am Heart Journal 1976; 92:723–729.

198 Fareed J, Hoppensteadt DA, Iqbal O, et al. Upregulation of monocyte chemotatic, protein-1 and CD-40 ligand in cancer and its modulation by a LMWH, enoxaparin. Observations from the Oncenox study [abstr]. Blood 2003; 102(11):552a.

199 Fareed D, Bick R, Bacher P, et al. Blood levels of nitric oxide, C-reactive protein and TNF-α are upregulated in patients with malignancy-associated hypercoagulable state: pathophysiologic implications. Pathophysiol Haemost Thromb 2003; 33(suppl 1):69–76.

200 Fareed D, Iqbal O, Tobu M, Hoppensteadt DA, Fareed J. Blood levels of nitric oxide, C-Reactive protein and TNF-α are upregulated in patients with malignancy-associated hypercoagulable state: pathophysiologic implications. ICATH 2004; 10(4):357–364.

201 Wun T, Law L, Harvey D, Sieracki B, Scudder SA, Ryu JK. Increased incidence of symptomatic venous thrombosis in patients with cervical carcinoma treated with concurrent chemotherapy, radiation and erythropoietin. Cancer 2003; 98(7):1514–1520.

202 http://www.rxlist.com/cgi/generic/epoietin_ad.htm. Dated 9th October, 2003.

203 Fuste B, Serradell M, Escolar G, et al. Erythropoietin triggers a signaling pathway in endothelial cells and increases the thrombogenicity of their extracellular matrices in vitro. Thromb Haemost 2002; 88:678–685.

204 Pixley RA, De La Cadena R, Page JD, et al. The contact system contributes to hypotension but not disseminated intravascular coagulation in lethal bacteremia: in vivo use of a monoclonal anti-factor XII antibody to block contact activation in baboons. J Clin Invest 1993; 92:61–68.

205 Bennett B, Oxnard SC, Douglas AS, et al. Studies on anti-haemophilic factor (AHF, factor VIII) during labor in normal women, in patients woth premature separation of the placenta, and in a patient with von Willebrand's disease. J Clin Lab Med 1974; 84:851–860.

206 Greer IA. Thrombosis in pregnancy: maternal and fetal issues. Lancet 1999; 353:1258–1265.

207 Williamson TH. Central retinal vein occlusion: what's the story? Br J Ophthalmol 1997; 81:698–704.

208 Bearman SI. The syndrome of hepatic venoocclusive disease after marrow transplantation. Blood 1995; 85:3005–3020.

209 Ulutin ON. Antithrombotic effect and clinical potential of defibrotide. Semin Thromb Hemost 1993; 19:186–191.

210 Richardson PG, Elias AD, Krishnan A, et al. Treatment of severe veno-occlusive disease with defibrotide: compassionate use results in response without significant toxicity in a high risk population. Blood 1998; 92:737–744.

211 Zucker-Franklin D, Cao YZ. Megakaryocytes of human immunodeficiency virus-infected individuals express viral RNA. Proc Natl Acad Sci USA 1989; 86:5595–5599.

212 Viale P, Pagani L, Alberici F. Clinical features and prognostic factors of HIV-associated thrombotic microangiopathies. Eur J Haematol 1998; 60:262–263.

213 Johnson BF, Manzo RA, Bergelin RO, et al. Relationship between changes in the deep venous system and the development of the postthrombotic syndrome after an acute episode of lower limb deep vein thrombosis: a one to six year follow-up. J Vasc Surg 1995; 21:307–313.

214 Killewich LA, Bedford GR, Beach KW, et al. Spontaneous lysis of deep venous thrombi: rate and outcome. J Vasc Surg 1989; 9:89–97.

215 Horlocker TT, Heit JA. Low molecular weight heparin: biochemistry, pharmacology, perioperative prophylaxis regimens, and guidelines for regional anesthetic management. Anesth Analg 1997; 85:874–885.

216 Schroeder DR. Statistics: detecting a rare adverse drug reaction using spontaneous reports. Reg Anesth Pain Med 1998; 23(suppl 2):183–189.

217 Bergquist D, Lindblad B, Matzsch T. Low molecular weight heparin for thromboprophylaxis and epidural/spinal anesthesia: is there a risk? Acta Anesthesiol Scand 1992; 36:605–609.

218 Tryba M. European practice guidelines: thromboembolism prophylaxis and regional anesthesia. Reg Anesth Pain Med 1998; 23(suppl 12):178–182.

219 Collins R, Scrimgeour A, Yusuf S, Peto R. Reduction in fatal pulmonary embolism and venous thrombosis by perioperative administration of subcutaneous heparin. Overview of results of randomized trials in general, orthopedic, and urologic surgery. N Engl J Med 1988; 318:1162–1173

220 Clagett GP, Reisch JS. Prevention of venous thromboembolism in general surgical patients. Results of meta-analysis. Ann Surg 1988; 208:227–240.

221 Bergentz SE. Dextran in the prophylaxis of pulmonary embolism. World J Surg 1978; 2:19–25.

222 Colditz GA, Tuden RL, Oster G. Rates of venous thrombosis after general surgery: combined results of ranomised clinical trials. Lancet 1986; 2(8499):143–146.

223 Nicolaides A, Bergquist D, Hull R. International Concensus Statement. Prevention of Venous Thrombosis. London, UK: Med-Orion Publishing Co., 1997.

224 Fareed J, Hoppensteadt DA, Bick RL. Management of thrombotic and cardiovascular disorders in the new millennium. Clin Appl Thromb Hemost 2003; 9(2):101–108.

225 Fareed J, Hoppensteadt DA. The management of thrombotic and cardiovascular disorders in the 21st century. In: Sasahara AA, Loscalzo J, eds. New Therapeutic Agents in Thrombosis and Thrombolysis, 2nd ed. New York, NY: Marcel Dekker, Inc., 2002:687.

226 Dalen JE, Hirsh J, Guyatt GH. Sixth ACCP consensus conference on antithrombotic therapy. Chest 2001; 119(1):1S–370S.

227 Gallus AS. Anticoagulants in the prevention of venous Thromboembolism. Bailliere's Clin Haematol 1990; 3(3):651–84.

2

Principles of antiplatelet therapy

Raul Altman, Alejandra Scazziota,
and María de Lourdes Herrera

Introduction

Although sealing vascular disruption is the main physiological activity of platelets, they are multifunctional cells and participate in several other processes that are of increasing interest. Besides arresting bleeding by the hemostatic plug, platelets have an important role in other physiological (recruitment of other blood cells, endothelial integrity, wound healing, inflammation) or pathological processes (atherosclerosis, inflammation, transplant rejection) (1).

Hemostasis is a physiological process for preventing hemorrhage, and platelets are crucial for its normal development. Normal endothelium is thrombo-resistant and platelets or other blood cells do not interact with endothelial cells. After endothelial injury, platelet adhere to exposed subendothelium, and under this condition, they are activated by agonists locally released and stimulate thrombin formation, contributing to the hemostatic clot. Under other circumstances, mainly in artery disease, tissue factor (TF) expressed by vascular cells upon plaque rupture activates platelets and leads to pathological thrombosis and vessel occlusion (2).

Platelets trigger hemostasis by accelerating the activation of the coagulation cascade by binding FXI via the receptor glycoprotein Ib/IX/V (GPIb/IX/V) and by providing a phospholipids surface for the assembly of the prothrombinase complex (FVa:FXa). A stronger stimulus through TF/activated aFVII (TF/aFVII) complex, in certain hemorheological conditions, triggers thrombosis.

Platelets in normal hemostasis

Platelets the smallest of the human blood cells are released from megakaryocytes in the bone marrow as anucleated fragments into the circulation.

Resting platelets are discoid with homogeneously distributed granules and surrounded by a bilamellar plasma membrane that extends through an open canalicular system into the cytoplasm (Fig. 1). Coating the inner surface of the platelet membrane is a network of cross-linked actin filaments, the cytoskeleton, which regulates the shape of resting platelets. The calcium pool, which is mobilized during platelet activation, and the enzymes involved in prostaglandin synthesis are localized in the dense tubular system that lies in contact to the open canalicular system. Dispersed in the cytoplasm, there are

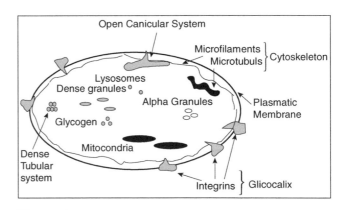

Figure 1

Platelet morphology in resting platelets. The platelet can be envisioned as composed of three primary zones: *peripheral zone* consists of an extramembranous glycocalyx, where there are adsorbed plasmatic proteins and the external domain of the integrin receptors. Inside of this zone is a plasmatic membrane similar to other trilamellar cellular plasma membranes. Under the membrane is an open canalicular system. The *sol–gel zone* consists of microtubules and microfilaments, the contractile proteins (cytoskeleton), and the dense tubular system. The *organelles zone* consists of dense bodies, α-granules, mitochondria, lysosomes, glycogen granules, and the dense tubular system.

mitochondria, glycogen particles, lysosomes, and α- and dense granules. The α-granules contain platelet factor 4 (PF4), β-thromboglobulin, fibronectin, vitronectin, thrombospondin (TSP), von Willebrand factor (vWF), platelet-derived growth factor (PDGF), coagulation factors such as fibrinogen, and factors V, VII, XI, and XIII, and protease inhibitors such as protein C, plasminogen activator inhibitor-1 (PAI-1), and TF pathway inhibitor (TFPI). Dense bodies liberate serotonin, adenosine diphosphate (ADP), and calcium. Some of the proteins contained in α-granules are synthesized by megakaryocytes, but others are endocytosed from the plasma (3).

When a vessel wall is damaged, platelets form the primary hemostatic plug to repair the site of a vascular lesion. Under conditions of physiological flow, the mechanism of a platelet immobilization at sites of injury is a complex multistep process. It requires platelet adhesion to the subendothelium and platelet–platelet interactions (recruitment and aggregation). In this process, activated platelets suffer a change in the assembly of cytoskeleton proteins resulting in shape change with the formation of pseudopodia. Further, the granules centralize, fuse with the plasma membrane, and secrete a variety of physiological agents such as ADP, serotonin, epinephrine, and thromboxane A_2 (TXA_2), which activate more platelets and attract them to the damaged vessel wall. The activation of platelets is associated with the binding of fibrinogen to its receptor, GPIIb/IIIa (integrin $\alpha_{IIb}\beta_3$), essential for platelet aggregation. Simultaneously, thrombin generation occurs, triggered by activated platelets' procoagulant activity, with the final formation of a stable platelet–fibrin plug (4).

Platelet adhesion

The adhesion of platelets to the subendothelial matrix via specific adhesive GPs is the initial step in primary hemostasis. Binding of platelets to the matrix results in rapid (Fig. 2) morphological conversion of platelets from flat discs to spiny spheres.

The GPIb/IX/V complex is the platelet receptor that mediates the deposition of platelets on the subendothelium involving an interaction with the high molecular weight multimeric plasma protein vWF. GPIb/IX/V is constitutively expressed on the platelet surface with approximately 25,000 copies per platelet. vWF does not bind appreciably to platelets in the circulation, but vWF bounded to collagen of the subendothelium enables its binding to the platelet receptor GPIb/V/IX, leading to the formation of firm bonds and platelet capture at the sites of collagen exposure (5). Conformational changes that occur in the GPIb/V/IX or vWF molecule modulate these interactions.

Platelet–collagen interactions are believed to have the greatest significance at the medium and high shear rates found in arteries and diseased vessels. The binding between immobilized vWF and GPIb/IX/V is reversible and slows the

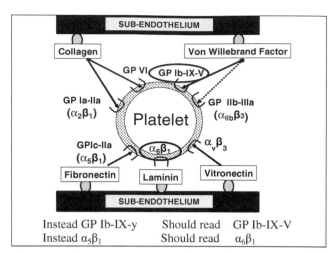

| Instead GP Ib-IX-y | Should read | GP Ib-IX-V |
| Instead $\alpha_5\beta_1$ | Should read | $\alpha_6\beta_1$ |

Figure 2

Main receptors involved in platelet adhesion. Most of the platelet receptors are heterodimers of α and β-subunits named integrins that are normally present as inactive form at resting platelets. β_1-integrins are $\alpha_2\beta_1$ (GPIa/IIa, collagen receptor); $\alpha_5\beta_1$ (fibronectin receptor), and $\alpha_6\beta_1$ (laminin receptor). β_3-integrins are $\alpha_{IIb}\beta_3$ (GPIIb/IIIa) and $\alpha_V\beta_3$ which share ligands (fibrinogen, fibronectin, von Willebrand factor, and vitronectin).

platelet temporarily near the injured vessel but is insufficient to stable adhesion, so at very high shear rates another receptor that is a membrane integrin, the GPIIb/IIIa, serves as an alternative adhesion substrate to vWF.

Collagen types III and I are strongly platelet-adhesive and thrombus-forming components of the vascular subendothelium also induce the exposure of procoagulant phosphatidylserine on platelets. Collagen fibers are exposed after endothelial injury and platelets adhere directly by collagen receptors GPIa/IIa (integrin $\alpha_2\beta_1$) and GPVI and indirectly by collagen-bound vWF by GPIb/V/IX and GPIIb/IIIa (integrin $\alpha_{IIb}\beta_3$) receptors (6).

However, for this to take place, at least one of these integrins must undergo conversion to the high affinity conformation in response to inside-out signals. This activation is induced by the immunoglobulin receptor GPVI. Thus, firm adhesion on collagen under high shear requires intracellular signals from GPVI (7).

The other macromolecular constituents of the exposed extracellular matrix, vitronectin, fibronectin, and laminin, have their own receptors on the platelet surface (Fig. 2) (8).

In flowing blood, red blood cells tend to stream to the center of the vessel lumen, whereas platelets distribute to the lumen periphery, so GPIb/IX/V complex mediates the rolling of cells and maintains surface contact, slowing down the platelets on the vessel wall. The binding between immobilized vWF and GPIb/IX/V is reversible and slows the platelet temporarily near the injured blood vessel (3).

Stimulation of platelets as a result of adhesion leads to spreading, activation of GPIIb/IIIa, enabling binding of soluble fibrinogen leading to platelet aggregation, and granule secretion.

Platelet aggregation

The central platelet receptor in aggregation is the GPIIb/IIIa (integrin $\alpha_{IIb}\beta_3$) linking activated platelets through fibrinogen bridges. GPIIb/IIIa supports platelet-to-platelet interaction and the dimeric structure of fibrinogen enables cross-linking adjacent activated platelets. The GPIIb/IIIa is one of the most abundant platelet surface receptors, perhaps 40,000 to 50,000 copies per platelet (5), 80% on its surface. It recognizes at least four adhesive proteins: fibrinogen, vWF, fibronectin, and vitronectin, which contain the three amino acids Arg-Gly-Asp (RGD sequence) for binding to the specific site in the GPIIb/IIIa receptor. The same as other integrins, GPIIb/IIIa is an heterodimer of α and β-subunits, which is normally present in an inactive form at resting state where it does not bind soluble fibrinogen or vWF. The binding of immobilized vWF to GPIb leads to a change in the fibrinogen recognition site of GPIIb/IIIa such that it can mediate irreversible platelet aggregation (9). In addition, G-proteins, intracellular calcium, protein kinases, and other proteins produce changes in the actin cytoskeleton, which allow GPIIb/IIIa complex to turn into the activated conformation required for ligand binding (inside-out signaling). Once bound to the ligand, the GPIIb/IIIa suffers additional conformational changes, which lead to phosphorylation of tyrosines of the cytoplasmatic GPIIb/IIIa chain tail (outside-in signaling) that results in high affinity binding sites for fibrinogen (10).

Activated platelets release granule components (platelet secretion), which stimulate additional circulating platelets that are recruited to form aggregates. Calcium mobilization leads to the release of α and dense granule components. The granules centralize and fuse with the plasma membrane via exocytosis with secretion of the granule content. Various GPs, such as P-selectin (CD62P), are exclusively localized on the α-granule membrane of resting platelets; upon secretion, the α-granule membrane fuses with the plasma membrane and exposes CD62P on the platelet surface (11).

P-selectin and other activation-dependent GPs, including CD40 ligand (CD40L), mediate platelet binding to neutrophils and monocytes (12). In this manner, platelets recruit leukocytes and T-cells into the growing plug. Platelet–monocyte aggregates play a role in enhancing formation of atherosclerotic plaques by the mechanisms described subsequently.

Platelet activity is controlled by a variety of surface receptors that regulate various functions. Platelet receptors are affected by several agonists (stimulus) and adhesive proteins. In general, binding of agonists to their receptors induce a complex cascade of signals that triggers to distinct processes: (*i*) platelets activation and granule release and (*ii*) the capacity of the platelet to bind to other adhesive proteins leading to the formation of thrombus (Fig. 3) (13).

The enzymes responsible for the platelet metabolism are distributed in different platelet structures. For example, the plasma membrane contains adenylate cyclase; in contrast, phospholipase (PL) A2, diglycerol lipase, cyclooxygenase

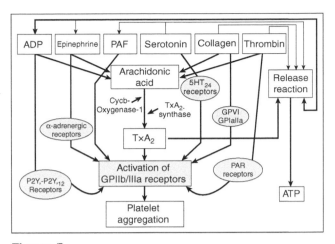

Figure 3

Agonist stimulation of platelet receptors induces various internal signaling pathways transduced from the membrane into the cytoplasm, which result in platelet receptors GPIIb/IIIa activation.

(COX), and thromboxane synthase are restricted to the intracellular dense tubular and granules membranes.

Platelet agonists ligation to its specific receptors leads to production and release of several intracellular messenger molecules such as calcium, products of the PLC, and COX.

Many platelet agonists, such as ADP, TXA_2, epinephrine, serotonin, and thrombin, interact with specific transmembrane receptors that are coupled to G-proteins, initiating several signaling pathways that lead to PLC activation ending in platelets shape change and granule secretion (Fig. 4).

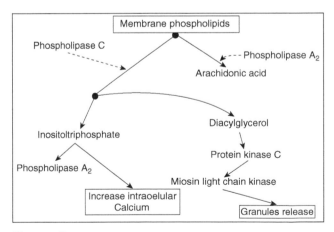

Figure 4

Phospholipase (PL) C catalyzes the hydrolysis of phosphatidyl inositolbiphosphate to inositoltriphosphate and diacylglycerol (DAG). IP3 induces the mobilization of calcium from the dense tubular system activating PLA_2. DAG activates a protein kinase C by a myosin-light-chain kinase, which is associated with phosphorylation of myosin light chain responsible for the shape change and granule secretion.

Thromboxane A_2 is synthesized in platelets following the release of arachidonic acid from phospholipid in the inner membrane leaflet by PLA_2. Arachidonic acid is subsequently metabolized by COX-1 that catalyzes the conversion of arachidonic acid to prostaglandin G_2 (PGG_2) and prostaglandin H_2 (PGH_2) unstable intermediates. TXA_2 synthase processes PGH_2 to produce TXA_2. TXA_2 has a half-life of 30 seconds (Fig. 5), promotes platelet aggregation, is a potent vasoconstrictor, and induces the proliferation of vascular smooth-muscle cells. TXA_2 receptors mediate, through a G-protein, the stimulation of PLC with the increase of inositol 1,4,5 triphosphate (IP3) and diacylglycerol (DAG) (14).

The former induces an increase in cytosolic concentration of calcium, whereas the latter activates a protein kinase C. Low-dose aspirin inhibits platelet COX-1 and induces a long-lasting inhibition of platelets aggregation (15).

This hemostatic/prothrombotic process is counterbalanced by vascular prostacyclin (PGI_2) derived predominantly from COX-2 activity and nitric oxide (NO) released from endothelial cells. In vascular endothelial cells, COX-2 produces primarily PGI_2 that inhibits platelet aggregation, induces vasodilation, inhibits the proliferation of vascular smooth-muscle cells, and is less susceptible to inhibition by low doses of aspirin. PGI_2 and NO induce an intracellular increase of second messengers. NO inhibits platelet function by stimulation of a soluble guanylyl cyclase to produce cGMP.

PGI_2 exerts its inhibitory activity by increasing cyclic adenosine monophosphate (cAMP) formation via adenylate cyclase, which stimulates phosphorylation of a cytoskeleton integrin protein-associated vasodilator-stimulated phosphoprotein (VASP), which prevents GPIIb–IIIa activation (16).

The other metabolic pathway derived from arachidonic acid is through the activity of the lypoxygenase-12 (2-LOX) (Fig. 5). 2-LOX converts arachidonic acid (AA) to 12-hydroperoxy-5,8,10,14-eicosatetraenoic acid (12-HPETE) that is rapidly reduced by peroxidases to the stable 12-hydroxy-5,8,10,14-eicosatetraenoic acid (12-HETE). In contrast to the prostaglandins, the products of the LOX are molecules that stimulate neutrophil chemotaxis and mediate hypersensitivity and inflammatory reactions as will be discussed subsequently. For example, platelet-derived 12-HPETE stimulates leukotriene production in leukocytes. Conversely, the formation of 12-HETE in platelets is inhibited by leukocyte-derived 5-HETE and 15-HETE.

Platelet agonists

Physiological effect at the site of an endothelial damage is the conjoint activity of several agonists from exposed subendothelium, released during platelet activation, coming from red or white cells or from activation of clotting mechanisms of the surrounding plasma.

Thrombin is a multifunctional serine protease involved in the cleavage of fibrinogen to fibrin and in the activation of a variety of cell types, including platelets and endothelial cells (17).

Thrombin and collagen are the strongest platelet agonists. Thrombin signaling is mediated by a family of G protein-coupled receptors, termed protease-activated receptors (PARs). Four PARs have been identified (PAR-1 through PAR-4); PAR-1, PAR-3, and PAR-4 are thrombin receptors (18). PAR-2 can be activated by trypsin and tryptase, but not by thrombin (19).

Current evidence suggests that thrombin activates human platelets by cleaving and activating PAR-1 and PAR-4 (20). Cleavage of human PAR-4 requires a higher concentration of thrombin than those for the cleavage of PAR-1.

Thrombin signaling might result in activation of PLC and phosphatidyl inositol 3-kinase (PI3K), which results in increasing the cytosolic calcium concentration and inhibiting cAMP formation. GPIb has also a thrombin-binding site; the complex thrombin–GPIb cleaves a GPV, which is an inhibitor of platelet function. The final result of these signaling events is platelet activation.

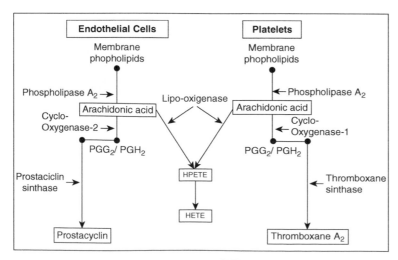

Figure 5

Arachidonic acid derived from membrane phospholipids is a 20-carbon fatty acid containing four double bonds. It is converted by cytosolic prostaglandin H synthase to the unstable intermediates prostaglandin G_2 and prostaglandin H_2 (PGH_2). The synthases are termed cyclooxygenases (COXs) and exist in two forms, COX-1 mainly in platelets and COX-2 mainly in endothelial cells. Subsequently, synthase acts on PGH_2 to form thromboxane A_2 or protacyclin, transient biological products that induce platelet aggregation or inhibition, respectively.

Adenosine diphosphate. In response to this agonist, platelets shape change, release granule contents, produce TXA_2, activate the fibrinogen receptor, and aggregate. As other weak agonists, ADP triggers the TXA_2 formation and the release of granule contents that reinforces aggregation.

There are three important ADP receptors on the platelet surface (16). The $P2X_1$ inotrophic receptor is responsible for rapid influx of calcium into the cytosol. The $P2Y_1$ receptor mediates mobilization of calcium through activation of PLC and shape change. The $P2Y_{12}$ receptor is coupled to adenyl cyclase inhibition mediated by a G-protein with subsequent decrease in the cAMP. The decrease in cAMP stimulates dephosphorylation of VASP that is closely correlated with the GPIIb/IIIa activation.

$P2Y_{12}$ receptor is required for complete aggregation response to ADP. Nevertheless, both (Fig. 6) receptors interact to lead the full response. ADP potentiates platelet secretion and irreversible aggregation. Enzymatic conversion of released ADP to inactive AMP by endothelial ecto-ADPase limits platelet activation by ADP. Thienopyridines (ticlopidine, clopidogrel, prasugrel, cangrelor) are used for inhibiting ADP-induced platelet function in the prevention of acute coronary events.

Epinephrine activates platelets through the α-adrenergic receptor coupled to a G-protein receptor. It is proposed that this agonist shares with ADP the $P2Y_{12}$ receptor signaling (16).

Serotonin [5-hydroxytryptamine (5-HT)], a well-known strong vasoconstrictor, binds to the G-protein-coupled 5HT2A receptor and amplifies, together with ADP, the platelet response. In addition, serotonin may play a procoagulant role in augmenting the retention of procoagulant proteins, such as fibrinogen and TSP, on the platelet surface (21). *Collagen* involves signaling by the major collagen receptors GPIa/IIa and GPVI. The signaling via GPVI is associated with an Fc-receptor γ-chain. Cross-linking of GPVI with Fc-receptor γ-chain leads to phosphorylation of the nonreceptor tyrosine kinase and activation of PLC. Recently, it has been revealed that GPIa/IIa may couple to many of the same intracellular signaling molecules such as GPVI (7).

The above-mentioned agonists are important factors in platelets activation and in the thrombotic process and many of the receptors are targets in the development of drugs for thrombosis prevention (Table 1).

Platelets in the cell-based model of hemostasis

The classical models of clotting cascades describe the sequential activation of clotting factors initiated by contact factors (Hageman factor, high molecular weight kininogen, and prekallikrein) or by the exposure of TF complexed with FVII. The TF–FVIIa complex activates the clotting cascade, which leads to platelets activation and thrombin generation.

Hemostasis is the specific response to vessel wall disruption, and platelets are primary factors in hemostasis and in acute arterial thrombosis. They adhere within seconds to the exposed subendothelial cells. Under this circumstance, platelets activated by agonists released at the site of endothelial injury increase thrombin generation (22). After activation, platelets also release the contents of intracellular granules and produce the externalization of membrane phosphatidylserine through the flip-flop mechanism (23), which will support the function of the prothrombinase complex. This is a local, not progressive, process because, as mentioned by Hemker and Béguin (24), clotting starts when 10 to 20 nmol/L of thrombin is formed and the faster initial thrombin activity could be safe for patients and important for hemostasis. Moreover, this local clotting mechanism and clot formation are limited by the little amount of exposed TF in a relatively small area, by dilution of activators in the blood

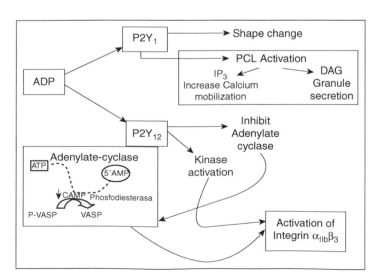

Figure 6

There are three important ADP receptors on the platelet surface. The $P2X_1$ is related with the rapid influx of calcium into the cytosol; the $P2Y_1$ mediates mobilization of calcium through activation of phospholipase C and shape change, and the $P2Y_{12}$ receptor is coupled to adenyl cyclase inhibition mediated by a G-protein with subsequent decrease of the cyclic adenosine monophosphate (cAMP). The decrease of cAMP stimulates dephosphorylation of vasodilator-stimulated phosphoprotein that is closely correlated with the GPIIb/IIIa activation. Thienopyridines compounds promote platelet inhibition mainly by blocking the $P2Y_{12}$ receptor.

Table 1   Inflammatory modulators expressed by platelets

NO. Inhibits platelet function and modifies monocytes, endothelial cells, and vascular smooth-muscle cells activity

PF4, CXCL4. Belongs to inflammatory cytokines family, mediates the relationship between monocytes and endothelial cells, induces neutrophil adhesion and secondary granule exocytosis, and influences macrophages adhesion to endothelial cell by triggering monocyte arrest in atherosclerotic arteries

CD40L. Are important in inflammation and contributes significantly to the recruitment of inflammatory cells to damaged endothelium in vivo. Also present in lymphocytes B-cells, monocytes, macrophages, and endothelial cells. Regulate macrophage and smooth-muscle cells of the vascular wall. Induce cytokines secretion of endothelial cells

PDGF. Induces proliferation of smooth-muscle cells of vascular wall

RANTES. Is the most efficient arrest chemokine. Influences macrophages adhesion to endothelial cell

TGF-β. Inhibits the production of pro-inflammatory mediators in vitro and in vivo. Stimulates biosynthesis of smooth-muscle cells in vascular wall

TSP-1. Matricellular protein released from activated platelets. Induces the expression of VCAM-1 and ICAM-1 on endothelium. Increases monocyte attachment

PSGL-1. Mediates the rolling of leukocytes on the endothelial cells allowing the recruitment of leukocytes to the inflamed tissue

JAMs. Members of an immunoglobulin subfamily expressed by leukocytes, platelets, and endothelial cells, regulates leukocyte/platelet/endothelial cell interactions in the immune system, and promotes inflammatory vascular responses

Abbreviations: CD40L, CD40 ligands; JAMs, junctional adhesion molecules; NO, nitric oxide; PDGF, platelet-derived grown factor; PF4, platelet factor 4; P-selectin glycoprotein ligand-1; RANTES, regulated on activation, normal T-cell expressed and secreted; TGF-β, transforming growth factor-β; TSP-1, thrombospondin-1; PSGL-1.

stream, by TFPI that locally inhibits TF/FVIIa activity, and by other natural coagulation inhibitors. This model of hemostasis (Fig. 7) is in line with the cell-based model of coagulation (25).

One controversial issue is whether TF is present in platelets or TF circulates in blood in the form of cell-derived microparticles (2). Nevertheless, although platelets could not contain TF, they could generate thrombin through a TF-independent mechanism (25).

On the contrary, in arterial thrombosis where inflammation promotes atheroma rupture, higher TF levels in atheroma, also expressed by monocytes and macrophage-derived foam cells, would be several times greater and, through enhancement of TF/FVIIa complex, will produce a strong platelets activation and thrombin generation. Blood flow changes (stasis) into a partial or total occluded vessel prevent activated factors and formed thrombin from dilution and together with platelet-erythrocyte interaction promotes thrombus to grow.

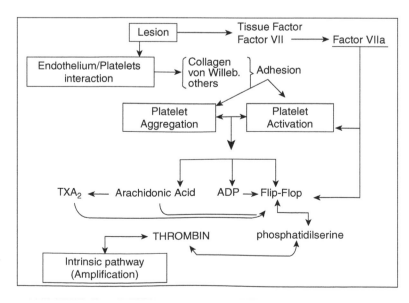

Figure 7
Platelet participation in normal hemostasis. The hemostatic plug is the specific response to external vessel lesion and depends on the extent of vessel wall damage, the specific interaction between endothelial cells and activated platelets, release of the contents of platelets intracellular granules in response to activation, the conjoint activity of activated factor VII and platelet agonists, and the "open conditions" of blood flow. After activation, platelets also produce the externalization of membrane phosphatidylserine through the flip-flop mechanism that will support the function of the prothrombinase complex ending in thrombin generation and local clot formation.

Based on the differences between hemostasis and thrombosis mechanisms, which, even though similar, are developing through different routes, the practical point related to antithrombotic therapies is that increased concentrations of antithrombotic drugs will affect thrombosis as well as hemostasis but, as the latter is a weaker process than the former, any important increase in anticoagulant potential will produce a bleeding tendency before stopping thrombosis (26).

Whether inhibition of TF will prevent acute arterial disease-associated thrombosis, where a lower possibility of bleeding can be expected, is a point that deserves to be investigated.

Platelet's contribution to inflammation and atherosclerosis

Arterial disease and blood clotting are associated with platelet activation that can occur from one or more different stimuli. Patients with acute coronary syndromes have increased interactions between platelets and leukocytes (heterotypic aggregates) that contribute to atherothrombosis (13).

It is now widely accepted that atherosclerosis is a chronic inflammatory arterial disease associated with risk factors, platelet, and other blood cells activities and their interactions with subendothelial cells. Activated platelets release active components from citosol and induce the externalization of phosphatidylserine through the flip-flop mechanism (23) that supports the function of the prothrombinase complex ending in thrombin generation.

Platelets are considered as the key factors in arterial thrombosis; recent studies indicate that they have an important regulatory role as the source of inflammatory mediators and directly initiate (Fig. 8) an inflammatory response of the vessel wall. Platelet and leukocyte recruitment on subendothelial cells is the early mechanism of vascular inflammatory damage. After vascular injury denudation of the endothelium and platelet adhesion, other blood cells are recruited: erythrocytes release ADP and leukocyte infiltration occurs by their interaction with adhered platelets and fibrin. Additionally, leukocyte binding to platelets allows the recruitment of leukocytes and monocytes and constitutes a bridge between inflammation, thrombosis, and atherosclerosis.

There are multicellular interactions that are important in inflammatory processes and in vascular remodeling. Activated platelets induce endothelial cells to secrete chemokines and to express adhesion molecules, indicating that platelets could initiate an inflammatory (Table 1) response of the vessel wall. Activated platelets promote leukocyte binding to inflamed or atherosclerotic lesions (27,28). Cell adhesion molecules (CAMs) are responsible for leukocyte–endothelium interactions. It plays a crucial role in inflammation and atherogenesis. Vascular CAM-1 (VCAM-1) and intracellular CAM-1 (ICAM-1) promote monocyte recruitment to sites of injury and constitute a critical step in inflammation and in atherosclerotic plaque development. TSP-1, a matricellular protein released in abundance from activated platelets and accumulated in sites of vascular injury, induces the expression of VCAM-1 and ICAM-1 on endothelium and significantly increases the monocyte attachment (29).

Leukocyte–platelet interaction is mediated in part by the β2-integrin Mac-1 (CD11b/CD18) and its counter-receptor on platelets; GPIbα is important in mediating leukocyte adhesion to a thrombus and leukocyte recruitment to a site of vascular injury (30). In this regard, recently described junctional adhesion molecules (JAMs) are members of an immunoglobulin subfamily expressed by leukocytes, platelets, and endothelial cells that regulate leukocyte/platelet/endothelial cell interactions in the immune system (31). Among these, JAM-1 is a platelet receptor involved in platelet adhesion and antibody-induced platelet aggregation and JAM-3, also called JAM-C, was described as a counter-receptor on platelets for the leukocyte β2-integrin Mac-1, which mediates leukocyte–platelet interactions and neutrophil transmigration and promotes inflammatory vascular responses (32).

Platelet-derived chemokines CCL5 [regulated on activation, normal T-cell expressed and secreted (RANTES)] and CXCL4 (PF4) influence macrophages adhesion to endothelial cell by triggering monocyte arrest in atherosclerotic arteries. RANTES was the most efficient arrest chemokine (33). PF4 induced neutrophil adhesion and secondary granule exocytosis.

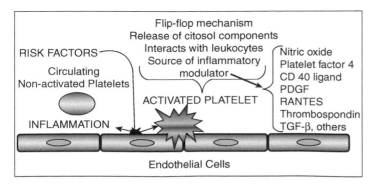

Figure 8

Disrupted endothelium initiates hemostatic or thrombotic process with platelet adhesion, activation, and aggregation. Activated platelets release active components from citosol, induce the externalization of phosphatidylserine through the flip-flop mechanism, have a regulatory role as the source of inflammatory mediators, and interact with circulating white cells. *Abbreviations*: PDGF, plated derived growth factor; RANTES, regulated on activation, normal T-cell expressed and secreted; TGF-β, transforming growth factor-β.

CD40 ligand (CD40L) is a cell-surface molecule that is expressed on activated T-cells and platelets. Platelet CD40L and its receptor CD40 are important in inflammation and contribute significantly to the recruitment of inflammatory cells to damaged endothelium in vivo (34). CD40L is a trimeric, transmembrane protein structurally related to the cytokine tumor necrosis factor-α present in lymphocytes, B-cells, monocytes, macrophages, and endothelial cells. Interaction of CD40L on T-cells with CD40 on B-cells is one of the determinants in the function of the humoral immune system and generates signals for the recruitment and extravasation of leukocytes at the site of injury. In patients with unstable coronary artery disease, elevation of soluble CD40L levels indicated an increased risk of cardiovascular events (35).

Polymorphonuclear leukocyte adhesion to activated platelets is important for leukocyte recruitment at sites of damage and this is supported by P-selectin expressed on the surface of activated platelets to the leukocyte receptor, P-selectin GP ligand-1 (PSGL-1) (36). PSGL-1 mediates the rolling of leukocytes on the endothelial cells allowing the recruitment of leukocytes to the inflamed tissue, initiates intracellular signals during leukocytes activation, and upregulates the transcriptional activity of colony stimulating factor-1 (CSF-1) increasing the endogenous expression of CSF-1.

Under shear flow conditions, there is a preferential recruitment of platelets by monocytes relative to neutrophils (37), an important point since the early development of lesions follows the invasion of the intima by monocytes, with transformation of monocyte-derived macrophages into foam cells when oxidized low-density lipoproteins are taken by monocytes contributing to the formation of atherosclerotic lesions. Macrophages release proteolytic enzymes called metalloproteinases, a group of zinc-dependent endopeptidases, which break down collagen in the fibrous cap, inducing its rupture and the release of TF into the blood near to atheroma. TF, expressed by macrophage-derived foam cells within atherosclerotic plaques and TF activity related substances, will enhance thrombin generation inducing thrombosis. Local thrombin generation not only results in a mixed fibrin/platelets clot but thrombin itself has pro-inflammatory activity and highlights the interaction between inflammation, thrombosis, and atherosclerosis.

Thrombin also activates platelets and other cells via cleavage of PARs, specifically by PAR-1 and PAR-4, expressed, besides platelets, by other cells including endothelial cells and smooth-muscle cells (38). Within each of these cells, PAR signaling can impact the initiation, progression, and complications of atherosclerosis.

Other inflammatory mediators, activated macrophages, T-lymphocytes, and mast cells also attach themselves to the endothelium and lead to the release of additional mediators, (adhesion molecules, cytokines, chemokines, growth factors), with important roles in atherogenesis. Also platelet's P-selectin induces TF and cytokine expression from monocytes (39).

Lastly, eicosanoids are important pro-inflammatory mediators derived from membrane metabolism. PLA_2 plays a key role in the production of eicosanoids, derived from arachidonic acid of the phospholipids contained in the cell membrane (40,41). As mentioned earlier, arachidonic acid is liberated from the membrane-bound phospholipids by several forms of PLA_2 and is the substrate for COX-1, COX-2, and 12-lipoxygenases (LOX) involved in vascular inflammation.

Besides 12-LOX in platelets, the 5-LOX isoforms are constitutive in neutrophils. Evidences indicate that LOXs are involved in inflammation diseases and in atherosclerosis. 5-LOX is the enzyme that catalyzes the formation of leukotrienes with potential role for leukocytes and platelets interaction and inflammation. After platelet and leukocyte stimulation, products of both COX-1 and 5-LOX pathways increase. COX-1 activity derivatives increase the vascular permeability mediated by prostaglandins and produce platelet aggregation mediated by TXA_2. The product of the lipoxygenase pathway, 5-oxo-6,8,11,14-eicosatetraenoic acid (5-Oxo-ETE), induces leukocyte chemotaxis and inflammation. 5-Oxo-ETE is formed by the oxidation of 5S-hydroxy-ETE (5-HETE) by 5-hydroxyeicosanoid dehydrogenase (5-HEDH), a microsomal enzyme found in leukocytes and platelets (42).

Leukotrienes increase vascular permeability, wall recruitment of leukocytes, endothelial-cell dysfunction, proliferation of smooth-muscle cells, immune reactivity and mediated vascular inflammation, and atherosclerosis (43).

COX-2 are mainly involved in PGI_2 formation and in the inflammatory process. COX-2 is inducible, for example, by pro-inflammatory cytokines and growth factors, implying a role for COX-2 in both inflammation and the control of cell growth. It promotes early atherosclerotic lesion formation in LDL receptor-deficient mice in vivo, and COX-2 is the enzyme responsible for most of the metabolism of arachidonic acid in the macrophage.

In conclusion, we have described how platelets initiate and participate in the hemostatic and thrombotic processes, as well as many of the multiple interactions of platelet with endothelial cells and with other blood cells, and their role in inflammation and atherosclerosis. From a practical point of view, these liaisons indicate that platelet inhibition could prevent thrombosis as well as inflammation and atherosclerosis. These potential properties have resulted in antiplatelets drugs being most commonly used as remedies for the prevention of acute arterial syndromes (Table 2). Although the main and most investigated activity of platelet inhibitors (aspirin, thienopyridines family, and GPIIb/IIIa inhibitors) is their capacity to affect platelet aggregation, they really are drugs with pluripotential effects that could contribute to their antithrombotic activities (44,45). On the way are antiplatelet combinations and new therapies for preventing platelet adhesion and activation (Table 2).

Other target has been also used for acute thrombotic prevention. Selective COX-2 inhibitors are effective

Table 2   Effects of different molecules on platelet function used to reduce the risk of thrombosis

Drugs	Main activity
Aspirin and other nonsteroidal anti-inflammatory drugs	Dose-related blockade of COX-1 and COX-2. Inhibit platelets PGG_2, PGH_2, and TXA_2 and endothelial PGI_2 formation
TXA_2 synthase inhibitors and receptor antagonist (BM 573, picotamide, terbogrel)	Inhibit TXA_2 formation and blocks platelet TXA_2 effects
Thienopyridines (ticlopidina, clopidogrel, prasugrel, cangrelor, AZD6140)	Inhibit platelet activation by preventing binding of ADP with it receptors, mainly $P2Y_{12}$
Inhibitors of phosphodiesterase (dipyridamole, cilostazol) prasugrel, cangrelor, AZD6140)	Increase platelet cAMP-inhibiting platelet aggregation. Dipyridamole also prevents the uptake of adenosine
Inhibitor of platelet vWF receptors	Inhibits the link of vWF with their platelet receptor GPIb inhibiting platelet adhesion
Blockade of fibrinogen γ-chain	Inhibits fibrinogen link to their platelets receptors
Blockers/inhibitors of platelets receptors GP IIb/IIIa (integrin $\alpha IIb\beta 3$) (abciximab, tirofiban, eptifibatide)	Prevent the link of fibrinogen with platelet receptors inhibiting platelet aggregation in front of different agonists
PAR antagonist	Inhibits thrombin. Potent potential effect for inhibiting platelet aggregation
Collagen-GPVI inhibitors	Inhibit platelet adhesion to subendothelium
PGI_2 analog/mimetic (epoprostenol, FR181157) Sildenafil	Inhibits platelet aggregation Inhibits type-5 phosphodiesterase and reduces platelet activation

Note: Several of the described drugs are still under development (currently in phase 2 or phase 3 trial) and not yet available in the pharmaceutical market for human use. Others, such as sildenafil, reduce platelets activity but, to our knowledge, no specific trial is under way. Although not included in the table, also direct thrombin inhibitor (melagatran, dabigatran) in high dose prolongs bleeding time, indicating that by effect of a strong inhibition of thrombin activity, probably at concentrations exceeding the dose that inhibited thrombosis, relationships between platelet and endothelial cells could be modified toward an hemorrhage tendency.

Abbreviations: ADP, adenosine diphosphate; cAMP, cyclic adenosine monophosphate; COX-1, cyclooxygenase-1; COX-2, cyclooxygenase-2; GP, glycoprotein; PAR, protease activated receptor; PGG_2, prostaglandin G_2; PGH_2, prostaglandin H_2; PGI_2, prostacyclin; TXA2, thromboxane A_2; vWF, von Willebrand factor.

anti-inflammatory agents and even if some of them appear to prevent coronary events (46), others increase the cardiovascular risk because of their inhibitory effect on endothelial PGI_2 synthesis without affecting TXA_2-dependent platelet function, although mechanisms unrelated to thromboxane production cannot be discarded (47). Additional trials and new combining strategies will be required to assess the effects of selective COX-2 inhibitors (48). The ongoing chapters deal with these important issues.

References

1   Gordon JL, Milner AJ. Blood platelets as multifunctional cells. In: Gordon JL, ed. Platelets in Biology and Pathology, ch. 1. New York: Elsevier/North-Holland Biomedical Press, 1976:3–22.

2   Mackman N. Role of tissue factor in hemostasis, thrombosis, and vascular development. Arterioscler Thromb Vasc Biol 2004; 24:1015–1022.

3   Ramasamy I. Inherited bleeding disorders: disorders of platelet adhesion and aggregation. Crit rev Oncol Hematol 2004; 49: 1–35.

4   Zwaal R, Schroit AJ. Pathophysiologic implications of membrane phospholipid asymmetry in blood cell. Blood 1997; 89:1121–1132.

5   Jurk K, Kehrel, B. Reliability of platelet function tests and drug monitoring platelets: physiology and biochemistry. Semin Thromb Hemost 2005; 31:381–392.

6   Kuijpers MJ, Schulte V, Oury C, et al. Facilitating roles of murine platelet glycoprotein Ib and alphaIIb beta3 in phosphatidylserine exposure during vWF-collagen-induced thrombus formation. J Physiol 2004; 558:403–415.

7   Nieswandt B, Watson S. Platelet–collagen interaction: is GPVI the central receptor? Blood 2003; 102:449–461.

8   Schmitz G, Rothe G, Ruf A, et al. European Working Group on clinical cell analysis: consensus protocol for the flow cyometric characterisation of platelet function. Thromb Haemost 1998; 79:885–896.

9   Shattil S, Newman P. Integrins: dynamic scaffolds for adhesion and signalling in platelets. Blood 2004; 104:1606–1615.

10   Lahav J, Jurk K, Hess O, et al. Sustained integrin ligation involves extracellular free sulfhydryls and enzymatically catalyzed disulfide exchange. Blood 2002; 100:2472–2478.

11   Furie B, Furie BC, Flaumenhaft R. A journey with platelet Pselectin: the molecular basis of granule secretion, signalling and cell adhesion. Thromb Haemost 2001; 86:214–221.

12 Andre P, Prasad KS, Denis CV, et al. CD40L stabilizes arterial thrombi by a beta 3 integrin-dependent mechanism. Nat Med 2002; 8:247–252.

13 Freedman J. Molecular regulation of platelet dependent thrombosis. Circulation 2005; 112:2725–2734.

14 Brass LF. Thrombin and platelet activation. Chest 2003; 124:18s–25s.

15 Patrono C, García Rodríguez LA, Landolfi R, Baigent C. Low-dose aspirin for the prevention of atherothrombosis. N Engl J Med 2005; 353:2373–2383.

16 Geiger J, Brich J, Höning-Liedl M, et al. Specific impairment of human platelet $P2Y_{AC}$ ADP receptor-mediated signalling by the antiplatelet drug Clopidogrel. Arterioscler Thromb Vasc Biol 1999; 19:2007–2011.

17 Minami T, Sugiyama A, Wu SQ, et al. Thrombin and phenotypic modulation of the endothelium. Arterioscler Thromb Vasc Biol 2004; 24:41–53.

18 Ishihara H, Connolly AJ, Zeng D, et al. Protease-activated receptor 3 is a second thrombin receptor in humans. Nature 1997; 386:502–506.

19 Luque A, Carpizo DR, Iruela-Arispe ML. ADAMTS1/METH1 inhibits endothelial cell proliferation by direct binding and sequestration of VEGF 165. J Biol Chem 2003; 278: 23656–23665.

20 Coughlin SR. Thrombin signalling and protease-activated receptors. Nature 2000; 407:258–264.

21 Dale GL, Friese P, Batar P, et al. Stimulated platelets use serotonin to enhance their retention of procoagulant proteins on the cell surface. Nature 2002; 415:175–179.

22 Altman R, Scazziota A, Rouvier J, Gonzalez C. Effect of sodium arachidonate on thrombin generation through platelet activation—inhibitory effect of aspirin. Thromb Haemost 2000; 84:1109–1112.

23 Lentz BR. Exposure of platelet membrane phosphatidylserine regulates blood coagulation. Prog Lipid Res 2003; 42:423–438.

24 Hemker HC, Béguin S. Thrombin generation in plasma: its assessment via the endogenous thrombin potential. Thromb Haemost 1995; 74:134–138.

25 Monroe DM, Hoffman M, Oliver JA, Roberts HR. A possible mechanism of action of activated factor VII independent of tissue factor. Blood Coagul Fibrinolysis 1998; 9(suppl 1):S15–S20.

26 Alexander KP, Chen AY, Roe MT, et al. Excess dosing of antiplatelet and antithrombin agents in the treatment of non-ST-segment elevation acute coronary syndromes. JAMA 2005; 294:3108–3116.

27 Rainger GE, Buckley C, Simmons DL, Nash GB. Neutrophils rolling on immobilised platelets migrate into homotypic aggregates after activation. Thromb Haemost 1998; 79:1177–1183.

28 Eriksson EE. Mechanisms of leukocyte recruitment to atherosclerotic lesions: future prospects. Curr Opin Lipidol 2004; 15:553–558.

29 Narizhneva NV, Razorenova OV, Podrez EA, et al. Thrombospondin-1 up-regulates expression of cell adhesion molecules and promotes monocyte binding to endothelium. FASEB J 2005; 19:1158–1160.

30 Chavakis T, Santoso S, Clemetson KJ, et al. High molecular weight kininogen regulates platelet-leukocyte interactions by bridging Mac-1 and glycoprotein Ib. J Biol Chem 2003; 278:45375–45381.

31 Naik UP, Eckfeld K. Junctional adhesion molecule 1 (JAM-1). J Biol Regul Homeost Agents 2003; 17:341–347.

32 Chavakis T, Keiper T, Matz-Westphal R, et al. The junctional adhesion molecule-C promotes neutrophil transendothelia l migration in vitro and in vivo. J Biol Chem 2004; 279:55602–55608.

33 Baltus T, von Hundelshausen P, Mause SF, Buhre W, Rossaint R, Weber C. Differential and additive effects of platelet-derived chemokines on monocyte arrest on inflamed endothelium under flow conditions. J Leukoc Biol 2005; 78:435–441.

34 Buchner K, Henn V, Grafe M, de Boer OJ, Becker AE, Kroczek RA. CD40 ligand is selectively expressed on CD4+ T cells and platelets: implications for CD40-CD40L signalling in atherosclerosis. J Pathol 2003; 201:288–295.

35 Heeschen C, Dimmeler S, Hamm CW, et al. CAPTURE Study Investigators. Soluble CD40 ligand in acute coronary syndromes. N Engl J Med 2003; 348:1104–1111.

36 Ba XQ, Chen CX, Xu T, Cui LL, Gao YG, Zeng XL. Engagement of PSGL-1 upregulates CSF-1 transcription via a mechanism that may involve Syk. Cell Immunol 2005; 237:1–6

37 Ahn KC, Jun AJ, Pawar P, et al. Preferential binding of platelets to monocytes over neutrophils under flow. Biochem Biophys Res Commun 2005; 329:345–355.

38 Coughlin R, Camerer E. Participation in inflammation. J Clin Invest 2003; 111:25–27.

39 Celi A, Pellegrini G, Lorenzet R, et al. P-selectin induces the expression of tissue factor on monocytes. Proc Natl Acad Sci U S A 1994; 91:8767–8771.

40 Dwyer J H, Allayee H, Dwyer KM, et al. Arachidonate 5-lipoxygenase promoter genotype, dietary arachidonic acid, and atherosclerosis. N Engl J Med 2004; 350:29–37.

41 Coffey MJ, Jarvis GE, Gibbins JM, et al. Platelet 12-lipoxygenase activation via glycoprotein VI. Involvement of multiple signaling pathways in agonist control of H(P)ETE synthesis. Circ Res 2004; 94:1598–1605.

42 Powell WS, Rokach J. Biochemistry, biology and chemistry of the 5-lipoxygenase product 5-oxo-ETE. Prog Lipid Res 2005; 44:154–183.

43 Lotzer K, Spanbroek R, Hildner M, et al. Differential leukotriene receptor expression and calcium responses in endothelial cells and macrophages indicate 5-lipoxygenase-dependent circuits of inflammation and atherogenesis. Arterioscler Thromb Vasc Biol 2003; 23:E32–E36.

44 Judge HM, Buckland RJ, Holgate CE, Storey RF. Glycoprotein IIb/IIIa and P2Y12 receptor antagonists yield additive inhibition of platelet aggregation, granule secretion, soluble CD40L release and procoagulant responses. Platelets 2005; 16: 398–407.

45 Altman R, Luciardi HL, Muntaner J, Herrera RN. The antithrombotic profile of aspirin. Aspirin resistance, or simply failure? Thromb J 2004; 2:1.

46 Altman R, Luciardi HL, Muntaner J, et al. Efficacy assessment of meloxicam, a preferential cyclooxygenase-2 inhibitor, in acute coronary syndromes without ST-segment elevation: the Nonsteroidal Anti-Inflammatory Drugs in Unstable Angina Treatment-2 (NUT-2) pilot study. Circulation 2002; 106: 191–195.

47 Jones SC. Relative thromboembolic risks associated with COX-2 inhibitors. Ann Pharmacother 2005; 39:1249–1259.

48 Grosser T, Fries S, Fitzgerald AG. Biological basis for the cardiovascular consequences of COX-2 inhibition: therapeutic challenges and opportunities. J Clin Invest 2006; 116:4–15.

3

Glycoprotein IIb/IIIa inhibitors

Sanjay Kaul

Platelet glycoprotein IIb/IIIa (GPIIb/IIIa) receptor inhibitors are widely used to prevent thrombotic vascular events, especially in patients with acute coronary syndromes (ACS) or in those undergoing intravascular interventional procedures. The purpose of this chapter is to evaluate the quality and magnitude of the clinical trial evidence in support of their use. In addition, key issues regarding their optimal application in clinical practice will be discussed.

thrombus formation is the key initiating factor in occlusive vascular disease; (*ii*) the GPIIb/IIIa receptor is a key element in the final common pathway leading to platelet aggregation and consequently platelet thrombus formation; (*iii*) the GPIIb/IIIa receptor is platelet specific; and (*iv*) inhibition of the GPIIb/IIIa receptor inhibits platelet aggregation without interfering in platelet adhesion, thereby reducing the risk of occurrence of serious bleeding.

Platelet physiology and the rationale for glycoprotein IIb/IIIa inhibitors

GPIIb/IIIa receptor is a major platelet integrin that plays a central role in platelet aggregation (1,2). It is uniquely and abundantly expressed on the platelet surface (~50,000–80,000 copies) with an additional internal pool in α-granules that can be rapidly mobilized to the platelet surface upon activation (1,2). Although GPIIb/IIIa has no ligand-binding activity in unstimulated platelets, it undergoes a conformational change upon platelet activation allowing it to bind to its ligands, fibrinogen and von Willebrand factor. Both ligands have multiple binding sites for activated GPIIb/IIIa and thereby induce platelet aggregation by cross-linking adjacent platelets (1,2). Activation of this integrin is considered the "common final pathway" since all the signaling pathways utilize this molecule at the last step toward aggregation (1,2) (Fig. 1).

Several experimental observations provide the rationale for blockade of GPIIb/IIIa receptors as a desirable therapeutic strategy in ischemic cardiovascular disease (3): (*i*) platelet

Pharmacology of glycoprotein IIb/IIIa inhibitors

Three intravenous GPIIb/IIIa inhibitors are currently available for clinical use: abciximab, tirofiban, and eptifibatide (4–7). Their mechanisms of action, important differences in pharmacology as well as approved indications and dosing regimens are listed in Table 1.

Abciximab is the Fab fragment of a chimeric human–mouse monoclonal antibody directed against the human GPIIb/IIIa receptor. It is a nonspecific blocker exhibiting cross-reactivities with vitronectin and the leukocyte integrin Mac-1, with a tight receptor binding and slow (~48 hours) reversibility of platelet inhibition after cessation of treatment (4,5). The pharmacodynamic and clinical significance of the cross-reactivities is, however, not entirely clear. Tirofiban is a tyrosine derivative, nonpeptide mimetic of the RGD (Arg-Gly-Asp) recognition sequence (4,5). Eptifibatide is a cyclic heptapeptide based on the KGD (Lys-Gly-Asp) sequence of the snake venom barbourin, a natural disintegrin (4,5). Both eptifibatide and tirofiban are highly selective inhibitors of the GPIIb/IIIa receptor with rapid onset of action, short half-lives, and

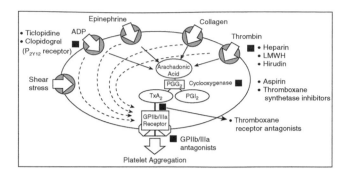

Figure 1

Platelet activation cascade in response to different agonists and the site of action of different antiplatelet agents.

recovery of platelet function within two to four hours after cessation of treatment (4,5). Target receptor blockade of >80% is required for a pharmacodynamic effect of these inhibitors (4,5).

Clinical evaluation of glycoprotein IIb/IIIa inhibitors

These agents have been tested in various conditions where platelet activation plays a major role, in particular in patients undergoing percutaneous coronary intervention (PCI), patients admitted with ACS, and patients receiving thrombolytic therapy for acute myocardial infarction (MI) (Fig. 2).

Glycoprotein IIb/IIIa inhibitors and percutaneous coronary intervention

Several large placebo-controlled randomized trials have evaluated adjunctive therapy with GPIIb/IIIa inhibitors in a broad cross-section of patients undergoing PCI (8–16): two trials focused on high-risk [acute MI, unstable angina (UA)] PCI [EPIC (8), RESTORE (9)], one selected refractory UA patients (CAPTURE) (10), five trials enrolled patients undergoing elective or urgent PCI with a wide array of interventional devices such as angioplasty, atherectomy, or stenting [EPILOG (11), Initiation Management Predischarge Process for Assessment of Carvedilol Therapy (IMPACT)-II (12), EPISTENT (13), ESPRIT (14), ISAR-REACT (15)], and one trial concentrated on early PCI in patients with ACS (ISAR-REACT 2) (16). Aside from CAPTURE where the study drug was administered for 18 to 24 hours prior to PCI and one hour thereafter, the study drug

was administered as a bolus immediately before coronary intervention, followed by infusions at 12 hours (abciximab) and 18 to 36 hours (eptifibatide or tirofiban). The primary outcome measure in these trials was a composite endpoint (typically death, nonfatal MI, or target vessel reintervention) with major bleeding as secondary safety endpoint. Follow-up ranged from 48 hours (ESPRIT) to 30 days in the rest. The primary results reported for these trials are summarized in Table 2.

Reductions in ischemic endpoints were observed in all trials except ISAR-REACT (15) with beneficial effects ranging from a minimum of 13% risk reduction in IMPACT II (12) to a maximum of 54% risk reduction in EPILOG (11). Post hoc analyses suggest a treatment effect by subgroup (observed in high-risk patients such as those with cardiac biomarker elevation, ST depression on electrocardiogram angiographically complex lesion or visible thrombus, diabetes, or history of prior antiplatelet treatment), time to treatment (greater benefit in patients treated earlier), and by endpoint (soft endpoints of periprocedural biomarker elevation and urgent reintervention being reduced to a much greater degree compared to hard endpoints of Q-wave MI or death) (6,8–16). The lack of treatment benefit observed in RESTORE and IMPACT II have been attributed to suboptimal doses of study drug (6,9,12). However, had the RESTORE investigators used urgent, instead of any, target vessel revascularization (TVR) (consistent with the endpoint used in abciximab trials), a nearly statistically significant treatment effect would have been observed in favor of tirofiban [24% relative risk reduction (RRR), $P = 0.052$] (6,9). This finding underscores the impact of choice of endpoints on overall results.

Bleeding complications were doubled with GPIIb/IIIa blockade in early studies (8,10). However, the use of weight-adjusted low dose of heparin [activated clotting time (ACT) target of 200–250 seconds] and optimal management of vascular access site (rapid sheath removal within four to

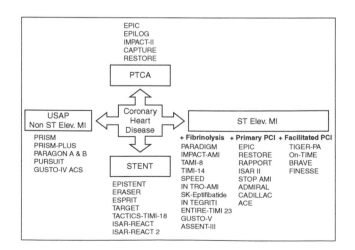

Figure 2

Randomized clinical trials evaluating glycoprotein IIb/IIIa inhibitors in different clinical settings.

Table 1   Comparison of platelet glycoprotein IIb/IIIa inhibitors

	Abciximab (ReoPro)	Tirofiban (aggrastat)	Eptifibatide (integrilin)
Structure	Antibody Fab fragment	Nonpeptide mimetic	Cyclic heptapeptide
Molecular weight	47.6 kDa	0.495 kDa	0.832 kDa
Receptor specificity	Nonspecific (GPIIb/IIIa, Vitronectin, Mac-1)	Specific for GPIIb/IIIa	Specific for GPIIb/IIIa
Receptor binding	Long acting, high affinity	Short acting, low affinity	Short acting, low affinity
Mechanism of receptor inhibition	Irreversible; steric hindrance and conformational change	Reversible; competitive inhibition (RGD recognition sequence)	Reversible; competitive inhibition (KGD recognition sequence)
Plasma half-life	10–30 min	~2 hr	~2.5 hr
Platelet function recovery	Slow (~48 hr)	Fast (2–4 hr)	Fast (2–4 hr)
Elimination route	Senescent platelets (RES)	Renal (70%) > hepatic (30%)	Renal (50%)
FDA-approved indication	Adjunct to PCI; early (<24 hr) PCI in ACS	Medical management of ACS	Adjunct to PCI; medical management of ACS
FDA-approved dose	PCI: 0.25 mg/kg IV bolus pre-PCI 0.125 mcg/kg/min (max. 10mcg/min) IV infusion x 12 hr post-PCI ACS with planned PCI: 0.25 mg/kg IV bolus 10 mcg/min IV infusion × 18–24 hr pre-PCI and × 1 hr post-PCI*	ACS: 0.4 mcg/kg/min IV infusion × 30 min; 0.1 mcg/kg/min × 48–108 hr	PCI: 180 mcg/kg IV bolus pre-PCI 2.0 mcg/kg/min IV infusion Second 180 mcg/kg bolus after 10 min. Infusion continues until hospital discharge or for 18–24 hr post PCI (whichever comes first) ACS: 180 mcg/kg IV bolus 2 mcg/kg/min (max 15 mg/hr) × 72—96 hr
Dosage adjustment	NA	CrCl <30 mL/min: decrease bolus rate and infusion rate by 50%	SCr >2.0 mg/dL: decrease infusion to 1.0 mcg/kg/min; SCr >4.0 mg/dL or requires hemodialysis (contraindicated)

Abbreviations: ACS, acute coronary syndromes; GP, glycoprotein; PCI, percutaneous coronary intervention.

six hours) in the latter studies (11,13,14) were crucial in substantially reducing the bleeding complications. In general, treatment with GPIIb/IIIa inhibitors increases the rate of major bleeding by 1%, thrombocytopenia (<100,000/mm^3) by 1%, and profound thrombocytopenia (<50,000/mm^3) by 0.4% (6). Intracerebral hemorrhage is an uncommon complication of GPIIb/IIIa inhibitors occurring in <0.2% of patients (6).

Glycoprotein IIb/IIIa inhibitors in unstable angina and non-ST elevation myocardial infarction

Systematic use of GPIIb/IIIa inhibitors in addition to standard treatment with aspirin and unfractionated heparin has been studied in six large randomized trials in patients with ACS of UA and non-ST elevation MI (NSTEMI) who were managed predominantly with medical management: two with tirofiban [PRISM (17), PRISM-PLUS (18)], one with eptifibatide (PURSUIT) (19), two with lamifiban [PARAGON-A (20), PARAGON-B (21)], and one with abciximab (GUSTO-IV ACS) (22).

Table 3 summarizes the primary results of these trials. Overall the use of GPIIb/IIIa inhibitors was associated with a modest, but significant reduction in the primary endpoint in PRISM, PRISM-PLUS, and PURSUIT. Treatment benefit was confined to early time points in PRISM (48 hours) and PRISM-PLUS (seven days), but not sustained at 30 days (17,18). In contrast, treatment with eptifibatide reduced the incidence of composite endpoint by 1.5% absolute risk difference (ARD) in PURSUIT which was observed within four days and maintained for 30 days without attenuation or amplification (19).

Table 2   Randomized clinical trials of platelet glycoprotein IIb/IIIa inhibitors during percutaneous coronary intervention

Trial	Clinical setting	Number of patients	PEP	Follow-up	PEP rate (%) New	PEP rate (%) Control	Risk ratio (95% CI)	Major bleeding (%) New	Major bleeding (%) Control	Risk ratio (95% CI)
EPIC (8)	Abciximab in high-risk PCI	2099	Death, MI, UR	30 day	8.3	12.8 (11.2)	0.68 (0.45–0.89)	14.0	7.0	2.12 (1.52–2.95)
RESTORE (9)	Tirofiban in high-risk PCI	2139	Death, MI, any TVR	30 day	10.3	12.2	0.85 (0.67–1.07)	5.3	3.7	1.42 (0.96–2.11)
CAPTURE (10)	Abciximab in PCI in UA	1265	Death, MI, UR	30 day	11.3	15.9	0.71 (0.53–0.94)	3.8	1.9	2.02 (1.02–4.00)
EPILOG (11)	Abciximab in elective or urgent PCI	2792	Death, MI, UR	30 day	5.2	11.7	0.46 (0.33–0.964)	3.8	3.1	1.23 (0.76–2.00)
IMPACT II (12)	Eptifibatide in elective or urgent PCI	4010	Death, MI, UR	30 day	9.2, 9.9[a]	11.4	0.81 (0.65–1.01) 0.87 (0.70–1.09)[a]	5.1	4.8	1.13 (0.82–1.54)[b]
EPISTENT (13)	Abciximab in elective or urgent PCI	2399	Death, MI, UR	30 day	5.3	10.8	0.49 (0.34–0.70)	2.1	1.4	1.57 (0.74–3.34)
ESPRIT (14)	Eptifibatide in non-urgent PCI	2064	D, MI, UR, bailout GPI use	48hr	6.6	10.5	0.63 (0.47–0.84)	1.3	0.4	3.2 (1.05–9.78)
ISAR-REACT (15)	Abciximab inL nonurgent PCI	2159	D, MI, UR	30 day	4.2	4.0	1.05 (0.78–1.58)	1.1	0.7	1.50 (0.62–3.66)
ISAR-REACT 2 (16)	Abciximab in high-risk PCI	2022	D, MI, UR	30 day	8.9	11.9	0.75 (0.58–0.97)	1.4	1.4	1.00 (0.50–2.08)

[a]High-dose lamifiban.
[b]Based on red blood cell transfusion.
Abbreviations: MI, myocardial infarction; PCI, percutaneous coronary intervention; PEP, primary endpoint; TVR, target vessel revascularization; UR, urgent reintervention.

Table 3   Randomized clinical trials of platelet glycoprotein IIb/IIIa inhibitors in medical management of unstable angina and NSTEMI

Trial	GPI	Number of patients	PEP	Follow-up	PEP rate (%)		Risk ratio (95% CI)	Major bleeding (%)		Risk ratio (95% CI)
					New	Control		New	Control	
PRISM (17)	Tirofiban x 48 hr	3232	Death, MI, RA	48 hr 30 day	3.8 15.9	5.6 17.1	0.68 (0.48–0.93) 0.93 (0.80–1.09)	0.37	0.37	1.00 (0.32–3.09)
PRISM-PLUS (18)	Tirofiban x >48 hr	1915	Death, MI, RA	7 day 30 day	12.9	17.9	0.72 (0.57–0.91) 0.83 (0.68–1.01)	4.0	3.0	1.33 (0.79–2.25)
PURSUIT (19)	Eptifibatide x <72 hr	10,948	Death, MI	30 day	14.2	15.7	0.91 (0.83–1.00)	9.0	10.5	1.16 (1.03–1.32)
PARAGON A (20)	Lamifiban low dose x 3–5 day Lamifiban high dose x 3–5 day	2282	Death, MI	30 day	10.6 12.0	11.7	0.90 (0.68–1.20) 1.02 (0.78–1.34)	3.0 6.0	3.0	1.00 (0.57–1.77) 1.97 (1.21–3.22)
PARAGON B (21)	Lamifiban x <72 hr	5225	Death, MI, RA	30 day	11.8	12.8	0.92 (0.80–1.07)	1.3 14.0[a]	0.9 11.7[a]	1.46 (0.86–2.47) 1.20 (1.04–1.39)[a]
GUSTO IV-ACS (22)	Abciximab 24 hr Abciximab 48 hr	7800	Death, MI	30 day	9.1 8.2	8.0	1.02 (0.85–1.22) 1.13 (0.95–1.35)	0.6 1.0	0.3	2.29 (0.94–5.56) 3.69 (1.61–8.50)

[a]Coronary artery bypass graft-related bleeding.
Abbreviations: GP, glycoprotein; MI, myocardial infarction; PEP, primary end-point; RA, refractory angina.

The GUSTO IV-ACS trial demonstrated no clinical benefit with abciximab (Table 3). Paradoxically, a statistically significant increase in mortality was observed at the end of 48 hours abciximab infusion (0.9% vs. 0.3% placebo; $P = 0.006$) (22). No subgroup benefited from abciximab; in fact, those with body weight <75 kg, low baseline troponin, or elevated baseline C-reactive protein (CRP) had excess mortality at one year with abciximab (23). The precise reasons for the negative findings in GUSTO IV-ACS are not clear but may be related to: (*i*) enrollment of low-risk patients (only 30% patients had ST depression and troponin elevation), (*ii*) lack of power (due to low event rate of 8% instead of projected 11%); (*iii*) dosing and the degree of platelet inhibition (maintenance dose based on 12-hour infusion derived from PCI studies may have been insufficient); (*iv*) lack of intervention—less than 2% underwent early revascularization; or (*v*) simply due to play of chance. Major bleeding was significantly increased in PURSUIT [it reported coronary artery bypass graft (CABG)-related bleeding], both PARAGON trials, and in the 48-hour-infusion arm of GUSTO-IV ACS trial.

A meta-analysis from Boersma et al. (24) showed an overall modest 1% ARD treatment effect of GPIIb/IIIa inhibitors on death and MI (Table 4). The treatment was particularly robust in 19% of patients undergoing intervention (PCI or CABG) within five days (3% ARD, RRR 0.79; 95% confidence interval: 0.68–0.91) and those with troponin elevations [risk reduction of 0.84 (0.70–1.30) vs. 1.17 (0.94–1.44) in troponin-negative patients]. However, the interaction of GPIIb/IIIa inhibitors with troponin elevation or revascularization was not tested in a randomized fashion (except in GUSTO-IV ACS), thereby weakening the clinical implication of these findings.

Table 4   Randomized clinical trials of platelet glycoprotein IIb/IIIa inhibitors during reperfusion therapy for acute ST-elevation myocardial infarction

Trial	Reperfusion strategy	Number of patients	PEP	Follow-up	PEP rate (%)		Risk ratio (95% CI)	Major bleeding (%)		Risk ratio (95% CI)
					New	Control		New	Control	
RAPPORT (49)	Abciximab + PCI versus PCI	483	Death, MI, TVR	6 mo 30 day	28.2 13.3	28.1 16.1	1.00 (0.76–1.34) 0.82 (0.53–1.27)	NA	NA	NA
ISAR II (50)	Abciximab + PCI versus PCI	401	Death, MI, TLR	30 day	5.0	10.5	0.47 (0.23–0.98)	3.5	4.5	0.77 (0.29–2.04) (RBC Tx)
ADMIRAL (51)	Abciximab + PCI versus PCI	300	Death, MI, uTVR	30 day	6.0	14.6	0.41 (0.20–0.87)	0.7	0	Not estimable
CADILLAC (52)	Abciximab + PTCA versus PTCA Abciximab + Stent versus Stent	1046 1036	Death, MI, TVR, stroke	6 mo 6 mo	16.5 10.2	20.0 11.5	0.82 (0.63–1.06) 0.89 (0.62–1.26)	NA	NA	NA
ACE (53)	Abciximab + PCI versus PCI	400	Death, MI, TVR, stroke	30 day 6 mo	4.5 10.2	10.5 11.5	0.43 (0.20–0.91) 0.89 (0.51–1.56)	3.5	3.0	1.17 (0.40–3.41)
GUSTO-V (55)	Abciximab + reteplase + heparin versus reteplase + heparin	16,588	Death	30 day	5.6	5.9	0.95 (0.84–1.08)	1.1	0.5	2.13 (1.48–3.06)
ASSENT-3 (56)	Abciximab + half-dose TNK + UFH versus full-dose TNK + UFH Abciximab + half-dose TNK + UFH versus full-dose TNK + Enox	6095	Death, MI, RA	30 day	11.4 11.1	15.4 11.4	0.72 (0.61–0.84) 0.97 (0.81–1.15)	4.3 4.3	2.2 3.0	2.00 (1.40–2.85) 1.42 (1.03–1.96)

Abbreviations: MI, myocardial infarction; PCI, percutaneous coronary intervention; PEP, primary end-point; RA, refractory angina; TLR, target lesion revascularization; TVR, target vessel revascularization; TNK, tenecteplase; UFH, Unfractionated heparin; UR, urgent reintervention.

Variability of glycoprotein IIb/IIIa inhibitor treatment effect in coronary intervention versus medical management

There appears to be heterogeneity in the magnitude of treatment effect associated with GPIIb/IIIa inhibitors in the interventional trials compared to the medical management trials with substantial attenuation of treatment effect in the latter. This variability has been attributed to the inherent diversity of patient acuity and the uncertain timing of thrombotic events within these populations—treatment being more effective when the timing is more precisely known as in PCI-induced vascular injury compared to spontaneous injury in ACS (7,25). However, a critical analysis of the trials summarized in Figure 3A to C reveals important insights.

Figure 3A demonstrates the results of a pooled analysis from CAPTURE (where all patients underwent PCI 18 to 24 hours after abciximab treatment), as well as the subgroup of

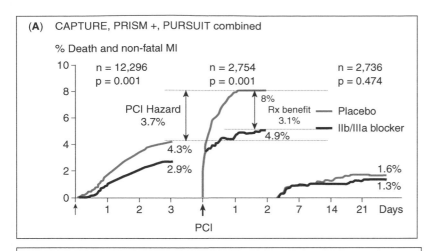

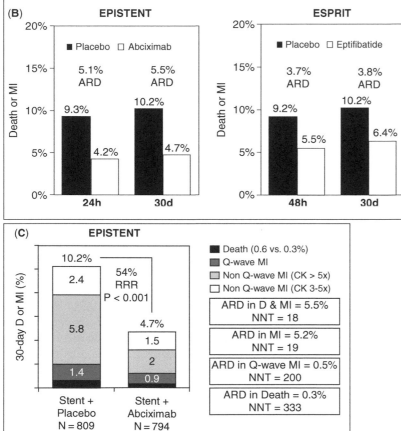

Figure 3
(A) Pooled data from CAPTURE, PRISM-PLUS, and PURSUIT trials of unstable angina showing the impact of glycoprotein (GP) IIb/IIIa inhibitors on death or myocardial infarction during medical therapy alone (*left*), during and immediately after percutaneous coronary intervention (PCI) (*middle*), and 2 to 30 days after PCI. (B) Data from the EPISTENT and ESPRIT trials demonstrating the impact of GPIIb/IIIa inhibitor treatment on death or myocardial infarction at 24 to 48 hours and at 30 days. (C) Data from the EPISTENT trial demonstrating the impact of abciximab treatment on death and type of myocardial infarction. *Abbreviation*: ARD, absolute risk difference; EPISTENT, evaluation of platelet inhibition in stent; ESPRIT, enhanced suppression of the platelet IIb/IIIa receptor with integrilin therapy; MI, myocardial infarction; NNT, number needed to treat.

patients undergoing PCI in PURSUIT and PRISM-PLUS following treatment with GPIIb/IIIa inhibitors (26). Although a modest clinical benefit began to accrue during the medical stabilization phase prior to PCI (an ARD of 1.4% in death or nonfatal MI at 72 hours), a more pronounced reduction was observed immediately post-PCI (ARD = 3.1%, representing nearly 70% of the overall benefit). Few events occurred more than two days after PCI, and no additional treatment effect was apparent up to 30-day follow-up. The sudden increase in risk observed in the control arm post-PCI (from 4.3% to 8.0%, ARD = 3.7%) represents the typical "PCI

hazard" associated with platelet embolization and microvascular occlusion, manifest predominantly as periprocedural biomarker (CK-MB or troponin) elevation. Treatment with GPIIb/IIIa inhibitors markedly abrogates this "short-lived" risk with little or no incremental impact on clinical outcomes. Thus, periprocedural events, marked mostly by biomarker elevations, drive the benefit associated with GPIIb/IIIa inhibitors. The findings of no treatment benefit with abciximab in GUSTO-IV ACS (in which <2% of patients underwent early revascularization) help support these observations (22).

Additional supportive evidence comes from analysis of death or MI event rates in EPISTENT and ESPRIT trials shown in Figure 3B. First, the in-hospital incidence of death or MI was ~9% in both trials, a number which is markedly higher than the 1% to 2% figure that is often quoted to the patients during informed consent. This discrepancy in event rates is driven by inclusion of periprocedural biomarker elevation criterion for MI in clinical trials compared to the "unequivocal" Q-wave criterion for MI in clinical practice. Second, over 90% of these events at 30 days in the placebo arm were evident by day 1 (EPSTENT) or 2 (ESPRIT), underscoring the fact that the event rates in both these trials were driven by biomarker elevations (measured for 24 hours or 48 hours post-PCI as mandated by protocol). Third, nearly 93% of treatment benefit with abciximab accrued by day 1 in EPSTENT (5.1% out of 5.5%) and over 97% of treatment benefit with eptifibatide occurred by day 2 in ESPRIT (3.7% out of 3.8%), suggesting that the majority of benefit with GPIIb/IIIa inhibitor is derived primarily from reducing periprocedural MIs. In EPISTENT trial, 86% of the treatment effect observed at 30 days (4.7% out of 5.5% ARD) was driven by reduction in non-Q-wave MIs defined by CK (not CK-MB) elevation >3 × upper limit of normal (ULN) (Fig. 3C). Mortality and Q-wave MI benefit were very modest: 0.3% and 0.5% ARD corresponding to an NNT of 333 and 200, respectively.

From these lines of evidence, it is apparent that the most likely reason for variability between interventional and medical management trials appears to be related to the frequency of early revascularization (100% in the former vs. <20% in the latter) and the utilization of periprocedural biomarker elevation criterion for MI. Thus, treatment benefit associated with GPIIb/IIIa inhibitor is observed very early and is primarily driven by reduction in postprocedural biomarker elevation, the least robust but the most prevalent component of the composite endpoint with little benefit on death or Q-wave MI.

Based on these data, there is insufficient evidence to warrant unconditional treatment with GPIIb/IIIa inhibitor. Consequently, the earlier Class I recommendation for "upstream" medical management of ACS with these agents was appropriately downgraded to Class IIa (level of evidence A without clopidogrel and B with clopidogrel) (27). Class I (level of evidence A) recommendation is reserved only for high-risk ACS patients undergoing early PCI strategy (27) and Class II for elective PCI, especially in diabetics (level of evidence B) (28).

Prognostic significance of cardiac biomarker release after percutaneous coronary intervention and the impact of glycoprotein IIb/IIIa inhibitor treatment

A large number of studies have shown that mild-to-moderate elevations of biochemical markers of myocardial damage

(CK, CK-MB) are detected in 10% to 20% of cases after PCI, but the clinical significance of these findings remains highly contentious (29). Interpretations have ranged from a direct cause-and-effect association between any level of periprocedural CK-MB elevation and subsequent mortality to the biomarker elevations being an epiphenomenon (statistical confounder), that is, a marker of high risk such as atheroma burden, plaque vulnerability, nonresponsiveness to antiplatelet therapy, or inflammatory status (29). The inconsistent conclusions may be due to potential methodological limitations of the published reports, such as study design (retrospective or post hoc evaluations vs. prospective studies) (selected subsets vs. the general population), lack of statistical power, sampling bias (higher frequency of biomarker sampling leading to positive associations), patient selection, and variable duration of follow-up (29). Increased susceptibility to ventricular arrhythmias via microreentrant circuits generated in areas of discrete microinfarction (detected by MRI technique), comprising of coronary collaterals, and microvascular circulation dysfunction have been speculated to be potential mechanisms responsible for adverse prognosis after CK-MB elevation (29).

If periprocedural CK-MB elevation is causally linked to increased mortality, then GPIIb/IIIa inhibitors that reduce these "events" should also reduce mortality. This is not consistently borne out by critical examination of the evidence. In the EPISTENT trial, the first and the only PCI trial to claim a mortality benefit with abciximab, there was no relation between periprocedural CK-MB elevation and mortality (30). In a pooled analysis of abciximab PCI studies, Anderson et al. (31) reported that periprocedural CK-MB elevation explained only 18% of the abciximab mortality benefit. Similar findings were also reported from pooled analysis of EPIC, EPILOG, and EPISTENT (maximum follow-up) where only 8% of mortality benefit could be explained by CK-MB elevation (32). In the TARGET trial, despite significant reductions in frequency of periprocedural CK-MB elevation for abciximab compared with tirofiban, the six-month or one-year mortality rates were virtually identical (33). Similarly, despite 23 excess non-Q-Wave MIs (primarily defined by periprocedural CK-MB elevation) in the bivalirudin arm of REPLACE-2 trial, 13 fewer deaths were observed in this group compared to GPIIb/IIIa inhibitor arm (34). Smaller molecules have been shown to reduce periprocedural CK-MB elevations, but have no effect on long-term mortality. This dissociation between rates of periprocedural CK-MB elevation and mortality has also been observed in non-GPIIb/IIIa inhibitor trials [BOAT (35), FRISC-II (36)] and fails to support CK-MB as a surrogate marker for mortality. These findings call into question the clinical relevance of biomarker elevations and whether they should be used routinely in clinical practice. Such a recommendation should ideally be justified based on the following criteria: (i) a consensus threshold criterion for definition of MI—currently, there are no standard criterion for what would constitute a clinically significant periprocedural MI with

ESC/ACC guidelines recommending any elevation of troponin or CK-MB >1 × ULN (37), FDA utilizing CK-MB elevation >2–3 × ULN for regulatory approval, and others advocating CK-MB elevation >5–8 × ULN (28,38); (ii) informed consent from patients should clearly state a 9% to 10% in-hospital risk of death or MI complicating elective PCI; and (iii) patients with biomarker elevations should be managed as aggressively as those with Q-wave MIs (careful monitoring, prolonged length of stay, and so on). These are seldom followed in current clinical practice and are unlikely to be adopted in the near future for obvious reasons.

Glycoprotein IIb/IIIa inhibitors in ST elevation myocardial infarction

Pharmacological and mechanical reperfusion strategies have substantially improved mortality and morbidity associated with STEMI over the last two decades. However, despite successful recanalization, suboptimal myocardial reperfusion may occur as a result of thrombotic reocclusion (from fibrinolysis-induced platelet activation) or distal embolization (associated with PCI-induced platelet activation), resulting in unfavorable outcomes. Interest in improving reperfusion success while reducing hemorrhagic complications has led to studies of GPIIb/IIIa inhibitors in three different settings in the treatment of STEMI: (i) as adjunctive therapy during primary PCI; (ii) as adjunctive therapy with low-dose fibrinolytic therapy alone; and (iii) as adjunctive therapy with low-dose fibrinolytic therapy preceding PCI (facilitated PCI). Support for these strategies comes from the early observation that abciximab reduces platelet aggregate size ("disaggregating" effect), increasing both fibrin accessibility and the rate of fibrinolysis ("dethrombotic" effect) (39,40). Although several phase I and phase II studies (41–48) have demonstrated acceptable safety and improved arterial patency [thrombolysis in myocardial infarction (TIMI) flow grade and TIMI frame count] and myocardial perfusion (ST segment resolution, and myocardial blush grade) achieved with all of these agents, extensive studies evaluating clinical outcomes are limited to abciximab.

The results of the large randomized studies with abciximab are summarized in Table 5 and they show inconsistent treatment effects (49–53). The primary composite endpoint was significantly reduced in three out of the five primary PCI trials (ISAR-2, ADMIRAL, ACE), mostly driven by reductions in urgent TVR. Benefits were sustained long-term in ADMIRAL and ACE and reduction in clinical outcomes were paralleled by improvements in pre-PCI coronary artery patency, post-PCI angiographic outcomes, and left ventricular function in ADMIRAL (51). In contrast, the benefit of abciximab seen in earlier trials was not confirmed in the largest study (CADILLAC), either with angioplasty or with stenting (52). The divergent

findings may be related to differences in study design (blinded assessment in ADMIRAL where pre-PCI treatment with abciximab was allowed in 26% of patients compared to unblinded assessment in CADILLAC where pre-PCI treatment was not allowed) and patient risks (higher risk enrolled in the former which may explain the higher mortality of 5% vs. 2% in CADILLAC). In a meta-analysis that included all five trials, abciximab therapy in patients undergoing primary PCI was associated with significant reductions in mortality at 30 days (2.4% vs. 3.4% with placebo) (Table 4) and at 6 to 12 months (4.4% vs. 6.2%) and in reinfarction at 30 days (1.0% vs. 1.9%); there was no increase in bleeding (Table 4) (54).

In contrast to the primary PCI trials, and despite promising preliminary angiographic data, the results with adjunctive use of abciximab with half-dose fibrinolysis have failed to demonstrate a mortality effect in individual trials (Table 5) (55–57) or in a pooled analysis (Table 5) (54). Furthermore, the rate of bleeding episodes (Tables 4 and 5) and the need for transfusion are significantly increased including intracerebral bleeding in patients over the age of 75 (58). Thus, the role of adjunctive GPIIb/IIIa inhibitor treatment during fibrinolysis remains uncertain.

With regard to facilitated PCI, two phase II trials with tirofiban provided preliminary evidence of improved angiographic benefit (59,60). In the BRAVE trial, however, despite improved TIMI III patency observed with half-dose reteplase and full-dose abciximab, no significant reductions in infarct size or mortality were observed; and bleeding was increased, although nonsignificantly (61). The results of the ongoing FINESSE trial will provide additional important information regarding the efficacy and safety of these agents for facilitated PCI.

From these data, it can be concluded that adjunctive GPIIb/IIIa inhibitor therapy for STEMI is associated with a significant reduction in 30-day and long-term mortality in patients treated with primary angioplasty but not in those receiving fibrinolysis. However, inconsistencies in efficacy data and the uncertainty associated with a higher risk of bleeding complications, particularly in association with other antithrombotic agents such as clopidogrel, make the assertion of benefit somewhat tenuous, thereby resulting in a Class IIa or IIb ACC/AHA guideline recommendation (62).

Oral glycoprotein IIb/IIIa inhibitors

The efficacy of chronic therapy with oral GPIIb/IIIa inhibitors has been assessed in five major randomized placebo-controlled trials (EXCITE, OPUS, SYMPHONY, SYMPHONY II, and BRAVO) (63,64). These agents were associated with a statistically significant increase in mortality in three out of the five trials. A meta-analysis of these trials (n = 45,523) demonstrated a significant increase in mortality (2.8% vs. 2.1% for placebo, odds ratio 1.35, 95% confidence interval: 1.15–1.61), mostly

Table 5 Meta-analytic estimates of efficacy and safety of platelet glycoprotein IIb/IIIa inhibitors at 30 days

Clinical outcome	D, MI, or UR [OR (95% CI)]	D or MI [OR (95% CI)]	Death [OR (95% CI)]	MI [OR (95% CI)]	Reintervention [OR (95% CI)]	Major bleeding [OR (95% CI)]
Elective or urgent PCI (88); N = 19 trials, N = 20,137	0.65 (0.59–0.72) NNT = 28 (22–36)	NA	0.69 (0.53–0.90) NNT = 322 (175–2000)	0.63 (0.56–0.70) NNT = 43 (34–60)	NA	1.26 (1.09–1.46) NNH = 76 (54–127)
ACS (24); N = 6 trials, N = 31,402	0.98 (0.93–1.02) NNT = 65 (38–233)	0.91 (0.85–0.99) NNT = 99 (58–341)	0.91 (0.81–1.03) NNT = 396 (149-α)	0.90 (0.83–0.98) NNT = 133 (74–658)	0.99 (0.94–1.03) NNT =70 (40–289)	1.62 (1.36–1.97) NNH = 87 (68–122)
STEMI (PCI + fibrinolysis) (54); N = 11 trials, N = 27,115	NA	NA	0.97 (0.87–1.08) NNT = 371 (124-α)	0.63 (0.54–0.73) NNT = 80 (61–116)	NA	1.51 (1.15–1.98) NNH = 50 (40–66)
STEMI (primary PCI only) (54); N = 8 trials, N = 3949	NA	NA	0.68 (0.47–0.99) NNT = 102 (49-α)	0.56 (0.33–0.94) NNT = 115 (62–779)	NA	1.16 (0.85–1.59) NNH = 160 (53-α)
STEMI (fibrinolysis only) (54); N = 3 trials, N = 23,166	NA	NA	1.00 (0.90–1.12) NNT = 5499 (161-α)	0.64 (0.54–0.75) NNT = 79 (59–120)	NA	1.77 (1.55–2.03) NNH = 48 (38–63)

Abbreviations: D, death; MI, myocardial infarction; NNH, numbers needed to harm; NNT, numbers needed to treat; PCI, percutaneous coronary intervention; STEMI, ST-elevation myocardial infraction; UR, urgent reintervention.

due to excess vascular deaths (63). In addition, a nonsignificant trend toward an increase in the incidence of MI was also observed. Oral GP IIb/IIIa therapy was also associated with a small but significant increase in major bleeding (4% vs. 2.4%, odds ratio 1.74) and a small but significant decrease in urgent revascularization (2.8% vs. 3.6%, odds ratio 0.77). The unfavorable benefit–risk profiles of the oral agents have lead to their discontinuation.

Although the precise mechanism for the increased risk of death due to oral platelet GPIIb/IIIa inhibition is not known, a number of potential mechanisms have been proposed (63,64): (*i*) subthreshold inhibition (<80%) of the IIb/IIIa receptor (as a result of intra-individual and interindividual pharmacokinetic variability) may promote shedding of platelet CD40 ligand, thereby inducing a prothrombotic and proinflammatory effect; (*ii*) potentiation of platelet activation via P-selectin expression; (*iii*) promotion of apoptosis via modulation of caspase enzymes; (*iv*) genetic predisposition—polymorphism in the GPIIIa polypeptide (PIAI/A2) of the IIb/IIIa receptor may identify patients at increased mortality risk after oral GPIIb/IIIa inhibitor therapy.

Key issues regarding glycoprotein IIb/IIIa inhibitor use in clinical practice

Based on the available evidence, several key issues emerge regarding the use of GPIIb/IIIa inhibitors that may be of importance to the practicing clinician.

Are there differences among the glycoprotein IIb/IIIa inhibitors?

Although all agents reduce ischemic risk in the setting of PCI, there is some heterogeneity in the magnitude and durability of treatment effect (6). Indirect comparison suggests that the reduction in ischemic complications in the setting of PCI appears to be greater for abciximab (~40% clinically important reduction) compared to the small molecules (Table 2). This has been attributed to abciximab's unique pharmacological properties of prolonged receptor blockade and nonspecific blockade of other receptors including the vitronectin and Mac-1 receptor, which may play an important role in modulating platelet-mediated thrombin generation, cell adhesion and proliferation, and inflammation (3–6). A direct head-to-head comparison has been performed in one trial (TARGET), which compared abciximab with tirofiban (33). A 1.6% absolute reduction in the rate of ischemic complications (mostly driven by periprocedural biomarker elevation) was observed at one month in favor of abciximab, primarily in patients with ACS undergoing PCI. By six months of follow-up, however, there was no significant difference in the combined or the individual endpoints between the two drugs (0.4% ARD), indicating no persistent advantage of abciximab over tirofiban. A likely contributor may be less potent GPIIb/IIIa blockade early on with suboptimal tirofiban dose used in the trial. With the exception of CAPTURE trial, the acute benefits of abciximab appear to persist over the long term. However, the biological plausibility of this phenomenon (the so-called "plaque passivation") remains uncertain. To date, there have been no large direct comparisons between abciximab and eptifibatide or between the small molecules in clinical trials.

In contrast to the putative superiority of abciximab in PCI, its role in medical stabilization therapy for ACS was seriously challenged by the findings of GUSTO-IV ACS trial, resulting in a Class III (contraindicated) recommendation. On the other hand, small molecules are recommended as Class II indication for medical management of ACS.

The bleeding potential is similar among the agents. However, thrombocytopenia, particularly profound thrombocytopenia (platelet count <50,000 mm^{-3}) occurs with a two- to four-fold higher frequency with abciximab (0.4–1.0%) compared with eptifibatide (0–0.2%) or tirofiban (0.1–0.3%) (6). The exact mechanism of this difference is not clear. However, immune complex-mediated reaction (due to an anamnestic response to the humanized chimeric antibody) may contribute to rapid precipitation of thrombocytopenia with abciximab (6). Platelet counts should, therefore, be measured early (within the first one to four hours) after administration of these agents and followed for the duration of therapy. Platelet transfusion should be considered for profound thrombocytopenia with or without serious bleeding (6).

Who is most likely to benefit with glycoprotein IIb/IIIa inhibitor treatment?

Although a retrospective analysis of three trials [CAPTURE (65), PRISM (66), PARAGON-B (67)] demonstrated

GPIIb/IIIa inhibitor to be particularly beneficial among patients admitted with elevated levels of cardiac troponin, this finding was not confirmed in GUSTO IV ACS where cardiac troponin levels were prospectively evaluated. In TACTICS-TIMI 18 study, the superiority of early invasive over early conservative strategy was limited to high-risk patients with troponin elevation and TIMI risk score of 5 to 7 (68). Similar observations were also observed in ISAR-REACT 2 study, where abciximab benefit was confined to troponin-positive patients with ACS (16). Thus, treatment with a GPIIb/IIIa inhibitor should be considered in high-risk patients with ACS and an elevated troponin level, who are scheduled for early revascularization.

What is the optimal timing of glycoprotein IIb/IIIa inhibitor therapy?

Whether the timing of GPIIb/IIIa inhibitor therapy makes any difference on efficacy and safety has been explored retrospectively in six randomized STEMI trials (three with abciximab and three with tirofiban) (69). In a pooled analysis of these trials, "upstream" (prior to transfer to the catheterization laboratory) administration of GPIIb/IIIa inhibitor appeared to improve coronary patency and resulted in favorable trends for clinical outcomes compared to "downstream" (in cath lab) administration. However, the timing of administration was neither randomized nor prespecified. Thus, the suggestion that these drugs may be most beneficial with early (preferably prehospital) treatment of patients in the first hours of acute STEMI awaits confirmation in prospective randomized investigations.

The EVEREST pilot trial of 93 patients with high-risk NSTE-ACS compared upstream tirofiban with downstream high bolus dose tirofiban and downstream abciximab 10 minutes before PCI (70). The results showed that upstream tirofiban regimen was associated with better tissue-level perfusion, both before and after intervention, and less postprocedural troponin release compared with downstream treatment. The open-label ACUITY trial prospectively assessed upstream versus cath-lab administration of GPIIb/IIIa inhibitors in 9207 intermediate- to high-risk ACS patients (71). Preliminary results indicate that upstream therapy was noninferior for the net clinical benefit endpoint (ischemic events plus major bleeding), had fewer ischemic events but did not meet the criteria for noninferiority, and significantly increased bleeding compared with delayed administration. The results of the ongoing EARLY ACS trial, a randomized, double blind, clinical trial comparing upstream double-bolus eptifibatide with downstream selective use in high-risk NSTE-ACS patients will further clarify the role of timing with these agents (72).

What is the optimal type, dose and duration of conjunctive heparin therapy?

Unfractionated heparin remains the anticoagulant of choice with GPIIb/IIIa inhibitor treatment being used in over 90% of patients with ACS in the United States. Several phase II and phase III trials have assessed the safety and efficacy of combined low molecular weight heparin (LMWH) and GPIIb/IIIa inhibitors [ACUTE II (73), NICE-3 (74), GUSTO-IV ACS (75), INTERACT (76), A-to-Z (77), and SYNERGY (78)]. Results indicate that with few exceptions (SYNERGY) combination therapy did not result in an excess of non-CABG major bleeding (~2%) and that patients receiving this combination could safely undergo PCI without significantly diminished efficacy compared to unfractionated heparin.

During PCI, low-dose, weight-adjusted heparin (initial bolus of 70 U/kg, maintenance dose adjusted to maintain an activated ACT of ≥200 seconds) is safe and effective with abciximab therapy. Postprocedural heparin does not provide incremental benefit and bleeding risk can be significantly mitigated by removing the vascular access sheaths within two to four hours after the procedure (6). The optimal dose of heparin with eptifibatide appears to be a loading dose of 60 U/kg and maintenance dose adjusted to maintain an ACT of 200 to 250 seconds (14). The optimal intensity or duration of heparin therapy for medical management of ACS remains unresolved (7).

Does monitoring of platelet inhibition improve efficacy and safety of glycoprotein IIb/IIIa inhibitors?

The level of platelet inhibition achieved with GPIIb/IIIa inhibitors varies widely among patients undergoing PCI. The GOLD multicenter study conducted with a bedside machine showed that patients having less than 95% inhibition at the 10-minute time point had a greatest incidence of in-hospital major cardiac events (14.4%) when compared with those with ≥95% platelet inhibition (6.4%; $P = 0.006$) (79). This approach to identify the therapeutic level of inhibition of GPIIb/IIIa-binding activity could potentially improve the efficacy and reduce the bleeding complications. However, larger controlled studies are needed before routine point-of-care testing can be recommended in clinical practice.

When should glycoprotein IIb/IIIa inhibitors be stopped prior to coronary artery bypass graft?

The primary concern is the increased risk of preoperative bleeding in patients requiring emergent CABG after administration of GPIIb/IIIa inhibitor. In general, elective CABG can be safely accomplished four to six hours following cessation of infusion of tirofiban and eptifibatide and >48 hours after abciximab infusion. Prophylactic platelet transfusion is generally not recommended to overcome the bleeding potential of the small molecules, but may be considered (especially at the time of coming off bypass) if CABG is performed within 48 hours of abciximab treatment (6).

Can glycoprotein IIb/IIIa inhibitors be re-administered?

Re-administration might be an issue for abciximab, due to its inherent immunogenicity. Human antichimeric antibody is detectable in about 5% to 6% patients receiving abciximab therapy, but no antibodies have been observed in response to the small molecules. In practice, re-administration registry of 500 patients showed similar safety and efficacy for repeat administration when compared with first time administration (80). No reports of hypersensitivity or anaphylactic reactions were reported with abciximab re-administration. Thus, these agents can be safely re-administered with careful monitoring of platelet counts, especially with abciximab therapy.

Do glycoprotein IIb/IIIa inhibitors prevent restenosis?

A significant 26% risk reduction in the need for TVR at six months observed in the EPIC trial led to the speculation that abciximab may reduce clinical restenosis given its unique "magical" property of inhibiting vitronectin and Mac-1 receptors (79). A careful examination reveals that most of the TVR benefit occurred within six weeks, likely reflecting impact on "abrupt closure" after angioplasty rather than "restenosis" (81). Subsequent studies involving objective angiographic [RESTORE (82), EPISTENT (83,84), ESPRIT (85)] and intravascular ultrasound (ERASER) (86) assessments failed to demonstrate any antirestenotic effect with any of the three agents. Subgroup analysis in EPISTENT demonstrated a significant restenosis benefit in diabetics (83,84). However, there were significant baseline imbalances in favor of abciximab, interaction term was not statistically significant ($P = 0.06$), patients were not randomized according to diabetes status, and statistical analysis was not adjusted for multiple comparisons (84). All of these limitations preclude drawing any clinically meaningful inferences. In contrast, abciximab was associated with a reduction in angiographic restenosis rates and TVR in diabetic patients in the ISAR-SWEET trial (87). Compounding these data, there is not even a trend towards benefit for diabetics with other GPIIb/IIIa inhibitors (85). Thus, there is little objective and consistent evidence for prevention of restenosis with GPIIb/IIIa inhibitors.

Do glycoprotein IIb/IIIa inhibitors improve survival?

None of the individual trials have primarily evaluated mortality benefit with GPIIb/IIIa inhibitors. Because mortality associated with elective PCI is rare (1–2% at one year), such a trial would require a large number of patients for sufficient power, thus making such an assessment cost-prohibitive. In the absence of trials assessing mortality, meta-analyses may provide some useful, albeit exploratory, information. Four large meta-analyses have been reported thus far: two in patients undergoing PCI (88,89), one in patients undergoing medical management for ACS (24), and one in patients with STEMI (54) (Table 4). A modest (<0.5% ARD), but statistically significant, survival benefit was observed only in the PCI meta-analyses, with short-term (30 day) benefit evident in both meta-analyses and long-term benefit (6–12 months) observed in one (86). Estimates of NNT to save one life are consistently in the range of >320 for the three main indications (Table 4).

None of the individual trials demonstrated mortality benefit at any time point except EPISTENT (reportedly a prespecified secondary endpoint), which showed reduced mortality at one year (30). Notable points worth mentioning regarding EPISTENT results include the following: (*i*) total, but not cardiac, mortality was significantly reduced (from 2.4% to 1%, $P = 0.037$ vs. from 1.2% to 0.6%, $P = 0.2$); (*ii*) mortality was not related to periprocedural CK-MB elevation or markers of embolization; (*iii*) abciximab appeared to protect against sudden cardiac death; (*iv*) statistical analysis was not adjusted for multiple comparisons and would not have met the significance criterion of an adjusted P-value threshold of 0.017; (*v*) one cancer death in the placebo arm made the difference between significance and nonsignificance; (*vi*) mortality was assessed at four time points (30 days, six months, one year, and three years), yet statistically significant differences were observed only at one year with loss of

significance at longer follow-up (suggesting the likelihood of a play of chance) (30,32,83). In contrast to the 57% reduction in EPISTENT trial, mortality was significantly increased with abciximab at 48 hours (22) and at one year (especially in patients with elevated CRP) in GUSTO-IV ACS (23). Moreover, in the stented subgroup in CADILLAC, abciximab treatment was associated with a 56% increased relative risk in mortality (from 3.2% to 5.0%, $P = 0.15$) (52). Despite a greater absolute risk difference (1.8% increase vs. 1.4% decrease in EPISTENT), the difference in CADILLAC was not statistically significant, likely due to a smaller sample size. In the pooled analysis of the EPIC, EPILOG, and EPISTENT trials of 1462 patients with diabetes, abciximab treatment reduced the one-year all-cause mortality rate from 4.5% to 2.5% ($P = 0.03$) (90). In contrast, in the ISAR-SWEET trial, treatment with abciximab was not associated with a reduction in mortality in 701 diabetic patients—the one-year mortality rates were 4.8% in the abciximab group and 5.1% in the placebo group ($P = 0.86$) (87). Thus, the mortality data with GPIIb/IIIa inhibitors are conflicting and equivocal, limited by methodological deficiencies and unclear mechanistic insights.

Are there suitable alternatives to glycoprotein IIb/IIIa inhibitors?

Two candidates have recently emerged as suitable alternatives to GPIIb/IIIa inhibitors in patients undergoing elective or urgent PCI: clopidogrel (a P2Y12 receptor antagonist) and bivalirudin (a direct thrombin antagonist). In ISAR-REACT, no differences were observed in efficacy and safety outcomes (except for an increase in need for transfusion) with abciximab compared to placebo in low to intermediate-risk patients undergoing PCI and pretreated with clopidogrel (600 mg loading dose two hours prior to PCI) (15). Similar findings were observed in diabetic patients undergoing PCI (ISAR SWEET) (87). In a recent trial in high-risk patients with UA/NSTEMI undergoing PCI (ISAR-REACT 2), treatment with abciximab reduced adverse events on top of pretreatment with 600 mg of clopidogrel, especially in patients with elevated troponin levels, without increased bleeding complications (16). These data suggest that pretreatment with a high loading dose of clopidogrel might be an acceptable alternative to GPIIb/IIIa inhibitors in low-risk patients undergoing PCI, but not in high-risk troponin-positive patients.

In REPLACE-2, treatment with bivalirudin plus provisional GPIIb/IIIa inhibitors was noninferior to heparin plus routine GPIIb/IIIa in patients undergoing urgent or elective PCI with respect to the combined efficacy plus safety endpoint. However, the noninferiority conclusion depended more on

Table 6   American College of Cardiology/American Heart Association guideline recommendations for platelet glycoprotein IIb/IIIa inhibitors

Indication	Class I (highly recommended)	Guideline recommendation		Class III (not recommended)
		Class II (generally recommended)		
		a (Leaning towards)	b (Leaning away)	
STEMI UA/NSTEMI		Abciximab (LOE B)	Eptifibatide or tirofiban (LOE C)	
PCI (Early invasive Rx)				
Without clopidogrel	Abciximab, eptifibatide, or tirofiban (LOE A) in high-risk patients			
With clopidogrel		Abciximab, eptifibatide, or tirofiban (LOE B)		
Medical (Early conservative Rx)				
Without clopidogrel		Eptifibatide or tirofiban (LOE A)		Abciximab
With clopidogrel		Eptifibatide or tirofiban (LOE B)		Abciximab
Elective PCI				
Without clopidogrel		Abciximab, eptifibatide, or tirofiban (LOE B)		
With clopidogrel		Abciximab, eptifibatide, or tirofiban (LOE B)		

Abbreviations: PCI, percutaneous coronary intervention; STEMI, ST-elevation myocardial infraction.

safety (43% odds reduction in major bleeding) than efficacy (9% odds increase) (34). The PROTECT-TIMI-30 study, comparing eptifibatide plus either heparin or enoxaparin versus bivalirudin alone in ACS patients undergoing PCI, also favored bivalirudin with improved coronary flow reserve (primary endpoint of the study) and reduced major bleeding (91). The ACUITY trial evaluated the optimum treatment of patients with moderate to high-risk ACS undergoing PCI (71). In this study, 13,819 such patients were randomized to one of three arms: unfractionated heparin or enoxaparin plus routine GPIIb/IIIa inhibitor; bivalirudin plus routine GPIIb/IIIa inhibitor; or bivalirudin with provisional GPIIb/IIIa inhibitor. The results showed that the bivalirudin with provisional GPIIb/IIIa inhibitor group performed the best, particularly in patients pretreated with clopidogrel. However, like REPLACE-2, the conclusion of noninferiority in ACUITY depended more upon safety (47% relative risk reduction in bleeding) than efficacy (7% relative risk increase in ischemic events). Other potential limitations that might call into question the enthusiastic claims that bivalirudin may be a substitute for standard therapy with heparin plus GPIIb/IIIa inhibitors include the open-label nature

of the study (which might introduce biases, thereby confounding the results), the liberal noninferiority margin (25% proportional difference used in ACUITY exceeding the margins used in contemporary noninferiority trials), and lack of per-protocol analysis (intention-to-treat analysis being biased towards noninferiority) (92).

Summary and conclusions

Platelet GPIIb/IIIa inhibitors represent a novel class of therapeutic agents that reduce the rate of postprocedure ischemic complications when given parenterally with some variability in the magnitude and durability of treatment effect among the agents tested. Treatment effect is achieved early with every modality of revascularization. Bleeding risk is increased with these agents but may be minimized by reduction and weight adjustment of concomitant heparin dosing and early removal of vascular access sheaths. In contrast to the benefit seen with PCI, the efficacy of these agents in the medical treatment of

ACS is substantially reduced. There are important differences in the pharmacokinetic, pharmacodynamics, and mechanism of action of the three approved inhibitors. However, the clinical significance of these differences is not clear. Cost-effective analyses of these agents generally fall within the range of economically attractive therapies. Oral GPIIb/IIIa inhibitors have been discontinued because they increase mortality and bleeding.

A critical examination of the data reveals that the benefit of GPIIb/IIIa inhibitors is primarily driven by reduction in the need for urgent revascularization secondary to abrupt closure after suboptimal results of angioplasty and atherectomy (not relevant in the stent era) and reduction in periprocedural MI as defined by biomarker elevation criterion. The link between biomarker reduction and late mortality as well as the proposed mechanisms is speculative and awaits clinical and pathophysiological clarification. There is little impact on the hard endpoint of Q-wave MI and conflicting effects have been observed on mortality. There is no convincing evidence for other purported benefits on restenosis, plaque stabilization, inflammation, and "passivation." The most rational and evidence-based use of these agents is during early invasive strategy in high-risk troponin-positive patients with ACS for which it carries the imprimatur of Class I (level of evidence A) recommendation of the ACC/AHA treatment guidelines. For all other indications, the guidelines recommend these agents as Class II except for abciximab which is contraindicated (Class III recommendation) in the medical management of ACS. Finally, newer therapies (clopidogrel and bivalirudin) may potentially offer similar benefit with less bleeding and lower cost in appropriate settings.

References

1 Plow EF, Ginsberg MH. Cellular adhesion: GPIIb-IIIa as a proto-typic adhesion receptor. Prog Hemost Thromb 1989; 9:117.

2 Lefkovits J, Plow EF, Topol EJ. Platelet glycoprotein IIb/IIIa receptors in cardiovascular medicine. N Engl J Med 1995; 332:1553–1559.

3 Coller BS. Platelet GPIIb/IIIa antagonists: the first anti-integrin receptor therapeutics. J Clin Invest 1997; 99:1467–1471.

4 Coller BS: Blockade of platelet GP IIb/IIIa receptors as an antithrombotic strategy. Circulation 1995; 92:2373–2380.

5 Topol EJ, Byzova TV, Plow EF. Platelet GP IIb-IIIa blockers. Lancet 1999; 353:227–231.

6 Lincoff MA, Califf RM, Topol EJ. Platelet glycoprotein IIb/IIIa inhibitors in coronary artery disease. J Am Coll Cardiol 2000; 284:1549–1558.

7 Bhatt DL, Topol EJ. Current role of platelet glycoprotein IIb/IIIa inhibitors in acute coronary syndromes. JAMA 2000; 35:1103–1115.

8 The EPIC Investigators. Use of a monoclonal antibody directed against the platelet glycoprotein IIb/IIIa receptor in high-risk angioplasty. N Engl J Med 1994; 330:956–961.

9 The RESTORE Investigators. Effects of platelet glycoprotein IIb/IIIa blockade with tirofiban on adverse cardiac events in patients with unstable angina or acute myocardial infarction undergoing coronary angioplasty. Circulation 1997; 96:1445–1453.

10 The CAPTURE Investigators. Randomised placebo-controlled trial of abciximab before and during coronary intervention in refractory unstable angina: the CAPTURE Study. Lancet 1997; 349:1429–1435.

11 The EPILOG Investigators. Platelet glycoprotein IIb/IIIa receptor blockade and low-dose heparin during percutaneous coronary revascularization. N Engl J Med 1997; 336:1689–1696.

12 The IMPACT-II Investigators. Randomized placebo-controlled trial of effect of eptifibatide on complications of percutaneous coronary intervention: the IMPACT-II. Lancet 1997; 349:1422–1428.

13 The EPISTENT Investigators. Randomized placebo-controlled and balloon-angioplasty-controlled trial to assess safety of coronary stenting with use of platelet glycoprotein-IIb/IIIa blockade. Lancet 1998; 352:87–92.

14 The ESPRIT Investigators. Novel dosing regimen of eptifi-batide in planned coronary stent implantation (ESPRIT): a randomised, placebo-controlled trial. Lancet 2000; 356:2037–2044.

15 Kastrati A, Mehilli J, Schuhlen H, et al. Intracoronary stenting and antithrombotic regimen-rapid early action for coronary treatment study investigators. A clinical trial of abciximab in elective percutaneous coronary intervention after pretreat-ment with clopidogrel. N Engl J Med 2004; 350:232–238.

16 Kastrati A, Mehilli J, Neumann FJ, et al. Abciximab in patients with acute coronary syndromes undergoing percutaneous coronary intervention after clopidogrel pretreatment: the ISAR-REACT 2 randomized trial. JAMA 2006; 295:1531–1538.

17 The PRISM Investigators. A comparison of aspirin plus tirofiban with aspirin plus heparin for unstable angina. N Engl J Med 1998; 338:1498–1505.

18 The PRISM-PLUS Investigators. Inhibition of the platelet glyco-protein IIb/IIIa receptor with tirofiban in unstable angina and non-Q-wave myocardial infarction. N Engl J Med 1998; 338:1488–1497.

19 The PURSUIT Trial Investigators. Investigators. Inhibition of platelet glycoprotein IIb/IIIa with eptifibatide in patients with acute coronary syndromes. N Engl J Med 1998; 339:436–443.

20 The PARAGON Investigators. International, randomised, controlled trial of lamifiban (a platelet glycoprotein IIb/IIIa inhibitor), heparin, or both in unstable angina. Circulation 1998; 97:2386–395.

21 The PARAGON B Investigators. Randomized, placebo-controlled trial of titrated intravenous lamifiban for acute coronary syndromes. Circulation 2002; 105:316–321.

22 The GUSTO-IV ACS Investigators. Effect of glycoprotein IIb/IIIA receptor blocker abciximab on outcome of patients with acute coronary syndromes without early revasculariza-tion: the GUSTO-IV ACS randomized trial. Lancet 2001; 357:1915–1924.

23 Ottervanger JP, Armstrong PW, Barnathan ES, et al. Long-term results after the glycoprotein IIb/IIIa inhibitor abciximab in

unstable angina. One-year survival in the GUSTO-IV ACS Trial. Circulation 2003; 107:437.

24 Boersma E, Harrington R, Moliterno D, et al. Platelet glycoprotein IIb/IIIa inhibitors in acute coronary syndromes: A meta-analysis of all major randomised clinical trials. Lancet 2002; 359:189–198.

25 Chew DP, Moliterno DJ. A critical appraisal of platelet glycoprotein IIb/IIIa inhibition. J Am Coll Cardiol 2000; 36:2028–2035.

26 Boersma E, Akkerhuis KM, Theroux P, et al. Platelet glycoprotein IIb/IIIa receptor inhibition in non-ST-elevation acute coronary syndromes: early benefit during medical treatment only, with additional protection during percutaneous coronary intervention. Circulation 1999; 100:2045–2048.

27 Braunwald E, Antman EM, Beasley JW, et al. ACC/AHA guidelines for the management of patients with unstable angina and non-ST-segment elevation myocardial infarction: executive summary and recommendations. A Report of the American College of Cardiology/American Heart Association Task Force on Practice Guidelines. Available at: http:// www.american-heart.org/downloadable/heart/1016214837537UANSTEMI 2002Web.pdf. Accessed July 7, 2006.

28 Smith SC, Feldman TE, Hirshfeld JW, et al. ACC/AHA/SCAI 2005 guideline update for percutaneous coronary intervention. A Report of the American College of Cardiology/American Heart Association Task Force on Practice Guidelines. Available at: http://content.onlinejacc.org/cgi/content/full/47/1/216. Accessed July 7, 2006.

29 Bhatt DL, Topol EJ, Cutlip DE, Kuntz RE. Controversies in cardiovascular medicine: does creatinine kinase-MB elevation after percutaneous coronary intervention predict outcomes in 2005? Circulation 2005; 112:906–923.

30 Topol EJ, Mark DB, Lincoff MA, et al. Outcomes at 1 year and economic implications of platelet glycoprotein IIb/IIIa blockade in patients undergoing coronary stenting: Results from a multicenter randomized trial. Lancet 1999; 354:2019–2024.

31 Anderson KM, Califf RM, Stone GW, et al. Long-term mortality benefit with abciximab in patients undergoing percutaneous coronary intervention. J Am Coll Cardiol 2001; 37:2059–2065.

32 Topol EJ, Lincoff AM, Kereiakes DJ, et al. Multi-year follow-up of abciximab therapy in three randomized, palcebo-controlled trials of percutaneous coronary revascularization. Am J Med 2002; 113:1–6.

33 Topol EJ, Moliterno DJ, Herrmann HC, et al. Comparison of two platelet glycoprotein IIb/IIIa inhibitors, tirofiban and abciximab, for the prevention of ischemic events with percutaneous coronary revascularization. N Engl J Med 2001; 344:1888–1894.

34 Lincoff AM, Kleiman NS, Kereiakes DJ, et al. REPLACE-2 investigators. Long-term efficacy of bivalirudin and provisional glycoprotein IIb/IIIa blockade vs heparin and planned glycoprotein IIb/IIIa blockade during percutaneous coronary revascularization. JAMA 2004; 292:696–703.

35 Baim D, Cutlip D, Sharma S, et al. Final results of the balloon vs. optimal atherectomy trial (BOAT). Circulation 1998; 97:322–331.

36 Lagerqvist BO, Husted S, Kontny F, et al. A long-term perspective on the protective effects of an early invasive strategy in unstable coronary artery disease. Two-year follow-up of the FRSIC-II invasive study. J Am Coll Cardiol 2002; 40:1902–1914.

37 Alpert JS, Thygesen k, Antman E, et al. Myocardial infarction redefined. A consensus document of The Joint European Society of Cardiology/American College of Cardiology Committee for the redefinition of myocardial infarction. J Am Coll Cardiol 2000; 36:959–969.

38 Stone GW, Mehran R, Dangas G, et al. Differential impact on survival of electrocardiographic Q-wave versus enzymatic myocardial infarction after percutaneous intervention. A device-specific analysis of 7174 patients. Circulation 2001; 104:642–647.

39 Cannon CP. Overcoming thrombolytic resistance. Rationale and initial clinical experience combining thrombolytic therapy and glycoprotein IIb/IIIa receptor inhibition for acute myocardial infarction. J Am Coll Cardiol 1999; 34:1395.

40 Collet JP, Montalescot G, Lesty C, et al. Effects of abciximab on the architecture of platelet-rich clots in patients with acute myocardial infarction undergoing primary coronary intervention. Circulation 2001; 103:2328.

41 The Paradigm Investigators. Combining thrombolysis with the platelet glycoprotein IIb/IIIa inhibitor lamifiban: results of the Platelet Aggregation Receptor Antagonist Dose Investigation and Reperfusion Gain in Myocardial Infarction (PARADIGM) trial. J Am Coll Cardiol 1998; 32:2003.

42 Ohman EM, Kleiman NS, Gacioch G, et al. Combined accelerated tissue-plasminogen activator and platelet glycoprotein IIb/IIIa integrin receptor blockade with integrilin in acute myocardial infarction. Results of a randomized, placebo-controlled, dose-ranging trial. Circulation 1997; 95:846.

43 Antman EM, Giugliano RP, Gibson MC, et al., for the TIMI 14 Investigators. Abciximab facilitates the rate and extent of thrombolysis: result of the thrombolysis in myocardial infarction (TIMI) 14 trial. Circulation 1999; 99:2720.

44 de Lemos JA, Antman EM, Gibson CM, et al. Abciximab improves both epicardial flow and myocardial reperfusion in ST-elevation myocardial infarction: Observations from the TIMI 14 Trial. Circulation 2000; 101:239.

45 Gibson CM, de Lemos JA, Murphy SA, et al. Combination therapy with abciximab reduces angiographically evident thrombus in acute myocardial infarction: a TIMI 14 substudy. Circulation 2001; 103:2550.

46 The Assessment of the Safety and Efficacy of the New Thrombolytic regimen (ASSENT)–3 Investigators. Trial of abciximab with and without low-dose reteplase for acute myocardial infarction. Strategies for Patency Enhancement in the Emergency Department (SPEED) Group. Circulation 2000; 101:2788.

47 Brener SJ, Zeymer U, Adgey AA, Vrobel TR. Eptifibatide and low-dose tissue plasminogen activator in acute myocardial infarction. The integrilin and low-dose thrombolysis in acute myocardial infarction (INTRO AMI) trial. J Am Coll Cardiol 2002; 39:377.

48 Giugliano RP, Roe MT, Harrington RA, Gibson CM. Combination reperfusion therapy with eptifibatide and reduced-dose tenecteplase for ST-elevation myocardial infarction. Results of the integrilin and tenecteplase in acute myocardial infarction (INTEGRITI) Phase II Angiographic urial. J Am Coll Cardiol 2003; 41:1251.

49 Brener SJ, Barr LA, Burchenal JEB, et al., on behalf of the ReoPro and Primary PTCA Organization and Randomized Trial (RAPPORT) Investigators. Randomized, placebo-controlled trial

of platelet glycoprotein IIb/IIIa blockade with primary angioplasty for acute myocardial infarction. Circulation 1998; 98:734.

50 Neumann FJ, Kastrati A, Schmitt C, et al. Effect of glycoprotein IIb/IIIa receptor blockade with abciximab on clinical and angiographic restenosis rate after the placement of coronary stents following acute myocardial infarction. J Am Coll Cardiol 2000; 35:915.

51 Montalescot G, Barragan P, Wittenberg O, et al., for the ADMIRAL Investigators. Platelet glycoprotein IIb/IIIa inhibition with coronary stenting for acute myocardial infarction. N Engl J Med 2001; 344:1895.

52 Stone GW, Grines CL, Cox DA, et al. Comparison of angioplasty with stenting, with or without abciximab, in acute myocardial infarction. N Engl J Med 2002; 346:957.

53 Antoniucci D, Rodriguez A, Hempel A, et al. A randomized trial comparing primary infarct artery stenting with or without abciximab in acute myocardial infarction. J Am Coll Cardiol 2003; 42:1879.

54 De Luca G, Suryapranata H, Stone GW, et al. Abciximab as adjunctive therapy to reperfusion in acute ST-segment elevation myocardial infarction: a meta-analysis of randomized trials. JAMA 2005; 293:1759.

55 Topol EJ. Reperfusion therapy for acute myocardial infarction with fibrinolytic therapy or combination reduced fibrinolytic therapy and platelet glycoprotein IIb/IIIa inhibition: the GUSTO V randomized trial. Lancet 2001; 357:1905.

56 Efficacy and safety of tenecteplase in combination with enoxaparin, abciximab, or unfractionated heparin: the ASSENT-3 randomized trial in acute myocardial infarction. Lancet 2001; 358:605.

57 Lincoff AM, Califf RM, Van De Werf F, et al. Mortality at 1 year with combination platelet glycoprotein IIb/IIIa inhibition and reduced-dose fibrinolytic therapy vs conventional fibrinolytic therapy for acute myocardial infarction: GUSTO V randomized trial. JAMA 2002; 288:2130.

58 Savonitto S, Armstrong PW, Lincoff AM, et al. Risk of intracranial haemorrhage with combined fibrinolytic and glycoprotein IIb/IIIa inhibitor therapy in acute myocardial infarction. Dichotomous response as a function of age in the GUSTO V trial. Eur Heart J 2003; 24:1807.

59 Lee DP, Herity NA, Hiatt BL, et al. Adjunctive platelet glycoprotein IIb/IIIa receptor inhibition with tirofiban before primary angioplasty improves angiographic outcomes: results of the TIrofiban Given in the Emergency Room before Primary Angioplasty (TIGER-PA) pilot trial. Circulation 2003; 107:1497.

60 van't Hof AW, Ernst N, de Boer MJ, et al. Facilitation of primary coronary angioplasty by early start of a glycoprotein 2b/3a inhibitor: results of the ongoing tirofiban in myocardial infarction evaluation (On-TIME) trial. Eur Heart J 2004; 25:837.

61 Kastrati A et al., for the Bavarian Reperfusion Alternatives Evaluation (BRAVE) study investigators. Early administration of reteplase plus abciximab versus abciximab alone in patients with acute myocardial infarction referred for percutaneous coronary intervention—a randomized controlled trial. JAMA 2004; 291:947–954.

62 Antman EM, Anbe DT, Armstrong PW, et al. ACC/AHA 2004 Guidelines for the Management of Patients With ST-Elevation Myocardial Infarction. A Report of the American College of Cardiology/American Heart Association Task Force on Practice Guidelines. Available at www.acc.org/ clinical/guidelines/stemi/index.pdf. Accessed July 7, 2006.

63 Chew DP, Bhatt DL, Topol EJ. Oral glycoprotein IIb/IIIa inhibitors: why don't they work? Am J Cardiovasc Drugs 2001; 1:421–428.

64 Quinn MJ, Plow EF, Topol EJ. Platelet glycoprotein IIb/IIIa inhibitors recognition of a two-edged sword? Circulation 2002; 106:379–385.

65 Hamm CW, Heeschen C, Goldmann B, et al. Benefit of abciximab in patients with refractory unstable angina in relation to serum troponin T levels. N Eng J Med 1999; 340:1623–1629.

66 Heeschen C, Hamm CW, Goldmann B, et al. Troponin concentrations for stratification of patients with acute coronary syndromes in relation to therapeutic efficacy of tirofiban. Lancet 2000; 354:1727–1762.

67 Newby LK, Ohman EM, Christenson RH, et al. Benefit of glycoprotein IIb/IIIa inhibition in patients with acute coronary syndromes and troponin T-positive status: the PARAGON-B troponin-T substudy. Circulation 2001; 103:2891–2896.

68 Cannon CP, Weintraub WS, Demopoulos LA, et al. Comparison of early invasive and conservative strategies in patients with unstable coronary syndromes treated with the glycoprotein IIb/IIIa inhibitor tirofiban. N Engl J Med 2001; 344:1879–1887.

69 Montalescot G, Borentain M, Payot L, Collet JP, Thomas D. Early vs late administration of glycoprotein IIb/IIIa inhibitors in primary percutaneous coronary intervention of acute ST-segment elevation myocardial infarction: a meta-analysis. JAMA 2004; 292:362–366.

70 Bolognese L, Falsini G, Liistro F, et al. Randomized comparison of upstream tirofiban versus downstream high bolus dose tirofiban or abciximab on tissue-level perfusion and troponin release in high-risk acute coronary syndromes treated with percutaneous coronary interventions: the EVEREST trial. J Am Coll Cardiol 2006; 47:522–528.

71 Stone GW, McLaurin BT, Cox DA, Bertrand ME, Lincoff AM, et al. ACUITY investigators. Bivalirudin for patients with acute coronary syndrome. New Engl J Med 2006; 355:2203–2216.

72 Giugliano RP, Newby LK, Harrington RA, et al. The early glycoprotein IIb/IIIa inhibition in non–ST-segment elevation acute coronary syndrome (EARLY ACS) trial: a randomized placebo controlled trial evaluating the clinical benefits of early front-loaded eptifibatide in the treatment of patients with non-ST-segment elevation acute coronary syndrome—study design and rationale. Am Heart J 2005; 149:994–1002.

73 Cohen M. Initial experience with the low-molecular-weight heparin, enoxaparin, in combination with the platelet glycoprotein IIb/IIIa blocker, tirofiban, in patients with non-ST segment elevation acute coronary syndromes. J Invasive Cardiol 2000; 12(suppl E):E5–E9; discussion E25–E28.

74 Ferguson JJ, Anrman EM, Bates ER, et al. Combining enoxaparin and glycoprotein IIb/IIIa antagonists for the treatment of acute coronary syndromes: final results of the National Investigators Collaborating on Enoxaparin-3 (NICE-3) study. Am Heart J 2003; 146:628–634.

75 James S, Armstrong P, Califf R, et al. Safety of abciximab combined with dalteparin in treatment of acute coronary syndromes. Eur Heart J 2002; 23:1538–1545.

76 Goodman SG, Fitchett D, Armstrong PW, et al., for the Integrilin and Enoxaparin Randomized Assessment of Acute Coronary Syndrome Treatment (INTERACT) trial investigators. Randomized

evaluation of the safety and efficacy of enoxaparin versus unfractionated heparin in high-risk patients with non-ST-segment elevation acute coronary syndromes receiving the glycoprotein IIb/IIIa inhibitor eptifibatide. Circulation 2003; 107:238–244.

77   Blazing MA, de Lemos JA, White HD, et al., for the A to Z Investigators. Safety and efficacy of enoxaparin vs unfractionated heparin in patients with non-ST-segment elevation acute coronary syndromes who receive tirofiban and aspirin: A randomized controlled trial. JAMA 2004; 292:55–64.

78   SYNERGY Trial Investigators. Enoxaparin vs unfractionated heparin in high-risk patients with non-ST-segment elevation acute coronary syndromes managed with an intended early invasive strategy: primary results of the synergy randomized trial. JAMA 2004; 292:45–54.

79   Steinhubl SR, Talley JD, Braden GA, et al. Point-of-care measured platelet inhibition correlates with a reduced risk of an adverse cardiac event after percutaneous coronary intervention: results of the GOLD (AU-Assessing Ultegra) multicenter study. Circulation 2001; 103:2572–2578.

80   Madan M, Kereiakes DJ, Hermiller JB, et al. Efficacy of abciximab readministration in coronary intervention. Am J Cardiol 2000; 85:435–440.

81   Topol EJ, Califf RM, Weisman HS, et al. Reduction of clinical restenosis following coronary intervention with early administration of platelet IIb/IIIa integrin blocking antibody. Lancet 1994; 343:881–886.

82   Gibson CM, Goel M, Cohen DJ, et al., for the RESTORE Investigators. Six-month angiographic and clinical follow-up of patients prospectively randomized to receive either tirofiban or placebo during angioplasty in the RESTORE trial. J Am Coll Cardiol 1998; 32:28.

83   Lincoff AM, Califf RM, Moliterno DJ, et al. Complementary clinical benefits of coronary artery stenting and blockade of platelet glycoprotein IIb/IIIa receptors. New Engl J Med 1999; 341:319–327.

84   Marso SP, Lincoff AM, Ellis SG, et al. Optimizing the percutaneous interventional outcomes for patients with diabetes mellitus: results of the EPISTENT (Evaluation of platelet IIb/IIIa inhibitor for stenting trial) diabetic substudy. Circulation 1999; 100:2477–2484.

85   O'Shea JC, Buller CE, Cantor WJ, et al. Long-term efficacy of platelet glycoprotein IIb/IIIa integrin blockade with eptifibatide in coronary stent intervention. JAMA 2002; 287:618.

86   The ERASER Investigators. Acute platelet inhibition with abciximab does not reduce in-stent restenosis (ERASER study). Circulation 1999; 100:799.

87   Mehilli J, Kastrati A, Schuhlen H, et al. Randomized clinical trial of abciximab in diabetic patients undergoing elective percutaneous coronary interventions after treatment with a high loading dose of clopidogrel. Circulation 2004; 110:3627–3635.

88   Karvouni E, Katritsis DG, Ioannidis JP. Intravenous glycoprotein IIb/IIIa receptor antagonists reduce mortality after percutaneous coronary interventions. J Am Coll Cardiol 2003; 41: 26–32.

89   Kong DF, Hasselblad V, Harrington RA, et al. Meta-analysis of survival with platelet glycoprotein IIb/IIIa antagonists for percutaneous coronary interventions. Am J Cardiol 2003; 92:651–655.

90   Bhatt DL, Marso SP, Lincoff AM, Wolski KE, Ellis SG, Topol EJ. Abciximab reduces mortality in diabetics following percutaneous coronary intervention. J Am Coll Cardiol 2000; 35:922–928.

91   Gibson CM, Morrow DA, Murphy SA, et al. A randomized trial to evaluate the relative protection against post-percutaneous coronary intervention microvascular dysfunction, ischemia and inflammation among antiplatelet and antithrombotic agents. The PROTECT-TIMI-30 trial. J Am Coll Cardiol 2006; 47: 2364–2373.

92. Kaul S, Diamond GA. Making sense of noninferiority: a clinical and statistical perspective on its application to cardiovascular clinical trails. Prog in Cardio Dis 2007; 49:284–299.

4

Adenosine diphosphate receptor inhibitors

Michel E. Bertrand

Introduction

Platelet aggregation is central to the process of vascular thrombotic occlusion, and over the last 20 years several pharmacological and clinical studies have clearly demonstrated that antiplatelet drugs play a major role in the management of vascular thrombosis. The antiplatelet triallists' collaboration performed a meta-analysis of 142 trials that included more than 73,000 patients, and the analysis clearly demonstrated that antiplatelet drugs reduce by 27% the risk of a composite outcome of vascular death, myocardial infarction (MI), and ischemic stroke. This benefit was consistent over a wide range of clinical manifestations. Platelet aggregation is induced via a very complex system (Fig. 1) of which three pathways are really essential: the cycloxygenase pathway, which is irreversibly blocked by aspirin; the adenosine diphosphate (ADP) receptor pathway, which is also irreversibly blocked by thienopyridines; and a group of compounds including monoclonal antibody and small peptides blocking the final common pathway, that is, the GpIIb/IIIa receptors.

Adenosine diphosphate receptors

Platelet activation by ADP and adenosine triphosphate (ATP) is a key player in hemostasis and thrombosis. Several receptors are involved, and there are a number of drugs that target these receptors (1). The P2X1 receptor is an ATP-gated channel but its role is not yet well defined.

The P2Y1 and P2Y12 receptors are 2 G protein-coupled, which selectively contributes to platelet aggregation. The P2Y1 receptor is responsible for ADP-induced platelet shape changes and transient aggregation, whereas the

P2Y12 receptor is responsible for the completion and amplification of the ADP stimulus, including thromboxane A_2 (TXA_2), thrombin, and collagen. This receptor was cloned in 2001 and its role in platelet aggregation by ADP is now well established, based on the action of selective inhibitors, gene targeting in mice, and human genetic evidence. Current agents ticlopidine, clopidogrel, cangrelor, prasugrel, and AZD-6140 target the P2Y12 receptor. Thienopyridines (ticlopidine, clopidogrel, and prasugrel) irreversibly inactivate the PY212 receptor via the covalent binding of an active metabolite produced by the liver. Cangrelor and AZD-6140 are competitive antagonists.

Structure of adenosine diphosphate receptor inhibitors

There are several drugs, but only the first two in the following list are available on the market.

1. Ticlopidine (Ticlid® Sanofi-Aventis) which is the Chloro-2 Benzyl-5 Tetrahydro-4,5,6,7 Thieno[3,2-C]Pyridine Chlorhydrate. Ticlopidine differs from clopidogrel by the presence of a radical H instead of CO_2CH_3 in the molecule.
2. Clopidogrel (SR 25990) (Plavix® Sanofi-Aventis) is the hydrogen sulfate salt of the S enanthiomer of methyl 2-(2-chlorophenyl)-2-[4,5,6,7-tetrahydrothieno(3,4-c)pyridine-5-yl] acetate. Its molecular formula is C16H16ClNO2S, H_2SO_4 (molecular weight of 419.9) (Fig. 2).
3. Prasugrel (CS-747, LY 640315)(Eli Lilly) is a thienopyridine under development that antagonizes the P2Y12

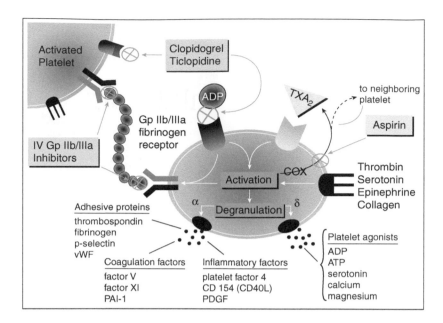

Figure 1
Platelet aggregation: different pathways of activation. *Abbreviations*: ADP, adenosine diphosphate; ATP, adenosine triphosphate; COX, cyclooxygenase; PAI, plasminogen activator inhibitor; PDGF, platelet derived growth factor.

receptor. This compound induces rapid and efficient generation of an active metabolite.

4. Cangrelor (Astra Zeneca) is a P2T(P2YADP) purino-receptor antagonist and platelet aggregation inhibitor. This derivative is suitable for IV injection. The company is developing derivatives of this compound. Plasma half-life is five minutes and it achieves 90% inhibition of platelet aggregation with recovery 20 minutes after the end of the infusion.

5. AZD6140 is an orally active, directly acting cyclopenthyl-triazolopyrimidine that reversibly blocks the P2Y12 receptor.

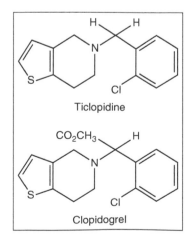

Figure 2
Chemical structure of ticlopidine and clopidogrel.

Mechanism of action: pharmacokinetic profile

Thienopyridines irreversibly inhibit ADP binding to the platelet surface purinergic receptor, P2Y12 (2). Structural analysis suggests that irreversible modification of the ADP-receptor site is caused by disulfide bridge formation between reactive thiol groups and a cysteine residue of the P2Y12 receptor (3). This explains the irreversible activity of clopidogrel on platelet function, an important clinical matter for hemorrhagic risk.

Thienopyridines are inactive in vitro. Absorbed in the upper gastrointestinal tract, clopidogrel is converted to an active metabolite by the hepatic cytochrome P450 system (3,4).

Peak levels of the principal metabolite, SR 26334 (which represents 85% of the circulating drug-related compound), occur one hour after oral administration: The pharmacokinetics are linear across a range from 50 to 150 mg of clopidogrel (5,6). The elimination half-life of this metabolite is approximately eight hours after single or multiple dose administration. SR 26334 is transformed in SR 25990 (the S oxide is still inactive), and the rearrangement of this compound leads to 2-oxo-clopidogrel. Finally, the active metabolite is generated by hydrolysis (Fig. 3).

Clopidogrel induces a maximum of 60% inhibition of ADP-induced aggregation after three to five days if administered without a loading dose. Bleeding time is significantly prolonged with this agent, reaching a maximum of 1.5- to 2-fold over baseline at three to seven days (7,8). Like aspirin, clopidogrel induces a permanent defect in a platelet protein, recoverable only by new platelet synthesis, allowing a

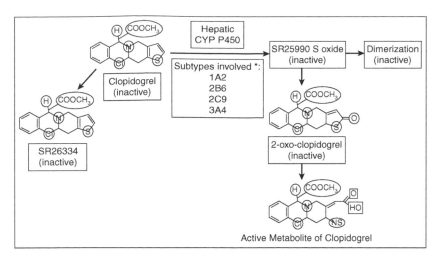

Figure 3
Clopidogrel and Cytochrome P 450 relationship.

repeated once-daily regimen with low doses despite a short chemical half-life. Recovery of platelet function, to produce new platelets (9,10), requires three to five days.

Dose

Clopidogrel inhibits platelet aggregation in a dose-dependent fashion. Several studies have shown that a loading dose of clopidogrel results in a much more rapid onset of platelet inhibition than that achieved by regular low doses (11), and recommended loading doses in acute coronary syndromes (ACS) management are 300 mg followed by 75 mg once daily.

A single dose of 400 mg induces 40% inhibition of platelet aggregation two hours later (12), and the level of platelet inhibition can be maintained with a daily dose of 75 mg. However, larger loading doses (450–600 mg) have been used in recent studies (13). Two recent trials have clearly addressed this matter. In the ALBION study, Montalescot and coworkers have demonstrated that a loading dose of 600 mg of clopidogrel achieves a better level of platelet inhibition than

a leading dose of 300 mg. A higher loading dose of 900 mg further increases, but nonsignificantly, platelet-level inhibition. Kastrati (14) and von Beckerath (15) found somewhat similar results. Currently, the faster action of a high loading dose (>300 mg) is recognized, suggesting that these doses would be particularly useful in the management of ACS.

Synergistic effects and interaction

Concomitant administration of aspirin does not significantly modify the ADP-platelet aggregation by clopidogrel, but clopidogrel potentiates the effects of aspirin on collagen-induced platelet aggregation (16): Figure 4 shows in a rabbit experimental model that aspirin + clopidogrel significantly reduces thrombus formation as expressed by the decrease of flow.

The transformation of SR26334 (inactive) in SR 25990 depends on different subtypes of the hepatic cytochrome P450 (CYP P450): Subtypes 1A2, 2B6, 2C9, and 3A4 are

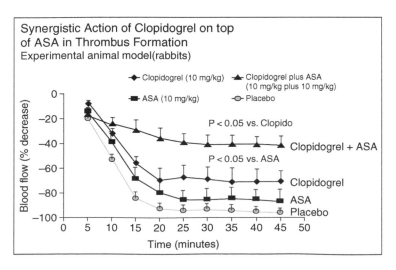

Figure 4
Synergistic effects of Clopidogrel and aspirin in thrombus formation. *Abbreviation*: ASA, acetylsalicylic acid. *Source*: From Ref. 16.

involved. In 2003, Lau et al. (17–19) suggested that atorvastatin, another CYP3A4 substrate, might competitively inhibit this activation and concluded that the use of a statin not metabolized by CYP3A4 may be warranted in patients treated with clopidogrel. However, these results have not been confirmed: statins in general, and atorvastatin in particular, seem not to affect the ability of clopidogrel to inhibit platelet function in patients undergoing coronary stenting (20). In addition, a number of studies conducted in patients of CAPRIE, CLASSICS, and CREDO receiving a statin have demonstrated that there was no clinical interaction between statins and clopidogrel (21). These post hoc analysis of placebo-controlled studies do not support the concept of a potential negative interaction when coadministering a CYP3A4-metabolized statin with clopidogrel.

Side effects—contra-indications

In addition to the risk of bleeding, which will be detailed in the different studies, thienopyridines are able to cause skin disorders (rashes or prurit) and gastrointestinal disorders (diarrhea). In the CLASSICS study, these side effects were observed in 8.2% of patients treated with ticlopidine and in 3.5% of those taking clopidogrel treatment. The most serious problem was related to hematologic disorders: neutropenia or thrombocytopenia. These disorders are much less frequent with clopidogrel than with ticlopidine: 0.04% of neutropenia in the CAPRIE study and 0.05% in the CURE trial. Thrombotic thrombocytopenic purpura are exceptional: one for 200,000 patients.

Thienopyridines are contraindicated in patients with allergy and hypersensitivity to the drug, in case of very severe hepatic insufficiency and, of course, in case of hemorrhagic disease: bleeding ulcer or intracranial hemorrhage.

Clopidogrel resistance

The term resistance is questionable because it has been used to indicate failure of the drug to prevent the condition for which it has been prescribed, or the failure to obtain a biological effect. In the first case, the recurrent event might also be related to the evolution of the disease; for the second, pharmacological resistance depends on the quality and reliability of biological assays. A number of proposed biological tests for assessment of platelet inhibition demonstrates that any of them is really satisfactory. For clopidogrel, vasodilator-stimulated phosphoprotein (239) phosphorylation assessment has been proposed as more specific, but recent data suggest a total lack of sensitivity (22). There are several studies, conducted in a limited number of patients, showing dose- and time-dependent variability and suggesting

some relation with clinical outcome (23,24). However, most have been conducted with optical platelet aggregometry and have to be reproduced in larger datasets. More recently, Serebruany (25) showed that the response to clopidogrel follows a bell-shaped curve, suggesting a Gaussian distribution. Defined by standard deviations less than and greater than the mean, the prevalence of hypo- and hyper-responsiveness in these patients was 4.2% and 4.8%, respectively. This shows that individuals receiving clopidogrel have a wide variability in response that follows a normal distribution. Clinical trials are needed to define whether hyporesponders to clopidogrel are at increased risk for thrombotic events and whether hyper-responders are at increased risk for bleeding. This is a necessary step to define clopidogrel resistance.

Indications

ADP receptor inhibitors might be used in patients with coronary artery disease, in neurology, and in angiology. This chapter will mainly consider indications of ticlopidine and clopidogrel since these are the only two drugs currently available in the market.

Thienopyridines in cardiology

There are three main indications for thienopyridines: ACS, interventional cardiology, and secondary prevention of coronary artery disease.

Acute coronary syndromes

Clopidogrel is indicated in the two types of ACS: with or without persistent ST-segment elevation.

Acute coronary syndromes without persistent ST-segment elevation: Clopidogrel has been investigated in ACS patients treated with aspirin (75–325mg) in a large clinical trial (CURE) (26) of 12,562 patients. Patients hospitalized within 24 hours after the onset of symptoms with electrocardiographic changes or cardiac enzyme rise were randomized to a loading dose of 300mg of clopidogrel followed by 75mg once daily versus placebo for a median of nine months. The first primary outcome (cardiovascular death, nonfatal MI, or stroke) was significantly reduced from 11.4% to 9.3% (ARR 5 2.1%, relative risk, 0.80; 95% CI: 0.72–0.90; P , 0.001). The rate of each component also tended to be lower in the clopidogrel group, but the most important difference was observed in the rates of MI (ARR 5 1.5%, relative risk, 0.77; 95% CI: 0.67–0.89). The rate of refractory ischemia during initial hospitalization decreased significantly (P 5 0.007) from 2.0% to 1.4% (ARR 5 0.6%, relative risk, 0.68; 95% CI: 0.52–0.90) but did not significantly differ after discharge (7.6% in both groups). Major bleeding was significantly more common in the clopidogrel group (3.7% vs. 2.7%, 11%, relative risk, 1.38; 95% CI: 1.13–1.67; P 5 0.001); the number of patients who required transfusion of two or more units was higher in the clopidogrel group than in the placebo group (2.8% vs. 2.2%, P 5 0.02). Major bleedings were approximately as frequent during early treatment (,30 days) as later (.30 days after randomization) (2.0% and 1.7%, respectively). Minor bleedings were significantly higher in the clopidogrel group than in the placebo group (5.1% versus 2.4%, P ,0.001).

Slightly fewer patients in the clopidogrel group underwent coronary revascularization (36% vs. 36.9%). Nevertheless, 1822 patients of the clopidogrel group underwent bypass surgery. Overall, there was no significant increase of major bleeding episodes after coronary artery bypass graft (CABG) (1.3% vs. 1.1%). But in the 912 patients who did not stop study medication until five days before surgery, the rate of major bleeding was higher in the clopidogrel group (9.6% vs. 6.3%, P = 0.06).

A clear increase in bleeding risk occurred as the dose of aspirin increased from ≤100 mg to 100–300 mg to >300 mg in both placebo-treated (2.0%, 2.2%, 4.0% major bleeds, respectively) and clopidogrel-treated patients (2.5%, 3.5%, 4.9%). There was no clear evidence in CURE or in the antiplatelet triallist's collaboration of improved outcome with higher doses of aspirin. Thus it is recommended that clopidogrel be used in conjunction with maintenance doses of ≤100 mg aspirin.

In 2005 the results of a phase 2, randomized, dose-ranging, double-blind safety trial (JUMBO-TIMI 26I) (27) of prasugrel versus clopidogrel in 904 patients undergoing elective or urgent percutaneous coronary intervention (PCI) were published. The primary endpoint of the trial was clinically significant (TIMI major plus minor): non-CABG-related bleeding events in prasugrel- versus clopidogrel-treated patients. Hemorrhagic complications were infrequent, with no significant difference between patients treated with prasugrel or clopidogrel in the rate of significant bleeding (1.7% vs. 1.2%; hazard ratio, 1.42; 95% CI: 0.40, 5.08). In prasugrel-treated patients, there was an insignificant lower incidence of the primary efficacy composite endpoint (30-day major adverse cardiac events) and of the secondary endpoints (MI, recurrent ischemia, and clinical target vessel thrombosis).

A new trial of 13,800 patients with ACS (TRITON-TIMI 38) is now ongoing.

Acute coronary syndromes with ST-segment elevation

The CLARITY (28–30) ($n = 3491$) and COMMIT (31) ($n = 45,852$) trials have tested the use of clopidogrel with lytic therapy in ST elevation ACS. The primary endpoint of CLARITY was a composite of occluded infarct related artery (TIMI grade flow 0/1) on predischarge angiogram, or death, or MI by hospital discharge if no angiography was performed. This study demonstrated a highly significant reduction in the frequency of occluded arteries (clopidogrel 15.0%, placebo 21.7%; 95% CI: 0.53–0.76; $P < 0.0001$). The TIMI grade flow 0/1 was significantly decreased from 18.4% to 11.7% (RRR = 0.59; 95% CI: 0.48–0.72; $P < 0.001$). As a result, at 30 days, there was a significant reduction ($P = 0.02$) of major clinical events (death, MI, or recurrent ischemia requiring urgent revascularization). There was no significant excess in TIMI major bleedings or intracranial hemorrhage in patients receiving fibrinolytic agents.

COMMIT or CCS-2 (31), conducted in China and without a loading dose of clopidogrel, tried to determine whether adding clopidogrel to acetylsalicylic acid (ASA) can produce a further reduction in mortality and the risk of vascular events in hospital for patients admitted with ST-elevation MI (STEMI).

A large cohort of patients ($n = 46,000$) with STEMI (<24 hours) was enrolled. There was a highly significant reduction in the risk of death (8.1% death vs. 7.5%, a 7% relative risk reduction (RRR), $P = 0.03$) and of death or re-MI or stroke (9% RRR, $P = 0.002$).

There was no significant increase in the risk of fatal or transfused bleeding.

Thus for every 1000 MI patients treated in hospital for about two to three weeks, clopidogrel might save 70 lives.

Clopidogrel will therefore be part of acute treatment for STEMI and should be administered at the first medical contact.

Thienopyridines and interventional cardiology

Coronary stenting: In the early 1990s, two trials were launched comparing ticlopidine given before percutaneous transluminal coronary angioplasty versus placebo [therapeutic angiogenesis by cell transplantation (TACT) trial (32) and White (33)]. The rate of major acute complications was significantly lower in the ticlopidine group than in the placebo group. When stent implantation was more frequently performed, one of the investigators (P. Barragan) of the TACT study (34,35) continued the TACT protocol and to prepare the patients with ticlopidine and aspirin. Surprisingly, the Barragan group had a very low rate of stent thrombosis. The first French registry published in 1995 (36) confirmed these results. Later in 1996, Karrillon et al. (37), in a second registry, definitively established the interest of a two-pronged antiplatelet approach by ticlopidine combined with aspirin. Finally, four randomized trials demonstrated the superiority of this aggressive antiplatelet management over traditional, full anticoagulation with coumadin or other antivitamin K. [ISAR (38), FANTASTIC (39), STARS (40), and MATTIS (41) studies].

The CLASSICS (42) trial, conducted on 1020 patients, compared ticlopidine and clopidogrel (LD300 mg/75 mg/day) on top of aspirin. It appeared that clopidogrel + aspirin was superior to ticlopidine + aspirin on the primary endpoint (a composite of major peripheral or bleeding complications, neutropenia, thrombocytopenia, or early discontinuation of the study drug for noncardiac adverse events): 9.1% versus 2.9% ($P < 0.001$). The same results were obtained for the secondary endpoints at 28 days (total mortality, major cardiac events, combined cardiac mortality, MI, and target lesion revascularization). Later, a meta-analysis of randomized trial registries showed clearly the superiority of clopidogrel over ticlopidine: mortality rate at one month follow-up (FU) was significantly lower with clopidogrel (0.48% vs. 1.09%, $P = 0.001$), and the rate of MI was significantly decreased (2–1.2%, $P = 0.002$) (43).

Thus, clopidogrel (LD300 mg + 75 mg/day for one month) is the standard of care after bare metallic stent implantation.

The results of the RAVEL trial comparing a drug-eluting stent (e-cypher coated with sirolimus) versus a bare metallic stent were presented in 2001. Aspirin + clopidogrel was given for two months without acute and subacute thrombosis. Nevertheless, fearing late stent thrombosis, it was admitted that the dual antiplatelet treatment had to be prolonged for three months after sirolimus stent implantation and for six months after paclitaxel stent implantation. Later, in a larger population from clinical randomized trials and registries it was observed that the rate of stent thrombosis was similar after bare metallic stent and coated stent.

Clopidogrel as a pretreatment to percutaneous coronary interventions

This indication was considered in three trials. The first was the PCI-CURE study (44) ($n = 2658$ patients), a prespecified subgroup analysis of CURE. This trial studied the benefit of pretreatment with clopidogrel (median 10 days) before PCI. At one-month follow-up, there was a significant ($P = 0.04$) reduction of cardiovascular death and MI (from 4.4% to 2.9%).

The second trial (CREDO) (45) was performed in 2116 patients randomized in two groups. One group received before PCI clopidogrel (LD300 mg/75 mg/day) + aspirin and the other group received only aspirin. Since most of the patients (one-third of stable angina and two-thirds of ACS) received a stent, both groups received open label clopidogrel + aspirin for one month after the procedure. At one month follow-up, there was only a nonsignificant trend (6.3% vs. 8.33% of death + MI + stroke) in favor of clopidogrel + aspirin. However, the results depend mainly on the duration of pretreatment. If given for more than six hours, there is significant benefit (5.8% vs. 9.4%, $P = 0.005$). Later, it was established that ASA + clopidogrel should be given for more than 13 hours to induce a significant benefit at one month follow-up.

The third trial was a subgroup analysis of the CLARITY (29) trial performed in acute MI. It was demonstrated that in STEMI patients, treated with fibrinolytic and who underwent PCI during the hospitalization period ($n = 1863$ patients), the dual antiplatelet treatment was able to reduce major vascular events (death, MI, and stroke) from 12% to 7.5% (RRR = 0.59 95% CI: 0.43–0.81; $P = 0.001$). Thus, the treatment with clopidogrel + aspirin of 43 STEMI patients followed by PCI prevents one major vascular event.

Long-term treatment with clopidogrel

ACS represents a prothrombotic state not just confined to the culprit lesion, with evidence of a pan coronary process and generalized platelet activation. Multiple vulnerable plaques in nonculprit vessels have been identified by angioscopy or intravascular ultrasound in ACS. Protracted treatment with clopidogrel induces antiplatelet activity that provides early benefits, and may limit thrombotic events within the following months. In the CURE study, the curves of major vascular events continue to diverge and showed an additional benefit from one-month follow-up to one year.

In the PCI-CURE trial, the study drug (placebo or clopidogrel) was again administered for an average of eight months. Further analysis of cardiovascular events before and after PCI showed that clopidogrel caused a highly significant 31% reduction in cardiovascular death or MI. Prolonged clopidogrel treatment for 12 months was examined in the CREDO study. From one to 12 months there was a further 41% relative risk reduction of the combined risk of death, MI, or stroke. More recent cost analyses (46–48) confirm the economic as well as clinical gain from this long-term strategy.

However, we have no data to support the concept of prolonged (>1 year) dual antiplatelet treatment except in patients who underwent vascular brachytherapy for in-stent re-stenosis. Due to the lack of re-endothelialization, this small group of patients should receive the dual treatment for life (49,50).

The CHARISMA trial (51) enrolled 15,603 patients with either cardiovascular disease or multiple risk factors followed for a median of 28 months. Overall, the dual antiplatelet regimen (aspirin + clopidogrel) was not significantly more effective than aspirin alone in reducing the rate of death, MI or stroke from cardiovascular causes.

Clopidogrel and secondary prevention of coronary artery disease

CAPRIE (52) was a randomized, blinded, international study designed to assess the relative efficacy of clopidogrel

(75 mg once daily) and aspirin (325 mg once daily) in reducing the risk of a composite outcome cluster of ischemic stroke, MI, or vascular death. The study population ($n = 19,185$ patients) comprised subgroups of patients with atherosclerotic vascular disease (recent ischemic stroke, recent MI, or symptomatic peripheral arterial disease). Patient follow-up was done for one to three years.

The results showed that patients treated with clopidogrel had an annual 5.32% risk of ischemic stroke, MI, or vascular death compared with 5.83% with aspirin (RRR = 8.7% in favor of clopidogrel, $P = 0.045$). There were no major differences in terms of safety.

The benefit of clopidogrel was consistent across the different subgroups but was particularly important in high-risk patients: in patients with prior CABG (53), 75 mg of clopidogrel compared to aspirin reduced the risk of vascular events (vascular death, MI, stroke, rehospitalization) from 22.3% to 15.9%. Similar results were obtained in diabetic patients (54) (reduction from 21.5% to 17.7%) of this endpoint and a reduction from 23.8% to 20.4% in patients with a history of MI or stroke.

Thus, clopidogrel has to be considered a safe alternative to aspirin for secondary prevention in patients with stable coronary artery disease. It should be given to all patients with coronary artery disease and who have either a contraindication or intolerance to aspirin.

Thienopyridine and atrial fibrillation

The burden and risks due to atrial fibrillation (AF) are high. The prevention of arterial emboli and particularly cerebral emboli implies oral anticoagulation (OAC). However, anticoagulant therapies are associated with a greater risk of major bleeding complications, have many contraindications, and are burdensome to patients. Aspirin, while somewhat effective, does not provide optimal protection for patients unable to take OAC. Since clopidogrel and ASA have shown additive benefit when used together, the combination might be more effective than ASA alone and as effective as OAC. The goal of the ACTIVE study was to investigate the efficacy and safety of clopidogrel + aspirin in patients with AF, compared with standard antithrombotic therapy (OAC therapy when warfarin is indicated).

The study design included three comparisons: ACTIVE W, ACTIVE A, and ACTIVE I in 14,000 patients. (Maximum follow-up was for 48 months). The primary endpoint was the time to first vascular event (stroke, MI, vascular death, systemic emboli). ACTIVE W arm was halted when 6600 patients were enrolled because there a clear benefit from warfarin treatment compared to clopidogrel + aspirin: 3.63% of vascular events versus 5.64% ($P = 0.0002$). Subgroup analysis showed that these disappointing results were observed in patients on warfarin prior to study (HR = 1.5, $P = 0.0006$), but there was no difference between the two strategies—when the patients were not on warfarin prior to study (HR = 1.32, $P = 0.17$). Nevertheless, further results are awaited from the ACTIVE-A arm (ASA or ASA + clopidogrel) in patients who cannot or would not take OAC.

Cardiological indications of clopidogrel are summarized in Table 1.

Thienopyridines and neurology

The results obtained in the CAPRIE trial showing that clopidogrel was superior to aspirin, particularly in high-risk patients, led researchers to consider whether addition of aspirin to

Table 1	Indications of clopidogrel			
Indication	Dose	Duration	Study
NST-segment elevation ACS	LD300 mg/75 mg/day	9 mo	CURE
ST-segment elevation ACS	LD300 mg/75 mg/day		CLARITY, COMMIT
All PCI	LD 300/75 mg/day	1 Yr	CREDO
Bare metallic stenting	LD 300/75 mg/day	1 mo	CLASSICS
Drug eluting stent (Sirolimus)	LD 300/75 mg/day	3 mo	SIRIUS
Drug eluting stent (Paclitaxel)	LD 300/75 mg/day	6 mo	TAXUS
Secondary prevention of CAD	75 mg/day	3 Yr	CAPRIE
History of ischemic stroke	75 mg/day	3 Yr	CAPRIE
Peripheral vessel disease	75 mg/day	3 Yr	CAPRIE

Abbreviations: ACS, acute coronary syndromes; CAD, coronary artery disease; PCI, percutaneous coronary intervention.

clopidogrel could have a greater benefit than clopidogrel alone in the prevention of vascular events in patients who had recently had an ischemic stroke or transient ischemic attack and at least one additional vascular risk factor. This was the goal of the MATCH study (55): a cohort of 7559 patients was randomized in two groups. The first received aspirin (75 mg/day) + clopidogrel 75 mg/day and the other received clopidogrel alone (75 mg/day). The primary endpoint was a composite of vascular death (including hemorrhagic death) + MI + ischemic stroke. There was an insignificant trend at 18-month follow-up in favor of aspirin + clopidogrel: 16% in the dual antiplatelet group and 17% in the clopidogrel group (RRR = 6.4%, $P = 0.244$). However, life-threatening bleeding rates were higher in the aspirin + clopidogrel group than in the clopidogrel alone group. Major bleeding also increased in the aspirin + clopidogrel group.

Thus, it appears that adding aspirin to clopidogrel in these vascular high-risk patients is not associated with a reduction of major vascular events, but results in higher risk of life-threatening and major bleeding. It is important to note the difference with cardiological trials where the comparator was aspirin alone, whilst in the MATCH study (55) the comparator was clopidogrel alone. Nevertheless, it appears that in patients with a history of cerebrovascular accident, the combination of aspirin + clopidogrel is not recommended.

Thienopyridines and peripheral vessel disease

Although peripheral arterial disease (PAD) is a risk marker for widespread atherothrombosis, the condition is under-diagnosed and under-treated. Clopidogrel offers significant benefit in PAD patients, and the CAMPER trial (56) was designed to assess whether clopidogrel on top of standard therapy (including ASA) could further improve long-term benefit after peripheral vascular interventions (angioplasty or surgery). Clopidogrel on top of standard therapy, including ASA, may have the potential to maintain the patency of lower limb arteries after peripheral angioplasty. CAMPER (56) is a randomized, double-blind, prospective, multicenter (100 U.S. centers) study ofthousands of patients who, showing objective evidence of PAD, have had successful peripheral angioplasty (with or without stenting). The maximum follow-up will be 30 months and the primary endpoints will be arterial patency.

Conclusions

ADP receptor inhibitors play a major role in the management of ACS; in interventional cardiology before and after stent implantation and in secondary prevention. Clopidogrel certainly heralds a major advance in the management of atherothrombosis.

A number of questions are still to be resolved, particularly the matter of long-term treatment. This topic is not only a major issue for the clinical outcome of patients with atherosclerotic disease but also from the economic standpoint. Finally, in the future, new ADP receptor blockers will have to be considered and compared to currently available thienopyridines.

References

1   Gachet C, Hechler B. The platelet P2 receptors in thrombosis. Semin Thromb Hemost 2005; 31:162–167.

2   Foster CJ, Prosser DM, Agans JM, et al. Molecular identification and characterization of the platelet ADP receptor targeted by thienopyridine antithrombotic drugs. J Clin Invest 2001; 107:1591–1598.

3   Savi P, Pereillo JM, Uzabiaga MF, et al. Identification and biological activity of the active metabolite of clopidogrel. Thromb Haemost 2000; 84:891–896.

4   Savi P, Labouret C, Delesque N, Guette F, Lupker J, Herbert JM. P2y(12), a new platelet ADP receptor, target of clopidogrel. Biochem Biophys Res Commun 2001; 283:379–383.

5   Caplain H, Donat F, Gaud C, Necciari J. Pharmacokinetics of clopidogrel. Semin Thromb Hemost 1999; 25(suppl 2): 25–28.

6   Lins R, Broekhuysen J, Necciari J, Deroubaix X. Pharmacokinetic profile of 14C-labeled clopidogrel. Semin Thromb Hemost 1999; 25(suppl 2):29–33.

7   Gachet C, Cazenave JP, Ohlmann P, et al. The thienopyridine ticlopidine selectively prevents the inhibitory effects of ADP but not of adrenaline on cAMP levels raised by stimulation of the adenylate cyclase of human platelets by PGE1. Biochem Pharmacol 1990; 40:2683–2687.

8   Mills DC, Puri R, Hu CJ, et al. Clopidogrel inhibits the binding of ADP analogues to the receptor mediating inhibition of platelet adenylate cyclase. Arterioscler Thromb 1992; 12:430–436.

9   Di Minno G, Cerbone AM, Mattioli PL, Turco S, Iovine C, Mancini M. Functionally thrombasthenic state in normal platelets following the administration of ticlopidine. J Clin Invest 1985; 75:328–338.

10 Boneu B, Destelle G. Platelet anti-aggregating activity and tolerance of clopidogrel in atherosclerotic patients. Thromb Haemost 1996; 76:939–943.

11 Savcic M, Hauert J, Bachmann F, Wyld PJ, Geudelin B, Cariou R. Clopidogrel loading dose regimens: kinetic profile of pharmacodynamic response in healthy subjects. Semin Thromb Hemost 1999; 25(suppl 2):15–19.

12 Herbert J, Frehel E, Vallee E, Kieffer G, Gouy D. Clopidogrel, a novel antiplatelet and antithrombotic agent. Cardiovasc Drug Rev 1993; 11:180–198.

13 Seyfarth HJ, Koksch M, Roethig G, et al. Effect of 300- and 450-mg clopidogrel loading doses on membrane and soluble

P-selectin in patients undergoing coronary stent implantation. Am Heart J 2002; 143:118–123.

14 Kastrati A, von Beckerath N, Joost A, Pogatsa-Murray G, Gorchakova O, Schomig A. Loading with 600 mg clopidogrel in patients with coronary artery disease with and without chronic clopidogrel therapy. Circulation 2004; 110: 1916–1919.

15 von Beckerath N, Taubert D, Pogatsa-Murray G, Schomig E, Kastrati A, Schomig A. Absorption, metabolization, and antiplatelet effects of 300-, 600-, and 900-mg loading doses of clopidogrel: results of the ISAR-CHOICE (Intracoronary Stenting and Antithrombotic Regimen: Choose Between 3 High Oral Doses for Immediate Clopidogrel Effect) Trial. Circulation 2005; 112:2946–2950.

16 Herbert JM, Dol F, Bernat A, Falotico R, Lale A, Savi P. The antiaggregating and antithrombotic activity of clopidogrel is potentiated by aspirin in several experimental models in the rabbit. Thromb Haemost 1998; 80:512–518.

17 Lau WC, Waskell LA, Watkins PB, et al. Atorvastatin reduces the ability of clopidogrel to inhibit platelet aggregation: a new drug-drug interaction. Circulation 2003; 107:32–37.

18 Lau WC, Carville DG, Bates ER. Clinical significance of the atorvastatin-clopidogrel drug-drug interaction. Circulation 2004; 110:e66–e67; author reply e66–e67.

19 Lau WC, Gurbel PA, Watkins PB, et al. Contribution of hepatic cytochrome P450 3A4 metabolic activity to the phenomenon of clopidogrel resistance. Circulation 2004; 109:166–171.

20 Serebruany VL, Midei MG, Malinin AI, et al. Absence of inter-action between atorvastatin or other statins and clopidogrel: results from the interaction study. Arch Intern Med 2004; 164:2051–2057.

21 Saw J, Steinhubl SR, Berger PB, et al. Lack of adverse clopido-grel-atorvastatin clinical interaction from secondary analysis of a randomized, placebo-controlled clopidogrel trial. Circulation 2003; 108:921–924.

22 Hezard N, Metz D, Garnotel R, et al. Platelet VASP phospho-rylation assessment in clopidogrel-treated patients: lack of agreement between Western blot and flow cytometry. Platelets 2005; 16:474–481.

23 Matetzky S, Shenkman B, Guetta V, et al. Clopidogrel resis-tance is associated with increased risk of recurrent atherothrombotic events in patients with acute myocardial infarction. Circulation 2004; 109:3171–3175.

24 Nguyen TA, Diodati JG, Pharand C. Resistance to clopidogrel: a review of the evidence. J Am Coll Cardiol 2005; 45:1157–1164.

25 Serebruany VL, Steinhubl SR, Berger PB, Malinin AI, Bhatt DL, Topol EJ. Variability in platelet responsiveness to clopidogrel among 544 individuals. J Am Coll Cardiol 2005; 45:246–251.

26 Yusuf S, Zhao F, Mehta SR, Chrolavicius S, Tognoni G, Fox KK. Effects of clopidogrel in addition to aspirin in patients with acute coronary syndromes without ST-segment elevation. N Engl J Med 2001; 345:494–502.

27 Wiviott SD, Antman EM, Winters KJ, et al. Randomized comparison of prasugrel (CS-747, LY640315), a novel thienopyridine P2Y12 antagonist, with clopidogrel in percuta-neous coronary intervention: results of the Joint Utilization of Medications to Block Platelets Optimally (JUMBO)-TIMI 26 trial. Circulation 2005; 111:3366–3373.

28 Sabatine MS, McCabe CH, Gibson CM, Cannon CP. Design and rationale of Clopidogrel as Adjunctive Reperfusion Therapy-Thrombolysis in Myocardial Infarction (CLARITY-TIMI) 28 trial. Am Heart J 2005; 149:227–233.

29 Sabatine MS, Cannon CP, Gibson CM, et al. Addition of clopi-dogrel to aspirin and fibrinolytic therapy for myocardial infarction with ST-segment elevation. N Engl J Med 2005; 352:1179–1189.

30 Sabatine MS, Cannon CP, Gibson CM, et al. Effect of clopi-dogrel pretreatment before percutaneous coronary intervention in patients with ST-elevation myocardial infarction treated with fibrinolytics: the PCI-CLARITY study. JAMA 2005; 294:1224–1232.

31 COMMIT collaborative group. Addition of Clopidogrel to aspirin in 45852 patients with acute myocardial infarction: randomized placebo controlled trial. Lancet 2005; 366: 1607–1621.

32 Bertrand ME, Allain H, Lablanche J. A randomized trial of ticlopidine vs. placebo for prevention of acute closure and restenosis after PTCA: The TACT study. Circulation 1990; 82:190.

33 White C, Chaitman B, Knudtson M, Chisholm R. Antiplatelet agents are effective in reducing the acute ischemic complica-tions of angioplasty but do not prevent restenosis: results from the ticlopidine trial. Coron Artery Dis 1991; 2:757–767.

34 Barragan P, Sainsous J, Silvestri M, et al. Pilot study of the efficacy of ticlopidine in early patency of coronary endopros-theses. Arch Mal Coeur Vaiss 1994; 87:1431–1437.

35 Barragan P, Sainsous J, Silvestri M, et al. Ticlopidine and subcu-taneous heparin as an alternative regimen following coronary stenting. Catheter Cardiovasc Diagn 1994; 32:133–138.

36 Van Belle E, McFadden EP, Lablanche JM, Bauters C, Hamon M, Bertrand ME. Two-pronged antiplatelet therapy with aspirin and ticlopidine without systemic anticoagulation: an alternative therapeutic strategy after bailout stent implantation. Coron Artery Dis 1995; 6:341–345.

37 Karrillon GJ, Morice MC, Benveniste E, et al. Intracoronary stent implantation without ultrasound guidance and with replacement of conventional anticoagulation by antiplatelet therapy. 30-day clinical outcome of the French Multicenter Registry. Circulation 1996; 94:1519–1527.

38 Schomig A, Neumann FJ, Kastrati A, et al. A randomized comparison of antiplatelet and anticoagulant therapy after the placement of coronary-artery stents. N Engl J Med 1996; 334:1084–1089.

39 Bertrand ME, Legrand V, Boland J, et al. Randomized multi-center comparison of conventional anticoagulation versus antiplatelet therapy in unplanned and elective coronary stent-ing. The full anticoagulation versus aspirin and ticlopidine (fantastic) study. Circulation 1998; 98:1597–1603.

40 Leon MB, Baim DS, Popma JJ, et al. A clinical trial comparing three antithrombotic-drug regimens after coronary-artery stenting. Stent Anticoagulation Restenosis Study Investigators. N Engl J Med 1998; 339:1665–1671.

41 Urban P, Macaya C, Rupprecht HJ, et al. Randomized evalua-tion of anticoagulation versus antiplatelet therapy after coronary stent implantation in high-risk patients: the multicen-ter aspirin and ticlopidine trial after intracoronary stenting (MATTIS). Circulation 1998; 98:2126–2132.

42 Bertrand ME, Rupprecht HJ, Urban P, Gershlick AH, Investigators FT. Double-blind study of the safety of clopidogrel with and without a loading dose in combination with aspirin compared with ticlopidine in combination with aspirin after coronary stenting: the clopidogrel aspirin stent international cooperative study (CLASSICS). Circulation 2000; 102:624–629.

43 Bhatt DL, Bertrand ME, Berger PB, et al. Meta-analysis of randomized and registry comparisons of ticlopidine with clopidogrel after stenting. J Am Coll Cardiol 2002; 39:9–14.

44 Mehta SR. Aspirin and clopidogrel in patients with ACS undergoing PCI: CURE and PCI-CURE. J Invasive Cardiol 2003; 15(suppl B):17B–20B; discussion 20B–21B.

45 Steinhubl SR, Berger PB, Mann JT III, et al. Early and sustained dual oral antiplatelet therapy following percutaneous coronary intervention: a randomized controlled trial. JAMA 2002; 288:2411–2420.

46 Lindgren P, Stenestrand U, Malmberg K, Jonsson B. The long-term cost-effectiveness of clopidogrel plus aspirin in patients undergoing percutaneous coronary intervention in Sweden. Clin Ther 2005; 27:100–110.

47 Lindgren P, Jonsson B, Yusuf S. Cost-effectiveness of clopidogrel in acute coronary syndromes in Sweden: a long-term model based on the CURE trial. J Intern Med 2004; 255:562–570.

48 Cowper PA, Udayakumar K, Sketch MH Jr, Peterson ED. Economic effects of prolonged clopidogrel therapy after percutaneous coronary intervention. J Am Coll Cardiol 2005; 45:369–376.

49 Waksman R, Ajani AE, Pinnow E, et al. Twelve versus six months of clopidogrel to reduce major cardiac events in patients undergoing gamma-radiation therapy for in-stent restenosis: Washington Radiation for In-Stent restenosis Trial (WRIST) 12 versus WRIST PLUS. Circulation 2002; 106: 776–778.

50 Waksman R, Ajani AE, White RL, et al. Prolonged antiplatelet therapy to prevent late thrombosis after intracoronary gamma-radiation in patients with in-stent restenosis: Washington Radiation for In-Stent Restenosis Trial plus 6 months of clopidogrel (WRIST PLUS). Circulation 2001; 103:2332–2335.

51 Bhatt DL, Topol EJ. Clopidogrel added to aspirin versus aspirin alone in secondary prevention and high-risk primary prevention: rationale and design of the Clopidogrel for High Atherothrombotic Risk and Ischemic Stabilization, Management, and Avoidance (CHARISMA) trial. Am Heart J 2004; 148: 263–268.

52 CAPRIE Steering Committee. A randomised, blinded, trial of clopidogrel versus aspirin in patients at risk of ischaemic events (CAPRIE). Lancet 1996; 348:1329–1339.

53 Bhatt DL, Chew DP, Hirsch AT, Ringleb PA, Hacke W, Topol EJ. Superiority of clopidogrel versus aspirin in patients with prior cardiac surgery. Circulation 2001; 103:363–368.

54 Bhatt DL, Marso SP, Hirsch AT, Ringleb PA, Hacke W, Topol EJ. Amplified benefit of clopidogrel versus aspirin in patients with diabetes mellitus. Am J Cardiol 2002; 90:625–628.

55 Diener HC, Bogousslavsky J, Brass LM, et al. Aspirin and clopidogrel compared with clopidogrel alone after recent ischaemic stroke or transient ischaemic attack in high-risk patients (MATCH): randomised, double-blind, placebo-controlled trial. Lancet 2004; 364:331–337.

56 Belch JJ, Topol EJ, Agnelli G, et al. Critical issues in peripheral arterial disease detection and management: a call to action. Arch Intern Med 2003; 163:884–892.

5

Phosphodiesterase inhibitors: dipyridamole and cilostazol

James J. Ferguson

Introduction

Two drugs are often included as part of the antiplatelet armamentarium: dipyridamole and cilostazol. Dipyridamole has been available clinically for about the last 40 years and played an important role as adjunctive therapy in the early days of surgical and percutaneous intervention. Cilostazol is a more recent addition to our pharmacologic options, has an established role in the management of peripheral arterial disease, and has gained a more recent attention with favorable new data in reducing restenosis following coronary stenting.

A frequently cited mechanism of action for these agents is phosphodiesterase (PDE) inhibition and the associated antiplatelet effects that accompany increases in intracellular cyclic adenosine monophosphate (cAMP). In fact, the effects of these drugs go far beyond their direct effect on PDE inhibition or platelet function. This chapter discusses: (*i*) cyclic nucleotides, PDE, and PDE inhibitors; (*ii*) the mechanisms of action of dipyridamole and cilostazol; (*iii*) drug issues; and (*iv*) current clinical applications for dipyridamole and cilostazol, including recent clinical trials that may have changed our perception of the possible utility of these agents for percutaneous intervention.

Cyclic nucleotides, phosphodiesterase, and phosphodiesterase inhibitors

In the late 1950s, biologists came to appreciate the importance of cyclic nucleotides and began to delve deeper into their regulation. In 1958, Sutherland and Rall (1) described a cyclic adenine ribonucleotide, 3′,5′-cyclic adenosine

monophosphate, or cAMP, which is formed in response to stimuli such as glucagon and epinephrine. It was subject to endogenous breakdown or hydrolysis and was found to play a pivotal role as a second messenger within cells, linking actions on the surface (via membrane receptors) with internal biologic mechanisms within cells.

Substances such as fluoride and caffeine were shown to inhibit the breakdown of cAMP. In addition, the medicinal use of caffeine, the oldest known PDE inhibitor, was described originally by Satler in 1860 (2) as a treatment for asthma. Attention then turned to more fully elucidating the biology of cyclic nucleotides (3). With the recognition of the importance of the cyclic nucleotides came further rapid advances in our understanding of their regulation. In the early 1970s, a number of investigators showed that the PDE activity could be fractionated; there turned out to be a number of distinct PDE subtypes specific to different tissues and with unique biological activities (4,5). There are now at least 11 major families of PDE that have been described (6) (Table 1), with more than 50 distinct isoforms, in addition to a number of more selective PDE inhibitors that have been developed in different therapeutic areas, including heart failure, coagulation, allergy and immunology, and erectile dysfunction. Nonselective inhibitors in common use include caffeine, theophylline, pentoxifylline, and methylxanthine.

PDEs are generally differentiated on the basis of their substrate specificity and how they are regulated. They consist of three main functional domains: a regulatory C-terminus (probably involved in the actions of PDE-specific kinases), a central catalytic domain, and a regulatory N-terminus (involved in the allosteric regulation of substrate binding and phosphorylation and membrane targeting).

As shown in Figure 1, the cyclic nucleotides cAMP and 3′,5′ guanosine cyclic monophosphate (cGMP) are formed by the action of adenyl cyclase (AC) or guanylyl cyclase (GC) on their

Table 1   Human phosphodiesterase enzyme families

Family	Characteristics	Tissue distribution
PDE1	CaU/calmodulin-stimulated	Heart, brain, lung, smooth muscle
PDE2	cGMP-stimulated	Adrenal, heart, lung, liver, platelets
PDE3	cGMP-inhibited; cAMP-selective	Heart, lung, liver, platelets, adipose tissue, immunocytes
PDE4	cAMP-specific; cGMP-insensitive	Sertoli cells, kidney, brain, liver, lung, immunocytes
PDE5	cGMP-specific	Lung, platelets, smooth muscle
PDE6	cGMP-specific	Photoreceptors
PDE7	cAMP-specific, high-affinity	Skeletal muscle, heart, kidney, brain, pancreas, T lymphocytes
PDE8	cAMP-specific, IBMX-insensitive	Testes, eye, liver, skeletal muscle, heart, kidney, ovary, brain, Tlymphocytes
PDE9	cGMP-specific, IBMX-insensitive	Kidney, liver, lung, brain
PDE10	cGMP-specific; cAMP-selective	Testes, brain
PDE11	cGMP-sensitive; dual specificity	Skeletal muscle, prostate, kidney, liver, pituitary, salivary glands, testes

Abbreviation: IBMX, 3-isobutyl-l-methylxanthine.

respective triphosphates, adenosine triphosphate (ATP) or guanosine triphosphate (GTP) (6). AC and GC have multiple tissue-specific isoforms, each with a specific cellular and tissue distribution, discrete signal-transducing receptors, and specific regulators (such as calmodulin or phosphorylation). The actions of cAMP and cGMP occur via the cyclic nucleotide-dependent protein kinases cAK and cGK. These protein kinases consist of a tetramer comprising two regulatory subunits and two catalytic subunits. To activate these protein kinases, four molecules of the cyclic nucleotide bind to the two regulatory subunits. This changes the conformation of the protein kinase and disengages the two active catalytic subunits from the parent tetramer; these active catalytic subunits can then go on to phosphorylate other specific targets, including ion channels, signaling proteins, and transcription regulators (6). Thus, cyclic nucleotides play a

key role in multiple tissues and numerous regulatory pathways, each with distinct mechanistic characteristics.

The cyclic nucleotides are broken down by hydrolytic cleavage of their 3′ phosphodiester bond— this process is catalyzed by PDE and results in the formation of the respective inactive 5′-monophosphates, 5′-AMP or 5′-GMP. PDE inhibitors interfere with this breakdown, leading to the accumulation of cAMP and cGMP, respectively. Although the actions of PDE are very compartment-specific and tightly regulated, there can also be a crosstalk between compartments in the face of rapid shift in cyclic nucleotide concentrations. The cyclic nucleotide-signaling cascade can also interact with other key protein kinase and transcription pathways. Finally, cyclic nucleotide pathways are also significantly autoregulated and subject to either positive or negative feedback.

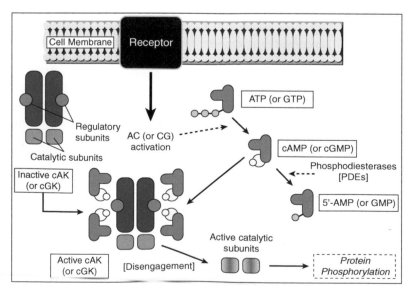

Figure 1

Generation, breakdown, and actions of cyclic nucleotides. cAMP and cGMP are formed by the action of adenyl cyclase or guanylyl cyclase on adenosine triphosphate or guanosine triphosphate. The actions of cAMP and cGMP occur via the protein kinases cAK and cGK. These protein kinases consist of a tetramer, with two regulatory subunits and two catalytic subunits, four molecules of cAMP or cGMP bind to the regulatory subunits, changing the conformation of the protein kinase and disengaging the two active catalytic subunits which can then go on to phosphorylate other specific targets. cAMP and cGMP are broken down by specific PDEs, thus limiting their actions. *Abbreviations*: AC, adenyl cyclase; AMP, adenosine monophosphate; ATP, adenosine triphosphate.

There are three primary PDEs that are found in platelets, PDE2, PDE3, and PDE5. Dipyridamole (in addition to the other actions noted subsequently) blocks PDE5, PDE6, PDE10, and PDE11; cilostazol blocks PDE3. These agents will be discussed in further detail subsequently.

Mechanisms of action
Dipyridamole

Dipyridamole is a drug with a number of mechanistic effects (Figs. 2 and 3). As noted earlier, it is a PDE inhibitor (most notably against PDE5, PDE6, PDE10, and PDE 11). It also stimulates the release of endogenous eicosanoids from the endothelium and has antioxidant properties. Most importantly, however, it also acts to inhibit the uptake and degradation of adenosine in the vasculature, effectively amplifying the biologic actions of endogenous adenosine (7–9).

Phosphodiesterase inhibition

As noted earlier, inhibition of PDE leads to the accumulation of intracellular cAMP and cGMP. There are also feedback mechanisms—high levels of cAMP may, in turn, have an indirect effect on endogenous factors such as prostacyclin and adenosine, which also serve to further increase the levels of cAMP. High levels of cyclic nucleotides have been shown to inhibit platelet aggregation in response to virtually all agonists. However, in the past, the direct antiplatelet activity of dipyridamole has been noted only at very high concentrations, above those usually achieved with oral therapy, and the ability

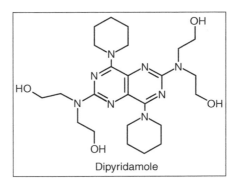

Figure 2
Chemical structure of dipyridamole.

of PDE inhibitors to directly affect platelet aggregation has been subject to question (10–12). It has also been noted (13,14) that the adenosine-related antiplatelet effects of dipyridamole are much more prominent in whole blood than in plasma. Moreover, the narrow view of dipyridamole as simply a vasodilator with antiplatelet properties is overly simplistic and somewhat inaccurate. Its therapeutic actions relate more to its effects on adenosine and the vascular wall than to its direct effect on platelets, coagulation, or blood flow.

The physiologic stimulus for guanylate cyclase is nitric oxide (NO). In response to physical forces, shear stress, or chemical stimuli (such as acetylcholine), endothelial cells release NO, which rapidly diffuses through the membrane, activates guanylate cyclase and increases cGMP. Thus, the cGMP-mediated effects of NO (such as platelet inhibition) can be potentiated by PDE inhibitors such as dipyridamole. Dipyridamole has also been shown to inhibit cAMP, although this effect only occurs at concentrations higher than those clinically achievable with oral therapy and may not be a direct effect. Nevertheless, high cGMP levels may also indirectly

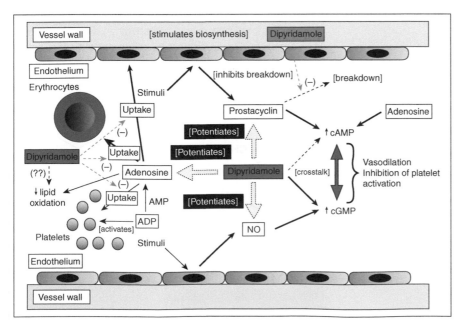

Figure 3
Mechanisms of action of dipyridamole. *Abbreviations*: ADP, adenosine diphosphate; AMP, adenosine monophosphate; cAMP, cyclic adenosine monophosphate; cGMP, guanosine cyclic monophosphate; NO, nitric oxide.

inhibit cAMP PDEs, yielding a net effect for dipyridamole of increasing both cAMP and cGMP. The latter effect will also amplify the effects of adenosine and prostacyclin.

Eicosanoid effects

The effect of dipyridamole to increase intracellular cAMP and cGMP may also have additional indirect potentiation of the platelet inhibitory effects of eicosanoids such as prosacyclin (PGI$_2$) and prostaglandin D$_2$, since these compounds themselves act to stimulate adenylate cyclase. Others have suggested that dipyridamole may also directly stimulate prostacyclin biosynthesis (15–17). By increasing cAMP, dipyridamole may also indirectly facilitate PGI$_2$ production, although cyclo-oxygenase-dependent generation of PGI$_2$ occurs in endothelial cells, but not in platelets. Other work has suggested that dipyridamole may protect PGI$_2$ synthetase from breakdown (18).

Antioxidant properties

Dipyridamole has also been shown to have antioxidant effects (19). Antioxidants act to remove harmful reactive-oxygen species and protect low-density lipoproteins (LDL) from oxidation; oxidized LDL plays a key role in the development and propagation of atherosclerosis. The antioxidant effects of dipyridamole may be both direct (by scavenging oxygen and hydroxyl radicals, inhibiting lipid peroxidation and oxidative modification of LDL) (20–22) and indirect (via adenosine, which reduces superoxide anion generation). Dipyridamole has been shown to be a more effective anioxidant than ascorbic acid, alpha-tocopherol, or probucol (22).

Inhibition of adenosine uptake

Adenosine, in addition to serving as a substrate for the generation of cAMP, plays a physiologic role as a platelet inhibitor and a vasodilator and may attenuate neutrophil-mediated damage to endothelial cells. Adenosine diphosphate (ADP)— a potent platelet agonist—is converted to adenosine, which is taken up rapidly by cells, especially erythrocytes and endothelial cells. A small proportion is metabolized to the aforementioned cyclic nucleotides. The remainder is broken down to inosine and subsequently to xanthine. Dipyridamole inhibits the active transport of adenosine into cells, but does not interfere with the passive diffusion. Since the platelet inhibitory effects of adenosine proceed via stimulation of adenylate cyclase, these effects can also be amplified by dipyridamole. In circulating blood, the largest amount of adenosine is found in red blood cells. This may, in part, help explain why dipyridamole is much more effective in whole blood than in plasma.

Cilostazol

Cilostazol is a PDE3 inhibitor and also is a drug with multiple mechanisms of action (23,24), some of which are directly platelet-related, and others of which exert their effects indirectly via endothelial cells (Figs. 4 and 5). As a PDE inhibitor, it increases the concentration of cyclic nucleotides within platelets and inhibits platelet aggregation in response to shear forces (via ADP) and a variety of agonists. Like other inhibitors of platelet activation, it blocks the expression and release of P-selectin, a key adhesion molecule on the membrane of platelet alpha granules that externalizes with activation, and plays an important role in the interactions between platelets, endothelial cells, and leukocytes. The effect of cilostazol on P-selectin expression appears to be additive to those of aspirin and clopidogrel (25).

Cilostazol has a number of additional indirect effects. Similar to dipyridamole, it enhances the actions of prostacyclin, although it has not been reported to directly increase prostacyclin release. Cilostazol also affects endothelial cells, specifically the release of cytokines, such as monocytic chemoattractant protein-1 (MCP-1), which appears to play an important role in the development and progression of atherosclerotic lesions (24). Cilostazol, like other PDE3 inhibitors, acts as a vasodilator.

Drug issues

Dipyridamole

Oral dipyridamole is available in two different forms. The first is dipyridamole USP (Persantine, Boehringer Ingelheim), which comes in 25, 50, and 75 mg tablets. The second is a combination product (Aggrenox, Boehringer Ingelheim) comprising 25 mg of aspirin and 200 mg of extended-release dipyridamole. Dipyridamole is metabolized in the liver and excreted via bile into the feces. Interestingly, Persantine is only FDA-approved "as an adjunct to coumarin anticoagulants in

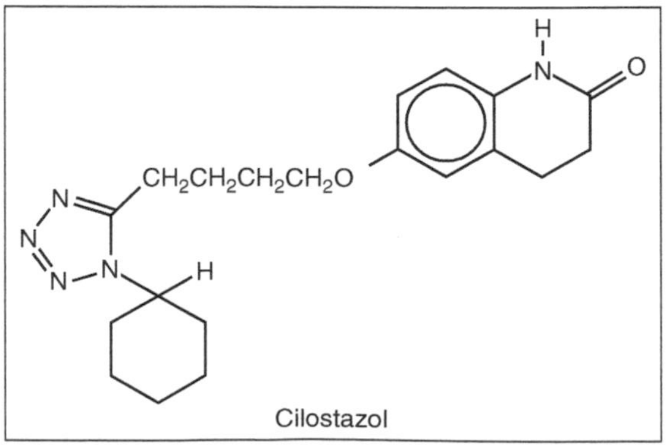

Figure 4
Chemical structure of cilostsazol.

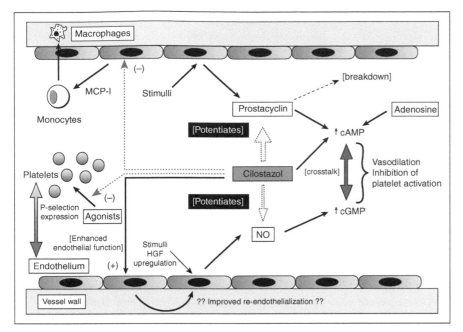

Figure 5
Mechanisms of action of cilostazol. *Abbreviations*: cAMP, cyclic adenosine monophosphate; cGMP, guanosine cyclic monophosphate; HGF, hepatocyte growth factor; MCP-I, monocyte chemoattractant protein-1; NO, nitric oxide.

the prevention of postoperative thromboembolic complications of cardiac valve replacement." The FDA-approved dosage of Persantine for this indication is 75 to 100 mg QID. Aggrenox is FDA-approved to "reduce the risk of stroke in patients who have had transient ischemia of the brain or completed stroke due to thrombosis." The FDA-approved dosage of aggrenox is one tablet twice daily. Both forms can be administered with or without food. The most common side effects are of gastrointestinal; dipyridamole has been associated with elevated hepatic enzymes and, rarely, hepatic failure. As a vasodilator, it should be used with caution in patients with low blood pressure. Dipyridamole also carries a warning for use in patients with severe coronary artery disease, although, as noted elsewhere, evidence for a "coronary steal" phenomenon with oral administration is lacking.

Cilostazol

Cilostazol (Pletal, Otsuka America) is a quinolone derivative that is FDA-approved for "the reduction of symptoms of intermittent claudication, as indicated by an increased walking distance." It is extensively metabolized by the cytochrome P-450 system (mainly 3A4 and 2C9), and the metabolites are excreted in the urine. It is available as 50 mg and 100 mg tablets; the recommended dose is 100 mg BID taken at least half an hour before or two hours after meals, since a high-fat meal significantly increases absorption. A dose of 50 mg BID can be considered when given with inhibitors of CYP3A4 (such as ketoconazole, erythromycin, or diltiazem) or CYP2C19 (such as omeprazole or grapefruit juice). The most common side effects are headache and diarrhea. Cilostazol

carries a labeled contraindication in patients with congestive heart failure (CHF) of any severity, largely as a consequence of problems that CHF patients have encountered with other PDE3 inhibitors, such as milrinone.

Clinical experience
Dipyridamole

Dipyridamole was first synthesized in 1959 (26). It entered clinical application as a coronary vasodilator in the 1960s and played an important role in the adjunctive pharmacologic regimens in the early days of coronary artery bypass surgery. At the time, the available antithrombotic options were limited, and the combination of aspirin and dipyridamole was shown to be superior in preserving early graft patency (27) and in maintaining vein graft patency over the longer term (28). With the development of balloon angioplasty, the aspirin–dipyridamole combination migrated into the world of interventional cardiology and also became part of the standard antithrombotic regimen for percutaneous transluminal coronary angioplasty (PTCA), in an era of few other options.

Schwartz et al. (29) examined the role of antiplatelet therapy in preventing restenosis following balloon angioplasty. They randomized 376 patients to receive either aspirin plus dipyridamole or placebo (similar to previous bypass studies). The active treatment arm received aspirin (330 mg) and dipyridamole (75 mg) three times daily for 24 hours prior to the procedure; eight hours before PTCA, the oral dipyridamole was replaced with intravenous dipyridamole (10 mg/hour for 24 hours)—the oral aspirin was continued;

16 hours after the procedure, the original oral combination was restarted and continued until follow-up angiography (four to seven months after PTCA or earlier if symptoms developed). Follow-up angiography was performed in 249 patients; restenosis was present in 37.7% of the treatment group and 38.6% of the placebo group. Of note, periprocedural myocardial infarctions (MIs) developed in 13 patients in the placebo group and three patients in the active group (6.9% vs. 1.6%; $P = 0.011$).

The further development of stents paralleled the clinical entry of the potent glycoprotein IIb/IIIa antagonists and the emergence of another antiplatelet option, thienopyridines, in the coronary interventional world. Interestingly, although dipyridamole was part of the existing "standard" for early balloon-expandable stents, it was not part of the control arm of Stent Anticoagulation Restenosis Study (STARS) (30) that established the role for the aspirin/thienopyridinde combination. With the rapid ensuing switch to aspirin and ticlopidine instead of oral anticoagulation, dipyridamole was subsequently largely ignored in interventional cardiology.

Although its role as an antiplatelet agent in interventional cardiology has been diminished with the emergence of other potent alternatives, two recent studies in the neurology field have highlighted the areas of renewed clinical interest, and there is an emerging appreciation that the potential clinical benefits of dipyridamole have little to do with its antiplatelet actions and much more to do with its other actions on the vascular wall.

After a number of earlier studies had suggested that dipyridamole did not add significantly to the benefits of aspirin in patients with transient ischemic attack (TIA) or stroke (31–36), the European Stroke Prevention Study-2 (ESPS-2) study (37) demonstrated that adding modified-release dipyridamole (a new formulation, 200 mg BID) to low dose (50 mg) daily aspirin significantly reduced vascular events in TIA and stroke patients. Later, the Management of Atherothrombosis with Clopidogrel in High-Risk Patients (MATCH) study (38) demonstrated that there was no benefit of clopidogrel plus aspirin in comparison to clopidogrel alone in a TIA/stroke population. Very recently, the European/Australasian Stroke Prevention in Reversible Ischemia Trial (ESPRIT) (39) study examined the benefits of dipyridamole plus aspirin versus aspirin alone for secondary prevention in 2739 patients with a history of TIA or stroke. Treatment was open label; during the study, 26% of the patients in the aspirin–dipyridamole group discontinued therapy, most frequently due to side effects (usually headache) compared with 13% of the aspirin alone group who discontinued their study medication—mainly for medical reasons such as new adverse outcome events. The primary endpoint (vascular death, nonfatal stroke, nonfatal MI, or major bleeding) was 13% in the aspirin–dipyridamole group and 16% in the aspirin alone group.

It is worth noting that the primary benefits of dipyridamole were related to cerebrovascular, and not cardiac, events. In neither ESPS-2 nor ESPRIT, were there any significant reductions in coronary events. Thus, at this point, dipyridamole does not appear to play a significant role in our therapeutic armamentarium for coronary intervention. It may have a role in the management of peripheral arterial disease, especially cerebrovascular disease. Nevertheless, the intriguing biology of the compound, and its myriad of effects on the vascular wall, both direct and indirect, raise the possibility of future—as-yet unexplored—clinical applications for cardiovascular disease. It is also worth noting that although intravenous dipyridamole is frequently used for provocative testing, there have been no reports of any coronary-steal-like incidents with oral administration of dipyridamole in any of the stroke studies (40).

Finally, purines such as caffeine (including dietary caffeine in coffee, tea, colas, and chocolate) and synthetic derivatives, such as theophylline, can interfere with the vascular actions of dipyridamole. These agents act to inhibit the adenosine A2A receptor, which serves to further emphasize the role of adenosine in the pharmacologic actions of dipyridamole (41–43). It has also been shown that this effect on A2A receptors is restricted to the vessel wall; the direct anti-aggregatory actions of dipyridamole are not blocked by purines and may, if anything, be enhanced by the indirect effect of purines to upregulate A2A receptors (44,45).

Cilostazol

Cilostazol is indicated for symptomatic relief of intermittent claudication (46,47). With recent attention focusing on new antiplatelet modalities in percutaneous coronary intervention, renewed interest in cilostazol has emerged. Although cilostazol has not been associated with the same increase in cardiac mortality noted with other PDE3 inhibitors used in patients with heart failure (such as milrinone), it is not recommended for use in patients with coexistent heart failure.

Two recent provocative studies have suggested that there may indeed be a role for yet another antiplatelet agent in interventional cardiology. Again, like dipyridamole, the benefits of cilostazol may have relatively little to do with its direct antiplatelet effect, and more to do with other more complex and more indirect mechanisms of action. As noted previously, one study has documented incremental inhibition of P-selectin expression when cilostazol was added to aspirin and clopidogrel (25). Another study documented that cilostazol alone did not significantly affect bleeding times, and adding cilostazol to aspirin and clopidogrel did not increase bleeding times (48,49). There appears to be some disconnection between its effect on platelet activation and P-selectin expression, and its affect on platelet function and bleeding times.

Lee et al. (50) examined the clinical effect of triple antiplatelet therapy with cilostazol (200 mg load, 100 mg BID), aspirin, and a thienopyridine (ticlopidine or clopidogrel) versus dual antiplatelet therapy with aspirin and a thienopyridine alone in 2012 patients undergoing successful coronary stenting. The primary endpoint of the study was the composite of death, MI, target lesion revascularization (TLR), or stent thrombosis at 30 days. The composite primary endpoint was not significantly different between groups, although there was a significantly lower incidence of stent thrombosis with triple therapy (0.1% vs. 0.5% with dual therapy; $P = 0.024$) and a significantly lower incidence of TLR with triple therapy (0.1% vs. 0.5% with dual therapy; $P = 0.024$). Major bleeding and overall adverse events were not significantly different between groups.

A second recent study was the CREST trial (51), which randomized 705 patients following successful stent implantation to either aspirin alone or aspirin plus cilostazol (100 mg BID) for six months (all patients got clopidogrel, 75 mg/day for 30 days following the procedure). As shown in Table 2, at six months, the minimal luminal diameter (by qualitative coronary angiography) was significantly higher in the cilostazol group (1.77 mm vs. 1.62 mm; $P = 0.01$); binary restenosis was also significantly reduced (22.0% vs. 34.5%; $P = 0.002$). This effect on restenosis appeared most prominent in higher-risk patients, including diabetics, and patients with lesions in smaller vessels, longer lesions, and left anterior descending lesions. There were no significant differences in bleeding between groups.

Both of these studies were conducted in the era of bare-metal stents. More recent attention has focused on a higher incidence of late thrombotic events in patients who have received drug-eluting stents (DES), particularly when the intense antiplatelet regimen is interrupted, even long term. The BASKET-LATE (52) study showed a significantly higher incidence of late MI in DES patients whose dual antiplatelet regimen was stopped at six months rather than continued long term. Given these concerns, drugs that provide incremental benefit in reducing thrombotic events, particularly with no significant increase in bleeding complications, may have substantial potential benefit, although this will have to be confirmed prospectively with appropriately designed and powered clinical trials.

The restenosis benefit is also intriguing, but, in all likelihood, has nothing to do with the antiplatelet actions of cilostazol, and may relate more to its effects on cytokine release from endothelial cells and smooth muscle cells. There is also preliminary evidence suggesting that cilostazol may speed the process of endothelialization (53). Again, with DES and their well-documented difficulties with endothelialization (54,55), this is a potentially very important future application that will require prospective testing in clinical trials.

Summary

Both dipyridamole and cilostazol have multiple direct and indirect mechanisms of action. Their direct effects on PDE and direct platelet inhibitory effects are probably less important than the indirect effects and the potentiating effect that they may have on other important pathways (adenosine, NO, and prostacyclin with dipyridamole; prostacyclin, P-selectin expression, and endothelial function with cilostazol). Dipyridamole largely came into use in interventional cardiology as a carry-over from bypass surgery; recent data suggest significant benefit in cerebrovascular disease. Cilostazol is used in patients with intermittent claudication, and recent data has shown a role in reducing restenosis in bare-metal stents. Neither drug seems to be associated with an increase in bleeding complications when superimposed on the combination of aspirin and clopidogrel. Given recent concerns that have arisen regarding the efficacy of (and potential need for) long-term antiplatelet therapy in patients with drug-eluting stents, these agents may find renewed use as we move our

Table 2 Quantitative angiographic outcomes at 6 months in CREST

	Placebo	Cilostazol	Signif
MLD preprocedure (mean)	0.87 mm	0.83 mm	0.21
MLD postprocedure (In-stent)	2.78 mm	2.76 mm	0.58
MLD postprocedure (In-segment)	2.36 mm	2.30 mm	0.23
MLD at 6 months (In-stent)	1.73 mm	1.86 mm	0.05
MLD at 6 months (In-segment)	1.62 mm	1.77 mm	0.01
Late loss (In-stent)	1.06 mm	0.91	0.01
Late loss (In-segment)	0.75 mm	0.57 mm	<0.01
Restenosis (binary)	34.5%	22.0%	0.002
DM	37.7%	17.7%	0.01
Small vessels	39.8%	19.3%	0.02
Long lesions	46.6%	29.9%	0.04
LAD	39.8%	19.3%	0.001

Abbreviations: DM, diabetes mellitus; LAD, left anterior descending artery; MLD, minimal lumen diameter.

attention from being narrowly focused on the platelet and coagulation to the much broader target of the vascular wall and endothelial function.

References

1 Sutherland EW, Rall TW. Fractionation and characterization of a cyclic adenine ribonucleotide formed by tissue particles. J Biol Chem 1958; 232:1077–1091.

2 Parsson CGA. On the medical history of xanthines and other remedies for asthma: a tribute to HH Satler. Thorax 1985; 40:881–886.

3 Antonoff RS, Ferguson JJ. Photoaffinity labeling with cyclic nucleotides. J Biol Chem 1974; 249:3319–3321.

4 Francis SH, Turko IV, Corbin JD. Cyclic nucleotide phosphodiesterases: relating structure and function. Prog Nucleic Acid Res Mol Biol 2000; 65:1–52.

5 Conti M, Jin SL. The molecular biology of cyclic nucleotide phosphodiesterases. Prog Nucleic Acid Res Mol Biol 1999; 63:1–38.

6 Essayan DM. Cyclic nucleotide phosphodiesterases. J Allergy Clin Immunol 2001; 108:671–680.

7 Fitzgerald G. Dipyridamole. N Engl J Med 1987; 316: 1247–1257.

8 Eisert WG. Dipyridamole. In: Michelson A, ed. Platelets. London: Academic Press, 2002:803–815.

9 Schaper W. Dipyridamole, an underestimated vascular protective drug. Cardiovasc Drugs Ther 2005; 19:357–363.

10 Tsien W-H, Sheppard H. The lack of correlation between inhibition of platelet aggregation and cAMP level. Fed Proc 1981; 40:809.

11 Ban G, Brereton GC, Fulwood M, et al. Effect of prosaglandin E, alone and incombination with theophylline or aspirin on collagen induced platelet aggregation and on platelet nucleotides including adenosine 3':5'-cyclic monophosphate. Biochem J 1970; 120:709–718.

12 Lam SC-T, Guccione MA, Packham MA, et al. Effect of cAMP phosphodiesterase inhibitors on ADP-induced shape change, cAMP and nucleoside diphosphokine activity of rabbit platelets. Thromb Haemost 1982; 47:90–95.

13 Gresele P, Zoja C, Deckmyn H, et al. Dipyridamole inhibits platelet aggregation in whole blood. Thromb Haemost 1983; 50:852–856.

14 Gresele P, Arnout J, Deckmyn H, et al. Mechanism of the antiplatelet action of dipyridamole in whole blood; Modulation of adenosine concentration and activity. Thromb Haemost 1986; 55:12–18.

15 Masotti G, Poggesi L, Galanti G, et al. Stimulation of prostacyclin by dipyridamole. Lancet 1979; 1:1412.

16 Blass K.E, Block H-U, Forster W, et al. Dipyridamole: a potent stimulator of prostacyclin (PGI$_2$) biosynthesis. Br J Pharmacol 1980; 68:71–73.

17 Neri Serneri GG, Mosotti G, Poggesi L, et al. Enhanced prostacycin production by dipyridamole in man. Eur J Clin Pharmacol 1981; 21:9–15.

18 Marnett LJ, Siedlik PH, Ochs RC, et al. Mechanism of prostaglandin H synthase and prostacyclin synthase by the antithrombotic and antimetastatic agent, nafazatrom. Mol Pharmacol 1984; 26:328–335.

19 Juliano L, Pedersen JZ, Rotilio G, et al. A potent chain-breaking antioxidant activity of the cardiovascular drug dipyridamole. Free Radic Biol Med 1995; 18:239–247.

20 Juliano L, Violi F, Ghiselli A, et al. Dipyridamole inhibits lipid peroxidation and scavenges oxygen radicals. Lipids 1989; 24:430–33.

21 Selly M, Czeti AL, McGuiness JA, et al. Dipyridamole inhibits the oxidative modification of low density lipoprotein. Atherosclerosis 1994; 111:91–97.

22 Juliano L, Colavita AR, Camastra, et al. Protection of low density lipoprotein oxidation at chemical and cellular level by the antioxidant drug dipyridamole. Br J Pharmacol 1996; 119:1438–1446.

23 Goto S. Cilostazol: potential mechanism of action for antithrombotic effects accompanied by a low rate of bleeding. Atheroscler Suppl 2006; 6:3–11.

24 Moriishita R. A scientific rationale for the CREST trial results: Evidence for the mechanism of action of cilostazol in restanosis. Atheroscler Suppl 2006; 6:41–46.

25 Ahn JC, Song WH, Kwon JA, et al. Effects of cilostazol on platelet activation in coronary stenting patients who already treated with aspirin and clopidogrel. Korean J Int Med 2004; 19:230–236.

26 Kadatz R. Die pharmakologischen Eigenschaften der neuen koronarerweiternden substanz 2,5-Bis(diethanolamino)-4,8-dipiperidino-pyrimide (5,5-d) pyrimidin. Arzneim Forsch 1959; 9:39.

27 Chesebro JH, Clementsw IP, Fuster V, et al. A platelet-inhibitor drug trial in coronary-artery bypass operation: Benefit of early perioperative dipyridamole and aspirin therapy on early postoperative vein-graft patency. N Engl J Med 1982: 307:73–78.

28 Chesebro JH, Fuster V, Elveback LR, et al. Effect of dipyridamole and aspirin on late vein-graft patency after coronary bypass operations. N Engl J Med 1984: 310:209–214.

29 Schwartz L, Bourassa MG, Lesperance J, et al. Aspirin and dipyridamole in the prevention of restenosis after percutaneous transluminal coronary angioplasty. N Engl J Med 1988; 318: 1714–1719.

30 Leon MS, Baim DS, Popma JJ, et al. A clinical trial comparing three antithrombotic drug regimens after coronary artery stenting. N Engl J Med 1998; 339:1665–1671.

31 Algra A, van Gijn J, Koudstaal PJ. Secondary prevention after cerebral ischemia of presumed arterial origin: Is aspirin still the touchstone? J Neurol Neurosurg Psychiatry 1999; 66:557–559.

32 Ameican-Canadian Co-operative Study Group. Persantine aspirin trial in cerebral ischemia, part II: endpoint results. Stroke 1985; 16:406–415.

33 Bousser MG, Eschwege E, Haganau M, et al. "AICLA" controlled trial of aspirin and dipyridamole in the secondary prevention of athero-thrombotic cerebral ischemia. Stroke 1983; 14:5–14.

34 Guiraud-Chaumeil B, Rascol A, David J, et al. Prevention des recidives des accidents vasculaires cerebraux ischemiques par les anti-agregants plaquettaires: resultants d'un essai therapique controle de 3 ans. Rev Neurol (Paris) 1982; 138:367–385.

35 Kaye JA. A trial to evaluate the relative roles of dipyridamole and aspirin in the prevention of deep vein thrombosis in stroke patients. Bracknell, Boehringer Ingelheim (Internal Report), 1990.

36 De Schryver ELLM, Algra A, van Gijn J. Cochrane review: dipyridamole for preventing major vascular events in patients with vascular disease. Stroke 2003; 34:2072–2080.

37 Diener HC, Cunha L, Forbes C, Sivenius J, Smets P, Lowenthal A. European stroke prevention study 2. Dipyridamole and acetylsalicylic acid in the secondary prevention of stroke. J Neurol Sci 1996; 143:1–13.

38 Diener HC, Bogousslavsky J, Brass LM, et al. Aspirin and clopidogrel compared with clopidogrel alone after recent ischaemic stroke or transient ischemic attack in high-risk patients (MATCH): randomized, double-blind, placebo-controlled trial. Lancet 2004; 364:331–337.

39 ESPRIT Study Group. Aspirin plus dipyridamole versus aspirin alone after cerebral ischemia of arterial origin (ESPRIT): Randomised controlled trial. Lancet 2006; 367:1665–1673.

40 Diener HC. Antiplatelet drugs in secondary prevention of stroke: lessons from recent trials. Neurology 1997; 49:S75–S81.

41 Juhran W, Voss EM, Dietmann K, et al. Pharmacological effects on coronary reactive hyperemia in conscious dogs. Naunyn-Schmiedebergs Arch Exp Pathol Pharmakol 1971; 269:32–47.

42 Curnish RR, Berne RM, Rubio R. Effect of aminophylline on myocardial reactive hyperemia. Proc Soc Exp Biol Med 1972; 141:593–598.

43 Schaumann W, Juhran W, Dietmann K. Antagonism of circulation effect of adenosine by theophylline. Arzneimittelforschung 1970; 20:372–377.

44 Varani K, Portaluppi F, Gessi S, et al. Dose and time effects of caffeine in take on human platelet adenosine A2A receptors. Circulation 2000; 285:102–107.

45 Duffy S, Vita JA, Holbrook M, et al. Effect of acute and chronic tea consumption on platelet aggregation in patients with coronary heart disease. ATVB 2001; 21:1084–1090.

46 Thompson PD, Zimet R, Forbes WP, et al. Meta-analysis of results from eight randomized, placebo-controlled trials on hthe effects of cilostazol on patients with intermittent claudication. Am J Cardiol 2002; 90:1314–1319.

47 Hankey GJ, Norman PE, Eikelboom JW. Medical treatment of peripheral arterial disease. JAMA 2006; 295:547–553.

48 Comerota AJ. Effect on platelet function of cilostazol, clopidogrel, and aspirin, each alone or in combination. Atheroscler (suppl) 2006; 6:13–19.

49 Wilhite DB, Comerota AJ, Schmieder FA, et al. Managing PAD with multiple platelet inhibitors: The effect of combination therapy on bleeding time. J Vasc Surg 2003; 38:710–713.

50 Lee S-W, Park S-W, Hong M-K, et al. Triple versus dual antiplatelet therapy after coronary stenting: impact on stent thrombosis. J Am Coll Cardiol 2005; 46:1833–1837.

51 Douglas JS, Holmes DR, Kereiakes DJ, et al. Coronary stent restenosis in patients treated with Cilostazol. Circulation 2005; 112:2826–2832.

52 Pfisterer ME. BASKET-LATE. Oral Presentation, ACC Scientific Sessions 2006, Atlanta, GA, March 14, 2006.

53 Aoki M, Morishita R, Hayashi S, et al. Inhibition of neointimal formation after balloon injury by cilostazol, accompanied by improvement of endothelial dysfunction iand induction of hepatocyte growth factor in rat diabetes model. Diabetologia 2001; 44:1032–1042.

54 Joner M, Finn AV, Farb A, et al. Pathology of drug-eluting stents in humans: Delayed healing and late thrombotic risk. J Am Coll Cardiol 2006; 48:193–202.

55 Kotani J, Awata M, Nanto S, et al. Incomplete neointimal coverage of sirolimus-eluting stents: Angioscopic findings. J Am Coll Cardiol 2006; 47:2108–2111.

6

Heparin, low molecular weight heparin

Raphaelle Dumaine and Gilles Montalescot

Introduction

Endothelial denudation, plaque disruption, and implantation of stents during percutaneous coronary interventions (PCIs) are systematically followed by platelet activation and deposition and mural thrombus formation. Such phenomena may lead to acute or subacute stent thrombosis, distal embolization, and vessel occlusion. The plaque disruption results in platelet activation and aggregation because of pathological contact between circulating blood procoagulant molecules and structures of the vessel wall such as fibronectin, collagen, and von Willebrand factor and in tissue factor and coagulation factor activation. Thrombin is a key enzyme of the coagulation cascade, as it controls the ultimate step: the conversion of fluid-phase fibrinogen into fibrin, which polymerizes into cross-linked fibrin polymers, forming the basis of the clot. Furthermore, thrombin sustains the clotting process by two mechanisms: amplification of its own production by activating the intrinsic pathway, particularly factors XI, IX, VIII, and X, and platelet activation. Thrombin binds to fibrin, fibrin degradation products, and subendothelial matrix and remains active once bound. However, bound thrombin cannot be inactivated by antithrombin–heparin complex (1). Thus, thrombin-rich clot represents a powerful reservoir of prothrombotic thrombin.

Unfractionated heparin (UFH) has long been the only thrombin inhibitor used during PCI. As will be developed further, several pharmacological characteristics limit the antithrombin activity of UFH and encourage the development of alternative antithrombin strategies.

This chapter discusses the evidence surrounding the comparison between low molecular weight heparins (LMWHs) and UFH during PCI.

Mechanisms of action

Thrombin has an active site and two exosites. Exosite I binds to its fibrin substrate, which is orientated toward the active site. Figure 1 compares the mechanisms of action of UFH and LMWH.

UFH binds to exosite 2, located on antithrombin, forming a ternary complex. This ternary complex is necessary for the inhibition of thrombin by antithrombin (Fig. 1A, left). Conversely to thrombin inhibition, inactivation of factor Xa does not require the formation of the ternary complex. UFH inhibits thrombin and factor Xa in the same proportion (the ratio of anti-Xa/IIa activity equals 1) (Fig. 1A, right). The interaction of the heparins (UFH and LMWH) with antithrombin is mediated by a unique pentasaccharide sequence, which is present in approximately one-third of the UFH chains (2).

In addition, UFH also binds simultaneously to fibrin and thrombin. The heparin–thrombin–fibrin complex lessens the ability of the heparin–antithrombin complex to inhibit thrombin and increases the affinity of thrombin for its fibrin substrate. This results in a protection of fibrin-bound thrombin from inactivation by the heparin-antithrombin complex (1) (Fig. 1B).

LMWHs result from the depolymerization of the UFH chains and contain ~20% of the chains, the critical pentasaccharide unit needed for their interaction with antithrombin (2). Converse to UFH, LMWH action is primarily directed against factor Xa, because most of the chains are not sufficiently long to form the ternary complex necessary for the inactivation of thrombin (<50% of the chains contain at least the 18 saccharide units needed for the formation of the ternary heparin–thrombin–antithrombin complex) (Fig. 1C). Depending on the LMWH, the antithrombin–anti-Xa activity ratio varies from 1.9 (tinzaparin) to 3.8 (enoxaparin) (2).

Unfractionated heparin

UFH has long been the only anticoagulant used during PCI. UFH is generally administered as weight-adjusted boluses under activated clotting time (ACT) guidance. The main limitation of use during PCI relies on the necessity of close monitoring of

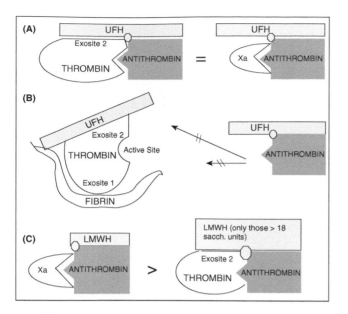

Figure 1

Mechanisms of action of unfractionated heparin and low molecular weight heparin. *Abbreviations*: LMWH, low molecular weight heparin; UFH, unfractionated heparin. *Source*: From Ref. 1.

between hemorrhagic and thrombotic risks remains vague, and highly dependent on the PCI setting (emergent setting/thrombus-rich lesions and elective setting/low thrombotic lesion). In a randomized study comparing a fixed dose of UFH (15,000 IU bolus) and a weight-adjusted UFH regimen (100 IU/kg), similar efficacy and safety outcomes were observed (4). Lower fixed doses (5000 or 2500 IU bolus) have also been used and do not seem to be associated with an increased thrombotic risk (5,6).

Prolonged UFH infusion after uncomplicated PCI is not recommended. In addition to issues regarding anticoagulation monitoring, UFH has several pharmacological limitations such as variable efficacy and stability, poor bioavailability, nonspecific protein binding, neutralization by platelet factor-4, and poor control of Von Willebrand factor release. These limitations, associated with a high incidence of heparin-induced thrombocytopenia, encouraged the development of alternative antithrombin strategies.

anticoagulant activity. Anticoagulant activity is assessed by ACT, which varies substantially in the presence of other comorbidities as well as with the devices used to measure ACT; higher ACT values (30–50 seconds) are observed using the Hemochron device than the HemoTec device (3).

Procedural anticoagulation monitoring is thus highly dependent on the device used to guide heparin administration (Table 1). In addition to this variability in ACT results, the optimal range of target ACT remains uncertain. Results from retrospective studies suggest that higher ACT values may be associated with less ischemic complications, but the balance

Low molecular weight heparins

Low molecular weight heparins in the setting of elective percutaneous coronary interventions

Pilot studies

When patients are not pretreated by any form of anticoagulation before reaching the catheter lab, rapid, effective, and predictable anticoagulation can be obtained with intravenous LMWH during PCI.

Table 1   Contemporary guidelines for unfractionated heparin use in patients undergoing percutaneous coronary intervention

	No concomittant GP IIb-IIIa inhibitors use	*Concomittant GP IIb-IIIa inhibitors use*
IV bolus	60–100 IU/kg	50–70 IU/kg
ACT to achieve	250–300 sec (HemoTec® device) 300–350 sec (Hemochron® device)	200 sec
Additional bolus if target ACT not achieved	2000—5000 IU	
Sheath removal	When ACT <180 sec	

Abbreviations: ACT, activated clotting time; GP, glycoprotein; IV, intravascular.
Source: From Ref. 3.

In a preliminary study, Choussat et al. (7) included 242 consecutive patients to receive a single intravascular (IV) bolus of enoxaparin (0.5 mg/kg) during elective PCI. A peak anti-Xa of >0.5 IU/mL was obtained in 97.5% of the population (Fig. 2); this dose allowed immediate sheath removal when used alone and did not require dose adjustment when used with a glycoprotein (GP) IIb–IIIa inhibitor.

This strategy has now been tested in multiple studies and in a meta-analysis of eight trials, making a randomized comparison between single bolus IV LMWH and UFH in PCI (8). There was a nonsignificant trend favoring LMWH with regard to both a combined efficacy [death/myocardial infarction (MI)/urgent revascularization] and hemorrhagic endpoints. When a further pooled analysis was performed, including data from all randomized trials and seven additional nonrandomized trials/registries, 3787 patients received LMWH and 978 received UFH, the composite efficacy endpoint occurred in 5.7% versus 7.5% ($P = 0.03$), major bleeding in 0.6% versus 1.8% ($P = 0.0001$), and all bleeding (major plus minor) in 3.7% versus 4.9% ($P = 0.09$) of patients who received LMWH and UFH, respectively (8). In this meta-analysis, the best outcome data were obtained with the 0.5 mg/kg IV dose.

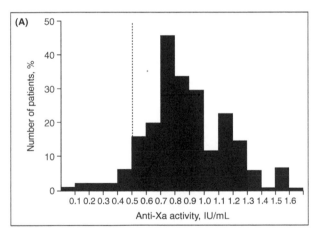

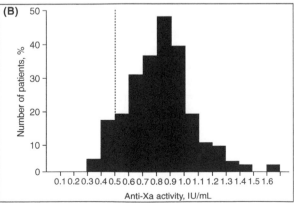

Figure 2

Distribution of anti-Xa activity levels at the beginning (A) and end (B) of percutaneous coronary intervention after a single intravascular dose of enoxaparin 0.5 mg/kg. *Source*: From Ref. 7.

Comparison between low molecular weight heparin and unfractionated heparin in elective percutaneous coronary intervention

These results were confirmed in the recent randomized STEEPLE trial. This study was a prospective, open-label, randomized trial including 3528 patients undergoing elective PCI. Patients were randomized to enoxaparin (0.5 or 0.75 mg/kg) or an ACT-adjusted UFH regimen, stratified by the operator's choice of GP IIb–IIIa inhibitor use. The primary endpoint was the incidence of noncoronary artery bypass graft (CABG)-related major and minor bleeding. Enoxaparin 0.5 mg/kg was associated with a significant 31% reduction in the primary endpoint when compared with UFH (6.0% vs. 8.7%, $P = 0.014$), and the 0.75 mg/kg dose was associated with a 24% reduction (6.6% vs. 8.7%, $P = 0.052$) meeting the criteria for noninferiority. There was a significant 57% reduction in major bleeding in both enoxaparin groups when compared with UFH.

The incidence of the quadruple endpoint of death/MI/urgent target revascularization/major bleeding at 30 days was similar among the three groups (7.2%, 7.9%, and 8.4% in the enoxaparin 0.5 mg/kg, enoxaparin 0.75 mg/kg, and UFH groups, respectively).

The sheath was immediately removed from the femoral site without excessive bleeding in the 0.5 mg/kg group.

Converse to UFH, the use of enoxaparin during PCI did not require anticoagulation monitoring, and there was no dose modification with concomitant GP IIb–IIIa receptor blockers administration (9).

Low molecular weight heparin in percutaneous coronary intervention for acute coronary syndrome

Preliminary studies

Current recommendations for antithrombin management of patients being treated with SC LMWH undergoing PCI suggest a transition to UFH with a bolus given immediately prior to intervention. In the setting of acute coronary syndromes (ACSs), this strategy demonstrated at least similar safety between UFH and enoxaparin, and similar or less ischemic events among patients treated with enoxaparin when compared with UFH-treated patients (10–12).

However, in spite of its logic and convenience, there is little literature regarding LMWH administration during PCI instead of UFH, in order to avoid anticoagulation change when transferring the patient to the cath lab.

Collet et al. examined the safety and efficacy of performing PCI in the setting of ACS on LMWH therapy without interruption of this treatment or additional anticoagulant therapy. The only rule was to perform PCI within eight hours of the last SC enoxaparin injection (when anti-Xa levels are close to the peak of activity). Four hundred and fifty-one consecutive patients with ACS received at least 48 hours of treatment with SC LMWH (enoxaparin 1 mg/kg/12 hours SC) in the coronary care unit, and 65% of the patients underwent coronary angiography within eight hours of the morning SC injection. PCI was performed in 28% of the patients, with no further enoxaparin and no UFH during PCI. Mean anti-Xa activity at the time of catheterization was in the therapeutic range (0.98 ± 0.03 IU/mL) and >0.5 IU/mL in 97.6% patients. No in-hospital acute vessel closure or urgent revascularization following PCI was observed. Death/MI at 30 days occurred in 3.0% in the PCI group, but 6.2% in the whole population, and in 10.8% of patients not undergoing catheterization. The 30-day major-bleeding rates were similar: 0.8% in the PCI group and 1.3% in the group of patients managed medically (13).

In the NICE-3 study (14), 661 ACS patients were treated with enoxaparin SC 1 mg/kg plus abciximab, eptifibatide, or tirofiban at standard doses. Two strategies were combined for the transition from the ward to the catheter laboratory: no interruption and no addition of enoxaparin for PCI within eight hours of the last SC injection and an additive IV bolus of 0.3 mg/kg when PCI was performed between 8 and 12 hours of the last SC injection. The major bleeding rate was 4.5% and the in-hospital death/MI/urgent target vessel revascularization rate was 5.7%.

Comparison between low molecular weight heparin and unfractionated heparin in percutaneous coronary intervention for acute coronary syndrome

Several randomized clinical trials have compared the efficacy and safety of LMWH and UFH among initially medically managed patients presenting with ACS (15–18). Among those, enoxaparin was the only LMWH to demonstrate a significant and sustained benefit over UFH; in the meta-analysis of the thrombolysis in MI (TIMI) 11B and ESSENCE trials, enoxaparin was associated with a significant reduction of death and MI at 8, 14, and 43 days (OR 0.77, 95% CI: 0.62–0.95; OR 0.79, 95% CI: 0.65–0.96; and OR 0.82, 95% CI: 0.69–0.97, respectively) (19).

More recently, safety and efficacy of these two antithrombin regimens have been compared among patients receiving up-to-date antithrombotic regimens, with tirofiban [A to Z (11), ACUTE II (10)] or eptifibatide [INTERACT (12)], and among patients undergoing an early invasive strategy [SYNERGY (20)].

In the ACUTE II trial (10), 525 patients with non-ST-segment elevation ACS and treated with tirofiban and aspirin were randomized to receive either UFH [5000 U bolus followed by an infusion of 1000 U/hour adjusted to a therapeutic activated partial thromboplastin time (aPTT), n = 210] or enoxaparin (1.0 mg/kg SC injection every 12 hours, n = 315) in a double-blind fashion during 24 to 96 hours. The primary safety endpoint of total bleeding incidence (TIMI major + TIMI minor + loss without any identified site) occurred among 4.8% versus 3.5% of patients receiving UFH versus enoxaparin (OR 1.4, 95% CI: 0.6–3.4). There was no difference in the incidence of death or MI between the UFH and enoxaparin groups (1.9% versus 2.5% and 7.1% versus 6.7%, respectively; P = NS for both). However, refractory ischemia and rehospitalization due to unstable angina occurred more often in the UFH, respectively, P < 0.05 for both).

The A to Z trial (phase A) was an open-label randomized noninferiority trial comparing enoxaparin (n = 2026) with weight- and aPTT-adjusted intravenous UFH (n = 1961) in non-ST-segment elevation ACS receiving aspirin and tirofiban (11). The prespecified criterion for noninferiority was met for the primary efficacy endpoint of death/MI/refractory ischemia at seven days (9.4% in the UFH group versus 8.4% in the enoxaparin group, HR 0.88, 95% CI: 0.71–1.08). When stratifying patients according to prerandomization treatment, the authors observed a trend toward a lower incidence of the primary endpoint in the enoxaparin arm when no prior anticoagulant had been administered (HR 0.77, 95% CI: 0.53–1.11, P = 0.38 for interaction). Enoxaparin was as safe as UFH regarding the incidence of TIMI minor or major bleeding (3.0% vs. 2.2%, P = NS).

The INTERACT trial was a randomized open-label trial comparing enoxaparin (n = 380) with intravenous aPTT-adjusted UFH (n = 366) in high-risk non-ST-segment elevation ACS receiving aspirin and eptifibatide (12). The primary safety endpoint of major non-CABG-related bleeding at 96 hours occurred significantly less often among enoxaparin-treated patients (1.8% vs. 4.6%, P = 0.03). Minor bleeding was more frequent in the enoxaparin group (30.3% vs. 20.8%, P = 0.003). The primary efficacy outcome of ischemia detected by continuous ECG monitoring was significantly less frequent in the enoxaparin group during the initial (14.3% vs. 25.4%, P = 0.0002) and subsequent (12.7% vs. 25.9%, P < 0.0001) 48-hour monitoring periods. Finally, death or MI at 30 days occurred significantly less among enoxaparin-treated patients (5% vs. 9%, P = 0.031).

The Superior Yield of the New Strategy of Enoxaparin Revascularization and GP IIb/IIIa Inhibitors (SYNERGY) trial (20) was a randomized, open-label, international trial comparing enoxaparin and UFH among 10,027 high-risk patients with non-ST-segment elevation ACS to be treated with an intended early invasive strategy. The incidence of the composite primary efficacy endpoint (death/MI at 30 days) was similar in enoxaparin and UFH-treated patients (14.0% vs. 14.5%, respectively, OR 0.96; 95% CI: 0.86–1.06). There was no difference in the rate of ischemic events between the two groups during PCI. The primary safety outcome was major bleeding or stroke. There was no difference between the two groups with respect to stroke incidence; the incidence of major bleeding was modestly increased in the enoxaparin group when using the TIMI bleeding classification (9.1% vs. 7.6%, $P = 0.008$) but not when using the GUSTO classification (2.7% vs. 2.2%, $P = 0.08$). The need for transfusions was similar among the two groups (17.0% vs. 16.0%, $P = 0.16$). When stratifying by prerandomization therapy, the benefit of enoxaparin was the highest among patients receiving either enoxaparin or no antithrombin therapy before randomization. The authors stated that "as a first-line agent in the absence of changing antithrombin therapy during treatment, enoxaparin appears to be superior to UFH without an increased bleeding risk" (20).

Data from various trials are becoming integrated into current recommendations. A recent expert consensus concluded that substantial evidence exists that patients receiving SC LMWH in the management of ACS can safely undergo cardiac catheterization and PCI and that concerns about transition of medical to interventional management "should not impede the upstream use of LMWH" (21). It was furthermore concluded that LMWH and GP IIb–IIIa antagonists can be safely used in combination without any apparent increase in the risk of major bleeding (21).

A pooled analysis was performed among 21,946 patients included in the six randomized trials comparing UFH and enoxaparin in the setting of non-ST-segment elevation ACS (22). Death at 30 days was similar for both antithrombin strategies (3.0% for both), but enoxaparin treatment was associated with lower incidence of death/MI at 30 days than UFH populations (10.1% vs. 11.0%; OR 0.91; 95% CI: 0.83–0.99; number needed to treat: 107). The benefit of enoxaparin was even higher among patients receiving no prerandomization antithrombin therapy (8.0% vs. 9.4%; OR 0.81; 95% CI: 0.70–0.94; number needed to treat: 72). No significant difference was found in blood transfusion (OR 1.01; 95% CI: 0.89–1.14) or major bleeding (OR 1.04; 95% CI: 0.83–1.30) at seven days after randomization.

In all these trials, enoxaparin was administered at the dose of 1 mg/kg SC every 12 hours, in order to achieve therapeutic anti-Xa levels. This is of importance as it has been demonstrated that low anti-Xa activity (<0.5 IU/mL) was an independent predictor of poor outcome among ACS patients; conversely, anti-Xa activity, within the target range of 0.5 to 1.2IU/mL, is not related to bleeding events (23). Among patients with impaired creatinine clearance (chronic kidney disease in elderly patients), the therapeutic range is achieved safely by reducing enoxaparin dose (24).

In ACS patients, LMWH has now been compared with newer anticoagulants such as direct thrombin inhibitors, such as bivalirudin [ACUITY trial (25)], and a pentasaccharide, such as fondaparinux [OASIS-5 and -6 trials (26,27)]. These new molecules appear to have similar efficacy as compared to enoxaparin and they may be safer with lower bleeding rates. The benefit and the indication of these newer and more costly anticoagulant agents in the catheterization laboratory remain to be determined.

Conclusion

LMWH is a safe and efficient alternative to UFH during PCI. From a practical point of view, a unique IV dose of 0.5 mg/kg enoxaparin is convenient, simple, and does not need adjustment for IIb–IIIa antagonist use nor for renal function. In addition, this unique dose requires no anticoagulant monitoring and allows an early sheath removal.

The convenience, safety, and efficacy of LMWHs have led many centers to use them as a standard of care for the treatment of ACS with or without ST-segment elevation, with no anticoagulant shift during PCI.

Emerging evidence suggests that other alternatives to UFH may be found among other therapeutic classes such as direct thrombin inhibitors: bivalirudin appears to be atleast as safe and effective as UFH in the setting of elective as well as emergent PCI. Other anticoagulant agents such as factor Xa inhibitors (fondaparinux) may be of interest in these settings and the results of ongoing trials should bring more definitive conclusions.

References

1 Weitz JI, Buller HR. Direct thrombin inhibitors in acute coronary syndromes: present and future. Circulation 2002; 105: 1004–1011.
2 Weitz JI. Low-molecular-weight heparins. N Engl J Med 1997; 337:688–698.
3 Popma JJ, Ohman EM, Weitz J, et al. Antithrombotic therapy in patients undergoing percutaneous coronary intervention. Chest 2001; 119:321S–336S.
4 Boccara A, Benamer H, Juliard JM, et al. A randomized trial of a fixed high dose vs a weight-adjusted low dose of intravenous heparin during coronary angioplasty. Eur Heart J 1997; 18:631–635.
5 Koch KT, Piek JJ, de Winter RJ, et al. Safety of low dose heparin in elective coronary angioplasty. Heart 1997; 77:517–522.
6 Kaluski E, Krakover R, Cotter G, et al. Minimal heparinization in coronary angioplasty–how much heparin is really warranted? Am J Cardiol 2000; 85:953–956.
7 Choussat R, Montalescot G, Collet JP, et al. A unique, low dose of intravenous enoxaparin in elective percutaneous coronary intervention. J Am Coll Cardiol 2002; 40:1943–1950.
8 Borentain M, Montalescot G, Bouzamondo A, et al. Low-molecular-weight heparin vs. unfractionated heparin in percutaneous coronary intervention: a combined analysis. Catheter Cardiovasc Interv 2005; 65:212–221.

9   Montalescot G and the STEEPLE investigators. The STEEPLE study: safety and efficacy of intravenous enoxaparin in elective percutaneous coronary intervention: an international randomized evaluation. European Society of Cardiology 2005 Hotline session.

10   Cohen M, Theroux P, Borzak S, et al. Randomized double-blind safety study of enoxaparin versus unfractionated heparin in patients with non-ST-segment elevation acute coronary syndromes treated with tirofiban and aspirin: the ACUTE II study. The antithrombotic combination using tirofiban and enoxaparin. Am Heart J 2002; 144:470–477.

11   Blazing MA, de Lemos JA, White HD, et al. Safety and efficacy of enoxaparin vs unfractionated heparin in patients with non-ST-segment elevation acute coronary syndromes who receive tirofiban and aspirin: a randomized controlled trial. JAMA 2004; 292:55–64.

12   Goodman SG, Fitchett D, Armstrong PW, et al. Randomized evaluation of the safety and efficacy of enoxaparin versus unfractionated heparin in high-risk patients with non-ST-segment elevation acute coronary syndromes receiving the glycoprotein IIb/IIIa inhibitor eptifibatide. Circulation 2003; 107:238–244.

13   Collet JP, Montalescot G, Lison L, et al. Percutaneous coronary intervention after subcutaneous enoxaparin pretreatment in patients with unstable angina pectoris. Circulation 2001; 103:658–663.

14   Ferguson JJ, Antman EM, Bates ER, et al. Combining enoxaparin and glycoprotein IIb/IIIa antagonists for the treatment of acute coronary syndromes: final results of the National Investigators Collaborating on Enoxaparin-3 (NICE-3) study. Am Heart J 2003; 146:628–634.

15   Antman EM, McCabe CH, Gurfinkel EP, et al. Enoxaparin prevents death and cardiac ischemic events in unstable angina/non-Q-wave myocardial infarction. Results of the thrombolysis in myocardial infarction (TIMI) 11B trial. Circulation 1999; 100:1593–1601.

16   Cohen M, Demers C, Gurfinkel EP, et al. A comparison of low-molecular-weight heparin with unfractionated heparin for unstable coronary artery disease. Efficacy and safety of subcutaneous enoxaparin in non-Q-wave coronary events study group. N Engl J Med 1997; 337:447–452.

17   Klein W, Buchwald A, Hillis SE, et al. Comparison of low-molecular-weight heparin with unfractionated heparin acutely and with placebo for 6 weeks in the management of unstable coronary artery disease. Fragmin in unstable coronary artery disease study (FRIC). Circulation 1997; 96:61–68.

18   Comparison of two treatment durations (6 days and 14 days) of a low molecular weight heparin with a 6-day treatment of unfractionated heparin in the initial management of unstable angina or non-Q wave myocardial infarction: FRAX.I.S. (FRAxiparine in Ischaemic Syndrome). Eur Heart J 1999; 20: 1553–1562.

19   Antman EM, Cohen M, Radley D, et al. Assessment of the treatment effect of enoxaparin for unstable angina/non-Q-wave myocardial infarction. TIMI 11B-ESSENCE meta–analysis. Circulation 1999; 100:1602–1608.

20   Ferguson JJ, Califf RM, Antman EM, et al. Enoxaparin vs unfractionated heparin in high-risk patients with non-ST-segment elevation acute coronary syndromes managed with an intended early invasive strategy: primary results of the SYNERGY randomized trial. JAMA 2004; 292:45–54.

21   Kereiakes DJ, Montalescot G, Antman EM, et al. Low-molecular-weight heparin therapy for non-ST-elevation acute coronary syndromes and during percutaneous coronary intervention: an expert consensus. Am Heart J 2002; 144:615–624.

22   Petersen JL, Mahaffey KW, Hasselblad V, et al. Efficacy and bleeding complications among patients randomized to enoxaparin or unfractionated heparin for antithrombin therapy in non-ST-Segment elevation acute coronary syndromes: a systematic overview. JAMA 2004; 292:89–96.

23   Montalescot G, Collet JP, Tanguy ML, et al. Anti-Xa activity relates to survival and efficacy in unselected acute coronary syndrome patients treated with enoxaparin. Circulation 2004; 110:392–398.

24   Collet JP, Montalescot G, Fine E, et al. Enoxaparin in unstable angina patients who would have been excluded from randomized pivotal trials. J Am Coll Cardiol 2003; 41:8–14.

25   Stone GW, Bertrand M, Colombo A, et al. Acute Catheterization and Urgent Intervention Triage strategY (ACUITY) trial: study design and rationale. Am Heart J 2004; 148:764–775.

26   Yusuf S, Mehta SR, Chrolavicius S, et al. Comparison of fondaparinux and enoxaparin in acute coronary syndromes. N Engl J Med 2006; 354:1464–1476.

27   Yusuf S, Mehta SR, Chrolavicius S, et al. Effects of fondaparinux on mortality and reinfarction in patients with acute ST-segment elevation myocardial infarction: the OASIS-6 randomized trial. JAMA 2006; 295:1519–1530.

7

Direct thrombin inhibition in percutaneous coronary intervention

Derek P. Chew, Sam J. Lehman, and Harvey D. White

Introduction

As a class of anticoagulants for the prevention of ischemic complications among patients undergoing percutaneous coronary intervention (PCI), the direct thrombin inhibitors have enjoyed a renewed interest, despite the fact that the development of these agents extends back over nearly two decades. These agents inhibit all the actions of thrombin by direct binding to this molecule, and in some cases, their action is limited by subsequent catalytic degradation by thrombin. Clinical evidence with these agents have been acquired in the context of balloon angioplasty as well as coronary stenting, across a spectrum of patient risk profiles and in conjunction with various antiplatelet agents, with the bulk of these data in the context of bivalirudin therapy. This chapter summarizes the basic physiology of thrombin and discusses each of the direct thrombin inhibitors with respect to their clinical pharmacology, indications, and clinical trial evidence in the context of PCI.

Thrombin physiology

As a serine protease, thrombin has a central role in thrombus formation (Fig. 1) (1). Vascular injury and inflammation result in the expression of tissue factor on the surface of endothelial cells and inflammatory cells. Interaction between tissue factor and factor VII leads to the initiation of the coagulation cascade, hence promoting the generation of thrombin from prothrombin. As a key factor in thrombosis, thrombin is responsible for the conversion of fibrinogen to fibrin and activation of factors V, VIII, and X, in addition to promoting platelet activation (2). With a short circulating half-life, the role of thrombin is normally tightly controlled by negative feedback mechanisms in the context of normal endothelium. These include the binding to thrombomodulin and protein C, which, in conjunction with protein S, inactivates the factors Va and VIIIa. In addition, this molecule promotes the release of tissue plasminogen activator. Thus, the effects of thrombin are usually confined to the local area of tissue injury.

The direct effects of thrombin on cellular structures are increasingly being appreciated. Acting via the protease-activated receptor (PAR)-1, thrombin promotes expression of P-selectin and CD 40 ligand on the surface of the platelets, and stimulates the release of adenosine diphosphate (ADP), serotonin, and thromboxane A2, as well as increased expression and activation of glycoprotein (GP) αIIb/β3 involved in fibrinogen and von Willebrand factor (vWF) binding and platelet aggregation (3,4). The effects on endothelial cells include the release of vWF and the upregulation of surface adhesion molecules enabling platelet and leukocyte adhesion. In response to thrombin, endothelial cells undergo conformational changes that allow transudation and edema formation. In the context of an intact endothelium, thrombin promotes vasodilation, but where the endothelium is denuded, local thrombin generation contributes to vasoconstriction. Evidence also suggests that thrombin promotes fibroblast cytokine production and is mitogenic (5). Hence, as a therapeutic target, thrombin has a critical role in orchestrating adverse local responses to balloon/stent local vascular injury.

A schematic of the structure of the thrombin molecule is presented in Figure 2. The important binding sites on the surface of the thrombin molecule include the catalytic site and two exosites (anionic and apolar) or substrate recognition sites. Whereas the catalytic site is responsible for the serine protease activity, the separate substrate recognition sites are involved in the binding of heparin, fibrinogen, and thrombomodulin (6). These sites serve as targets for the direct thrombin inhibitors.

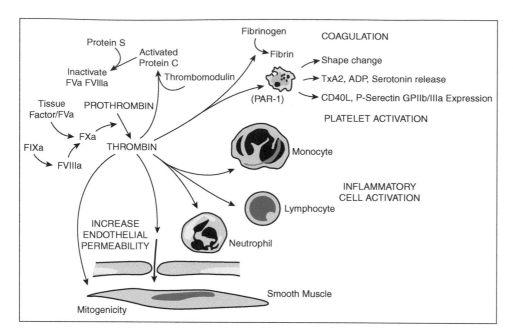

Figure 1
The role of thrombin in vascular injury. *Abbreviation*: ADP, adenosine diphosphate.

Pharmacology

Collectively, the direct thrombin inhibitors are prototypically represented by hirudin, the antithrombotic molecule found in the saliva of the medicinal leech (*Hirudo medicinalis*). This protein is a 65 amino acid molecule that forms a highly stable but noncovalent complex with thrombin (7). With two domains, the NH$_2$-terminal core domain and the COOH-terminal tail, the hirudin molecule inhibits the catalytic site and the anion-binding exosite in a two-step process. The first step is an ionic interaction that leads to a rearrangement of the thrombin–hirudin complex to form a tighter bond that is stoichiometrically 1:1 and irreversible. The apolar-binding site may also be involved in hirudin binding. This complex and

tight binding of hirudin to thrombin helps account for the highly specific effect of hirudin on thrombin, but none of the other serine proteases. As a group, the direct thrombin inhibitor molecules are small, in contrast to the indirect thrombin inhibitors, and consequently demonstrate greater efficacy for the inhibition of clot-bound thrombin, in addition to fluid-phase thrombin (8). Through recombinant DNA technology, recombinant hirudin (r-hirudin) has been produced in two forms, with and without sulfated Tyr63. In contrast to the naturally occurring molecule, the nonsulfated tyrosine appears to have a 10-fold lower affinity for thrombin.

The interaction between hirudin and thrombin forms the template for understanding and categorizing the other direct thrombin inhibitors. In broad terms, these have been divided into univalent and bivalent molecules. The univalent molecules, such as dabigatran, argatroban, and melagatran (and the oral prodrug, ximelagatran), inhibit only the catalytic site. Therefore, these agents inactivate only fibrin-bound thrombin. Of note, argatroban binds to the apolar-binding site adjacent to the catalytic site and provides competitive inhibition. Although the inhibition of thrombin with these agents is potent, binding with these agents is less robust than that observed with hirudin. Hence, dissociation occurs leaving some active thrombin available. The bivalent molecules, the natural and r-hirudin and bivalirudin, bind to the catalytic site and at least one of the exosites. However, while the interaction between hirudin and thrombin is irreversible, the inhibition provided by bivalirudin is more transient, by nature of its structure (9). Bivalirudin is a synthetic 20 amino acid molecule. Its two domains, which block the anion-binding exosite and catalytic sites, are linked by four glycine spacers. In contrast to the larger hirudin amino acid chain, bivalirudin's truncated structure leads to less avid ionic binding. In addition,

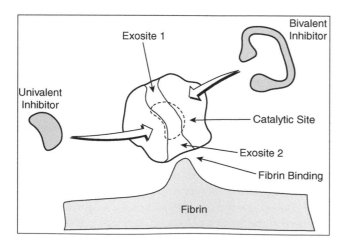

Figure 2
Thrombin-inhibitor pharmacology.

thrombin acts to cleave the bivalirudin molecule at the Arg-Pro bond of the NH_2-terminal extension, which releases the thrombin active site for further thrombotic activity. Several other direct thrombin inhibitors have been developed in addition to those discussed, but so far these have not found a clinical role in the catheterization laboratory.

Pharmacokinetics

An appreciation of the pharmacodynamic interactions between the various direct thrombin inhibitors provides an insight into the differences in pharmacokinetic behavior (10). All of these agents require parenteral administration with the exception of ximelagatran, which is converted to melagatran in the liver, and dabigatran. With the exception of argatroban, these agents are renally cleared, and clearance is attenuated in the setting of reduced renal function. In the setting of excessive dosing, these agents can be removed by hemofiltration. Argatroban's main route of elimination is through hepatic metabolism and dose reduction in the setting of hepatic dysfunction is required. However, renal function also influences dosing (11). Bivalirudin also undergoes proteolysis within the plasma, thus contributing to its shorter half-life and relatively constant elimination characteristics even among patients with mild to moderate renal impairment. Nevertheless, dose attenuation is required among patients with creatinine clearance <30 mL/min. A summary of the pharmacokinetic properties of these agents is presented in Table 1. No reversal agent has yet been developed for these agents, and in the context of active bleeding, nonspecific measures such as transfusion of blood productions, including fresh frozen plasma and local measures, are recommended. Hence, among patients undergoing PCI, the relatively short half-life of bivalirudin appears to be an advantage.

Monitoring direct thrombin inhibitors

As opposed to the low molecular weight heparins, the direct thrombin inhibitors prolong the activated clotting time (ACT) and the activated partial thromboplastin time (APTT) (12). Studies with bivalirudin demonstrate that this occurs in a dose-dependent manner, and at the doses used within the clinical trials, the prolongation of ACT observed was generally greater than that observed with heparin and heparin/GP IIb/IIIa inhibition combinations. However, less apparent is the relationship between the ACT level and ischemic or bleeding outcomes. As opposed to heparin therapy (13), a relationship between actual levels of ACT achieved and bleeding outcomes has not been described, and of note, despite higher ACT levels achieved with this agent, bleeding rates have been consistently lower than that observed with unfractionated heparin-based strategies.

Some evidence suggests that monitoring these agents with the ecarin clotting time (ECT) may be more appropriate. Measurements based on this test appear to better correlate with bivalirudin and hirudin levels (14). Whether levels based on this assay evolve to recommended targets for therapy remains to be established.

Indications and clinical evidence for the use of direct thrombin inhibitors in percutaneous coronary interventions

Although the role of these agents in the management of patients presenting with acute coronary syndromes (ACS)

Table 1	Thrombin-inhibition pharmacokinetics				
Characteristics	*Recombinant hirudins*	*Bivalirudin*	*Argatroban*	*Ximelagatran and melagatran*	*Dabigatran*
Route of administration	Intravenous, subcutaneous	Intravenous	Intravenous	Intravenous and subcutaneous (melagatran), oral (ximelagatran)	Oral
Plasma half-life	Intravenous (60 min) Subcutaneous (120 min)	25 min	45 min	Intravenous and subcutaneous (2–3 hr), oral (3–5 hr)	12 hr
Main site of clearance	Kidney	Kidney, liver, and other sites	Liver	Kidney	Kidney

remains contentious, the evidence in the setting of PCI is robust. The vast majority of these data are with bivalirudin, though consistent evidence also exists for some of the other direct thrombin inhibitors as subgroup analyses of ACS patients undergoing PCI (hirudin) and within special indications such as in the setting of heparin-induced thrombocytopenia syndrome (HITS) (argatroban).

Clinical evidence: hirudin

Initial studies of hirudin among patients undergoing PCI suggested an improvement in clinical outcomes (15,16). These initial reports lead to the conduct of the Hirudin in a European Trial Versus Heparin in the Prevention of Restenosis after PTCA (HELVETICA) trial that compared two dose regimens of hirudin with unfractionated heparin in patients with unstable angina in the context of balloon angioplasty (17). Randomization to intravenous hirudin was associated with a reduction in early cardiac events, but at seven-month follow-up (the primary endpoint), there was no difference in event-free survival or restenosis among the three treatment groups. In contrast to the observations with bivalirudin, a slight excess in bleeding was observed. Similarly, the angioplasty substudy among ST-elevation myocardial infarction (MI) patients of the Global Utilization of Strategies to Open Occluded Coronary Arteries IIb (GUSTO IIb) trial randomized 503 patients undergoing PCI to receive either hirudin or heparin (18). The primary endpoint of death, MI, or stroke at 30 days was reduced with hirudin by 23%, but this did not reach statistical significance. No excess in bleeding was observed. A nonrandomized analysis of all patients enrolled within GUSTO IIb (ST-elevation and non-ST-elevation) undergoing PCI while receiving treatment with either hirudin ($n = 672$) or heparin ($n = 738$) observed a reduction in 30 day MI (4.9% vs. 7.6%, $P = 0.04$) among the hirudin group (19). A nonsignificant excess in bleeding was observed. These data are consistent with a similar analysis from the OASIS-2 trial assessing the outcomes in 172 patients undergoing PCI within 72 hours of randomization (20). In this observational analysis, hirudin was associated with a lower rate of death or MI at 96 hours, (6.4% vs. 21.4%, OR 0.30; 95% CI: 0.36–0.81) and 35 days (6.4% vs. 22.9%, OR 0.25; 95% CI: 0.07–0.86). Hence, in meta-analysis of these data drawn from two PCI and nine ACS trials ($n = 35,970$), in conjunction with the data with bivalirudin and the univalent direct thrombin inhibitors, the direct thrombin inhibitors have been shown to be associated with lower rates of death or MI (OR 0.66; 95% CI: 0.48–0.91), in the context of PCI undertaken with 72 hours of randomization, with a reduction in bleeding driven by the benefits observed in the PCI trials (Fig. 3) (21). Attenuated benefit was observed when PCI was delayed after this time, with no benefit with these agents observed in the context of conservative management. Case reports also suggest that r-hirudin (lepirudin) may be used in patients with HITS undergoing PCI (22).

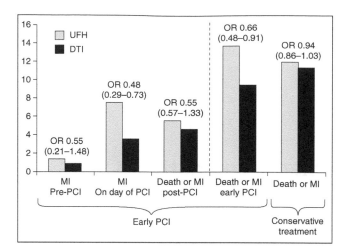

Figure 3
DTI meta-analysis. *Abbreviations*: DTI, direct thrombin inhibition; MI, myocardial infarction; OR, odds ratio; PCI, percutaneous coronary intervention; UFH, unfractionated heparin.

Clinical evidence: argatroban

To date, the role of argatroban in PCI has been inadequately studied. As an alternative to heparin among patients with HITS, a small case series suggests that this agent is safe (23,24). A small open labeled study of argatroban among patients treated with abciximab ($n = 150$) and eptifibatide ($n = 2$) suggests that the use of this agent in combination with GP IIb/IIIa inhibition is feasible (25). Definitive data demonstrating specific advantages over currently practiced strategies are still awaited.

Clinical evidence: bivalirudin

The initial clinical trial evidence supporting the use of bivalirudin was observed in the Bivalirudin Angioplasty Trial (BAT) (26,27). This study predated the use of coronary stents, GP IIb/IIIa inhibition, and the routine use of thienopyridines. A total of 4312 patients presenting for urgent or elective angioplasty were randomized to bivalirudin 1 mg/kg bolus and 2.5 mg/kg/hr infusion or high-dose unfractionated heparin. A subgroup of 741 post-MI patients underwent stratified randomization. At seven days, bivalirudin was associated with a 22% reduction (6.2% vs. 7.9%, $P = 0.039$) in the incidence of death, MI, or urgent revascularization, a 62% reduction (3.9% vs. 9.7%, $P < 0.001$) in major bleeding events, and a 44% reduction in the combination of bleeding and ischemic events. The suppression of ischemic and bleeding events was more striking among the post-MI patients with the triple ischemic endpoint being reduced by 46% by 90 days [odds ratio (OR) 0.54; 95% CI: 36–0.81, $P = 0.009$].

With the emerging development of the GP IIb/IIIa inhibitors, two smaller pilot studies were conducted. The CACHET A/B/C studies with 208 patients examined the role of bivalirudin in the context of either routine or provisional use of abciximab. Although this study was small, a reduction in bleeding events, without an increase in ischemic events was observed. In contrast, the randomized evaluation of PCI linking angiomax to reduced clinical events (REPLACE)-1 study randomized 1056 PCI patients to either 0.75 mg/kg and 1.75 mg/kg/hr or heparin 60 to 70 U/kg with GP IIb/IIIa inhibition (either abciximab, eptifibatide, or tirofiban) either provisionally, routinely, or not at all at the discretion of the clinician (28). Approximately 76% and 85% of patients in this study received a GP IIb/IIIa inhibitor and stent, respectively. Despite the liberal use of GP IIb/IIIa inhibition, a nonsignificant benefit favoring the use of bivalirudin was observed at 48 hours in terms of both ischemic and bleeding complications. These studies formed the basis of the contemporary pivotal study, REPLACE-2.

Published in 2003, the REPLACE-2 study enrolled 6010 patients undergoing elective or urgent PCI, randomizing them to bivalirudin (0.75 mg/kg and 1.75 mg/kg/hr IV) and provisional abciximab or eptifibatide versus the planned use of these agents and heparin (65 U/kg IV) in a double blind, double dummy manner (29). This study was designed as a noninferiority trial with respect to the commonly used "triple ischemic endpoint" of death, MI, or urgent revascularization by 30 days. In addition, noninferiority with respect to a "quadruple endpoint" of ischemia and bleeding was also examined. Mirroring the inclusion and exclusion criteria for the EPISTENT studies, (30) the major exclusions to this study were patients presenting with ST-elevation MI undergoing PCI for reperfusion, patients at significant risk of bleeding or those requiring dialysis. Consequently, approximately 50% of patients underwent PCI for an ACS, multivessel intervention was undertaken in ~15% of cases, and saphenous vein graft intervention occurred in 6% of patients. Provisional use of a GP IIb/IIIa inhibitor was permitted for a wide range of indications including coronary dissection, thrombus formation, unplanned stenting, slow flow, distal embolization, and ongoing clinical instability. GP IIb/IIIa inhibition was used in 7.5% of bivalirudin treated patients, and 5.2% of heparin/GP IIb/IIIa inhibition patients received provisional placebo ($P = 0.002$). Across the study, 86% of patients received pretreatment with a thienopyridine, and the vast majority of this was clopidogrel. Meeting the predefined noninferiority boundary, bivalirudin (and provisional GP IIb/IIIa inhibition) was associated with a nonsignificant excess in ischemic events (7.6% vs. 7.9%, OR 1.09; 95% CI: 0.90–1.32, $P = 0.40$). This difference was accounted for entirely by a small excess in CKMB-elevations 5 to 10 times the upper limit of normal, but in no other category. However, bleeding events were significantly reduced when evaluated by the thrombolysis in myocardial infarction (TIMI) criteria or the slightly broader protocol definition that included blood transfusion. Most of the bleeding benefit was evident as reduced

vascular access site events. Although not designed to evaluate mortality at 12 months, a lower point estimate for mortality in favor of the bivalirudin arm (1.6% vs. 2.5%, $P = 0.16$) was reassuring in that the nonsignificant excess in MI was not associated with an excess in mortality (31).

Hence in pooled analysis of the randomized clinical trial experience in PCI, including 11,638 patients (bivalirudin, 5861; heparin, 5777), bivalirudin was associated with a reduction in the incidence of death, MI, revascularization, and major bleeding (7.8% vs. 10.8%, $P < 0.001$) at 48 hours (32). Despite a very low event rate, a benefit in terms of mortality was observed (0.01% vs. 0.02%, $P = 0.049$), whereas reductions for major bleeding were substantial (2.7% vs. 5.8%, $P < 0.001$). Furthermore, given the lower overall costs of this agent and savings associated with reduced bleeding, the use of bivalirudin remains economically attractive (33).

In the recent ACUITY trial in moderate and high-risk patients ($n = 13,819$) with ACS undergoing an invasive strategy, patients were randomized to five arms: unfractionated heparin or LMWH + upstream GPIIb/IIIa inhibitors, unfractionated heparin or LMWH + in lab GPIIb/IIIa inhibitors, bivalirudin + upstream GPIIb/IIIa inhibitors, bivalirudin + in lab GPIIb/IIIa inhibitors alone, bivalirudin alone.

The primary endpoint was a composite of death, MI, or unplanned revascularization for ischemia plus major bleeding. The time from drug administration to angiogram was 5.3 hours.

Fifty-six percent of patients underwent PCI, 32% had medical therapy, and 12% had surgery. The primary endpoint showed noninferiority for the net clinical outcome: 11.7% heparin + IIb/IIIa groups versus 11.8% bivalirudin + IIb/IIIa groups, $P < 0.001$. The ischemic composite was 7.3% versus 7.7%, $P = 0.015$, for noninferiority and major bleeding was 5.7% versus 5.3%, $P < 0.001$ for noninferiority.

The results for bivalirudin group alone was 10.1% for the composite endpoint, $P < 0.0001$, 7.8% for the ischemic endpoint, $P = 0.32$, and 3.0% for major bleeding, $P < 0.001$ (all P-values for superiority). All causes of major bleeding were numerically lower with bivalirudin, except for intracranial hemorrhage, 0.07% versus 0.07%. Notably transfusions were less frequent with bivalirudin; 2.7% heparin + GP IIb/IIIa versus 1.6%, $P < 0.001$. Thus, the simpler regimen of bivalirudin alone resulted in significantly greater net clinical benefit (34).

Special groups
Decreased renal function

Among patients treated with direct thrombin inhibitors, several observational studies have sought to address known high-risk groups undergoing PCI. Although large-scale studies in ST-elevation MI are ongoing, observational data with bivalirudin suggest that the use of this agent is at least feasible, complementing the data with hirudin in the GUSTO IIb study (18,35). Both pooled analysis from the BAT, CACHET, and REPLACE-1 and an analysis from REPLACE-2 have demonstrated an increase in the risk of bleeding and ischemic events among patients with reduced renal function being treated with heparin and heparin/GP IIb/IIIa inhibition (36,37). In these analyses, the benefit of bivalirudin in relative terms was maintained, for both ischemic and bleeding events. Hence, in absolute terms, among patients with creatinine clearance <60 mL/min, bivalirudin is associated with a greater absolute benefit.

Diabetes

Patients with diabetes remain an important subgroup given the evidence supporting reduced revascularization and mortality associated with abciximab in these patients undergoing PCI (38). Compared with a strategy of heparin and GP IIb/IIIa inhibition, diabetic patients treated with bivalirudin experienced a numerically lower but nonsignificant late mortality at 12 months (2.3% vs. 3.9%, $P = NS$). No differences were observed with short-term bleeding and ischemic outcomes.

Heparin-induced thrombocytopenia syndrome

Bivalirudin may also have a particular role among patients with HITS (39). Among 52 patients studied, clinical success defined as the absence of death, q-wave infarction, or emergent CABG was achieved in 96% of patients. No patients experienced thrombocytopenia (platelet count $<50 \times 10^9$/L), suggesting that bivalirudin is a safe alternative to indirect thrombin inhibition among this high-risk group.

Drug-eluting stents, brachytherapy, and peripheral intervention

Several smaller studies have also explored the use of bivalirudin with drug-eluting stents, brachytherapy, and in peripheral intervention (40–42). Although lacking optimal comparative design, these studies appear to indicate a safety and efficacy profile comparable to that observed in the randomized clinical trials.

Combination therapies

Direct thrombin inhibition provides theoretical advantages for combination pharmacotherapies in PCI. Providing potent inhibition of thrombin-induced platelet activation, synergistic effects with agents blocking the activation and aggregation of platelets can be expected. Furthermore, these agents have not been shown to induce platelet activation in the same manner that has been observed with heparin (43). Although the majority of evidence with bivalirudin has focused on its role as an alternative to heparin and GP IIb/IIIa inhibition, the combination of bivalirudin and GP IIb/IIIa inhibition in a planned and provisional strategy also appears to be safe (28). Although not a randomized comparison, patients in the REPLACE-1 study receiving both bivalirudin and GP IIb/IIIa inhibition experienced a nonsignificant excess in bleeding events compared with those receiving bivalirudin alone, and ischemic events were nonsignificantly lower than heparin/GP IIb/IIIa inhibition treated patients in this pilot study. Although associated with lower rates of ischemic events, pretreatment with clopidogrel in the REPLACE-2 study did not impact the relative risk of ischemic events or the benefit with respect to bleeding associated with bivalirudin compared with heparin and GP IIb/IIIa inhibition (44).

Applications to interventional cardiology: when and why

Argatroban is indicated for HITS and bivalirudin is indicated for a wide range of clinical indications including patients undergoing elective PCI and those presenting with ACS. Specific evidence among patients undergoing catheter-based reperfusion for ST-elevation MI is currently lacking but is being addressed in ongoing trials. Bivalirudin has particular advantages among certain high-risk groups who are at increased risk of bleeding and ischemic events, such as the elderly, those presenting with anemia, and patients with moderate renal impairment. Evidence in the setting of more recent innovations in interventional practice such as drug-eluting stents, brachytherapy, and peripheral intervention do not suggest any variance with the benefit documented in clinical trials. The use of bivalirudin is cost-effective.

Conclusion

The direct thrombin inhibitors have theoretical advantages over the indirect anticoagulants that include more predictable dose–responses, and efficacy against clot bound thrombin. With bivalirudin, clinical trials suggest superiority compared with heparin alone and comparable outcomes when compared with heparin and GP IIb/IIIa inhibition strategies. Lower rates of bleeding and improved cost-effectiveness make bivalirudin a useful "work-horse" anticoagulant in the catheterization laboratory with more data among patients undergoing primary PCI eagerly awaited. Clinical evidence with other direct thrombin inhibitors remains limited, though their use is supported in the context of HITS.

References

1　White CM. Thrombin-directed inhibitors: pharmacology and clinical use. Am Heart J 2005; 149:S54–S60.

2　Becker RC, Spencer FA, Gibson M, et al. Influence of patient characteristics and renal function on factor Xa inhibition pharmacokinetics and pharmacodynamics after enoxaparin administration in non-ST-segment elevation acute coronary syndromes. Am Heart J 2002; 143:753–759.

3　Nappi J. The biology of thrombin in acute coronary syndromes. Pharmacotherapy 2002; 22:90S–96S.

4　Bates ER. Bivalirudin: an anticoagulant option for percutaneous coronary intervention. Expert Rev Cardiovasc Ther 2004; 2:153–162.

5　Zucker TP, Bonisch D, Muck S, et al. Thrombin-induced mitogenesis in coronary artery smooth muscle cells is potentiated by thromboxane A2 and involves upregulation of thromboxane receptor mRNA. Circulation 1998; 97:589–595.

6　Tulinsky A. Molecular interactions of thrombin. Semin Thromb Hemost 1996; 22:117–124.

7　Tsuda Y, Szewczuk Z, Wang J, et al. Interactions of hirudin-based inhibitor with thrombin: critical role of the IleH59 side chain of the inhibitor. Biochemistry 1995; 34:8708–8714.

8　Weitz JI, Leslie B, Hudoba M. Thrombin binds to soluble fibrin degradation products where it is protected from inhibition by heparin-antithrombin but susceptible to inactivation by antithrombin-independent inhibitors. Circulation 1998; 97:544–552.

9　Parry MA, Maraganore JM, Stone SR. Kinetic mechanism for the interaction of hirulog with thrombin. Biochemistry 1994; 33:14807–14814.

10　Di Nisio M, Middeldorp S, Buller HR. Direct thrombin inhibitors. N Engl J Med 2005; 353:1028–1040.

11　Arpino PA, Hallisey RK. Effect of renal function on the pharmacodynamics of argatroban. Ann Pharmacother 2004; 38:25–29.

12　Cheneau E, Canos D, Kuchulakanti PK, et al. Value of monitoring activated clotting time when bivalirudin is used as the sole anticoagulation agent for percutaneous coronary intervention. Am J Cardiol 2004; 94:789–792.

13　Brener SJ, Moliterno DJ, Lincoff AM, et al. Relationship between activated clotting time and ischemic or hemorrhagic complications: analysis of 4 recent randomized clinical trials of percutaneous coronary intervention. Circulation 2004; 110:994–998.

14　Casserly IP, Kereiakes DJ, Gray WA, et al. Point-of-care ecarin clotting time versus activated clotting time in correlation with bivalirudin concentration. Thromb Res 2004; 113:115–121.

15　van den Bos AA, Deckers JW, Heyndrickx GR, et al. Safety and efficacy of recombinant hirudin (CGP 39 393) versus heparin in patients with stable angina undergoing coronary angioplasty. Circulation 1993; 88:2058–2066.

16　Hafner G, Rupprecht HJ, Luz M, et al. Recombinant hirudin as a periprocedural antithrombotic in coronary angioplasty for unstable angina pectoris. Eur Heart J 1996; 17:1207–1215.

17　Serruys PW, Herrman J-PR, Simon R, et al. A comparison of hirudin with heparin in the prevention of restenosis after coronary angioplasty. N Engl J Med 1995; 333:757–763.

18　The Global Use of Strategies to Open Occluded Coronary Arteries in Acute Coronary Syndromes (GUSTO IIb) Angioplasty Substudy Investigators. A clinical trial comparing primary coronary angioplasty with tissue plasminogen activator for acute myocardial infarction. N Engl J Med 1997; 336:1621–1628.

19　Roe MT, Granger CB, Puma JA, et al. Comparison of benefits and complications of hirudin versus heparin for patients with acute coronary syndromes undergoing early percutaneous coronary intervention. Am J Cardiol 2001; 88:1403–1406.

20　Mehta SR, Eikelboom JW, Rupprecht HJ, et al. Efficacy of hirudin in reducing cardiovascular events in patients with acute coronary syndrome undergoing early percutaneous coronary intervention. Eur Heart J 2002; 23:117–123.

21　Sinnaeve PR, Simes J, Yusuf S, et al. Direct thrombin inhibitors in acute coronary syndromes: effect in patients undergoing early percutaneous coronary intervention. Eur Heart J 2005; 26:2396–2403.

22　Manfredi JA, Wall RP, Sane DC, et al. Lepirudin as a safe alternative for effective anticoagulation in patients with known heparin-induced thrombocytopenia undergoing percutaneous coronary intervention: case reports. Catheter Cardiovasc Interv 2001; 52:468–472.

23　Matthai WH Jr. Use of argatroban during percutaneous coronary interventions in patients with heparin-induced thrombocytopenia. Semin Thromb Hemost 1999; 25(suppl 1):57–60.

24　Lewis BE, Matthai WH Jr, Cohen M, et al. Argatroban anticoagulation during percutaneous coronary intervention in patients with heparin-induced thrombocytopenia. Catheter Cardiovasc Interv 2002; 57:177–184.

25　Jang IK, Lewis BE, Matthai WH Jr, et al. Argatroban anticoagulation in conjunction with glycoprotein IIb/IIIa inhibition in patients undergoing percutaneous coronary intervention: an open-label, nonrandomized pilot study. J Thromb Thrombolysis 2004; 18:31–37.

26　Bittl JA, Strony J, Brinker JA, et al. Treatment with bivalirudin (hirulog) as compared with heparin during coronary angioplasty for unstable or postinfarction angina. N Engl J Med 1995; 333:764–769.

27　Bittl JA, Chaitman BR, Feit F, et al. Bivalirudin versus heparin during coronary angioplasty for unstable or postinfarction angina: final report reanalysis of the Bivalirudin Angioplasty Study. Am Heart J 2001; 142:952–959.

28　Lincoff AM, Bittl JA, Kleiman NS, et al. Comparison of bivalirudin versus heparin during percutaneous coronary intervention (the Randomized Evaluation of PCI Linking Angiomax to Reduced Clinical Events [REPLACE]-1 trial). Am J Cardiol 2004; 93:1092–1096.

29 Lincoff AM, Bittl JA, Harrington RA, et al. Bivalirudin and provisional glycoprotein IIb/IIIa blockade compared with heparin and planned glycoprotein IIb/IIIa blockade during percutaneous coronary intervention: REPLACE-2 randomized trial. JAMA 2003; 289:853–863.

30 The EPISTENT Investigators. Randomised placebo-controlled and balloon-angioplasty-controlled trial to assess safety of coronary stenting with use of platelet glycoprotein-IIb/IIIa blockade. Lancet 1998; 352:87–92.

31 Lincoff AM, Kleiman NS, Kereiakes DJ, et al. Long-term efficacy of bivalirudin and provisional glycoprotein IIb/IIIa blockade vs heparin and planned glycoprotein IIb/IIIa blockade during percutaneous coronary revascularization: REPLACE-2 randomized trial. JAMA 2004; 292:696–703.

32 Ebrahimi R, Lincoff AM, Bittl JA, et al. Bivalirudin vs heparin in percutaneous coronary intervention: a pooled analysis. J Cardiovasc Pharmacol Ther 2005; 10:209–216.

33 Cohen DJ, Lincoff AM, Lavelle TA, et al. Economic evaluation of bivalirudin with provisional glycoprotein IIb/IIIa inhibition versus heparin with routine glycoprotein IIb/IIIa inhibition for percutaneous coronary intervention: results from the REPLACE-2 trial. J Am Coll Cardiol 2004; 44:1792–1800.

34 Stone GW, McLaurin BT, Cox DA, et al. Bivalirudin for patients with acute coronary syndromes. N Engl J Med 2006; 355: 2203–2216.

35 Stella JF, Stella RE, Iaffaldano RA, et al. Anticoagulation with bivalirudin during percutaneous coronary intervention for ST-segment elevation myocardial infarction. J Invasive Cardiol 2004; 16:451–454.

36 Chew DP, Bhatt DL, Kimball W, et al. Bivalirudin provides increasing benefit with decreasing renal function: a meta-analysis of randomized trials. Am J Cardiol 2003; 92:919–923.

37 Chew DP, Lincoff AM, Gurm H, et al. Bivalirudin versus heparin and glycoprotein IIb/IIIa inhibition among patients with renal impairment undergoing percutaneous coronary intervention (a subanalysis of the REPLACE-2 trial). Am J Cardiol 2005; 95:581–585.

38 Gurm HS, Sarembock IJ, Kereiakes DJ, et al. Use of bivalirudin during percutaneous coronary intervention in patients with diabetes mellitus: an analysis from the randomized evaluation in percutaneous coronary intervention linking angiomax to reduced clinical events (REPLACE)-2 trial. J Am Coll Cardiol 2005; 45:1932–1938.

39 Mahaffey KW, Lewis BE, Wildermann NM, et al. The anticoagulant therapy with bivalirudin to assist in the performance of percutaneous coronary intervention in patients with heparin-induced thrombocytopenia (ATBAT) study: main results. J Invasive Cardiol 2003; 15:611–616.

40 Dangas G, Lasic Z, Mehran R, et al. Effectiveness of the concomitant use of bivalirudin and drug-eluting stents (from the prospective, multicenter BivAlirudin and Drug-Eluting STents [ADEST] study). Am J Cardiol 2005; 96:659–663.

41 Allie DE, Hebert CJ, Lirtzman MD, et al. A safety and feasibility report of combined direct thrombin and GP IIb/IIIa inhibition with bivalirudin and tirofiban in peripheral vascular disease intervention: treating critical limb ischemia like acute coronary syndrome. J Invasive Cardiol 2005; 17:427–432.

42 Kuchulakanti P, Wolfram R, Torguson R, et al. Bivalirudin compared with IIb/IIIa inhibitors in patients with in-stent restenosis undergoing intracoronary brachytherapy. Cardiovasc Revasc Med 2005; 6:154–159.

43 Keating FK, Dauerman HL, Whitaker DA, Sobel BE, Schneider DJ. Increased expression of platelet P-selectin and formation of platelet-leukocyte aggregates in blood from patients treated with unfractionated heparin plus eptifibatide compared with bivalirudin. Thromb Res 2006; 118:361–369.

44 Saw J, Lincoff AM, Desmet W, et al. Lack of clopidogrel pretreatment effect on the relative efficacy of bivalirudin with provisional glycoprotein IIb/IIIa blockade compared to heparin with routine glycoprotein IIb/IIIa blockade: a REPLACE-2 substudy. J Am Coll Cardiol 2004; 44:1194–1199.

8

Clinical application of direct antithrombin inhibitors in acute coronary syndrome

Shunji Suzuki, Hikari Watanabe, Takefumi Matsuo, and Masanori Osakabe

Introduction

Percutaneous coronary intervention (PCI) such as coronary angioplasty and stent implantation has become a worldwide routine strategy for coronary arterial occlusive diseases. Along with the recognition that thrombus formation is very likely to be involved in acute coronary syndrome (ACS), selection of the optimal anticoagulant is becoming essential to achieve reliable anticoagulation for successful PCI.

Although unfractionated heparin (UFH) has long been used as the standard anticoagulant with great potency, there are some therapeutic dilemmas in its use. Given the availability of new anticoagulants and to address these clinical considerations, the choice of the anticoagulant should take into account the individual patient's condition.

Heparin

The anticoagulant action of heparin was discovered by McLean in 1916, and it has since been the landmark anticoagulant therapy employed in clinical practice. The most common preparation of heparin is UFH (molecular weight: 5000 to 30,000 Da) which is a mixture of mucopolysaccharides derived from porcine intestinal mucosa. Among the various pathways affected by UFH, the main action is to accelerate the inhibitory effects of antithrombin on thrombin and factors Xa, Va, and VIIa.

The American College of Cardiology and the American Heart Association recommend that UFH should be given during a PCI procedure to achieve an activated clotting time (ACT) of 250 to 350 seconds [200 seconds if glycoprotein (GP) IIbIIIa receptor inhibitor is given] with a weight-adjusted bolus dose,

70 to 100 U/kg (50–70 U/kg if GPIIbIIIa receptor inhibitors is given) (1). Similar guidelines have been issued from the European Society of Cardiology (2). In a multicenter prospective study in Japan, patients underwent a successful PCI received UFH of 4980 ± 1754 (mean ± SD) U at an activated partial thromboplastin time (aPTT) ratio of 2.4 ± 1.8 (mean ± SD). Empirically, lower dose has been used in Japan (3).

Despite the excellence of UFH as an anticoagulant, several problems occur during PCI. Following vascular injury by PCI which disrupts the endothelium and subendothelium, the resultant generation of thrombin may not be sufficiently minimized with UFH. Recently, the additional use of GPIIb/IIIa inhibitors for the purpose of suppressing platelet activation during PCI has in some situations been recommended to address this problem of UFH. For these reasons, it has not been concluded whether heparin is the optimal anticoagulant to support successful PCI (4).

Inter-individual difference in anticoagulation

UFH acts directly on platelets to promote platelet aggregation and releases platelet factor 4 (PF4) from the endothelium. PF4 binds UFH and neutralizes its anticoagulant action (5). Furthermore, UFH induces the release of tissue factor pathway inhibitor (TFPI) from platelets and endothelial cells into the circulation. One of the major effects of UFH is the release of free-type TFPI, which strongly inhibits FVIIa tissue factor. Therefore, the anticoagulant actions of UFH vary depending on the individual patient and are influenced by the level of PF4, antithrombin, and histidine-rich GP.

No inhibition of fibrin/clot-bound thrombin

Due to its large molecular size in comparison with direct thrombin inhibitors (DTIs), UFH is unable to penetrate into fibrin clot and to inhibit thrombin trapped in a clot. Hence, its anticoagulant activity is limited only to the inhibition of thrombin in the process of thrombi formation.

Heparin resistance

The conventional dosing regime of UFH aims to maintain aPTT values within 1.5 to 2.5 times the baseline value. If aPTT 1.5-fold or above the baseline is not obtained when dosing with 35,000 U/day of UFH, this condition is regarded as heparin resistance. Heparin resistance presents in various clinical settings and, in particular, is closely associated with decreased antithrombin-III (AT-III). Since UFH accelerates its antithrombin action in the presence of AT-III, a lower level of AT-III attenuates such action. Once the AT-III level in the blood falls to 60% of the usual levels, a dose of 35,000 U/day or greater UFH is required to prolong aPTT to attain the therapeutic range. The absence of AT-III is observed in congenital or acquired clinical events (sepsis, multiple trauma, burn injury, malignant tumor, and extracorporeal circulation). When UFH is administered to those patients, careful monitoring of the AT-III level is needed because AT-III is consumed during the use of UFH. If AT-III decreases to 60% or below, the risk of venous thrombosis increases.

Heparin cofactor II (HC-II), unlike AT-III, is not a core factor. However, the thrombin neutralization rate is further accelerated by the mediation of dermatan and heparan sulfate. Normally, when vascular injury occurs in the subendothelium and dermatan sulfate increases, HC-II deserves the effects of thrombin neutralization. When coronary artery angioplasty was performed with UFH in a patient with congenital HC-II deficiency, recurrent restenosis occurred in a very short period; however, subsequent angioplasty with argatroban, a direct thrombin inhibitor, did not result in restenosis (6). With the reduced level of HC-II, even with a normal/adequate level of AT-III, UFH could not inhibit sufficiently fibrin-bound thrombin generated during a PCI procedure. It is possible that restenosis might be predicted in situations where there is a lower than normal level of AT III and/or HC-II. UFH does not demonstrate an adequate anticoagulant action without these cofactors.

Heparin-induced thrombocytopenia and platelet stimulation

Heparin-induced thrombocytopenia (HIT) is a serious adverse drug reaction to heparin (Fig. 1). HIT is caused by the

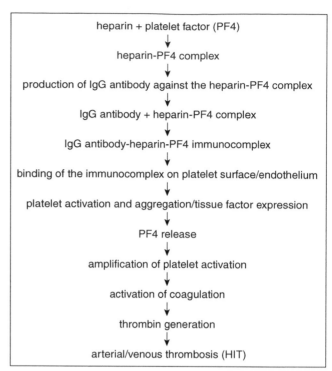

heparin + platelet factor (PF4)
↓
heparin-PF4 complex
↓
production of IgG antibody against the heparin-PF4 complex
↓
IgG antibody + heparin-PF4 complex
↓
IgG antibody-heparin-PF4 immunocomplex
↓
binding of the immunocomplex on platelet surface/endothelium
↓
platelet activation and aggregation/tissue factor expression
↓
PF4 release
↓
amplification of platelet activation
↓
activation of coagulation
↓
thrombin generation
↓
arterial/venous thrombosis (HIT)

Figure 1

Model of the pathogenesis of heparin-induced thrombocytopenia (HIT). Heparin forms heparin/platelet factor 4 (PF4) complex in vivo. Thereafter, autoantibodies (HIT antibodies) against this complex are generated and further form an immune complex. This immune complex binds to the Fc receptor on the surface of platelets, which are activated, leading to further secretion of PF4 and platelet aggregation. The activated platelets also produce microparticles which amplify thrombin generation. Moreover, released PF4 is also responsive to heparan sulfate on the endothelium to form a complex. HIT antibodies also bind to this complex and induce not only endothelial damage but also the expression of tissue factor on endothelial cells. Platelet activation and thrombin generation are mainly pathogenic in a hypercoagulable state at the onset of HIT. *Abbreviation*: HIT, heparin-induced thrombocytopenia.

transient production of autoantibodies (HIT antibodies) following heparin administration. HIT antibodies are generated against antigen of PF4-heparin complex approximately 5 to 10 days after the first exposure to heparin. HIT antibodies are composed of immunoglobulin G (IgG) primarily, and also IgA and IgM. After the generation of HIT antibodies, complications of thrombocytopenia and arterial/venous thrombi may be observed. The pathogenicity of thrombus formation is suspected as follows: first, HIT antibodies activate platelets through FcγIIIa receptor and release microparticles from it, second, the antibodies bind to the heparan sulfate–PF4 complex on endothelial cells, and finally, the endothelium is activated, expressing tissue factor and producing thrombogenic activation (7). As UFH is used routinely in PCI, attention should be paid to the risk of HIT. HIT is unavoidable as long as UFH is employed in PCI procedures (3,8–10). Unfortunately, HIT-associated complications are not always properly recognized in cardiovascular events. Such failure of recognition happens in the following way: (*i*) the use of oral antiplatelet agents masks the signs and symptoms, (*ii*) heparin is administered for only a short period and most HIT is underestimated, and (*iii*) the level of HIT antibodies becomes undetectable during the long period of non-use of heparin between previous PCI and subsequent cardiac interventions.

Some patients with acute myocardial infarction (AMI) are found to have HIT antibodies "career state of HIT antibodies" regardless of previous heparin usage. In those patients, early-onset HIT has been observed, which occurs within a very short period after UFH administration during PCI even if it is the initial exposure to UFH (10). Once HIT antibodies are generated after the exposure to UFH, the antibodies do not disappear for approximately 100 days after the cessation of UFH. If UFH intervention is resumed while the antibodies remain, HIT may readily develop as "rapid-onset type of HIT" (11). Thrombotic complications are highly anticipated following the abrupt onset of HIT in patients who have been exposed recently to UFH.

In some patients carrying HIT antibodies, "delayed-onset type of HIT" occurs a couple of days to several weeks after the cessation of heparin therapy (12,13). Recently, thanks to more sophisticated equipment, the post-PCI hospitalization period has become shorter. Nevertheless, it is alarming that patients treated with UFH for PCI have a potential risk of HIT onset after hospital discharge.

All interactions between UFH and platelets are complex and only partially elucidated, but it is known that heparin itself stimulates platelets via a platelet-binding domain of heparin (14). In the therapeutic range, UFH induces the release of *P*-selectin and activates GPIIb/IIIa receptors when adenosine diphosphate (ADP) or thrombin receptor agonist peptide stimulates platelet responsibility, and then enhances platelet aggregation (15,16). Even in healthy individuals, agonist-induced platelet aggregation is often enhanced when heparin is added.

Polymorphonuclear leukocyte elastase

Polymorphonuclear leukocyte elastase as a marker of leukocyte activation is a GP with a molecular weight of about 30,000, and there are three isozymes. It has a biological role in host defense mechanisms, but it sometimes induces abnormal blood coagulation and injury of the vascular intima. In particular, polymorphonuclear leukocyte elastase has a strong deteriorating effect on fibrinolytic enzymes and antithrombin and induces hypercoagulability in the presence of UFH. In high level of polymorphonuclear leukocyte elastase in ACS, an anticoagulant effect of heparin is presumably attenuated owing to degradation of heparin-induced AT-III activity.

Options of other anticoagulants for percutaneous coronary intervention

UFH has long been used empirically as a conventional anticoagulant for PCI procedures; however, no placebo-controlled studies have been conducted to confirm the efficacy and safety of UFH in patients undergoing PCI (Fig. 2). Thus, in daily practice, at a catheter laboratory, UFH is used without evidence.

The pathogenic mechanism of ACS is that coronary arteriosclerotic plaques rupture and erode leading to thrombosis. Once injury to the coronary endothelial cells occurs, collagen and von Willebrand factor exposed to subendothelial matrix adhere to platelets. Consequently, these platelets are

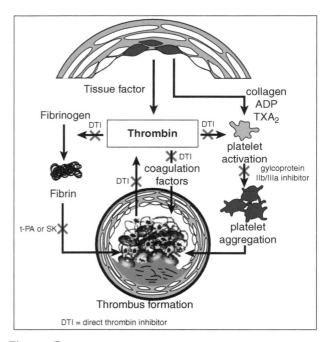

Figure 2

Critical role of thrombin in thrombogenesis. Thrombin plays a critical and central role in thrombogenesis through platelet activation, fibrin generation, and clot stabilization at the site of arterial disruption, which are caused by percutaneous coronary intervention or plaque rupture in acute coronary syndromes. Tissue factor released at the site of vessel injury or plaque rupture activates coagulation, resulting in the generation of small amounts of thrombin. The small amount of thrombin activates platelets and other coagulation factors, which amplifies this process and causes an explosive burst of thrombin generation. Furthermore, thrombin is the most potent physiological activator of platelets. The morphology of platelets changes and then adheres to the site of the damaged vessel. Activated platelets recruit additional platelets by synthesizing thromboxan A_2 and releasing adenosine diphosphate. Platelet activation induces conformational changes in glycoprotein IIb/IIIa receptor resulting in platelet aggregation. Clotting factors form a stable thrombus on the surface of aggregated platelets. *Abbreviation*: DTI, direct thrombin inhibitor.

activated leading to platelet adhesion. Tissue factors exposed on the damaged endothelium and subendothelial matrix and released into blood circulation trigger an extrinsic pathway activation, which leads to thrombin generation and then fibrin clot formation (17,18). And also, as a key factor of thrombotic events, share stress to vascular wall by arterial flow results in tissue factor expression on endothelial cells, release of procoagulant factors from activated platelets and finally thrombin generation. Anticoagulation using DTIs may be a better option in patients with ACS undergoing PCI or not.

In the meta-analysis with 11 randomized studies, anticoagulant effects in ACS and PCI were compared between a direct antithrombin agent and UFH. The direct thrombin inhibitor showed better outcome in death or myocardial infarction than UFH (19). DTIs are expected to be an alternative to UFH for PCI.

Direct thrombin inhibitors

DTIs (Fig. 3, Table 1) have been developed to overcome the drawbacks of UFH therapy and aim to effectively inhibit thrombin without involving antithrombin. Thrombin plays a critical role in thrombogenesis through platelet activation, fibrin generation, and clot stabilization at the site of endothelial disruption. Thrombin generation also occurs following endothelial injury due to physical pressure during angioplasty. Furthermore, increased thrombin generation is found to be a trigger at the onset of ACS. Therefore, DTIs have been investigated to see if they can achieve greater clinical efficacy than that of conventional UFH therapy (20–22).

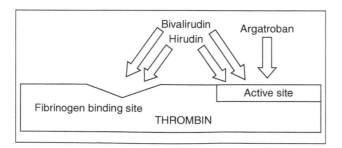

Figure 3

Pharmacologic differences between hirudin, argatroban, and bivalirudin. Hirudin and bivalirudin are bivalent direct thrombin inhibitors. They bind to both the active site and the fibrinogen binding site. Argatroban is a univalent inhibitor and binds to the active site only (no fibrinogen binding site). Hirudin is an irreversible inhibitor, while argatroban and bivalirudin exhibit reversible binding. After binding to thrombin, bivalirudin is cleaved by thrombin at the active site, restoring thrombin activity (80).

Argatroban

Argatroban (Table 2) is a selective direct thrombin inhibitor discovered by Okamoto et al. in 1978 in Japan. In the United States, argatroban is licensed as an anticoagulant for the prophylaxis and treatment of thrombosis in patients with HIT as well as for patients with or at risk for HIT undergoing PCI check. In some European countries, including Sweden and Germany, argatroban is also available for anticoagulation in adult patients with HIT. In Japan, the approved indications are for use in patients with chronic arterial occlusion, in hemodialysis patients with a deficiency or a decrease in AT-III levels, and in patients with acute cerebral thrombosis. With its arginine-based structure and molecular weight of 527 Da, argatroban binds directly to the active site of thrombin with an inhibitory constant (K_i) of 0.04 μM. It shows no inhibitory effects on serine protease inhibitors such as trypsin, plasmin, and factor Xa, but is highly selective for thrombin and exerts its anticoagulant action independent of AT-III and HC-II as cofactors.

Pharmacodynamically, argatroban can bind to both free and fibrin- or clot-bound thrombin. Its inhibitory action on bound thrombin is much greater than those of UFH or hirudin (23). As argatroban reversibly binds to thrombin, the likelihood of significant hemorrhagic events is reduced. Argatroban strongly inhibits thrombin-induced platelet aggregation (24), but does not cause platelet stimulation, which is commonly observed in heparin. In patients with HIT undergoing PCI (25) or dialysis (26), argatroban has been used as an alternative to UFH. Owning to its low molecular weight and synthetic nature, argatroban does not cause biological antibodies (27). For anticoagulation therapy in patients with a high polymorphonuclear leukocyte elastase level, argatroban is more effective than heparin plus AT-III (28).

The metabolism of argatroban is via hepatic hydroxylation and aromatization by cytochrome enzymes CYP3A4/5 and elimination via biliary excretion (29); however, argatroban is not altered by its concomitant use with erythromycin (a CYP3A4/5 inhibitor), which suggests no significant drug–drug interaction (30). In hepatically impaired patients, argatroban clearance is decreased four-fold and so dose reduction and careful monitoring are required (31). Argatroban can be used as a substitute for UFH in HIT patients with renal insufficiency requiring hemodialysis treatment (32).

Argatroban in percutaneous coronary intervention

During a PCI procedure, thrombin generation in the vessels damaged by the manipulation cannot be suppressed by UFH but can be by argatroban (4,33).

The feasibility and safety of argatroban in combination with GPIIb/IIIa inhibition were studied in 152 patients who

Table 1 Characteristics of unfractionated heparin and direct thrombin inhibitors

	UFH	Argatroban	Lepirudin	Bivalirudin
Nature	Mixture of mucopolysaccharide	Synthetic arginine analog	Recombinant protein	Synthetic peptide
Molecular weight	5000–30,000 Da	527 Da	6980 Da	2180 Da
Antithrombotic action	Thrombin ≈ Xa	Thrombin	Thrombin	Thrombin
		Fibrin-bound, free-thrombin	Fibrin-bound, free-thrombin	Fibrin-bound, free-thrombin
Thrombin inhibition	Irreversible	Reversible	Irreversible	Reversible
Necessary cofactor	AT III · HC II	No	No	No
Half-life	60 min	40–50 min	80 min	25 min
Target aPTT (x baseline)	x 1.5–2.5	x 1.5–3.0	x 1.5–2.5	x 1.5–3.0
Antidote	Protamin	No	No	No
Elimination	Liver (Kidney)	Liver	Kidney	Kidney
Platelet stimulation	++	—	—	—
Interaction with PF-4	++	—	—	—
Thrombocytopenia	++	—	—	—
Trigger for HIT	++	—	—	—
Antigenecity	+	—	+[a]	+
Approved indication				
Prophylaxis of HIT		US, EU	—	—
Treatment of HIT		US, EU	US, EU	—
PCI in HIT		US	—	US
PCI		—	—	US, EU

[a]Readministration could lead to anaphylaxis.

Abbreviations: aPTT, activated partial thromboplastin time; AT, antithrombin; HC, heparin cofactor; HIT, heparin-induced thrombocytopenia; PCI, percutaneous coronary intervention; PF, platelet factor; UFH, unfractionated heparin.

underwent PCI. The integrin GPIIb/IIIa receptor on platelets is the final common pathway of platelet aggregation. PCI was performed in patients receiving argatroban to achieve an ACT of 275 to 325 seconds in combination with predominantly abciximab (a Fab fragment of the chimeric human-murine monoclonal antibody against the GPIIb/IIIa receptor) or eptifibatide (a synthetic cyclic heptapeptide with high specificity for the GPIIb/IIIa receptor). The primary endpoint, a composite of cardiovascular adverse events at 30 days, occurred in four patients. Two patients experienced major bleeding, one a retroperitoneal bleed and the other a groin hematoma. This trial shows that adequate anticoagulation can be achieved with a combination of a reduced dose of argatroban and a GPIIb/IIIa inhibitor, and moreover, this combination of treatment was well tolerated with an acceptable bleeding risk in patients undergoing PCI (34).

Argatroban as adjunctive therapy to thrombolytics in acute myocardial infarction

In the Myocardial Infarction with Novastan and Tissue-Plasminogen Activator (MINT) trial, a comparative trial of effects of UFH and argatroban on reperfusion by tissue-plasminogen activator (t-PA) was carried out in 125 patients with AMI (Table 3). Three treatment regimens were tested: UFH, low-dose argatroban and high-dose argatroban. A dose-dependent benefit over UFH in achieving Thrombolysis in Myocardial Infarction (TIMI) grade 3 flow at 90 minutes after thrombolytic therapy was observed: $P = 0.20$: between low-dose argatroban versus UFH, $P = 0.13$: between high-dose argatroban versus UFH. The incidence of the composite

Table 2   Pharmacodynamics and pharmacokinetics of argatroban

Pharmacology	*Competitively and reversibly inhibits thrombin*
Pharmacokinetics	
Half-life	40–50 min
Elimination	CYP 3A4/5 Hepatic[a]
Metabolism/hepatic impairment	1/4 reduction of starting dose
Renal dysfunction	No dose modification
Pharmacodynamic effects on aPTT and ACT	
HIT	Continuous infusion starting with 2 μg/kg/min. aPTT is monitored 2 hr after start of infusion and infusion rate is adjusted to aPTT 1.5–3.0 times baseline not to exceed aPTT 100 sec and 10 μg/kg/min
PCI in HIT	A bolus of 350 μg/kg given over 3–5 min following by continuous infusion with 25 μg/kg/min. ACT is monitored 5–10 min after bolus dose is completed. If ACT <300 sec another bolus dose of 150 μg/kg is given and infusion is increased to 30 μg/kg/min. If ACT >450 sec infusion rate is reduced to 15 μg/kg/min[b]

[a]CYP 3A4/5: liver microsomal cytochrome P450 enzymes 3A4/5.

[b]The dose was reduced to 250 or 300 μg/kg bolus followed by 15 mg/kg/min infusion to achieve ACT of 275 to 325 seconds when GPIIb/IIIa inhibitors was co-administrated in non-HIT patients undergoing PCI.

Abbreviations: aPTT, activated partial thromboplastin time; ACT, activated clotting time; HIT, heparin-induced thrombocytopenia; PCI, percutaneous coronary intervention.

endpoint of cardiovascular adverse events at day 30 was numerically lower in both argatroban groups than in the heparin group ($P = 0.23$) (35).

The Argatroban in Acute Myocardial Infarction (ARGAMI) trial was conducted to compare the effects of argatroban and UFH as adjunctive therapy to t-PA in patients with AMI. One hundred and twenty seven patients were randomized to either the UFH group or the argatroban group. Patency rate at 90 minutes was not significantly different between the two groups (36).

ARGAMI-2 was conducted to compare the effects of UFH and low and high doses of argatroban as adjunctive therapy to t-PA or streptokinase (SK) in 1200 patients with AMI. At the interim analysis, the low-dose argatroban group was discontinued due to the lack of efficacy. No statistically significant difference was observed in mortality or any other primary efficacy endpoints between the UFH and high-dose argatroban groups (37).

Dose description of argatroban

The dose regimens for HIT and PCI in HIT patients are presented in Table 2. In the patients with HIT, it is recommended that argatroban is administered as a continuous intravenous infusion starting at 2 μg/kg/min. The dose was adjusted to attain an aPTT of 1.5 to 3.0 times the baseline,

but not exceeding 100 seconds (38,39). aPTT should be checked two hours after the initiation of argatroban to confirm that the desired aPTT range is achieved. The initial dose of argatroban should be one-fourth for patients with moderate hepatic impairment.

However, it has been reported that the initial dose of 2.0 μg/kg/min led to excessive anticoagulation even in patients with normal hepatic function (40,41). In some patients in cardiothoracic intensive care units or with metastatic cancer, a dose reduction could be proposed. In the ongoing investigator's initiated trial for HIT in Japan, lower initial dose of 0.7 μg/kg/min is used (42). Empirically lower doses are used in Japan than in Europe or United States.

As an anticoagulant for patients with or at risk for HIT undergoing PCI, the recommended dosage is a bolus of 350 μg/kg/min followed by a continuous infusion of 25 μg/kg/min. ACT should be checked 5 to 10 minutes after the bolus dose is completed. The PCI procedure may proceed when the ACT is greater than 300 seconds. When the ACT is less than 300 seconds, an additional bolus dose of 150 μg/kg should be administered, the infusion dose increased to 30 μg/kg/min, and the ACT checked 5 to 10 minutes later. When the ACT is greater than 450 seconds, the infusion rate should be decreased to 15 μg/kg/min, and the ACT again checked 5 to 10 minutes later. Once an adequate therapeutic ACT of between 300 and 450 seconds has been achieved, this infusion dose should be continued for the duration of the

Table 3 Clinical trials of argatroban in acute myocardial infarction with thrombolytics

Trial (reference)	Target population	Number of patients	Dose regimen	Results
MINT (35)	AMI with tPA	125	Argatroban (100 μg/kg bolus + 1 or 3 μg/kg/min infusion) vs. UFH (70 U/kg bolus + 15 U/kg/hr infusion)	Efficacy: non-significant benefit in TIMI 3 flow in argatroban. Safety: no difference in rate of major bleeding
ARGAMI (36)	AMI with tPA	127	Argatroban (100 μg/kg bolus + 3 μg/kg/min infusion) vs. UFH (5000 U bolus + 1000 U/hr infusion)	Efficacy: no difference in angiographic patency. Safety: no difference in rate of bleeding
ARGAMI-2 (37)	AMI with tPA or SK	1200	Argatroban (60 μg/kg bolus + 2 μg/kg/min or 120 μg/kg bolus + 4 μg/kg/min infusion) vs. UFH (5000U bolus + 1000U/hr infusion)	Efficacy: no difference in mortality. Safety: no difference in rate of major bleeding

Abbreviations: AMI, acute myocardial infarction; ARGAMI, argatroban in acute myocardial infarction; MINT, myocardial infarction with novastan and tissue plasminogen activator; SK, streptokinase; TIMI, thrombolysis in myocardial infarction; tPA, tissue plasminogen activator; UFH, unfractionated heparin.

procedure. When a patient requires anticoagulation after the procedure, argatroban may be continued, but at a lower infusion dose, such as the dose for HIT.

Thrombin-specific inhibitors also prolong the prothrombin time/international normalized ratio (INR). Thus, careful monitoring should be employed during transition from argatroban to oral anticoagulant. The dose of argatroban should be reduced to 2 μg/kg/min to predict the INR on oral anticoagulant alone. When the INR reaches four on combination therapy, argatroban can be discontinued and an INR on oral anticoagulant alone should lie in the range 2.0 – 3.7. The INR should be measured four to six hours again after the stop of argatroban (43,44). In the investigator's initiated trial in Japan, argatroban is to be stopped when the INR on combination therapy reaches 2.5 to 3.0 (42).

Monitoring of argatroban

Anticoagulation with argatroban is easily controlled with minimal inter-patient differences, but monitoring is recommended for safety use. aPTT and ACT are correlated predictably with doses up to 40 μg/kg/min infusion. This therefore allows the flexible use of aPTT and/or ACT depending on the clinical setting (45).

A dose-proportional curve was also noted in ecarin clotting time (ECT) (46). ECT is measured based on the conversion from prothrombin to meizothrombin mediated by ecarin, the venom of the snake. Thrombin inhibitors can inhibit

meizothrombin converting fibrinogen to fibrin. ECT may be used as an index of the plasma level of argatroban in patients undergoing PCI (46,47). However, aPTT is used to monitor argatroban for doses used in the management of HIT type II as this test is widely available and understood by both specialists and general physicians. In the case of PCI, ACT is used as it is familiar to interventionalists and allows real-time monitoring at the cath lab.

Hirudin

Hirudin, a protease inhibitor originally existing in the salivary glands of the medicinal leech, *Hirudo medicinalis*, is a single-chain polypeptide consisting of 65 amino acid residues (molecular weight: approximately 7000). Hirudin inhibits selectively thrombin but not factor Xa and binds to thrombin (1:1) to form an irreversible complex. Hirudin exerts better anticoagulation than UFH because it inhibits both fibrin-bound thrombin and free thrombin in circulation. Hirudin does not stimulate platelets unlike heparin so that it can be used in patients with HIT (48). There are two forms of recombinant hirudin, lepirudin, and desirudin. In Europe and the United States, one of the recombinant hirudins, lepirudin, was approved for anticoagulation in patients with HIT and associated thromboembolic disease.

Lepirudin has been reported to generate antihirudin antibodies in 40% or more of treated patients after infusion for more than five days. These antibodies may affect the enhancement and/or reduction of coagulation cascade. Occasionally this leads to drug accumulation because a lepirudin–immunoglobulin complex is formed and renal clearance of the drug is delayed. Fatal anaphylaxis has been reported in patients who received a repeat intravenous bolus administration of lepirudin after an interval of a few months (49). Since hirudin is excreted by the kidneys, dose reduction and careful monitoring are needed for patients with renal insufficiency.

Hirudin in percutaneous coronary intervention

In the Hirudin in European Trial Versus Heparin in the Prevention of after PTCA (HELVETICA) trial, 1141 patients with unstable angina undergoing PCI were randomized to one of the following three groups: UFH or two dose regimens of hirudin. The primary endpoint of event-free survival at seven months was not significantly different in the three groups, but hirudin groups showed a significant relative risk reduction ($P = 0.023$) in the endpoint of early events occurring within 96 hours after PCI. The incidences of hemorrhagic complications were not different among the three groups (50).

Hirudin as adjunctive therapy to thrombolytics in acute myocardial infarction

Hirudin has been studied extensively in ACS (Table 4). The TIMI 5 trial was conducted in 246 patients with AMI to compare the efficacy of UFH and hirudin as adjunctive therapy to t-PA (51). In the hirudin group, the rate of recanalization to achieve TIMI 3 coronary flow without death or reinfarction was greater than that in the UFH group ($P = 0.07$). No inter-group difference in the incidence of major hemorrhage was observed. In TIMI 6, the effects of UFH and hirudin were compared in 193 patients with AMI in combination with SK. The results of both groups were similar for both safety and efficacy endpoints (52).

In the Global Use of Strategies to Open Occluded Coronary Arteries (GUSTO)-IIb trial, the effects of UFH and hirudin in combination with either t-PA or SK were compared in 3289 patients with AMI (53). When dosed in combination with SK, the benefit of hirudin over UFH was observed in the clinical efficacy endpoint with the same levels of bleeding complications. In the TIMI 9b trial, 3002 patients with AMI were dosed with hirudin or UFH in combination with t-PA or SK, but no difference between the groups was observed in the clinical efficacy endpoint up to 30 days after administration (54). The administration of UFH or hirudin was not initiated

during thrombolytic therapy but within 60 minutes after the completion of thrombolytics, which might have masked the difference between the groups.

Dose description of hirudin

Lepirudin is indicated for anticoagulation in patients with HIT and thrombosis. The registered dose is 0.4 mg/kg for bolus and the infusion rate is started from 0.15 mg/kg/h, which can be adjusted to obtain an aPTT of 1.5 to 2.5 times the baseline, and the aPTT should be checked every four hours until steady state is achieved. Lepirudin is also reported to be an effective anticoagulant for patients with isolated HIT when administered at lower doses of 0.10 mg/kg/hr adjusted by aPTT without the initial bolus (55).

Upon transition to oral anticoagulants, the dose of lepirudin should be reduced to attain prolongation of the aPTT by 1.5. When coumarin derivatives are initiated, lepirudin should be continued for four to five days and discontinued when the INR stabilizes within the target range.

Monitoring of hirudin

Hirudin treatment has been monitored by aPTT and frequent aPTT monitoring is required in patients with renal impairment, serious liver injury, or an increased risk of bleeding (56). Stricter dose adjustment is required in renal impairment patients. ECT may be a more appropriate marker, particularly for high-dose hirudin (57).

Bivalirudin (formerly hirulog)

Through the investigation of several hirudin-based analogs, bivalirudin has been developed. Bivalirudin is approved as an anticoagulant for patients undergoing PCI in the United States and Europe. Recently, the FDA has approved an extension to the indication, namely for HIT patients undergoing PCI.

Bivalirudin is a synthetic 20-amino acid compound. The molecular weight is 2180 Da and the plasma half-life is 25 minutes. Bivalirudin can bind to both fibrin-bound thrombin and free thrombin. Dose reduction in proportion to the creatinine level is necessary in patients with renal insufficiency.

Bivalirudin, like hirudin, interacts with both the active site and fibrinogen-binding site. Once bivalirudin binds to thrombin, however, its amino-terminal domain binding to the active site is cleaved, leading to the recovery of catalytic activities of thrombin. Although the carboxy terminal domain remains bound to the fibrinogen binding site, this interaction is weak. Thus, bivalirudin shows a short duration of thrombin inhibition. Some researchers have suggested that higher doses of bivalirudin can be used with less bleeding owing to this

Table 4 Clinical trials of hirudin in acute myocardial infarction with thrombolytics

Trial (reference)	Target population	Number of patients	Dose regimen	Results
TIMI 5 (51)	AMI with tPA	246	Hirudin (0.15 mg/kg bolus + 0.05 mg/kg/hr infusion. 0.1 mg/kg bolus + 0.1 mg/kg/hr infusion. 0.3 mg/kg bolus + 0.2 mg/kg/hr infusion, or 0.6 mg/kg bolus + 0.2 mg/kg/hr infusion) vs. UFH 5000 U bolus + 1000 U/hr infusion	Efficacy: non-significant benefit in TIMI 3 flow in hirudin. Safety: no difference in rate of major bleeding
TIMI 6 (52)	AMI with SK	193	Hirudin (0.15 mg/kg bolus + 0.05 mg/kg/hr infusion, 0.3 mg/kg bolus + 0.1 mg/kg/hr infusion, or 0.6 mg/kg bolus + 0.2 mg/kg/hr infusion) vs. UFH 5000 U bolus + 1000 U/hr infusion	Efficacy: no effect. Safety: no difference in rate of major bleeding
TIMI 9b (54)	AMI with tPA or SK	3002	Hirudin (0.1 mg/kg bolus + 0.1 mg/kg/hr infusion) vs. UFH 5000 U bolus + 1000 U/hr infusion	Efficacy: comparable. Safety: comparable
GUSTO IIb (53)	AMI with tPA or SK	3289	Hirudin (0.1 mg/kg bolus + 0.1 mg/kg/hr infusion) vs. UFH 5000 U bolus + 1000 U/hr infusion	Efficacy: benefit of hirudin with SK but no benefit with t-PA. Safety: no difference in rate of bleeding

Abbreviations: AMI, acute myocardial infarction: GUSTO, Global Use of Strategies to Open Occluded Coronary Arteries: SK, streptokinase: TIMI, thrombolysis in myocardial infarction: tPA, tissue plasminogen activator: UFH, unfractionated heparin.

temporary inhibition of the thrombin catalytic site (58). However, bivalirudin's shorter duration of action could induce rebound hypercoagulability on the cessation of antithrombin therapy (59).

The molecular weight of bivalirudin is smaller than that of hirudin. Therefore, it is unlikely to cause anaphylactic responses; however, bivalirudin has been reported to show cross-reactivity to anti-lepirudin antibodies. Caution is required when administering bivalirudin to patients previously treated with lepirudin (60).

Bivalirudin in percutaneous coronary intervention

Bivalirudin was studied at five doses in 291 patients undergoing coronary angioplasty (61). The incidence of hemorrhagic complications was markedly low during this trial. It was demonstrated that bivalirudin could be an alternative anticoagulant to UFH in preventing transient complications during coronary angioplasty.

Further to the above pilot trial, the Bivalirudin Angioplasty Trial (BAT) was designed. In this trial, 4098 patients undergoing PCI for their unstable or postinfarction angina were randomly assigned to either a bivalirudin or a UFH treatment arm in a double-blind manner. Bivalirudin did not significantly decrease the incidence of the above primary endpoints in the entire trial population when compared with UFH (62).

The data from BAT were subsequently reanalyzed (63). The endpoints, incidences of death, myocardial infarction or repeat revascularization with a contemporary definition, were compared between bivalirudin and UFH at 7, 90, and 180 days after PCI in the entire intention-to-treat cohort of 4312 patients, whereas the original report analyzed the per-protocol population. The incidence of the combined endpoints of death, myocardial infarction or repeat revascularization was significantly lower with bivalirudin than with heparin ($P = 0.039$). The significant difference between bivalirudin and UFH for the combined endpoints persisted at 90 days ($P = 0.012$), but not at 180 days ($P = 0.153$). The bleeding rate was significantly lower in the bivalirudin group than the UFH group as in the original analysis ($P < 0.001$).

In the Randomized Evaluation in Percutaneous Coronary Intervention Linking Angiomax to Reduced Clinical Events (REPLACE)-2 (64), bivalirudin with the provisional use of GPIIb/IIIa inhibitors and UFH with the planned use of GPIIb/IIIa inhibitors were compared in 6010 patients undergoing urgent or elective PCI. In this trial, both in primary and secondary clinical efficacy endpoints, noninferiority was shown statistically. In the incidence of major bleeding events, a significant reduction was observed in the bivalirudin group compared with the UFH group ($P < 0.001$). The median ACT five minutes after the trial drug bolus was longer in the bivalirudin group (358 seconds) versus UFH (317 seconds). A follow-up trial to one year showed that the clinical outcome of bivalirudin with provisional GPIIb/IIIa inhibitors was comparable with that of heparin with planned GPIIb/IIIa inhibition (65,67).

These data suggest that bivalirudin could be used routinely as a substitute for heparin during PCI. Bivalirudin achieves approximately the same clinical effect as heparin when used in PCI, and there may be an early advantage in the high-risk subgroup of patients with postinfarction angina.

Bivalirudin as adjunctive therapy to thrombolytics in acute myocardial infarction

The Hirulog Early Reperfusion or Occlusion (HERO) trial was conducted in patients with AMI to investigate the effects of bivalirudin in combination with SK and aspirin (Table 5) (66). Four hundred and twelve patients who presented with onset of ST elevation within 12 hours were randomized in a double-blind manner to one of three adjunctive anticoagulation regimens, UFH, low-dose or high-dose bivalirudin. The primary endpoint of TIMI grade 3 flow occurred in 48% of patients in the high-dose bivalirudin group, 46% of those in the low-dose bivalirudin group, and 35% of those in the UFH group (UFH vs. bivalirudin groups; $P = 0.023$). There was no significant difference in the incidence of clinical efficacy events.

In the HERO-2 trial, bivalirudin and UFH were compared as adjunctive therapy to SK in patients with AMI. In the primary endpoint of mortality, there was no difference (10.8% with bivalirudin vs. 10.9% with heparin, $P = 0.85$), although the incidence of reinfarction was significantly lower in the bivalirudin groups ($P = 0.001$) (67).

Dose description of bivalirudin

The clinically recommended dose of bivalirudin was originally 1.0 mg/kg bolus followed by infusion at 2.5 mg/kg/hr for four hours. After the REPLACE-2 trial, the dose was reduced to 0.75 mg/kg bolus followed by an infusion of 1.75 mg/kg/hr for the duration of the PCI procedure, which is the dosage approved in the United States and Europe. The postprocedural infusion can be continued for up to four hours. It is recommended that ACT should be measured five minutes after bolus dosing, where ACT is expected to be 320 to 400 seconds, and a second bolus of 0.3 mg/kg should be administered if needed [if ACT is less than 225 seconds according to the EMEA Sm PC (68)]. Bivalirudin shows a linear correlation between the dose or plasma concentration and

---

Table 5   Clinical trials of bivalirudin in acute myocardial infarction with thrombolytics

Trial (reference)	Target population	Number of patients	Dose regimen	Results
HERO (66)	AMI with SK	412	Bivalirudin (0.125 mg/kg bolus + 0.25 mg/kg/hr infusion for 12 hr + 0.125 mg/kg/hr for 60 hr or 0.25 mg/kg bolus + 0.5 mg/kg/hr infusion for 12 hr + 0.25 mg/kg/hr for 60 hr) vs. UFH (5000 U bolus + 1000–1200 U/hr infusion for 60 hr)	Efficacy: significant benefit in TIMI3 flow in bivalirudin groups; safety: lower rate of major bleeding in bivalirudin groups
HERO-2 (67)	AMI with SK	17073	Bivalirudin (0.25 mg/kg bolus + 0.5 mg/kg/hr infusion for 12 hr and then, 0.25 mg/kg/hr for 36 hr) vs. UFH (5000 U bolus + 800–1000 U/hr infusion)	Efficacy: no difference; safety: no difference in rate of severe bleeding

Abbreviations: AMI, acute myocardial infarction; HERO, hirulog early reperfusion or occlusion; SK, streptokinase; TIMI, thrombolysis in myocardial infarction; UFH, unfractionated heparin.

anticoagulation (ACT) (69,70). From systematic review of the relationship between dose, ACT and the clinical effects of bivalirudin, an ACT of 300 seconds or more provides adequate anticoagulation; in other words, no increase in clinical benefit is obtained with higher ACT levels and the incidence of bleeding was independent of ACT levels (71). The infusion dose should be reduced and ACT should be carefully monitored in patients with renal impairment (68,72).

Hemorrhagic risk of DTIs vs. unfractionated heparin

The use of DTIs as adjunctive therapy to thrombolytics has been extensively studied in comparison with UFH. Therefore, the risk of bleeding of DTI versus UFH could be evaluated from the results of these trials conducted in a substantial number of patients.

The first trials with hirudin were terminated prematurely due to the high incidence of bleeding events (73–75). In the subsequent trials using a reduced dose of hirudin, the bleeding rate decreased to the level observed with UFH (54,76).

Bleeding rates were compared between DTIs and UFH in thrombolytic trials of AMI when DTIs exerted similar anticoagulant efficacy to UFH. Differences in bleed rates and 95% confidence intervals are shown in Figure 4. The difference in bleeding rate was significant in one of the bivalirudin trials (HERO). An absolute risk reduction of 13% was obtained in the HERO trial as the maximum and −0.2% in the HERO-2 trial as the minimum. Since the significant reduction of bleeding rate was not observed in the other eight trials, the bleeding risks of DTIs are said to be similar to those of UFH. To avoid unexpected bleeding events, monitoring of the drugs is necessary in the same manner as for UFH. Overall, these data show that the risk for bleeding with DTIs is no greater than that with UFH.

Alternative anticoagulant for heparin-induced thrombocytopenia patients undergoing percutaneous coronary intervention

PCI induces endothelial injury and plaque disruption, causing platelet activation, subsequent release of PF4 which is a heparin-induced antigen, thrombin generation, and an inflammatory response (Table 6). The addition of aspirin to UFH is used routinely to overwhelm the activation of platelets and the subsequently stimulated coagulation system. In a comparative trial between argatroban and UFH, inflammatory, hemostatic, and

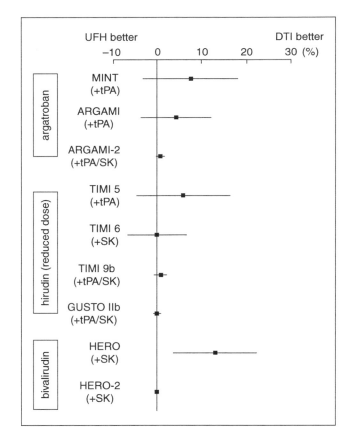

Figure 4

Bleeding rate difference between DTIs and unfractionated heparin (UFH) in nine thrombolytic trials of acute myocardial infarction. The difference in rate of major bleeding is shown when the DTI as an adjunctive therapy to thrombolytics showed similar efficacy to UFH. Aspirin was used to suppress activated platelet function in all trials. Black squares and bars indicate the point estimates and the intervals of 95% confidence of the rate differences in each trial. A different definition for bleeding classification was applied to the following trials: hemorrhagic stroke and hematoma greater than 5 cm in the ARGAMI trial and severe bleeding in the GUSTO IIb and HERO-2 trials. *Abbreviations*: ARGAMI, argatroban in acute myocardial infarction; DTI, direct thrombin inhibitor; HERO, hirulog early reperfusion or occlusion; GUSTO, Global Use of Stratigies to Open Occluded Coronary Arteries; SK, streptokinase; UFH, unfractionated protein.

endothelium-derived markers changed in patients with stable angina undergoing PCI. Both drugs had no effects on the PCI-induced inflammatory response, but argatroban appeared more effective in inhibiting thrombin and preventing antithrombin consumption during and after a PCI procedure (33).

In HIT patients undergoing PCI, combination of argatroban and aspirin was administered as an alternative to UFH and obtained reliable anticoagulation (77). Argatroban has been evaluated in three multicenter, open-label, prospective trials in 91 patients in a total of 112 procedures with or at risk for HIT undergoing PCI (25). In these studies, argatroban was administered as a bolus of 350 μg/kg followed by an infusion

Table 6 Alternative anticoagulants in percutaneous coronary intervention in heparin-induced thrombocytopenia

Drug	Dose regimen	Monitoring	Characteristics	Approved countries	Trial (reference)
Argatroban	350 μg/kg bolus + 25 μg/kg/min during procedure	Target ACT 300–450 sec	Low bleeding risk No antigenicity	US	ARG 216/310/311, n = 91 (76)
Hirudin	0.4 mg/kg bolus + 0.10–0.24 mg/kg/hr for 24 hr or/ + 0.04 mg/kg/hr for 24 hr	Target aPTT 60–100 sec	High bleeding risk Antibody formation (≈40%)	—	n = 25 (77)
Bivalirudin	0.75 mg/kg bolus + 1.75 mg/kg/hr for 4 hr during procedure	Target ACT 350 sec	Low bleeding risk Antibody formation (<1.0%)	US	ATBAT, n = 52 (78)

Abbreviations: ACT, activated clotting time; aPTT, activated partial thromboplastin time.

of 25 μg/kg/min, adjusted to achieve an ACT of 300 to 450 seconds. Argatroban was found to be a safe and effective anticoagulant in HIT patients undergoing PCI without a significant increase in bleeding. On this basis, argatroban was approved by the FDA as an anticoagulant for patients with or at risk for HIT undergoing PCI. When used in combination with GPIIb/IIIa inhibitors, the dose of argatroban was reduced to a bolus of 250 or 300 μg/kg followed by a 15 μg/kg/min infusion to target lower ACT of about 300 seconds in non-HIT patients (34). Strict monitoring by ACT is required to avoid unexpected overdose of argatroban in intensive-care patients with hepatorenal failure, especially after cardiac surgery.

Hirudin has been used for anticoagulation in non-HIT patients undergoing PCI treatment (50). The molecular structure of drug is completely different from UFH, and the drug does not stimulate generation of HIT antibodies. Although theoretically hirudin might be employed as an alternative to UFH, it has not been studied in HIT patients undergoing PCI, because of its higher incidence of bleeding. In a trial with 25 HIT patients who underwent PCI and were enrolled after platelet recovery to greater than 50,000/μL, the drug was clinically and angiographically efficacious (78). However, generation of antibodies against hirudin was detected in about half of the hirudin-treated patients after five days of treatment. The antibodies could interfere with anticoagulant activity of the drug. Again, strict monitoring is necessary to avoid unexpected bleeding complications.

Bivalirudin is indicated as an anticoagulant for HIT patients undergoing PCI (79). In the Anticoagulant Therapy with Bivalirudin to Assist in the Performance of Percutaneous Coronary Intervention in Patients with Heparin-Induced Thrombocytopenia (ATBAT) trial, 52 patients undergoing PCI with current or previous HIT were enrolled. These included high-risk patients such as those with an increased risk of ischemic and bleeding complications, a higher population of women, a majority of patients with prior MI, and 21% reported a history of HITTS. The bivalirudin treatment appeared safe, and 98% of patients undergoing PCI had a successful procedure. One patient had major bleeding. Two dose regimens, high and low dosages, were used. Despite the relatively small number of patients, this trial suggests that bivalirudin in high-risk patients with HIT undergoing PCI may be used safely and with a good effect. The lowdose, a bolus of 0.75 mg/kg followed by an infusion of 1.75 mg/kg/hr during a procedure, is the one recommended for this indication.

Conclusion

UFH has been a valuable therapeutic option for ACS. UFH remains unsurpassed by any drugs discovered within the last century, and the prevention and treatment of ACS are still achieved by routine use of heparin. For heparin anticoagulation, careful monitoring is required due to the individual variation in efficacy and the risk of bleeding. To achieve improved efficacy and safety of heparin, new drugs such as low-molecular weight heparins and DTIs have been introduced, and new drugs are continuously studied. It has been delineated that platelet activation and subsequent thrombin generation are pathogenic for thrombus formation in ACS, and the neutralization of thrombin is crucial not only for the treatment of ACS but also for a successful PCI procedure. Three DTIs, argatroban, hirudin, and bivalirudin, have been studied to explore if these are better treatments than UFH in ACS and PCI. In the trials of DTIs as adjunctive therapy to thrombolytics in AMI, it is suggested that hemorrhagic complications of DTIs would be less or at least have the same frequency as those of UFH. Now the DTIs are anticipated to be alternatives to UFH, but they are still unrecognized and not used as frequently as UFH in ACS.

HIT is the most avoidable adverse reaction in heparin anticoagulation, but it is not uncommon in clinical settings and is often unrecognized. Platelet activation induced by heparin/PF4 complex antibodies and subsequent thrombin generation play a central role in the pathophysiology of HIT, which result in thrombocytopenia and the thrombotic complications of HIT. Patients with HIT should be treated with an alternative anticoagulant to avoid potentially fatal thrombotic complications. DTIs have been used for the treatment of HIT. In particular, argatroban has been also recommended to substitute for heparin in HIT patients undergoing PCI. One of the advantages of argatroban is that it does not generate anti-bodies. The other two DTIs generate more or less antibodies, leading to intricate anticoagulant action, especially antibodies for lepirudin are considered to be relevant to anaphylactic shock. As the number of aged patients with ACS and/or undergoing PCI is increased, heparin exposure is repeated and it promotes the generation of HIT antibodies and subsequently develops to HIT. Risk for HIT by re-exposure to heparin should be given careful attention to in the current clinical settings.

References

1   Smith SC, Feldman TE, Hirshfeld JW, et al. ACC/AHA/SCAI 2005 guideline update for percutaneous coronary intervention. *Circulation* 2006; 113:166–286.

2   Silber S, Albertsson P, Aviles FF, et al. Guidelines for percutaneous coronary interventions. Eur Heart J 2005; 26:804–847.

3   Matsuo T, Tomaru T, Kario K, et al. Incidence of heparin-PF4 complex antibody formation and heparin-induced thrombocytopenia in acute coronary syndrome. Thromb Res 2005; 115:475–481.

4   Sakamoto S, Hirase T, Suzuki S, et al. Inhibitory effect of argatroban on thrombin-antithrombin III complex after percutaneous transluminal coronary angioplasty. Thromb Haemost 1995; 74:801–802.

5   Young E, Prins M, Levine MN, et al. Heparin binding to plasma proteins, an important mechanism for heparin resistance. Thromb Haemost 1992; 67:639–643.

6   Matsuo T, Kario K, Sakamoto S, et al. Hereditary heparin cofactor II deficiency and coronary artery disease. Thromb Res 1992; 65:495–505.

7   Kelton JG, Sheridan D, Santos A, et al. Heparin-induced thrombocytopenia: laboratory studies. Blood 1988; 72:925–930.

8   Jang IK, Hursting MJ. When heparins promote thrombosis: review of heparin-induced thrombocytopenia. Circulation 2005; 111:2671–2683.

9   Nikolsky E, Dangas GD. Percutaneous interventions in patients with immune-mediated heparin-induced thrombocytopenia. Semin Thromb Hemost 2004; 30:305–314.

10   Suzuki S, Koide M, Sakamoto S, et al. Early onset of immunological heparin-induced thrombocytopenia in acute myocardial infarction. Blood Coagul Fibrinoly 1997; 8:13–15.

11   Warkentin TE, Kelton JG. Temporal aspects of heparin-induced thrombocytopenia. N Engl J Med 2001; 344: 1286–1292.

12   Wallis DE, Workman DL, Lewis BE, et al. Failure of early heparin cessation as treatment for heparin-induced thrombocytopenia. Am J Med 1999; 106:629–635.

13   Suzuki S, Sakamoto S, Okada T, et al. Acute myocardial infarction caused by delayed heparin-induced thrombocytopenia and acute immunoreaction due to re-exposure to heparin in a systemic lupus erythematosus patient with HIT antibodies. Clin Appl Thromb Hemost 2003; 9:341–346.

14   Eika C. On the mechanism of platelet aggregation induced by heparin, protamine and polybrene. Scand J Haematol 1972; 9:248–257.

15   Matsuo T, Matsuo M, Kario K, et al. Characteristics of heparin-induced platelet aggregates in chronic hemodialysis with long-term heparin use. Haemostasis 2000; 30:249–257.

16   Xiao Z, Theroux P. Platelet activation with unfractionated heparin at therapeutic concentrations and comparisons with a low-molecular weight heparin and with a direct thrombin inhibitor. Circulation 1998; 97:251–256.

17   Badimon L, Badimon JJ. Interaction of Platelet Activation and Coagulation. Atherosclerosis and Coronary Artery Disease. Philadelphia: Lippincott-Raven, 1996:639–656.

18   Davie EW, Fujikawa K, Kisiel W. The coagulation cascade. Initiation, maintenance, and regulation. Biochemistry 1991; 30:10363–10370.

19   The Direct Thrombin Inhibitor Trialists' Collaborative Group. Direct thrombin inhibitors in acute coronary syndromes: principal results of a meta-analysis based on individual patients' data. Lancet 2002; 359:294–302.

20   Yeh RW, Jang IK. Argatroban: Update. Am Heart J 2006; 151:1131–1138.

21   Weitz JI, Bates ER. Direct thrombin inhibitors in cardiac disease. Cardiovasc Toxicol 2003; 3:13–25.

22   Eriksson BI, Dahl OE. Prevention of venous thromboembolism following orthopaedic surgery: clinical potential of direct thrombin inhibitors. Drugs 2004; 64:577–595.

23   Berry CN, Girardot C, Lecoffre C, et al. Effects of the synthetic thrombin inhibitor argatroban on fibrin- or clot-incorporated thrombin: comparison with heparin and recombinant Hirudin. Thromb Haemost 1994; 72:381–386.

24   Kawai H, Yamamoto T, Hara H, et al. Inhibition of factor Xa-induced platelet aggregation by a selective thrombin inhibitor, argatroban. Thromb Res 1994; 74:185–191.

25   Lewis BE, Matthai WH Jr, Cohen M, et al. Argatroban anticoagulation during percutaneous coronary intervention in patients with heparin-induced thrombocytopenia. Catheter Cardiovasc Interv 2002; 57:177–184.

26   Matsuo T, Kario K, Chikahira Y, et al. Treatment of heparin-induced thrombocytopenia by use of argatroban, a synthetic thrombin inhibitor. Br J Haematol 1992; 82:627–629.

27   Walenga JM, Ahmad S, Hoppensteadt D, et al. Argatroban therapy does not generate antibodies that alter its anticoagulant activity in patients with heparin-induced thrombocytopenia. Thromb Res 2002; 105:401–405.

28   Suzuki S, Sakamoto S, Koide M, et al. Effective anticoagulation by argatroban during immunoadsorption therapy for malignant rheumatoid arthritis with a high polymorphonuclear leukocyte elastase level. Thromb Res 1995; 80:93–98.

29   Kondo LM, Wittkowsky AK, Wiggins BS. Argatroban for prevention and treatment of thromboembolism in heparin-induced thrombocytopenia. Ann Pharmacother 2001; 35:440–451.

30   Tran JQ, Di Cicco RA, Sheth SB, et al. Assessment of the potential pharmacokinetic and pharmacodynamic interaction between erythromycin and argatroban. J Clin Pharmacol 1999; 39:513–519.

31   Swan SK, Hursting MJ. The pharmacokinetics and pharmacodynamics of argatroban: effects of age, gender, and hepatic or renal dysfunction. Pharmacotherapy 2000; 20:318–329.

32   Matsuo T, Yamada T, Yamanashi T, et al. Choice of anticoagulant in a congenital antithrombin III (AT-III)-deficient patient with chronic renal failure undergoing regular haemodialysis. Clin Lab Haematol 1989; 11:213–219.

33   Suzuki S, Matsuo T, Kobayashi H, et al. Antithrombotic treatment (argatroban vs. heparin) in coronary angioplasty in angina pectoris: effects on inflammatory, hemostatic, and endothelium-derived parameters. Thromb Res 2000; 98:269–279.

34   Jang IK, Lewis BE, Matthai WH Jr, et al. Argatroban anticoagulation in conjunction with glycoprotein IIb/IIIa inhibition in patients undergoing percutaneous coronary intervention: an open-label, nonrandomized pilot study. J Thromb Thrombolysis 2004; 18:31–37.

35   Jang IK, Brown DFM, Giugliano RP, et al. A multicenter, randomized study of argatroban versus heparin as adjunc to tissue plasminogen activator (TPA) in acute myocardial infarction: myocardial infarction with Novastan and TPA (MINT) study. J Am Coll Cardiol 1999; 33:1879–1885.

36   Vermeer F, Vahanian A, Fels PW, et al. Argatroban and alteplase in patients with acute myocardial infarction: the ARGAMI study. J Thromb Thrombolysis 2000; 10:233–240.

37   Behar S, Hod H, Kaplinsky E, et al. Argatroban versus heparin as adjuvant therapy to thrombolysis for acute myocardial infarction: safety considerations-ARGAMI-2 study. Circulation 1998; 98:I-453–I-454.

38   Lewis BE, Wallis DE, Berkowitz SD, et al. Argatroban anticoagulant therapy in patients with heparin-induced thrombocytopenia. Circulation 2001; 103:1838–1843.

39   Lewis BE, Wallis DE, Leya F, et al. Argatroban anticoagulation in patients with heparin-induced thrombocytopenia. Arch Intern Med 2003; 163:1849–1856.

40   Reichert MG, MacGregor DA, Kincaid EH, et al. Excessive argatroban anticoagulation for heparin-induced thrombocytopenia. Ann Pharmacother 2003; 37:652–654.

41   Kubiak DW, Szumita PM, Fanikos JR. Extensive prolongation of aPTT with argatroban in an elderly patient with improving renal function, normal hepatic enzymes, and metastatic lung cancer. Ann Pharmacother 2005; 39:1119–1123.

42   Miyata S. Editorial comment to "Heparin-induced thrombocytopenia and treatment with thrombin inhibitors". Jpn J Thromb Hemost 2005; 16:621–622.

43   Harder S, Graff J, Klinkhardt U, et al. Transition from argatroban to oral anticoagulation with phenprocoumon or acenocoumarol: effects on prothrombin time, activated partial thromboplastin time, and ecarin clotting time. Thromb Haemost 2004; 91:1137–1145.

44   Sheth SB, DiCicco RA, Hursting MJ, et al. Interpreting the International Normalized Ratio (INR) in individuals receiving argatroban and warfarin. Thromb Haemost 2001; 85:435–440.

45   Swan SK, St Peter JV, Lambrecht LJ, et al. Comparison of anticoagulant effects and safety of argatroban and heparin in healthy subjects. Pharmacotherapy 2000; 20:756–770.

46   Callas D, Fareed J. Comparative anticoagulant effects of various thrombin inhibitors, as determined in the ecarin clotting time method. Thromb Res 1996; 83:463–468.

47   Ahmad S, Ahsan A, Iqbal O, et al. Pharmacokinetics and pharmacodynamics of argatroban as studied by HPLC and functional methods: implications in the monitoring and dosage-optimizations in cardiovascular patients. Clin Appl Thromb Hemost 1998; 4:243–249.

48   Greinacher A, Volpel H, Janssens U, et al. Recombinant hirudin (Lepirudin) provides safe and effective anticoagulation in patients with heparin-induced thrombocytopenia. A prospective study. Circulation 1999; 99:73–80.

49   Greinacher A, Lubenow N, Eichler P. Anaphylactic and anaphylactoid reactions associated with lepirudin in patients with heparin-induced thrombocytopenia. Circulation 2003; 108:2062–2065.

50   Serruys PW, Herrman J-P, Simon R, et al. A comparison of hirudin with heparin in the prevention of restenosis after coronary angioplasty. N Engl J Med 1995; 333:757–763.

51   Cannon CP, McCabe CH, Henry TD, et al. A pilot trial of recombinant desulfatohirudin compared with heparin in conjunction with tissue-type plasminogen activator and aspirin for acute myocardial infarction: results of the thrombolysis in myocardial infarction (TIMI) 5 trial. J Am Coll Cardiol 1994; 23:993–1003.

52   TIMI 6 Investigators. Initial experience with hirudin and streptokinase in acute myocardial infarction: results of the thrombolysis in myocardial infarction (TIMI) 6 trial. Am J Cardiol 1995; 75:7–13.

53   Metz BK, White HD, Granger CB, et al. Randomized comparison of direct thrombin inhibition versus heparin in conjunction with fibrinolytic therapy for acute myocardial infarction: results from the GUSTO-IIb trial. J Am Coll Cardiol 1998; 31:1493–1498.

54   Antman EM for the TIMI 9b Investigators. Hirudin in acute myocardial infarction: thrombolysis and thrombin inhibition in myocardial infarction (TIMI) 9b trial. Circulation 1996; 94:911–921.

55   Lubenow N, Eichler P, Lietz T, et al. Lepirudin for prophylaxis of thrombosis in patients with acute isolated heparin-induced thrombocytopenia: an analysis of three prospective studies. Blood 2004; 104:3072–3077.

56   Zeymer U, von Essen R, Tebbe U, et al. Frequency of "optimal anticoagulation" for acute myocardial infarction after thrombolysis with front-loaded recombinant tissue-type plasminogen activator and conjunctive therapy with recombinant hirudin (HBW 023). ALKK Study Group. Am J Cardiol 1995; 76:997–1001.

57   Potzsch B, Hund S, Madlener K, et al. Monitoring of recombinant hirudin: assessment of a plasma-based ecarin clotting time assay. Thromb Res 1997; 86:373–383.

58   Bates SM, Weitz JI. Direct thrombin inhibitors for treatment of arterial thrombosis: potential difference between bivalirudin and hirudin. Am J Cardiol 1998; 82:P12–P18.

59 Shah PB, Popma JJ, Piana RN. Bivalirudin in percutaneous coronay interventions and acute coronary syndromes: new concepts, new directions. Curr Interv Cardiol Rep 1999; 1:346–358.

60 Eichler P, Lubenow N, Strobel U, et al. Antibodies against lepirudin are polyspecific and recognize epitopes on bivalirudin. Blood 2004; 103:613–616.

61 Topol EJ, Bonan R, Jewitt D, et al. Use of a direct antithrombin, Hirulog, in place of heparin during coronary angioplasty. Circulation 1993; 87:1622–1629.

62 Bittl JA, Strony J, Brinker JA, et al. Treatment with bivalirudin (Hirulog) as compared with heparin during coronary angioplasty for unstable angina or postinfarction angina. N Engl J Med 1995; 333:764–769.

63 Bittl JA, Chaitman BR, Feit f, et al. Bivalirudin versus heparin during coronary angioplasty for unstable or postinfarction angina: final report reanalysis of the Bivalirudin Angioplasty Study. Am Heart J 2001; 142:952–959.

64 Lincoff AM, Bittl JA, Harrington RA, et al. Bivalirudin and provisional glycoprotein IIb/IIIa blockade compared with heparin and planned glycoprotein IIb/IIIa blockade during percutaneous coronary intervention: REPLACE-2 randomized trial. JAMA 2003; 289:853–863.

65 Lincoff AM, Kleiman NS, Kereiakes DJ, et al. Long-term efficacy of bivalirudin and provisional glycoprotein IIb/IIIa blockade vs heparin and planned glycoprotein IIb/IIIa blockade during percutaneous coronary revascularization: REPLACE-2 randomized trial. JAMA 2004; 292:696–703.

66 White HD, Aylward PE, Frey MJ, et al. Randomized, double-blind comparison of Hirulog versus heparin in patients receiving streptokinase and aspirin for acute myocardial infarction (HERO). Circulation 1997; 96:2155–2161.

67 The Hirulog and Early Reperfusion or Occlusion (HERO) -2 Trial Investigators. Thrombin-specific anticoagulation with bivalirudin versus heparin in patients receiving fibrinolytic therapy for acute myocardial infarction: the HERO-2 randomised trial. Lancet 2001; 358:1855–1863.

68 Angiox: EMEA Summary of Product Characteristics. 2006 September.

69 Sciulli TM, Mauro VF. Pharmacology and clinical use of bivalirudin. Ann Pharmacother 2002; 36:1028–1041.

70 Reed MD, Bell D. Clinical pharmacology of bivalirudin. Pharmacotherapy 2002; 22(part2):105S–111S.

71 Lui HK. Dosage, pharmacological effects and clinical outcomes for bivalirudin in percutaneous coronary intervention. J Invasive Cardiol 2000; 12(suppl F):41F–52F.

72 The Medicines Company. Angiomax US label. 2005 December.

73 The Global Use of Strategies to Open Occluded Coronary Arteries (GUSTO IIa) Investigators. Randomized trial of intravenous heparin versus recombinant hirudin for acute coronary syndromes. Circulation 1994; 90:1631–1637.

74 Antman E for the TIMI 9A Investigators. Hirudin in acute myocardial infarction: safety report from the Thrombolysis and Thrombin Inhibition in Myocardial Infarction (TIMI) 9A Trial. Circulation 1994; 90:1624–1630.

75 Neuhaus KL, von Essen R, Tebbe U, et al. Safety observations from the pilot phase of the randomized r-hirudin for improvement of thrombolysis (HIT-III) study. Circulation 1994; 90:1638–1642.

76 GUSTO II b Investigators. A comparison of recombinant hirudin with heparin for the treatment of acute coronary syndromes. N Engl J Med 1996; 335:775–782.

77 Suzuki S, Sakamoto S, Koide M, et al. Effective anticoagulation by argatroban during coronary stent implantation in a patient with heparin-induced thrombocytopenia. Thromb Res 1997; 88:499–502.

78 Cochran K, DeMartini TJ, Lewis BE, et al. Use of lepirudin during percutaneous vascular interventions in patients with heparin-induced thrombocytopenia. J Invas Cardiol 2003; 15: 617–621.

79 Mahaffey KW, Lewis BE, Wildermann NM, et al. The anticoagulant therapy with bivalirudin to assist in the performance of percutaneous coronary intervention in patients with heparin-induced thrombocytopenia (ATBAT) study: main results. J Invasive Cardiol 2003; 15:611–616.

80 Pifarre R, Scanlon PJ. Evidence-Based Management of the Acute Coronary Syndrome. Philadelphia: Hanley & Belfus, 2001:132.

9

Oral antithrombin drugs

Brigitte Kaiser

Introduction

Improved understanding of the molecular mechanisms of blood coagulation has led to the development of new anticoagulants for the prevention and treatment of thromboembolic disorders in order to overcome the limitations of existing anticoagulants. These limitations include the need for coagulation monitoring and subsequent dose adjustment for vitamin K antagonists (Table 1), the difficulty of continuing prophylaxis out of hospital due to require parenteral administration for heparins, and the risk of heparin-induced thrombocytopenia (1). Various new anticoagulants target specific coagulation enzymes or different steps in the coagulation cascade, that is, the initiation of coagulation by factor VIIa/tissue factor (FVIIa/TF), its propagation by factors IXa, Xa and their cofactors, and the thrombin-mediated fibrin formation (2). The serine proteinase thrombin is the central enzyme in the coagulation pathway. It catalyzes the conversion of fibrinogen to fibrin by cleaving the peptide bond between arginine and glycine in the fibrinogen sequence Gly-Val-Arg-Gly-Pro-Arg, activates the factors V, VIII, and XIII, and strongly stimulates platelet aggregation. Besides its procoagulant activities, thrombin also exhibits anticoagulant properties via the activation of the protein C pathway. Because of its pivotal role in the coagulation process, thrombin has been a target for the development of specific and selective inhibitors for many years (3). Intensive structure-based design over the last 20 years resulted in the development of numerous direct thrombin inhibitors (TIs), most of which have been peptidomimetic compounds that mimic the fibrinogen sequence interacting with the active site of thrombin (4). The new TIs bind directly to thrombin and block its interaction with different thrombin substrates. At present, the most important TIs that have been extensively evaluated for clinical use are the bivalent inhibitors, hirudin and bivalirudin, which interact with both the active site and the exosite-1 of thrombin in an irreversible and reversible manner,

respectively, as well as argatroban, which reversibly binds to the active site. Unfortunately because of their chemical structures, these new agents are not sufficiently absorbed after oral administration and have to be administered parenterally. Thus, they are less suitable for long-term anticoagulation. The development of orally effective, direct TIs seems to be a promising alternative to the existing direct or indirect anticoagulants for long-term use in patients with thromboembolic disorders. However, the design of those new drugs is difficult because different physicochemical properties are required for either the binding of a compound to the active site of thrombin or its absorption from the gastrointestinal tract (5). At present, various oral direct TIs are reported to be under development, of which ximelagatran and dabigatran etexilate are in a more advanced stage of clinical development (6,7).

Ximelagatran

Chemistry

Ximelagatran (Exanta®) was the first oral TI and the first new oral anticoagulant to become available since the development of warfarin more than 50 years ago. Ximelagatran is a prodrug of the small-molecule noncovalent tripeptidomimetic direct TI melagatran, which mimics the D-Phe-Pro-Arg sequence. Melagatran has a strong basic amidine structure, a free carboxylic acid, and, in addition, a less basic amine function, implying that it will be positively charged under physiological conditions, and thus it exhibits poor bioavailability and absorption upon oral dosing. Chemical modification of the melagatran molecule by N-hydroxylation at the amidine function and inclusion of an ethyl group at the carboxylic acid structure leads to the development of the double prodrug ximelagatran (Fig. 1). Ximelagatran is 170 times more

Table 1 Comparison of vitamin K antagonists (warfarin sodium) with oral direct thrombin inhibitors (melagatran/ximelagatran)

Warfarin sodium	Melagatran/Ximelagatran
Reduces synthesis of clotting factors (II, VII, IX, and X, protein C and S)	Targeted specificity for thrombin; direct competitive and reversible inhibition of both free and clot-bound thrombin
Slow onset and offset of action	Rapid onset of action, rapid reversal of thrombin inhibition after cessation of therapy (dependent on plasma concentration and elimination half-life)
Large interindividual dosing differences	Predictable and reproducible pharmacokinetic and pharmacodynamic profile
Multiple drug and food interactions	No interactions with food and alcohol, only low potential for drug interactions
Individual dose adjustment required	Use of fixed-dose regimens, no dose adjustment
Need for frequent and careful monitoring	No routine monitoring of the anticoagulant effect; control of liver enzymes at long-term therapy
Reversal of anticoagulation with vitamin K or with plasma or clotting factors replacement	No antidote available
Once daily oral administration	Twice daily oral administration

lipophilic than melagatran and uncharged at intestinal pH, resulting in a much better penetration of the gastrointestinal barrier, and thus an increased bioavailability (8–10). Melagatran binds rapidly, reversibly, and competitively to the active site of thrombin with a K_i value of 0.002 μmol/L. It has a high selectivity for α-thrombin; except for trypsin, the K_i value for thrombin is at least 300-fold lower than for other serine proteases involved in blood coagulation and fibrinolysis (11).

Pharmacodynamics

Melagatran inhibits both thrombin activity and its generation and it effectively inactivates free and clot-bound thrombin with similar high potency (8,12–16). Using routine coagulation assays, clotting times in human plasma are prolonged to twice the control value at low concentrations of melagatran, that is, at 0.010, 0.59, and 2.2 μmol/L for thrombin time, activated partial thromboplastin time, and prothrombin time, respectively. The IC_{50} value for thrombin-induced platelet aggregation is 0.002 μmol/L. Inhibition of fibrinolysis is not observed at concentrations below the upper limit of the proposed therapeutic concentration interval (<0.5 μmol/L) (11). The antithrombotic effectiveness of ximelagatran was demonstrated in different species using experimental models of venous (9,17,18) and arterial (16,19–22) thromboembolism, as an adjunct in coronary artery thrombolysis (23), and in animal models of disseminated intravascular coagulation (24). In healthy volunteers, melagatran was effective in

inhibiting thrombus formation at low and high shear rates in an ex vivo model of human arterial thrombosis (25). In experimental models, ximelagatran was at least as effective as warfarin in the prevention of thrombus formation, but with a wider separation between antithrombotic effects and bleeding (7,21).

Pharmacokinetics

Studies on the pharmacokinetic behavior of ximelagatran and melagatran have been carried out in animal species (26), as well as in healthy volunteers (26,27), orthopedic surgery patients (28,29), patients with deep venous thrombosis (DVT) (30), and volunteers with severe renal impairment (31) and mild-to-moderate hepatic impairment (32). After oral administration, ximelagatran is rapidly absorbed from the small intestine and undergoes rapid biotransformation to the active agent melagatran. The absorption of ximelagatran is at least 40% to 70% in rats, dogs, and humans, whereas the bioavailability of melagatran following oral administration of ximelagatran is 5% to 10% in rats, 10% to 50% in dogs, and about 20% in humans. The reason for the lower bioavailability of melagatran is a first-pass metabolism of ximelagatran with subsequent biliary excretion of the formed metabolites (26). After absorption, ximelagatran is rapidly bioconverted to its active form melagatran via two minor intermediates, that is, ethyl-melagatran, which is formed by reduction of the hydroxyamidine, and N-hydroxy-melagatran, which is formed by hydrolysis of the ethyl ester. Both intermediates

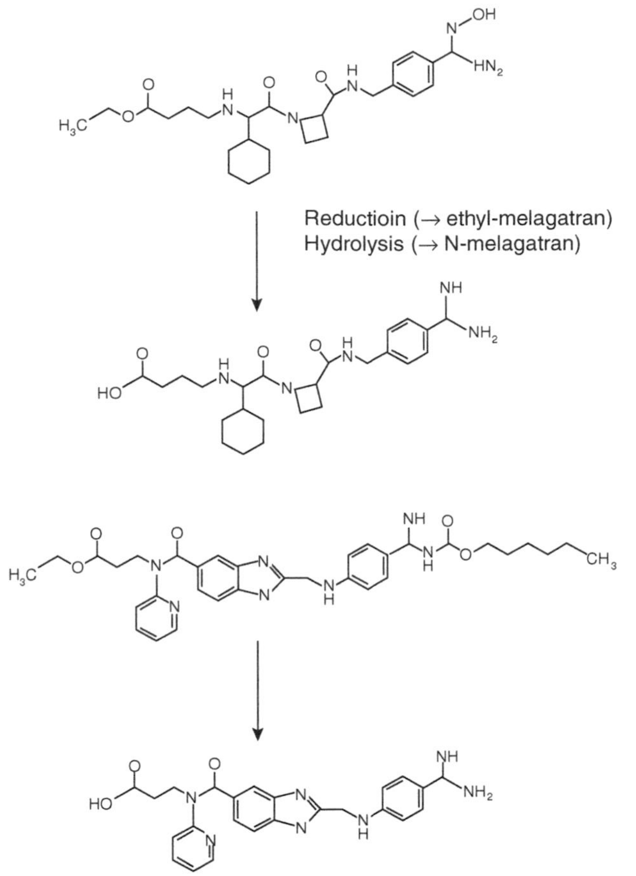

Figure 1
Chemical structures of the thrombin inhibitors, melagatran and dabigatran, and their orally effective prodrugs, ximelagatran and dabigatran etexilate. *Source*: From Refs. 4, 26, 33, 68.

are subsequently metabolized to melagatran. Ethyl-melagatran is an active metabolite but due to its low plasma concentration, it unlikely contributes to the anticoagulant action of ximelagatran (9,26,27). Biotransformation of ximelagatran and its intermediates is catalyzed by several enzyme systems located in microsomes and mitochondria of liver, kidney, and other organs (33).

Intravenously injected melagatran has a relatively low plasma clearance, a small volume of distribution, and a short elimination half-life. Its oral absorption is low and highly variable. In contrast, ximelagatran is rapidly absorbed after oral administration and then metabolized to melagatran. The plasma concentration of melagatran after oral dosing with ximelagatran declines in a mono-exponential manner with a plasma half-life of four to five hours. Melagatran is primarily excreted unchanged in urine; the renal clearance correlates well with the glomerular filtration rate (Table 2). Only trace amounts of ximelagatran are renally excreted; the major compound in urine and feces is melagatran. In feces of all species, appreciable quantities of ethyl-melagatran are recovered, suggesting a reduction of the hydroxyamidine group of ximelagatran in the gastrointestinal tract (26). In contrast to vitamin K antagonists, the potential of melagatran for drug–drug interactions is very low (34–36). Pharmacokinetic interactions between melagatran and various other drugs mediated via the most common drug-metabolizing

enzymes of the CYP 450 system have not been observed (37). Concomitant intake of food or alcohol does not alter the bioavailability of melagatran which also shows only low inter- and intraindividual variability (38–40). The pharmacokinetic/pharmacodynamic profile of ximelagatran and its active form melagatran is consistent across a broad range of different patient populations and is unaffected by gender, age, body weight, ethnic origin, obesity, and mild-to-moderate hepatic impairment (39,41–43). In patients with severe renal impairment, excretion of melagatran is delayed, resulting in longer half-life, increased plasma concentrations, and stronger and prolonged anticoagulation (31). Mild-to-moderate hepatic impairment has no influence on the pharmacokinetics and pharmacodynamics of melagatran, thus requiring no dose adjustment in those patients (32). After oral administration, neither ximelagatran nor its two intermediates and only trace amounts of melagatran were detected in milk of breastfeeding women (44).

Clinical studies

Oral direct TIs have a promising role in the management of venous thromboembolism and other associated medical conditions (3,7,45–48). Ximelagatran has been successfully

Table 2   Pharmacokinetic parameters of melagatran after oral administration of ximelagatran in various species

	Human	Rat	Dog
Oral dose of ximelagatran[a]	50 mg (105 μmol)	40 μmol/kg	40 μmol/kg
Oral absorption in all species			
Melagatran		Low and highly variable 40–70%	
Ximelagatran			
Bioavailability (%)	19 ± 6	13 ± 3	50 ± 13
Maximum melagatran plasma concentration (C_{max}) (μmol/L)	0.36 ± 0.03	2.16 ± 0.22	15.9 ± 5.0
Time to reach C_{max} (t_{max}) (hr)	1.85 ± 0.78	0.80 ± 0.27	1.13 ± 0.6
Elimination half-life ($t_{1/2}$) (hr)[b]	3.6 ± 0.7	1.4 ± 0.4	11 ± 3
Elimination half-life ($t_{1/2}$) (hr)[c]	1.6 ± 0.2	0.4 ± 0.03	1.2 ± 0.2
Plasma clearance[c]	145 ± 15 mL/min	15.8 ± 2.1 mL/min/kg	7.0 ± 1.0 mL/min/kg
Volume at distribution (V_{ss})[c]	17.3 ± 1.7 L	0.37 ± 0.02 L/kg	0.36 ± 0.04 L/kg
Renal clearance	120 mL/min	23.1 mL/min/kg	4.37 mL/min/kg
Excretion of melagatran (%)[c]			
Urine	82.6 ± 3.9	65.9 ± 3.5	42.5 ± 7.8
Feces	5.7 ± 2.2	24.3 ± 4.3	38.9 ± 15.5
Excretion of ximelagatran (%)[b]			
Urine	25.2 ± 4.3	21.3 ± 1.9	22.6 ± 2.4
Feces	71.1 ± 4.5	71.3 ± 1.1	66.9 ± 3.1

[a]$n = 5$ for humans and rats; $n = 4$ for dogs.
[b]Measured after oral administration at the aforementioned doses.
[c]Measured after IV administration of melagatran at 2.3 mg (5.3 μmol) in humans and 2 μmol/kg in dogs and male rats.
Source: From Ref. 26.

studied in large phase III trials in various clinical settings (49–52). Based on its predictable pharmacokinetic and pharmacodynamic properties without significant time- and dose-dependencies, ximelagatran can usually be administered in fixed doses without the need for individualized dosing or coagulation monitoring. Ximelagatran is effective and well-tolerated for the prevention of venous thromboembolism in high-risk orthopedic patients after hip and knee replacement surgery (EXPRESS = EXpanded PRophylaxis Evaluation Surgery Study; EXULT = EXanta Used to Lessen Thrombosis; METHRO = MElagatran for THRombin inhibition in Orthopedic surgery) (29,53–56). Ximelagatran is also effective in the acute treatment of venous thromboembolism and long-term secondary prevention of recurrent venous thromboembolism (THRIVE = THRombin Inhibitor in Venous thromboEmbolism) (57–59), for the prevention of stroke in patients with nonvalvular atrial fibrillation (SPORTIF = Stroke Prevention using an ORal Thrombin Inhibitor in atrial Fibrillation) (60–64), and in the prevention of

major cardiovascular events after myocardial infarction (ESTEEM = Efficacy and Safety of the oral Thrombin inhibitor ximelagatran in combination with aspirin, in patiEnts with rEcent Myocardial damage) (65). A survey of the phase III clinical trials with ximelagatran is given in Table 3. The different clinical trials demonstrated at least comparable efficacy of ximelagatran and warfarin; in terms of prevention of primary events, bleeding, and mortality, the oral TI may offer a promising alternative to the vitamin K antagonist. Together with the convenience of fixed oral dosing and the consistent and predictable anticoagulation, with no need for coagulation monitoring, ximelagatran has a great potential as a new option for long-term prophylaxis and therapy of thromboembolic disorders.

Although clinical trials indicated that ximelagatran can potentially be used in clinical indications, the Food and Drug Administration recently refused to approve ximelagatran over concerns about liver toxicity. In clinical trials, in 6% to 10% of patients, raised aminotransferase levels were observed during

Table 3 Clinical phase III trials with ximelagatran

Study	Indication	Study design	Interventions		Number of patients		Reference
			Ximelagatran	Control	Ximelagatran	Control	
SPORTIF III	Stroke prevention in nonvalvular atrial fibrillation	Open-label	36 mg twice daily for at least 12 months	Warfarin, target INR. 2.0–3.0	1704	1703	(60,83)
SPORTIF V	Stroke prevention in nonvalvular atrial fibrillation	Double-blind	36 mg twice daily for at least 12 months	Warfarin, target INR. 2.0–3.0	1960	1962	(61,83)
THRIVE II and IV	Acute therapy for proximal DVT	Randomized double-blind	36 mg twice daily for 6 months	Enoxaparin (1 mg/kg s.c. twice daily) + warfarin (INR. 2.0–3.0)	1240	1249	(57)
THRIVE III	Extended secondary prevention of DVT	Randomized double-blind	24 mg twice daily for 18 months	Placebo for 18 months	612	611	(58,59,84)
METHRO III	Hip and knee replacement	Randomized double-blind	Melagatran 3 mg s.c. 4–12 hrs after surgery; then ximelagatran 24 mg twice daily for 8–11 days	Enoxaparin 40 mg s.c. once daily for 8–11 days starting 12 hrs before surgery	1399	1389	(54)
EXPRESS	Hip and knee replacement	Randomized double-blind	Melagatran 2 mg s.c. immediately before surgery. melagatran 3 mg s.c. 8 hrs after surgery, then ximelagatran 24 mg twice daily	Enoxaparin 40 mg s.c. once daily for 8–11 days starting 12 hrs before surgery	1410	1425	(53)
EXULT A	Knee replacement	Randomized double-blind	Ximelagatran 24 mg or 36 mg twice daily for 7–12 days, initiated 12 hr after surgery	Warfarin initiated evening after surgery and adjusted to INR 2.5	614 (24 mg), 629 (36 mg)	608	(56)
EXULT B	Knee replacement	Randomized double-blind	Ximelagatran 24 mg or 36 mg twice daily for 7–12 days, initiated morning after surgery	Warfarin initiated evening after surgery and adjusted to INR 2.5	1151	1148	(85)

Note: SPORTIF II and IV, THRIVE I, METHRO I, METHRO II, and ESTEEM were dose-guiding studies.

Abbreviations: DVT, deep venous thrombosis; ESTEEM. Efficacy and Safety of the oral Thrombin inhibitor ximelagatran in combination with aspirin. in patiEnts with rEcent Myocardial damage: EXPRESS. EXpanded PRophylaxis Evaluation Surgery Study; EXULT. EXanta Used to Lessen Thrombosis; INR. international normalized ratio; s.c.. subcutaneous; METHRO. MElagatran for THRombin inhibition in Orthopedic surgery; SPORTIF. Stroke Prevention using an ORal Thrombin Inhibitor in atrial Fibrillation; THRIVE. THRombin Inhibitor in Venous thromboEmbolism.

Source: From Refs. 29, 55, 63, 65, 86.

long-term use (>35 days) of ximelagatran. The increase in levels of alanine aminotransferase (more than three-fold over the upper level of normal) occurred one to six months after initiation of therapy, but in 96% of patients, recovery was confirmed regardless of continuation of therapy or not (66). Although the true clinical significance of these findings remains unclear at this time, it likely requires regular liver function monitoring. Furthermore, because melagatran is renally eliminated, dose adjustment will be required in patients with renal impairment. Finally, there is no known antidote for the reversal of ximelagatran's effect, though it is much shorter-acting than warfarin (67).

Dabigatran etexilate

Dabigatran etexilate is another promising oral TI which is being evaluated in experimental and clinical studies, although the presently available data are still limited and not as comprehensive as for ximelagatran and its active form melagatran.

Chemistry, pharmacodynamics, and pharmacokinetics

Dabigatran etexilate (BIBR 1048) is the orally active double prodrug of the small molecule, direct TI dabigatran (BIBR 953 ZW) (Fig. 1). Dabigatran belongs to a new structural class of nonpeptidic inhibitors employing a trisubstituted benzimidazole as the central scaffold and 4-amidinophenylalanine as a mimetic of arginine (68). Dabigatran is a specific, competitive, and reversible inhibitor of thrombin which exhibits a strong thrombin inhibitory activity (K_i = 4.5 nM), as well as a high selectivity to thrombin; the K_i value for other serine proteases except trypsin (K_i = 50 nM) is at least 400-fold higher (68). Dabigatran also shows a favorable activity profile in vivo, following intravenous administration into rats. Because of its highly polar, zwitterionic nature, its oral absorption is insufficient. From a number of synthesized prodrugs, dabigatran etexilate exhibited strong and long-lasting anticoagulant effects after oral administration into different animal species, and thus was chosen for clinical development (68).

After oral administration, dabigatran etexilate is rapidly converted to dabigatran. In healthy volunteers, dabigatran was well-tolerated and primarily renally excreted. The absolute oral bioavailability of dabigatran etexilate is not reported, but urinary excretion of dabigatran amounted to 3.5% to 5%. This indicates a low oral bioavailability, as 80% of dabigatran is cleared renally (7). Cytochrome P450 isoenzymes are not involved in the metabolism of dabigatran and the compound neither induces nor inhibits cytochrome P450 isoenzyme

activity. Dabigatran is conjugated to activated glucuronic acid to form an acylglucuronide conjugate (69). Following oral administration of dabigatran etexilate in healthy volunteers, the median time to reach maximum concentration (t_{max}) was 2 hours and the mean terminal half-life ($t_{1/2}$) was 8.7 hours. Coadministration of food delayed the absorption with increasing t_{max} to four hours. In the majority of patients undergoing total hip replacement, dabigatran etexilate was also well-tolerated and adequately absorbed. However, there was a high interindividual variability in the AUC (area under the plasma concentration–time curve), C_{max} (maximum plasma concentration), and t_{max} (median t_{max} six hours) (69).

Clinical studies

An open-label, dose-escalating safety study, BISTRO I, was conducted in 314 patients with total hip replacement surgery. Dabigatran etexilate was given orally at doses from 12.5 to 300 mg twice daily or 150 and 300 mg once daily administered 4 to 8 hours after surgery for 6 to 10 days. The TI demonstrated an acceptable safety profile with a therapeutic window above 12.5 mg and below 300 mg twice daily, as well as a satisfactory antithrombotic potential. Only two patients with reduced renal clearance suffered bleeding from multiple sites at the highest dose (70). The dose-dependent effectiveness and safety of dabigatran etexilate was also demonstrated in the BISTRO II study, a double-blind study in patients undergoing total hip or knee replacement. Dabigatran etexilate given at doses of 50, 150, and 225 mg twice daily or 300 mg once daily starting 1 to 4 hours after surgery and continuing for 6 to 10 days was compared to enoxaparin 40 mg subcutaneous (s.c.) once daily starting 12 hours prior to surgery (71). At present, various phase II and phase III clinical trials with oral dabigatran etexilate are mainly in the stage of recruiting patients (72). The different studies will investigate the (i) efficacy and safety of three doses of dabigatran etexilate in preventing venous thromboembolism in patients with total knee replacement surgery (placebo controlled), administered 11 to 14 days postoperatively; (ii) dabigatran etexilate as long-term anticoagulant therapy for stroke and systemic embolism prevention in patients with nonvalvular atrial fibrillation (RE-LY study, two blinded doses of dabigatran etexilate with open-label warfarin); (iii) efficacy and safety of two different dabigatran etexilate dose regimens compared to enoxaparin (30 mg sc twice daily) in patients with primary elective total knee replacement surgery; (iv) efficacy and safety of two different dose regimens of dabigatran etexilate compared to enoxaparin (40 mg once daily) for 6 to 10 days in the prevention of venous thromboembolism in patients with total knee replacement surgery (RE-MODEL) and for 28 to 35 days in patients with total hip replacement surgery (RE-NOVATE). The PETRO Extension Trial (PETRO-Ex) is a follow-up treatment study of patients with atrial fibrillation who have been previously treated with BIBR 1048.

Other direct oral thrombin inhibitors

Current pharmaceutical research is focused on the design of novel anticoagulants with improved pharmacologic and clinical profiles that offer benefits over traditional therapies. Specific progress has been made in the development of small molecule factor Xa and TIs that are characterized by a predictable pharmacological profile, oral formulation, and decreased need for coagulation monitoring. Most of the newly developed oral TI are in a less advanced stage of development; they are mainly undergoing preclinical testing, and some compounds are in phase I clinical trials (73). The potential role of many of the new inhibitors as clinically useful antithrombotic agents still remains to be evaluated.

Clinical indications for oral thrombin inhibitors

Clinical studies with oral direct TIs demonstrated that these drugs are effective and promising agents for the prevention and therapy of various thromboembolic disorders. The simplicity of drug administration and their benefits over established therapeutic strategies suggest that they will find increasing use in clinical practice for various indications (2,3,7,45,74).

Patients undergoing major orthopedic surgery, such as total hip or knee replacement, are at high risk of venous thromboembolism. DVT may lead to life-threatening pulmonary embolism, disabling morbidity in the form of the post-thrombotic syndrome, and risk of recurrent thrombotic events. Oral direct TIs are expected to represent an effective, safer, and/or more convenient alternative to vitamin K antagonists, low molecular weight heparins, or unfractionated heparin for the prevention of venous thrombosis after major orthopedic surgery, as well as for acute therapy and secondary prevention of DVT (47,75–77).

Atrial fibrillation is increasing in incidence in developed countries and, because of the risk of embolic stroke, most patients require continuous anticoagulation. A large number of patients with atrial fibrillation are currently treated with vitamin K antagonists. Results of clinical trials in patients with atrial fibrillation indicate that oral direct TIs may become potential drugs for the prevention of embolic stroke and may replace warfarin (62,78,79–81).

Patients with acute coronary syndromes such as acute myocardial infarction and unstable angina remain at risk for recurrent myocardial ischemia despite therapy with antiplatelet agents and heparin. Although first clinical trials indicate a possible use of oral direct TIs for the prevention of cardiovascular events in patients after acute myocardial infarction, the presently available data are still limited and it has not yet been demonstrated that oral TIs are more efficacious and safer for long-term use after acute coronary syndromes than the established drugs (48,82).

Conclusions

The central position of thrombin in the coagulation cascade has made it a popular target for the discovery of novel antithrombotic agents, and several direct TIs are currently under development or even in clinical use for certain indications. The ultimate goal of most research program and drug optimization strategies is to develop an oral anticoagulant that overcomes the interactions, safety concerns, and the need for monitoring that limits the use of vitamin K antagonists. Structure-based design resulted in the development of orally bioavailable, small-molecule, direct TIs; among them, ximelagatran and dabigatran etexilate are the furthest along in clinical development. Although highly effective as an anticoagulant and safe with regard to bleeding, ximelagatran has been associated with liver function abnormalities the importance of which needs resolution. Dabigatran etexilate is much earlier in development and is currently of unproven value. A number of other oral direct serine proteinase inhibitors with distinct pharmacological profiles are presently undergoing preclinical and clinical testing and it is highly likely that alternatives to conventional anticoagulants and especially to warfarin will be available in the near future.

References

1   Hawkins D. Limitations of traditional anticoagulants. Pharmacotherapy 2004; 24:62S–65S.

2   Hirsh J, O'Donnell M, Weitz JI. New anticoagulants. Blood 2005; 105:453–463.

3   Gurm HS, Bhatt DL. Thrombin, an ideal target for pharmacological inhibition: a review of direct thrombin inhibitors. Am Heart J 2005; 149:S43–S53.

4   Kikelj D. Peptidomimetic thrombin inhibitors. Pathophysiol Haemost Thromb 2003; 33:487–491.

5   Hauptmann J, Sturzebecher J. Synthetic inhibitors of thrombin and factor Xa: from bench to bedside. Thromb Res 1999; 93:203–241.

6   Nutescu EA, Shapiro NL, Chevalier A, et al. A pharmacologic overview of current and emerging anticoagulants. Cleve Clin J Med 2005; 72(suppl 1):S2–S6.

7   Gustafsson D. Oral direct thrombin inhibitors in clinical development. J Intern Med 2003; 254:322–334.

8   Gustafsson D, Elg M. The pharmacodynamics and pharmacokinetics of the oral direct thrombin inhibitor ximelagatran and its active metabolite melagatran: a mini-review. Thromb Res 2003; 109(suppl 1):S9–S15.

9   Gustafsson D, Nystrom J, Carlsson S, et al. The direct thrombin inhibitor melagatran and its oral prodrug H 376/95:

intestinal absorption properties, biochemical and pharmacodynamic effects. Thromb Res 2001; 101:171–181.

10 Crowther MA, Weitz JI. Ximelagatran: the first oral direct thrombin inhibitor. Expert Opin Investig Drugs 2004; 13:403–413.

11 Gustafsson D, Antonsson T, Bylund R, et al. Effects of melagatran, a new low-molecular-weight thrombin inhibitor, on thrombin and fibrinolytic enzymes. Thromb Haemost 1998; 79:110–118.

12 Bostrom SL, Dagnelid E, Hansson GF, et al. Inhibition of thrombin-induced feedback activation of factor V: a potential pathway for inhibition of thrombin generation by melagatran. Blood Coagul Fibrinolysis 2004; 15:25–30.

13 Bostrom SL, Hansson GF, Kjaer M, et al. Effects of melagatran, the active form of the oral direct thrombin inhibitor ximelagatran, and dalteparin on the endogenous thrombin potential in venous blood from healthy male subjects. Blood Coagul Fibrinolysis 2003; 14:457–462.

14 Bostrom SL, Hansson GF, Sarich TC, et al. The inhibitory effect of melagatran, the active form of the oral direct thrombin inhibitor ximelagatran, compared with enoxaparin and r-hirudin on ex vivo thrombin generation in human plasma. Thromb Res 2004; 113:85–91.

15 Sarich TC, Wolzt M, Eriksson UG, et al. Effects of ximelagatran, an oral direct thrombin inhibitor, r-hirudin and enoxaparin on thrombin generation and platelet activation in healthy male subjects. J Am Coll Cardiol 2003; 41:557–564.

16 Mattsson C, Sarich TC, Carlsson SC. Mechanism of action of the oral direct thrombin inhibitor ximelagatran. Semin Vasc Med 2005; 5:235–244.

17 Carlsson S, Elg M, Mattsson C. Effects of ximelagatran, the oral form of melagatran, in the treatment of caval vein thrombosis in conscious rats. Thromb Res 2002; 107:163–168.

18 Carlsson S, Elg M. The effects of ximelagatran and warfarin on the prophylaxis of a caval vein thrombosis and bleeding in the anaesthetized rat. Blood Coagul Fibrinolysis 2005; 16:245–249.

19 Mehta JL, Chen L, Nichols WW, et al. Melagatran, an oral active-site inhibitor of thrombin, prevents or delays formation of electrically induced occlusive thrombus in the canine coronary artery. J Cardiovasc Pharmacol 1998; 31:345–351.

20 Schersten F, Wahlund G, Bjornheden T, et al. Melagatran attenuates fibrin and platelet deposition in a porcine coronary artery over-stretch injury model. Blood Coagul Fibrinolysis 2003; 14:235–241.

21 Elg M, Gustafsson D, Carlsson S. Antithrombotic effects and bleeding time of thrombin inhibitors and warfarin in the rat. Thromb Res 1999; 94:187–197.

22 Klement P, Carlsson S, Rak J, et al. The benefit-to-risk profile of melagatran is superior to that of hirudin in a rabbit arterial thrombosis prevention and bleeding model. J Thromb Haemost 2003; 1:587–594.

23 Mattsson C, Bjorkman JA, Abrahamsson T, et al. Local proCPU (TAFI) activation during thrombolytic treatment in a dog model of coronary artery thrombosis can be inhibited with a direct, small molecule thrombin inhibitor (melagatran). Thromb Haemost 2002; 87:557–562.

24 Elg M, Gustafsson D. A combination of a thrombin inhibitor and dexamethasone prevents the development of experimental disseminated intravascular coagulation in rats. Thromb Res 2006; 117:429–437.

25 Sarich TC, Osende JI, Eriksson UG, et al. Acute antithrombotic effects of ximelagatran, an oral direct thrombin inhibitor, and r-hirudin in a human ex vivo model of arterial thrombosis. J Thromb Haemost 2003; 1:999–1004.

26 Eriksson UG, Bredberg U, Hoffmann KJ, et al. Absorption, distribution, metabolism, and excretion of ximelagatran, an oral direct thrombin inhibitor, in rats, dogs, and humans. Drug Metab Dispos 2003; 31:294–305.

27 Eriksson UG, Bredberg U, Gislen K, et al. Pharmacokinetics and pharmacodynamics of ximelagatran, a novel oral direct thrombin inhibitor, in young healthy male subjects. Eur J Clin Pharmacol 2003; 59:35–43.

28 Eriksson UG, Mandema JW, Karlsson MO, et al. Pharmacokinetics of melagatran and the effect on ex vivo coagulation time in orthopaedic surgery patients receiving subcutaneous melagatran and oral ximelagatran: a population model analysis. Clin Pharmacokinet 2003; 42:687–701.

29 Eriksson BI, Arfwidsson AC, Frison L, et al. A dose-ranging study of the oral direct thrombin inhibitor, ximelagatran, and its subcutaneous form, melagatran, compared with dalteparin in the prophylaxis of thromboembolism after hip or knee replacement: METHRO I. MElagatran for THRombin inhibition in Orthopaedic surgery. Thromb Haemost 2002; 87:231–237.

30 Cullberg M, Eriksson UG, Wahlander K, et al. Pharmacokinetics of ximelagatran and relationship to clinical response in acute deep vein thrombosis. Clin Pharmacol Ther 2005; 77:279–290.

31 Eriksson UG, Johansson S, Attman PO, et al. Influence of severe renal impairment on the pharmacokinetics and pharmacodynamics of oral ximelagatran and subcutaneous melagatran. Clin Pharmacokinet 2003; 42:743–753.

32 Wahlander K, Eriksson-Lepkowska M, Frison L, et al. No influence of mild-to-moderate hepatic impairment on the pharmacokinetics and pharmacodynamics of ximelagatran, an oral direct thrombin inhibitor. Clin Pharmacokinet 2003; 42:755–764.

33 Clement B, Lopian K. Characterization of in vitro biotransformation of new, orally active, direct thrombin inhibitor ximelagatran, an amidoxime and ester prodrug. Drug Metab Dispos 2003; 31:645–651.

34 Sarich TC, Schutzer KM, Dorani H, et al. No pharmacokinetic or pharmacodynamic interaction between atorvastatin and the oral direct thrombin inhibitor ximelagatran. J Clin Pharmacol 2004; 44:928–934.

35 Sarich TC, Schutzer KM, Wollbratt M, et al. No pharmacokinetic or pharmacodynamic interaction between digoxin and the oral direct thrombin inhibitor ximelagatran in healthy volunteers. J Clin Pharmacol 2004; 44:935–941.

36 Fager G, Cullberg M, Eriksson-Lepkowska M, et al. Pharmacokinetics and pharmacodynamics of melagatran, the active form of the oral direct thrombin inhibitor ximelagatran, are not influenced by acetylsalicylic acid. Eur J Clin Pharmacol 2003; 59:283–289.

37 Bredberg E, Andersson TB, Frison L, et al. Ximelagatran, an oral direct thrombin inhibitor, has a low potential for cytochrome P450-mediated drug-drug interactions. Clin Pharmacokinet 2003; 42:765–777.

38 Sarich TC, Johansson S, Schutzer KM, et al. The pharmacokinetics and pharmacodynamics of ximelagatran, an oral direct

thrombin inhibitor, are unaffected by a single dose of alcohol. J Clin Pharmacol 2004; 44:388–393.

39 Wolzt M, Sarich TS, Eriksson UG. Pharmacokinetics and pharmacodynamics of ximelagatran. Semin Vasc Med 2005; 5:245–253.

40 Wolzt M, Sarich TS, Eriksson UG. Low potential for interactions between melagatran/ximelagatran and other drugs, food, or alcohol. Semin Vasc Med 2005; 5:254–258.

41 Johansson LC, Frison L, Logren U, et al. Influence of age on the pharmacokinetics and pharmacodynamics of ximelagatran, an oral direct thrombin inhibitor. Clin Pharmacokinet 2003; 42:381–392.

42 Johansson LC, Andersson M, Fager G, et al. No influence of ethnic origin on the pharmacokinetics and pharmacodynamics of melagatran following oral administration of ximelagatran, a novel oral direct thrombin inhibitor, to healthy male volunteers. Clin Pharmacokinet 2003; 42:475–484.

43 Sarich TC, Teng R, Peters GR, et al. No influence of obesity on the pharmacokinetics and pharmacodynamics of melagatran, the active form of the oral direct thrombin inhibitor ximelagatran. Clin Pharmacokinet 2003; 42:485–492.

44 Hellgren M, Johansson S, Eriksson UG, et al. The oral direct thrombin inhibitor, ximelagatran, an alternative for anticoagulant treatment during the puerperium and lactation. Bjog 2005; 112:579–583.

45 Weitz JI, Bates SM. New anticoagulants. J Thromb Haemost 2005; 3:1843–1853.

46 Linkins LA, Weitz JI. Pharmacology and clinical potential of direct thrombin inhibitors. Curr Pharm Des 2005; 11:3877–3884.

47 Agnelli G. Clinical potential of oral direct thrombin inhibitors in the prevention and treatment of venous thromboembolism. Drugs 2004; 64(suppl 1):47–52.

48 Wallentin L. Prevention of cardiovascular events after acute coronary syndrome. Semin Vasc Med 2005; 5:293–300.

49 Colwell C, Mouret P. Ximelagatran for the prevention of venous thromboembolism following elective hip or knee replacement surgery. Semin Vasc Med 2005; 5:266–275.

50 Schulman S. The role of ximelagatran in the treatment of venous thromboembolism. Pathophysiol Haemost Thromb 2005; 34(suppl 1):18–24.

51 Halperin JL. Ximelagatran: oral direct thrombin inhibition as anticoagulant therapy in atrial fibrillation. J Am Coll Cardiol 2005; 45:1–9.

52 Brighton TA. The direct thrombin inhibitor melagatran/ximelagatran. Med J Aust 2004; 181:432–437.

53 Eriksson BI, Agnelli G, Cohen AT, et al. The direct thrombin inhibitor melagatran followed by oral ximelagatran compared with enoxaparin for the prevention of venous thromboembolism after total hip or knee replacement: the EXPRESS study. J Thromb Haemost 2003; 1:2490–2496.

54 Eriksson BI, Agnelli G, Cohen AT, et al. Direct thrombin inhibitor melagatran followed by oral ximelagatran in comparison with enoxaparin for prevention of venous thromboembolism after total hip or knee replacement. Thromb Haemost 2003; 89:288–296.

55 Eriksson BI, Bergqvist D, Kalebo P, et al. Ximelagatran and melagatran compared with dalteparin for prevention of venous thromboembolism after total hip or knee replacement: the METHRO II randomised trial. Lancet 2002; 360:1441–1447.

56 Francis CW, Berkowitz SD, Comp PC, et al. Comparison of ximelagatran with warfarin for the prevention of venous thromboembolism after total knee replacement. N Engl J Med 2003; 349:1703–1712.

57 Fiessinger JN, Huisman MV, Davidson BL, et al. Ximelagatran vs low-molecular-weight heparin and warfarin for the treatment of deep vein thrombosis: a randomized trial. J Am Med Assoc 2005; 293:681–689.

58 Schulman S, Wahlander K, Lundstrom T, et al. Secondary prevention of venous thromboembolism with the oral direct thrombin inhibitor ximelagatran. N Engl J Med 2003; 349:1713–1721.

59 Schulman S, Lundstrom T, Walander K, et al. Ximelagatran for the secondary prevention of venous thromboembolism: a complementary follow-up analysis of the THRIVE III study. Thromb Haemost 2005; 94:820–824.

60 Olsson SB. Stroke prevention with the oral direct thrombin inhibitor ximelagatran compared with warfarin in patients with non-valvular atrial fibrillation (SPORTIF III): randomised controlled trial. Lancet 2003; 362:1691–1698.

61 Albers GW, Diener HC, Frison L, et al. Ximelagatran vs warfarin for stroke prevention in patients with nonvalvular atrial fibrillation: a randomized trial. J Am Med Assoc 2005; 293:690–698.

62 Lip GY, Edwards SJ. Stroke prevention with aspirin, warfarin and ximelagatran in patients with non-valvular atrial fibrillation: A systematic review and meta-analysis. Thromb Res 2006; 118:321–333.

63 Petersen P, Grind M, Adler J. Ximelagatran versus warfarin for stroke prevention in patients with nonvalvular atrial fibrillation. SPORTIF II: a dose-guiding, tolerability, and safety study. J Am Coll Cardiol 2003; 41:1445–1451.

64 Albers GW. Stroke prevention in atrial fibrillation: pooled analysis of SPORTIF III and V trials. Am J Manag Care 2004; 10:S462–S469; discussion S469–S473.

65 Wallentin L, Wilcox RG, Weaver WD, et al. Oral ximelagatran for secondary prophylaxis after myocardial infarction: the ESTEEM randomised controlled trial. Lancet 2003; 362:789–797.

66 Lee WM, Larrey D, Olsson R, et al. Hepatic findings in long-term clinical trials of ximelagatran. Drug Saf 2005; 28:351–370.

67 Dager WE, Vondracek TG, McIntosh BA, et al. Ximelagatran: an oral direct thrombin inhibitor. Ann Pharmacother 2004; 38:1881–1897.

68 Hauel NH, Nar H, Priepke H, et al. Structure-based design of novel potent nonpeptide thrombin inhibitors. J Med Chem 2002; 45:1757–1766.

69 Stangier J, Eriksson BI, Dahl OE, et al. Pharmacokinetic profile of the oral direct thrombin inhibitor dabigatran etexilate in healthy volunteers and patients undergoing total hip replacement. J Clin Pharmacol 2005; 45:555–563.

70 Eriksson BI, Dahl OE, Ahnfelt L, et al. Dose escalating safety study of a new oral direct thrombin inhibitor, dabigatran etexilate, in patients undergoing total hip replacement: BISTRO I. J Thromb Haemost 2004; 2:1573–1580.

71 Eriksson BI, Dahl OE, Buller HR, et al. A new oral direct thrombin inhibitor, dabigatran etexilate, compared with enoxaparin for prevention of thromboembolic events following total hip or knee replacement: the BISTRO II randomized trial. J Thromb Haemost 2005; 3:103–111.

72 www.ClinicalTrials.gov.

73 Saiah E, Soares C. Small molecule coagulation cascade inhibitors in the clinic. Curr Top Med Chem 2005; 5: 1677–1695.

74 Di Nisio M, Middeldorp S, Buller HR. Direct thrombin inhibitors. N Engl J Med 2005; 353:1028–1040.

75 Busti AJ, Bussey HI. The role of oral direct thrombin inhibitors in the treatment of venous thromboembolism. Pharmacotherapy 2004; 24:184S–189S.

76 Hawkins D. The role of oral direct thrombin inhibitors in the prophylaxis of venous thromboembolism. Pharmacotherapy 2004; 24:179S–183S.

77 Eriksson H. Treatment of venous thromboembolism and long-term prevention of recurrence: present treatment options and ximelagatran. Drugs 2004; 64(suppl 1):37–46.

78 Olsson SB, Halperin JL. Prevention of stroke in patients with atrial fibrillation. Semin Vasc Med 2005; 5:285–292.

79 Wittkowsky AK, Kenyon KW. The role of oral direct thrombin inhibitors in atrial fibrillation. Pharmacotherapy 2004; 24:190S–198S.

80 Sinnaeve PR, Van de Werf FJ. Will oral antithrombin agents replace warfarin? Heart 2004; 90:827–828.

81 Reiffel JA. Will direct thrombin inhibitors replace warfarin for preventing embolic events in atrial fibrillation? Curr Opin Cardiol 2004; 19:58–63.

82 Granger CB, Weaver WD. Reducing cardiac events after acute coronary syndromes. Rev Cardiovasc Med 2004; 5(suppl 5):S39–S46.

83 Halperin JL. Ximelagatran compared with warfarin for prevention of thromboembolism in patients with nonvalvular atrial fibrillation: Rationale, objectives, and design of a pair of clinical studies and baseline patient characteristics (SPORTIF III and V). Am Heart J 2003; 146:431–438.

84 Eriksson H, Lundstrom T, Wahlander K, et al. Prognostic factors for recurrence of venous thromboembolism (VTE) or bleeding during long-term secondary prevention of VTE with ximelagatran. Thromb Haemost 2005; 94:522–527.

85 Colwell CW Jr, Berkowitz SD, Lieberman JR, et al. Oral direct thrombin inhibitor ximelagatran compared with warfarin for the prevention of venous thromboembolism after total knee arthroplasty. J Bone Joint Surg Am 2005; 87:2169–2177.

86 Eriksson H, Wahlander K, Gustafsson D, et al. A randomized, controlled, dose-guiding study of the oral direct thrombin inhibitor ximelagatran compared with standard therapy for the treatment of acute deep vein thrombosis: THRIVE I. J Thromb Haemost 2003; 1:41–47.

10

Rationale for direct factor Xa inhibitors in acute coronary syndromes

Volker Laux and Markus Hinder

Acute coronary syndromes (ACS) are a major cause of morbidity and mortality. They are characterized by intracoronary thrombus formation at the site of atherosclerotic plaques. Coronary thrombosis is the underlying mechanism in the transition from stable angina to the unstable angina (UA) syndrome, characterized by embolization of the developed thrombus and atherosclerotic plaque rupture.

Pathophysiology of acute coronary syndromes

Generally, the pathophysiology of ACS can be divided into four phases: (*i*) the development of the atherosclerotic plaque, (*ii*) plaque rupture, (*iii*) acute ischemia, and (*iv*) long-term risk of recurrent ischemia (1). Thrombus formation on the atherosclerotic plaque leads to partial or total obstruction of the vessel, with subsequent thromboembolism representing the acute event. The presence of thrombi on atherosclerotic plaques has been demonstrated at autopsies and on angiographic and atherectomy specimens from patients with UA (2–5). Biomarkers of ongoing thrombosis (e.g., platelet activation, thrombin generation, and thrombin activity) indicate the central role of the coagulation and the platelet system. Atherosclerosis and thrombosis in arterial conditions are closely connected and form the clinical picture of atherothrombosis. Five pathophysiological processes contribute to the development of an acute atherothrombotic event (6): nonocclusive thrombus on the pre-existing plaque, dynamic obstruction of a coronary vessel (e.g., spasm), progressive mechanical obstruction, inflammatory and infection processes, and secondary UA.

Coronary vasoconstriction has been demonstrated for major epicardial coronary arteries (7) and for the small intramural coronary resistance vessels (8) and may occur because of local vasoconstrictors derived from platelets present in the thrombus, such as serotonin, thromboxane A_2, and thrombin.

Current management of acute coronary syndromes

ACS can be classified into UA, myocardial infarction (MI) without ST-segment elevation [non-ST-elevation MI (NSTEMI)], or STEMI. The presence of cardiac troponin in ACS indicates worse prognosis than the absence of troponin (9).

Diagnosis and risk stratification in ACS is closely connected. Depending on the presence or absence of ST-elevation together with other risk factors, patients will undergo reperfusion therapy [thrombolysis, primary percutaneous coronary intervention (PCI)], coronary angiography, or pharmacological treatment. In NSTEMI, there exist two major strategies: an early invasive strategy in which all patients routinely undergo cardiac angiography for potential PCI or coronary artery bypass grafting (CABG) and an early conservative strategy consisting of medical treatment for lower risk patients.

The pharmacological treatment options for ACS include agents that either reduce oxygen demand (beta blockers) or increase oxygen supply (nitrates, potassium channel activators, calcium channel blockers) to the heart and antiplatelet (aspirin, ADP-receptor antagonists, GPIIb/IIIa receptor blockers) and antithrombin therapy (unfractionated heparin, low molecular weight heparin, direct thrombin inhibitors) (10).

Role of biomarkers in acute coronary syndromes

Several biomarkers describe the severity of ACS and can be used as a guidance for clinical risk stratification. The decrease of the cardiac enzymes CK and CK-MB have been regarded for a long time as the gold standard for diagnosis of MI (11). However, it has been observed in histological specimens that small damages of myocardial cells do not necessarily increase CK-MB (12). With the isolation of cardiac isoforms of the troponins, it has been demonstrated that troponin T (TnT) and troponin I (TnI) are well suited for diagnosis of ACS (13,14). In contrast to CK-MB, troponins are also sensitive to minimal myocardial cell necrosis. The magnitude of the increase of these myocardium-specific enzymes reflects the extent of the myocardial damage.

Biomarkers that are involved in the early stages of the pathogenetic process can be used to identify patients at risk (Fig. 1). One of the key players in thrombogenesis is thrombin, which is involved not only in the coagulation part of the thrombus formation but also promotes platelet aggregation. The formation of thrombin from prothrombin after activation by prothrombinase can be measured by means of prothrombin fragment 1 + 2 (F1 + 2), a small activation peptide of 32 amino acids. F1 + 2 represents the "factor Xa activity" in vivo. The physiological reaction of inactivation of thrombin through irreversible binding to antithrombin III to its catalytic site is used for a second sensitive test of thrombin generation, the thrombin–antithrombin complex assay (T-AT). The proteolytic activity of thrombin on fibrinogen is described by the release of fibrinopeptide A (FpA), a 16-amino acid peptide from fibrinogen's Aα-chain, and fibrinopeptide B (FpB) with 14 amino acids from fibrinogen Bβ-chain. FpA is a useful biomarker for thrombin activity and often used for diagnosis of the ACS and its progression. The Bβ 15 to 42-related peptides are small peptide cleavage products released by the action of plasmin on fibrinogen and represent a sensitive indicator of fibrinolytic activity. Plasma D-dimers are generated when the endogenous fibrinolytic system degrades fibrin. They consist of two identical subunits that are derived from two fibrin molecules. D-dimers are indicative of cross-linked fibrin in contrast to fibrinogen cleavage products.

The majority of patients with MI and UA have high plasma levels of FpA (15–17). FpA is also found in the urine of these patients (18). These data correlate with clinical findings in angiographic and pathologic studies demonstrating the importance of intracoronary thrombosis (19). In TIMI-5, the main levels for F1 + 2, FpA, TAT, and Bβ1-42 were elevated in patients with ST-elevation (20), clearly reflecting an activation of the coagulation cascade in MI. Moreover, in this study it could be demonstrated that FpA and TAT levels were associated with increased mortality. In about 50% of ACS patients, abnormally high plasma levels of F1 + 2 and FpA were found during the acute phase of the disease (21). However, no difference was found between patients with UA and acute MI, indicating that F1 + 2 and FpA are not dependent on the nature of the thrombus (22).

Procoagulant activity and thrombus-associated thrombin activity have also been demonstrated during coronary interventions measuring plasma levels of F1 + 2 (23) or FpA (24). Interestingly, FpA also increased despite maximal anticoagulation with heparin. The correlation between increased FpA plasma levels and increased incidence of complications and ischemic events indicated the involvement of heparin-resistant thrombin activity into the failure of the intervention (25). Beneath the activation of the coagulation system, it has been demonstrated that platelet activation in the coronary sinus of patients undergoing coronary intervention is significant (26).

Standard therapy for acute coronary syndromes

The involvement of platelets and the coagulation system in the development of ACS indicate that both antiplatelets and anticoagulants are possible approaches for pharmacological treatment (Fig. 2).

The benefit of acetylsalicylic acid (ASA), an inhibitor of cyclooxygenase-1, in decreasing death or MI in patients has been clearly demonstrated, and its use is recommended in all patients with UA (27–29).

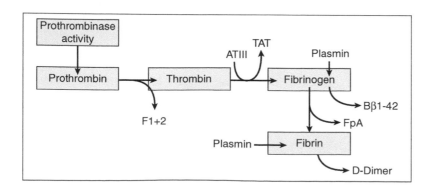

Figure 1
Coagulation derived biomarker in acute coronary syndromes.

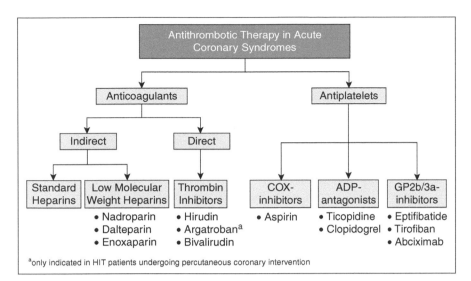

Figure 2

Currently existing antithrombotic therapy in acute coronary syndromes. *Abbreviations*: ADP, adenosine diphosphate; COX, cyclooxygenase; GP2b/3a, glycoprotein 2b/3a.

Antagonists of the ADP P_2Y_{12} receptor, ticlopidine and its safer successor clopidogrel, are also potent inhibitors of platelet aggregation and have demonstrated their efficacy alone and on top of ASA in numerous in clinical studies. The results of the CAPRIE study, a large study involving 19,185 patients with recent MI, stroke, or established peripheral arterial disease (PAD) demonstrated an 8.7% overall risk reduction versus ASA in the combined endpoints of the first occurrence of MI, stroke, or other vascular death (30).

The CURE trial investigated the efficacy and safety of clopidogrel in 12,562 patients when administered together with aspirin in patients with ACS (UA or non–Q-wave MI). The combination demonstrated a 20% relative risk reduction in the combined endpoints of MI, stroke, or cardiovascular death compared with placebo (31).

The inhibition of platelet–platelet interaction can be achieved with antagonists of the integrin glycoprotein (GP) IIb/IIIa receptor, which is the platelet receptor for fibrinogen (32). Three types of GPIIb/IIIa antagonists have been developed, which compete with fibrinogen to occupy the receptors: a monoclonal antibody (abciximab), a cyclic heptapeptide (eptifibatide), and nonpeptide mimetics (tirofiban, lamifiban). A large number of multi-center trials have been performed with GPIIb/IIIa antagonists in ACS including PCI (EPIC, CAPTURE, EPILOG, EPISTENT, IMPACT-II, PURSUIT, RESTORE, PRISM, PRISM-PLUS) (33) and indicate that inhibition of GPIIb/IIIa is effective in decreasing the risk of acute clinical events in patients where there is a higher risk of an occluding clot forming, for example, in patients undergoing PCI. Although the GPIIb/IIIa antagonists have been shown to effectively reduce the major outcome, they have a high liability for increased risk of bleeding. Therefore, different alternatives are currently being tested, including the front-loaded regimen of clopidogrel and also new anticoagulants with an indirect platelet inhibition potential beneath the anticoagulant function.

The presence of markers of thrombin generation, thrombin activity, and fibrin (fibrinogen) degradation indicates that coagulation is involved in the pathophysiology of ACS. To prevent the development of fibrin during the coagulation process, antithrombin therapy is recommended. Heparinoids bind to antithrombin III, thereby accelerating inhibition of clotting factors IIa and Xa by antithrombin III. Unfractionated heparins (UFH) inhibit FXa and FIIa at a ratio of 1:1, whereas low-molecular-weight heparins (LMWH) preferentially inhibit FXa at a ratio of 2:1 to 4:1 (34).

The recommendation for UFH is based on documented efficacy in many older mid-sized trials. Meta-analyses showed a clear reduction in MI and death, but at the cost of an increase in major bleeding rates (35,36). The advantages of LMWH over unfractionated heparin include a better bioavailability, a stronger and longer anti-Xa activity, less platelet activation, and no need for monitoring. A major drawback of standard heparin therapy is the potential risk of heparin-induced thrombocytopenia, which is considerably reduced with LMWH (37).

In the ESSENCE trial, the LMWH enoxaparin led to a relative risk reduction of 15% to 16% in the rate of death, MI, or refractory ischemia as compared to unfractionated heparin at 30 days in UA/NSTEMI patients (38). Nadroparin [FRAXIS study (39)] and dalteparin [FRIC study (40)] did not demonstrate superiority against unfractionated heparin. Human pharmacokinetic data indicate that these differences in clinical efficacy might be explained by different elimination half-lives of antifactor Xa activity (dalteparin: 2.8 hours, nadroparin: 3.7 hours, enoxaparin 4.1 hours) (41).

Several direct thrombin inhibitors have been studied in NSTEMI and STEMI patients and were compared to unfractionated heparin. In the GUSTO IIb- and OASIS-2 trial (42,43), hirudin was studied versus heparin in patients with ACS. Despite early benefits, no statistical significance could be demonstrated at 30 days. Together with the OASIS-1 data, a combined analysis indicated a 22% relative risk reduction in cardiovascular death or MI at 72 hours, 17% at 7 days, and 10% at 35 days (42).

A comprehensive meta-analysis comprising different thrombin inhibitors (hirudin, bivalirudin, efegatran, argatroban) indicates a superiority of direct thrombin inhibition over unfractionated heparin for the prevention of death or MI in patients with ACS including STEMI (44). Hirudin has been approved for patients with heparin-induced thrombocytopenia; however, it is not approved specifically for ACS (45).

The direct thrombin inhibitor bivalirudin is a synthetic, 20 amino acid peptide that binds reversibly to the active site and to the substrate recognition site of thrombin. Cleavage of the inhibitor by thrombin results in the recovery of the active site (46). In the REPLACE-2 trial, bivalirudin, with GP IIb/IIIa inhibition on a provisional basis for complications during PCI, was compared with unfractionated heparin plus planned Gp IIb/IIIa blockade in patients undergoing urgent or elective PCI. The primary composite endpoint was 30-day incidence of death, MI, urgent repeat revascularization, or in-hospital major bleeding. Bivalirudin with provisional Gp IIb/IIIa blockade demonstrated noninferiority to heparin plus planned Gp IIb/IIIa blockade during contemporary PCI. Moreover, bivalirudin was associated with less bleeding (47).

Role of coagulation factor Xa in acute coronary syndromes

Coagulation factor X is a vitamin K-dependent GP and the zymogen of factor Xa. Factor Xa plays a central role in coagulation because it is located at the convergence point of the intrinsic and extrinsic pathway. Factor X is activated by excision of a small peptide from its heavy chain by either the extrinsic tenase complex (tissue factor–factor VIIa) or by the intrinsic tenase complex (factor VIIIa–factor IXa). Together with its cofactor, coagulation factor Va, factor Xa forms the prothrombinase complex, which converts prothrombin into thrombin in a process requiring several binding steps (Fig. 3). The prothrombinase complex is generated on a phospholipid surface, which is provided by platelets during activation. In the unactivated state, platelets do not express significant amounts of phosphatidylserine. During activation, phosphatidylserine is

translocated from the inner to the outer leaflet of the platelet membrane (48). This outward phosphatidylserine shuttle is accompanied by an increased ability of the platelets to enhance the prothrombin–thrombin conversion by factor Xa, in the presence of factor Va and calcium (49). Factor V is stored in platelet α-granules (50) and activated after secretion during platelet activation by factor Xa (51,52). After the Xa/Va complex is formed, thrombin formation occurs, which results in a rapid acceleration of procoagulant activity (53). The procoagulant activity within a clot primarily depends on the formation of thrombin induced by the prothrombinase complex on the platelet surface (54,55). This prothrombinase activity can also be demonstrated on pathological thrombi from patients with arterial thrombosis. In a balloon-induced arterial injury study in rabbits, bound prothrombinase activity to injured segments was detected within 15 minutes and it induced activation of prothrombin for 96 hours (56). These data indicate that inhibition of factor Xa within the prothrombinase complex is a valid concept to treat or prevent arterial thrombosis and might be superior to the current established therapy.

Preclinical data for factor Xa inhibitors

In contrast to unfractionated heparin, the factor Xa inhibitor tick anticoagulant peptide (TAP) effectively inhibited coronary arterial thrombosis in a canine electrolytic injury model (57). TAP was also effective in inhibition of the procoagulant properties of whole blood clots in vitro; however, it was stated that TAP might be not optimal due to its slow binding kinetics (54). Meanwhile, several low molecular weight direct factor Xa inhibitors are in clinical development (Table 1), some of them specifically for the treatment and secondary prevention of ACS. DX-9065a, ZK-807834 and otamixaban have been intensively characterized in vitro and in vivo and are in clinical investigations for the treatment of acute arterial thrombosis.

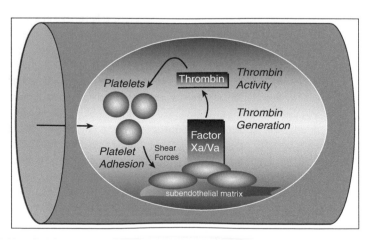

Figure 3

Schematic view of the role of coagulation factor Xa in arterial thrombosis. After endothelial injury, platelets adhere to the subendothelial matrix. The procoagulant activity of the arterial clot can be attributed to the formation of the prothrombinase complex on the platelet surface which cleaves prothrombin and produces thrombin. Thrombin subsequently acts as a strong agonist of further platelet aggregation.

Table 1 Direct factor Xa inhibitors in clinical development

Name	Company	Clinical phase
BAY 59-7939	BayerHealthcare	III
Otamixaban	Sanofi-Aventis	II
BMS-562247	Bristol-Myers Squibb	II
LY-517717	Eli Lilly	II
ZK-807834	Berlex/Schering	II
DU-176b	Daiichi Sankyo	II
YM-150	Astellas	II
DX-9065a	Daiichi	II
KFA-1982	Kissei	I
TC-10	Teijin	I

The compounds potently inhibit factor Xa in vitro with reversible binding kinetics and are able to inhibit not only free but also prothrombinase-bound factor Xa (Ki 41 nM, 0.11 nM, and 0.5 nM, respectively) (58–60). In contrast, no direct effect on platelet aggregation has been described (60–62). Antithrombotic activity in arterial and venous thrombosis models has been demonstrated and it has a reduced effect on hemorrhage in comparison to standard therapy (58,60,63). Factor Xa inhibitors are able to reduce the endogenous thrombin potential in platelet-poor as well as in platelet-rich plasma (64,65). Thus, thrombin generation seems to be a suitable biomarker for clinical evaluation and has been evaluated in phase I studies (66,67).

In preclinical models of ACS, factor Xa inhibitors have been investigated and compared to standard treatments. Otamixaban was compared to bivalirudin in a Folts model in pigs (68). Both treatments were effective in inhibiting cyclic flow variations as indicators of unstable coronary artery thrombosis. In contrast to bivalirudin, otamixaban did not prolong bleeding times, indicating a larger therapeutic window for factor Xa inhibition. Moreover, ZK-807834 (69) and otamixaban (70) were able to reduce reocclusion rates on top of thrombolytic therapy in dogs as compared to unfractionated heparin and achieved better reocclusion rates than the former.

Clinical data on direct factor Xa inhibitors in acute coronary syndromes

The first evidence for the ex vivo antithrombotic effects of a direct factor Xa inhibitor in humans was provided in the Badimon chamber (71). Healthy volunteers received escalating intravenous doses of DX-9065a with and without concomitant aspirin. Porcine tunica media served as thrombogenic surface in the flow chamber. DX-9065a alone and in combination with aspirin significantly inhibited thrombus formation in this ex vivo assay at low and high shear rates. These data suggest that inhibitors of factor Xa can be considered efficacious antithrombotic agents to prevent the acute complications of thrombosis.

Other phase I studies investigated the effects of the coadministration of the direct factor Xa inhibitor otamixaban with aspirin and tirofiban on both anticoagulation and platelet inhibition (72,73). It was demonstrated that the factor Xa inhibitor alone had no effect on ex vivo platelet aggregation and both platelet inhibitors alone did not change anticoagulation global and factor Xa-specific coagulation parameters. Equally important, the studies showed that both therapeutically relevant principles in the treatment of ACS, that is, anticoagulation and platelet-inhibition, are maintained following the co-administration of otamixaban with the platelet inhibitors.

The XANADU-1B trial investigated for the first time the pharmacokinetics, pharmacodynamics, and the safety profile of the direct factor Xa inhibitor DX-9065a after 72 hours intravenous infusion in patients with stable coronary disease (74). A dose- and concentration-dependent increase of anti-FXa activity, international normalized ratio (INR), and activated partial thromboplastin time (aPTT) was observed. However, the classical measurements of anticoagulant activity, PT, INR, and aPTT, correlated less well with plasma concentrations during the early infusion time compared with the later time points. Anti-Fxa activity revealed a strong correlation with plasma concentrations, indicating a close relationship between these two parameters. The compound was well tolerated: no major or minor bleeding (according to the TIMI criteria) and no serious adverse effect occurred during the infusion period of 72 hours. In the highest dose group, a small, nonsignificant increase in GUSTO-minor bleeding was observed. Significant correlations between plasma concentrations, prothrombin fragment F1 + 2 and D-dimer could be observed within this study, indicating a reduction of thrombin generation and the formation of fibrin by means of factor Xa inhibition (75).

The XANADU-PCI trial (76) was performed to investigate the pharmacokinetics, the effect on coagulation markers, and the preliminary efficacy and safety of four different doses of DX-9065a during PCI. Patients undergoing elective, native-vessel PCI were randomized to four escalating DX-9065a doses/concentrations. Infusion was stopped at completion of the PCI. All patients were treated concomitantly with aspirin and clopidogrel; in most cases GPIIb/IIIa receptor antagonists were also administered. Dose levels I–III were designed to achieve drug concentrations of DX-9065a of >75 ng/mL, >100 ng/mL, and >150 ng/mL, respectively. Dose level IV was comparable to stage III regimen but included patients recently given heparin. Arterial sheaths were removed one to two hours after the procedure or at the time of measurement of activated clotting time (ACT) <170 seconds. INRs were 1.9, 2.6, 3.2, and 3.8 in the four levels, and anti-FXa levels were 0.33, 0.36, 0.45, and 0.62 U/mL, respectively. Dose level II was stopped after occurrence of one serious thrombotic event suspicious of insufficient anticoagulation. A close correlation between plasma concentration and INR or anti-FXa activity could be demonstrated. In general, ischemic and bleeding events were rare. However, probably due to the small population size ($n = 175$), no clear relation to the DX-9065a dose could be observed. The authors of the study concluded that elective PCI is feasible using direct FXa inhibition for anticoagulation.

In the XANADU-ACS trial (77), 402 patients with ACS were randomized to unfractionated heparin, low-dose DX-9065a, or high-dose DX-9065a. The primary end-point was the composite of death, MI, urgent revascularization, or ischemia on continuous ST-segment monitoring. These patients were representative for a high-risk ACS population. More than 80% of them had MI. Nearly all patients received aspirin, more than 75% received clopidogrel or ticlopidine, and over 60% received GP IIb/IIIa inhibitors. Ninety-eight percent underwent catheterization, 55% PCI, and 17% CABG. According to Rajagopal and Bhatt (78), the trial population represented a realistic ACS population with state-of-the-art care. The anti-FXa activity increased during infusion in the low/high dose DX-9065a groups from 0.09/0.10 to 0.23/0.41 U/mL (in the heparin group from 0.14 to 0.44 U/mL). Whole-blood INRs increased to approximately 2.0 with low-dose DX-9065a and to 2.5 with high-dose DX-9065a (1.5 with heparin).

The primary efficacy endpoint occurred with similar frequency in all treatment groups. In the patients treated with high-dose DX-9065a, a tendency for lower rates of clinically important endpoints was observed. Major or minor bleeding rates were similar among patients in the heparin and high-dose DX-9065a group, but lower in patients in the low-dose DX-9065a group. It can be concluded that direct inhibition of factor Xa is an attractive alternative to currently available anticoagulants in ACS.

A further direct factor Xa inhibitor, otamixaban, is currently being investigated in the SEPIA-PCI trial in patients undergoing nonurgent PCI in comparison to heparin (78).

Conclusions

ACSs are a major cause of morbidity and mortality. They are characterized by intracoronary thrombus formation at the site of atherosclerotic plaques resulting in UA and MI. Although effective treatments and procedures are available, patients remain at high risk of reinfarction and death.

In addition to the presently available treatments, a new concept is evolving that targets and inhibits the prothrombinase multienzyme complex on the platelet surface thus inhibiting further thrombin generation in arterial thrombosis.

New small molecule FXa inhibitors currently in development are able to enter the clot/prothrombinase complex and inhibit free and bound factor Xa regarded as the key enzyme in ACS. Although direct FXa inhibitors do not inhibit platelet aggregation, they abolish platelet-dependent thrombus formation in canine coronary thrombosis. Thus, direct inhibition of FXa may have higher efficacy and better risk/benefit profile than existing antithrombotic therapies in the treatment and prevention of ACS.

References

1 Gelfand EV, Cannon CP. Acute coronary syndromes. In: Colman RW et al., eds. Hemostasis and Thrombosis: Basic Principles and Clinical Practice. Philadelphia: Lippincott, Williams and Wilkins, 2006:1387–1404.

2 Davies MJ. The composition of coronary-artery plaques. N Engl J Med 1997; 336:1312–1314.

3 Harrington RA, Califf RM, Holmes DR Jr, et al. Is all unstable angina the same? Insights from the Coronary Angioplasty Versus Excisional Atherectomy Trial (CAVEAT-I). Am Heart J 1999; 137:227–233.

4 Silva JA, White CJ, Collins TJ, et al. Morphologic comparison of atherosclerotic lesions in native coronary arteries and saphenous vein grafts with intracoronary angioscopy in patients with unstable angina. Am Heart J 1998; 136:156–163.

5 Nesto RW, Waxman S, Mittleman MA, et al. Angioscopy of culprit coronary lesions in unstable angina pectoris and correlation of clinical presentation with plaque morphology. Am J Cardiol 1998; 81:225–228.

6 Braunwald E. Unstable angina: an etiologic approach to management. Circulation 1998; 98:2219–2222.

7 Prinzmetal M, Kennamer R, Merliss R, et al. A variant form of angina pectoris. Am J Med 1959; 27:375.

8 Bottcher M, Botker HE, Sonne H, et al. Endothelium-dependent and -independent perfusion reserve and the effect of L-arginine on myocardial perfusion in patients with syndrome X. Circulation 1999; 99:1795–1801.

9 Hamm CW, Goldmann BU, Heeschen C, et al. Emergency room triage of patients with acute chest pain by means of rapid testing for cardiac troponin T or troponin I. N Engl J Med 1997; 337(23):1648–1653.

10 Bertrand ME, Simoons ML, Fox KA, et al. Task force on the management of acute coronary syndromes of the European Society of Cardiology. Management of acute coronary syndromes in patients presenting without persistent ST-segment elevation. Eur Heart J 2002; 23:1809–1840.

11 Joint International Society and Federation of Cardiology/World Health Organization Task Force on Standardization of Clinical Nomenclature. Nomenclature and criteria for diagnosis of ischemic heart disease. Circulation 1979; 59:607–609.

12 Falk E. Unstable angina with fatal outcome: dynamic coronary thrombosis leading to infarction and/or sudden death: autopsy evidence of recurrent mural thrombosis with peripheral embolization culminating in total vascular occlusion. Circulation 1985; 71:699–708.

13 Gerhardt W, Nording G, Ljungdahl L. Can troponin T replace CK-MB mass as "goldstandard" for acute myocardial infarction ("AMI")? Scand J Clin Lab Invest 1999; 59(suppl 230):83–89.

14 Wu AH, Apple FS, Gibler WB, et al. National Academy of Clinical Biochemistry Standards of Laboratory Practice: recommendations for the use of cardiac markers in coronary artery diseases. Clin Chem 1999; 5:1104–1121.

15 Neri Serneri GG, Gensini GF, Abbate R, et al. Is raised plasma fibrinopeptide A a marker of acute coronary insufficiency? Lancet 1980; II:982.

16 Theroux P, Latour JG, Leger-Gautier C, et al. Fibrinopeptide A plasma levels and platelet factor 4 levels in unstable angina pectoris. Circulation 1987; 75:156–162.

17 Van Hulsteijn H, Kolff J, Briet E, et al. Fibrinopeptide A and ß-thromboglobulin in patients angina pectoris and acute myocardial infarction. Am Heart J 1984; 107:39–45.

18 Ardissino D, Gamba MG, Merlini PA, et al. Fibrinopeptide A excretion in urine: a marker of cumulative thrombin activity in stable versus unstable angina patients. Am J Cardiol 1991; 68:58B–63B.

19 Fuster V, Badimon L, Badimon JJ, et al. Mechanism of disease: the pathogenesis of coronary artery disease and the acute coronary syndromes. N Engl J Med 1994; 326:242–250.

20 Scharfstein JS, Abendschein DR, Eisenberg PR, et al. Usefulness of fibrinogenolytic and procoagulant markers during thrombolytic therapy in predicting clinical outcomes in acute myocardial infarction. TIMI-5 Investigators. Thrombolysis in myocardial infarction. Am J Cardiol 1996; 78:503–510.

21 Merlini PA, Bauer KA, Oltrona L, et al. Persistent activation of the coagulation mechanism in unstable angina and myocardial infarction. Circulation 1994; 90:61–68.

22 Mizuno K, Satumora K, Miyamoto A, et al. Angioscopic evaluation of coronary artery thrombi in acute coronary syndromes. N Engl J Med 1992; 326:287–291.

23 Haskel EJ, Prager NA, Sobel BE, et al. Relative efficacy of antithrombin compared with antiplatelet agents in accelerating coronary thrombolysis and preventing early reocclusion. Circulation 1991; 83:1048–1056.

24 Marmur JD, Merlini PA, Sharma SK, et al. Thrombin generation in human coronary arteries after percutaneous transluminal balloon angioplasty. J Am Coll Cardiol 1994; 24:1484–1491.

25 Oltrona L, Eisenberg PR, Lasala JM, et al. Association of heparin resistant thrombin activity with acute ischemic complications of coronary interventions. Circulation 1996; 94:2064–2071.

26 Gasperetti CM, Gonias SL, Gimple LW, et al. Platelet activation during coronary angioplasty inhumans. Circulation 1993; 88:2728–2734.

27 Theroux P, Ouimet H, McCans J, et al. Aspirin, Heparin or both to treat unstable angina. New Engl J Med 1988; 319:1105–1111.

28 Theroux P, Waters D,Qiu S, et al. Aspirin versus heparin to preventmyocardial infarction during the acute phase of unstable angina. Circulation 1993; 88:2045–2048.

29 Cairns JA, Singer J, Gent M, et al. One year mortality outcomes of all coronary and intensive care unit patients with acute myocardial infarction, unstable angina or other chest pain in Hamilton, Ontario, a city of 375,000 people. Can J Cardiol 1989; 5:239–246.

30 CAPRIE Steering Committee. A randomised, blinded, trial of clopidogrel versus aspirin in patients at risk of ischemic events (CAPRIE). Lancet 1996; 348:1329–1339.

31 The Clopidogrel in Unstable angina to prevent Recurrent Events (CURE) Trial Investigators. Effects of clopidogrel in addition to aspirin in patients with acute coronary syndromes without ST-segment elevation. N Engl J Med 2001; 345:494–502.

32 Coller BS. Platelet GPIIb/IIIa antagonists: the first anti-integrin receptor therapeutics. J Clin Invest 1997; 99:1467–1471.

33 Bennett JS. Novel platelet inhibitors. Annu Rev Med 2001; 52:161–184.

34 McCart GM, Kayser SR. Therapeutic equivalency of low-molecular-weight heparins. Ann Pharmacother 2002; 36:1042–1057.

35 Cohen M, Adams PC, Parry G, et al. Combination antithrombotic therapy in unstable rest angina and non-Q-wave infarction in nonprior aspirin users. Primary end points analysis from the ATACS trial. Antithrombotic Therapy in Acute Coronary Syndromes Research Group. Circulation 1994; 89:81–88.

36 Oler A, Whooley MA, Oler J, et al. Adding heparin to aspirin reduces the incidence of myocardial infarction and death in patients with unstable angina. A meta-analysis. JAMA 1996; 276:811–815.

37 Walenga JM, Jeske WP, Prechel MM, et al. Decreased prevalence of heparin-induced thrombocytopenia with low-molecular-weight heparin and related drugs. Semin Thromb Hemost 2004; 30(suppl 1):69–80.

38 Cohen M, Demers C, Gurfinkel EP, et al. A comparison of low molecular weight heparin with unfractionated heparin for unstable coronary artery disease. Efficacy and Safety of Subcutaneous Enoxaparin in Non-Q-wave Coronary Events Study Group. N Engl J Med 1997; 337:447–452.

39 The FRAXIS Study Group. Comparison of two treatment durations (6 days and 14 days) of a low molecular weight heparin with a 6-day treatment of unfractionated heparin in the initial management of unstable angina or non-Q-wave myocardial infarction: FRAXIS (fraxiparine in acute ischaemic syndrome). Eur Heart J 1999; 20:1553–1562.

40 Klein W, Buchwald A, Hillis SE, et al. Comparison of low molecular weight heparin with unfractionated heparin acutely and with placebo for 6 weeks in the management of unstable coronary artery disease. Fragmin in Unstable Coronary Artery Disease Study (FRIC). Circulation 1997; 96:61–68.

41 Collignon F, Frydman A, Caplain H, et al. Comparison of the pharmacokinetic profiles of three low-molecular mass heparins – dalteparin, enoxaparin and nadroparin administered subcutaneously in healthy volunteers (doses for prevention of thromboembolism). Thromb Haemost 1995; 73:630–640.

42 Gusto IIB Investigators. A comparison of recombinant hirudin with heparin for the treatment of acute coronary syndromes. The Global Use of Strategies to Open Occluded Coronary Arteries (GUSTO) IIb Investigators. N Engl J Med 1996; 335:775–782.

43 Fox KA. Implications of the Organization to Assess Strategies for Ischemic Syndromes-2 (OASIS-2) Study and the results in the context of other trials. Am J Cardiol 1999; 84:26M–31M.

44 Direct Thrombin Inhibitors Trialist's Collaborative Group. Lancet 2002; 359:294–302.

45 Bertrand ME, Simoons ML, Fox KAA, et al. Management of acute coronary syndromes in patients presenting without persistent ST-segment elevation. Eur Heart J 2002; 23:1809–1840.

46 Bates SM, Weitz JI. The mechanism of action of thrombin inhibitors. J Invasive Cardiol 2000; 12(suppl):F27–F32.

47 Lincoff AM, Bittl JA, Harrington RA, et al. Bivalirudin and provisional glycoprotein IIb/IIIa blockade compared with heparin and planned glycoprotein IIb/IIIa blockade during percutaneous coronary intervention. JAMA 2003; 289:853–863.

48 Hoffman M, Monroe DM III. A cell-based model of hemostasis. Thromb Haemost 2001; 85:958–965.

49 Bevers EM, Comfurius P, Zwaal RF. Changes in membrane phospholipid distribution during platelet activation. Biochim Biophys Acta 1983; 736:57–66.

50 Tracy PB, Eide LL, Bowie EJ, et al. Radioimmunoassay of factor V in human plasma and platelets. Blood 1982; 60:59–63.

51 Foster WB, Nesheim ME, Mann KG. The factor Xa-catalyzed activation of factor V. J Biol Chem 1983; 258:13970–13977.

52 Monkovic DD, Tracy PB. Functional characterization of human platelet released factor V and its activation by factor Xa and thrombin. J Biol Chem 1990; 265:17132–17140.

53 Mann KG. The coagulation explosion. Ann N Y Acad Sci 1994; 714:265–269.

54 Eisenberg PR, Siegel JE, Abendschein DR, et al. Importance of factor Xa in determining the procoagulant activity of whole-blood clots. J Clin Invest 1993; 91:1877–1883.

55 McKenzie CR, Abendschein DR, Eisenberg PR. Sustained inhibition of whole-blood clot procoagulant activity by inhibition of thrombus-associated factor Xa. Arterioscler Thromb Vasc Biol 1996; 16:1285–1291.

56 Ghigliotti G, Waissbluth AR, Speidel C, et al. Prolonged activation of prothrombin on the vascular wall after arterial injury. Arterioscler Thromb Vasc Biol 1998; 18:250–257.

57 Lynch JJ Jr, Sitko GR, Lehman ED, et al. Primary prevention of coronary arterial thrombosis with the factor Xa inhibitor rTAP in a canine electrolytic injury model. Thromb Haemost 1995; 74:640–645.

58 Becker RC, Alexander J, Dyke CK, et al. Development of DX-9065a, a novel direct factor Xa antagonist, in cardiovascular disease. Thromb Haemost 2004; 92:1182–1193.

59 Post JM, Sullivan ME, Abendschein D, et al. Human in vitro pharmacodynamic profile of the selective Factor Xa inhibitor ZK-807834 (CI-1031). Thromb Res 2002; 105:347–352.

60 Chu V, Brown K, Colussi D, et al. Pharmacological characterization of a novel factor Xa inhibitor, FXV673. Thromb Res 2001; 103:309–324.

61 Posta JM, Sullivana ME, Abendschein D, et al. Human in vitro pharmacodynamic profile of the selective Factor Xa inhibitor ZK-807834 (CI-1031). Thromb Res 2002; 105:347–352.

62 Morishima Y, Tanabe K, Terada Y, et al. Antithrombotic and hemorrhagic effects of DX-9065a, a direct and selective factor Xa inhibitor: comparison with a direct thrombin inhibitor and antithrombin III-dependent anticoagulants. Thromb Haemost 1997; 78:1366–1371.

63 Abendschein DR, Baum PK, Martin DJ, et al. Effects of ZK-807834, a novel inhibitor of factor Xa, on arterial and venous thrombosis in rabbits. J Cardiovasc Pharmacol 2000; 35:796–805.

64 Gerotziafas GT, Elalamy I, Chakroun T, et al. The oral, direct factor Xa inhibitor—BAY 59-7939—inhibits thrombin generation in vitro after tissue factor pathway activation. J Thromb Haemost 2005; 3(suppl 1):P2295.

65 Lorenz M, Stamm S, Hinder M, et al. Inhibition of thrombin generation by Otamixaban (XRP0673), a direct and selective factor Xa inhibitor. J Thromb Haemost 2005; 3(suppl 1):P0716.

66 Harder S, Graff J, von Hentig N, et al. Effects of BAY 59-7939, an innovative, oral, direct Factor Xa inhibitor, on thrombin generation in healthy volunteers. Pathophysiol Haemost Thromb 2003; 33(suppl 2):PO078.

67 Paccaly A, Ozoux ML, Chu V, et al. Pharmacodynamic markers in the early clinical assessment of otamixaban, a direct factor Xa inhibitor. Thromb Haemost 2005; 94:1156–1163.

68 Just M, Lorenz M, Skrzipczyk HJ, et al. Otamixaban, a direct factor Xa inhibitor, more potently inhibits experimental coronary thrombosis than bivalirudin, a direct thrombin inhibitor. J Thromb Haemost 2005; 3(suppl 1):P0115.

69 Abendschein DR, Baum PK, Verhallen P, et al. A novel synthetic inhibitor of factor Xa decreases early reocclusion and improves 24-h patency after coronary fibrinolysis in dogs. J Pharmacol Exp Ther 2001; 296:567–572.

70 Rebello SS, Bentley RG, Morgan SR, et al. Antithrombotic efficacy of a novel factor Xa inhibitor, FXV673, in a canine model of coronary artery thrombolysis. Br J Pharmacol 2001; 133:1190–1198.

71 Shimbo D, Osende J, Chen J, et al. Antithrombotic effects of DX-9065a, a direct factor Xa inhibitor: a comparative study in humans versus low molecular weight heparin. Thromb Haemost 2002; 88:733–738.

72 Hinder M, Paccaly A, Frick A, et al. Anticoagulant and antiplatelet effects are maintained following coadministration of otamixaban, a direct factor Xa inhibitor, with tirofiban in healthy volunteers. Thromb Haemost 2005; 93:794–795.

73 Hinder M, Frick A, Rosenburg R, et al. Anticoagulant and antiplatelet effects are maintained following coadministration of otamixaban, a direct factor Xa inhibitor, and acetylsalicylic acid. Thromb Haemost 2006; 95:224–228.

74 Dyke CK, Becker RC, Kleiman NS, et al. First experience with direct factor Xa inhibition in patients with stable coronary disease: a pharmacokinetic and pharmacodynamic evaluation. Circulation 2002; 105:2385–2391

75 Becker RC, Alexander JH, Dyke C, et al. Effect of the novel direct factor Xa inhibitor DX-9065a on thrombin generation and inhibition among patients with stable atherosclerotic coronary artery disease. Thromb Res 2006; 117:439–446.

76 Alexander JH, Dyke CK, Yang H, et al. Initial experience with factor-Xa inhibition in percutaneous coronary intervention: the XaNADU-PCI Pilot. J Thromb Haemost 2004; 2(2):234–241.

77 Alexander JH, Yang H, Becker RC, et al. First experience with direct, selective factor Xa inhibition in patients with non-ST-elevation acute coronary syndromes: results of the XaNADU-ACS Trial. J Thromb Haemost 2005; 3:439–447.

78 Rajagopal V, Bhatt DL. Factor Xa inhibitors in acute coronary syndromes: moving from mythology to reality. J Thromb Haemost 2005; 3:436–438.

11

Combined anticoagulant and antiplatelet therapy

Harry L. Messmore, Erwin Coyne, Meghan Businaro, Omer Iqbal, William Wehrmacher, and Walter Jeske

Introduction

To understand the evolution of therapy of the acute coronary syndrome (ACS), which includes unstable angina, acute myocardial infarction, and interventional therapy—percutaneous coronary intervention (PCI), it is most useful to trace the historical events that provided a rationale for the use of anticoagulant and antiplatelet drugs. The focus of this chapter is upon the explosion in knowledge of the physiology of the hemostatic mechanism and will trace the rational development of therapy based upon the pathophysiology of the ACS over the past 40 years.

History

The 1912 paper by James Herrick set the stage for the subsequent use of antithrombotic drugs to treat ACS. In his landmark paper, he reviewed the clinical and pathological findings of this disorder that had been published over the preceding 70 years (1). He correlated clinical history and physical findings with anatomic pathology. He included studies of experimental coronary occlusion in animals. These published animal studies reproduced the human clinical and pathologic features of the disorder, but the means used to reproduce the human syndrome consisted of ligations of main coronary arteries or their branches. This did not take into account the fact that human cases usually had lesions in several coronary artery sites, which restricted collateral flow in some cases. The anatomic description of the lesions in the

human at autopsy included partial occlusion of coronary arteries by atherosclerosis including thrombi. Some cases had total occlusion by plaque alone. (Herrick's personal observation included one classic clinical case of death due to coronary occlusion that had a fresh red thrombus in the proximal left coronary artery at a site of severe narrowing on autopsy.) The entire clinical course was 52 hours. In all his report, he offered convincing evidence that thrombosis was a major mechanism of coronary occlusion in such cases. No experiments were carried out on animals until 26 years later.

The discovery of heparin by McClean four years after Herrick's report made it possible to consider antithrombotic therapy for ACS (2). Solandt and Best were the first to carry out such experiments using animal models, primarily dogs. Theirs was one of the few laboratories to have heparin available, an early product developed by Best and coworkers at the Connaught Laboratories associated with the University of Toronto in Canada. In their experiments, they produced coronary thrombosis using chemical injury to the endothelium thereby inducing coronary thrombosis in approximately 20 hours. Pretreatment with parenteral heparin in doses to prolong the whole blood clotting time to approximately three times normal for the dog prevented early death due to myocardial infarction as compared with untreated controls. Electrocardiographic monitoring showed a diminution of the R-wave, which was similar to that seen in controls in which the coronary arteries were ligated. This report was published in 1938 (3).

It was a remarkable coincidence that Irving S. Wright, a prominent internist and vascular specialist, experienced deep vein thrombosis following an appendectomy in 1938, and

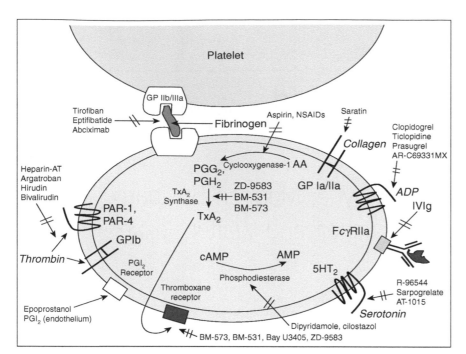

Figure 1
Sites of action of currently approved and experimental antiplatelet drugs. Antiplatelet drugs are capable of inhibiting platelet activation by blocking cell surface receptors and inhibiting the generation of bioactive substances. Platelet aggregation is potently inhibited by blocking fibrinogen binding to GP IIb/IIIa. The sites of action of currently used and experimental (bold) antiplatelet agents are depicted. *Abbreviations*: AA, arachidonic acid; AT, antithrombin; GP, glycoprotein; 5HT, serotonin; IVIg, intravenous immunoglobulin; NSAID, nonsteroidal anti-inflammatory drug; PAR, protease activated receptor; PG, prostaglandin; Tx, thromboxane.

shortly thereafter in the same year was consulted by a 31-year-old man with extensive bilateral migratory thrombophlebitis involving both legs, veins of the abdominal wall, and mesentery. Dr. Wright was able to obtain heparin from the Toronto group to administer to this patient. A remarkable recovery occurred. The heparin had to be stopped eventually because the available supply was exhausted. A few months later there was a recurrence of the venous thrombosis in the patient in association with adult mumps. Heparin was resumed and continued until the newly discovered dicumarol became available for clinical use on a compassionate basis in 1941 (4,5). Dr. Karl Link and coworkers of the University of Wisconsin and their clinical collaborators at the Mayo Clinic had recently published this discovery (5). Dr. Wright and his associates along with Link and his group in Wisconsin and physicians at the Mayo Clinic in Rochester, Minnesota developed guidelines for the clinical use of dicumarol (6). A laboratory monitoring system called the prothrombin time, discovered by Armand Quick (7) in 1935 was introduced for clinical use. Investigators in Canada, the United States, and Sweden showed that both heparin and warfarin were reasonably safe and effective anticoagulants for human use (8). James et al. (9) showed that its effect could be neutralized by the injection of vitamin K. There were never any randomized clinical trials of heparin for thrombotic disorders until 1960 when it was shown that it was clearly superior to placebo for the treatment of pulmonary embolism (10). At this point, the empiric approach to therapy with heparin began to become more rational based upon in-depth basic science studies of the physiology of the hemostatic system and of the pathology of the vascular lesions of atherosclerosis.

Physiology of platelets and endothelium

Basic studies beginning in the 1960s and continuing to the present have shown that the endothelial cell is metabolically active, providing components of the coagulation systems such as tissue plasminogen activator, tissue factor pathway inhibitor (TFPI), von Willebrand Factor (vWF), and vasodilator substances such as nitric oxide (NO) and prostacyclin (PGI_2). These substances are elaborated under the influence of stimuli from the coagulation enzymes such as thrombin and from platelet factors such as PGG_2 (Fig. 1). Tissue factor may be generated on the surface of the endothelial cells by specific stimuli as are surface receptors for cytokines and adhesion molecules for leukocytes, platelets and activated coagulation factors. vWF produced in the endothelial cells and in megakaryocytes attaches to the subendothelium at sites of injury or plaque rupture. High-molecular-weight multimers of vWF induce thrombosis in arterioles when the enzyme ADAMTS 13 is decreased on a hereditary or an acquired basis [thrombotic thrombocytopenic purpura (TTP)] (11,12).

Pathophysiology of plaque rupture

The rupture of a subendothelial plaque into the vascular lumen is a major factor in the initiation of thrombosis by causing a platelet-rich thrombus to develop at that site. The persistence of this thrombus at the site is promoted by

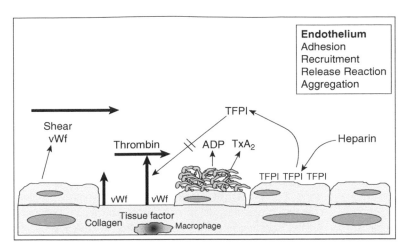

Figure 2
Formation of thrombus at the site of endothelial damage. Von Willebrand factor exposed at sites of endothelial damage acts to bind platelets to the vessel wall. Tissue factor, expressed on subendothelial tissue and cytokine-primed macrophages, acts to generate thrombin, which activates platelets and produces fibrin. TFPI, normally present on the endothelial surface, can be released by heparins and can inhibit tissue factor-induced thrombin generation.
Abbreviations: ADP; adenosine disphosphate; TFP1, tissue factor pathway inhibitor.

vascular narrowing due to the atherosclerotic process. High shear rates at that point promote the binding of vWF to the platelet surface and to the subendothelial connective tissue. Thrombin is simultaneously generated at the site, converting fibrinogen to fibrin that binds the platelets into a mass that further occludes the vessel. The release of thromboxane A_2 (TXA$_2$) from the platelets causes aggregation of adjacent platelets and it causes adenosine diphosphate (ADP) to be released from platelet-dense granules. TXA$_2$ is a potent vasoconstrictor further narrowing the coronary vessels. In Figure 2, the interaction of platelets with damaged endothelium is depicted, showing key endothelial and platelet release factors. Lipid-laden macrophages are the major components of the plaque and when the endothelial cells and the fibrous cap covering the plaque are disrupted, tissue factor is generated at the site as well as platelet-derived growth factor, promoting further fibrin deposition, platelet aggregation, and proliferation of smooth muscle cells. Leukocytes attracted to the vicinity may also release TXA$_2$, enhancing vasospasm that is partially reversed by the synthesis of NO by the endothelial cells. (As thrombin is generated it also "feeds back" to factor V and FVIII, activating them and accelerating the process of coagulation.) Thrombin also cleaves FXIII that cross-links the fibrin strands rendering them somewhat resistant to lysis by plasmin. Thrombin also binds to thrombomodulin on the endothelium that activates protein C, an inhibitor of the coagulation process. Another action of thrombin is to activate thrombin activatable fibrinolysis inhibitor also known as procarboxypeptidase. The process we have just described occurs at the site of plaque rupture, an autochthonous (local) process that is not easily modulated by antithrombotic drugs, and which may in fact be caused by heparin or low molecular weight heparin (LMWH) in the heparin-induced thrombocytopenia (HIT) syndrome (11–15).

In Figure 1, the platelet is shown to have multiple surface receptors, multiple organelles, and biochemical pathways that facilitate its communication and interaction with the environment. These receptors and biochemical pathways are each potential targets for anticoagulant and antiplatelet drugs. (Blocking single enzymes and single platelet receptors by various drugs only partially blocks platelet function.) When glycoprotein (GP) IIb/IIIa is blocked, platelet–platelet interaction is blocked, which has a more profound inhibitory effect on thrombus formation than the blocking of other sites. Thus, inhibition of GPIIb/IIIa may be highly effective but is also a great risk for bleeding (14–16).

Pharmacology of the anticoagulant and antiplatelet drugs

Anticoagulants

Anticoagulants are essential to the management of the ACS. The anticoagulants in current clinical use include heparin, LMWH, fondaparinux, bivalirudin, lepirudin, and argatroban. Recent studies of fondaparinux (OASIS 5–Michelangelo Trial) show it to be undergoing trials effective in non-ST-elevation myocardial infarction and therefore it is included in this anticoagulant group (17).

Heparin is a glycosaminoglycan extracted from animal tissues (porcine mucosa, beef lung, etc.). It is a mixture of molecules having a mean molecular weight of 15,000 Da. A pentasaccharide sequence found in approximately one third of the molecules binds to antithrombin in mammalian blood, enhancing its inhibitory effects on the enzymes thrombin, factor Xa, factor VIIa, and factor IXa. The reaction is reversible, heparin being released after the antithrombin molecule binds to the procoagulant enzymes. Heparin binds to platelets, platelet factor-4 (which neutralizes it), histidine-rich GP, vWF, and a number of other proteins. Its half-life is about one hour in the circulation (18). Antibodies to heparin bound to PF4 and other positively charged proteins cause severe thrombotic problems in less than 1% to 3% of patients treated for five days or more (19). Hemorrhage related to circulating blood levels is the major side effect of heparin, occurring in about 6% of patients given therapeutic doses, but major bleeding occurs in less than 1% (18). It is poorly absorbed by the oral route. Its bioavailability is relatively low by the subcutaneous route that must therefore be dose adjusted according to laboratory test results, which is the case with intravenous heparin as well (18).

LMWHs are derivatives of standard heparin in which reduction of the mean molecular weight of the original heparin has been chemically reduced from a mean of 15,000 Da to a mean of approximately 5000 Da. To accomplish this, heparin molecules are treated with nitrous acid, heparinases, or benzylation and alkaline hydrolysis. The resultant product has the intact pentasaccharide sequence in at least one-third of the molecules and interaction with antithrombin is preserved in those molecules. Interactions and binding to platelets, proteins in the blood and endothelium is less than that of heparin. This property is advantageous because it permits prediction of circulating blood levels for a given subcutaneous dose. Monitoring of blood levels is unnecessary except in patients with significant renal impairment. A major difference is in the binding of the LMWH to factors Xa and thrombin when it is complexed to antithrombin. (Many of the molecules lack enough sugar moieties (<18) to bind to thrombin and AT, simultaneously precluding the inhibition of thrombin.) Factor Xa inhibition is not a problem. The resultant anti-Xa/IIa ratio is variable depending upon the method of degradation, but is 4:1, 3:1, or 2:1, for example, depending upon the manufacturing process. Each of these are unique drugs and mimic the properties of heparin to varying degrees. Their properties are the same as heparin but they manifest these properties to varying degrees as compared with heparin and with each other. They, like heparin, do not inhibit factor Xa or thrombin bound to fibrin in thrombi (18). Comparison of these properties is shown in Table 1.

Fondaparinux is a chemically synthesized pentasaccharide that mimics the antithrombin-binding site of heparin and LMWH. Its molecular size (1728 Da) is too small to bind to thrombin molecules while it is bound to antithrombin. Therefore, it is a pure anti-Xa inhibitor. It binds very little to platelets, proteins, or endothelium and is excreted in the urine. It does not form a complex with PF4 or other positively charged molecules. It is not neutralizable by protamine sulfate. Recent clinical trials have resulted in FDA approval for prophylaxis of deep vein thrombosis in orthopedic surgery. It has been shown to be effective and safe for the treatment of pulmonary embolism (20,21) and ACS (non-ST-elevation MI) (OASIS 5—Michelangelo Trial) (17).

Bivalirudin is a direct thrombin inhibitor that has found utility for reducing the rate of acute reocclusion in patients treated with PCI. It is preferential to heparin in PCI when HIT is present. This drug is a derivative of hirudin, which is a dedicated thrombin inhibitor with no other in vivo activities of significance. The molecule is semisynthetic; the C-terminal of hirudin is linked by a polyglycine spacer to the tetrapeptide region of the N-terminal that reacts with the thrombin active site (22). It is monitored by the activated clotting time test. Its pharmacologic properties are shown in Table 1.

Hirudin is a direct thrombin inhibitor marketed in a recombinant form (lepirudin). It is a protein derived from a salivary gland of the medicinal leech. It binds tightly to exosite 1 and the apolar site near the catalytic site. It is used as a substitute for

Table 1 Pharmacologic properties of anticoagulant and antiplatelet drugs used to treat ACS

Drug	Target	Route	Lab monitoring	Reference
Aspirin	Cox-1	Oral	No	16
Clopidogrel	ADP-R	Oral	No	16
Tirofiban	GPIIb/IIIa	IV	No	16
Eptifibatide	GPIIb/IIIa	IV	No	16
Abciximab	GPIIb/IIIa	IV	No	16
LMWH	Xa, IIa	SC	No	18
Fondaparinux	Xa	SC	No	18
Heparin	Xa, IIa	IV	Yes	18
Bivalirudin	IIa	IV	Yes	25
Argatroban	IIa	IV	Yes	24
Lepirudin	IIa	IV	Yes	25

Abbreviations: ADP, adenosine diphosphate; Cox-1, cyclooxygenase; GPIIb/IIIa, glycoprotein; IV, intravenous; IIa, factor IIa-thrombin; SC, subcutaneous; Xa, factor Xa.

heparin or LMWH in patients who have HIT where the risk of thrombosis is high. Laboratory monitoring of the anticoagulant effects of the parenterally administered drug is necessary. The activated partial thromboplastin time (APTT) or the ecarin clotting time tests may be used for this purpose but only the APTT has been clinically evaluated for HIT (Table 1) (23).

Argatroban is a synthetic arginine derivative that is a competitive inhibitor of the action of thrombin on fibrinogen. It is given parenterally and monitored by the APTT test. It has a short half-life. It is nonantigenic. It is approved for use in HIT and has undergone trials for PCI in some patients (Table 1) (24).

Antiplatelet drugs

Aspirin is a direct-acting antiplatelet drug. (Its prolonged duration of action after therapy is discontinued will be discussed below under clinical use of the combination of anticoagulant and antiplatelet drugs.) A summary of its pharmacology is in Table 1.

GP IIb/IIIa Inhibitors

These direct-acting inhibitors bind to the IIb/IIIa GPs that are expressed on the platelet surface when platelets are activated. Three such drugs are in routine clinical use (16).

1. 7E3 monoclonal antibody to GPIIb/IIIa (abciximab) is very useful as an antiplatelet drug in high-risk ACSs and PCI. It can be used in conjunction with reduced levels of heparin and with aspirin (Table 1). Patients may uncommonly experience sudden severe thrombocytopenia within the early hours of treatment as a side effect.
2. Eptifibatide (Integrelin), a cyclic heptapeptide based on a peptide sequence in snake venom, is a GPIIb/IIIa inhibitor used in conjunction with heparin and aspirin for the treatment of ACS or in PCI, with or without stenting and clopidogrel (Table 1).
3. Tirofiban (Aggrastat) is a nonpeptide antagonist of the GPIIb/IIIa receptor. It is administered intravenously. Its properties are shown in Table 1. It is used in ACS for unstable angina and in PCI along with aspirin and heparin.

Thienopyridines

The thienopyridines include clopidogrel, ticlopidine, and prosugel. Clopidogrel is the only member of this class in clinical use at this time. A second generation of this drug, Prosugel, is undergoing trials (27). Ticlopidine is not used

because of its propensity to cause TTP. Clopidogrel is a prodrug that must be converted to an active drug in the liver. It binds to and blocks the ADP receptor on platelets, a measurable effect lasting at least five days. An initial loading dose is necessary if prompt action is desired, otherwise a maintenance dose of three to seven days will be necessary before the platelet function is optimally impaired. Resistance to clopidogrel has been reported. This can be detected by platelet aggregometry utilizing ADP as the agonist (16,25).

Combined anticoagulant and antiplatelet therapy

In Figure 3, an abbreviated coagulation cascade beginning with tissue factor is flanked by drugs that inhibit the coagulation enzymes and platelet function. The action of these drugs on platelets may be direct, as in the case of aspirin where the action is directed to a platelet enzyme or to a receptor as in the case of clopidogrel. Heparin, LMWH, and thrombin inhibitors act indirectly by blocking the agonist thrombin. The effect of aspirin and clopidogrel lasts for several days after the drug has been withdrawn but the effect of heparin, LMWH, and thrombin inhibitors disappear in minutes to hours after the drug is withdrawn. Patients on aspirin and/or clopidogrel may bleed if taken to surgery on an emergency basis. The GPIIb/IIIa inhibitor abciximab may also have a prolonged effect (16). Resistance to aspirin and synthetic IIb/IIIa inhibitors have been described (16). Patients with unstable angina are at varying risk for thrombosis and it has been determined that the higher risk patient requires a combination of anticoagulants and antiplatelet agents. LMWH has largely replaced standard heparin in most treatment regimens with the exception of PCI. Direct thrombin inhibitors have been given in clinical trials (25). A newer drug, fondaparinux, a synthetic LMWH, which is a factor Xa inhibitor undergoing clinical trial (17). Idraparinux, a longer acting version of fondaparinux, is being developed (26).

Clinical use of the combination of anticoagulant and antiplatelet drugs

The combination of heparin and aspirin for the treatment of ACS began in the 1980s. Aspirin had been synthesized by the Bayer Pharmaceutical Company in 1895 and marketed as an analgesic and antipyretic drug. Approximately 60 years later, it was found to enhance the bleeding tendency observed in known hemorrhagic disorders (1956) and to prolong the bleeding time of normals in 1964 (27,28). During this period, the morphology of platelets and their ultrastructure was being intensively studied, and the biochemistry of platelet aggregation induced by ADP was described (29). By 1970, the effect of aspirin on platelets was shown to be via the acetylation of cyclooxygenase, an enzyme that converts arachidonic acid to prostaglandin (16). This was an irreversible effect that lasted for the life of the platelets. Generation of TXA_2 and the prostaglandins, PGG_2 and PGH_2, was blocked. Thus the production of PGI_2 by the endothelium was temporarily blocked. Vane (30) discovered the effect on prostaglandin synthesis in 1971. He was awarded the Nobel prize for that work in 1982. Some of the more relevant biochemical pathways within the platelets are shown in Figure 1. (It is to be noted that the agonists thrombin, collagen, and ADP acting on their respective receptors are clinically the most relevant.) It is important to note the feedback pathway of platelet polyphosphate and platelet microparticles (Fig. 3) on the coagulation cascade and the specific enhancement of FV activity and the suppression of TFPI by the polyphosphates, as well as the contributions of platelet microparticles to enhance the coagulation pathway activity. Polyphosphate release from activated platelets is not blocked by aspirin (31).

Most of the clinical studies devoted to the treatment of unstable angina during the 1970s were devoted to comparing the medical therapy of this disorder with coronary artery bypass graft surgery. The medical arm of these studies did not include heparin (32). It was controversial as to whether heparin improved the major outcome criteria of myocardial infarction, revascularization, and death. Beta-blockers, nitroglycerin, oxygen, and bed rest were standard therapy. (Beginning in 1980s, the aspirin trials began, followed in the late 1980s by the combination of aspirin and heparin.) In 1981, a study showed the incidence of myocardial infarction to be only 3% in aspirin-treated patients as compared with 15% in the control group (33). These findings were confirmed in studies by Lewis et al. and Cairns et al. (32,33), showing a very clear benefit of aspirin without heparin. In these studies, the dose of aspirin varied from 325 mg twice daily to four times daily. Other investigators showed that doses as low as 80 mg/day were as effective in blocking cyclooxygenase, as were doses of 160 and 325 mg or more (16). However, the lower doses did not reach peak effect as early as did the higher doses, prompting the initial use of the higher doses.

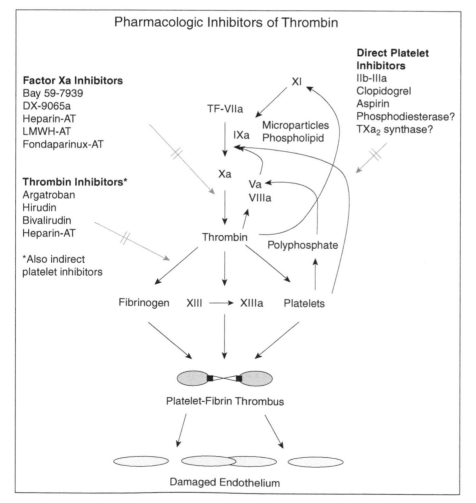

Figure 3

Pharmacologic inhibitors of thrombin. Thrombin is a key enzyme in the hemostatic system in that it leads to the formation of fibrin strands and is a potent stimulus for platelet activation. Thrombin inhibitors, factor Xa inhibitors, and antiplatelet drugs act at different points in the hemostatic system to regulate the amount of thrombin that is generated.

(A very important study by Theroux et al. (34) in 1988 was the first to demonstrate the use of aspirin in combination with in ACS.) It was shown in the study that the incidence of all major endpoints was significantly reduced to 3.3% with aspirin, 0.8% with heparin, and 1.6% with a combination. The incidence of serious bleeding was not prohibitive. The fact that the combination of aspirin and heparin was better than aspirin alone but worse than heparin alone could be taken as evidence for using heparin alone, but subsequent studies showed that a rebound in the acute ischemic events occurred when heparin was stopped unless the aspirin was continued (34). Subsequent studies combining two or more antiplatelet drugs with heparin or LMWH gave better results than heparin and aspirin in the moderate- and high-probability patients and in PCI (27).

The modern era (1990 and beyond) has seen many new antiplatelet drugs become available for clinical use along with newer anticoagulants. The motivation for developing these drugs has been the perceived need for a broader inhibition of platelet function and of the coagulation system in patients with ST-elevation with or without Q-waves and the perception that PCI, particularly with stent placement, required the more potent IIb/IIIa inhibitors along with aspirin and clopidogrel in order to more completely suppress procoagulant tendencies in these patients. The currently available anticoagulant drugs for use in ACS and PCI are shown in Table 1. Note that the thienopyridines and the several IIb/IIIa inhibitors have become available and are being selectively used in higher risk patients. Bleeding risks are greater with the IIb/IIIa inhibitors when used in combination with heparin, but are reasonably safe when the heparin dose is reduced. When the acute reocclusion rate is high, they are required (27). Among the anticoagulant drugs, the LMWHs developed during the 1980s have replaced heparin for use in unstable angina based upon greater bioavailability with dosing that is more predictable than with heparin and with less tendency to cause HIT. One disadvantage of the LMWHs is their tendency to reach unpredictably high blood levels in patients with renal insufficiency. Furthermore, a reliable antidote is not available for patients who bleed (18). Protamine sulfate neutralizes the antithrombin effects of LMWHs but is unable to block the anti-Xa activity (18).

The numerous clinical trials that have been widely published and that are summarized in other chapters of this textbook attest to the need for combination drug therapy in the ACS. It is to be expected that results obtained in clinical practice will vary somewhat from those found in clinical trials but on balance it is important to treat patients in accordance with guidelines derived from clinical trials unless there are contraindications or relative risks. It is not possible to state that a given drug is more effective or safer than another drug without a head-to-head clinical trial of the drug in question.

Factors that the practicing clinicians can control better than in some clinical trials include ascertaining the fact that the patient is in fact taking or being given the drug in the appropriate doses and that appropriate monitoring is carried out and acted upon in a timely manner. This is not always the case as shown in a recent study (35).

We have attempted to find evidence for gender differences that could alter the information we have provided in this chapter but we could not find reliable human studies in this regard. This does not include differences that may exist in the endothelium or in the coronary artery anatomy or in the pathophysiology of atherosclerosis, but refers to effectiveness of antiplatelet and anticoagulation drugs as compared to the opposite sex.

Future antithrombotic agents

There are a number of additional targets that may lead to effective antithrombotic therapy in ACS. In terms of anticoagulants, the concepts of agents that have dual inhibitor sites such as the one we find in heparin but that lack in some of its undesirable qualities could be very useful. The same concept may apply to drugs that have both anticoagulant and antiplatelet properties. It is quite probable that inhibitors of tissue factor as well as of the platelet ADP receptor when combined with aspirin might be very effective. An ability to block the feedback action of the polyphosphates released from platelets upon activation is also an attractive aim (Fig. 3).

Several in-depth reviews of this subject have been recently-published (36,37).

References

1   Herrick J. Certain clinical features of sudden obstruction of the coronary arteries. Trans Am Assoc Phys 1912; 27:100–116.

2   McClean J. The thromboplastic action of cephalin. Am J Physiol 1916; 41:250–257.

3   Solandt DY and Best CH. Heparin and coronary thrombosis in experimental animals. Lancet 1938; ii:130–132.

4   Best CH. Preparation of heparin and its use in the first clinical cases. Circulation 1959; 19:79–86.

5   Wright IS. Experience with anticoagulants. Circulation 1959; 29:110–115.

6   Link KP. The discovery of dicumarol and its sequels. Circulation 1959; 19:97–107.

7   Quick AJ. The thromboplastin reagent for the determination of prothrombin. Science 1940; 92:113–114.

8   Butt HR, Allen EV, Bollman JL. A preparation from spoiled sweet clover (3,3')-methylene-bis-(4 hydroxycoumarin) which prolongs coagulation and prothrombin time of the blood: preliminary report of experimenta and clinical studies. Proc Staff Meet Mayo Clin 1941; 16:388–395.

9   James DF, Bennett IL Jr, Scheinberg P, et al. Clinical studies on dicumarol hypoprothrombinemia and vitamin K preparations. Int Med 1949; 83:632–652.

10 Barritt DW, Jordan SC. Anticoagulant drugs in the treatment of pulmonary embolism. A controlled trial. Lancet 1960; 1: 1309–1312.

11 Kroll MH, Rezendiz JC. Mechanism of platelet activation. In: Loscalzo J, Schafer A, eds. Thrombosis and Hemorrhage. 3rd ed. Philadelphia: Lippincott Williams, 2003:187–205.

12 Rosenberg RD, Aird WC. Vascular bed specific hemostasis and hypercoagulable states. N Engl J Med 1999; 340:1555–1564.

13 Kraegel AH, Reddy SC, Willes H, et al. Morphometric analysis of the composition of coronary arterial plaques in isolated unstable angina pectoris with pain at rest. Am J Cardiol 1990; 66:562–567.

14 Fuster V, Lewis A. Connor memorial lecture. Mechanisms leading to myocardial infarction. Insight from studies of vascular biology. Circulation 1994; 90:2126–2146.

15 Sakharov DV, Plow EF, Rifken DC. On the mechanism of the antithrombin activity of plasma carboxypeptidase B. J Biol Chem 1997; 272:14477–14482.

16 Patrono C, Coller B, FitzGerald GA, et al. Platelet active drugs. The relationship among dose, effectiveness and side effects. Chest 2004; 126(suppl):234S–264S.

17 Michelangelo OASIS 5 Steering Committee. Design and rationale of the MICHELANGELO Organization to Assess Strategies in acute Ischemic Syndrome (OASIS)-5 trial. Am Heart J 2005; 150:1107.

18 Hirsh J, Raschke R. Heparin and low molecular weight heparin. Chest 2004; 126(suppl):188S–203S.

19 Warkentin T, Greinacher A. Heparin-induced thrombocytopenia. Chest 2004; 126(suppl):311S–337S.

20 Buller HR, Davidson BL, Decausus H, et al. Fondaparinux or enoxaparin for the initial treatment of symptomatic deep vein thrombosis: a randomized trial. Ann Int Med 2004; 140:867–873.

21 The Matisse Investigators. Subcutaneous fondaparinux versus intravenous unfractionated heparin in the initial treatment of pulmonary embolism. N Engl J Med 2003; 349: 1695–1702.

22 Weitz JI, Hirsh J, Samama M. New anticoagulant drugs. Chest 2004; 126:265S–286S.

23 Lubenow N, Greinacher A. Management of patients with heparin-induced thrombocytopenia: focus on recombinant hirudin. J Thromb Thrombolysis 2000; 10:S47–S57.

24 Iqbal O, Ahmad S, Lewis BE, et al. Monitoring of argatroban in ARG310 study: potential recommendations for its use in interventional cardiology. Clin Appl Thrombosis/Hemostasis 2002; 8(3):217–224.

25 Becker RC. Hirudin-based anticoagulant strategies for patients with suspected heparin-induced thrombocytopenia undergoing percutaneous coronary interventions and bypass grafting. J Thromb Thrombolysis 2000; 10:S59–S68.

26 Herbert JM, Herault JP, Bernat A, et al. Biochemical and pharmacological properties of SANORG 34000, a potent long-acting pentasaccharide. Blood 1998; 91:4197–4205.

27 Harrington RA, Becker RC, Ezekowitz M, et al. Antithrombotic therapy for coronary artery disease. Chest 2004; 126(suppl): 513S–548S.

28 Stuart MJ. The post aspirin bleeding time. A screening test evaluating hemostatic disorders. Br J Haematol 1979; 43: 649–656.

29 Born GVR. Aggregation of blood platelets by adenosine diphosphate. Nature 1962; 94:927–929.

30 Vane JR. Inhibition of prostaglandin synthesis as a mechanism of action for aspirin-like drugs. Nat New Biol 1971; 231: 232–235.

31 Smith SA, Mutch NJ, Baskar D, et al. Polyphosphate modulates blood coagulation and fibrinolysis. Proc Natl Acad Sci USA 2006; 103:903–908.

32 Lewis HD Jr, Davis JW, Archebald DG, et al. Protective effects of aspirin against acute myocardial infarction and death in men with unstable angina: results of a veterans administration cooperative study. N Engl J Med 1983; 309: 396–403.

33 Cairns JA, Gent M, Singer J, et al. Aspirin, sulfinpyrazone or both in unstable angina: results of a Canadian multicenter trial. N Engl J Med 1985; 313:1369–1375.

34 Theroux P, Ouimet H, Mc Cans J, et al. Aspirin, heparin or both to treat unstable angina. N Engl J Med 1988; 319: 1105–1111.

35 Raschke R, Hirsh J, Guildry JR. Suboptimal monitoring and dosing of unfractionated heparin in comparative studies with low-molecular weight heparin. Ann Int Med 2003; 138:720–723.

36 Messmore HL, Jeske W, Wehrmacher W. Antiplatelet agents: current drugs and future trends. Hematol Oncol Clin N Am 2005; 19:89–117.

37 Pipe SW. The promise and challenges of bioengineered recombinant clotting factors. J Thromb Haemost 2005; 3(8): 1692–1701.

12

Fibrinolytic therapy

Freek W. A. Verheugt

Acute myocardial infarction has become the largest mortality and morbidity problem of health care in the West. Epidemiology, pathophysiology, diagnosis, and treatment of acute myocardial infarctions were studied and developed gradually after Einthoven invented electrocardiography in 1901. Since acute myocardial infarction in patients presenting with ST-elevation is caused by a thrombotic occlusion of a major epicardial coronary artery, the largest step taken forward in the causal treatment of acute myocardial infarction has been in the introduction of reperfusion therapy.

The key element of benefit with reperfusion therapy is the time taken to complete it [thrombolysis in myocardial infarction (TIMI) flow grade 3]. The benefit of this strategy rises exponentially, the earlier the therapy is initiated (Fig. 1). The highest number of lives are saved by reperfusion therapy when it is used within the first hour after symptom onset thus creating a window of opportunity (golden hour) (1). Clearly and logically, the mechanism of this benefit relates in maximizing myocardial salvage by early restoration of adequate coronary blood flow, resulting in the preservation of left ventricular function, and thereby enhancing both early and long-term survival.

According to the principle of the infarct wavefront, a brief interruption of blood flow is associated with a small infarct size. The temporal dependence of the beneficial effect of coronary reperfusion has also been characterized by multiple metrics, including positron emission tomography (2). Irrespective of the methodology, however, the relationship between the duration of symptoms and the infarct size remains consistent.

The exponential curve illustrating the benefit of reperfusion therapy upon mortality and myocardial salvage has major implications on the timing of undertaking the treatment. Fibrinolytic therapy is less beneficial and contraindications are more stringent the later a patient is presented and the smaller the size of the area at risk. Consequently, reducing the delays will have a much more positive return in patients presenting early compared to those presenting late (3). These considerations have provided a strong incentive for the initiation of very early reperfusion therapy, including the use of prehospital fibrinolysis (4), which shortens the treatment time by about an hour and improves clinical outcome compared to inhospital therapy. Unfortunately, patient delay is still the main factor and does not seem to be influenced by public campaigns (5). On the other hand, fibrinolytic therapy can be initiated in the prehospital setting.

Two major forms of reperfusion therapy are available: fibrinolytic therapy and primary coronary intervention. This review mainly addresses the former.

Mechanism of fibrinolysis

Fibrinolytic agents (Table 1) aim at plasminogen activation at the site of the thrombotic occlusion (Fig. 2) during the early hours of acute transmural myocardial infarction. Besides lysis of fibrinogen, plasmin also splits several important clotting factors, such as prothrombin. When prothrombin is split, thrombin generation occurs and this has strong procoagulant effects. Although the procoagulant effect of fibrinolysis can be diminished by the concomitant heparin therapy, the nature of this therapy with its unpredictable efficacy and bleeding risk makes unsure the complete abolishment of the procoagulant effect of fibrinolytic therapy. Guidelines advice an intravenous bolus of 60U/kg to a maximum of 4000 U unfractionated heparin followed by a continuous infusion for at least 48 hours, with a target activated partial thromboplastin time (aPTT) of 50 to 70 seconds, measured 3, 6, 12, and 24 hours after the first dose. Finally, aspirin must be given immediately with a loading dose of 200 to 300 mg, followed by a maintenance dose of 75 to 160 mg daily.

Indications for fibrinolysis

Since most patients with ST-elevation acute coronary syndrome have acutely occluded vessels (6), fibrinolytic

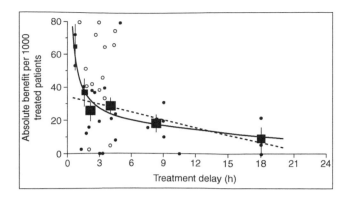

Figure 1
Relationship of time to treatment with early mortality in fibrinolytic therapy for acute myocardial infarction. *Source:* From Ref. 1.

therapy is indicated in most cases if primary balloon angioplasty cannot be done within 90 minutes of the first medical contact (7). Only a few patients with acute coronary syndrome without ST-elevation have a total thrombotic coronary occlusion. Therefore, in such patients reperfusion therapy is not indicated and may be even harmful through its procoagulant effect. In several trials on fibrinolytic therapy in acute coronary syndrome, bleeding and thrombotic complications have made this therapy unpopular (8).

The indication for fibrinolytic therapy has to be weighed against the absolute or relative contraindications. The earlier the patient is presented and the larger the area at risk recorded in the presenting electrocardiogram, the more beneficial fibrinolytic therapy is, and more contraindications are relative. The later the patient is presented and the smaller the area at risk, the less fibrinolytic therapy is beneficial and the more contraindications are stringent.

Table 1 Available fibrinolytic agents
Nonfibrin specific
Streptokinase
Anisoylated plasminogen streptokinase complex (anistreplase)
Urokinase
Fibrin specific
Recombinant tissue plasminogen activator (or alteplase)
TNK t-PA (tenecteplase)
Reteplase

The risks of fibrinolysis

The major risk of fibrinolytic therapy is in its inherent bleeding complications. The most severe bleeding complication is the occurrence of intracerebral hemorrhage. This is seen in about 0.5% of patients treated with fibrinolysis. Risk factors for the development of cerebral bleeding following fibrinolytic therapy are low body weight (<65 kg), female sex, hypertension, and the use of oral anticoagulants prior to fibrinolysis. Other bleeding complications are gastrointestinal bleeding and hemorrhage following arterial punctures. In most cases, these bleeding complications can be managed conservatively and have a rather good prognosis. A second problem after fibrinolytic therapy is the occurrence of reocclusion (9). Reocclusion is seen after fibrinolysis in about 10% of cases in hospital and about 30% in the following year. So far, only parenteral and oral anticoagulation have proven to be effective against reocclusion (10,11). Finally, fibrinolytic agents may be immunogenic. This is especially seen with streptokinase and streptokinase-derived agents like anistreplase. The recombinant endogenous plasminogen activator, the tissue plasminogen activator (rt-PA), or alteplase, has a low incidence of immunologic reactions and can be given to patients with streptokinase allergy or in patients who have had streptokinase before. Currently, there are mutants of rt-PA that can be given as single bolus (TNK-tPA, or tenecteplase). This has the major advantage of ease of administration: for example, in an ambulance.

The cost of fibrinolytic agents is considerable: streptokinase costs about US $100, and rt-PA and its mutants about US $2000. However, these agents have different early (90 minutes) recanalization rates: over 50% for front-loaded tissue rt-PA versus only 30% to 35% for streptokinase. Since early patency is correlated with early survival (12), the initial cost of the thrombolytic drug alone is not important. Patients who present early with a large myocardial infarction benefit more from a drug with a high early patency rate than patients presenting late with a small myocardial infarction.

Patients without ST-segment elevation usually do not have an acute coronary occlusion. Therefore, they will not benefit by thrombolytic therapy, but do have the risk of its complications.

Alternatives to fibrinolytic therapy

The clear alternative to fibrinolytic therapy in the reperfusion strategy of ST-segment elevation acute myocardial infarction is primary coronary angioplasty. This therapy has a clinical benefit over the optimal thrombolytic strategy: front-loaded rt-PA or tenecteplase (13). The major drawback of primary angioplasty is its limited availability and treatment delay. The

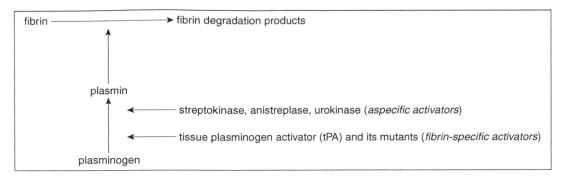

Figure 2
Mechanism of fibrinolytic drugs.

delay is caused by preparation of the catheterization labora-tory and mobilization of personnel to perform the procedure. Moreover, when patients have to be transferred for primary angioplasty, the delay can be considerable. The initial cost of primary angioplasty is higher than that of thrombolytic ther-apy, but the patency achieved is superior to thrombolytic therapy: up to 90% (14). The risk of thrombolytic therapy is higher than that of primary angioplasty, since cerebral bleed-ing is absent with primary angioplasty. During the treatment delay, patients may be treated with a thrombolytic to speed up reperfusion prior to angioplasty (facilitated angioplasty). However, the trials evaluating this therapy show better preangioplasty patency but no benefit over plain primary angioplasty, and bleeding is significantly increased (15). Also lower doses of fibrinolytic agents alone or in combination with platelet glycoprotein receptor antagonists failed to improve outcome.

References

1 Boersma E, Maas AC, Deckers JW, Simoons ML. Early throm-bolytic therapy in acute myocardial infarction: reappraisal of the golden hour. Lancet 1996; 348:771–775.

2 Bergmann SR, Lerch RA, Fox KAA, et al. Temporal depen-dence of beneficial effects of coronary thrombolysis characterized by positron emission tomography. Am J Med 1982; 73:573–580.

3 Gersh BJ, Stone GW, White HD, Holmes DR. Pharmacological facilitation of primary percutaneous coronary intervention for acute myocardial infarction: is the slope of the curve the shape of the future? JAMA 2005; 293:979–986.

4 Morrison LJ, Verbeek PR, McDonald AC, Sawadsky BV, Cook DJ. Mortality and prehospital thrombolysis for acute myocar-dial infarction. JAMA 2000; 283:2686–2692.

5 Lupker RV, Raczynski JM, Osganian S, et al. Effect of a commu-nity intervention in patient delay and emergency medical service use in acute coronary heart disease: the Rapid Early

Action for Coronary Treatment (REACT). JAMA 2000; 284:60–67.

6 DeWood MA, Spores J, Notske R, et al. Prevalence of total coronary occlusion during the early hours of transmural myocardial infarction. N Engl J Med 1980; 303:897–902.

7 Van de Werf F, Ardissino D, Betriu A, et al. Management of acute myocardial infarction in patients presenting with ST-elevation. Eur Heart J 2003; 24:28–66.

8 TIMI-IIIB Investigators. Effects of tissue plasminogen activator and a comparison of early invasive and conservative strategies in unstable angina and non-Q-wave myocardial infarction: results of the TIMI-IIIB trial. Circulation 1994; 89:1545–1556.

9 Verheugt FWA, Meijer A, Lagrand WK, Van Eenige MJ. Reocclusion: the flip side of coronary thrombolysis. J Am Coll Cardiol 1996; 27:766–773.

10 Ross AM, Molhoek P, Lundergan C, et al. Randomized comparison of enoxaparin, a low molecular weight heparin, with unfractionated heparin adjunctive to tissue plasminogen activator thrombolysis and aspirin: second trial of Heparin and Aspirin Reperfusion Therapy (HART II). Circulation 2001; 104:648–652.

11 Brouwer MA, Van den Bergh PJPC, Vromans RPJW, et al. Aspirin plus medium intensity coumadin versus aspirin alone in the prevention of reocclusion after successful thrombolysis for suspected acute myocardial infarction: results of the APRI-COT-2 study. Circulation 2002; 106:659–665.

12 Stone GW, Cox D, Gracia E, et al. Normal flow (TIMI-3) before mechanical reperfusion therapy is an independent determinant of survival in acute myocardial infarction: results from the primary angioplasty in myocardial infarction trials. Circulation 2002; 104:636–641.

13 Keeley EC, Boura JA, Grines CL. Primary coronary angioplasty versus intravenous fibrinolytic therapy for acute myocardial infarction: a quantitative review of 23 randomised trials. Lancet 2003; 361:13–20.

14 Grines CL, Serruys PW, O'Neil WW. Fibrinolytic therapy: is it a treatment of the past? Circulation 2003; 107:2538–2542.

15 Keeley EC, Boura JA, Grines CL. Comparison of primary and facilitated percutaneous coronary intervention for ST-elevation myocardial infarct: quantitative review of randomized trials. Lancet 2006; 367:579–588.1

13

Resistance to antiplatelet drugs

Paul A. Gurbel and Udaya S. Tantry

Introduction

Acute coronary syndromes (ACSs) are major causes of morbidity and mortality around the world. The common underlying pathological events during ACS are endothelial denudation and formation of occlusive thrombus. Platelets are not only central to thrombotic processes (the platelet hypothesis), but also play an important role in atherosclerosis, coagulation, and inflammation (1,2). Platelets are small anucleate subcellular fragments that circulate freely in the blood in the normal physiological state. However, disruption of the normal protective nature of the endothelium occurs during ACSs and percutaneous coronary intervention (PCI), exposing the subendothelial matrix. Transient binding of platelet surface receptors, glycoprotein (GP) Ib-IX-V and GPVI to von Willebrand's factor and collagen, respectively, present in the subendothelial matrix facilitates initial platelet adhesion to the vessel wall. Subsequent intracellular signaling events trigger platelet activation, granule secretion, and finally the activation of GPIIb/IIIa receptors (final common pathway). Binding of fibrinogen and vWF to the activated GPIIb/IIIa receptor facilitates irreversible platelet aggregation and further recruitment of platelets (3–5). Thrombin is initially generated through tissue factor released from the vessel wall and is another primary agonist responsible for platelet activation. Platelet activation leads to the activation of phospholipase A_2 (PLA_2), which cleaves membrane phospholipids to release arachidonic acid. Arachidonic acid is converted to thromboxane A_2 (TxA_2) by sequential actions of cycloxygenase-1 and thromboxane synthase present in platelets. Secreted TxA_2 binds to a specific Gq-coupled thromboxane receptor (TP) and activates and recruits surrounding platelets as a positive feedback mechanism (6). Adenosine diphosphate (ADP) released from dense granules activates surrounding platelets via autocrine and paracrine mechanisms by binding to specific G-protein-coupled purinergic receptors, $P2Y_{12}$ and $P2Y_1$ (1,3). Concomitant activation of both purinergic receptors is needed for complete aggregation by ADP. However, the binding of ADP to the $P2Y_{12}$ receptor and subsequent intracellular signaling pathways are predominantly responsible for the activation of the GPIIb/IIIa receptor (4,7). Thus, ADP and TxA_2 amplify platelet activation processes and recruitment of platelets during stable thrombus generation. In addition, platelet activation also results in the expression of adhesion molecules, especially P-selectin and CD40 ligand (CD40L) on the platelet surface. These molecules play an important role in the heterotypic aggregation of platelets with leukocytes, inflammation and amplification of thrombin generation (Fig. 1) (8–10).

Rationale for antiplatelet therapy

Experiments in animal models and autopsy studies have demonstrated the primary involvement of platelets during thrombus formation and plugging of microvasculature (11,12). Increased expression of platelet surface molecules and heightened platelet reactivity have been demonstrated in patients with ACS and during PCI (2,13,14). High platelet reactivity has been associated with stent thrombosis, restenosis, inflammation, myocardial infarction (MI), and other ischemic events (15–22). Platelet activation and high platelet reactivity have also been associated with diabetes, hypertension, and hyperlipidemia (23–25). Therefore, the rationale for antiplatelet therapy is to prevent the development of occlusive thrombus formation, to arrest the procoagulant activity and inflammatory processes, to promote disaggregation of platelets, and finally to facilitate the reperfusion of occluded blood vessels. The determination of optimal platelet inhibition is dependent on the degree of ischemic risk and is counterbalanced by the risk of bleeding.

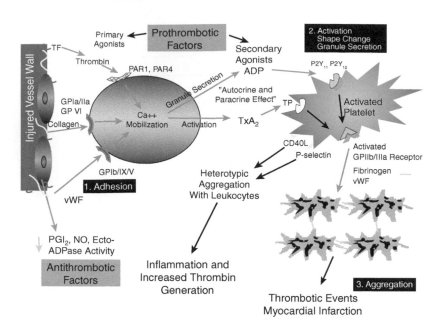

Figure 1

(*See color plate.*) Role of platelet activation and aggregation in cardiovascular diseases. Binding of primary (collagen, Thrombin, and vWF) and secondary (ADP, TxA2, etc.) agonists to specific receptors leads to final activation of GPIIb/IIIa receptors and irreversible platelet aggregation. *Abbreviations*: ADP, adenosine diphosphate; CD40L, CD40 ligand; ExctoADPase, ectoadenosine diphosphatase; GP, glycoprotein; NO, nitric oxide; PAR1 and PAR4, protease-activated thrombin receptors; PGI2, prostaglandin I2; TF, tissue factor; TxA2, thromboxane A2; P2Y1, P2Y12, ADP receptors; vWF, von Willebrand factor.

Resistance to antiplatelet drugs

Large-scale clinical trials have demonstrated the central role of platelet inhibition by antiplatelet agents in the primary treatment of ACS, in the prevention of complications during and after PCI, and in the long-term treatment of cardiovascular disease. Effective platelet inhibition immediately before and during PCI attenuates the development of in-hospital and postdischarge thrombotic complications (26–30). Extensive laboratory evaluations of the platelet response to aspirin or clopidogrel have not studied in these large-scale clinical trials. Despite the well-documented overall clinical efficacy of antiplatelet therapy, response variability and nonresponsiveness have been demonstrated for aspirin and clopidogrel treatment based on the ex vivo laboratory evaluation of the platelet response (31–33). This phenomenon has also been described as "resistance," "hyporesponsiveness," or "treatment failure" (Box 1).

Thrombosis is a multifactorial process that involves multiple pathways of platelet activation and factors other than platelets. Therefore, we believe that treatment failure is a poor definition since certain vascular complications are unrelated to platelet-specific mechanisms and hence antiplatelet drugs may not have any effect in these clinical conditions (34). Moreover, the underlying pathobiology may differ between clinical disease entities in atherothrombotic disease. Aspirin may be effective in certain disease states through shear-dependent mechanisms, whereas clopidogrel or GPIIb/IIIa blockers may be effective in preventing other atherothrombotic complications through shear-independent mechanisms (35,36). Finally, since multiple agonists activate platelets, clinical ischemic events can occur despite complete drug-induced inhibition of a particular pathway of activation. It is

Box 1 Definition of antiplatelet resistance	
Antiplatelet Drug Nonresponsiveness/ target Resistance	= Failure to Inhibit
Antiplatelet Drug Nonresponsiveness/ Resistance	≠ Clinical Failure
No single pathway mediates all thrombotic events—multiple pathways of platelet activation	

our opinion that resistance to a specific antiplatelet agent as measured by ex vivo testing is best indicated by persistent activity of the target despite treatment with the specific antiplatelet agent that inhibits the target. This definition also implies that patients are receiving sufficient dosing to produce optimal drug levels for inhibition of the target. Therefore, the occurrence of clinical events during treatment (treatment failures) with a specific antiplatelet agent should not be regarded as "resistance" to the therapeutic agent (37).

Aspirin

Mechanism of action

Aspirin is the most economical and effective antiplatelet drug prescribed for the treatment of cardiovascular and cerebrovascular (CV) diseases. Initially, Vane et al. (38)

demonstrated that aspirin inhibits prostaglandin generation (TxA$_2$) in platelets and has a potent antiplatelet effect. This antiplatelet effect is due to irreversible acetylation of a serine residue (Ser529) on COX-1 in platelets that prevents the binding of arachidonic acid to the catalytic site of cyclooxygenase (39,40). In addition, aspirin elicits anti-inflammatory effects by inhibiting the COX-2-dependent synthesis of other prostaglandins in endothelial and inflammatory cells (26). Because the inhibitory effects of aspirin on the COX-1 enzyme is 50- to 100-fold more potent than those on the COX-2 enzyme, COX-2-related effects are comparatively low using the doses recommended for patients with cardiovascular diseases (26). However, aspirin has been demonstrated to inhibit collagen- induced inhibition in a modest dose-dependent manner (41). Additional antithrombotic effects of aspirin include antioxidant, anti-inflammatory, and antiatherosclerotic effects on endothelial cells and leukocytes (42). These additional effects of aspirin may contribute to antithrombotic properties in preventing cardiovascular events (Fig. 2).

Aspirin is rapidly absorbed; peak plasma concentrations are achieved within 40 minutes; and significant platelet inhibition is observed within an hour. Although the plasma half-life is 20 minutes, irreversible binding and the lack of de-novo protein synthesis in platelets results in COX-1 inhibition for the life span of platelets (~10 days). The stable metabolite of TxA$_2$, can be measured in plasma or urine and is a specific indicator of platelet response to aspirin therapy (43,44).

The extensive analyses of primary and secondary clinical trials have indicated that aspirin treatment is associated with a 20% to 44% reduction in cardiovascular adverse events (26,27). Based on the results of these trials, the US Preventive Services Task Force (USPSTF) recommends that low-dose aspirin (81 mg/day) should be administered in patients whose 5-year risk of a first CV event is ≥3% and whose 10-year risk is ≥6%. Whenever rapid and complete inhibition of platelet aggregation is desired, such as in the setting of acute MI, unstable angina, or PCI, a 160 to 325 mg aspirin-loading dose is favored (45). The Antithrombotic Trialists' Collaboration (ATC), the European Society of Cardiology (ESC) Committee for practice guidelines, the American College of Chest physicians, and the American Heart Association/American College of Cardiology (AHA/ACC) guidelines recommended aspirin therapy to prevent atherothrombotic complications (26, 27,46,47).

Aspirin resistance

Despite the well-recognized effect of aspirin in inhibiting arachidonic acid-induced platelet aggregation, other major activation pathways through ADP and thrombin are unaffected, except at low agonist concentrations (Fig. 2). Elevated levels of collagen, ADP, and thrombin can stimulate platelet aggregation independent of the thromboxane pathway. Thromboxane, unlike collagen and thrombin, is not involved in the primary activation of platelets. These properties may limit the efficacy of aspirin in preventing thrombosis in patients with ACS (5).

Earlier, Mehta et al. (48) in 1978 reported that about 30% of patients with coronary artery disease (CAD) had minimal inhibition (unchanged bleeding time) of platelet function by aspirin therapy. Since then, numerous studies evaluated the efficacy of aspirin therapy using various laboratory methodologies to demonstrate the phenomenon of aspirin "resistance." Since the target of aspirin is COX-1, resistance to aspirin is indicated by persistent activity of COX-1 in the presence of aspirin therapy. In cases where excessive bone marrow stimulation is present creating young platelets with high COX-2 activity, arachidonic acid stimulation may produce aggregation despite adequate COX-1 inhibition.

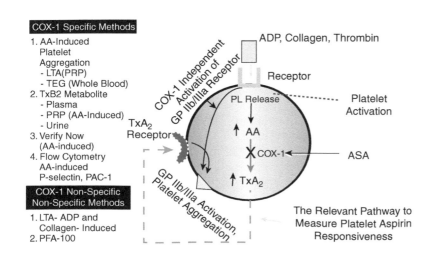

Figure 2

(*See color plate.*) Mechanism of action of aspirin and laboratory evaluation of aspirin responsiveness. *Abbreviations*: AA, arachidonic acid; ADP, adenosine diphosphate; ASA, aspirin; COX-1 and COX-2, cyclooxygenase isoenzymes; GP, glycoprotein; LTA, light transmission aggregometry; platelet function analyzer-100; TxA2, thromboxane A2; TxB2, metabolite of TxA2; PRP, platelet-rich plasma; TEG, thrombelastography; Tx, thromboxane; PFA-100.

Laboratory evaluation of aspirin resistance

The laboratory evaluation of platelet response to aspirin therapy has demonstrated response variability and nonresponsiveness. Based on different ex vivo methods, studies have shown wide variability in the prevalence of aspirin resistance (<1–54.7%) (45,49–58) (Table 1). Potential reasons for these discrepancies include (i) wide variability in the criteria to define aspirin resistance, (ii) variability in the methods to measure responsiveness, (iii) the timing of the laboratory test after aspirin treatment, (iv) the duration of aspirin treatment, and (v) the dose of aspirin administered.

Platelet response to aspirin may vary over the course of time. Decreased inhibition of platelet COX-1 was observed in some patients chronically treated with aspirin (59). Use of agonists such as ADP, epinephrine, or collagen that can aggregate platelets in the presence of complete COX-1 inhibition and therefore do not isolate COX-1 activity may overestimate the prevalence of aspirin nonresponsiveness. Moreover, point-of-care assays similarly employ methods based on platelet responses induced by epinephrine, ADP, or collagen. Finally, the relevance of these methods to the in vivo response to aspirin is unknown. More specific methods that indicate the degree of COX-1 activity include arachidonic acid-induced platelet aggregation and the measurement of the stable metabolite of TxA_2 following aspirin therapy in urine and plasma (43,44,60–62). Thus, there are important limitations in the specificity of the widely used laboratory methods. A validated criterion to prove the concept of aspirin resistance has not yet been established. Nevertheless, recent studies have correlated laboratory measurements of aspirin resistance in patients taking aspirin to the occurrence of thrombotic events, indicating a potential link between the measurement of ex vivo platelet function and in vivo events.

Mechanism of aspirin resistance

There are many potential mechanisms responsible for the occurrence of aspirin resistance or nonresponsiveness. Many of these studies reporting aspirin resistance have employed methods that did not isolate COX-1 inhibition and/or used treatment failure as their definition for aspirin resistance. Cigarette smoking, noncompliance, transient expression of COX-2 in newly formed platelets, and extra-platelet sources of PGG_2/PGH_2 (endothelial cells, monocytes/macrophages) may contribute to an attenuated clinical response to aspirin (63–66). Erythrocytes may attenuate the effect of aspirin by enhancing the prothrombotic effects of platelets and this property may contribute to aspirin resistance (67). Concomitant use of ibuprofen inhibits the irreversible binding of aspirin to COX-1 (68). Increased platelet turnover soon after surgical operations may influence the response of aspirin, and studies have found that aspirin resistance is increased transiently soon after cardiac surgery (69,70). Finally, genetic polymorphisms of the COX-1 gene or GPIIb/IIIa may contribute to variability in the platelet response to aspirin therapy and the occurrence of aspirin resistance (71,72).

Clinical relevance of aspirin resistance

In an earlier study, Grotemeyer et al. measured platelet aggregates in stroke patients after a 500 mg aspirin dose and found that 30% of patients had a platelet reactivity index greater than 1.25. These patients were defined as aspirin resistant. At a follow-up of two years with 500 mg aspirin treatment three times daily, aspirin-resistant patients had a 10-fold increase in the risk of recurrent vascular events as compared to aspirin-sensitive patients (44% vs. 4.4%, $P < 0.001$) (51). Using a whole blood aggregometry method to evaluate aspirin resistance, Mueller et al. (62) found an 87% increase in the incidence of reocclusion in "aspirin-resistant" patients who underwent peripheral balloon angioplasty and were treated with 100 mg aspirin daily for 18 months. Using a more COX-1-specific method by measuring urinary thromboxane metabolite levels, among patients enrolled in Heart Outcomes Prevention Evaluation (HOPE) trial for aspirin responsiveness, Eikelboom et al. (44) found that the risk of MI, stroke, or cardiovascular death was greatest in patients with the highest quartile of urinary thromboxane levels. Gum et al. found a 5% incidence of aspirin resistance in patients with stable cardiovascular disease taking 325 mg aspirin daily for up to 2.5 years. These investigators included the classic method of arachidonic acid-induced platelet aggregation in their definition of resistance. Aspirin resistance was associated with a significant increase in the composite endpoint of death, MI, or stroke (53,54). Recently, Chen et al. used a point-of-service assay employing cationic propyl gallate as the agonist to determine the incidence of aspirin resistance in patients with CAD scheduled for nonurgent PCI. Among 151 patients, 19.2% of patients met the criteria of aspirin resistance. Despite treatment with clopidogrel and heparin, aspirin resistance was associated with ~2.9-fold increase in the occurrence of myonecrosis (elevated serum CKMB levels) (56) (Table 2).

Table 1 Aspirin resistance studies

Investigators	n	ASA dose (mg/day)	Time	Method	Criteria for aspirin resistance	%AR	Comments
Hurlen et al. (49)	143	AMI 75–160	2–24 hr	PAR	PAR < 0.82 PAR < 0.82 after additional ASA	9.8 1.4	No clinical relevance
Buchanan et al. (50)	40	CABG 325		Bleeding time Platelet TxA$_2$, 12-HETE and platelet adhesion	No prolongation of bleeding time above baseline	43	Increased 12-HETE and platelet adhesion associated with AR
Buchanan et al. (51)	287	CABG 325	24 hr 2 yr follow-up	Bleeding time	No prolongation of bleeding time above baseline	54.7	AR associated with no change in thrombotic event rate
Grotemeyer et al. (52)	180	Stroke 1500	1 yr follow-up	Platelet reactivity (PR)	Normal PR index (>1.25) at 2 or 12 hr	33.3	40% of AR patients had major endpoints (MI, stroke, and death)
Gum et al. (53,54)	325	Stable CAD 325	≥ 7 days 2 yr follow-up	LTA- AA and ADP PFA-100 collagen/ ADP or collagen/EPI	> 70% ADP-induced aggregation + AA (0.5 mg/ml) induced >20% after ASA. Normal (<193 sec) collagen/EPI closure time after ASA	5.5 9.5	AR associated with 3 × higher risk (death, MI, CVA)
Eikelboom et al. (44) (HOPE Study)	488	75–325 follow-up	5 yr follow-up	Urinary 11-dehydro TxA$_2$	Elevated urinary 11-dehydro TxA$_2$ - Upper quartile	25	Upper quartile had 1.8 × higher risk (MI, stroke, CVA)
Wang et al. (55)	422	Stable CAD 81–325	≥ 7 days	RPFA	ARU > 550	23	Patients with a history of CAD had twice the odds of being AR
Chen et al. (56)	151	Non-urgent PCI 81–325	≥ 7 days	RPFA Myonecrosis (CK-MB +TnI)	ARU > 550	19.2	AR associated with 2.9-fold increase in myonecrosis
Gonzalez-Conejero et al. (57)	24	HS 100 and 500	2 wk	PA – 1 mM AA or 10 ug/ml Collagen. 11-dehydro TxA$_2$. PFA-100. genotyping	< 300 sec closer time	33.3 (100 mg) 0 (500 mg)	AR can be overcome by increased dose of aspirin
Tantry et al. (58)	*223*	*PCI 325*	*Long-term*	*LTA -1 mM AA*	*> 50% aggregation*	*< 1.0*	

Abbreviations: AA, arachidonic acid; AMI, acute myocardial infarction; AR, aspirin resistance; ASA, aspirin; CABG, coronary artery bypass graft surgery; CAD, coronary artery disease; CK-MB, creatinine kinase-MB; CVA, cerebrovascular accident; EPI, epinephrine; HS, healthy subjects; LTA, light transmittance aggregometry; mm, millimolar; PAR, platelet activity ratio; PCI, percutaneous coronary intervention; PR, platelet reactivity; RPFA, rapid platelet function analyzer; T$_x$A$_2$, thromboxane A$_2$.
Source: From Ref. 5.

Table 2   Clinical relevance of aspirin resistance

Investigators	n	Patients	Method	Results
Grotmeyer et al. (52)	180	CVA	Platelet aggregates	10 × increase in vascular events
Mueller et al. (62)	100	PVD	Platelet aggregation (whole blood)	87% increase in incidence of reocclusion
Eikelboom et al. (44)	976	HOPE trial	Urinary TxB$_2$	Increase in MI/stroke/death with increase in TxB$_2$
Gum et al. (53,54)	325	Stable CAD	Platelet aggregation (LTA)	3.12 × increase in MI/stroke/death
Chen et al. (56)	151	PCI	RPFA	2.9 × increase in myocardial necrosis

Abbreviations: CAD, coronary artery diseases; CVA, cerebrovascular accident; HOPE, heart outcomes prevention evaluation; LTA, light transmittance aggregometry; MI, myocardial infarction; PCI, percutaneous coronary intervention; PVD, peripheral vascular diseases; RPFA, rapid platelet function analyzer; TxB$_2$, thromboxane B$_2$.
Source: From Ref. 5.

Therapeutic intervention for aspirin resistance

Initial studies have suggested that the inhibition of COX-1 by aspirin can reach saturable levels (>95% inhibition) with a 100 mg daily dose (26,73,74). A higher dose (>75–325 mg/day) is not clearly associated with an increased clinical benefit but may be accompanied by an elevated risk of bleeding (26,27). In a recent study, normal volunteers were found to be resistant to aspirin treatment (100 mg/day) as determined by the platelet function analyzer (PFA-100), a device that measures shear-induced platelet aggregation. However, an increased dose of aspirin (325 mg/day) was effective in overcoming aspirin resistance as measured by PFA-100 (57). Similarly, it has been reported by measuring serum thromboxane B$_2$ (TxB$_2$) levels and arachidonic acid-induced platelet aggregation that low-dose (75 mg/day) aspirin treatment is not sufficient to completely inhibit the platelet COX-1 activity in some stable cardiovascular patients. Complete inhibition of arachidonic acid-induced aggregation by the addition of exogenous aspirin to platelets indicated that a higher dose might be needed in select patients (75).

In a recent study, aspirin response was measured by arachidonic acid-induced aggregation in platelet-rich plasma using standard light transmittance aggregometry (LTA) and in whole blood using thrombelastography (TEG) in patients undergoing elective coronary stenting treated with 325 mg daily aspirin. About 3.5% patients were found to be noncompliant with aspirin therapy and all responded well to in-hospital treatment. Only one patient met the aspirin-resistance criteria (>20% arachidonic acid-induced aggregation). Thus, a higher dose and strict compliance to the therapy can effectively overcome the occurrence of "aspirin resistance" in selected patients (58). Dual antiplatelet therapy with aspirin and P2Y$_{12}$ blockers may improve clinical outcomes in those infrequent patients who are truly resistant to aspirin (58).

Clopidogrel

The thienopyridines, ticlopidine and clopidogrel, are effective inhibitors of platelet aggregation. Clopidogrel was compared to aspirin therapy in patients with atherosclerotic vascular disease in the CAPRIE trial and was associated with superior protection against thrombotic events (28). Earlier, ticlopidine had been extensively used in the treatment of patients with cardiovascular disease. However, the more favorable side effect profile of clopidogrel has led to its establishment as the thienopyridine of choice. Since clopidogrel and aspirin inhibit platelet aggregation through different pathways, dual antiplatelet therapy provides complementary and additive benefits compared to either agent alone (2,5).

Mechanism of action

Clopidogrel is absorbed from the intestine and extensively converted by the hepatic cytochrome P450 (CYP) 3A4 to an active thiol metabolite (76,77). This short-lived active metabolite irreversibly binds to the P2Y$_{12}$ receptor through a disulfide bridge linking the reactive thiol group and two cysteine residues (cys17 and cys270) present in the extracellular domains of the P2Y$_{12}$ receptor. This permanent binding of the metabolite to the P2Y$_{12}$ receptor results in effective blockade of ADP-induced platelet activation and aggregation (78). The importance of P2Y$_1$ in pathological conditions, as well as efficiency of P2Y$_1$ receptor antagonist as an antiplatelet agent remain unclear (Fig. 3) (79).

Ex vivo measurements of platelet aggregation induced by ADP, and low concentrations of collagen and thrombin are decreased after clopidogrel treatment. Little information is available on the effect of clopidogrel treatment on arachidonic acid metabolism or arachidonic acid-induced platelet aggregation (5). By attenuating ADP-induced platelet activation, clopidogrel also inhibits the expression of P-selectin and CD-40L and the formation of heterotypic aggregates. The latter effect results in the attenuation of inflammatory processes, as indicated by reduced release of C-reactive protein and tumor necrosis factor (80,81). In addition, attenuation of thrombin generation by clopidogrel has also been reported (82–84).

Based on large clinical trials, a 300 mg clopidogrel-loading dose with a 75 mg clopidogrel daily dose, in addition to an 81 to 325 mg aspirin daily dose, had been considered the gold standard to prevent adverse cardiovascular events following PCI. However, recent studies employing a 600 mg loading dose have been conducted and use of this loading dose has increased (47).

Laboratory evaluation of platelet response to clopidogrel treatment

Since clopidogrel specifically inhibits one of two ADP receptors, ex vivo measurement of ADP-induced platelet aggregation by LTA is the most commonly used laboratory method to evaluate clopidogrel responsiveness. LTA is a cumbersome, time-consuming method that requires trained technicians. In this method, maximum platelet aggregation in response to 5 and 20 μM ADP is determined in platelet-rich plasma before and after treatment with clopidogrel. Patients with an absolute difference in aggregation of ≤10% have been considered nonresponders or "resistant"; those with 10% to 20% considered semi-responders; and those with ≤30% are considered responders (85,86). Recently, ex vivo "final" platelet aggregation measured at six minutes following stimulation by ADP was proposed as a better measure of clopidogrel response than maximum aggregation (87).

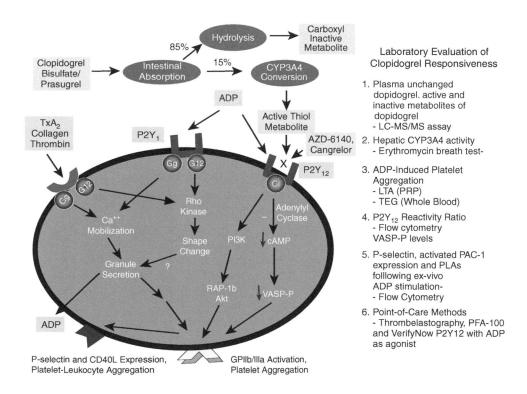

Figure 3

(*See color plate.*) Mechanism of action of clopidogrel and laboratory evaluation of clopidogrel nonresponsiveness. *Abbreviations*: ADP, adenosine diphosphate; CYP3A4, hepatic cytochrome 3A4; Gai2, G12, and Gq, G family protein-associated platelet receptors; GP, glycoprotein; IP3, P2Y1, and P2Y12, ADP receptors; LS-MS/MS, liquid chromatography-mass spectrometry; LTA, light transmittance aggregometry; TxA2, thromboxane A2; PFA-100, platelet function analyzer-100; PLA, platelet-leukocyte aggregation; PI3K, phosphoionisitol-3-kinase; PRP, platelet-rich plasma; TEG, thromelastography; VASP-P, vasodilator stimulated phosphoprotein-phospohrylated. *Source*: From Ref. 115.

Flow cytometric determinations of P-selectin and activated GPIIb/IIIa receptor expression following ADP stimulation have been used to assess platelet inhibition by clopidogrel. Flow cytometry is also a cumbersome method and requires sophisticated instrumentation and well-trained technicians. The phosphorylation state of vasodilator-stimulated phosphoprotein (VASP) is a specific intracellular marker of clopidogrel-induced $P2Y_{12}$ receptor inhibition and can also be measured by flow cytometry. Permeation of the membrane and the use of monoclonal antibodies specific for phosphorylated VASP are required in this method (15,88).

The TEG using the platelet mapping assay with ADP as the agonist, and the recently developed VerifyNow™ P2Y12 assay have been proposed as reproducible point-of-care methods to assess platelet inhibition by clopidogrel (21,89,90). These methods are undergoing investigation in clinical studies.

Clinical studies of clopidogrel response variability

Similar to other drugs, response variability and nonresponsiveness have been demonstrated for clopidogrel. In an earlier study, marked response variability to clopidogrel treatment (300 mg loading dose followed by 75 mg per day maintenance dose) following stent implantation was demonstrated by LTA and changes in the expression of activation-dependent markers following stimulation with ADP. A certain percentage of patients were found to have no demonstrable antiplatelet effect (85). In this study, 63% of patients were resistant to clopidogrel treatment at two hours, 30% were resistant at day 1 and day 5 post-stenting, and 15% were resistant at day 30 post-stenting (Fig. 4). Therefore, clopidogrel "resistance" in this study appeared to be time dependent. In addition, post-stenting platelet reactivity to ADP was greater than pre-stenting in a certain proportion of these patients. These patients were regarded as having "heightened" platelet reactivity to ADP. The phenomenon of clopidogrel "resistance" has been confirmed by multiple investigators and is now variously described as "nonresponsiveness," "hyporesponsiveness," or "clopidogrel resistance." (Table 3) (85,86,91–95).

Clopidogrel nonresponsiveness is also dependent on dose. In the largest pharmacodynamic study comparing 300 and 600 mg clopidogrel-loading doses, treatment with a 600 mg loading dose during PCI reduced clopidogrel nonresponsiveness to 8% compared to 28% to 32% with a 300 mg loading dose (Fig. 5). Moreover, the latter study demonstrated a narrower response profile, following treatment with 600 mg clopidogrel (86).

Despite the well-documented clinical efficacy of dual antiplatelet therapy of clopidogrel and aspirin, it has been repeatedly demonstrated that a certain percentage of patients may not be protected by this regimen and may suffer recurrent ischemic events, including stent thrombosis.

Mechanism of clopidogrel nonresponsiveness

The mechanisms responsible for clopidogrel response variability are incompletely defined. Pharmacokinetic and pharmacodynamic differences in clopidogrel metabolism have been proposed to explain variable platelet inhibition.

Pharmacokinetic mechanisms

Inadequate production of the active metabolite to sufficiently block the $P2Y_{12}$ receptor may be responsible for clopidogrel nonresponsiveness. Poor bioavailability may be due to reduced intestinal absorption of clopidogrel, decreased conversion to the active metabolite, or drug–drug interactions at the CYP3A4 level. In recent studies, measurement of active and inactive metabolites of clopidogrel suggested that intestinal absorption was the primary factor affecting the production of active metabolite (96,97). A ceiling effect in unchanged clopidogrel and clopidogrel metabolite levels and platelet inhibition with a 600 mg loading dose in patients undergoing stenting was observed and no additional effect was seen with a 900 mg loading dose (97). The same authors suggested that in only selected patients hepatic conversion was a determinant factor in nonresponsiveness, following treatment with a 600 mg loading dose (98).

However, convincing evidence supporting the pivotal role of hepatic CYP3A4 activity in mediating the antiplatelet effect of clopidogrel comes from the work of Lau et al. Their studies have demonstrated that the activity of CYP3A4 by using the radioactive erythromycin breath test is directly related to the extent of platelet inhibition induced by clopidogrel (76,99). Pharmacologic manipulation of CYP3A4 activity with stimulators such as rifampin and St. Johns wort enhanced the inhibitory effect of clopidogrel, whereas agents that inhibited CYP3A4 activity such as erythromycin attenuated the effect of clopidogrel (99). Atorvastatin, unlike statins that are not metabolized by CYP3A4, compete with clopidogrel for the active site of CYP3A4 and may affect clopidogrel active metabolite levels. Lau et al. (99) have demonstrated that atorvastatin attenuates platelet inhibition by clopidogrel. However, retrospective analyses of clinical trials have found no evidence of an atorvastatin drug–drug interaction (100,101). It has been suggested that a 600 mg clopidogrel-loading dose may be

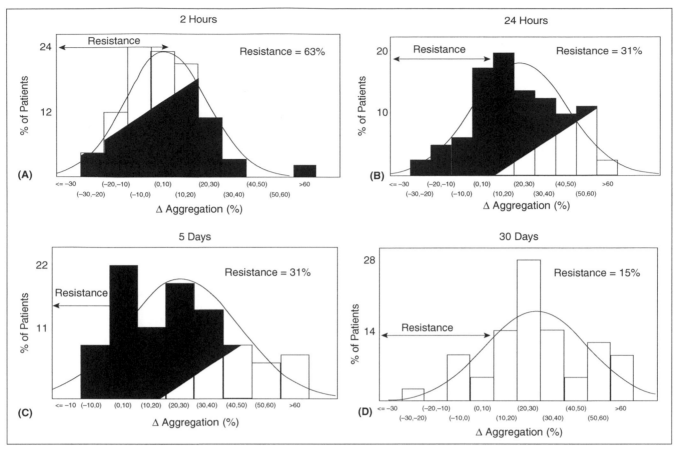

Figure 4

Relationship between frequency of patients and absolute change in aggregation [D aggregation (%)] in response to 5mM ADP at two hours (**A**), 24 hours (**B**), 5 days (**C**), and 30 days (**D**) after stenting. D Aggregation (%) is defined baseline aggregation (%) minus post-treatment aggregation (%). Resistance, as defined herein, is D aggregation # 10%. Resistance is present in those patients subtended by double-headed arrow. *Curves* represent normal distribution of data. *Source*: From Ref. 85.

effective in overcoming the drug–drug interaction between clopidogrel and statins (102).

Pharmacodynamic mechanisms

Suboptimal platelet response to clopidogrel may be due to an increased number of platelet P2Y$_{12}$ receptors or polymorphism of platelet receptors. Genetic polymorphisms of platelet GPIIb/IIIa, GPIa/IIa, or P2Y$_{12}$ receptors have been reported to affect platelet function and may influence clopidogrel response variability (103–105). Recently, it was reported that an increased percentage of patients with peripheral arterial disease have the P2Y$_{12}$ receptor H2 haplotype (104). However, in another study, the relation of this haplotype to clopidogrel responsiveness could not be demonstrated (105). Since the relation

of genetic polymorphisms to clopidogrel responsiveness is inconclusive, further studies are required to establish a correlation between receptor polymorphisms and clopidogrel nonresponsiveness.

It has been shown that patients with diabetes exhibit platelet activation and increased reactivity to agonists. The heightened platelet reactivity may be related to the increased prevalence of nonresponders and occurrence of ischemic events reported in patients with diabetes (106,107). It has also been reported that patients with a high body mass index (BMI) exhibited a suboptimal platelet response with the standard 300 mg loading dose (108).

All of the data mentioned earlier strongly support insufficient metabolite generation as the primary explanation for nonresponsiveness rather than genetic polymorphisms of platelet receptors or intracellular signaling mechanisms. The latter mechanisms may be relevant in those patients who may remain resistant and with high platelet reactivity to ADP even after treatment with high doses of clopidogrel.

Table 3   Clopidogrel resistance studies

Investigators	n	Patients	Clopidogrel dose (mg, load/qd)	Definition of clopidogrel resistance	Time	Incidences (%)
Gurbel et al. (85)	92	PCI	300/75	5 and 50 μM ADP-induced aggregation <10% absolute change	24 hr	31–35
Jaremo et al. (91)	18	PCI	300/75	ADP-induced fibrinogen binding <40% of baseline	24 hr	28
Muller et al. (92)	119	PCI	600/75	5 and 50 μM ADP-induced aggregation <10% relative change	4 hr	5–11
Mobley et al. (93)	50	PCI	300/75	1 μM ADP-induced aggregation, TEG and Ichor PW: <10% absolute inhibition	Pre and post	30
Lepantalo et al. (89)	50	PCI	300/75	2 or 5 μM AD-induced aggregation and PFA-100 10% inhibition and 170s	2.5 hr	40
Serebruany et al. (94)	544	Heterogeneous population	300 loading dose	5 μM ADI-induced aggregation, 2 standard deviation below mean	Up to 30 days	4.2
Angiolillo et al. (95)	48	PCI	300/75	6 μM ADP-induced aggregation <40% inhibition	10, 4 and 224 hr	44
Matetzky et al. (16)	60	STEMI	300/75	5 μM ADP-induced aggregation and CPA <10% inhibition	Daily for 5 days	25
Gurbel et al. (86)	190	PCI	300 or 600/75	5 and 20 μM ADI-induced aggregation <10% absolute inhibition	24 hr	28–32 with 300 mg 8 with 600 mg

Abbreviations: AD, adenosine diphosphate; CPA, cone and platelet analyzer; PCI, percutaneous coronary interventions; PFA, platelet function analyzer; TEG, thrombelastography.
Source: From Ref. 5.

Clinical relevance of clopidogrel nonresponsiveness and high post-treatment platelet reactivity

Limited data are available to link clopidogrel nonresponsiveness to the occurrence of thrombotic events. Matetzky et al. studied clopidogrel responsiveness in patients undergoing stenting for acute ST-elevation MI. They found that patients who exhibited the highest quartile of ADP-induced aggregation had a 40% probability for a recurrent cardiovascular event within six months (16). Moreover, it has been reported that some clopidogrel nonresponders have low pretreatment reactivity to ADP, whereas some responders have high post-treatment reactivity to ADP. Given these observations, the evaluation of thrombotic risk based on platelet inhibition may be flawed and either overestimate or underestimate the risk in selected patients. Therefore, the most reliable predictor of thrombotic risk may be the measurement of post-treatment platelet reactivity (109,110). In the PREPARE POST-STENTING study (Platelet reactivity in patients and recurrent events post-stenting), patients suffering a recurrent ischemic event within six months of the procedure had high post-stent platelet reactivity to ADP compared to patients without ischemic events (21). In the CLEAR PLATELETS and CLEAR

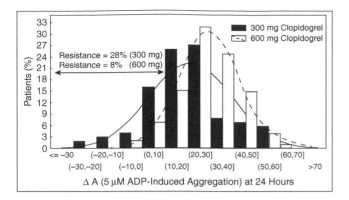

Figure 5
Distribution of the absolute change in 5 μM ADP-induced aggregation (Δ aggregation) and incidence of clopidogrel resistance in patients treated with 300 and 600 mg clopidogrel-loading dose. All of the patients under double-headed arrow meet the definition of clopidogrel resistance. The distribution is shifted rightward and narrower in the 600 mg group indicating greater inhibition (responsiveness to clopidogrel) and lower incidence of resistance. Source: From Ref. 86.

PLATELETS-Ib studies, a 600 mg loading dose was associated with increased platelet inhibition compared to a 300 mg loading dose. In turn, increased platelet inhibition was accompanied by a decrease in the release of myocardial necrosis and inflammation (19,20). In a very recent study of 106 patients undergoing stenting, high post-treatment platelet reactivity was asso-ciated with an increased risk of recurrent cardiovascular events (22).

Three small studies suggest that despite standard clopido-grel treatment, high platelet reactivity may be a risk factor for stent thrombosis. Barragan et al. (88) demonstrated high $P2Y_{12}$ receptor reactivity as measured by VASP phosphoryla-tion levels in patients with stent thrombosis. In the recent CREST (Clopidogrel effect on platelet reactivity in patients with stent thrombosis) study, platelet function was evaluated in patients with and without stent thrombosis by using platelet aggregation, stimulated expression of active GPIIb/IIIa expression, and the $P2Y_{12}$ reactivity ratio measured by VASP phosphorylation (15). Elevated levels of all of these measurements were observed in patients with stent thrombosis, indicating that the $P2Y_{12}$ receptor was inade-quately inhibited (15). Finally, Ajzenberg et al. (17) observed increased shear-induced platelet aggregation in patients with stent thrombosis compared to patients without stent thrombosis who were on dual antiplatelet therapy and to normal controls who were not on dual antiplatelet therapy. Prasugrel is a new thienopyridine derivative that produces more potent platelet inhibition, and a rapid onset of action. The latter properties may provide a superior alternative to clopidogrel, with less response variability and a decreased prevalence of nonresponsiveness (111). All of these small studies support that insufficient inhibition of $P2Y_{12}$ receptors by clopidogrel therapy and high post-treatment platelet reac-tivity are pivotally related to the occurrence of stent thrombosis and recurrent ischemic events following PCI.

Therapeutic interventions for clopidogrel nonresponsiveness

In recent clinical studies, a 600 mg clopidogrel-loading dose was associated with a higher level of platelet inhibition and lower incidence of nonresponsiveness when compared to a 300 mg dose (19,20,86). Moreover, a 600 mg clopidogrel-loading dose was associated with a narrower response profile (86). Kastrati et al. (112) found that patients achieved addi-tional platelet inhibition when a 75 mg/day clopidogrel maintenance dose was followed by an additional 600 mg loading dose. In the CLEAR PLATELETS and CLEAR PLATELETS-Ib studies, a 600 mg loading dose was associated with increased platelet inhibition compared to a 300 mg clopi-dogrel-loading dose (19,20).

Standardized methods to quantify ex vivo clopidogrel responsiveness and criteria to define nonresponsiveness and high post-treatment platelet reactivity are still lacking. In order to firmly link high platelet reactivity and poor clopidogrel responsiveness to the occurrence of adverse ischemic events, a standard methodology is mandatory. These advances will facilitate the conduction of large-scale clinical trials. High loading doses may be considered for selected patients, but its superiority and associated risk profile compared to standard dose has to be established in large-scale clinical trials. Despite these limitations, the current ACC/AHA guidelines for PCI provide a Class IIa recommen-dation that "a regimen of greater than 300 mg is reasonable to achieve higher levels of antiplatelet activity more rapidly." Finally, the ACC/AHA guidelines provide a Class IIb recom-mendation that "in patients in whom subacute thrombosis may be catastrophic or lethal ... platelet aggregation studies may be considered and the dose of clopidogrel increased to 150 mg per day if less than 50% inhibition of platelet aggre-gation is demonstrated" (47).

New $P2Y_{12}$ receptor antagonists are undergoing investiga-tion. AZD 6140 (Astra-Zeneca; Södertälje, Sweden) and cangrelor (Medicines Company; Parsippany, NJ, U.S.A.) are reversible, direct, and potent inhibitors. AZD 6140 is an oral $P2Y_{12}$ inhibitor, whereas cangrelor is administered parentally. Both of these agents exhibit more consistent and greater platelet inhibition compared to clopidogrel (113–115). The short onset and offset of action makes cangrelor an appealing adjunctive antiplatelet agent during PCI when maximum and rapid platelet inhibition of ADP-induced aggregation is required (115). Prasugrel (Eli Lily and Company Indianapolis, IL, and

Sankyo Co. Ltd. Tokyo, Japan) is a new thienopyridine derivative that produces more potent platelet inhibition, and a rapid onset of action. The latter properties may provide a superior alternative to clopidogrel, with less response variability and a decreased prevalence of nonresponsiveness (111).

Conclusions

Reports of high incidences of aspirin resistance may be due to laboratory measurements based on nonspecific methods that do not isolate the response of platelet COX-1 to aspirin or due to an inadequate dose required to fully inhibit the COX-1 in selected patients. Clopidogrel nonresponsiveness is a consistent phenomenon observed in research studies conducted at multiple medical centers around the world. Data from small studies support that patients with high ex vivo platelet reactivity to ADP during and after percutaneous intervention may be at greatest risk for subsequent ischemic events.

However, at this time, there are no uniformly established methods to quantify ex vivo platelet reactivity after clopidogrel and aspirin treatment or the extent of platelet inhibition by clopidogrel and aspirin. Therefore, specific treatment recommendations for patients exhibiting high platelet reactivity during clopidogrel or aspirin therapy or who have poor platelet inhibition by clopidogrel or aspirin are not established. A higher aspirin dose ($\geq$325 mg/day) and strict compliance to therapy may effectively overcome the occurrence of "aspirin resistance" in selected patients. A clopidogrel maintenance dose of 150 mg may be considered in patients exhibiting clopidogrel nonresponsiveness. In the near future, new P2Y$_{12}$ receptor blockers will likely overcome the limitations of clopidogrel.

Demonstration of nonresponsiveness to antiplatelet agents in certain patients by laboratory methods indicate that treating all patients with the same dose may not be advisable, and that a patient-specific antiplatelet treatment strategy is needed to achieve maximum benefit of antiplatelet treatment (5,111). Finally, the so-called "resistance" to antiplatelet drugs will be more meaningful only when a standardized user-friendly laboratory method to isolate the effect of the drug is available, and only after a strong relation of laboratory "resistance" to the occurrence of adverse clinical outcomes is established in large-scale clinical trials. Routine measurement of platelet function in patients with cardiovascular disease should become the standard of care leading toward the future of personalized antithrombotic treatment strategies determined by the critical pathways influencing thrombotic risk in the individual patient. Finally, measurement of platelet function in isolation ignores the critical influences of coagulation and platelet–fibrin interactions in determining individual thrombotic risk (21). Future risk assessment strategies will likely employ methods that measure platelet–coagulation pathway crosstalk.

References

1 Strukova S. Blood coagulation-dependent inflammation. Coagulation-dependent inflammation and inflammation-dependent thrombosis. Front Biosci 2006; 11:59–80.

2 Gurbel PA, Bliden KP, Hayes KM, Tantry U. Platelet activation in myocardial ischemic syndromes. Expert Rev Cardiovasc Ther 2004; 2:535–545.

3 Jackson SP, Nesbitt WS, Kulkarni S. Signaling events underlying thrombus formation. J Thromb Haemost 2003; 1: 1602–1612. Review.

4 Ruggeri ZM. Platelets in atherothrombosis. Nat Med 2002; 8:1227–1234.

5 Tantry US, Bliden KP, Gurbel PA. Resistance to antiplatelet drugs: current status and future research. Expert Opin Pharmacother 2005; 6:2027–2045.

6 Li Z, Zhang G, Le Breton GC, Gao X, Malik AB, Du X. Two waves of platelet secretion induced by thromboxane A2 receptor and a critical role for phosphoinositide 3-kinases. J Biol Chem 2003; 278:30,725–30,731.

7 Dorsam RT, Tuluc M, Kunapuli SP. Role of protease-activated and ADP receptor subtypes in thrombin generation on human platelets. J Thromb Haemost 2004; 2:804–812.

8 Gawaz M. Role of platelets in coronary thrombosis and reperfusion of ischemic myocardium. Cardiovasc Res 2004; 61: 498–511.

9 Samara WM, Gurbel PA. The role of platelet receptors and adhesion molecules in coronary artery disease. Coron Artery Dis 2003; 14:65–79.

10 van der Meijden PE, Feijge MA, Giesen PL, Huijberts M, van Raak LP, Heemskerk JW. Platelet P2Y12 receptors enhance signalling towards procoagulant activity and thrombin generation. A study with healthy subjects and patients at thrombotic risk. Thromb Haemost 2005; 93:1128–1136.

11 Davies MJ, Thomas AC, Knapman PA, Hangartner JR. Intramyocardial platelet aggregation in patients with unstable angina suffering sudden ischemic cardiac death. Circulation 1986; 73:418–427.

12 Furie B, Furie BC. Thrombus formation in vivo. J Clin Invest 2005; 115:3355–3362.

13 Gurbel PA, Kereiakes DJ, Dalesandro MR, Bahr RD, O'Connor CM, Serebruany VL. Role of soluble and platelet-bound P-selectin in discriminating cardiac from noncardiac chest pain at presentation in the emergency department. Am Heart J 2000; 139:320–328.

14 Matsagas MI, Geroulakos G, Mikhailidis DP. The role of platelets in peripheral arterial disease: therapeutic implications. Ann Vasc Surg 2002; 16:246–258.

15 Gurbel PA, Bliden KP, Samara W, et al. Clopidogrel effect on platelet reactivity in patients with stent thrombosis: results of the CREST Study. J Am Coll Cardiol 2005; 46:1827–1832.

16 Matetzky S, Shenkman B, Guetta V, et al. Clopidogrel resistance is associated with increased risk of recurrent atherothrombotic events in patients with acute myocardial infarction. Circulation 2004; 109:3171–3175.

17 Ajzenberg N, Aubry P, Huisse MG, et al. Enhanced shear-induced platelet aggregation in patients who experience subacute stent thrombosis: a case-control study. J Am Coll Cardiol 2005; 45:1753–1756.

18 Gurbel PA, Zaman K, Bliden KP, Tantry US. Maximum clot strength is a novel and highly predictive indicator of restenosis: a

potential future measure to determine who needs antiproliferative therapy and how much. J Am Coll Cardiol 2006; 47:43B.

19 Gurbel PA, Bliden KP, Zaman KA, Yoho JA, Hayes KM, Tantry US. Clopidogrel loading with eptifibatide to arrest the reactivity of platelets: results of the clopidogrel loading with eptifibatide to arrest the reactivity of platelets (CLEAR PLATELETS) study. Circulation 2005; 111:1153–1159.

20 Gurbel PA, Bliden KP, Tantry US. The effect of clopidogrel with and without eptifibatide on tumor necrosis factor-alpha and C-reactive protein release after elective stenting: Results of the CLEAR PLATELETS-Ib study. J Am Coll Cardiol 2006; 48:2186–2191.

21 Gurbel PA, Bliden KP, Guyer K, et al. Platelet reactivity in patients and recurrent events post-stenting: results of the PREPARE POST-STENTING Study. J Am Coll Cardiol 2005; 46:1820–1826.

22 Cuisset T, Frere C, Quilici J, et al. High post-treatment platelet reactivity identified low-responders to dual antiplatelet therapy at increased risk of recurrent cardiovascular events after stenting for acute coronary syndrome. J Thromb Haemost 2006; 4:542–549.

23 Watala C. Blood platelet reactivity and its pharmacological modulation in (people with) diabetes mellitus. Curr Pharm Des 2005; 11:2331–2365. Review.

24 Preston RA, Jy W, Jimenez JJ, et al. Effects of severe hypertension on endothelial and platelet microparticles. Hypertension 2003; 41:211–217.

25 Sener A, Ozsavci D, Oba R, Demirel GY, Uras F, Yardimci KT. Do platelet apoptosis, activation, aggregation, lipid peroxidation and platelet-leukocyte aggregate formation occur simultaneously in hyperlipidemia? Clin Biochem 2005; 38:1081–1087.

26 Patrono C, Coller B, Dalen JE, et al. Platelet-active drugs: the relationships among dose, effectiveness, and side effects. Chest 2001; 119 (suppl 1):39S–63S.

27 Antithrombotic Trialists' Collaboration. Collaborative meta-analysis of randomised trials of antiplatelet therapy for prevention of death, myocardial infarction, and stroke in high risk patients. Brit Med J 2002; 324:71–86.

28 CAPRIE Streerin Committee. A randomised, blinded, trial of clopidogrel versus aspirin in patients at risk of ischaemic events (CAPRIE). CAPRIE Steering Committee. Lancet 1996; 348: 1329–1339.

29 Yusuf S, Zhao F, Mehta SR, Chrolavicius S, Tognoni G, Fox KK; Clopidogrel in Unstable Angina to Prevent Recurrent Events Trial Investigators. Effects of clopidogrel in addition to aspirin in patients with acute coronary syndromes without ST-segment elevation. N Engl J Med 2001; 345:494–502.

30 Steinhubl SR, Berger PB, Mann JT III, et al.; CREDO Investigators. Clopidogrel for the reduction of events during observation. Early and sustained dual oral antiplatelet therapy following percutaneous coronary intervention: a randomized controlled trial. J Am Med Assoc 2002; 288:2411–2420.

31 Campbell CL, Steinhubl SR. Variability in response to aspirin: do we understand the clinical relevance? J Thromb Haemost 2005; 3:665–669.

32 Gurbel PA. Clopidogrel response variability and drug resistance. Haematologica 2004; 897 (suppl 7):9–11.

33 Patrono C. Aspirin resistance: definition, mechanisms and clinical read-outs. J Thromb Haemost 2003; 1:1710–1713.

34 Waller BF. Nonatherosclerotic coronary heart disease. In: Alexander RW, Schlant RC, Fuster V, eds. Hurst's the Heart. 9th ed. New York: McGraw Hill, 1998:1197–1240.

35 Sakariassen KS, Hanson SR, Cadroy Y. Methods and models to evaluate shear-dependent and surface reactivity-dependent antithrombotic efficacy. Thromb Res 2001; 104:149–174. Review.

36 Patrono C. Prevention of myocardial infarction and stroke by aspirin: different mechanisms? different dosage? Thromb Res 1998; 92:S7–S12.

37 Michelson AD, Catteneo M, Eikelboom JW, et al. Aspirin resistance: position paper of the working group on aspirin resistance, platelet physiology subcommittee of the scientific and standardization committee, International society on thrombosis and haemostasis. J Thromb Haemost 2005; 3: 1309–1311.

38 Vane Jr. Inhibition of prostaglandin syntheses as a mechanism of action for aspirin-like drugs. Nat New Biol 1971; 231:232–235.

39 Roth GJ, Stanford N, Majerus PW. Acetylation of prostaglandin synthase by aspirin. Proc Natl Acad Sci USA 1975; 72:3073–3077.

40 Loll PJ, Picot D, Garavito RM. The structural basis of aspirin activity inferred fron the crystal structure of inactivated prostaglanding H2 synthase. Nat Struct Biol 1995; 2:637–643.

41 Tantry U, Gurbel PA, Bliden KP, DiChiara J. Inconsistency in the prevalence of platelet aspirin resistance as measured by COX-1 non-specific assays in patients treated with 81, 162, and 325 mg aspirin. J Am Coll Cardiol 2006; 47:290A.

42 Awtry EH, Loscalzo J. Aspirin. Circulation 2000; 101:1206–1218. Review.

43 Catella F, Healy D, Lawson JA, FitzGerald GA. 11-Dehydrothromboxane B2: a quantitative index of thromboxane A2 formation in the human circulation. Proc Natl Acad Sci USA 1986; 83:5861–5865.

44 Eikelboom JW, Hirsh J, Weitz JI, Johnston M, Yi Q, Yusuf S. Aspirin-resistant thromboxane biosynthesis and the risk of myocardial infarction, stroke, or cardiovascular death in patients at high risk for cardiovascular events. Circulation 2002; 105: 1650–1655.

45 Hennekens CH. Update on aspirin in the treatment and prevention of cardiovascular disease. Am J Manag Care 2002; 8(22 suppl):S691–S700. Review.

46 Patrono C, Bachmann F, Baigent C, et al.; European Society of Cardiology. Expert consensus document on the use of antiplatelet agents. The task force on the use of antiplatelet agents in patients with atherosclerotic cardiovascular disease of the European society of cardiology. Eur Heart J 2004; 25: 166–181.

47 Smith SC Jr, Feldman Te, Hirshfeld JW Jr, Jacobs AK. American College of Cardiology American Heart Association Task Force on practice guidelines. ACC/AHA/SCAI writing committee to update 2001 guidelines for percutaneous coronary intervention. ACC/AHA/SCAI 2005 guidelines update for percutaneous coronary intervention: a report of the American College of Cardiology/American Heart Association Task Force on practice guideline (ACC/AHA/SCAI writing committee to update 2001 guidelines for percutaneous coronary intervention). Circulation 2006; 113:e166–e286.

48 Mehta J, Mehta P, Burger C, Pepine CJ. Platelet aggregation studies in coronary artery disease. Past 4. Effect of aspirin. Atherosclerosis 1978; 31:169–175.

49   Hurlen M, Seljeflot I, Arnesen H. The effect of different antithrombotic regimens on platelet aggregation after myocardial infarction. Scand Cardiovasc J 1998; 32:233–237.

50   Buchanan MR, Brister SJ. Individual variation in the effects of ASA on platelet function: implications for the use of ASA clinically. Can J Cardiol 1995; 11:221–227.

51   Buchanan MR, Schwartz L, Bourassa M, Brister SJ, Peniston CM; BRAT Investigators. Results of the BRAT study—a pilot study investigating the possible significance of ASA nonresponsiveness on the benefits and risks of ASA on thrombosis in patients undergoing coronary artery bypass surgery. Can J Cardiol 2000; 16:1385–1390.

52   Grotemeyer KH, Scharafinski HW, Husstedt IW. Two-year follow-up of aspirin responder and aspirin nonresponder. A pilot-study including 180 post-stroke patients. Thromb Res 1993; 71:397–403.

53   Gum PA, Kottke-Marchant K, Poggio ED, et al. Profile and prevalence of aspirin resistance in patients with cardiovascular disease. Am J Cardiol 2001; 88:230–235.

54   Gum PA, Kottke-Marchant K, Welsh PA, White J, Topol EJ. A prospective, blinded determination of the natural history of aspirin resistance among stable patients with cardiovascular disease. J Am Coll Cardiol 2003; 41:961–965.

55   Wang JC, Aucoin-Barry D, Manuelian D, et al. Incidence of aspirin nonresponsiveness using the Ultegra Rapid Platelet Function Assay-ASA. Am J Cardiol 2003; 92:1492–1494.

56   Chen W-H, Lee P-Y, Ng W, et al. Aspirin resistance is associated with a high incidence of myonecrosis after non-urgent percutaneous coronary intervention despite clopidogrel pretreatment. J Am Coll Cardiol 2004; 43:1122–1126.

57   Gonzalez-Conejero R, Rivera J, Corral J, Acuna C, Guerrero JA, Vicente V. Biological assessment of aspirin efficacy on healthy individuals: heterogeneous response or aspirin failure? Stroke 2005; 36:276–280.

58   Tantry US, Bliden KP, Gurbel PA. Overestimation of platelet aspirin resistance detection by thrombelastograph platelet mapping and validation by conventional aggregometry using arachidonic acid stimulation. J Am Coll Cardiol 2005; 46:1705–1709.

59   Pulcinelli FM, Riondino S, Celestini A, et al. Persistent production of platelet thromboxane A2 in patients chronically treated with aspirin. J Thromb Haemost 2005; 3:2784–2789.

60   Eikelboom JW, Hankey GJ. Failure of aspirin to prevent atherothrombosis: potential mechanisms and implications for clinical practice. Am J Cardiovasc Drugs 2004; 4:57–67.

61   Maree AO, Fitzgerald DJ. Aspirin and coronary artery disease. Thromb Haemost 2004; 92:1175–1181.

62   Mueller MR, Salat A, Stangl P, et al. Variable platelet response to low-dose ASA and the risk of limb deterioration in patients submitted to peripheral arterial angioplasty. Thromb Haemost 1997; 78:1003–1007.

63   Tsiara S, Elisaf M, Mikhailidis DP. Influence of smoking on predictors of vascular disease. Angiology 2003; 54:507–530.

64   Rocca B, Secchiero P, Ciabattoni G, et al. Cyclooxygenase-2 expression is induced during human megakaryopoiesis and characterizes newly formed platelets. Proc Natl Acad Sci USA 2002; 99:7634–7639.

65   Marcus AJ, Weksler BB, Jaffe EA, Broekman MJ. Synthesis of prostacyclin from platelet-derived endoperoxides by cultured human endothelial cells. J Clin Invest 1980; 66:979–986.

66   Weber AA, Zimmermann KC, Meyer-Kirchrath J, Schror K. Cyclooxygenase-2 in human platelets as a possible factor in aspirin resistance. Lancet 1999; 353:900.

67   Valles J, Santos MT, Aznar J, et al. Erythrocyte promotion of platelet reactivity decreases the effectiveness of aspirin as an antithrombotic therapeutic modality: the effect of low-dose aspirin is less than optimal in patients with vascular disease due to prothrombotic effects of erythrocytes on platelet reactivity. Circulation 1998; 97:350–355.

68   Catella-Lawson F, Reilly MP, Kapoor SC, et al. Cyclooxygenase inhibitors and the antiplatelet effects of aspirin. N Engl J Med 2001; 345:1809–1817.

69   Zimmermann N, Wenk A, Kim U, et al. Functional and biochemical evaluation of platelet aspirin resistance after coronary artery bypass surgery. Circulation 2003; 108: 542–547.

70   Payne DA, Jones CI, Hayes PD, Webster SE, Ross Naylor A, Goodall AH. Platelet inhibition by aspirin is diminished in patients during carotid surgery: a form of transient aspirin resistance? Thromb Haemost 2004; 92:89–96.

71   Schafer AI. Genetic and acquired determinants of individual variability of response to antiplatelet drugs. Circulation 2003; 108:910–911.

72   O'Donnell CJ, Larson MG, Feng D, et al.; Framingham Heart Study. Genetic and environmental contributions to platelet aggregation: the Framingham heart study. Circulation 2001; 103:3051–3056.

73   De Caterina R, Giannessi D, Boem A, et al. Equal antiplatelet effects of aspirin 50 or 324 mg/day in patients after acute myocardial infarction. Thromb Haemost 1985; 54:528–532.

74   DUTCH group. A comparison of two doses of aspirin (30 mg vs. 283 mg a day) in patients after a transient ischemic attack or minor ischemic stroke. The Dutch TIA Trial Study Group. N Engl J Med 1991; 325:1261–1266.

75   Maree AO, Curtin RJ, Dooley M, et al. Platelet response to low-dose enteric-coated aspirin in patients with stable cardiovascular disease. J Am Coll Cardiol 2005; 46:1258–1263.

76   Lau WC, Gurbel PA, Watkins PB, et al. Contribution of hepatic cytochrome P450 3A4 metabolic activity to the phenomenon of clopidogrel resistance. Circulation 2004; 109:166–171.

77   Savi P, Combalbert J, Gaich C, et al. The antiaggregating activity of clopidogrel is due to a metabolic activation by the hepatic cytochrome P450-1A. Thromb Haemost 1994; 72:313–317.

78   Ding Z, Kim S, Dorsam RT, Jin J, Kunapuli SP. Inactivation of the human P2Y12 receptor by thiol reagents requires interaction with both extracellular cysteine residues, Cys17 and Cys270. Blood 2003; 101:3908–3914.

79   Gachet C. Regulation of platelet functions by p2 receptors. Annu Rev Pharmacol Toxicol 2006; 46:277–300.

80   Hermann A, Rauch BH, Braun M, Schror K, Weber AA. Platelet CD40 ligand (CD40L)—subcellular localization, regulation of expression, and inhibition by clopidogrel. Platelets 2001; 12:74–82.

81   Xiao Z, Theroux P. Clopidogrel inhibits platelet-leukocyte interactions and thrombin receptor agonist peptide-induced platelet activation in patients with an acute coronary syndrome. J Am Coll Cardiol 2004; 43:1982–1988.

82   Di Nisio M, Bijsterveld NR, Meijers JC, Levi M, Buller HR, Peters RJ. Effects of clopidogrel on the rebound hypercoagulable state after heparin discontinuation in patients with acute coronary syndromes. J Am Coll Cardiol 2005; 46: 1582–1583.

83 Evangelista V, Manarini S, Dell'Elba G, et al. Clopidogrel inhibits platelet-leukocyte adhesion and platelet-dependent leukocyte activation. Thromb Haemost 2005; 94:568–577.

84 Gurbel PA, Bliden KP, Guyer K, Aggarwal N, Tantry US. Delayed thrombin-induced platelet-fibrin clot generation by clopidogrel: a new dose-related effect demonstrated by thrombelastography in patients undergoing coronary artery stenting . J Am Coll Cardiol 2006; 47:16B.

85 Gurbel PA, Bliden KP, Hiatt BL, O'Connor CM. Clopidogrel for coronary stenting: response variability, drug resistance, and the effect of pretreatment platelet reactivity. Circulation 2003; 107:2908–2913.

86 Gurbel PA, Bliden KP, Hayes KM, Yoho JA, Herzog WR, Tantry US. The relation of dosing to clopidogrel responsiveness and the incidence of high post-treatment platelet aggregation in patients undergoing coronary stenting. J Am Coll Cardiol 2005; 45:1392–1396.

87 Labarthe B, Theroux P, Angioi M, Ghitescu M. Matching the evaluation of the clinical efficacy of clopidogrel to platelet function tests relevant to the biological properties of the drug. J Am Coll Cardiol 2005; 46:638–645.

88 Barragan P, Bouvier JL, Roquebert PO, et al. Resistance to thienopyridines: clinical detection of coronary stent thrombosis by monitoring of vasodilator-stimulated phosphoprotein phosphorylation. Catheter Cardiovasc Interv 2003; 59:295–302.

89 Lepantalo A, Virtanen KS, Heikkila J, Wartiovaara U, Lassila R. Limited early antiplatelet effect of 300 mg clopidogrel in patients with aspirin therapy undergoing percutaneous coronary interventions. Eur Heart J 2004; 25:476–483.

90 Von beckerath N, Pogasta-Murray G, Wieczorek A Schomig A, Kastrati A. Correlation between platelet response units measured with a point-of-care test and ADP-induced platelet aggregation assessed with conventional optical aggregometry. ESC 2005; P2936 (abstract)

91 Jaremo P, Lindahl TL, Fransson SG, Richter A. Individual variations of platelet inhibition after loading doses of clopidogrel. J Intern Med 2002; 252:233–238.

92 Muller I, Besta F, Schulz C, Massberg S, Schonig A, Gawaz M. Prevalence of clopidogrel non-responders among patients with stable angina pectoris scheduled for elective coronary stent placement. Thromb Haemost 2003; 89:783–787.

93 Mobley JE, Bresee SJ, Wortham DC, Craft RM, Snider CC, Carroll RC. Frequency of nonresponse antiplatelet activity of clopidogrel during pretreatment for cardiac catheterization. Am J Cardiol 2004; 93:456–458.

94 Serebruany VL, Steinhubl SR, Berger PB, Malinin AI, Bhatt DL, Topol EJ. Variability in platelet responsiveness to clopidogrel among 544 individuals. J Am Coll Cardiol 2005; 45:246–251.

95 Angiolillo DJ, Fernandez-Ortiz A, Bernardo E, et al. Identification of low responders to a 300-mg clopidogrel loading dose in patients undergoing coronary stenting. Thromb Res 2005; 115:101–108.

96 Taubert D, Kastrati A, Harlfinger S, et al. Pharmacokinetics of clopidogrel after administration of a high loading dose. Thromb Haemost 2004; 92:311–316.

97 von Beckerath N, Taubert D, Pogatsa-Murray G, Schomig E, Kastrati A, Schomig A. Absorption, metabolization, and antiplatelet effects of 300-, 600-, and 900-mg loading doses of clopidogrel: results of the ISAR-CHOICE (Intracoronary Stenting and Antithrombotic Regimen: Choose Between 3 High Oral Doses for Immediate Clopidogrel Effect) Trial. Circulation 2005; 112:2946–2950.

98 von Beckerath N, Taubert D, Pogatsa-Murray G, et al. A patient with stent thrombosis, clopidogrel-resistance and failure to metabolize clopidogrel to its active metabolite. Thromb Haemost. 2005; 93:789–791.

99 Lau WC, Waskell LA, Watkins PB, et al. Atorvastatin reduces the ability of clopidogrel to inhibit platelet aggregation: a new drug-drug interaction. Circulation 2003; 107:32–37.

100 Saw J, Steinhubl SR, Berger PB, et al. Lack of adverse clopidogrel-atorvastatin clinical interaction from secondary analysis of a randomized, placebo-controlled clopidogrel trial. Circulation 2003; 108:921–924.

101 Wienbergen H, Gitt AK, Schiele R, et al.; MITRA PLUS Study Group. Comparison of clinical benefits of clopidogrel therapy in patients with acute coronary syndromes taking atorvastatin versus other statin therapies. Am J Cardiol 2003; 92:285–288.

102 Gorchakova O, von Beckerath N, Gawaz M, et al. Antiplatelet effects of a 600 mg loading dose of clopidogrel are not attenuated in patients receiving atorvastatin or simvastatin for at least 4 weeks prior to coronary artery stenting. Eur Heart J 2004; 25:1898–1902.

103 Beer JH, Pederiva S, Pontiggia L. Genetics of platelet receptor single-nucleotide polymorphisms: clinical implications in thrombosis. Ann Med 2000; 32:10–14.

104 Fontana P, Gaussem P, Aiach M, Fiessinger JN, Emmerich J, Reny JL. P2Y12 H2 haplotype is associated with peripheral arterial disease: a case-control study. Circulation 2003; 16:108:2971–2973.

105 Von Beckerath N, von Beckerath O, Koch W, Eichinger M, Schomig A, Kastrati A. P2Y12 gene H2 haplotype is not associated with increased adenosine diphosphate-induced platelet aggregation after initiation of clopidogrel therapy with a high loading dose. Blood Coagul Fibrinolysis 2005; 16:199–204.

106 Ferroni P, Basili S, Falco A, Davi G. Platelet activation in type 2 diabetes mellitus. J Thromb Haemost 2004; 2:1282–1291.

107 Angiolillo DJ, Fernandez-Ortiz A, Bernardo E, et al. Platelet function profiles in patients with type 2 diabetes and coronary artery disease on combined aspirin and clopidogrel treatment. Diabetes 2005; 54:2430–2435.

108 Angiolillo DJ, Fernandez-Ortiz A, Bernardo E, et al. Platelet aggregation according to body mass index in patients undergoing coronary stenting: should clopidogrel loading-dose be weight adjusted? J Invasive Cardiol 2004; 16:169–174.

109 Samara WM, Bliden KP, Tantry US, Gurbel PA. The difference between clopidogrel responsiveness and posttreatment platelet reactivity. Thromb Res 2005; 115:89–94.

110 Tantry US, Bliden KP, Gurbel PA. What is the best measure of thrombotic risks—pretreatment platelet aggregation, clopidogrel responsiveness, or posttreatment platelet aggregation? Catheter Cardiovasc Interv 2005; 66:597.

111 Tantry US, Bliden KP, Gurbel PA. Prasugrel. Expert Opin Investigative Drugs 2006; 15:1627–1633.

112 Kastrati A, von Beckerath N, Joost A, Pogatsa-Murray G, Gorchakova O, Schomig A. Loading with 600 mg clopidogrel in patients with coronary artery disease with and without chronic clopidogrel therapy. Circulation 2004; 110:1916–1919.

113 Peters G, Robbie G, Single dose pharmacokinetics and pharmacodynamics of AZD6140—an oral reversible ADP receptor antagonist (abstr). Haematologica 2004; 89:14–15.

114 Greenbaum AB, Grines CL, Bittl JA, Becker RC. Initial experience with an intravenous P2Y12 platelet receptor antagonist in patients undergoing percutaneous coronary intervention: results from a 2-part, phase II, multicenter, randomized, placebo- and active-controlled trial. Am Heart J 2006; 151:689, e1–e689, e10.

115 Wiviott SD, Antman EM, Winters KJ, et al. JUMBO-TIMI 26 Investigators. Randomized comparison of prasugrel (CS-747, LY640315), a novel thienopyridine P2Y12 antagonist, with clopidogrel in percutaneous coronary intervention: results of the Joint Utilization of Medications to Block Platelets Optimally (JUMBO)-TIMI 26 trial. Circulation 2005; 28:111:3366–3373.

14

Lipid-lowering agents

Andrew M. Tonkin and Omar Farouque

Atherosclerosis depends on the interplay between genetic, behavioral, and environmental factors. However, the landmark INTERHEART study (1) and other large-scale population studies have established that over a life course this is a largely preventable process. The INTERHEART study showed that approximately 85% of the variation in rates of myocardial infarction (MI) was associated with nine risk factors. Of these, population-attributable risk both for older and younger subjects was highest for the ratio of apolipoprotein B/apolipoprotein A_1. This ratio is a measure of atherogenic particle number [apolipoprotein B, superior to low-density lipoprotein (LDL) cholesterol concentration alone] and antiatherogenic particles [apolipoprotein A_1, reflecting high-density lipoprotein (HDL) cholesterol]. Elevated blood cholesterol, considered to be greater than 147 mg/dL (3.8 mmol/L), was also found to be the leading risk factor for coronary heart disease (CHD), and estimated to account for more than half of cases worldwide in the recent World Health Report (2).

Epidemiology

There is clear epidemiologic evidence of a continuous (log linear) relation between cholesterol levels and the risk of CHD events and mortality, both within communities and when comparing different populations (3). Although it has been estimated that each 1% decrement in total cholesterol is associated with a 2% to 3% decrease in CHD risk, regression dilution bias underestimates the strength of the association. From the meta-analysis of international studies, it has been suggested that each 10% decrement in total cholesterol is associated with 38% reduction in CHD events (4).

Overview of clinical trials

Older primary prevention trials had often been undertaken in cohorts at low absolute risk of CHD events. The initial secondary prevention studies had typically involved patients with elevated cholesterol levels. In addition, these older trials had tested diet and previous lipid-lowering agents, which only lowered cholesterol by an average of approximately 10% (5). As a consequence, these trials were typically underpowered and had not shown a clear reduction in all-cause mortality. There had been good evidence that lipid-modifying therapy could prevent fatal and nonfatal CHD events (5). However, there were some concerns that noncardiovascular events particularly related to cancers and violence or trauma could be increased. In summary, there was considerable uncertainty about the overall effects of treatment.

Attitudes to lipid-modifying therapy have been changed particularly by the large-scale clinical trials of statins, which have been published over the last decade. The statins competitively inhibit 3-hydroxy-3-methylglutaryl-coenzyme A reductase, the enzyme that catalyses the rate-limiting step in cholesterol biosynthesis in the liver (6). The reduction in cholesterol synthesis by HMG CoA reductase inhibition triggers increased expression of LDL cholesterol receptors on hepatic cells that clear circulating LDL cholesterol and its precursor. Statins have other effects. They are associated with a relatively smaller increase in HDL cholesterol concentrations and modest reductions in triglyceride concentrations (7). The beneficial effects of statins may also involve nonlipid-modifying mechanisms by an effect on inflammatory responses, atherosclerotic plaque stability, endothelial function, and thrombosis (8). These pleiotropic effects of statins may have particular importance following acute coronary syndromes and will be discussed further. These large-scale

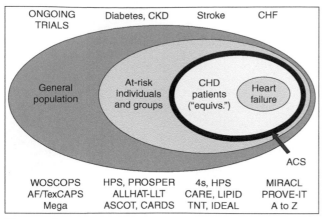

Figure 1
Major large-scale trials of statins. *Abbreviations*: ACS, acute coronary syndrome; CHD, coronary heart disease; CHF, congestive heart failure; CKD, chronic kidney disease.

trials have also established the overall safety of the agents in clinical use at this time.

Figure 1 indicates the major large-scale trials of statins and their key features are summarized in Table 1. The trials can be categorized according to population subgroups in which they have been undertaken:

1. In the general population for primary prevention of CHD: The West of Scotland Coronary Prevention Study (WOSCOPS) (9), Air Force/Texas coronary atherosclerosis Prevention study (AFCAPS/TexCAPS) (10), and the completed but unpublished MEGA study in Japan (A. Nakamura, presented to AHA Scientific Sessions, November 2005).

2. In high-risk individuals and groups: people with clinical evidence of macrovascular disease other than CHD, the Heart Protection Study (HPS) (11); with diabetes, the HPS and Collaborative Atorvastatin Diabetes Study (CARDS) (12); the elderly, Prospective Study of Pravastatin in the Elderly at Risk (PROSPER) (13) or with hypertension, Antihypertensive and Lipid-Lowering Treatment to Prevent Heart Attack Trial (ALLHAT) (14) and Anglo-Scandinavian Cardiac Outcomes Trial (ASCOT) (15).

3. In patients with known CHD: the 4S (16), Cholesterol and Recurrent Events (CARE) (17) and Long-term Intervention with Pravastatin in Ischemic Disease (LIPID) (18) studies, HPS (11), Treating to New Targets (TNT) (19), and the incremental decrease in endpoints through aggressive lipid lowering (IDEAL) (20) study.

4. Patients enrolled early after acute coronary syndromes: Myocardial Ischemia Reduction with Aggressive Cholesterol Lowering (MIRACL) (21), Fluvastatin On Risk

Table 1 Design features (A) and major cardiovascular endpoints (B) in controlled trials of statin therapy

(A)

Trial	Prevention strategy	Drug	Number of patients and sex	Age (years)	Baseline cholesterol level (mmol/L)	Follow-up (years)	Primary endpoint
WOSCOPS	Primary	Pravastatin	6595, M	45–64	≥6.5	4.9	CHD events
AFCAPS/ TexCAPS	Primary	Lovastatin	5608, M 997, F	45–73 55–73	4.6–6.8	5.2	CHD events
ASCOT-LLA	Primary	Atorvastatin	8363, M 1942, F	40–79	≤6.5	3.3	CHD death and nfMI
ALLHAT	Primary	Pravastatin	5304, M 5051, F		LDL 2.6–4.9	4.8	All-cause mortality
4S	Secondary	Simvastatin	3617, M 827, F	35–70	5.5–8.0	5.4	Total mortality
CARE	Secondary	Pravastatin	3583, M 576, F	21–75	<6.2	5.0	CHD events
LIPID	Secondary	Pravastatin	7498, M 1516, F	31–75	4.0–7.0	6.0	CHD mortality
HPS	Primary and secondary	Simvastatin	15,454, M 5082, F	40–80	>3.5	5.0	Vascular events
PROSPER	Primary and secondary	Pravastatin	2804, M 3000, F	70–82	4.0–9.0	3.2	CHD death, nfMI, stroke

(Continued)

Table 1   Design features (A) and major cardiovascular endpoints (B) in controlled trials of statin therapy (*Continued*)

(B)[a]

Trial and treatment	CHD mortality %	Total mortality %	MI (fatal and nonfatal) %	UAP %	CABG %	PCI %	Coronary revascularization	Stroke %
WOSCOPS								
Placebo	1.9	4.1	6.5	—	2.5	—		1.4
Pravastatin	1.3[b]	3.2	4.6[c]	—	1.7[d]	—		1.4
AFCAPS/TexCAPS								
Placebo	0.9	2.3	5.6	5.1	9.3	—		—
Pravastatin	0.6	2.4	3.3[d]	3.5[b]	6.2[c]	—		—
ASCOT-LLA								
Placebo	3.0[e]	4.1		0.5				2.4
Atorvastatin	1.9[c]	3.6		0.4				1.7[b]
ALLHAT								
Usual care	3.9	14.9						0.4
Pravastatin	3.7	15.3						0.4
4S								
Placebo	8.5	11.5	15.2	14.9	17.2	—		4.3
Simvastatin	5.0[c]	8.2[c]	9.0[d]	13.3	11.3[c]	—		2.7
CARE								
Placebo	5.7	9.4	10.0	17.3	10.0	10.5		3.8
Pravastatin	4.6	8.7	7.5[d]	15.2	7.5	8.3		2.6
LIPID								
Placebo	8.3	14.1	10.3	24.6	11.6	15.7		4.5
Pravastatin	6.4[d]	11.0	7.4[c]	22.3[d]	9.2[c]	13.0		3.7
HPS								
Placebo	6.9	14.7	5.6	10.0			7.1	5.7
Simvastatin	5.7[c]	12.9[c]	3.5[c]	8.6[c]			5.0[c]	4.3[c]
PROSPER								
Placebo	4.2	10.5	8.7				1.6	7.3
Pravastatin	3.3[b]	10.3	7.7				1.3	7.1

[a]The primary endpoint differed between studies. Also, because of different definitions of CHD events, it is inappropriate to present the numbers needed to treat to prevent an event to allow comparisons between the trials.

[b]*P* < 0.05.

[c]*P* < 0.001.

[d]*P* < 0.01.

[e]Includes nonfatal MI.

Abbreviations: ALLHAT, Antihypertensive and Lipid-Lowering Treatment to Prevent Heart Attack Trial; AFCAPS/TexCAPS, Air Force/Texas Coronary Atherosclerosis Prevention Study; ASCOT-LLA, Anglo-Scandinavian Cardiac Outcomes Trial-Lipid Lowering Arm; CABG, coronary artery bypass grafting; CARE, Cholesterol and Recurrent Events; CHD, coronary heart disease; F, female; HPS, Heart Protection Study; LIPID, Long-Term Intervention with Pravastatin in Ischemic Disease; M, male; MI, myocardial infarction; nfMI, nonfatal myocardial infarction; PCI, percutaneous coronary intervention; PROSPER, Pravastatin in Elderly Individuals at Risk of Vascular Disease; UAP, unstable angina pectoris; WOSCOPS, West of Scotland Coronary Prevention Study.

Diminishment after Acute Myocardial Infarction (FLORIDA) (22), Pravastatin in Acute Coronary Treatment (PACT) (23), Pravastatin or Atorvastatin Evaluation and Infection Therapy—Thrombolysis in Myocardial Infarction 22 (PROVE-IT TIMI 22) (24), and A to Z (25) studies.

The major features of treatment guidelines concern indications for treatment, the particular treatments to be used, and in the case of biomedical risk factors, target levels following intervention. Figure 2 shows how these aspects are informed by clinical trials. In particular, net benefit depends on the absolute risk reduction (related to both baseline risk and relative risk reduction) and safety of the treatment. The greater the risk of the patient group or individual for future events, the greater is the absolute risk reduction with therapy (Fig. 3). Health policy decisions are informed not only by outcome data but also by cost-effectiveness analyses. Cost-effectiveness in turn relates to the absolute benefits that are observed.

with previous acute MI whose cholesterol levels were lower (<242 mg/dL, 6.2 mmol/L) than in subjects enrolled in 4S. The LIPID study (18) took these observations further by demonstrating a reduction in all-cause mortality and all major cardiovascular events in patients who were stable after either acute MI or unstable angina and whose cholesterol levels at baseline were in an "average" range for patients (155–271 mg/dL, 4.0–7.0 mmol/L).

The HPS (11) provided further important answers. Among 20,536 patients aged 40 to 80 years with CHD, cerebrovascular or peripheral arterial disease or diabetes, simvastatin reduced all-cause mortality from 14.7% to 12.9% ($P = 0.0003$). The reduction in vascular events was similar and significant in important prespecified subgroups. These included those in whom there had been residual uncertainty, including patients with manifestations of vascular disease other than CHD, women, those aged over 70 years at baseline, and those with LDL or total cholesterol levels less than 3.0 or 5.0 mmol/L (116 or 193 mg/dL), respectively.

Treatment in patients with known coronary artery disease

Patients with clinical evidence of coronary heart disease or other vascular diseases

The 4S (16) was a landmark study which demonstrated that among patients with previous acute MI, simvastatin decreased not only CHD events but also CHD and all-cause mortality. The CARE study (17) extended these findings by demonstrating that pravastatin reduced subsequent CHD events in patients

Patients with stroke and peripheral arterial disease

The 4S (16), CARE (17), and LIPID (18) studies demonstrated a reduction in stroke in patients with known CHD. However, manifest CHD was necessary for inclusion in these trials. The HPS (11) showed a reduction in subsequent vascular events (but not recurrent stroke) in patients who had previous stroke but no previous clinical manifestations of CHD—from 23.6% to 18.7% ($P = 0.001$). At this time, guidelines usually support statin therapy in patients with previous stroke, although it is noted that stroke patients included in HPS were younger, less likely to be hypertensive, and differed in other features from usual stroke patients.

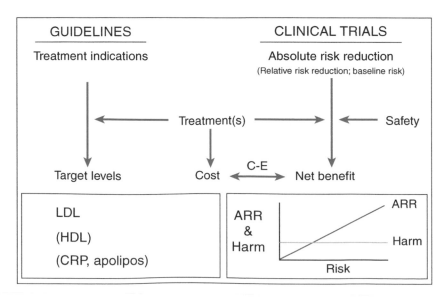

Figure 2
Major features of treatment guidelines and clinical trials. *Abbreviations*: CRP, C-reactive protein; HDL, high-density lipoprotein; LDL, low-density lipoprotein.

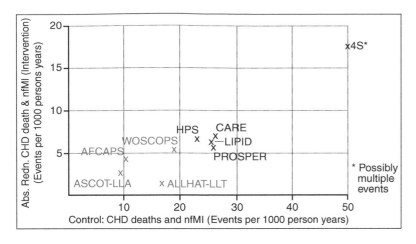

Figure 3
Absolute reduction in risk of coronary heart disease death and nonfatal myocardial infarction in landmark large-scale statin trials depends on rates of events in control limbs of the trials. *Abbreviations*: CHD, coronary heart disease; nfMI, nonfatal myocardial infarction.

Similarly in HPS, simvastatin reduced vascular events over five years from 30.5% to 24.7% ($P < 0.0001$) in patients with manifest peripheral arterial disease but no CHD. Patients with peripheral arterial disease are at very high risk of future CHD events and stroke and an aggressive approach to therapy is indicated, irrespective of cholesterol level.

People with diabetes

There are now substantial data on the benefits of statins in people with diabetes. In the HPS, among 5963 individuals with diabetes, major vascular events were reduced by simvastatin from 25.1% to 20.2% ($P < 0.0001$) (26). Among the subgroup of 2912 people with diabetes without prior vascular disease, the rate of major cardiovascular events was reduced from 13.5% to 9.3% ($P = 0.0003$).

The CARDS randomized 2838 people with Type 2 diabetes plus retinopathy, microalbuminuria, hypertension, or smoking and no history of macrovascular disease to receive either atorvastatin or placebo. Atorvastatin reduced the combined primary endpoint of major CHD events, revascularization, or stroke from 9.0% to 5.8% over 4.5 years ($P = 0.001$) (12).

Should all people with diabetes receive a statin? The answer is an emphatic yes in those who already have CHD, stroke, or peripheral arterial disease. Guidelines differ on whether all those with diabetes but no clinical vascular disease should also be treated. This is recommended in many countries, whereas others suggest an individual approach based on the estimated risk of future events.

Target low-density lipoprotein cholesterol level

In an analysis of the landmark randomized controlled trials, the Cholesterol Treatment Triallists Collaboration has shown a linear relationship between the reduction in cardiovascular events and amount of LDL cholesterol lowering (27). This is shown in Figure 4. For example, each 1.0 mmol/L reduction in LDL cholesterol was associated with a 13% reduction in all-cause mortality. More recent trials have specifically tested whether or

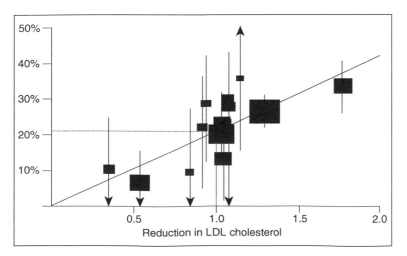

Figure 4
Proportional effects on major vascular events by mean difference in low-density lipoprotein cholesterol. *Abbreviation*: LDL, low-density lipoprotein. *Source*: From Ref. 27.

not achieving lower levels of LDL cholesterol translates to increased benefit. Some of these studies (19,20) have been performed in stable CHD patients, whereas others have been undertaken in patients randomized early after onset of an acute coronary syndrome as discussed later in the chapter (24,25).

The TNT study compared atorvastatin 10 or 80 mg daily in 10,001 subjects with stable CHD who had achieved an LDL cholesterol less than 130 mg/dL (3.4 mmol/L) during open-label run-in with atorvastatin 10 mg daily (19). Those assigned 10 mg atorvastatin in the double-blind phase achieved a mean LDL cholesterol of 101 mg/dL (2.6 mmol/L) compared to a mean LDL cholesterol of 77 mg/dL (2.0 mmol/L) on 80 mg atorvastatin. Over a median follow-up of 4.9 years, the primary endpoint, a composite of CHD death, nonfatal nonprocedure-related MI, resuscitation after cardiac arrest or fatal or nonfatal stroke was reduced from 10.9% to 8.7% with more aggressive LDL cholesterol lowering ($P < 0.001$).

The IDEAL study included 8888 subjects with stable CHD (20). The trial had an open-label design with blinded endpoint evaluation. During treatment, those randomized to receive 20 or 40 mg simvastatin daily had a mean LDL cholesterol of 104 mg/dL (2.7 mmol/L) compared to an LDL cholesterol of 81 mg/dL (2.1 mmol/L) in those assigned 80 mg atorvastatin daily. There was an insignificant risk reduction in the primary endpoint, a composite of coronary death, hospitalization for nonfatal MI, or cardiac arrest with resuscitation from 10.4% in the simvastatin group to 9.3% in the atorvastatin group ($P = 0.07$), after a median follow-up of 4.8 years. However, a significant reduction in some secondary endpoints was noted in the high dose atorvastatin arm, including nonfatal MI, major cardiovascular events (any primary event or stroke), and any coronary event (any primary event, coronary revascularization, or hospitalization for unstable angina). Use of any treatment in usual practice should consider the balance between benefit and harm with an intervention. In each of these trials, some side effects were more common in those on the more intensive LDL-lowering regimen. However, the risk of rhabdomyolysis is very low, although increased with higher statin doses. Overall, the body of data is consistent and supports a target LDL cholesterol of less than 2.0 mmol/L in known CHD patients. A similar conclusion has been reached by the National Cholesterol Education Program—Adult Treatment Panel who suggested that a target LDL cholesterol of 70 mg/dL (1.8 mmol/L) is a very reasonable therapeutic option in very high-risk patients (28).

High-density lipoprotein cholesterol

Robust epidemiologic evidence has identified an inverse relationship between HDL-cholesterol levels and CHD risk. Indeed, HDL-cholesterol is included in the Framingham CHD risk prediction scores (29). HDL-cholesterol protects against atherosclerosis by enhancing reverse cholesterol transport, inhibition of LDL cholesterol oxidation in the atherosclerotic plaque, and anti-inflammatory effects by inhibiting monocyte adhesion to the vascular endothelium (30).

The Veterans Affairs HDL-cholesterol Intervention Trial (VA-HIT) included 2531 men with documented CHD and low-serum HDL-cholesterol concentrations (mean 40 mg/dL), but without elevated LDL cholesterol (mean 111 mg/dL) (31). Treatment with gemfibrozil, 1200 mg/day, for five years resulted in a significant reduction in the risk for death from CHD or nonfatal MI, from 21.7% in the placebo group to 17.3% in the gemfibrozil group ($P = 0.006$). This was associated with a 4% reduction in total cholesterol, a 6% increase in HDL-cholesterol, and a 31% reduction in serum triglycerides, compared with placebo. Gemfibrozil did not decrease LDL cholesterol. Although triglyceride reduction was the largest lipid change, triglyceride levels at baseline or on treatment did not predict CHD levels. Multivariate analysis showed that the incidence of CHD events decreased by 11% for each 5 mg/dL (0.13 mmol/L) increase in HDL-cholesterol concentrations. In gemfibrozil-treated patients, HDL-cholesterol was the only significant predictor of CHD events, but the decrease in CHD events was greater than could be explained by changes in HDL-cholesterol alone.

At this time in clinical practice, the role of fibrates is particularly in combination therapy with a statin. Monitoring of creatine phosphokinase levels is appropriate because of the very small, although increased risk of rhabdomyolysis.

In addition, a recent study in which reconstituted HDL was infused into human subjects after acute coronary syndromes showed a significant reduction in plaque volume in the coronary arteries as assessed by intravascular ultrasound (32).

Triglycerides

It is now recognized that elevated plasma triglyceride levels also predict future events, independent of the levels of other lipid subfractions (33). It is also known that when triglyceride levels are raised to levels above 130 mg/dL (1.5 mmol/L), the predominant LDL phenotype is more atherogenic small dense LDL particles rather than large buoyant LDL particles (34). This is particularly relevant in the context of diabetes and the metabolic syndrome. Apolipoprotein B measures the total number of atherogenic lipid particles, including very LDL cholesterol and chylomicrons, as well as LDL (34). In this context, it is important that a number of studies have demonstrated that apolipoprotein B is superior to LDL cholesterol and also non-HDL cholesterol in predicting future risk of atherosclerotic events (35,36). It might be anticipated that future guidelines will ascribe greater importance to apolipoprotein B that also does not require fasting samples, and particularly in those individuals who have elevated triglyceride levels.

Other targets

Atherosclerosis including acute coronary syndromes is an inflammatory process (37). Among biomarkers of inflammation, most attention and data has focused on C-reactive protein (CRP), which have been reported to be independently related to risk of future CHD events (38). Moreover, in the PROVE-IT TIMI 22 study, CRP levels at 30 days after treatment were not only independent of LDL cholesterol levels at that time but outcomes were improved in those who achieved not only an LDL cholesterol level of < 70 mg/dL (1.8 mmol/L) but also CRP levels less than 2 mg/L (39). However, uncertainties still remain and at this time it is considered premature to include CRP levels as a specific target.

Lipid-lowering following acute coronary syndromes

Several randomized clinical trials of lipid lowering therapy with statins have been conducted in patients with acute coronary syndromes (Table 2). The first of these trials was the MIRACL study, which enrolled 3086 subjects (baseline total cholesterol <7–8 mmol/L) with unstable angina or non-Q-wave MI and randomized them to atorvastatin 80 mg daily or placebo within 96 hours of hospital admission (21). Mean LDL cholesterol levels at the end of the study were 135 mg/dL (3.5 mmol/L) in the placebo group and 72 mg/dL (1.9 mmol/L) in the atorvastatin group. The primary endpoint of death, nonfatal MI, cardiac arrest with resuscitation, or recurrent ischemia requiring hospitalization occurred in 17.4% of the placebo group compared to 14.8% of the atorvastatin group ($P = 0.048$) at four months. The difference in the primary endpoint was driven by a reduction in recurrent ischemia in the atorvastatin group (6.2% vs. 8.4%; $P = 0.02$) without any significant change in the other elements of the composite endpoint.

The FLORIDA study recruited 540 patients with MI and a total cholesterol level of <6.5 mmol/L and randomized them to either fluvastatin 80 mg daily or placebo at a median time of eight days after symptom onset (22). The primary composite endpoint of the study was ischemia on ambulatory electrocardiogram monitoring or a major clinical event defined as death,

Table 2	Summary of published randomized statin trials in acute coronary syndromes						
Trial	*Therapy*	*Comparator*	*Number of patients*	*Follow-up*	*Primary endpoint (composite)*	*LDL-C on treatment*	*Outcome for primary endpoint*
MIRACL	Atorvastatin 80 mg (ACS < 24 hr)	Placebo	3086	4 mo	Death, nfMI, cardiac arrest, hospitalization for recurrent ischemia	1.9 mmol/L vs. 3.5 mmol/L	14.8% atorvastatin vs. 17.4% placebo ($P = 0.048$)
FLORIDA	Fluvastatin 80 mg (ACS < 24 hr)	Placebo	540	1 yr	Ischemia on AECG, death, recurrent MI or ischaemia, revascularization	2.7 mmol/L vs 3.9 mmol/L	33% fluvastatin vs. 36% placebo ($P = 0.24$)
PACT	Pravastatin 20/40 mg (ACS < 24 hr)	Placebo	3408	1 mo	Death, MI, hospitalization for UAP	Not reported	11.6% pravastatin vs. 12.4% placebo ($P = 0.48$)
PROVE-IT TIMI 22	Atorvastatin 80 mg (ACS < 10 days)	Pravastatin 40 mg	4162	2 yr	Death, MI, hospitalization for UAP, revascularization or stroke	1.60 mmol/L vs. 2.46 mmol/L	22.4% atorvastatin vs. 26.3% pravastatin ($P = 0.005$)
A to Z (Z phase)	Simvastatin 40 mg for 4 mo then 80 mg (ACS < 5 days)	Placebo for 4 mo then simvastatin 40 mg	4497	2 yr	Cardiovascular death, nfMI, readmission for ACS, stroke	1.71 mmol/L vs. 2.10 mmol/L at 2 yr	14.4% simvastatin vs. 16.7% placebo/ simvastatin ($P = 0.14$) at 2 yr

Abbreviations: ACS, acute coronary syndrome; AECG, ambulatory electrocardiogram; FLORIDA, fluvastatin on risk diminishment after acute myocardial infarction; MI, myocardial infarction; MIRACL, myocardial ischemia reduction with aggressive cholesterol lowering; nfMI, nonfatal myocardial infarction; PACT, pravastatin in acute coronary treatment; PROVE-IT TIMI 22, pravastatin or atorvastatin evaluation and infection therapy—thrombolysis in myocardial infarction 22; UAP, unstable anginapectoris.

recurrent MI, or recurrent ischemia requiring hospitalization or revascularization. In this negative trial, which was underpowered for clinical events, there was no difference in the composite endpoint at 12 months (36% placebo arm vs. 33% fluvastatin arm; $P = 0.24$). Mean LDL cholesterol in the fluvastatin group was 103 mg/dL (2.7 mmol/L) compared to 149 mg/dL (3.9 mmol/L).

The PACT study was designed to examine the efficacy of pravastatin given within 24 hours of the onset of unstable angina or MI. The aim was to recruit 10,000 patients, but the study was stopped early by the sponsor after 3408 patients had been enrolled, thus it was underpowered. In the early phase of the study, pravastatin 20 mg daily was compared with placebo, although the dose of pravastatin was later increased to 40 mg daily. There was no statistical difference in the primary endpoint of death, recurrent MI, or rehospitalization for unstable angina at one month (11.6% pravastatin arm vs. 12.4% placebo arm; $P = 0.48$).

The PROVE-IT TIMI-22 trial compared 40 mg pravastatin and 80 mg atorvastatin daily in 4162 patients randomized within 10 days of an acute coronary syndrome (24). Unlike MIRACL, FLORIDA, and PACT where planned coronary revascularization was an exclusion criterion, 69% of trial participants had already had percutaneous coronary intervention (PCI) prior to randomization. This reflects contemporary clinical practice. Treatment in other regards would also be seen as standard accepted therapy. Median LDL cholesterol during treatment was 95 mg/dL (2.46 mmol/L) and 62 mg/dL (1.60 mmol/L) for those on 40 mg pravastatin and 80 mg atorvastatin, respectively ($P < 0.001$). Over a mean of 24 months follow-up, there was a significant reduction in the primary endpoint (a composite of all-cause death, MI, unstable angina requiring rehospitalization, revascularization more than 30 days after randomization, and stroke) from 26.3% in the less intensively treated group to 22.4% in those randomized to 80 mg atorvastatin ($P = 0.005$). As in the MIRACL study, the benefit of intensive lipid lowering with high dose atorvastatin was evident early ($P = 0.07$ at 30 days).

The A to Z trial compared early initiation of an intensive statin regimen (40 mg daily of simvastatin for one month, then 80 mg simvastatin daily) with delayed initiation of a less intensive regimen (placebo for four months, then 20 mg simvastatin daily) in 4497 patients following acute coronary syndromes (25). In this study, 44% of patients underwent PCI prior to randomization, and mean LDL cholesterol at eight months was 63 mg/dL (1.63 mmol/L) compared to 77 mg/dL (1.99 mmol/L) in those assigned to the more and less intensive treatment, respectively. There was a nonsignificant reduction in the primary endpoint, a composite of cardiovascular death, nonfatal MI, readmission for acute coronary syndrome and stroke over a 24-month follow-up, from 16.7% to 14.4% with intensive treatment ($P = 0.14$). However, there was a significant reduction in this primary endpoint in the period of 4 to 24 months during follow-up.

A number of observational studies also support the early administration of statins in the high-risk subset of patients with acute coronary syndromes (40–42). These data are consistent with the findings of randomized trials, which indicate that early administration of intensive lipid-lowering therapy with statins leads to improved clinical outcomes within months. Currently, the data favors the use of high dose atorvastatin based on the findings of MIRACL and PROVE-IT TIMI-22 studies. Moreover, the results of PACT and A to Z studies do not support an early clinical advantage for moderate intensity statin therapy. Whether there is any difference in clinical endpoints between statins prescribed at high dose is unknown, as there have not been any prospective head-to-head comparisons in this setting.

Despite the large body of evidence supporting the use of lipid-lowering therapy in patients with CHD, these drugs remain underutilized. Data from the U.S. National Registry of Myocardial Infarction 3 (NRMI-3) reveal that lipid-lowering therapy was part of the discharge prescription in only 32% of patients presenting with acute MI (43). There are advantages to initiating therapy early, as the likelihood that an acute coronary syndrome patient will use lipid-lowering therapy in the medium- to long-term is enhanced when these agents are begun in-hospital (44). Encouragingly, there has been an increase in the usage of lipid-lowering therapy over recent years, although there is still room for considerable improvement (45,46).

Lipid-dependent and pleiotropic effects of statins

Several mechanisms have been put forth to explain the remarkable clinical benefits observed with statin therapy. These include lipid-dependent and lipid-independent (or pleiotropic) effects. In view of the strong association between atherogenic lipoproteins and CHD, the traditional thinking has been that the potent LDL cholesterol lowering effect of statins was the explanation for the reduction in clinical events in the large trials. Indeed, LDL cholesterol lowering may result in a reduction of proatherogenic oxidized LDL particles, and have salutary effects on endothelial function (47,48), platelet function (49,50), vascular inflammation (48), and the slowing of atherosclerotic lesion progression (51,52).

In recent years, there has been great interest in the pleiotropic effects of statins (Table 3). Many of these effects have been attributed to HMG-CoA reductase inhibition and the subsequent impairment in the synthesis of isoprenoid intermediates, which are downstream products of the cholesterol biosynthetic pathway. As a consequence, isoprenylation of proteins involved in intracellular signaling may be prevented, resulting in a variety of effects, such as an increase in bioavailability of endothelium-derived nitric oxide (53).

Table 3 Pleiotropic effects of statins

Beneficial effects	Proposed mechanisms
Improved endothelial vasodilator function	Increased nitric oxide production
	Prevents downregulation of endothelial nitric oxide synthase
	Decreased synthesis of endothelin-1
Anti-inflammatory effects	Reduced endothelial and soluble adhesion molecules
	Reduced CD40 expression and CD40-related activation of vascular cells
	Reduced leukocyte–endothelial cell interactions
	Reduced C-reactive protein levels and proinflammatory cytokines
	Inhibition of LDL oxidation
	Reduced cytotoxicity of T-lymphocytes
	Inhibition of proinflammatory T helper 1 cell development and augmentation of anti-inflammatory T helper 2 cell development
Plaque stabilization	Reduced oxidized LDL uptake
	Decreased matrix metalloproteinases
	Increased tissue inhibitor of metalloproteinase 1
	Increased collagen and fewer inflammatory cells in atherosclerotic plaque
Antithrombotic effects	Reduced tissue factor expression and thrombin generation
	Reduced platelet reactivity
	Increased t-PA and decreased plasminogen activator inhibitor-1
Other effects	Increased circulating endothelial progenitor cells

Abbreviation: LDL, low-density lipoprotein.
Source: From Refs. 8, 54–56, 79, 95–113.

There is debate in the literature about the relative importance of lipid-dependent mechanisms versus pleiotropic effects of statins. Several lines of evidence suggest that the pleiotropic effects of statins are clinically relevant:

1. The earlier appearance of clinical benefit in statin lipid-lowering trials compared to nonstatin lipid-lowering trials despite significant reductions in LDL cholesterol.
2. The early clinical benefits observed in statin trials of acute coronary syndrome patients (MIRACL and PROVE-IT TIMI-22) where coronary vascular inflammation, thrombosis, and unstable plaque are critical pathophysiologic elements that may be positively modified by statins compared to the more delayed benefits observed in statin trials of patients with stable coronary artery disease.
3. The rapid improvement of peripheral endothelial vasodilator function in studies of subjects given statin drugs before changes in serum cholesterol are observed (54,55). In an elegant randomized study in patients with chronic heart failure, simvastatin improved endothelial function but ezetimibe did not despite a similar change in LDL cholesterol (56).
4. The reduction in stroke observed in long-term statin trials despite the lack of association between cholesterol levels and stroke in most epidemiological and observational studies.

Adding to the controversy, however, a recent meta-regression analysis demonstrated that the reduction in CHD risk can be explained by the degree of LDL cholesterol lowering alone without having to invoke alternative lipid-independent mechanisms (57). One of the difficulties in resolving this issue is that some of the biologic effects ascribed to statin pleiotropy may be accounted for by LDL cholesterol lowering. Moreover, experimental studies indicate differences between statins in their lipid-independent effects. Our current state of knowledge precludes a firm conclusion to be made on the potential clinical significance of the well-documented pleiotropic effects of statins. From a practical perspective, the goal of lipid-lowering therapy should be in attaining recommended lipid targets as discussed earlier.

Specific issues relating to percutaneous coronary intervention

Randomized clinical trials

The Atorvastatin Versus Revascularization (AVERT) study compared aggressive lipid-lowering therapy with PCI in 341 low-risk patients with single or double vessel coronary disease who had mild angina or were asymptomatic (58). Subjects with LDL cholesterol levels of 115 mg/dL (≥3.0 mmol/L) were randomized to atorvastatin 80 mg daily or PCI followed by usual lipid-lowering care. On-treatment LDL cholesterol was 77 mg/dL (1.99 mmol/L) in the atorvastatin group and 119 mg/dL (3.08 mmol/L) in the angioplasty group. There was a strong trend to reduction in the primary endpoint, which was a composite of coronary and cerebrovascular ischemic events in the atorvastatin arm at 18 months (13% vs. 21%), and this was driven mainly by fewer hospitalizations for unstable angina. The atorvastatin arm had a longer time to a first ischemic event ($P = 0.03$); however, those in the angioplasty arm had better relief of anginal symptoms (improvement in 54% vs. 41%; $P = 0.009$). Bare-metal stents were used in only 30% of lesions treated with PCI, which is not reflective of present day practice.

The Lescol Intervention Prevention Study (LIPS) randomized 1677 patients with coronary disease and total cholesterol levels between 135 and 270 mg/dL (3.5–7.0 mmol/L) to fluvastatin 40 mg twice daily or placebo at hospital discharge after successful completion of their first PCI (59). The study was designed to examine the clinical efficacy of statin therapy in the post-PCI setting and the primary endpoint was a composite of cardiac death, nonfatal MI, and coronary revascularization. The mean baseline LDL cholesterol in the study population was 132 mg/dL (3.4 mmol/L). Bare-metal stents were used in just over 60% of patients. The primary endpoint occurred in 21% of the fluvastatin group and 27% in the placebo group over a median follow-up of 3.9 years ($P = 0.01$). The event-free survival curves began to diverge at 1.5 years. The benefits of statin therapy were observed in patients with acute coronary syndromes and also those with diabetes (60,61). The median reduction in LDL cholesterol levels was 27% with fluvastatin at six weeks compared to a 11% increase in the placebo group. In a further analysis where

clinical restenosis events (target vessel reinterventions) in the first six months were excluded, the event-free survival curves began to diverge at about six months (59). It is possible that similar early advantages may be observed with the combination of statin therapy and drug-eluting stents, which have minimized the problem of restenosis. As in the case with acute coronary syndromes, long-term compliance with therapy is also enhanced if lipid-lowering therapy is initiated in-hospital after PCI (62).

Prescription of aggressive lipid-lowering therapy and PCI should not be seen as competing strategies but rather complementary treatment modalities with different aims in patients with coronary artery disease. The large-scale Clinical Outcomes Utilizing Revascularization and Aggressive Drug Evaluation (COURAGE) trial will examine this issue further by randomizing patients with coronary artery disease to aggressive medical therapy alone (including lipid-lowering) or PCI with aggressive medical therapy.

Use of intravascular ultrasound

A recent trend in lipid-lowering clinical trials is the use of serial intravascular ultrasound (IVUS) studies with automated pull-back to quantitate coronary atheroma burden. Plaque burden can be measured at different time points using volumetric analysis of a specific coronary segment, as determined by predetermined landmarks such as side branches, and is highly reproducible (63). This methodology has superseded the use of angiography in evaluating the impact of pharmacologic interventions on plaque progression or regression, as in the following clinical trials. In the apoliprotein A-1 Milano trial, weekly infusions of a recombinant HDL particle over a five-week period resulted in a reduction in mean atheroma volume (32). In the Reversal of Atherosclerosis with Aggressive Lipid Lowering (REVERSAL) randomized trial, intensive lipid-lowering with atorvastatin 80 daily was compared to moderate intensity lipid-lowering with pravastatin 40 mg daily (52). On-treatment LDL cholesterol was 79 mg/dL (2.05 mmoL) versus 110 mg/dL (2.85 mmol/L), respectively. Median atheroma volume decreased by 0.4% in the atorvastatin arm, but increased by 2.7% in the pravastatin arm over an 18-month period.

Peri-procedural myocardial infarction

Cardiac enzyme elevation (creatine kinase-MB, cardiac troponin) may occur on average in 20% to 30% of patients after PCI and is associated with adverse clinical outcomes in the short- and long-term (64). Magnetic resonance imaging studies have demonstrated that these elevations are due to myocardial microinfarcts (65,66). The pathophysiology of this complication may include distal embolization of plaque and thrombotic debris, vasoconstriction, and inflammation (64).

Retrospective studies indicate that statin pretreatment is an independent predictor for survival at six months after PCI, and that this benefit begins to emerge as early as one month after PCI (67). Recent randomized trials indicate that these agents reduce the incidence of postprocedural MI. Pasceri et al. (68) randomized 153 patients to atorvastatin 40 mg daily or placebo seven days before elective PCI. Elevations of markers of myocardial injury above the upper limit of normal were significantly lower in the statin arm compared to placebo (CK-MB 12% vs. 35%, $P = 0.001$; troponin I 20% vs. 48%, $P = 0.0004$; myoglobin 22% vs. 51%, $P = 0.0005$). Briguori et al. (69) randomized 451 patients to statin treatment (atorvastastin, pravastatin, simvastatin or fluvastatin) or no statin treatment at least three days before PCI. The occurrence of large non-Qwave MI was reduced in the statin arm from 15.6% to 8% ($P = 0.012$). Potential mechanisms of benefit may relate to the pleiotropic effects of statins on thrombosis, plaque stability, endothelial function, and inflammation.

Potential interaction of HMG-CoA reductase inhibitors and clopidogrel

Clopidogrel is a thienopyridine antiplatelet agent that irreversibly inhibits the platelet $P2Y_{12}$ adenosine diphosphate receptor. It is a critical part of the regimen used to prevent stent thrombosis, and like statin drugs is often prescribed to patients with coronary artery disease. In vitro studies show that clopidogrel is metabolized to its active form in the liver through the cytochrome P450 3A4 enzyme (70), as are some statins such as atorvastatin, simvastatin, and lovastatin, raising the theoretic possibility of drug interactions. In an ex vivo platelet function study, Lau et al. (70) showed that clopidogrel was a less effective inhibitor of platelet aggregation when administered with atorvastatin, but not pravastatin, which is not significantly metabolized by the cytochrome P450 system. A subsequent post hoc analysis of the Clopidogrel for the Reduction of Events During Observation (CREDO) trial showed that the clinical benefits of clopidogrel were similar regardless of whether the statin used was metabolised by cytochrome P450 3A4 or not (71). Further reassurance was provided by a prospective study examining 19 different platelet characteristics in patients undergoing coronary stenting, which found that statins did not attenuate the antiplatelet effects of clopidogrel (72).

Coronary blood flow after primary percutaneous coronary intervention

There is evidence that coronary blood flow is improved in patients pretreated with statins after acute infarct PCI (73,74). Celik et al. (74) found that Thrombolysis In Myocardial Infarction (TIMI) frame counts were lower, implying better coronary blood flow, in patients who underwent successful acute infarct PCI and were taking atorvastatin for ≥ 6 months compared to patients not taking statins. Iwakura et al. found a lower incidence of coronary no-reflow in patients on chronic statin therapy compared to those not taking statin after successful MI (9.1% vs. 34%; $P = 0.003$). Multivariate analysis indicated that statin pretreatment was a protective factor against no-reflow. In this study, the statin-treated patients also had better wall motion, smaller left ventricular dimensions and ejection fraction (73). These studies suggest that statin therapy may help to preserve coronary microvascular function in the setting of acute infarct PCI.

Contrast-induced nephropathy

Contrast-induced nephropathy has been defined as an increase in serum creatinine of at least 25% or an absolute increase in serum creatinine of at least 0.5 mg/dL within 48 to 72 hours of iodinated contrast administration and is associated with significant morbidity and mortality (75). Important risk factors include diabetes mellitus, chronic renal insufficiency, administration of large volumes of high osmolar contrast agents, and intravascular volume depletion. Numerous pharmacologic preventive measures have been studied, but consistent benefits have not been demonstrated. In a recent large retrospective study, preprocedural statin therapy was independently associated with a lower risk of contrast nephropathy and nephropathy requiring dialysis (76).

Coronary endothelial dysfunction after drug-eluting stenting

Recent studies have demonstrated evidence for coronary endothelial dysfunction after drug-eluting stenting. Togni et al. (77) studied coronary endothelial function in 25 patients six months after stent deployment and found paradoxic exercise-induced vasoconstriction in coronary segments adjacent to sirolimus-eluting stents, but vasodilation in patients with bare-metal stents. Similarly, Hofma et al. (78) noted a pronounced vasoconstrictor response to intracoronary acetylcholine in the coronary segment immediately distal to sirolimus-eluting stents at six months, but not in patients receiving bare-metal stents. The mechanisms, clinical relevance, and therapeutic implications of these finding are uncertain. Given the salutary effects of statins in improving coronary and peripheral endothelial vasomotor function (54–56,79), it is conceivable that they may have a beneficial role in this setting.

Restenosis after percutaneous coronary intervention

Restenosis in the era of balloon angioplasty and bare-metal stenting was regarded as the primary limitation of PCI, often necessitating repeat revascularization procedures. Mechanisms included varying degrees of elastic recoil, neointimal hyperplasia, and negative arterial remodeling stimulated by direct injury to vascular cellular elements, inflammation, and thrombosis (80). The dramatic effect of drug-eluting stents in reducing restenosis has sidelined efforts to lower restenosis using systemic pharmacologic therapies.

The majority of studies examining the impact of lipid-lowering therapies on restenosis were performed in the pre-stent era. Most studies demonstrate a lack of association among serum lipids, lipoprotein subfractions, plasma levels of oxidized LDL, and restenosis (81,82). Similarly, the larger prospective trials indicate the statin therapy does not prevent restenosis after balloon angioplasty (83–85). There are conflicting data on the role of statins in preventing bare-metal instent restenosis with some (86), but not all studies indicating an antirestenotic effect (87).

Other drugs that have an impact on serum lipids have also been examined. Probucol pretreatment has been shown to lower the rate of restenosis after balloon angioplasty in clinical trials (88,89). Although its lipid-lowering effect is due to an increase in the fractional catabolic rate of LDL cholesterol (90), its antirestenotic effect is believed to be related to other properties, including inhibition of LDL oxidation, promotion of endothelial regeneration, and anti-inflammatory effects (91). However, probucol is not widely available due to its ability to lower HDL-cholesterol and concerns relating to proarrhythmia.

Fibrates also have properties that may be beneficial in preventing restenosis beyond lipid lowering. Activation of peroxisome proliferative activated receptor (PPAR)-alpha may result in suppression of inflammation and reduction in restenosis after coronary balloon angioplasty in animal models (92); however, clinical data are lacking. Omega-3 fatty acids have modest effects on lowering triglycerides and raising HDL-cholesterol. A meta-analysis of 12 randomized trials in the balloon angioplasty era showed that pretreatment with omega-3 fatty acids did not have a significant impact on reducing restenosis (93).

Bioengineered stents and endothelial progenitor cells

In a preliminary study, Aoki et al. (94) reported the feasibility of deploying a bioengineered stent coated with murine monoclonal anti-human CD34 antibodies to capture CD34 1 endothelial progenitor cells in humans. The aim of this stent is to enhance re-endothelialization after stent implantation. Atorvastatin 40 mg daily and simvastatin 10 mg daily have been shown to increase the number of circulating endothelial progenitor cells in humans within four weeks (56,95). This property of statins may have a potential therapeutic use if used in conjunction with bioengineered stents.

Conclusion

An extremely robust evidence base supports the essential role of statins among cardiovascular therapies in CHD patients. Benefits relate to the magnitude of LDL cholesterol lowering and an overview of trials are consistent with a target LDL cholesterol of 2 mmol/L (77 mg/dL). Pleiotropic effects independent of LDL cholesterol lowering may be particularly relevant in the context of acute coronary syndromes. In addition, there is increasing evidence for other beneficial effects of statins in patients undergoing PCI.

References

1   Yusuf S, Hawken S, Ounpuu S, et al. Effect of potentially modifiable risk factors associated with myocardial infarction in 52 countries (the INTERHEART study): case-control study. Lancet 2004; 364:937–952.

2   World Health Organization. The World Health Report 2002— Reducing Risks, Promoting Healthy Life. Geneva: World Health Organization, 2002.

3   Law MR, Wald NJ, Thompson SG. By how much and how quickly does reduction in serum cholesterol concentration lower risk of ischaemic heart disease? BMJ 1994; 308:367–372.

4   Law MR. Lowering heart disease risk with cholesterol reduction: evidence from observational studies and clinical trials. Eur Heart J Suppl 1999; 1(suppl S):S3–S8.

5   Muldoon MF, Manuck SB, Matthews KA. Lowering cholesterol concentrations and mortality: a quantitative review of primary prevention trials. BMJ 1990; 301:309–314.

6   Endo A, Tsujita Y, Kuroda M, Tanzawa K. Inhibition of cholesterol synthesis in vitro and in vivo by ML-236A and ML-236B, competitive inhibitors of 3-hydroxy-3-methylglutaryl-coenzyme A reductase. Eur J Biochem 1977; 77:31–36.

7   Maron DJ, Fazio S, Linton MF. Current perspectives on statins. Circulation 2000; 101:207–213.

8   Rosenson RS, Tangney CC. Antiatherothrombotic properties of statins: implications for cardiovascular event reduction. JAMA 1998; 279:1643–1650.

9   Shepherd J, Cobbe SM, Ford I, et al. Prevention of coronary heart disease with pravastatin in men with hypercholesterolemia. West of Scotland Coronary Prevention Study Group. N Engl J Med 1995; 333:1301–1307.

10   Downs JR, Clearfield M, Weis S, et al. Primary prevention of acute coronary events with lovastatin in men and women with average cholesterol levels: results of AFCAPS/TexCAPS. Air Force/Texas Coronary Atherosclerosis Prevention Study. JAMA 1998; 279:1615–1622.

11   Heart protection study Collaborative Group MRC/BHF Heart Protection Study of cholesterol lowering with simvastatin in 20,536 high-risk individuals: a randomised placebo-controlled trial. Lancet 2002; 360:7–22.

12   Colhoun HM, Betteridge DJ, Durrington PN, et al. Primary prevention of cardiovascular disease with atorvastatin in type 2 diabetes in the Collaborative Atorvastatin Diabetes Study (CARDS): multicentre randomised placebo-controlled trial. Lancet 2004; 364:685–696.

13   Shepherd J, Blauw GJ, Murphy MB, et al. Pravastatin in elderly individuals at risk of vascular disease (PROSPER): a randomised controlled trial. Prevention of coronary heart disease with pravastatin in men with hypercholesterolemia. West of Scotland Coronary Prevention Study Group. Lancet 2002; 360:1623–1630.

14   The ALLHAT Officers and Coordinators for the ALLHAT Collaborative Research Group. Major outcomes in moderately hypercholesterolemic, hypertensive patients randomized to pravastatin vs usual care: the Antihypertensive and Lipid-Lowering Treatment to Prevent Heart Attack Trial (ALLHAT-LLT). JAMA 2002; 288:2998–3007.

15   Sever PS, Dahlof B, Poulter NR, et al. Prevention of coronary and stroke events with atorvastatin in hypertensive patients who have average or lower-than-average cholesterol concentrations, in the Anglo-Scandinavian Cardiac Outcomes Trial-Lipid Lowering Arm (ASCOT-LLA): a multicentre randomised controlled trial. Lancet 2003; 361:1149–1158.

16   Scandinavian Simvastatin Survival Study Group. Randomised trial of cholesterol lowering in 4444 patients with coronary heart disease: the Scandinavian Simvastatin Survival Study (4S). Lancet 1994; 344:1383–1389.

17   Sacks FM, Pfeffer MA, Moye LA, et al. The effect of pravastatin on coronary events after myocardial infarction in patients with average cholesterol levels. Cholesterol and Recurrent Events Trial investigators. N Engl J Med 1996; 335:1001–1009.

18   The Long-Term Intervention with Pravastatin in Ischaemic Disease (LIPID) Study Group. Prevention of cardiovascular events and death with pravastatin in patients with coronary heart disease and a broad range of initial cholesterol levels. N Engl J Med 1998; 339:1349–1357.

19   LaRosa JC, Grundy SM, Waters DD, et al. Intensive lipid lowering with atorvastatin in patients with stable coronary disease. N Engl J Med 2005; 352:1425–1435.

20   Pedersen TR, Faergeman O, Kastelein JJ, et al. High-dose atorvastatin vs usual-dose simvastatin for secondary prevention after myocardial infarction: the IDEAL study: a randomized controlled trial. JAMA 2005; 294:2437–2445.

21   Schwartz GG, Olsson AG, Ezekowitz MD, et al. Effects of atorvastatin on early recurrent ischemic events in acute coronary syndromes: the MIRACL study: a randomized controlled trial. JAMA 2001; 285:1711–1718.

22   Liem AH, van Boven AJ, Veeger NJ, et al. Effect of fluvastatin on ischaemia following acute myocardial infarction: a randomized trial. Eur Heart J 2002; 23:1931–1937.

23   Thompson PL, Meredith I, Amerena J, Campbell TJ, Sloman JG, Harris PJ. Effect of pravastatin compared with placebo initiated within 24 hours of onset of acute myocardial infarction or unstable angina: the Pravastatin in Acute Coronary Treatment (PACT) trial. Am Heart J 2004; 148:e2.

24   Cannon CP, Braunwald E, McCabe CH, et al. Intensive versus moderate lipid lowering with statins after acute coronary syndromes. N Engl J Med 2004; 350:1495–1504.

25   de Lemos JA, Blazing MA, Wiviott SD, et al. Early intensive vs a delayed conservative simvastatin strategy in patients with acute coronary syndromes: phase Z of the A to Z trial. JAMA 2004; 292:1307–1316.

26   Collins R, Armitage J, Parish S, Sleigh P, Peto R. MRC/BHF Heart Protection Study of cholesterol-lowering with simvastatin in 5963 people with diabetes: a randomised placebo-controlled trial. Lancet 2003; 361:2005–2016.

27   Baigent C, Keech A, Kearney PM, et al. Efficacy and safety of cholesterol-lowering treatment: prospective meta-analysis of data from 90,056 participants in 14 randomised trials of statins. Lancet 2005; 366:1267–1278.

28   Grundy SM, Cleeman JI, Merz CN, et al. Implications of recent clinical trials for the National Cholesterol Education Program Adult Treatment Panel III guidelines. Circulation 2004; 110:227–239.

29   Wilson PW, D'Agostino RB, Levy D, Belanger AM, Silbershatz H, Kannel WB. Prediction of coronary heart disease using risk factor categories. Circulation 1998; 97:1837–1847.

30   Barter PJ. Cardioprotective effects of high-density lipoproteins: the evidence strengthens. Arterioscler Thromb Vasc Biol 2005; 25:1305–1306.

31   Robins SJ, Collins D, Wittes JT, et al. Relation of gemfibrozil treatment and lipid levels with major coronary events: VA-HIT: a randomized controlled trial. JAMA 2001; 285:1585–1591.

32   Nissen SE, Tsunoda T, Tuzcu EM, et al. Effect of recombinant ApoA-I Milano on coronary atherosclerosis in patients with acute coronary syndromes: a randomized controlled trial. JAMA 2003; 290:2292–2300.

33   Patel A, Barzi F, Jamrozik K, et al. Serum triglycerides as a risk factor for cardiovascular diseases in the Asia-Pacific region. Circulation 2004; 110:2678–2686.

34   Barter PJ, Ballantyne CM, Carmena R, et al. Apo B versus cholesterol in estimating cardiovascular risk and in guiding therapy: report of the thirty-person/ten-country panel. J Intern Med 2006; 259:247–258.

35   Walldius G, Jungner I, Holme I, Aastveit AH, Kolar W, Steiner E. High apolipoprotein B, low apolipoprotein A-I, and improvement in the prediction of fatal myocardial infarction (AMORIS study): a prospective study. Lancet 2001; 358:2026–2033.

36   Pischon T, Girman CJ, Sacks FM, Rifai N, Stampfer MJ, Rimm EB. Non-high-density lipoprotein cholesterol and apolipoprotein B in the prediction of coronary heart disease in men. Circulation 2005; 112:3375–3383.

37   Libby P. Inflammation in atherosclerosis. Nature 2002; 420:868–874.

38   Ridker PM, Wilson PW, Grundy SM. Should C-reactive protein be added to metabolic syndrome and to assessment of global cardiovascular risk? Circulation 2004; 109:2818–2825.

39 Ridker PM, Morrow DA, Rose LM, Rifai N, Cannon CP, Braunwald E. Relative efficacy of atorvastatin 80 mg and pravastatin 40 mg in achieving the dual goals of low-density lipoprotein cholesterol >70 mg/dl and C-reactive protein >2 mg/l: an analysis of the PROVE-IT TIMI-22 trial. J Am Coll Cardiol 2005; 45:1644–1648.

40 Aronow HD, Topol EJ, Roe MT, et al. Effect of lipid-lowering therapy on early mortality after acute coronary syndromes: an observational study. Lancet 2001; 357:1063–1068.

41 Fonarow GC, Wright RS, Spencer FA, et al. Effect of statin use within the first 24 hours of admission for acute myocardial infarction on early morbidity and mortality. Early withdrawal of statin therapy in patients with non-ST-segment elevation myocardial infarction: national registry of myocardial infarction. Use of lipid-lowering medications at discharge in patients with acute myocardial infarction: data from the National Registry of Myocardial Infarction 3. Am J Cardiol 2005; 96:611–616.

42 Stenestrand U, Wallentin L. Early statin treatment following acute myocardial infarction and 1-year survival. JAMA 2001; 285:430–436.

43 Fonarow GC, French WJ, Parsons LS, Sun H, Malmgren JA. Use of lipid-lowering medications at discharge in patients with acute myocardial infarction: data from the National Registry of Myocardial Infarction 3. Circulation 2001; 103:38–44.

44 Smith CS, Cannon CP, McCabe CH, Murphy SA, Bentley J, Braunwald E. Early initiation of lipid-lowering therapy for acute coronary syndromes improves compliance with guideline recommendations: observations from the Orbofiban in Patients with Unstable Coronary Syndromes (OPUS-TIMI 16) trial. Am Heart J 2005; 149:444–450.

45 Newby LK, LaPointe NM, Chen AY, et al. Long-term adherence to evidence-based secondary prevention therapies in coronary artery disease. Circulation 2006; 113:203–212.

46 Alexander KP, Roe MT, Chen AY, et al. Evolution in cardiovascular care for elderly patients with non-ST-segment elevation acute coronary syndromes: results from the CRUSADE National Quality Improvement Initiative. J Am Coll Cardiol 2005; 46:1479–1487.

47 Tamai O, Matsuoka H, Itabe H, Wada Y, Kohno K, Imaizumi T. Single LDL apheresis improves endothelium-dependent vasodilatation in hypercholesterolemic humans. Circulation 1997; 95:76–82.

48 Selwyn AP, Kinlay S, Libby P, Ganz P. Atherogenic lipids, vascular dysfunction, and clinical signs of ischemic heart disease. Circulation 1997; 95:5–7.

49 Lacoste L, Lam JY, Hung J, Letchacovski G, Solymoss CB, Waters D. Hyperlipidemia and coronary disease. Correction of the increased thrombogenic potential with cholesterol reduction. Circulation 1995; 92:3172–3177.

50 Nofer JR, Tepel M, Kehrel B, et al. Low-density lipoproteins inhibit the Na H antiport in human platelets. A novel mechanism enhancing platelet activity in hypercholesterolemia. Circulation 1997; 95:1370–1377.

51 Callister TQ, Raggi P, Cooil B, Lippolis NJ, Russo DJ. Effect of HMG-CoA reductase inhibitors on coronary artery disease as assessed by electron-beam computed tomography. N Engl J Med 1998; 339:1972–1978.

52 Nissen SE, Tuzcu EM, Schoenhagen P, et al. Effect of intensive compared with moderate lipid-lowering therapy on progression of coronary atherosclerosis: a randomized controlled trial. JAMA 2004; 291:1071–1080.

53 Rikitake Y, Liao JK. Rho GTPases, statins, and nitric oxide. Circ Res 2005; 97:1232–1235.

54 Laufs U, Wassmann S, Hilgers S, Ribaudo N, Bohm M, Nickenig G. Rapid effects on vascular function after initiation and withdrawal of atorvastatin in healthy, normocholesterolemic men. Am J Cardiol 2001; 88:1306–1307.

55 John S, Schneider MP, Delles C, Jacobi J, Schmieder RE. Lipid-independent effects of statins on endothelial function and bioavailability of nitric oxide in hypercholesterolemic patients. Am Heart J 2005; 149:473.

56 Landmesser U, Bahlmann F, Mueller M, et al. Simvastatin versus ezetimibe: pleiotropic and lipid-lowering effects on endothelial function in humans. Circulation 2005; 111:2356–2363.

57 Robinson JG, Smith B, Maheshwari N, Schrott H. Pleiotropic effects of statins: benefit beyond cholesterol reduction? A meta-regression analysis. J Am Coll Cardiol 2005; 46:1855–1862.

58 Pitt B, Waters D, Brown WV, et al. Aggressive lipid-lowering therapy compared with angioplasty in stable coronary artery disease. Atorvastatin versus Revascularization Treatment Investigators. N Engl J Med 1999; 341:70–76.

59 Serruys PW, de Feyter P, Macaya C, et al. Fluvastatin for prevention of cardiac events following successful first percutaneous coronary intervention: a randomized controlled trial. JAMA 2002; 287:3215–3222.

60 Arampatzis CA, Goedhart D, Serruys PW, Saia F, Lemos PA, de Feyter P. Fluvastatin reduces the impact of diabetes on long-term outcome after coronary intervention—a Lescol Intervention Prevention Study (LIPS) substudy. Am Heart J 2005; 149:329–335.

61 Lee CH, de Feyter P, Serruys PW, et al. Beneficial effects of fluvastatin following percutaneous coronary intervention in patients with unstable and stable angina: results from the Lescol intervention prevention study (LIPS). Heart 2004; 90:1156–1161.

62 Aronow HD, Novaro GM, Lauer MS, et al. In-hospital initiation of lipid-lowering therapy after coronary intervention as a predictor of long-term utilization: a propensity analysis. Arch Intern Med 2003; 163:2576–2582.

63 Mintz GS, Nissen SE, Anderson WD, et al. American college of cardiology clinical expert consensus document on standards for acquisition, measurement and reporting of intravascular ultrasound studies (IVUS). A report of the American college of cardiology task force on clinical expert consensus documents. J Am Coll Cardiol 2001; 37:1478–1492.

64 Herrmann J. Peri-procedural myocardial injury: 2005 update. Eur Heart J 2005; 26:2493–2519.

65 Ricciardi MJ, Wu E, Davidson CJ, et al. Visualization of discrete microinfarction after percutaneous coronary intervention associated with mild creatine kinase-MB elevation. Circulation 2001; 103:2780–2783.

66 Selvanayagam JB, Porto I, Channon K, et al. Troponin elevation after percutaneous coronary intervention directly represents the extent of irreversible myocardial injury: insights from cardiovascular magnetic resonance imaging. Circulation 2005; 111:1027–1032.

67 Chan AW, Bhatt DL, Chew DP, et al. Early and sustained survival benefit associated with statin therapy at the time of percutaneous coronary intervention. Circulation 2002; 105:691–696.

68 Pasceri V, Patti G, Nusca A, Pristipino C, Richichi G, Di Sciascio G. Randomized trial of atorvastatin for reduction of myocardial damage during coronary intervention: results from the ARMYDA (Atorvastatin for Reduction of MYocardial Damage during Angioplasty) study. Circulation 2004; 110:674–678.

69 Briguori C, Colombo A, Airoldi F, et al. Statin administration before percutaneous coronary intervention: impact on periprocedural myocardial infarction. Eur Heart J 2004; 25:1822–1828.

70 Lau WC, Waskell LA, Watkins PB, et al. Atorvastatin reduces the ability of clopidogrel to inhibit platelet aggregation: a new drug-drug interaction. Circulation 2003; 107:32–37.

71 Saw J, Steinhubl SR, Berger PB, et al. Lack of adverse clopidogrel-atorvastatin clinical interaction from secondary analysis of a randomized, placebo-controlled clopidogrel trial. Circulation 2003; 108:921–924.

72 Serebruany VL, Midei MG, Malinin AI, et al. Absence of interaction between atorvastatin or other statins and clopidogrel: results from the interaction study. Arch Intern Med 2004; 164:2051–2057.

73 Iwakura K, Ito H, Kawano S, et al. Chronic pre-treatment of statins is associated with the reduction of the no-reflow phenomenon in the patients with reperfused acute myocardial infarction. Eur Heart J 2006; 27:534–539.

74 Celik T, Kursaklioglu H, Iyisoy A, et al. The effects of prior use of atorvastatin on coronary blood flow after primary percutaneous coronary intervention in patients presenting with acute myocardial infarction. Coron Artery Dis 2005; 16:321–326.

75 Barrett BJ, Parfrey PS. Clinical practice. Preventing nephropathy induced by contrast medium. N Engl J Med 2006; 354:379–386.

76 Khanal S, Attallah N, Smith DE, et al. Statin therapy reduces contrast-induced nephropathy: an analysis of contemporary percutaneous interventions. The potential role of statins in contrast nephropathy. Am J Med 2005; 118:843–849.

77 Togni M, Windecker S, Cocchia R, et al. Sirolimus-eluting stents associated with paradoxic coronary vasoconstriction. J Am Coll Cardiol 2005; 46:231–236.

78 Hofma SH, van der Giessen WJ, van Dalen BM, et al. Indication of long-term endothelial dysfunction after sirolimus-eluting stent implantation. Eur Heart J 2006; 27:166–170.

79 Treasure CB, Klein JL, Weintraub WS, et al. Beneficial effects of cholesterol-lowering therapy on the coronary endothelium in patients with coronary artery disease. N Engl J Med 1995; 332:481–487.

80 Welt FG, Rogers C. Inflammation and restenosis in the stent era. Arterioscler Thromb Vasc Biol 2002; 22:1769–1776.

81 Segev A, Strauss BH, Witztum JL, Lau HK, Tsimikas S. Relationship of a comprehensive panel of plasma oxidized low-density lipoprotein markers to angiographic restenosis in patients undergoing percutaneous coronary intervention for stable angina. Am Heart J 2005; 150:1007–1014.

82 Jorgensen B, Simonsen S, Endresen K, et al. Luminal loss and restenosis after coronary angioplasty. The role of lipoproteins and lipids. Eur Heart J 1999; 20:1407–1414.

83 Bertrand ME, McFadden EP, Fruchart JC, et al. Effect of pravastatin on angiographic restenosis after coronary balloon angioplasty. The PREDICT Trial Investigators. Prevention of Restenosis by Elisor after Transluminal Coronary Angioplasty. J Am Coll Cardiol 1997; 30:863–869.

84 Serruys PW, Foley DP, Jackson G, et al. A randomized placebo-controlled trial of fluvastatin for prevention of restenosis after successful coronary balloon angioplasty; Final results of the fluvastatin angiographic restenosis (FLARE) trial. Effect of pravastatin on angiographic restenosis after coronary balloon angioplasty. The PREDICT Trial Investigators. Prevention of Restenosis by Elisor after Transluminal Coronary Angioplasty. Eur Heart J 1999; 20:58–69.

85 Weintraub WS, Boccuzzi SJ, Klein JL, et al. Lack of effect of lovastatin on restenosis after coronary angioplasty. Lovastatin Restenosis Trial Study Group. N Engl J Med 1994; 331:1331–1337.

86 Walter DH, Schachinger V, Elsner M, Mach S, Auch-Schwelk W, Zeiher AM. Effect of statin therapy on restenosis after coronary stent implantation. Am J Cardiol 2000; 85:962–968.

87 Petronio AS, Amoroso G, Limbruno U, et al. Simvastatin does not inhibit intimal hyperplasia and restenosis but promotes plaque regression in normocholesterolemic patients undergoing coronary stenting: a randomized study with intravascular ultrasound. Am Heart J 2005; 149:520–526.

88 Tardif JC, Cote G, Lesperance J, et al. Probucol and multivitamins in the prevention of restenosis after coronary angioplasty. Multivitamins and Probucol Study Group. N Engl J Med 1997; 337:365–372.

89 Yokoi H, Daida H, Kuwabara Y, et al. Effectiveness of an antioxidant in preventing restenosis after percutaneous transluminal coronary angioplasty: the Probucol Angioplasty Restenosis Trial. J Am Coll Cardiol 1997; 30:855–862.

90 Steinberg D. Studies on the mechanism of action of probucol. Am J Cardiol 1986; 57:16H–21H.

91 Lau AK, Leichtweis SB, Hume P, et al. Probucol promotes functional reendothelialization in balloon-injured rabbit aortas. Circulation 2003; 107:2031–2036.

92 Kasai T, Miyauchi K, Yokoyama T, Aihara K, Daida H. Efficacy of peroxisome proliferative activated receptor (PPAR)-alpha ligands, fenofibrate, on intimal hyperplasia and constrictive remodeling after coronary angioplasty in porcine models. Atherosclerosis 2005; 188:274–280.

93 Balk EM, Lichtenstein AH, Chung M, Kupelnick B, Chew P, Lau J. Effects of omega-3 fatty acids on coronary restenosis, intima-media thickness, and exercise tolerance: a systematic review. Atherosclerosis 2006; 184:237–246.

94 Aoki J, Serruys PW, van Beusekom H, et al. Endothelial progenitor cell capture by stents coated with antibody against CD34: the HEALING-FIM (Healthy Endothelial Accelerated Lining Inhibits Neointimal Growth-First In Man) registry. J Am Coll Cardiol 2005; 45:1574–1579.

95 Vasa M, Fichtlscherer S, Adler K, et al. Increase in circulating endothelial progenitor cells by statin therapy in patients with stable coronary artery disease. Circulation 2001; 103:2885–2890.

96 Kureishi Y, Luo Z, Shiojima I, et al. The HMG-CoA reductase inhibitor simvastatin activates the protein kinase Akt and promotes angiogenesis in normocholesterolemic animals. Nat Med 2000; 6:1004–1010.

97 Hernandez-Perera O, Perez-Sala D, Navarro-Antolin J, et al. Effects of the 3-hydroxy-3-methylglutaryl-CoA reductase inhibitors, atorvastatin and simvastatin, on the expression of endothelin-1 and endothelial nitric oxide synthase in vascular endothelial cells. J Clin Invest 1998; 101:2711–2719.

98 Ridker PM, Rifai N, Pfeffer MA, Sacks F, Braunwald E. Long-term effects of pravastatin on plasma concentration of C-reactive protein. The Cholesterol and Recurrent Events (CARE) Investigators. Circulation 1999; 100:230–235.

99 Pruefer D, Scalia R, Lefer AM. Simvastatin inhibits leukocyte-endothelial cell interactions and protects against inflammatory processes in normocholesterolemic rats. Arterioscler Thromb Vasc Biol 1999; 19:2894–2900.

100 Seljeflot I, Tonstad S, Hjermann I, Arnesen H. Reduced expression of endothelial cell markers after 1 year treatment with simvastatin and atorvastatin in patients with coronary heart disease. Atherosclerosis 2002; 162:179–185.

101 Mulhaupt F, Matter CM, Kwak BR, et al. Statins (HMG-CoA reductase inhibitors) reduce CD40 expression in human vascular cells. Cardiovasc Res 2003; 59:755–766.

102 Koh KK, Son JW, Ahn JY, et al. Comparative effects of diet and statin on NO bioactivity and matrix metalloproteinases in hypercholesterolemic patients with coronary artery disease. Arterioscler Thromb Vasc Biol 2002; 22:e19–e23.

103 Rezaie-Majd A, Maca T, Bucek RA, et al. Simvastatin reduces expression of cytokines interleukin-6, interleukin-8, and monocyte chemoattractant protein-1 in circulating monocytes from hypercholesterolemic patients. Arterioscler Thromb Vasc Biol 2002; 22:1194–1199.

104 Suzumura K, Yasuhara M, Tanaka K, Suzuki T. Protective effect of fluvastatin sodium (XU-62-320), a 3-hydroxy-3-methylglutaryl coenzyme A (HMG-CoA) reductase inhibitor, on oxidative modification of human low-density lipoprotein in vitro. Biochem Pharmacol 1999; 57:697–703.

105 Blanco-Colio LM, Munoz-Garcia B, Martin-Ventura JL, et al. 3-hydroxy-3-methylglutaryl coenzyme A reductase inhibitors decrease Fas ligand expression and cytotoxicity in

activated human T lymphocytes. Circulation 2003; 108: 1506–1513.

106 Hakamada-Taguchi R, Uehara Y, Kuribayashi K, et al. Inhibition of hydroxymethylglutaryl-coenzyme a reductase reduces Th1 development and promotes Th2 development. Circ Res 2003; 93:948–956.

107 Crisby M, Nordin-Fredriksson G, Shah PK, Yano J, Zhu J, Nilsson J. Pravastatin treatment increases collagen content and decreases lipid content, inflammation, metalloproteinases, and cell death in human carotid plaques: implications for plaque stabilization. Circulation 2001; 103:926–933.

108 Li DY, Chen HJ, Mehta JL. Statins inhibit oxidized-LDL-mediated LOX-1 expression, uptake of oxidized-LDL and reduction in PKB phosphorylation. Cardiovasc Res 2001; 52:130–135.

109 Fuhrman B, Koren L, Volkova N, Keidar S, Hayek T, Aviram M. Atorvastatin therapy in hypercholesterolemic patients suppresses cellular uptake of oxidized-LDL by differentiating monocytes. Atherosclerosis 2002; 164:179–185.

110 Solem J, Levin M, Karlsson T, Grip L, Albertsson P, Wiklund O. Composition of coronary plaques obtained by directional atherectomy in stable angina: its relation to serum lipids and statin treatment. J Intern Med 2006; 259:267–275.

111 Undas A, Brummel-Ziedins KE, Mann KG. Statins and blood coagulation. Arterioscler Thromb Vasc Biol 2005; 25:287–294.

112 Casani L, Sanchez-Gomez S, Vilahur G, Badimon L. Pravastatin reduces thrombogenicity by mechanisms beyond plasma cholesterol lowering. Thromb Haemost 2005; 94:1035–1041.

113 Wiesbauer F, Kaun C, Zorn G, Maurer G, Huber K, Wojta J. HMG CoA reductase inhibitors affect the fibrinolytic system of human vascular cells in vitro: a comparative study using different statins. Br J Pharmacol 2002; 135:284–292.

15

Improving the diagnosis and management of high blood pressure in the cardiac patient

Clarence E. Grim

There is nothing that cardiologists (and all other practitioners) do that is more cost effective than accurately diagnosing and managing high blood pressure (BP). Lowering BP reduces risk from all causes of death by at least 20%, as well as deaths due to all forms of cardiovascular (by 25–50%) and renal diseases (by 50%). And the older the patient, the greater the benefit. Therefore, cardiologists must be skilled in diagnosing and controlling the BP to defined goals in all patients before and after the onset of coronary artery disease and its treatments.

This chapter highlights a common BP measurement error made by cardiologists, demonstrates how to validate automated device accuracy in the individual patient, and discusses a systematic approach to bringing the difficult patient's BP to goal. The key concept that is developed here is that the control of BP is always an individual experiment in the individual patient, as we currently have no good way to predict which drug or drugs will work best in each patient. The stepwise "combination of combinations" program that I set out has evolved over 40 years of practice in patients with difficult-to-manage high BP.

The cardiologist is frequently the referral resource for other practitioners who are having problems managing a patient's high BP but, in general, cardiologists have received little direct training or update in the evaluation and management of the difficult, hypertensive patient. Deficiencies in basic skills needed for the evaluation and treatment of these patients include a lack of attention to BP measurement during office visits by failing to use the recommended mercury manometer and the auscultatory technique, cessation of which diagnose and manage high BP to the highest level of accuracy. In many offices, the BP is measured while the patient is seated on the examining table (1), which falsely increases diastolic BP by about 7 mmHg and results in overdiagnosis and over-treatment of many patients. Over-treatment increases side effects, such as fatigue and dizziness, and the patient's dissatisfaction with the regimen and the practitioner, which can lead to stopping therapy.

Another common failure is neglecting to instruct the patient to measure BP at home in order to use this to guide therapy. Measuring BP at home allows the practitioner to make decisions based on many more samples of BP rather than relying on readings taken every few months in the office. This also leads to overdiagnosis and overtreatment in those who have office hypertension but normal BP at home. However, many office and home devices now utilize the oscillometric technique, which leads to serious inaccuracies in at least 50% of patients. When BP is measured with an automated device, office staff should document the accuracy of each device on each patient, as all automated devices make serious systematic errors in at least 50% of patients, ≥ 5 mmHg (2).

How to test the accuracy of an electronic blood pressure device

The American Heart Association (AHA) Guidelines 2005 state that "Accurate measurement of blood pressure is essential to classify individuals, to ascertain blood pressure related-risk and to guide management. The auscultatory technique with a trained observer and mercury manometer continues to be the method of choice in the office." The oscillometric method can be used for office measurement, but only devices independently validated according to standard protocols should be used, and individual calibration is recommended (3).

The beauty of the mercury manometer is that you can assess its accuracy by simply looking at it. If the mercury meniscus is at zero when there is no pressure in the cuff and the column moves smoothly with inflation and deflation it is accurate and can be used as the gold standard for pressure measurement. All other devices must be calibrated against a mercury manometer at regular intervals. Commercial electronic calibration manometers (such as the NETECH DigiMano) must be sent back to the manufacturer yearly for calibration against a mercury standard. Devices that pass the validation protocols of the American Association of Medical Instrumentation (AAMI) will have systematic errors of more than 5 mmHg in a substantial number of individual patients.

The calibration check of a nonmercury device requires two steps: (i) validation of the manometer in the device and (ii) validation of the ability of the device to estimate the pressure in an individual patient.

For an up-to-date list of validate devices go to http://www.bhsoc.org/bp_monitors/automatic.stm

Does the manometer in my nonmercury device record pressure accurately?

First, you must document whether the manometer of the device (electronic or aneroid) registers pressure accurately. Connect the device to be tested to the reference device (mercury, aneroid, or electronic) with a Y tube, as shown in Figure 1.

The Y tube transmits pressure equally to the reference device and the device to be tested. Using the bulb connected to the Y, pressure is increased to 300 mmHg and then lowered by 10 mmHg. Recording the pressure on each device validates the accuracy of the aneroid or electronic device. Any device that differs by more than 3 mmHg from the mercury or reference standard is considered to be out of calibration and should be removed from service.

Does this automated device estimate the pressure accurately enough in my patient?

The second step is to assess the error (if any) of the BP estimated by the automated device. This is done by simultaneous or by sequential readings.

Simultaneous readings

This is the preferred option. If the device can deflate at a constant rate of 2 to 3 mm/sec, one can do simultaneous readings. Record the BP by the auscultatory method as the automated device takes the BP. To be certain the automatic device inflates high enough to get an accurate pressure, you must obtain the palpated systolic pressure and then ensure that the automatic device inflates at least 30 mm above that. Then listen as the automatic device deflates and record the systolic and diastolic pressure you hear. After you have recorded your reading, record the reading from the automated device. This should be done at least three times and then analyzed as in Table 1.

Sequential readings

Many devices deflate too fast or in steps, and so you must use sequential readings. We recommend that this be done enough times to ensure that you have a good estimate of the BP recorded by the machine and the human observer. AAMI recommends that this be done at least five times. The averages are then calculated and compared. Your local guidelines should be used to assess whether the device is accurate enough to be used in your patient. An error of more than 5 mmHg and a

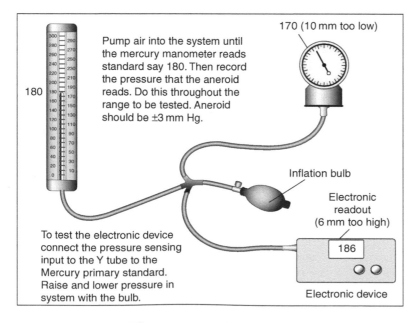

To test the electronic device connect the pressure sensing input to the Y tube to the Mercury primary standard. Raise and lower pressure in system with the bulb.

Pump air into the system until the mercury manometer reads standard say 180. Then record the pressure that the aneroid reads. Do this throughout the range to be tested. Aneroid should be ±3 mm Hg.

170 (10 mm too low)

Inflation bulb

Electronic readout (6 mm too high)

186

Electronic device

Figure 1
If using an electronic calibration standard, it is connected in place of the mercury manometer. You should test only one device at a time.

Table 1 How to test an automated blood pressure device against a trained and certified human observer using a mercury manometer and stethescope[a]

Reading	Human systolic	Human diastolic	Device systolic	Device diastolic	Systolic error	Diastolic error
1	156	90	150	95	−6	5
2	150	86	145	90	−5	4
3	146	82	140	87	−6	5
Average	151	86	145	91	−6	+5
					Mean error	
					−5.7	4.7
SD	4	3	4	3	0.5	0.5

[a]See text on how to set up in an Excel file.

standard deviation (SD) of more than 8 is generally considered unacceptable. Inform the patient and note this error in the patient's chart so others will be aware of it.

To use this table in an Excel spreadsheet, you enter three readings made by your trained observer and three made by the device. The mean error and its SD is calculated by using Excel functions. If the error is more than 5 mmHg, this device should not be used in this patient.

Failure to document these directional errors will also lead to decisions being made on the basis of only a single BP reading. Another important approach is to take a home reading and to use a systematic approach to the clinical and laboratory evaluation of the new patient to exclude secondary causes of high BP and to guide treatment. Finally, recent advances in the genetics of high BP need to be kept in mind while evaluating new patients and their families.

How to quickly bring blood pressure under control in the most difficult patient

In my experience, many cardiologists fail to recognize that secondary causes of high BP tend to be much higher in their referral practice and they miss important clues to secondary causes. Appendix I outlines a systematic approach to be certain that one is not missing secondary causes of high BP.

Blood pressure control before and after surgery or angiography

In contrast to older agents, which had much longer half lives, that are used to control BP this combination of combinations uses

agents that, except for diuretics, will lead to a rapid increase in BP if they are not given every 24 hours (Appendix 2). Therefore the agents should not be stopped on the night before or the day of interventional studies, as the BP may rapidly increase during or after the study and lead to complications, including hemorrhage around puncture sites or acute pulmonary edema.

When BP control is needed during interventional procedures, one can use intravenous nitrates or combined alpha-beta blockers such as labetalol. When these agents fail, I use Nipride, which I have never had fail to control the BP in patients with Cushing's, primary aldosteronism, renal artery stenosis, pheochromocytoma, and scleroderma with malignant hypertension.

In the postoperative state, BP control can be continued even if the patients are nil per os (NPO) as the medications can be crushed and given via a nasogastric tube.

Summary

This chapter discusses some key features for BP measurement and management in the office and the home and stresses the continued use of the mercury manometer as recommended by the newest AHA guidelines. A method to validate home and office device accuracy is detailed. Finally a stepwise "combination of combinations" approach to BP control in the difficult patient is reviewed, which can be used in the in- and outpatient setting.

References

1 Cushman WC, Cooper KM, Horne RA, Meydrech EF. Effect of back support and stethoscope head on seated blood pressure determinations. Am J Hypertens 1990; 3: 240–241.

2   Gerin W, Schwartz AR, Schwartz JE, et al. Limitations of current validation protocols for home blood pressure monitors for individual patients. Blood Press Monit 2002; 7(6):313–318.

3   Pickering TG, Hall JE, Appel LJ, et al. Part 1: blood pressure measurement in humans: a statement for professionals from the Subcommittee of Professional and Public Education of the American Heart Association Council on High Blood Pressure Research. Hypertension 2005; 45:142–161.

4   Grim CE. Evolution of diagnostic criteria for primary aldosteronism: why is it more common in "drug-resistant" hypertension today? Curr Hypertens Rep 2004; 6(6):485–492.

5   Grim CE. Management of malignant hypertension. Comprehensive Therapy 1980; 6:44–48.

6   Appel, LJ, Moore, TJ, Obarzanek, E, et al. A clinical trial of the effects of dietary patterns on blood pressure. DASH Collaborative Research Group. N Engl J Med 1997; 336:1117–1124; May 13–16, 1998.

Appendix 1

Secondary causes of high blood pressure (office clues)

1. Observe in the patient: cushing's, acromegaly, hyper–hypothyroid, neurofibromas, web neck, short 4th metacarpal, café-au-lait spots, swollen feet?
2. Listen to the patient:
2.1. Family history—low K, hypertension (HTN) pregnancy, early stroke in men (suggests some of the new single gene causing high BP), etc.
2.2. Medical history—low K; BP with pregnancy; birth control pills (BCP); licorice; over the counter (OTC) phrine; renal trauma; episodes of HTN inferring pheochromocytoma, that is, headache; hyperhidrosis; high heart rate; hypermetabolism; etc.
3. Smell the patient: alcohol (EtOH), tobacco, uremia?
4. Examine the patient: fundi, bruits, left ventricular hypertrophy (LVH), large kidneys, radial-femoral (R-F) pulse lag, edema?
5. Labs: lytes, blood urea nitrogen (BUN)/creatinine, urine albumin, plasma aldosterone/plasma renin ratio to screen for excess aldosterone or mineralocorticoid production, or renin for renal artery stenosis (RAS) or renin-secreting tumor.
6. Patient's education:
6.1. Teach self-BP. If they do not have one, have them get an Omron or AND device with right-sized cuff (arm circum >33, use large cuff).
6.2. Instruct on self-BP measurement: Shared Care video (sharedcareinc.com)—sit 5 minutes, take three readings, write them all down, and average the last two. Take BP in AM before taking treatment (RX) and any other time they feel like BP is high or they are dizzy.
6.3. Record in the book and bring in.
7. Dietary approaches to stopping hypertension (DASH) eating plan: Have the patient got the DASH Diet for Hypertension Book by Thomas Moore, read it, and use it for the 14-day test. They may wish to visit bloodpressureline@yahoogroups. com for support.
8. Review medications
8.1. If not on a diuretic, always use hydrochlorothiazide (HCTZ) half of 25 mg (costs $8–15/100). Have them buy this.
9. Change to a combination of combinations: Consider stopping all other RX and begin
9.1. Lotrel 2.5/10 bid, if on Norvasc, switch to Lotrel, and
9.2. Bisoprolol (BIS) 2.5/HCTZ 6.25 each AMor bid.
10. Titrate to get BP control: Have patient call with BPs in two to three days.

10.1. If not at goal, increase Lotrel two AM (and two PM and BIS to two AM, two PM—do this till at Lotrel 10/20 bid and BIS 10/6.25 bid.
10.2. If BP not at goal in four weeks, then add Minoxidil 5 mg every morning. Increase every few days by using 5 mg AM, 5 PM, 10 mg AM, 10 PM, etc. Patient needs to be weighed daily. If weight goes up, then add furosemide 40 bid and increase. If still edema, add metolazone 10 mg every morning.
10.3. Check for out eating your BP RX: 24-hour urine for Na/K/creatinine if the 24-hour sodium excretion is >1500 mg a day then tell patient they are not adhering to the DASH diet.
11. Diagnose drug resistant HTN, likely primary aldosteronism (4): If aldo/renin ratio is high, then add Spironolactone 50 mg/day and may increase to 400 mg/day. If gynecomastia, use Inspra 25 to 50/d. Consider adrenal computed tomography and adrenal vein aldo/cortisol with ACTH stim. If the family history (Hx) is positive for low K then do overnight dex test for aldo/cortisol and/or genotype for glucocorticoid remedial aldosteronism (GRA).
12. Look for other causes of HTN:
12.1. If you would do an angioplasty or an operation, do classical renal arteriogram—not MRA or nuclear scan; the only way to exclude renal artery stenosis as a cause of HTN is by selective transfemoral angiography to get details of main and branch renal arteries.
12.2. Pheochromocytoma: 24-hour urine for catecholamines, Na, K, and creatinine.

Appendix 2

How to get rapid blood pressure control in the hospital or in the clinic—the combination of combinations approach

The following protocol has been developed and modified over the last 30 years and has been very successful in bringing BP quickly under control in the hospital and in the outpatients' clinic. The physiological rational is based on the complex and redundant BP control systems that must be overcome to bring BP to goal. The basic concept is that the BP-regulatory control systems are designed to keep the pressure constant. Any attempt to block one system to lower the pressure activates the other systems that try to keep the pressure at its current set point. Thus, the regimen includes diuretics to get at the volume factor that is the key to all forms of high BP, beta blocker (BB) or other agents to block the SNS response to volume depletion and BP lowering, angiotension converting enzyme/angiotensin receptor blocker (ACE/ARB) l inhibition to counteract activation of this system with BP lowering, and finally agents that act directly on the vascular smooth muscle such as CCBs or minoxidil.

1. Immediate reduction needed: very rare. Nipride never fails (5). Take BP every two minutes. Infuse with pump Nipride (mix as per instructions). Double dose every two minutes till BP falls, then back down to 1/2 of last step up and adjust till at goal—usually takes about 30 minutes to stabilize. Add oral agents as given in the table.
2. If reduction not needed immediately: Take BP every hour and use a stepwise increase by using a combination of combinations. In the outpatient clinic, one can use this approach by stepping up the intensity of control every day or two, or even every week, if the patient or family member is measuring BP regularly.
3. Volume contol: Give HCTZ 25 po q 12 hours. If edema or Cr >2, use furosemide 40 q 12 hours. Leave orders that stress that you want the BP to be measured every hour and you want to increase meds as given in the table, every four to six hours. Always implement the DASH 1500-mg sodium diet as well (6).
4. Renin-angiotensin-aldosterone system (RAAS), calcium channel blocker (CCB), and BB: The combination of the drug Lotrel contains ACE and CCB, and the other combination is BIS and HCTZ.

	Diuretic	Lotrel	BIS/HCTZ
Step 1: 1st dose at 8 AM	25 HCTZ or 40 furosemide if (EGFR < 50)	2.5/10	2.5/6.25
Step 2: 2 PM	BP not at goal, give At goal repeat	5/10 2.5/10	5/6.25 2.5/6.25
Step 3: 8 PM	At goal Not at goal, repeat diuretic + increase other agents.	2.5/10 q 12 hr 5/20	2.5/6.25 q 12 hr 5/6.25
Step 4: 2 AM	Not at goal At goal	10/20 None	10/6.25 None
Step 5: 8 AM	At goal, −HCTZ 12.5 or 25 q AM Not at goal	Give last dose q AM Add Minoxidil 5	Give last dose q AM Lotrel 10/20 q AM BIS 10/6.25 q AM
Step 6: 2 PM	Not at goal At goal	Minoxidil 10 Minoxidil 5 mg q day	
Step 7: 8 PM	Not at goal At goal	Minoxidil 15 Minoxidil 10 q day	
Step 8: 2 AM	Not at goal At goal	Minoxidil 20 mg Minoxidil 20 mg q day	
Step 9: 8 AM	At goal, watch the weight for increase on Minoxidil. May need to add furosemide and metolazone	Repeat last dose of Minoxidil q day	Lotrel 10/20 q AM, BIS 10/6.25 q AM. Consider Lotrel 5/10 bid BIS 5/6.25 bid

Note: Others to add as outpatient: Spironolactone up to 300/day. Cough → ARB. Catapres if intolerant of BB.

Abbreviations: BB, beta blocker; BIS, bisoprolol; BP, blood pressure; EGFR, estimated glomerular filtration rate; HCTZ, hydrochlorothiazide.

16

Homocysteine regulators

Torfi F. Jonasson and Hans Ohlin

Introduction

Homocysteine is a nonprotein-building amino acid formed as a metabolite in the methionine cycle. It was first associated with disease in 1962 (1,2). Individuals with a mutation in cystathionine-β-synthase (CBS) develop classical homocystinuria with extremely elevated plasma tHcy (>100 μmol/L) (3). Homocystinuria is characterized by early atherosclerosis and thromboembolism as well as mental retardation and osteoporosis and is ameliorated by vitamin supplementation aimed at reducing the blood concentration of homocysteine (4).

Moderately elevated plasma homocysteine, defined as levels between 15 and 30 μmol/L (5), has emerged as a new risk factor for ischemic heart disease and stroke (6).

The metabolism of homocysteine

Homocysteine is formed as an intermediary amino acid in the methionine cycle (Fig. 1). Methionine is metabolized to s-adenosylmethionine (SAM), the methyl donor in most methylation reactions and essential for the synthesis of creatinine, DNA, RNA, proteins, and phospholipids. SAM is converted by methyl donation to s-adenosylhomocysteine (SAH), which is then hydrolyzed to homocysteine. SAH is an inhibitor of methyl group donation from SAM.

Homocysteine is eliminated via the trans-sulfuration pathway by conversion to cysteine in two steps.

The vitamin B_6-dependent enzyme CBS catalyzes the first step, in which homocysteine reacts with serine to form L-cystathionine. In the second step, L-cystathionine is converted to L-cysteine, a-ketobutyrate, and ammonia by the vitamin B_6-dependent enzyme cystathionase (7).

The trans-sulfuration pathway is present in the liver, kidneys, small intestine, and pancreas, where it is linked to the production of glutathione.

In the folate cycle, which is linked to the methionine cycle, homocysteine is remethylated to methionine by the vitamin B_{12}-dependent enzyme methionine synthase (MS), thereby completing the cycle. 5-Methyltetrahydrofolate (CH_3-THF) acts as a methyl donor in this reaction, which produces methionine and tetrahydrofolate (THF).

Continuing the folate cycle, THF reacts with serine to produce 5,10-methylenetetrahydrofolate, a reaction catalyzed by the vitamin B_6-dependent enzyme serine/glycine hydroxymethyltransferase.

5,10-Methylenetetrahydrofolate is then reduced to CH_3-THF by the vitamin B_2 (riboflavin)-dependent enzyme 5,10-methylenetetrahydrofolate reductase (MTHFR), using NADPH as cosubstrate. MTHFR is the key enzyme for diverting 5,10-methylentetrahydrofolate to methylation of homocysteine or to DNA synthesis though the conversion of uracil to thymidine.

Causes of elevated plasma concentrations of homocysteine

There are a number of enzyme disorders that cause plasma tHcy elevation (8–12); the two most important are discussed later.

CBS deficiency is inherited as an autosomal recessive trait. Homozygous individuals (1 in 200,000 births) have classical homocystinuria with extremely high plasma tHcy. The 677 C > T polymorphism in MTHFR is believed to be one of the most common causes of mildly elevated plasma tHcy. The frequency of the homozygous genotype is 11% to 15% in North Americans, 5% to 23% in Europeans, 11% in healthy Japanese populations, and only 2.5% in the Indian population in New Delhi (12–14). The polymorphism induces thermolability in the enzyme, resulting in defect remethylation of

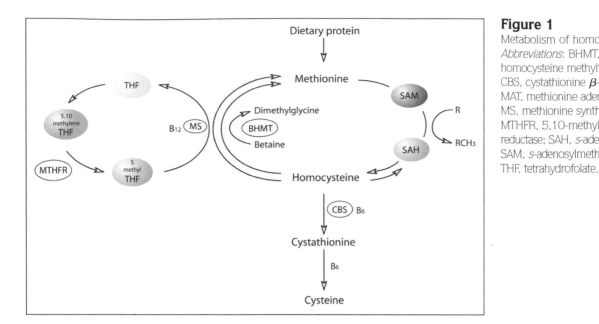

Figure 1
Metabolism of homocysteine.
Abbreviations: BHMT, betaine
homocysteine methyltransferase;
CBS, cystathionine β-synthase;
MAT, methionine adenosine transferase;
MS, methionine synthase;
MTHFR, 5,10-methylenetetrahydrofolate
reductase; SAH, s-adenosylhomocysteine;
SAM, s-adenosylmethionine;
THF, tetrahydrofolate.

homocysteine and increased plasma levels. The high plasma levels of tHcy caused by the 677 C > T polymorphism respond to folate supplementation (15).

As shown in the review of the homocysteine metabolism, vitamin B_{12}, vitamin B_6, and folate are important cofactors in the metabolic pathways for homocysteine elimination, and consequently, deficiencies of these vitamins are characterized by elevated plasma concentrations of tHcy. Hyperhomocysteinemia is also frequently found in diseases such as renal failure, rheumatic and auto-immune diseases, hypothyroidism, and malignancies. Several drugs are also known to increase plasma tHcy concentrations (16–24).

Homocysteine: a risk factor for cardiovascular disease

Many studies published during the last few decades have suggested that hyperhomocysteinemia is a risk factor for coronary artery disease (CAD), stroke, and thromboembolic disease. The Homocysteine Studies Collaboration meta-analysis of 30 studies concluded that elevated tHcy is a moderate risk factor for ischemic heart disease; a level 3 μmol/L lower reduces the risk with an odds ratio of 0.89 (95% CI = 0.83–0.96). The same was true for homocysteine as a risk factor for stroke (odds ratio = 0.81; 95%5CI = 0.69–0.95) (6). A meta-analysis of 40 studies of the MTHFR 677 C > T polymorphism demonstrated a mildly increased risk of coronary heart disease with an odds ratio of 1.16 (95% CI = 1.05–1.28) (25).

Homocysteine and extent of coronary artery disease

Several studies have demonstrated an association between plasma tHcy levels and extent of CAD in populations not exposed to fortification of flour products with folic acid, even after controlling for conventional risk factors (26,27). In contrast, Brilakis et al. (28) found no association between plasma tHcy and angiographic CAD in a North American population consuming cereal grain flour fortified with folic acid. Silberberg et al. (29) found an association between plasma folate and CAD independent of tHcy.

Possible mechanisms of action
Oxidative stress

In vitro studies have shown that homocysteine can undergo autoxidation, leading to the formation of oxygen free radicals (30–32). Homocysteine is involved in oxidative modification of low-density lipoprotein in vitro (33). Increased lipid peroxidation in humans with hyperhomocysteinemia has been reported (34,35). However, vitamin supplementation that resulted in substantial reduction of tHcy concentrations did not normalize either the homocysteine redox status or the increased lipid peroxidation in CAD patients (35,36).

Effects on nitrous oxide

Homocysteine decreases the bioavailability of nitrous oxide (NO) via a mechanism involving glutathione peroxidase (37). Tawakol et al. (38) reported that hyperhomocysteinemia is associated with impaired endothelium-dependent vasodilation in humans. Homocysteine impairs the NO synthase pathway both in cell culture (39) and in monkeys with hyperhomocysteinemia, by increasing the levels of asymmetric dimethylarginine (ADMA), an endogenous NO synthase inhibitor (40). Elevation of ADMA may mediate endothelial dysfunction during experimental hyperhomocysteinemia in humans (41). However, Jonasson et al. (42) did not find increased ADMA levels in patients with coronary heart disease and hyperhomocysteinemia, nor did vitamin supplementation have any effect on ADMA levels in spite of substantial plasma tHcy reduction.

Effects on coagulation

Subjects with homocystinuria suffer from thromboembolic events.

Epidemiological studies indicate that elevated plasma tHcy increases the risk of venous thromboembolism (43,44). In homocystinuria, the presence of the factor V Leiden mutation further increases the risk of thromboembolism (45). It has been proposed that hyperhomocysteinemia might interfere with the inhibition of activated factor V by activated protein C, possibly via similar effects as those caused by the factor V Leiden mutation (46,47). However, one in vitro study (48) and one large clinical study failed to demonstrate an association between hyperhomocysteinemia and activated protein C resistance (49).

Hcy has been shown to reduce binding of tPA to its endothelial cell receptor, annexin II, in cell cultures (50). Animal studies have indicated that elevated plasma tHcy could cause acquired dysfibrinogenemia, leading to the formation of clots that are abnormally resistant to fibrinolysis (51). Elevated plasminogen activator inhibitor and tHcy in patients with acute coronary syndrome have been shown to be associated with increased risk for major adverse cardiac events (MACE) after successful percutaneous coronary intervention (PCI) and stenting (52), whereas factor V Leiden mutation and lipoprotein (a) were not.

Inflammation

Several prospective studies have shown that markers of inflammation, such as sensitive C-reactive protein and serum amyloid A (S-AA), are predictors of increased risk for myocardial infarction, stroke, or peripheral vascular disease (53–56).

Increases in plasma S-AA levels have previously been reported in patients with coronary disease (57). S-AA and plasma intracellular adhesion molecule-1 were elevated in patients with CAD and hyperhomocysteinemia, but only S-AA decreased after vitamin supplementation (35). Homocysteine activates nuclear factor-kB in endothelial cells, possibly via oxidative stress (58), and increases monocyte chemoattractant protein-1 expression in vascular smooth muscle cells (59). Additionally, it stimulates interleukin-8 expression in human endothelial cultures (60). These inflammatory factors are known to participate in the development of atherosclerosis. Taken together, these reports suggest an association of elevated tHcy and low-grade inflammation in CAD.

Homocysteine and smooth muscle proliferation

Proliferative effects of homocysteine have been demonstrated in several in vitro studies. Brown et al. (61) found that homocysteine activates the MAP kinase signal transduction pathway in vascular smooth muscle cells.

Buemi et al. reported that the addition of Hcy to the medium of smooth muscle cells in tissue culture caused a significant increase in cell proliferation and death through apoptosis and necrosis. When folic acid was added to the culture medium, homocysteine concentrations in media were reduced and the effects of Hcy on the proliferation/apoptosis/necrosis balance of cells in culture were inhibited (62). Ozer et al. (63) showed that the MAPK kinase pathway is involved in DNA synthesis and proliferation of vascular smooth muscle induced by homocysteine.

Carmody et al. found that the addition of homocysteine to a culture of vascular smooth muscle cells resulted in a dose-dependent increase in DNA synthesis and cell proliferation, but vitamins B_6 and B_{12} alone did not substantially inhibit the effect of homocysteine. However, the addition of folic acid resulted in significant inhibition of DNA synthesis (64). Rosiglitazone has been shown to reduce serum tHcy levels, smooth muscle proliferation, and intimal hyperplasia in Sprague–Dawley rats fed a diet high in methionine (65).

The results of the in vitro studies are promising with respect to possible positive in vivo effects of vitamin supplementation. However, the recent results of large prospective clinical trials of vitamin supplementation have been disappointing; these results are further discussed later.

To conclude, hyperhomocysteinemia is associated with oxidative stress, inflammation, endothelial dysfunction, and dysfunction of coagulation in animals and in humans, but vitamin supplementation does not consistently normalize these changes in spite of large reductions in homocysteine. It still remains be seen whether homocysteine per se causes the pathological processes or whether it is simply an innocent bystander.

Vitamin therapy for prevention of cardiovascular disease

Three large-scale clinical trials of vitamin supplementation have been published. In the Vitamin Intervention for Stroke Prevention Study (VISP), 3680 adults with nondisabling cerebral infarction were randomized to either a high-dose vitamin formulation containing 25 mg pyridoxine, 0.4 mg cobalamin, and 2.5 mg folic acid or a low-dose formulation containing 200 μg pyridoxine, 6 μg cobalamin, and 20 μg folic acid. The mean reduction of tHcy was 2 μmol/L greater in the high-dose group than in the low-dose group. The primary outcome, the risk of ischemic stroke within two years, was 9.2% in the high-dose group and 8.8% in the low-dose group (risk ratio = 1.0; 95% CI = 0.8–1.3) (66).

The Norwegian Vitamin (NORVIT) trial included 3749 patients who had had an acute myocardial infarction within seven days before the start of the trial. The patients were randomly assigned in a two-by-two factorial design to receive one of the following four daily treatments: 0.8 mg folic acid, 0.4 mg vitamin B_{12}, and 40 mg vitamin B_6; 0.8 mg folic acid and 0.4 mg B_{12}; 40 mg vitamin B_6; or placebo. The mean total homocysteine level was reduced by 27% in patients given folic acid and B_{12}, but the treatment had no significant effect on the primary outcome, a composite of recurrent myocardial infarction, stroke, and sudden death due to coronary heart disease (risk ratio = 1.08; 95% CI = 0.93–1.25). Treatment with vitamin B_6 was not associated with any significant benefit. In the group given folic acid, vitamin B_{12}, and vitamin B_6, there was a trend toward an increased risk (relative risk = 1.22; 95% CI = 1.00–1.50; P = 0.05) (67).

In the Heart Outcomes Prevention Evaluation 2 (HOPE-2) study, 5522 patients aged 55 or older with vascular disease or diabetes were randomized to treatment with either placebo or a combination 2, 5 mg of folic acid, 50 mg vitamin B_6, and 1 mg vitamin B_{12}, for an average of five years. The primary outcome was a composite of death from cardiovascular causes, myocardial infarction, and stroke. Mean plasma homocysteine levels decreased by 2.4 μmol/L in the treatment group and increased by 0.8 μmol/L in the placebo group. The primary outcome occurred in 18.8% of patients assigned to active therapy and in 19.8% of those assigned to placebo (relative risk = 0.95; 95% CI = 0.84–1.07; P = 0.41) (68).

The results of these three large trials are consistent and lead to the conclusion that there is no clinical benefit from vitamin supplementation in patients with cardiovascular disease (CVD). As suggested by Loscalzo (69), the results indicate that either homocysteine is not a important atherogenic determinant or the vitamin therapy might have other adverse effects that offset its homocysteine-lowering effects, such as cell proliferation through synthesis of thymidine, hypermethylation of DNA, or increased methylation potential leading to elevated levels of ADMA.

Homocysteine and restenosis after percutaneous coronary intervention

Is homocysteine involved in the pathogenesis of restenosis? An association between homocysteine and restenosis is not unlikely, given the fact that homocysteine appears to induce inflammation, impair endothelial function, and stimulate smooth muscle proliferation; all these mechanisms are potentially implicated in the development of restenosis. However, the data regarding tHcy levels and the risk of restenosis after coronary angioplasty are conflicting. Some investigators found an increased risk of restenosis after PCI in patients with high plasma levels of homocysteine, especially in patients not treated with stents (70–72), whereas others did not find any increased risk either in patients with (73–75) or without stents (76).

Homocysteine-lowering therapy and restenosis after coronary angioplasty

In the Swiss Heart Study (77), 205 patients were randomly assigned after successful angioplasty to receive either placebo or a combination therapy of folic acid (1 mg), vitamin B_{12} (400 μg), vitamin B_6 (10 μg) or placebo. The primary endpoint was restenosis within six months, as assessed by quantitative coronary angiography. Angiographic follow-up was achieved in 177 patients. Vitamin treatment significantly decreased plasma tHcy levels from 11.1 to 7.2 μmol/L (P < 0.001). At follow-up, the minimal luminal diameter was significantly larger in the treatment group, 1.7 mm versus 1.45 mm (P = 0.02), and the degree of stenosis was less severe (39.9% vs. 48.2%, P = 0.01). The treatment group had a lower rate of restenosis (19.6% vs. 37.6%, P = 0.01) and less need for revascularization of the target lesion (10.8% vs. 22.3%, P = 0.047). A difference in treatment effect between stented and nonstented lesions was evident. In 101 lesions treated with balloon angioplasty only, vitamin treatment reduced the rate of restenosis from 41.9% to 10.3% (P < 0.001). In 130 stented lesions, only a nonsignificant trend to treatment effect was found; restenosis rate in the treatment group was 20.6% versus 29.9% with placebo (P = 0.32). However, the subgroups cannot readily be compared, since it was left to the discretion of the operator whether to use stents or not. Similar results were obtained in the subgroup of patients with small coronary arteries (<3 mm) (78). The authors suggest that vitamin therapy might be an attractive therapeutic alternative, especially in small coronary arteries that are considered less suited for stent therapy.

In an extension of the original study, including 553 patients after successful angioplasty, the clinical outcome of the combined vitamin therapy for six months was compared to placebo. After one year, the composite endpoint (death, nonfatal myocardial infarction, and need for revascularization) was significantly lower in patients treated with vitamin therapy (15.4% vs. 22.8%, $P = 0.03$), primarily due to a reduced rate of target lesion revascularization. The benefit was evident at the end of the six months and was maintained at 12 months after the angioplasty procedure. The findings remained unchanged after adjustment for potential confounders (78).

In contrast, the Folate After Coronary Intervention Trial (FACIT) demonstrated adverse effects of vitamin treatment in patients treated with coronary stenting (75). In this study, 636 patients who had undergone successful coronary stenting with bare metal stents were randomized to either vitamin therapy or placebo. In the vitamin group, 1 mg of folic acid, 5 mg of vitamin B_6 and 1 mg of B_{12} were given intravenously, followed by oral therapy. The 1, 2 mg dose of folate given orally was slightly higher than that previously used in the Swiss Heart Study (1 mg). The dose of B6, 48 mg, was higher than in the previous study (10 mg), while the B12 dose, 60 μg, was lower (400 μg). At the end of the six-month treatment, the study endpoints (minimal luminal diameter, late loss, and restenosis rate) were evaluated by means of quantitative coronary angiography. tHcy levels decreased significantly from a mean of 12.2 μmol/L at baseline to 9.0 μmol/L at six months in the folate group ($P<0.001$), but not in the pacebo group. At follow-up, the mean minimal diameter was smaller in the folate group than in the placebo group (1.59 vs. 1.74 mm, $P = 0.008$). Additionally, the restenosis rate tended to be higher in the folate group (34.5% vs. 26.5%, $P = 0.05$) (75). Folate therapy had adverse effects on the risk of restenosis in all subgroups except for women, patients with diabetes, and patients with markedly elevated tHcy levels ($\geq$15 μmol/L) at baseline. A clinical evaluation at 250 days did not reveal any significant difference between those patients receiving folate and those receiving placebo with regard to either incidence of death or rate of acute infarction in the target vessel. A trend toward more repeated target-vessel revascularizations was observed in the folate group (15.8% vs. 10.6%, $P = 0.05$).

The difference between the outcome of the Swiss Heart Study and that of FACIT illustrates how difficult it is to explain the results in terms of the biological effects of vitamin therapy. The positive results of the Swiss Heart Study seem to confirm the classical homocysteine hypothesis, which holds that homocysteine is an important atherosclerotic determinant and that lowering of homocysteine with vitamin therapy might reduce the rates of cardiovascular events. However, it is more difficult to explain the results of FACIT by an adverse effect of low plasma homocysteine, and consequently, a less simplistic perspective on the methionine–homocysteine metabolism and the multiple effects of folate, B_6, and B_{12} is needed.

The authors of FACIT point out that there might be a difference in the mechanisms of restenosis after balloon angioplasty and after stenting. Proliferation of smooth muscle cells and matrix formation are the most important mechanisms after stenting, whereas after balloon angioplasty thrombus formation and vascular remodeling are of predominant importance to the process of restenosis; and the latter changes are potentially more susceptible to homocysteine lowering. Apart from lowering homocysteine, folate plays a crucial role in the synthesis of DNA via the conversion of uracil to thymidine. Thus, administration of high doses of folate might have a proliferative effect in the vessel wall. Lowering of homocysteine will also decrease the concentration of SAH, which is an inhibitor of methyl donation from SAM, and consequently, folate therapy will increase methyl donation from SAM. Methylation of DNA is an epigenetic mechanism for modulating gene expression and may be involved in the pathogenesis of atherosclerosis (79). Thus, there are reasons to believe that folate therapy might have adverse effects, and that the outcome of folate therapy might depend on a balance between the possible benefits of homocysteine lowering and the potential adverse effects of folate. To complicate the matter even further, folate is also capable of improving endothelial function independently of changes in homocysteine: 5-MTHF can directly increase NO production and scavenge superoxide (80). Although the results of clinical trials of homocysteine-lowering therapy have generally been disappointing, they have certainly helped to raise the homocysteine hypothesis to a higher level of complexity.

In summary, there is abundant evidence both in vitro and in vivo that homocysteine plays an important role in the pathogenesis of atherosclerosis, possibly by promoting oxidative stress, inflammation, thrombosis, and endothelial dysfunction. Epidemiological studies have shown that hyperhomocysteinemia appears to be an independent risk factor for CVD. However, several studies have established that pathological changes in hyperhomocysteinemia, such as oxidative stress and inflammation, are not always corrected by homocysteine-lowering therapy, raising doubts as to whether mildly elevated tHcy levels in humans are noxious per se, or whether homocysteine is simply a innocent bystander to other causative mechanisms. The bystander concept is certainly supported by several recent large-scale clinical trials that have failed to show any clinical benefits of vitamin therapy in cardiovascular patients. However, it is also possible that vitamin therapy may have adverse effects which counteract any possible beneficial effect of homocysteine lowering. Data from the FACIT study support this notion by demonstrating increased restenosis following vitamin therapy after coronary stenting. At present, therapy with folate, B_6, and B_{12} cannot be recommended for the prevention of CVD; it may even be harmful in patients treated with coronary stenting. The results of the Swiss Heart Study do suggest that there may still be a case for vitamin therapy in patients treated with balloon angioplasty without stenting. However, given the overall negative results of vitamin therapy in clinical trials, this potential benefit must be confirmed by future studies before vitamin therapy can be recommended for this subgroup of patients.

References

1   Carson NA, Neill DW. Metabolic abnormalities detected in a survey of mentally backward individuals in Northern Ireland. Arch Dis Child 1962; 37:505–513.

2   Gerritsen T, Vaughn JG. Waisman HA. The identification of homocystine in the urine. Biochem Biophys Res Commun 1962;9: 493–496.

3   Mudd SH, Finkelstein JD, Irreverre F, Laster L. Homocytinuria: an enzymatic defect. Science 1964; 143:1443–1445.

4   Mudd SH, Skovby F, Levy HL, et al. The natural history of homocystinuria due to cystathionine beta-synthase deficiency. Am J Hum Genet, 1985; 37(1):1–31.

5   Kang SS, Wong PW, Malinow MR. Hyperhomocyst(e)inemia as a risk factor for occlusive vascular disease. Annu Rev Nutr 1992; 12:279–298.

6   Homocysteine Studies Collaboration. Homocysteine and risk of ischemic heart disease and stroke: a meta-analysis. JAMA 2002; 288(16):2015–2022.

7   Jacobsen DW. Biochemistry and metabolism. In: Robinson K, ed. Homocysteine and vascular disease. Dordrecht Netherlands: Kluwer Academic Publishers, 2000:15–39.

8   Goyette P, et al. Human methylenetetrahydrofolate reductase: isolation of cDNA, mapping and mutation identification [published erratum appears in Nat Genet 1994 Aug; 7(4):551]. Nat Genet 1994; 7(2):195–200.

9   Goyette P, et al. Seven novel mutations in the methylenetetrahydrofolate reductase gene and genotype/ phenotype correlations in severe methylenetetrahydrofolate reductase deficiency. Am J Hum Genet 1995; 56(5): 1052–1059.

10 Goyette P, et al. Severe and mild mutations in cis for the methylenetetrahydrofolate reductase (MTHFR) gene, and description of five novel mutations in MTHFR. Am J Hum Genet 1996; 59(6):1268–1275.

11 Kluijtmans LA, et al. Identification of four novel mutations in severe methylenetetrahydrofolate reductase deficiency. Eur J Hum Genet 1998; 6(3):257–265.

12 Weisberg I, et al. A second genetic polymorphism in methylenetetrahydrofolate reductase (MTHFR) associated with decreased enzyme activity. Mol Genet Metab 1998; 64(3): 169–172.

13 Nishio H, et al. A common mutation in methylenetetrahydrofolate reductase gene among the Japanese population. Jpn J Hum Genet 1996; 41(2):247–251.

14 Kumar J, et al. Homocysteine levels are associated with MTHFR A1298C polymorphism in Indian population. J Hum Genet 2005; 50(12)655–663.

15 Guttormsen AB, et al. Determinants and vitamin responsiveness of intermediate hyperhomocysteinemia (> or = 40 micromol/liter). The Hordaland Homocysteine Study. J Clin Invest 1996; 98(9):2174–2183.

16 Hultberg B, Andersson A, Sterner G. Plasma homocysteine in renal failure. Clin Nephrol 1993; 40(4):230–235.

17 Arnadottir M et al. The effect of high-dose pyridoxine and folic acid supplementation on serum lipid and plasma homocysteine concentrations in dialysis patients. Clin Nephrol 1993; 40(4):236–240.

18 Roubenoff R, et al. Abnormal homocysteine metabolism in rheumatoid arthritis. Arthritis Rheum 1997; 40(4):718–722.

19 Nedrebo BG, et al. Plasma total homocysteine levels in hyperthyroid and hypothyroid patients. Metabolism 1998; 47(1): 89–93.

20 Cheng TT, Chiu CK. Elevated homocysteine levels in patients with Raynaud's phenomenon secondary to systemic lupus erythematosus. Clin Rheumatol 2002; 21(3):251–254.

21 Vanizor Kural B, et al. Plasma homocysteine and its relationships with atherothrombotic markers in psoriatic patients. Clin Chim Acta 2003; 332(1–2):23–30.

22 Morgan SL, et al. Folic acid supplementation prevents deficient blood folate levels and hyperhomocysteinemia during longterm,low dose methotrexate therapy for rheumatoid arthritis: implications for cardiovascular disease prevention. J Rheumatol 1998; 25(3):441–446.

23 Arnadottir M, Hultberg B. Treatment with high-dose folic acid effectively lowers plasma homocysteine concentration in cyclosporine-treated renal transplant recipients. Transplantation 1997; 64(7):1087.

24 James GK, Jones MW, Pudek MR. Homocyst(e)ine levels in patients on phenytoin therapy. Clin Biochem 1997; 30(8): 647–649.

25 Klerk M, et al. MTHFR 677C– > T polymorphism and risk of coronary heart disease: a meta-analysis. JAMA 2002; 288(16): 2023–2031.

26 Yoo JH, et al. Moderate hyperhomocyst(e)inemia is associated with the presence of coronary artery disease and the severity of coronary atherosclerosis in Koreans. Thromb Res 1999; 94(1):45–52.

27 Genest JJ Jr, et al. Plasma homocyst(e)ine levels in men with premature coronary artery disease. J Am Coll Cardiol 1990; 16(5):1114–1119.

28 Brilakis ES, et al. Lack of association between plasma homocysteine and angiographic coronary artery disease in the era of fortification of cereal grain flour with folic acid. Atherosclerosis 2002; 165(2):375–381.

29 Silberberg JS, et al. Association between plasma folate and coronary disease independent of homocysteine. Am J Cardiol 2001; 87(8):1003–1004; A5.

30 Hultberg B, Andersson A, Isaksson A. Metabolism of homocysteine, its relation to the other cellular thiols and its mechanism of cell damage in a cell culture line (human histiocytic cell line U-937). Biochim Biophys Acta 1995; 1269(1):6–12.

31 Wall RT, et al. Homocysteine-induced endothelial cell injury in vitro: a model for the study of vascular injury. Thromb Res 1980; 18(1–2):113–121.

32 Heinecke JW, et al. Oxidation of low density lipoprotein by thiols: superoxide-dependent and -independent mechanisms. J Lipid Res 1993; 34(12):2051–2061.

33 Halvorsen B, et al. Effect of homocysteine on copper ion-catalyzed, azo compound-initiated, and mononuclear

cell-mediated oxidative modification of low density lipoprotein. J Lipid Res 1996; 37(7):1591–1600.

34 Voutilainen S, et al. Enhanced in vivo lipid peroxidation at elevated plasma total homocysteine levels. Arterioscler Thromb Vasc Biol 1999; 19(5):1263–1266.

35 Jonasson T, et al. Plasma homocysteine and markers for oxidative stress and inflammation in patients with coronary artery disease–a prospective randomized study of vitamin supplementation. Clin Chem Lab Med 2005; 43(6):628–634.

36 Jonasson T, Ohlin H, Andersson A, Arnadottir A, Hultberg B. Renal function excerts only a minor influence on high plasma homocysteine concentration in patients with acute coronary syndromes. Clin Chem Lab Med 2002; 40(2):137–142.

37 Upchurch GR Jr, et al. Homocyst(e)ine decreases bioavailable nitric oxide by a mechanism involving glutathione peroxidase. J Biol Chem 1997; 272(27):17012–17017.

38 Tawakol A, et al. Hyperhomocyst(e)inemia is associated with impaired endothelium-dependent vasodilation in humans. Circulation 1997; 95(5):1119–1121.

39 Stuhlinger MC, et al. Homocysteine impairs the nitric oxide synthase pathway: role of asymmetric dimethylarginine. Circulation 2001; 104(21):2569–2575.

40 Boger RH, et al. Plasma concentration of asymmetric dimethylarginine, an endogenous inhibitor of nitric oxide synthase, is elevated in monkeys with hyperhomocyst(e)inemia or hypercholesterolemia [In Process Citation]. Arterioscler Thromb Vasc Biol 2000; 20(6):1557–1564.

41 Boger RH, et al. Elevation of asymmetrical dimethylarginine may mediate endothelial dysfunction during experimental hyperhomocyst(e)inaemia in humans. Clin Sci (Colch) 2001; 100(2):161–167.

42 Jonasson TF, et al. Hyperhomocysteinaemia is not associated with increased levels of asymmetric dimethylarginine in patients with ischaemic heart disease. Eur J Clin Invest 2003; 33(7):543–549.

43 Cattaneo M, Martinelli I, Mannucci PM. Hyperhomocysteinemia as a risk factor for deep-vein thrombosis. N Engl J Med 1996; 335(13): 974–975; author reply 975–976.

44 den Heijer M, et al. Hyperhomocysteinemia as a risk factor for deep-vein thrombosis. N Engl J Med 1996; 334(12):759–762.

45 Mandel H, et al. Coexistence of hereditary homocystinuria and factor V Leiden-effect on thrombosis. N Engl J Med 1996; 334(12):763–768.

46 Undas A, et al. Homocysteine inhibits inactivation of factor Va by activated protein C. J Biol Chem 2000; 276(6):4389–4397.

47 Lentz SR, et al. Effect of hyperhomocysteinemia on protein C activation and activity. Blood 2002; 100(6):2108–2112.

48 Podda G, et al. No effect of fasting plasma total homocysteine on protein C activity in vitro. Blood 2003; 101(6):2446–2447.

49 Zarychanski R, Houston DS. Plasma homocysteine concentration is not associated with activated protein C resistance in patients investigated for hypercoagulability. Thromb Haemost 2004; 91(6):1115–1122.

50 Hajjar KA, et al. Tissue plasminogen activator binding to the annexin II tail domain. Direct modulation by homocysteine. J Biol Chem 1998; 273(16):987–993.

51 Sauls DL, Wolberg AS, Hoffman M. Elevated plasma homocysteine leads to alterations in fibrin clot structure and stability: implications for the mechanism of thrombosis in hyperhomocysteinemia. J Thromb Haemost 2003; 1(2):300–306.

52 Marcucci R, et al. PAI-1 and homocysteine, but not lipoprotein (a) nor thrombophilic polymorphism, are associated with the occurrence of major adverse cardiac events after successful coronary stenting. Heart 2005; 92(3):377–381.

53 Jousilahti P, et al. Association of markers of systemic inflammation, C reactive protein, serum amyloid A, and fibrinogen, with socioeconomic status. J Epidemiol Community Health 2003; 57(9):730–733.

54 Shishehbor MH, Bhatt DL, Topol EJ, Using C-reactive protein to assess cardiovascular disease risk. Cleve Clin J Med 2003; 70(7):634–640.

55 Lowe GD, The relationship between infection, inflammation, and cardiovascular disease: an overview. Ann Periodontol 2001; 6(1):1–8.

56 Horne BD, et al. Statin therapy, lipid levels, C-reactive protein and the survival of patients with angiographically severe coronary artery disease. J Am Coll Cardiol 2000; 36(6):1774–1780.

57 Fyfe AI, et al. Association between serum amyloid A proteins and coronary artery disease: evidence from two distinct arteriosclerotic processes. Circulation 1997; 96(9):2914–2919.

58 Au-Yeung KK, et al. Hyperhomocysteinemia activates nuclear factor-kappa B in endothelial cells via oxidative stress. Circ Res 2004; 94(1):28–36.

59 Wang G, Siow YL, Karmin O. Homocysteine stimulates nuclear factor kappaB activity and monocyte chemoattractant protein-1 expression in vascular smooth-muscle cells: a possible role for protein kinase C. Biochem J 2000; 352(Pt 3):817–826.

60 Geisel J, et al. Stimulatory effect of homocysteine on interleukin-8 expression in human endothelial cells. Clin Chem Lab Med 2003; 41(8):1045–1048.

61 Brown JC, Rosenquist TH, Monaghan DT, ERK2 activation by homocysteine in vascular smooth muscle cells. Biochem Biophys Res Commun 1998; 251(3):669–676.

62 Buemi M, et al. Effects of homocysteine on proliferation, necrosis, and apoptosis of vascular smooth muscle cells in culture and influence of folic acid. Thromb Res 2001; 104(3):207–213.

63 Kartal Ozer N, Taha S, Azzi A. Homocysteine induces DNA synthesis and proliferation of vascular smooth muscle cells by interfering with MAPK kinase pathway. Biofactors 2005; 24(1–4):193–199.

64 Carmody BJ, et al. Folic acid inhibits homocysteine-induced proliferation of human arterial smooth muscle cells. J Vasc Surg 1999; 30(6):1121–1128.

65 Murthy SN, et al. Rosiglitazone reduces serum homocysteine levels, smooth muscle proliferation, and intimal hyperplasia in Sprague–Dawley rats fed a high methionine diet. Metabolism 2005; 54(5):645–652.

66 Toole JF, et al. Lowering homocysteine in patients with ischemic stroke to prevent recurrent stroke, myocardial infarction, and death: the Vitamin Intervention for Stroke Prevention (VISP) randomized controlled trial. JAMA 2004; 291(5):565–575.

67 Bonaa KH, et al. Homocysteine lowering and cardiovascular events after acute myocardial infarction. N Engl J Med 2006.

68 Lonn E, Yusuf S, Arnold MJ, et al. Homocysteine lowering with folic acid and B vitamins in vascular disease. N Engl J Med 2006; 354(15):1567–1577.

69 Loscalzo J. Homocysteine trials––clear outcomes for complex reasons. N Engl J Med 2006; 354(15):1629–1632.

70 Morita H, et al. Homocysteine as a risk factor for restenosis after coronary angioplasty. Thromb Haemost 2000; 84(1):27–31.

71 Marcucci R, et al. Tissue factor and homocysteine levels in ischemic heart disease are associated with angiographically documented clinical recurrences after coronary angioplasty. Thromb Haemost 2000; 83(6):826–832.

72 Schnyder G, et al. Association of plasma homocysteine with restenosis after percutaneous coronary angioplasty. Eur Heart J 2002; 23(9):726–33.

73 Koch W, et al. Homocysteine status and polymorphisms of methylenetetrahydrofolate reductase are not associated with restenosis after stenting in coronary arteries. Arterioscler Thromb Vasc Biol 2003; 23(12):2229–2234.

74 Genser D, et al. Relation of homocysteine, vitamin B(12), and folate to coronary in-stent restenosis. Am J Cardiol 2002; 89(5):495–499.

75 Lange H, et al. Folate therapy and in-stent restenosis after coronary stenting. N Engl J Med 2004; 350(26): 2673–2681.

76 Wong CK, et al. Lack of association between baseline plasma homocysteine concentrations and restenosis rates after a first elective percutaneous coronary intervention without stenting. Heart 2004; 90(11):1299–1302.

77 Schnyder G, et al. Decreased rate of coronary restenosis after lowering of plasma homocysteine levels. N Engl J Med 2001; 345(22):1593–1600.

78 Schnyder G, et al. Effect of homocysteine-lowering therapy on restenosis after percutaneous coronary intervention for narrowings in small coronary arteries. Am J Cardiol 2003; 91(10):1265–1269.

79 Lund G, et al. DNA methylation polymorphisms precede any histological sign of atherosclerosis in mice lacking apolipoprotein E. J Biol Chem 2004; 279(28):29147–29154.

80 Doshi SN, et al. Folate improves endothelial function in coronary artery disease: an effect mediated by reduction of intracellular superoxide? Arterioscler Thromb Vasc Biol 2001; 21(7):1196–1202.

17

Role of systemic antirestenotic drugs and results of current clinical trials

Ron Waksman

Introduction

The introduction of balloon angioplasty to treat coronary atherosclerosis has created a difficult problem, namely restenosis. The interventional cardiology community and pharmaceutical and device industries are sparing no efforts to combat this problem, which continues to be a formidable challenge. Coronary stents have reduced its incidence to 20% to 30%, a reduction of 30% to 40% (1,2). The recent development of drug-eluting stents (DES) has further decreased but not eliminated the problem (3). Efforts to, therefore, overcome the challenge of restenosis—including research into newer mechanisms, targets, experimental and therapeutic agents, and clinical trials—are still actively pursued. This chapter discusses the oral agents tested in this area, trials conducted thus far and their results, its limitations, and future directions for this modality of treatment.

Why oral agents for restenosis?

The simplest answer is ease of administration. More importantly, there are several limitations to local delivery of drugs in the form of DES. The efficacy of these new devices depends on several variables, including the selection of an effective drug, its solubility, diffusion characteristics, release kinetics, arterial tissue concentration, retention, and whether the platform is polymer based or nonpolymeric. Local delivery of the drug in this manner may delay rather than prevent neointima. This is supported by preclinical studies that show impaired healing and neointimal catch-up (4). There is concern that neointimal growth will accelerate in response to the

non-biodegradable polymer coating after complete elution of the drug. These issues may rejuvenate investigations into systemic therapy, particularly with those agents that have shown positive results when administered locally, either as standalone therapy or as an adjunct to DES. Other reasons include, possibility of administration of oral agents over a longer period of time, in patients with multiple stent implantations, the ability to withdraw the drug in case of hypersensitivity or intolerance, and perhaps the lack of effects associated with DES such as subacute thrombosis, aneurysm formation, and the like.

Pathology of restenosis and targets for prevention

Atherosclerosis is a progressive, inflammatory condition of the vessel wall leading to accumulation of lipid and other materials causing lesion formation and lumen encroachment (5). Balloon angioplasty fractures these lesions and helps in re-establishing the lumen patency. Stents act as scaffolding and prevent elastic recoil and vascular remodeling (6,7). Although stents are effective in reducing restenosis by eliminating these two mechanisms, they cause restenosis by neointimal hyperplasia (NIH). Stents are associated with a prolonged, intense inflammatory state with recruitment of leukocytes, mainly monocytes. The initial events immediately after stent placement result in de-endothelialization and the deposition of a layer of platelets and fibrin at the injured site. Activated platelets express adhesion molecules such as P-selectin and glycoprotein (GP) Ibα, which attach to circulating leukocytes via platelet receptors. Under the influence of cytokines, leukocytes bind tightly to adhesion molecules via direct attachment to platelet receptors such as

GP Ibα. Cytokines released from smooth muscle cells (SMCs) and resident leukocytes induce migration of leukocytes across the platelet–fibrin layer and into the tissue. Growth factors are released from platelets, leukocytes, and SMCs, and influence the proliferation and migration of SMCs from the media into the denuded intimal area. The cell cycle consists of resting phase, G_0, G_1, S phase, and M phase. Once stimulated, the cell undergoes these phases and proliferates. The resultant neointima consists of SMCs, extracellular matrix, and macrophages recruited over several weeks. There is a shift toward fewer cellular elements with greater production of extracellular matrix followed by re-endothelialization of at least part of the injured vessel surface over time. The difference between restenosis that occurs as result of balloon angioplasty and that from stent implantation is mainly due to a longer duration and a more intense inflammatory response with stents. Therefore, it is intriguing to assume that targeting the release of these mediators, the inhibition of cell cycle, and migration of SMCs would reduce neointimal proliferation.

Studies in the last two decades tested several oral agents for their efficacy in decreasing restenosis, but only a few of them reported beneficial effects (8,9). Table 1 lists the drugs that failed to show consistent benefit in reducing restenosis. Although radiation therapy was successful in reducing in-stent restenosis, it failed to obtain a single-digit restenosis rate for de novo lesions, especially when coupled with stents, either as a

platform of the radioactive stent or as a catheter-based system. Nevertheless, the experimental work with vascular brachytherapy guided the direction for prevention of restenosis. The work focused primarily on antiproliferative therapy and intervention in the cell cycle. Based on the current understanding of the mechanism of restenosis, the pharmacological agents useful to treat restenosis are grouped into five classes:

1. anti-inflammatory and immunomodulators,
2. antiproliferative agents,
3. inhibitors of SMC migration,
4. agents promoting re-endothelialization, and
5. vitamins, antioxidants, and others.

Some of these agents have more than one action. For example, sirolimus is antiproliferative, but also carries anti-inflammatory properties and possesses immunoregulatory functions. Similarly, cilastozole has antiplatelet activity, but also inhibits SMC migration and directly inhibits intimal proliferation. Table 2 lists the drugs that have shown positive results in clinical trials and their mechanisms of action.

Anti-inflammatory and immunomodulators

Oral agents in this category include corticosteroids, nonsteroidal inflammatory drugs, statins, and tranilast.

Corticosteroids

Corticosteroids are potent anti-inflammatory agents, which also have immunosuppressive activity. Interleukins-1 and -6, secreted by activated macrophages, are powerful stimuli for SMC proliferation and hepatocyte stimulating factors inducing the production of acute-phase proteins including C-reactive protein (CRP). Accordingly, preprocedural high plasma levels of CRP and its persistent elevation of plasma levels following successful stent implantation have been found to predict the risk of restenosis (10,11). In the double-blind, randomized, placebo-controlled Inhibition of Metalloproteinase in a Randomized Exercise and Symptoms Study (IMPRESS), Versaci et al. (12) tested the effect of oral prednisone on the angiographic restenosis rate after successful stent implantation in patients with persistent elevation of systemic markers of inflammation after the procedure. Eighty-three patients who underwent successful stenting with CRP levels >0.5 mg/dL 72 hours after the procedure were randomized to receive oral prednisone or placebo for 45 days. The six-month restenosis rate and late loss were lower in the prednisone-treated patients than in the placebo-treated patients (7% vs. 33%, $P = 0.001$, and

---

Table 1   Oral agents that failed to reduce restenosis

Antiplatelet and antithrombotic drugs
    Aspirin, dipyridamole, ticlopidine
    Thromboxane A2 receptor antagonists—vapiprost and solutroban
        Omega-3 fatty acids
        Warfarin
Antiallergic drugs
    Tranilast
Growth factor antagonist
    Trapidil
    ACE inhibotors: cilazapril, fosinopril, enalapril
Nitric oxide donors
    Molsidomine
Antifibrotic drugs
    Colchicines
Lipid lowering drugs
    Lovastatin, fluvastatin, simvastatin
Vitamins
    Tocopherol
Serotonin antagonist
    Ketanserin
Antianginals
    Calcium channel blocker and beta-blockers

Table 2   Oral agents to treat coronary restenosis and the trials conducted

Oral agent	Principal mechanism of action	Trial	Results
Prednisolone	Anti-inflammatory	IMPRESS (12)	Significantly low restenosis and late loss
		IMPRESS II (13)	Lower MACE, recurrence of angina, and TVR
Pravastatin	Anti-inflammatory	REGRESS (24)	Lower binary restenosis at 2 years
Tranilast	Inhibits SMC migration and proliferation, decreases collagen synthesis	TREAT (25) TREAT-2 (26) PRESTO (27)	Lower restenosis Lower restenosis No difference
Sirolimus	Inhibition of CDK complexes, antiproliferative	ORBIT (32) ORAR (35) ORAR II (36)	Lower restenosis Lower restenosis Lower restenosis
PPAR-γ	Inhibitory action on SMC growth, migration and suppression of neointimal proliferation	Takagi et al. (40) (Troglitazone) Takagi et al. (41) (Pioglitazone) Choi et al. (43) (Rosiglitazone) Marx et al. (44) (Pioglitazone)	Reduced neointimal proliferation Reduced restenosis, TLR, and neointimal proliferation Lower restenosis and lower degree of diameter stenosis Significantly lower restenosis
Cilastozole	Inhibitory effect on SMC migration by inhibiting P-selectin release	ESPIRIT (45) Kimishirado (46) CREST (47)	Low restenosis Low restenosis and TLR Low restenosis
Folic acid	Reduction in plasma homocy steine levels	SWISS Heart Study (51)	Reduced TLR
Probucol	Antioxidant	MVT and Probucol Study Group (52) PART (53) CART (54)	Low restenosis Low TLR Less neointimal proliferation
Pemirolast	Inhibition of smooth muscle cell proliferation and migration	Ohsawa (55)	Low restenosis and neointimal hyperplasia
Sarprogrelate	Inhibits serotonin induced SMC proliferation	Fujita et al. (56)	Low restenosis
Valsartan	AT-II receptor antagonist, improved endothelial function	VAL-PREST (57)	Low restenosis and reintervention
Verapamil	Calcium channel blocker	VESPA (60)	Low restenosis

Abbreviations: CDK, cyclin-dependent kinase; CREST, cilostazol for restenosis trial; MACE, major adverse cardiac events; ORAR, oral rapamycin to prevent restenosis; ORBIT, oral rapamune to inhibit restenosis; PPAR, peroxisome proliferator-activated receptor; PRESTO, prevention of restenosis with tranilast and its outcomes; SMC, smooth muscle cell; TLR, target lesion revascularization; tREAT, Tranilast restenosis following angioplasty trials; TVR, target vessel failure.

0.39 ± 0.6 vs. 0.85 ± 0.6 mm, $P = 0.001$, respectively). The IMPRESS-II MVD study comprised 95 patients; 43 of whom received prednisone, and 52 received placebo. At 18-month follow-up, major adverse cardiac events (MACE), recurrence of angina, and target vessel failure (TVR) were considerably lower in the prednisone group compared to placebo (4.7% vs. 34.6%, 4.7% vs. 25%, and 7% vs. 27%, respectively) (13).

Three other randomized, placebo-controlled studies (14–16) investigated the influence of intravenous methyl prednisolone before angioplasty with negative results. In these studies, 1.0 g methyl prednisolone was infused intravenously

2 to 24 hours before planned percutaneous transluminal coronary angioplasty (PTCA) and stenting. In the M-Heart study, the infused prednisolone was followed by an oral prednisolone of 60 mg daily for one week. Angiographic restudy showed restenosis rates of 36% versus 40%, 40% versus 39%, and 17.5% versus 18.8% (P = NS) compared to placebo, in these studies, respectively. It is not surprising that these trials failed to show any benefit because restenosis is a slow and chronic inflammatory process and a single pulse dose of methyl prednisolone would not provide a durable effect.

Nonsteroidal anti-inflammatory agents

The proposed mechanism of action of nonsteroidal anti-inflammatory agents (NSAIDs) includes inhibition of prostaglandin synthesis in inflammatory cells, thus blocking monocyte adhesion, cell differentiation, proliferation, and angiogenesis (17). Although theoretically it is appealing to consider NSAIDs that reduce restenosis by interfering with the release of inflammatory substances, thus impairing migration of monocytes, data from animal experiments did not translate into clinical reality. Ebselen, a selenium-containing NSAID with additional antioxidant properties, was tested in 80 patients undergoing PTCA and was shown to be associated with lower restenosis compared to placebo (18.6% vs. 38.2%, P < 0.05) (9). Experimental data in animals, however, showed sulindac to be beneficial in reducing stenosis, but aspirin failed to show any benefit. This could be due to the inability of aspirin to inhibit cyclooxygenase (COX)-2. Further, sulindac has additional actions independent of COX activity such as inhibition of proliferation, induction of apoptosis, inhibition of peroxisome proliferator-activated receptor (PPAR)-δ, and increased formation of intracellular ceramide leading to the induction of apoptosis. These mechanisms have been postulated for other NSAIDs such as aspirin and for the new specific COX-2 inhibitors, as well. The main reasons NSAIDs are not tested in clinical trials are because of toxicity issues and that very high doses are required to achieve these effects in vivo.

Statins

Clinical efficacy of anti-inflammatory properties has been shown in several trials independent of their lipid-lowering effects (18,19). Statins reduce CRP levels and it is known that elevated CRP levels are associated with restenosis. Counter intuitively, however, several trials tested statins for restenosis prevention and were disappointing (20–23). The only trial that showed reduction in restenosis was the REGRESS trial (24), which used pravastatin 40 mg once daily for a period of two years. In this study, the binary restenosis assessed at two years was significantly lower in the pravastatin group as opposed to other trials, which assessed restenosis within six months. Importantly, stents were not used in this trial and positive remodeling at the end of two years may have contributed to better results. Overall, the role of statins to prevent restenosis remains unproven.

Tranilast

Tranilast is an antiallergic drug, which is a derivative of anthranilic acid that interferes with proliferation and migration of vascular medial SMCs. Tranilast also suppresses collagen synthesis in vascular medial SMCs. While the Tranilast Restenosis Following Angioplasty Trials (TREAT)-1 and -2 (25,26) reported reduction in restenosis, the large scale multicenter, double-blind, randomized, placebo-controlled Prevention of Restenosis with Tranilast and its Outcomes (PRESTO) Trial did not find any significant differences between Tranilast and placebo (27).

Antiproliferative drugs

Two different strategies to control neointimal proliferation after vascular injury are proposed. First is the cytostatic approach, which aims to control the regulation and expression of cell cycle-modulating proteins at any level along the pathway—modulating cell proliferation. Second, the cytotoxic approach—killing proliferating cells—has the disadvantage of induction of necrosis, which may contribute to vessel wall weakening. Among the antiproliferative agents proposed for this application are sirolimus and its analog everolimus and a variety of antineoplastic drugs such as actinomycin D, vincristine, doxorubicin, vinblastine, and the like.

Sirolimus (Rapamycin)

Sirolimus (Rapamycin, Rapamune®), a natural macrocyclic lactone, is a potent immunosuppressive agent. It was developed by Wyeth-Ayerst Laboratories (Philadelphia, Pennsylvania, U.S.A.) and approved by the Food and Drug Administration for the prophylaxis of renal transplant rejection in 1999 (28,29). Sirolimus has its roots in Easter Island, where an actinomycete streptomyces hygroscopicus was found that produced a novel macrolide antibiotic with potent antibiotic, potent antifungal, immunosuppressive, and antimitotic activities.

Sirolimus binds to an intracellular receptor protein and elevates p27 levels, which leads to inhibition of cyclin-dependent kinase (CDK) complexes, and ultimately induces cell-cycle arrest in the late G1 phase. It inhibits proliferation of both rat and human SMCs in vitro and reduces intimal thickening in models of vascular injury (29,30). Sirolimus inhibits

T lymphocyte activation and proliferation, which occurs in response to antigenic and cytokine stimulation; however, its mechanism is distinct from that of other immunosuppressants. Sirolimus also inhibits antibody production. In cells, sirolimus binds to the immunophilin, FK binding protein-12 (FKBP-12), to generate an immunosuppressive complex. This complex binds to and inhibits the activation of the mammalian target of rapamycin (mTOR), a key regulatory kinase. This inhibition suppresses cytokine-driven T-cell proliferation, inhibiting the phase progression of the cell cycle (30,31). The Oral Rapamune to Inhibit Restenosis (ORBIT) study was an open-label study of 60 patients with de novo lesions treated with bare metal stents in up to two vessels. After a loading dose of 5 mg, patients received a daily dose of 2 mg ($n = 30$) and 5 mg ($n = 30$) for 30 days. At six months' follow-up, late loss (0.6 ± 0.5 mm vs. 0.7 ± 0.5 mm; $P = $ NS), in-stent binary restenosis (7.1% vs. 6.9%; $P = $ NS), in-stent percent volume obstruction by intravascular ultrasound (IVUS) (29% vs. 24%; $P = $ NS), and clinically driven target lesion revascularization (TLR) (14.3% vs. 6.9%; $P = $ NS) were similar in 2- and 5 mg groups (32).

Brito et al., in a pilot study, tested the hypothesis that oral sirolimus is safe and effective to inhibit in-stent NIH and, therefore, effective to prevent and treat ISR. Twelve patients (18 lesions) with high risk for ISR, including eight ISR lesions, were incorporated. One day before the procedure, patients were given a 15 mg loading dose of oral sirolimus, followed by 5 mg daily for 28 days, with weekly whole blood level measurements. The four- and eight-month follow-up revealed an angiographic late loss of 0.40 ± 0.24 and 0.67 ± 0.45 mm ($P < 0.01$), respectively. At 24-month clinical follow-up, adverse events were one death (8.3%), two TLR (11.1%), and four TVR (22.2%) (33).

Oral rapamycin is absorbed rapidly and concentrations peak within one hour in the blood. A loading dose of three times the maintenance dose will achieve steady-state concentrations within 24 hours in most patients. The drug is metabolized by cytochrome p450 system and is well tolerated. In a pilot study, Rodriguez et al. (34) reported the results of the Oral Rapamycin to Prevent Restenosis (ORAR) trial in which 34 patients undergoing coronary stent therapy were treated with oral rapamycin (6 mg loading dose, followed by 2 mg daily) for one month after stent implantation for de novo and restenotic lesions. At six months, angiography showed a restenosis rate of 18.9% in de novo lesions and 50% in in-stent restenotic lesions. Interestingly, it was found that restenosis was 0% in patients with rapamycin levels >8 ng/mL. In ORAR I, Rodriguez et al. studied 76 patients with 103 de novo lesions treated percutaneously with bare stents who received a loading dose of oral rapamycin 6 mg followed by a daily dose of 2 mg during 28 days in phase I (49 arteries in 34 patients) and 2 mg/day of oral rapamycin plus 180 mg/day of diltiazem in phase II (54 arteries in 42 patients). In-stent restenosis in phase I was 19% compared with 6.2% in phase II ($P = 0.06$). Angiographic ISR in lesions of patients with rapamycin blood concentrations ≥ 8 ng/mL was 6.2% and with rapamycin concentrations <8 ng/mL was 22% ($P = 0.041$). Late loss was also significantly lower when rapamycin concentrations were ≥ 8 ng/mL (0.6 mm vs. 1.1 mm, $P = 0.031$). A Pearson's test showed a linear correlation between follow-up late loss and rapamycin blood concentration ($r = -0.826$, $P = 0.008$) (35).

In ORAR II, 100 patients were randomized to either oral rapamycin (6-mg loading dose given 2.7 hour before intervention followed by 3 mg/day for 14 days) plus diltiazem 180 mg/day or no therapy after the implantation of a coronary bare metal stent design. At nine months, the in-segment binary restenosis was reduced by 72% (11.6% rapamycin vs. 42.8% no-therapy group, $P = 0.001$) and the in-stent binary restenosis was reduced by 65% (12% rapamycin vs. 34.6% no-therapy group, $P = 0.009$). The in-segment late loss was also significantly reduced with oral therapy (0.66 vs. 1.13 mm, respectively; 43% reduction, $P < 0.001$). At one year, patients in the oral rapamycin group also showed a significantly lower incidence of target vessel revascularization (TVR) (8.3% vs. 38%, respectively, $P < 0.001$), TLR (7.6% vs. 37.2%, respectively, $P < 0.001$), and major adverse cardiovascular events (20% vs. 44%, respectively, $P = 0.018$) (36).

Sirolimus analogs and anti-immunosuppressive molecules

The initial success with sirolimus has led to the search of sirolimus analogs. Among these are everolimus (a new macrocylic triene derivative), ABT 578, and other anti-immunosuppressive compounds such as mycophenolic acid, cyclosporine, and tacrolimus, which inhibit proliferation via G1 arrest and reduce the immune response. Data from animal experiments suggest that oral everolimus administered for one month effectively inhibits NIH (37); however, human trials have not been conducted.

Thiozolidenediones

Thiozolidenediones are antidiabetic drugs known to have inhibitory action on SMC growth, migration, and suppression of neointimal proliferation (38,39). Drugs include rosiglitazone, troglitazone, and pioglitazone. Troglitazone and pioglitazone were tested in two separate studies involving noninsulin-dependent diabetic patients following coronary stent implantation and were shown to inhibit NIH by serial IVUS study (40,41). Accumulating evidence shows that this group of compounds reduces markers of endothelial cell activation and levels of CRP and fibrinogen levels even in coronary artery disease (CAD) patients without diabetes (42). Thus, these agents may be useful to treat restenosis in both diabetic and nondiabetic patients.

In their study, Choi et al. conducted a prospective, randomized, case-controlled trial involving 95 diabetic patients with CAD who were randomly assigned to either the control or rosiglitazone group (48 and 47 patients, respectively). Eighty-three patients (45 patients with 55 lesions in the control group, and 38 patients with 51 lesions in the rosiglitazone group) completed follow-up angiography. The rate of in-stent restenosis was significantly reduced in the rosiglitazone group compared with the control group (for stent lesions: 17.6% vs. 38.2%, $P = 0.030$). The rosiglitazone group had a significantly lower degree of diameter stenosis ($23.0\% \pm 23.4\%$ vs. $40.9\% \pm 31.9\%$, $P = 0.004$) compared with the control group (43).

In a randomized, placebo-controlled, double-blind trial, Marx et al. examined the effect of six-month pioglitazone therapy on neointima volume after coronary stenting in nondiabetic CAD patients. Fifty nondiabetic patients after coronary stent implantation were randomly assigned to pioglitazone (30 mg daily; pio) or placebo (control) treatment in addition to standard therapy and neointima volume was assessed by IVUS at the six-month follow-up. Pio treatment significantly reduced neointima volume within the stented segment, with $2.3 \pm 1.1 \, \text{mm}^3/\text{mm}$ in the pio group versus $3.1 \pm 1.6 \, \text{mm}^3/\text{mm}$ in controls ($P = 0.04$). Total plaque volume (adventitia–lumen area) was significantly lower at follow-up in the pio group ($11.2 \pm 3.2 \, \text{mm}^3/\text{mm}$) compared with controls ($13.2 \pm 4.2 \, \text{mm}^3/\text{mm}$; $P = 0.04$). Moreover, the binary restenosis rate was 3.4% in the pio group versus 32.3% in controls ($P < 0.01$) (44).

Inhibitors of SMC migration

Cilostazole

As previously mentioned, for SMC proliferation after coronary angioplasty, cell activation and cell-to-cell interaction of platelets and leukocytes mediated by adhesion molecules are considered to be important. Coronary stenting produces the release of an adhesion molecule, P-selectin, from α-granule of activated platelets. P-selectin-mediated platelet–leukocyte interaction has a crucial role in the development of stent restenosis. Cilostazol is an antiplatelet, antithrombotic, phosphodiesterase III inhibitor that by inhibiting P-selectin release has inhibitory effects on SMC migration. In addition, cilostazol may directly act to inhibit intimal hyperplasia.

Randomized trials conducted with cilostazol 200 mg daily have shown that it is effective in reducing restenosis (45–47). Douglas et al. undertook the Cilostazol for Restenosis Trial (CREST), a randomized, double-blind, placebo-controlled trial to determine whether cilostazol would reduce re-narrowing in patients after stent implantation in native coronary arteries. Seven hundred and five patients who had successful coronary stent implantation received, in addition to

aspirin, cilostazol 100 mg BID or placebo for six months; clopidogrel 75 mg daily was administered to all patients for 30 days. Restenosis was determined by quantitative coronary angiography at six months. Restenosis, defined as $\geq 50\%$ narrowing, occurred in 22.0% of patients in the cilostazol group and in 34.5% of the placebo group ($P = 0.002$), a 36% relative risk reduction was observed. Restenosis was significantly lower in cilostazol-treated diabetics (17.7% vs. 37.7%, $P = 0.01$) and in those with small vessels (23.6% vs. 35.2%, $P = 0.02$), long lesions (29.9% vs. 46.6%, $P = 0.04$), and left anterior descending coronary artery site (19.3% vs. 39.8%, $P = 0.001$) (47).

Strategies to promote healing and re-endothelialization

In contrast to the agents outlined earlier in this section that primarily inhibit biological activity, a strategy to promote healing and re-endothelialization, may indirectly reduce the trigger for proliferation and inflammation by rapidly restoring the injured endothelium and its functions. A number of studies have shown the role of endothelial growth factors (EGF), fibroblast growth factors (FGF), and vascular endothelial growth factors (VEGF) in modulating the re-endothelialization process (48–50). As yet, we do not have any oral formulations to test this strategy, however.

Vitamins, antioxidants, and other agents

Other drugs have claimed to potentially enhance healing and minimize the neointimal formation by various mechanisms. These include antioxidants with vitamins (51), probucol (52–54), antipruritic agent pemirolast (55), serotonin antagonist sarproglate (56), and angiotensin I receptor antagonist valsartan (57). Although individual trials failed to show any benefit, meta analysis of calcium channel blockers (58) and beta blockers (59) showed reduction in angiographic and clinical restenosis. Bestehorn et al. investigated the effect of oral verapamil on clinical outcome and angiographic restenosis after percutaneous coronary intervention (PCI). This randomized, double-blind trial included 700 consecutive patients with successful PCI of a native coronary artery. Patients received the calcium channel blocker verapamil, 240 mg twice daily for six months, or placebo. Late lumen loss was $0.74 \pm 0.70 \, \text{mm}$ with verapamil and $0.81 \pm 0.75 \, \text{mm}$ with placebo ($P = 0.11$). Compared with placebo, verapamil reduced the rate of restenosis $\geq 75\%$ [7.8% vs. 13.7%; RR 0.57 (95% CI 0.35–0.92); $P = 0.014$] (60).

Limitations of studies with oral agents

Table 3 summarizes the studies conducted with different oral agents and their restenosis rates. The majority of these trials included a small number of patients, and some failed to reproduce the same result on larger-scale trials. The reasons for failure of these trials include:

1. The long time span from balloon angioplasty to the stent era. As we previously alluded, the restenosis mechanisms are different between angioplasty and stenting.

2. Many of the trials involved a small number of patients, many times of <100. The results, therefore, were not reproducible in larger, multicenter trials such as the PRESTO trial.

3. The drug dosages needed to achieve sufficient levels to inhibit restenosis are higher than therapeutic doses or tolerable doses.

4. Bioavailability of the oral drugs depends on multiple factors including drug metabolism and drug interaction.

5. Our understanding of the pathological mechanisms of restenosis is constantly evolving and the targets of therapy are changing.

Table 3   Restenosis rates in various trials that showed positive results using oral agents

Oral agent	Trial	Number of patients	Restenosis (%) Drug	Control
Prednisolone	IMPRESS (12)	83	7.0	33.0
Pravastatin	REGRESS (23)	221	7.0	29.0
Tranilast	TREAT (25)	255	17.6	39.4
	TREAT-2 (26)	297	25.9	41.9
Sirolimus	ORBIT (32)	60	4.8	—
	ORAR (35)	34	18.9	—
	ORAR II (36)	100	11.6	42.8
Troglitazone	Takagi et al. (40)	52	NA	NA
Pioglitazone	Takagi et al. (41)	43	17.0	43.0
Rosiglitazone	Choi et al. (43)	95	17.6	38.2
Pioglitazone	Marx et al. (44)	50	3.4	32.3
Cilastozole	ESPIRIT (45)	117	5.4 (DCA + stent) 8.9 (DCA only)	—
	Kimishirado (46)	130	13.0	31.0
	CREST (47)	705	20.8	34.5
Folic acid	SWISS Heart Study (51)	553	9.9	16.0
Probucol	MVT and Probucol Study Group (52)	317	20.7	38.9
	PART (53)	101	5.0	12.0
	CART (54)	305	NA	NA
Pemirolast	Ohsawa (55)	84	15.0	34.1
Sarprogrelate	Fujita et al. (56)	79	4.3	28.6
Valsartan	VAL-PREST (57)	250	19.2	38.6
Verapamil	VESPA (60)	700	7.8	13.7

Abbreviations: CREST, cilostazol for restenosis trial; IMPRESS, Inhibition of metalloproteinase in a randomized exercise and symptoms study; ORAR, oral rapamycin to prevent restenosis; ORBIT, oral rapamune to inhibit restenosis; TREAT, tranilast restenosis following angioplasty trial.

Conclusion

In view of the DES limitations, there is a definite role for systemic therapy for restenosis. The focus of research involving oral agents for the treatment of restenosis is changing. While previous trials focused on antiplatelets, anticoagulants, lipid lowering, and concomitant potential of antianginals like calcium channel blockers and beta-blockers, newer trials are targeting inflammation, smooth muscle proliferation, and inhibition of cell proliferation. Oral agents may potentially have a great impact on the practical application for the treatment of restenosis. The analogy of clopidogrel therapy compared to heparin-coated stents in preventing subacute thrombosis supports this contention. At the present time, however, we do not have the answer as to what the ideal agents of choice are, the loading dose, maintenance dose and duration of therapy. From the available experience with oral agents, currently we surmise that a high loading dose of an antiproliferative drug followed by a tolerable maintenance dose for a short duration will suffice. Nevertheless, the dissemination and durability of DES—and their effects now proven to four years—have slowed enthusiasm for intensive research to explore a systemic or oral agent to compete with DES. Late thrombosis and the high cost of DES, however, will eventually initiate continued research for new compounds to be tested as potential substitutions for DES.

References

1   Fischman DL, Leon MB, Baim DS, et al. For the Stent Restenosis Study Investigators. A randomized comparison of coronary-stent placement and balloon angioplasty in the treatment of coronary artery disease. N Engl J Med 1994; 331: 496–501.

2   Serruys PW, de Jaegere P, Kiemeneij F, et al. For the BENES-TENT Study Group. A comparison of balloon-expandable-stent implantation with balloon angioplasty in patients with coronary artery disease. N Engl J Med 1994; 331: 489–495.

3   Waksman R. Drug-eluting stents: from bench to bed. Cardiovasc Radiat Med 2002; 3:226–241.

4   Farb A, Heller PF, Shroff S, et al. Pathological analysis of local delivery of paclitaxel via a polymer-coated stent. Circulation 2001; 104:473–479.

5   Ross R. Atherosclerosis: an inflammatory disease. N Engl J Med 1999; 340:115–126.

6   Mintz GS, Popma JJ, Pichard AD, et al. Arterial remodeling after coronary angioplasty a serial intravascular ultrasound study. Circulation 1996; 94:35–43.

7   Hoffmann R, Mintz GS, Dussaillant GR, et al. Patterns and mechanisms of in-stent restenosis: a serial intravascular ultrasound study. Circulation 1996; 94:1247–1254.

8   Faxon DP. Systemic drug therapy for restenosis, "de javu all over again". Circulation 2002; 06:2296–2298.

9   Mody VH, Durairaj A, Mehra AO. Pharmacological approaches to prevent restenosis. In: Faxon DP, ed. Restenosis: A Guide to Therapy. U.K.: Martin Dunite, 2001:97–112.

10   Gaspardone A, Crea F, Versaci F, et al. Predictive value of C-reactive protein after successful coronary artery stenting in patients with stable angina. Am J Cardiol 1998; 82:515–518.

11   Walter DH, Fichtlscherer S, Sellwig M, Auch-Schwelk W, SchächingerV, Zeiher M. Preprocedural C-reactive protein levels and cardiovascular events after coronary stent implantation. J Am Coll Cardiol 2001; 37:839–846.

12   Versaci F, Gaspardone A, Tomai F, et al. Immunosuppressive therapy for the prevention of restenosis after coronary artery stent implantation (IMPRESS Study). J Am Coll Cardiol 2002; 40:1935–1942.

13   Ribichini F. Final results of the IMPRESS-2 MVD study. Presented at Euro PCR 2005.

14   Stone GW, Rutherford BD, McConahay DR, et al. A randomized trial of corticosteroids for the prevention of restenosis in 102 patients undergoing repeat coronary angioplasty. Catheter Cardiovasc Diagn 1998; 18:227–231.

15   Pepine CJ, Hirshfeld JW, Macdonald RG, et al. A controlled trial of corticosteroids to prevent restenosis after coronary angioplasty. M-HEART Group. Circulation 1990; 81:1753–1761.

16   Lee CW, Chae JK, Lim HY. Prospective randomized trial of corticosteroids for the prevention of restenosis after intracoronary stent implantation. Am Heart J 1999; 138:60–63.

17   Masferrer JL, Needleman P. Anti-inflammatories for cardiovascular disease. Proc Natl Acad Sci USA 2000; 97:12400–12401.

18   Ridker PM, Rifai N, Pfeffer MA, et al. Inflammation, pravastatin, and the risk of coronary events after myocardial infarction in patients with average cholesterol levels: Cholesterol and Recurrent Events (CARE) Investigators. Circulation 1998; 98:839–844.

19   Albert MA, Danielson E, Rifai N, et al. Effect of statin therapy on C-reactive protein levels: the pravastatin inflammation/CRP evaluation (PRINCE). A randomized trial and cohort study. JAMA 2001; 286:64–70.

20   Weintraub WS, Boccuzzi SJ, Klein JL, et al. Lack of effect of lovastatin on restenosis after coronary angioplasty. Lovastatin Restenosis Trial Study Group. N Engl J Med 1994; 331:1331–1337.

21   Waksman R, Kosinski AS, Klein L, et al. Relation of lumen size to restenosis after percutaneous transluminal coronary balloon angioplasty. Lovastatin Restenosis Trial Group. Am J Cardiol 1996; 78:221–224.

22   Bertrand ME, McFadden EP, Fruchart JC, et al. Effect of pravastatin on angiographic restenosis after coronary balloon angioplasty. The PREDICT Trial Investigators. Prevention of Restenosis by Elisor after Transluminal Coronary Angioplasty. J Am Coll Cardiol 1997; 30:863–869.

23   Serruys PW, Foley DP, Jackson G, et al. A randomized placebo-controlled trial of fluvastatin for prevention of restenosis after successful coronary balloon angioplasty; final results of the fluvastatin angiographic restenosis (FLARE) trial. Eur Heart J 1999; 20:58–69.

24   Mulder HJ, Bal ET, Jukema JW, et al. Pravastatin reduces restenosis two years after percutaneous transluminal coronary angioplasty (REGRESS trial). Am J Cardiol 2000; 86:742–746.

25   Tamai H, Katoh O, Suzuki S. Impact of tranilast on restenosis after coronary angioplasty: Tranilast Restenosis Following Angioplasty Trial (TREAT) Am Heart J 1999; 138:968–975.

26 Tamai H, Katoh O, Yamaguchi T, et al. The impact of tranilast on restenosis after coronary angioplasty: Tranilast Restenosis Following Angioplasty Trial (TREAT-2). Am Hear J 2002; 143:506–513.

27 Holmes DR, Savage M, LaBlanche JM, et al. Results of Prevention of REStenosis with Tranilast and its outcomes (PRESTO) Trial. Circulation 2002; 106:1243–1250.

28 Marx SO, Marks AR. Bench to bedside: the development of rapamycin and its application to stent restenosis. Circulation 2001; 8:852–855.

29 Saunders RN, Metcalfe MS, Nicholson ML. Rapamycin in transplantation: a review of the evidence. Kidney Int 2001; 1:3–16.

30 Cao W, Mohacsi P, Shorthouse R, Pratt R, Morris RE. Effects of rapamycin on growth factor-stimulated vascular smooth muscle cell DNA synthesis. Inhibition of basic fibroblast growth factor and platelet-derived growth factor action and antagonism of rapamycin by FK506. Transplantation 1995; 3:390–395.

31 Poon M, Marx SO, Gallo R, Badimon JJ, Taubman MB, Marks AR. Rapamycin inhibits vascular smooth muscle cell migration. J Clin Invest 1996; 10:2277–2283.

32 Waksman R, Ajani AE, Pichard AD, et al. Oral Rapamune to Inhibit Restenosis study. Oral rapamycin to inhibit restenosis after stenting of de novo coronary lesions: the Oral Rapamune to Inhibit Restenosis (ORBIT) study. J Am Coll Cardiol 2004; 44:1386–1392.

33 Brito FS Jr, Rosa WC, Arruda JA, Tedesco H, Pestana JO, Lima VC. Efficacy and safety of oral sirolimus to inhibit in-stent intimal hyperplasia. Catheter Cardiovasc Interv 2005; 64:413–418.

34 Rodriguez AE, Alemparte MR, Vigo CF, et al. Pilot study of Oral Rapamycin to prevent Restenosis in patients undergoing coronary stent therapy: Argentina Single-Center Study (ORAR trial) J Inv Cardiol 2003;15:581–584.

35 Rodriguez AE, Rodriguez Alemparte M, Vigo CF, et al. Role of oral rapamycin to prevent restenosis in patients with de novo lesions undergoing coronary stenting: results of the Argentina single centre study (ORAR trial). Heart 2005; 91:1433–1437.

36 Rodriguez AE, Granada JF, Rodriguez-Alemparte M, et al. ORAR II Investigators. Oral rapamycin after coronary bare-metal stent implantation to prevent restenosis: the Prospective, Randomized Oral Rapamycin in Argentina (ORAR II) Study. J Am Coll Cardiol 2006; 47:1522–1529.

37 Farb A, John M, Acampado E, et al. Oral Everolimus Inhibits In-Stent Neointimal Growth. Circulation 2002; 106:2379–2384.

38 Law RE, Meehan WP, Xi XP, et al. Troglitazone inhibits vascular smooth muscle cell growth and intimal hyperplasia. J Clin Invest 1996; 98:1897–1905.

39 Phillips JW, Barringhaus KG, Sanders JM, et al. Rosiglitazone Reduces the Accelerated Neointima Formation After Arterial Injury in a Mouse Injury Model of Type 2 Diabetes Circulation 2003; 108:1994–1999.

40 Takagi T, Akasaka T, Yamamuro A, et al. Troglitazone Reduces Neointimal Tissue Proliferation After Coronary Stent Implantation in Patients With Non-Insulin Dependent Diabetes Mellitus. J Am Coll Cardiol 2000; 36:1529–1535.

41 Takagi T, Yamamuro A, Tamita K, et al. Pioglitazone reduces neointimal tissue proliferation after coronary stent implantation in patients with type 2 diabetes mellitus: an intravascular ultrasound scanning study. Am Heart J 2003; 146:E5.

42 Sidhu JS, Cowan D, Kaski JC. The effects of Rosiglitazone, a peroxisome proliferator activated receptor gamma agonist, on markers of endothelial cell activation, C-reactive protein, and fibrinogen levels in non-diabetic coronary artery disease patients. J Am Coll Cardiol 2003; 42:1757–1763.

43 Choi D, Kim SK, Choi SH, et al. Preventative effects of rosiglitazone on restenosis after coronary stent implantation in patients with type 2 diabetes. Diabetes Care 2004; 27:2654–2660.

44 Marx N, Wohrle J, Nusser T, et al. Pioglitazone reduces neointima volume after coronary stent implantation: a randomized, placebo-controlled, double-blind trial in nondiabetic patients. Circulation 2005; 112:2792–2798.

45 Tsuchikane E, Kobayashi T, Kobayashi T, et al. Debulking and stenting versus debulking only of coronary artery disease in patients treated with cilostazol (final results of ESPRIT). Am J Cardiol 2002; 90:573–578.

46 Kimishirado H, Inoue T, Mizoguchi K, et al. Randomized comparison of cilostazole versus ticlopdine hydrochloride for antiplatelt therapy after coronary stent implantation for prevention of late restenosis. Am Heart J 2002; 144: 303–308.

47 Douglas JS Jr, Holmes DR Jr, Kereiakes DJ, et al. Cilostazol for Restenosis Trial (CREST) Investigators. Coronary stent restenosis in patients treated with cilostazol. Circulation 2005; 112:2826–2832.

48 Van Belle E, Tio FO, Couffinhal T, Maillard L, Passeri J, Isner JM. Stent endothelialization. Time course, impact of local catheter delivery, feasibility of recombinant protein administration, and response to cytokine expedition. Circulation 1997; 2:438–448.

49 Van Belle E, Tio FO, Chen D, et al. Passivation of metallic stents after arterial gene transfer of phVEGF165 inhibits thrombus formation and intimal thickening. J Am Coll Cardiol 1997; 6:1371–1379.

50 Asahara T, Bauters C, Pastore C, et al. Local delivery of vascular endothelial growth factor accelerates reendothelialization and attenuates intimal hyperplasia in balloon-injured rat carotid artery. Circulation 1995; 11:2793–2801.

51 Schnyder G, Roffi M, Flammer Y, Pin R, Hess OM. Effect of Homocysteine-Lowering Therapy With Folic Acid, Vitamin B12, and Vitamin B6 on Clinical Outcome After Percutaneous Coronary Intervention: The Swiss Heart Study: A Randomized Controlled Trial. JAMA 2002; 288:973–979.

52 Tardif JC, Cote G, Lesperance J, et al. Probucol and multivitamins in the prevention of restenosis after coronary angioplasty. Multivitamins and Probucol Study Group. N Engl J Med 1997; 337:365–372.

53 Daida H, Kuwabara Y, Yokoi H, et al. Effect of probucol on repeat revascularization rate after percutaneous transluminal coronary angioplasty (from the Probucol Angioplasty Restenosis Trial [PART]). Am J Cardiol 2000; 86:550–552.

54 Tardif JC, Grégoire J, Schwartz L, et al. Effects of AGI-1067 and Probucol After PercutaneousCoronaryInterventions. Circulation 2003; 107:552–558.

55 Ohsawa H, Noike H, Kanai M, et al. Preventive effect of an antiallergic drug, pemirolast potassium, on restenosis after

stent placement: quantitative coronary angiography and intravascular ultrasound studies. J Cardiol 2003; 42:13–22.

56 Fujita M, Mizuno K, Ho M, et al. Sarpogrelate treatment reduces restenosis after coronary stenting. Am Heart J 2003; 145:E16.

57 Peters S, Gotting B, Trummel MJ, et al. Valsartan for prevention of restenosis after stenting of type B2/C lesions: the VAL-PREST trial. J Invasive Cardiol 2001; 13:93–97.

58 Dens J, Desmet W, Piessens J. An updated meta-analysis of calcium-channel blockers in the prevention of restenosis after coronary angioplasty Am Heart J 2003; 145:404–408.

59 Jackson JD, Muhlestein JB, Bunch TJ. β-Blockers reduce the incidence of clinical restenosis: Prospective study of 4840 patients undergoing percutaneous coronary revascularization Am Heart J 2003; 145:875–881.

60 Bestehorn HP, Neumann FJ, Buttner HJ, et al. Evaluation of the effect of oral verapamil on clinical outcome and angiographic restenosis after percutaneous coronary intervention: the randomized, double blind, placebo-controlled, multicenter Verapamil Slow-Release for Prevention of Cardiovascular Events After Angioplasty (VESPA) Trial. J Am Coll Cardiol 2004; 43:2160–2165.

18

Role of systemic antineoplasic drugs in the treatment of restenosis after percutaneous stent implantation

Alfredo E. Rodriguez

Introduction

Since the introduction of coronary angioplasty, restenosis of the target lesion has been the main limitation of this procedure.

Acute vessel recoil, chronic remodeling, and intimal hyperplasia were the mechanisms involved in this process (1–4). However, after the introduction of stents in the daily practice during interventional procedures, intimal hyperplasia became the mechanism associated in the pathophysiology of in-stent restenosis (5–9). Therefore, its prevention should be related with therapies that inhibit smooth muscle cell proliferation.

In recent years, drug-eluting stents (DES) (Sirolimus, Johnson & Johnson and Paclitaxel, Boston Scientific) have been associated with significant reduction of in-stent restenosis among patients undergoing percutaneous coronary interventions (PCI) in de novo lesions (10–17). Despite the fact that all these devices have shown that the stent polymeric coating is a good solution for storing drug and defining a release mechanism, several publications have raised concerns about long-term safety issues such as potential risk for late-stent thrombosis or inducing chronic inflammation in the coronary artery (18–22). The issue of late-stent thrombosis with DES is clearly not going away; it is possible due to the polymer or the delayed re-endothelialization consequent to long-term drug release. Long-term (indefinitely) dual antiplatelet therapy may be the answer; however, such medication reduces cost efficacy and may not cover the times when general surgical procedures are needed; it is likely that the patients will have an antiplatelet-dependent life. If systemic antirestenosis agents proved efficacious, and, therefore, antiplatelet needed, could be reduced to the bare metal stent in a one-month period.

Animal data suggest that the degree of neointimal proliferation formed after stent implantation is mediated by smooth muscle cell proliferation and occurs during the first two weeks after the initial vascular injury (24). The relative success of nonpolymeric based drug-delivery stents using short-time release of medications support the concept that sustained release of antiproliferative agents may not be necessary to maintain a biological effect (25). Several preclinical studies have demonstrated the ability of systemically administered sirolimus or its analogs in reducing smooth muscle cell proliferation occurring after vascular injury (24,26–28). Systemic use of rapamycin and its analog was associated, in animal data, with a significant reduction in intimal hyperplasia, but only recently, clinical studies were reported with oral administration (29–34).

Anti-inflammatory drugs in the treatment of restenosis

In the past, several clinical studies with corticosteroids failed to demonstrate a significant reduction in coronary restenosis after percutaneous transluminal coronary angioplasty (35,36). However, as we mentioned previously, after balloon angioplasty, there were other mechanisms involved in the pathophysiology of coronary restenosis (such as acute wall recoil or chronic remodeling) that explained the negative results of those studies (35,36).

In contrast, in the current stent era, experimental studies indicated that a marked activation of inflammatory cells at the site of stent struts play a key role in the process of neointimal proliferation and restenosis (37–40). Indeed, interleukins 1 and 6 secreted by activated macrophages are powerful stimuli for smooth muscle cell proliferation and restenosis (41,42).

These were the rationalities for the use of corticosteroids in clinical data in the prevention of restenosis (43).

Inhibition metalloproteinase randomized exercise and symptoms study I and II

In recent years, two multicenter experiments were conducted with oral prednisone therapy in patients undergoing coronary bare-metal stent implantation (44,45).

The randomized IMPRESS I study included nondiabetic patients with single discrete de novo stenosis in patients with C-reactive protein (CRP), elevated during 72 hours after PCI. Prednisone was given orally during 30 days after stent deployment.

The major findings of this study showed that patients treated with oral prednisone had a significant lower major adverse cardiac and cerebrovascular event (MACCE) ($P = 0.0063$), any target vessel revascularization ($P = 0.001$), and binary restenosis ($P = 0.001$) than those allocated in the placebo group. Twelve-month event-free survival rates were 93% and 65% in patients treated with prednisone and placebo, respectively (relative risk 0.18, 95% confidence intervals 0.05–0.61).

The rate of six-month restenosis was 7% versus 33% and late loss was 0.39 versus 0.85 mm ($P = 0.001$); both were significantly lower in oral prednisone-treated patients than in placebo-treated patients.

The following experience was reported for the same group of investigators: In IMPRESS II, they included a nonrandomized multi-vessel and multi-stent cohort of patients treated with oral prednisone. As the previous one, only patients with elevated CRP levels 48 hours after the PCI procedure were included. In this study, they compared with similar cohort-matched populations.

Major findings of IMPRESS II were a significant reduction of target vessel revascularization, MACCE, and restenosis. Event-free survival at 12 months was 93% in prednisone-treated patients versus 69.8% in control ($P = 0.006$).

Both studies showed an angiographic amount of late loss around 0.61 mm. Clinical and angiographic outcome of these two studies are described in Table 1.

These two experiences had a potential limitation, such as a highly selected population (nondiabetics), reference vessel size greater than 2.8 mm and results only applied in patients with persistently high CRP levels.

However, the favorable clinical and angiographic outcome demonstrated with both studies, taking into account that both were independent, non–industry-sponsored studies, offers promising results that may be an interesting alternative to more expensive therapies, such as DES therapy, and needs larger controlled evaluation in more complex subsets of patients.

Systemic immunosuppressive therapies in the treatment of restenosis: sirolimus and sirolimus analogs in experimental and clinical data

A number of animal data supported the use of systemic immunosuppressive therapies in reducing smooth muscle cell growth, the mediator of neointimal proliferation (26,37,38). Preclinical studies have demonstrated a significant reduction of neointimal proliferation after balloon injury in the porcine or rabbits model of restenosis, with the systemic use of rapamycin (26).

Gallo et al. (26) was the first who reported animal data showing a significant reduction of neointimal hyperplasia with the venous infusion of rapamycin.

More recently, with sirolimus analogs such as everolimus or with the use of nanoparticles of paclitaxel, a significant

Table 1 Clinical and angiographic follow-up of inhibition of metalloproteinase in a randomized exercise symptoms study I and study II

	IMPRESS Group (n = 41)	IMPRESS II Group (n = 43)
Reference diameter (mm)	3.18 ± 0.5	2.95 ± 0.99
Restenosis (%)	7	3.8
Late loss (mm)	0.39 ± 0.6	0.55 ± 0.38
Net gain (mm)	1.48 ± 0.7	—
Event free survival (%)	93	93
TVR (%)	7	7
MACCE (%)	7	7

Abbreviations: MACCE, major adverse cardiac and cerebrovascular events; TVR, target vessel revascularization.

reduction of neointimal hyperplasia in animal data is also shown (24,46).

However, systemic therapy with clinical data was related only with the use of oral rapamycin.

Rapamycin (Rapamune, Wyeth-Ayerst Laboratories) is a natural macrocyclic lactone with a potent immunosuppressive and antiproliferative effect that was approved by the Food and Drug Administration for the prophylaxis against renal transplant rejection.

The anti-inflammatory and antiproliferative effects of rapamycin were based on its ability to inhibit the target of rapamycin kinase, an essential component in the pathways of the cell cycle progression (20–24,26–28).

Several nonrandomized pilot studies in de novo lesions have been reported in recent years with the systemic use of rapamycin.

Clinical and angiographic results of the most important of these studies are described in Table 2. As we can see in the table, although there were some differences in the design of these studies, there were correlative findings from those trials, in terms of angiographic follow-up results and safety long-term outcome data.

First, there was a consistent benefit in clinical and angiographic binary restenosis data. As we can see in Table 2, in-stent restenosis of the two pilot studies, which comprised only de novo lesions, angiographic restenosis was in only a single digit of restenosis, with a late loss of around 0.6 mm. All these numbers represent, compared to the average restenosis rate of control arm from the more recent DES trials, a reduction of 81% of in-stent restenosis and a 42% reduction of late loss, and also represent a reduction of 90% of MACCE.

We can obtain several lessons from these pilot trials (30–34,47). First, the angiographic in-stent binary restenosis was lower than 10%. The ORBIT trial had 7% of in-stent binary restenosis and 0.60 mm of late loss.

This study also shows that a high maintenance dose did not improve angiographic follow-up results and in contrast was associated with higher side effects.

With 2 mg/day, ORBIT investigators (33) found 40% of minor and moderate side effects, compared with 66% with 5 mg/day for 30 days.

A small pilot trial from Brazil reporting 6.6% of in-stent restenosis with 0.61 mm of late loss and with no target lesion revascularization or any major events after two years of follow-up (47) also confirmed these positive results.

Second, side effects were minor or moderate in almost all studies and were reported among 30% to 80%, according to the maintenance doses used in the studies. At the present time, it is clear that one should not give a patient more than 2 or 3 mg/day as maintenance dose for more than 14 days (33). With high maintenance doses, similar final angiographic results were obtained but with poor tolerance, as we mentioned earlier in the ORBIT trial.

In patients with in-stent restenosis, the first pilot trial reported negative results in a small population of inpatients presenting restenosis after brachiterapy failure; however, of note, in this population, even with DES therapy, they also had negative results, some of them, such as those reported by the Thorax Center, with high incidence of restenosis and stent thrombosis (29,48).

The only randomized controlled data in this in-stent restenotic population were reported by the German group, the OSIRIS trial, which showed a significant reduction of clinical and angiographic parameters of restenosis ($P = 0.005$) using a loading dose of oral rapamycin of 12 mg started 48 hours before the PCI procedure, followed by 2 mg/day for seven days thereafter (32). Angiographic restenosis as needed for target lesion revascularization was reduced by 50% and 40%, respectively, with the use of oral sirolimus therapy (Table 2).

Table 2   Angiographic and clinical outcome at follow-up of oral rapamycin studies (published until 2005)

(5 mg)[b]	OSIRIS[a] (n = 99)	ORAR I[b] (n = 76)	ORBIT (2 mg)[b] (n = 30)	ORBIT (n = 30)
Binary Restenosis, (%)				
In-stent	—	6.2	7.1	6.9
In-lesion	22.1	10.4	4.8	6.9
Late Loss (mm)	0.49 ± 0.54	0.63 ± 0.22	0.60 ± 0.56	0.68 ± 0.56
Stent Thrombosis (%)	0	0	0	0
TVR (%)	15.2	15	16.7	20.6
MACCE (%)	18.2	20	24	20

[a]In-stent restenosis.
[b]De Novo Lesions.
Abbreviations: MACCE, major adverse cardiac and cerebrovascular events; ORAR, oral rapamycin to prevent restenosis; ORBIT, oral rapamune to inhibit restenosis; TVR, target vessel revascularization.

Oral rapamycin in de novo lesions: lessons learned from ORAR studies

Oral rapamycin to prevent restenosis I pilot trial

From December 2001 through February 2003, 76 patients with a clinical indication of PCI for a de novo lesion were included in this protocol. The procedures were performed in the cardiac Catheterization Laboratories at Otamendi Hospital in Buenos Aires, Argentina (30,34).

Among these 76 patients, 109 bare-coronary stents were deployed in 103 de novo lesions in an equal number of major native epicardial vessels. Patients with in-stent restenosis, bifurcation lesions, vein graft lesions, lesion length of >0.20 mm, acute myocardial infarction in the previous 72 hours, poor left ventricular function (ejection fraction <35%), renal failure defined as creatinine concentration of >2 mg, or under immunosuppressive treatment were excluded from the study.

In Phase I, rapamycin was given orally as a loading dose of 6 mg followed by a daily dose of 2 mg/day for 28 days, starting immediately after a successful stent deployment.

In Phase II, a daily dose of 180 mg of diltiazem was added—the diltiazem used together with oral rapamycin in renal transplant patients has been associated with high therapeutic blood concentration of rapamycin and lower side effects (11,12). (In Figure 1 we can see the study design and patient inclusion of both phases of this pilot study.)

It has been shown that coadministration of a single dose of diltiazem with rapamycin leads to higher rapamycin exposure. The mean whole blood rapamycin area under the plasma concentration in time curve increased by 60% and the maximum concentration increased by 43%. Coadministration also decreased the renal clearance of rapamycin, presumably by inhibiting the first-pass metabolism of rapamycin (12).

Rapamycin blood concentrations were measured in all patients. In Phase I, rapamycin blood concentration was measured in all patients after the third week of treatment. However, as the immunosuppressive effect of the drug was achieved during the first four days, in Phase II study, blood concentration of the drug was measured during the first week (7).

A lipid profile (cholesterol, high-density lipoprotein, low-density lipoprotein, and triglycerides) and complete blood count were determined before and after four weeks of treatment for all patients.

Results

Table 3 presents the baseline demographic, clinical, and angiographic characteristics of the patients. Mean age was 63 years. More than 60% of patients presented with unstable angina: 20% were diabetic, 23% had a previous AMI, and more than 80% had class B or C lesions according to the American College of Cardiology/American Heart Association classification.

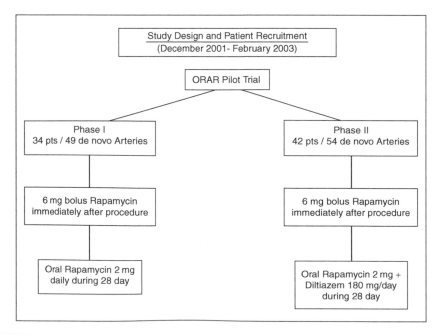

Figure 1

Study design and patient population of oral rapamycin to prevent restenosis pilot study.

Table 3 Baseline, clinical, and angiographic characteristics

Characteristics	Overall (76 pts/ 103 art)	≥8 ng/mL (44 pts/ 58 art)	<8 ng/mL (32 pts/ 45 art)	P
Female	6/76 (8%)	2/44 (4.5%)	4/32 (12.5%)	Ns
Hypertension	47/76 (62%)	23/44 (52%)	24/32 (75%)	Ns
High cholesterol	47/76 (62%)	28/44 (64%)	19/32 (59%)	Ns
Diabetes	15/76 (20%)	5/44 (11.3%)	10/32 (31%)	Ns
Stroke	0	0	0	Ns
Current smoker	18/76 (24%)	12/44 (27%)	6/32 (19%)	Ns
Previous AMI	17/76 (22.3%)	10/44 (23%)	7/32 (22%)	Ns
Unstable angina IIB- IIIB-C	52/76 (68.4%)	29/44 (66%)	24/32 (75%)	Ns
ACC/AHA morphology				
Type A	16/103 (16%)	8/58 (14%)	8/45 (18%)	Ns
Type B1	28/103 (27%)	15/58 (26%)	13/45 (29%)	Ns
Type B2	29/103 (28%)	17/58 (29%)	12/45 (27%)	Ns
Type C	30/103 (29%)	18/58 (31%)	12/45 (27%)	Ns
Target artery (%)				
LMCA	6/103 (6%)	4/58 (7%)	2/45 (4.4%)	Ns
LAD	57/103 (55%)	32/58 (55%)	25/45 (56%)	Ns
LCX	23/103 (22%)	12/58 (21%)	12/45 (27%)	Ns
RCA	17/103 (17%)	10/58 (17%)	6/45 (13%)	Ns

Abbreviations: AMI, acute myocardial infarction; LAD, left anterior descending; LCX, left circumflex; LMCA, left main coronary artery; RCA, right coronary artery; pt, patient.
Source: From Ref. 34.

In Phase II, after the first week of treatment, five patients who did not reach a sufficient blood concentration of the drug received an additional 1 mg of oral rapamycin (3 mg daily) plus diltiazem.

Hospital and 30-day results

All stents were deployed successfully. One patient, who developed subacute artery closure a few hours after the procedure, presented the only adverse event during hospitalization. During the first month, 19 patients (25%) had minor side effects, six patients in Phase I (18%) and 13 in Phase II (31%). Only three discontinued the medication (3.9%), one in Phase I and two in Phase II. The most frequent side effects were diarrhea (7.8%) and skin rash (9.2%).

There were no changes in white cell count or cholesterol concentration relative to baseline, whereas triglyceride concentrations tended to be higher than atbaseline ($P = 0.09$). Rapamycin blood concentration was significantly higher in Phase II than in Phase I (9.3 vs. 6.2 ng/mL, $P = 0.0002$).

Late clinical and angiographic follow-up

Clinical follow-up was obtained for all patients during the one year after PCI. Angiographic follow-up 6.8 ± 1.1 months after the procedure was available for 82% of the arteries treated (85 of 103), 90% in Phase I (44 of 49) and 76% (41 of 54) in Phase II.

During the one year of follow-up including in-hospital events, MACCE occurred in 15 of 76 of patients (20%):13 target-vessel revascularization, one repeat PCI and stenting in a nontarget vessel, and one myocardial infarction (this patient also had an emergency PCI after the initial procedure).

Angiographic binary restenosis in the follow-up angiogram was found in 15% (13 of 85). In-segment restenosis was 22% in Phase I versus 10% in Phase II ($P = 0.221$), whereas a trend to a lower in-stent restenosis in Phase II compared to Phase I (6.2% vs. 19%, $P = 0.066$) was found.

In Table 4, we can see quantitative coronary angiography data of the 85 lesions with follow-up angiography. At follow-up, the minimum luminal diameter (MLD) of lesions in patients with a high rapamycin blood concentration was

Table 4   Baseline and follow-up quantitative coronary angiography data

	Rapamycin blood concentration		
	≥8 ng/mL (n = 48)	<8 ng/mL (n = 37)	P Value
Reference diameter (mm)	3.0 (0.49)	3.15 (0.48)	NS
MLD post (mm)	2.79 (0.48)	2.9 (0.50)	NS
MLD follow-up (mm)	2.16 (0.62)	1.71 (0.59)	0.05
Late loss (mm)	0.60 90.56)	1.1 (0.61)	0.031
Net gain (mm)	1.4 (0.61)	1.0 (0.63)	0.021
In-stent restenosis	6.2%	22%	0.041
In-segment restenosis	10.4%	22%	NS

Data are mean (SD) or percentage.
Abbreviation: MLD, minimum luminal diameter.
Source: From Ref. 34.

significantly larger than in those with lower concentrations of the drug. The analysis of late loss and net gain with rapamycin concentrations also showed a significant difference in favor of lesions of patients with high rapamycin concentrations (Table 4). Angiographic binary in-stent restenosis was also significantly lower in the group with rapamycin high concentrations: (6.2% vs. 22%, $P = 0.041$). As we can see in Figure 2, Pearson's test showed a linear correlation between the late loss at the follow-up and rapamycin blood concentration ($r = 20.826$, $P = 0.008$) during the first week of treatment. Multivariate logistic regression analysis identified that reference vessel size (-2.206, $P = 0.008$) and

rapamycin blood concentration (-0.243, $P < 0.036$) were the only independent predictors of angiographic restenosis at follow-up.

Constructing a receiver operating characteristic (ROC) curve, which is a quantitative analysis, it showed that a rapamycin blood concentration of >8 ng/mL was the proper cutoff to define high blood concentration of the drug, and that it was in agreement with the mean rapamycin blood concentration in patients having no restenosis (7.9 ng/mL).

In conclusion, early high concentration of sirolimus in peripheral blood samples was strongly associated with low late loss and an optimal angiographic follow up results.

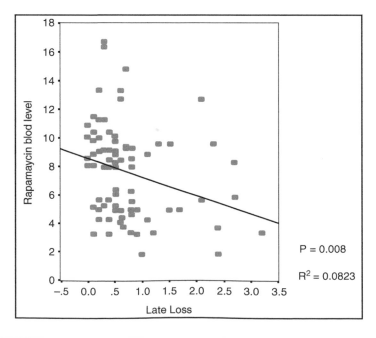

Figure 2
Pearson test demonstrating correlation among late loss and rapamycin blood concentration. *Source*: From Ref. 34.

Oral rapamycin to prevent restenosis II randomized trial

Patient population and study design

After the end of the pilot Phase I and II studies, we moved forward to a randomized trial. Thus, from September 2003 to September 2004, 100 patients with severe stenosis in de novo coronary artery were enrolled and included in the ORAR II randomized protocol (49).

Inclusion criteria were similar to our previous pilot study (34). Patients with clinical indication of percutaneous coronary revascularization were randomized if they had a de novo severe stenosis in a native coronary artery, a lesion suitable for stent, and a reference vessel size between 2.5 and 4.0 by visual estimation, and were a candidate for coronary bypass surgery. All the PCI procedures were performed at the Catheterization Laboratories at Otamendi Hospital and Sanatorio Las Lomas in Buenos Aires, Argentina.

Patients were excluded if they had acute myocardial infarction 48 hours prior to randomization, rapamycin allergy, clopidogrel, or aspirin intolerance, significant bleeding in the last six months, stroke or transient ischemic attack in the last 12 months, severe concomitant illness, recent major bleeding requiring transfusion, major blood dyscrasias, participation in another trial that does not allow a follow-up angiogram, patients with dyslipidemia of difficult treatment, patients with thrombocitopenic disease, patients with chronic total occlusion or in-stent restenosis lesions, and patients not amenable to sign the inform consent allowed to a follow-up angiogram. In contrast with the previous ORAR pilot, now, lesion length was not an exclusion criterion and multiple stents in the same vessel as well as overlapping stent were allowed.

The protocol of this nonindustry sponsor study was approved by the Ethics Committee of the Argentine Society of Cardiac Angiography and Interventions and by the Argentina National Regulatory Agency for Drug, Food, and Medical Technology (ANMAT). During the study, an Independent Safety Monitoring Committee adjudicated the clinical adverse events.

All eligible patients were randomized to control or oral rapamycin group. In the oral rapamycin arm, we modified the therapeutic scheme in relation to our previous pilot studies; patients in ORAR II received a loading dose of 6 mg, at least two hours before stent implantation, followed by 3 mg/day for a total of 14 days. Diltiazem sustained release 180 mg/day was added to a sirolimus regimen in order to achieve a higher sirolimus blood concentration (21). Blood samples were drawn to measure sirolimus blood levels and were taken at seven days after the oral loading dose of sirolimus, according to the second phase of our ORAR pilot trial. In addition, serum creatine, cholesterol, triglycerides, red and white blood cells, and platelet counts were measured before and at the end of sirolimus treatment. Coronary angiography was scheduled between six to nine months after the initial PCI procedure.

PCI was performed using standard techniques (6,30). All 100 patients received one or more identical close cell-stent design. The same stent design was used in order to avoid potential bias with stent selection in both groups. All patients received 325 mg/day of aspirin indefinitely and clopidogrel as a loading dose of 300 mg on the day of the procedure and 75 mg/day thereafter for one month. Statins were given to all patients indefinitely.

The primary endpoint of the study was to compare the angiographic binary restenosis rate and late loss determined by an independent core laboratory blinded to treatment allocation. Angiographic binary restenosis was defined as >50% residual stenosis in the target lesion in the follow-up angiography. In patients with multilesions, lesions were counted separately. Secondary endpoints were target lesion, target vessel revascularization, target vessel failure, and major adverse cardiovascular events. Target lesion and target vessel revascularization were performed in the presence of angiographic restenosis, and symptoms and signs of myocardial ischemia. A major adverse cardiovascular event was defined as death, myocardial infarction, stroke, and target vessel revascularization at one year of follow-up. Target vessel failure was defined as death, nonfatal myocardial infarction, and target vessel revascularization, during the entire follow-up period.

Results

Between September 2003 and September 2004, 100 patients were randomized, 50 patients in control (55 arteries and 59 lesions) and 50 patients in oral sirolimus arm (60 arteries and 66 lesions). A total of 132 stents were deployed, 61 in control and 71 in oral sirolimus; small-stent sizes (2.5 mm) were deployed in 44.7% of the lesions.

Baseline demographic, clinical, and angiographic characteristics between both groups are described in Table 5; treating diabetes was more frequent in oral sirolimus group ($P = 0.056$). Hospital and 30 days outcome in both groups was similar. During the course of treatment with oral sirolimus, 26% of the patients had side effects; however, none of them were major. The most frequent side effect was mouth ulceration (16%). Only two patients (3.9%) discontinued the treatment, three and eight days, respectively, after the first course of the doses. Overall adverse side effects of ORAR I and II, ORBIT, and OSIRIS are described in Table 6.

After rapamycin treatment, during the first 30 days, white blood counts showed a significant transient change; however, as we found previously in the ORAR pilot trial, severe leukopenia was not seen in any case.

Table 5   Baseline demographic, clinical, and angiographic characteristics

Characteristics	Oral sirolimus + BMS group (n =50)	Control group (n =50)	P value
Age (yrs)	64.6 ± 9.1	65.1 ± 8.3	Ns
Male sex (%)	88	94	Ns
Diabetes Mellitus (%)	24	8	0.056
Hyperlipidemia (%)	92	92	Ns
Hypertension (%)	92	82	Ns
Stroke (%)	0	0	Ns
Renal failure	0	0	Ns
Current Smoker (%)	24	18	Ns
Previous Myocardial Infarction (%)	22	38	Ns
Non Q type	0	0.5	Ns
Q type	22	36	Ns
Stable Angina	0	2	Ns
Unstable Angina	76	54	Ns
Target Artery (%)			
RCA	20	27.2	Ns
LAD	53.3	40	Ns
LCX	25	32.7	Ns
LM	1.6	0	Ns
MVD	86	88	Ns
ACC–AHA class (%)[a]			
A	4.5	5	Ns
B1	25.7	35.5	Ns
B2	46.9	39	Ns
C	22.7	20.3	Ns

[a]ACC denotes American College of Cardiology and AHA American Heart Association

Note: BMS, Standard Stent.

Abbreviations: BMS, bare metal stent; LAD, left anterior descending artery; LCX, left circumflex coronary artery; LM, left main; MVD, multiple vessel disease; RCA, right coronary artery.

Source: From Ref. 49.

Hospital and follow-up results of ORAR II randomized are described in Table 7. One-year clinical follow-up was obtained in all patients in both groups. After hospital discharge during the follow-up, there were two deaths (4%) in the control group (both cardiac), while two patients in oral sirolimus (4%) died during follow-up (one due to colon cancer and the other after an elective coronary bypass surgery). After hospital discharge, there was no documented nonfatal myocardial infarction or stroke in both the groups.

The rate of clinically driven target lesion or target vessel revascularization was significantly lower in oral sirolimus compared with control (Table 7). Target vessel revascularization was 5/60 (8.3%) versus 21/55 (38%), respectively ($P < 0.001$), and the target lesion revascularization was 5/66 (7.6%) versus 22/59 (37.2%), respectively ($P < 0.001$). Target vessel failure and major adverse cardiovascular events were also improved with oral sirolimus therapy ($P = 0.01$ and $P = 0.031$, respectively, Table 7).

Figure 3 shows the survival curves of freedom from target vessel revascularization (Fig. 3A) and freedom from major adverse cardiovascular events (Fig. 3A) showing significantly better outcome in those patients treated with oral sirolimus, that is, the numbers represent an 80% reduction of target vessel revascularization and 55% reduction of major adverse cardiovascular events compared to the control group.

Baseline and follow-up angiographic data are shown in Table 8. Clinically driven or per-protocol follow-up angiography at nine months was completed in 87% of the population (87 patients and 99 vessels). At 9 months, the binary in-stent restenosis rate per vessel was 12% for the rapamycin group and 34.6% for the control group ($P = 0.015$). The in-segment analysis showed a restenosis rate of 12% and 42.8% for the rapamycin and control group, respectively ($P = 0.001$). As shown in Figure 4, the use of oral rapamycin reduced the risk of binary restenosis by 65% within the stent and by 72% in the analysis segment. With the earlier mentioned numbers, the

Table 6 Side effects and drug discontinuation

Symptoms	ORAR I (n = 76)	ORAR II (n = 50)	ORBIT (n = 99)	OSIRIS[a] (2 mg) (n = 30)	ORBIT (5 mg) (n = 30)
Nausea and vomiting	1	0	0	2	1
Gum Sores	4	8	0	4	6
Diarrhea	6	3	1	5	6
Pneumonia	0	0	0	0	0
Rash	7	1	0	2	10
Leukopenia	0	0	0	0	2
Hepatic dysfunction	0	0	0	0	1
Fatigue	0	0	0	0	1
Elevated triglycerides	0	0	0	0	1
Fever	2	0	0	0	0
Constipation	2	0	0	0	0
Gastritis	1	0	0	0	0
Insomnia	1	0	0	0	0
Headache	1	0	0	0	0
Otitis	0	0	1	0	0
Allergic Reaction	1	0	2	0	0
Overall (%)	19 (25)	13 (26)	4(4)	13 (43)	20 (66)
Drug discontinuation (%)	3 (3.9)	2 (4)	4(4)	4 (13)	10 (33.3)

[a]Only severe side effects.

Table 7 Hospital and follow-up results of ORAR II

Variable	Oral sirolimus + BMS group (n = 50)	BMS group (n = 50)	P value
In-Hospital events (%)			
Death	0	0	Ns
Myocardial Infarction	4	2	Ns
Stroke	2	2	Ns
Target-lesion revascularization	0	0	Ns
Target-vessel revascularization	0	0	Ns
Target-vessel failure	4	2	Ns
Any major adverse cardiac and cardiovascular event	6	2	Ns
At follow-up (%)			
Death	4	4	Ns
Myocardial Infarction	4	2	Ns
Stroke	2	2	Ns
Target-lesion revascularization	7.6	37.2	<0.001
Target-vessel revascularization	8.3	38	<0.001
Target-vessel failure	18	44	0.009
Any major adverse cardiac and cardiovascular event	20	44	0.018

Abbreviation: BMS, bare metal stent.
Source: From Ref. 49.

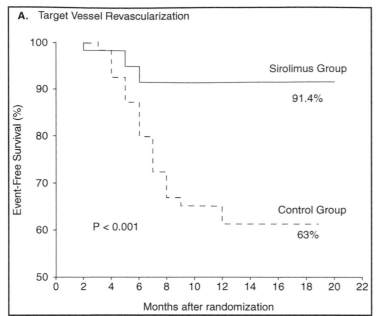

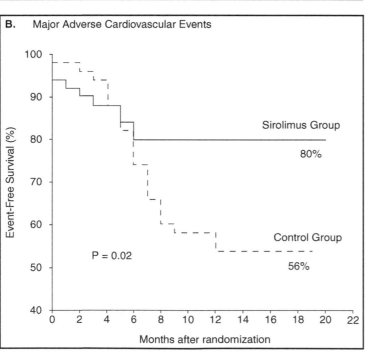

Figure 3
Event-free survival from target vessel revascularization (A) and major adverse cardiovascular events (B).

power of our study to detect differences between groups for restenosis was 0.81 per patient and 0.94 per vessel. The in-stent restenosis pattern in five patients in the oral rapamycin group who developed restenosis, was diffuse, but not proliferative or with total occlusion. The degree of restenosis in the control group showed that from 23 lesions with restenosis, a significant restenosis was present in 87%, including patients with proliferative or total closure. Thus, this finding explains the high rate of conversion to target lesion revascularization (TLR) in control group. With the oral therapy, in-stent late loss was reduced from 1.41 mm in control versus 0.73 mm in oral rapamycin group, and in-segment from 1.13 mm in control versus 0.66 mm in oral rapamycin group, meaning a reduction of 48% and 43% in-stent and in-segment late loss, respectively.

Multivariate analysis, (Table 9) showed that randomization to control group was the only independent predictor of restenosis (odds ratio OR 6.01; 95% Confidence Interval: 2.19–16.46) $P < 0.0001$. As we see in Table 8, compared with the control group, patients who received oral rapamycin had a significantly smaller amount of late loss [0.66 mm in the sirolimus group vs.

Table 8 Results of quantitative coronary angiography

Variable	Oral sirolimus + BMS group (n = 50)	BMS group (n = 50)	P value
Diameter of reference vessel (mm)	2.8 ± 0.63	2.81 ±0.45	1
Minimal luminal diameter (mm)			
Before procedure	1.03 ±0.43	0.98 ±0.48	0.571
After procedure	2.7 ±0.37	2.62 ±0.38	0.171
At 270 days	2.04 ± 0.70	1.47 ±0.76	0.0002
Stenosis (% of luminal diameter)			
Before procedure	66.5 ±12.2	65.68 ±14.66	0.755
After procedure	11.7 ±5.6	11.3 ±7.27	0.726
At 270 days	32.7 ±20.15	55.76 ±25.01	0.001
Lesion length (mm)	13.35 ±6.33	12.79 ±4.28	0.144
Stent length (mm)	15.7 ±2.62	16 ±2.78	0.149
Net gain (mm)	0.97 ±0.62	0.49 ±0.88	0.007
Late Luminal Loss (mm)	0.66 ±0.59	1.13 ±0.72	0.0002
Restenosis (%)*			
In-segment (n = 99)	12 (6/50)	42.8 (21/49)	0.001
In-stent (n = 99)	12 (6/50)	34.6 (17/49)	0.015

Abbreviation: BMS, bare metal stent.
Source: From Ref. 49.

1.13 mm in the control group (P = 0.0002)], resulting in greater luminal dimensions and a smaller degree of stenosis at follow-up. The relative reduction in the risk of restenosis among patients who received oral rapamycin was independent of diabetes mellitus status, vessel location, and the length and diameter of the lesion or stent.

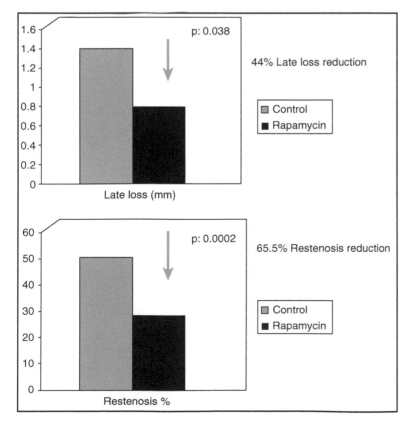

Figure 4
Relative reduction of late loss and binary restenosis in oral sirolimus and control group of oral rapamycin to prevent restenosis II randomized.

Table 9 Multivariate logistic regression analysis: predictors of restenosis of ORAR II randomized

Variable	Odds ratio	95% C.I.	P value
Rapamycin treatment	0.163	0.060–0.447	0.0002
Diabetes	0.401	0.084–1.915	0.252
Dislipidemia	0.570	0.225–1.444	0.236
Previous AMI	1.367	0.515–3.627	0.530
Unstable angina	0.596	0.252–1.406	0.237
Lesion class ACC/AHA			
A	0.893	0.089–8.945	0.923
B1	0.636	0.241–1.682	0.362
B2	1.493	0.632–3.527	0.360
C	0.988	0.365–2.673	0.981
Reference diameter <2.9 mm	2.334	0.963–5.66	0.061
Lesion length >15 mm	1.26	0.4–4.0	0.68
Right coronary artery	1.36	0.51–3.62	0.53
Left anterior descending coronary	0.42	0.16–1.06	0.06
Left circumflex coronary	1.75	0.69–4.44	0.23

Abbreviations: ACC/AHA, American College of Cardiology/American Heart Association; AMI, acute myocardial infarction; CI, confidence interval.

Clinical implications of the oral rapamycin to prevent restenosis randomized study

This prospective, randomized and controlled trial in patients with de novo lesions demonstrated a significant reduction of angiographic binary restenosis and late loss when patients were allocated to the oral sirolimus arm, and both the endpoints were determined by blind operators. Clinical safety and efficacy parameters of restenosis such as target vessel, target lesion revascularization, and Major Adverse Cardiovascular Events at follow-up were also significantly improved with oral sirolimus therapy. As we can see in Table 10, compared with control group, ORAR II active patients had a similar degree of reduction of in-stent restenosis, TLR, and MACCE than those obtained with DES in major recent randomized trials (49,50). Furthermore, those numbers are far from the average of in-stent and in-segment restenosis and late loss reported by control arm in recent DES trials. In fact, control arm of SIRIUS, C SIRIUS, E SIRIUS, and TAXUS IV reported an average of binary restenosis over 40% with 1.0 mm of late loss (12–14,17).

The population sample analyzed in the present study represents a relatively high-risk population involving B2/C lesions (~70%), small vessels (44.7%), and lesions longer than 18 millimeters (53%). Also, overlapping (7%) and multiple stent implantations per treated vessel (17%) were

Table 10 Reduction of binary restenosis, TLR, and MACCE. Comparison between randomized des trials and ORAR II study

Variable	Restenosis (%)	Restenosis reduction (%)	TLR (%)	TLR reduction (%)	MACCE (%)	MACCE reduction (%)
SIRIUS	9	75	4	75	8	62
E-SIRIUS	5.9	86	4	81	8	64
TAXUS II	11	75	4.7	62	11	50
TAXUS IV	7.9	70	3	73.5	8.5	43
TAXUS V	19	45	8.6	45	15	29
ORAR II	12	72	8.3	75	20	50

Abbreviations: DES, drug-eluting stents; MACCE, major adverse cardiac and cerebrovascular events; SIRIUS, E- SIRIUS, TAXUS II, TAXUS IV, TAXUS V, ORAR II; TVR, target vessel revascularization.

also allowed in the study. DES has been extensively studied in several randomized studies (10–17), and has been associated with a significant reduction of restenosis and late loss, compared to bare stents. In fact, late loss during the first year of follow-up showed only minor increase of minimal luminal diameter with DES therapy, and those numbers (10–17) are lower than the one presented here, meaning that local therapy achieved high immunosuppressive effects. However, this safety in the long-term outcome is not well defined, the incidence of stent thrombosis with DES appears to be higher than bare metal stents (BMS) in determined subset of patients, such as multiple vessel stenting, overlapping, bifurcations, unprotected left main, etc., and a call for caution has been recently reported (20). Furthermore, a nonrandomized comparison in similar patient/population treated with DES or BMS plus oral sirolimus demonstrated a one year similar safety/efficacy profile, but with a significant lower cost with the oral sirolimus therapy (51).

In our pilots and observational studies (30,34), we demonstrated that high sirolimus blood concentration was associated with a single digit restenosis rate and lower late loss, and there was a linear correlation between follow-up late loss and the sirolimus blood concentration measured during the first week, meaning that it was unnecessary to give the drug for more than 14 days after the procedure. In the ORAR II randomized study, the sirolimus oral administration scheme was different as was previously reported (27,31): the bolus was given two hours before intervention, the daily doses were 3 mg instead of 2 mg and only for 14 days. It is not clear when will be the ideal moment to begin the oral treatment. However taking into account that optimal immuno- suppressive effects of sirolimus were obtained after four days of treatment a preintervention loading doses will obtain better results—such was the case of the randomized OSIRIS and ORAR II trials.

In conclusion, this randomized study with oral rapamycin in patients with de novo lesions, treated with coronary bare-stent therapy, demonstrated a significant reduction of angiographic and clinical parameters of restenosis, suggesting that this strategy may be a cost-effective alternative (49,50) to DES therapy in a wide group of patients, such as those with reference vessel size more than 2.5 mm, nondiabetics, those with multiple vessel disease, and patients unable for long-term antiplatelet therapy. Furthermore, clinical and angiographic parameters of restenosis were significantly reduced with the oral therapy, even though the significance was greater in the presence of treated diabetes in the oral rapamycin patients.

Conclusions

Reduction of restenosis after stent implantation with DES therapy was one of the major breakthroughs in interventional cardiology in recent years. The routine use of DES has been associated with a significant reduction of clinical and angiographic parameters of restenosis in several larger controlled studies. In contrast, the use of systemic anti-inflammatory and immunosuppressive drugs to prevent restenosis after BMS implantation has only recently been clinically tested.

Small observational and randomized studies with oral prednisone and oral rapamycin have been demonstrated as reduction of clinical and angiographic parameters of restenosis. Although the studies are relatively small sample sized, these studies were conducted without economic support of the industry, which represents the major strength of all studies, conceived and performed without any conflict of interest.

The major advantages of the systemic approach to restenosis should be the relatively inexpensive and also powerful and safety method to reduce restenosis in selected group of patients. Oral rapamycin can also be used in determining high risk subsets of patients such as those with diabetes, bifurcations, and in-stent restenotic lesions, alone or in conjunction with DES. In insulin-dependant diabetic patients, oral rapamycin together with DES may help to reduce the still higher than acceptable risk of restenosis that is currently reported with DES.

However, larger controlled studies should be mandatory to put in perspective the role of this systemic approach in the prevention and knowledge of restenosis after stent implantation.

References

1 Rodríguez A, Santaera O, Larribau M, Sosa MI, Palacios IF. Early decrease in minimal luminal diameter after successful percutaneous transluminal coronary angioplasty predicts late restenosis. Am J Cardiol 1993; 71:1391–1395.

2 Rensing BJ, Hermans WRM, Beatt KJ, et al. Quantitative angiographic assessment of elastic recoil after percutaneous transluminal coronary angioplasty. Am J Cardiol 1990; 66:1039–1044.

3 Rodríguez A, Palacios I, Fernández M, Larribau M, Giraudo M, Ambrose J. Time course and mechanism of early luminal diameter loss after percutaneous transluminal coronary angioplasty. Am J Cardiol 1995; 76:1131–1134.

4 Mintz G, Popma J, Pichard A, et al. Arterial remodeling after coronay angioplasty. A serial intravascular ultrasound study. Circulation 1996; 94:35–44.

5 Kimura T, Nosaka H, Yokol H, Iwabuchi M, Nobuyoshi M. Serial angiographic follow-up after Palmaz-Schatz stent implantation comparison with conventional balloon angioplasty. J Am Coll Cardiol 1993; 21:1557–1563.

6 Rodríguez A, Santaera O, Larribau M, et al. Coronary stenting decreases restenosis in lesions with early loss in luminal diameter 24 hours after successful PTCA. Circulation 1995; 91:1397–1402.

7 Serruys PW, Jaegere P, Kiemeneij F, et al. for the BENESTENT Study Group. A comparison of balloon expandable stent

implantation with balloon angioplasty in patients with coronary artery disease. N Engl J Med 1994; 331:489–495.

8   Fischman D, Leon M, Baim D, et al. for the Stent Restenosis Study Investigators. A randomized comparison of coronary stent and balloon angioplasty in the treatment of coronary artery disease. N Engl J Med 1994; 331:496–501.

9   Rodríguez A, Ayala F, Bernardi V, et al. Optimal Coronary Balloon Angioplasty with Provisional Stenting Versus Primary Stent (OCBAS). Immediate and long-term follow-up results. J Am Coll Cardiol 1998; 32:1351–1357.

10 Sousa JE, Costa MA, Abizaid AC, et al. Sustained suppression of neointimal proliferation by sirolimus-eluting stents. One-year angiographic and intravascular ultrasound follow-up. Circulation. 2001; 104:2007–2011.

11 Morice MC, Serruys PW, Sousa JE, et al. A randomized comparison of sirolimus-eluting stent with a standard stent for coronary revascularization. N Eng J Med. 2002; 346: 1773–1780.

12 Moses JW, Leon MB, Popma JJ, et al. Sirolimus-eluting stents versus standard stents in patients with stenosis in a native coronary artery. N Engl J Med 2003; 349:1315–1323.

13 Schampaert E, Cohen EA, Schluter M, et al. The Canadian study of the sirolimus-eluting stent in the treatment of patients with long de novo lesions in small native coronary arteries (C-SIRIUS). J Am Coll Cardiol 2004; 43:1110–1115.

14 Schofer J, Schluter M, Gershlick AH, et al. Sirolimus-eluting stents for treatment of patients with long atherosclerotic lesions in small coronary arteries. Double-blind, randomized controlled trial. (E-SIRIUS). Lancet 2003; 362:1093–1099.

15 Grube E, Silber S, Hauptmann KE, et al. TAXUS I. Six- and twelve month results from a randomized, double-blind trial on a slow-release paclitaxel-eluting stent for de novo coronary lesions. Circulation 2003; 107:38–42.

16 Colombo A, Drzewiecki J, Banning A, et al. Randomized study to assess the effectiveness of slow- and moderate-release polymer based paclitaxel-eluting stents for coronary artery lesions. Circulation 2003; 108:788–794.

17 Stone GW, Ellis SG, Cox DA, et al. A polymer-based, paclitaxel-eluting stent in patients with coronary artery disease. N Engl J Med 2004; 350:221–231.

18 Virmani R, Guagliumi G, Farb A, et al. Localized Hypersensitivity and late coronary thrombosis secondary to a sirolimus-eluting stent. Should we be cautious? Circulation 2004; 109:701–705.

19 Mc Fadden E, Stabile E, Regar E, et al. Late thrombosis in drug-eluting coronary stent after discontinuation of antiplatelet therapy. Lancet 2004 364:1419–1421.

20 Rodriguez A, Mieres J, Fernandez-Pereira C, et al Coronary stent thrombosis in current drug eluting stent era: insights from ERACI III trial. J Am Coll Cardiol 2006; 47:205–207.

21 Bottiger Y, Sawe J, Brattstrom C, et al. Pharmacokinetic interaction between single oral dose of diltiazem and sirolimus in healthy volunteers. Cli Pharmacol 2001; 69:32–40.

22 Jhonson RW, Kreis H, Oberbauer R, et al. Sirolimus allows early cyclosporine withdrawal in renal transplantation resulting in improved renal function and lower blood pressure. Transplantation 2001; 72:777–786.

23 Mancini D, Pinney S, Burkhoff D, et al. Use of rapamycin slows progression of cardiac transplantation vasculopathy. Circulation. 2003; 108: 48–53. E-pub 2003 May 12.

24 Farb A, Jhon M, Acampado E, et al. Oral Everolimus inhibits in-stent neointimal growth. Circulation 2002; 106:2379–2384.

25 Park SJ, Shim WH, Ho DS, et al. A paclitaxel eluting stent for the prevention of coronary restenosis. N Engl J Med 2003; 348:1537.

26 Gallo R, Padurean A, Jayaraman T, et al. Inhibition of intimal thickening after balloon angioplasty in porcine coronary arteries by targeting regulators of the cell cycle. Circulation 1999; 99:2164–2470.

27 Poon M, Marx SO, Gallo R, et al. Rapamycin inhibits vascular smooth muscle cell migration. J Clin Invest 1996; 82:2277–2283.

28 Burke SE, Lubbers NL, Chen YW, et al. Neointimal formation after balloon-induced vascular injury in Yucatan minipigs is reduced by oral rapamycin. J Cardiovasc Pharmacol 1999; 33: 829–835.

29 Brara P, Moussavian M, Grise M, et al. Pilot Trial of oral rapamycin for recalcitrant restenosis. Circulation 2003, 107: 1722–1724.

30 Rodríguez A, Rodríguez Alemparte M, Vigo C, et al. Pilot study of oral rapamycin to prevent restenosis in patients undergoing coronary stent therapy. Argentina single center study. J Invas Cardiol 2003; 15:581–584.

31 Rodríguez A, Fernández Pereira C, Rodríguez Alemparte M. Oral rapamycin in the treatment of diffuse proliferative in-stent restenosis in a patient with small reference vessel. J Invas Cardiol 2003; 15:515–518.

32 Hausleiter J, Kastrati A, Mehilli J, et al. Randomized, double blind, placebo controlled trial of oral sirolimus for restenosis prevention in patients with in-stent restenosis. The oral sirolimus to inhibit recurrent in-stent stenosis trial (OSIRIS). Circulation 2004; 110:790.

33 Waksman R, Ajani A, Pichard A, et al. Oral Rapamycin to inhibit restenosis after stenting of de novo coronary lesions. The oral rapamune to inhibit restenosis (ORBIT) study. Jam Coll Cardiol 2004; 44:1386–1392.

34 Rodríguez A, Rodríguez Alemparte M, Vigo C, et al. Role of oral rapamycin to prevent restenosis in patients with de novo lesions undergoing coronary stent therapy. Results of the Argentina single center study (ORAR Trial). Heart 2005; 91:1433–1437.

35 Stone GW, Rutherford BD, McConahay DR, et al. A randomized trial of corticosteroids for the prevention of restenosis in 102 patients undergoing repeat coronary angioplasty. Cathet Cardiovasc Diagn 1989; 18:227–231.

36 Pepine CJ, Hirshfeld JW, MacDonald RG, et al. A controlled trial of corticosteroids to prevent restenosis after coronary angioplasty. Circulation 1990; 81:1753–1761.

37 Forrester JS, Fishbein M, Helfant R, Fagin J. A paradigm for restenosis based on cell biology: clues for the development of new preventive therapies. J Am Coll Cardiol 1991; 17: 758–769.

38 De Servi S, Mazzone A, Ricevuti G, et al. Granulocyte activation after coronary angioplasty in humans. Circulation 1990; 82:140–146.

39 Kornowoski R, Hong MK, Tio FO, Bramwell O, Wu H, Leon MB. In-stent restenosis: contributions of inflammatory responses and arterial injury to neointimal hyperplasia. J Am Coll Cardiol 1998; 31:224–230.

40 Pietersma A, Kofflard M, de Wit EA, et al. Late lumen loss after coronary angioplasty is associated with the activation status of circulating phagocytes before treatment. Circulation 1995; 91: 1320–1325.

41 Helle M, Boeije L, Pascaual-Salcedo D, Aarden L. Differential induction of interleukin-6 production by monocytes, endothelial cells and smooth muscle cells. Progr Clin Biol Res 1991; 367: 61–71.

42 Ikeda U, Ikeda M, Oohara T, et al. Interleukin-6 stimulates growth of vascular smooth muscle cells in a PDGF-dependent manner. Am J Physiol 1991; 250:1713–1717.

43 MacDonald RG, Panush RS, Pepine CJ. Rationale for use of glucocorticoids in modification of restenosis after percutaneous transluminal coronary angioplasty. Am J Cardiol 1987; 60: B56–B60.

44 Versaci F, Gaspardone A, Tomai F, et al. Immunosuppressive therapy for the prevention of restenosis after coronary artery stent implantation (IMPRESS Study) J Am Coll Cardiol 2002; 40:1935–1942.

45 Ribichini F, Tomai F, Ferrero V, et al. Immunosuppresive oral prednisone after percutaneous interventions in patients with multi-vessel coronary artery disease. The IMPRESS-2/MVD Study. EuroIntervention Journal 2005; 1:173–180.

46 Kolodgie FD, John M, Khurana C, et al. Sustained reduction of in-stent neointimal growth with the use of a novel systemic nanoparticle paclitaxel. Circulation 2002; 106: 1195–98.

47 Chaves AJ, Sousa AG, Mattos L, et al. Pilot study with an intensified oral sirolimus regimen for the prevention of in-stent restenosis in de novo lesions. Catheter Cardiovasc Interv 2005; 66:535–540.

48 Degertekin M, Regar E, Tanabe K, et al. Sirulimos-eluting stent for treatment of complexin-stent restenosis. J Am Coll Cardiol 2003; 41:184–189.

49 Rodriguez A, Granada J,Rodriguez-Alemparte M, et al. Oral rapamycin following coronary bare stent implantation to prevent restenosis: the prospective, randomized ORAR II (Oral Rapamycin in Argentina) Study. J Am Coll of Cardiol 2006; 18(17):1522–1529.

50 Rodriguez A, Fernandez-Pereira C, Rodriguez –Alemparte M. Oral rapamycin after bare metal stent implantation, Letter to Editor. Catheter Cardiovasc Interv 2006; 68:333–334.

51 Fernandez–Pereira C, Mieres J, Vigo C, et al. Cost effectiveness in patients treated with drug eluting stents vs bare metal stents and oral rapamycin [abstr]. Am J Cardiol 2006; 96: 7(suppl)–331.

19

Antioxidants

Umberto Cornelli

Introduction

Antioxidants represent a very large category of products because many chemical entities may have direct or indirect antioxidant activity.

The only official definition of antioxidants is related to "dietary antioxidants."

The definition proposed by the Panel on Dietary Antioxidants and Related Compounds of the Food and Nutrition Board is that "a dietary antioxidant is a substance in food that significantly decreases the adverse effects of reactive oxygen species (ROS), reactive nitrogen species (RNS), or both on normal physiological function in humans" (1).

ROS and RNS derived from physiological processes help either to produce energy and metabolites or to generate defenses against invasive microorganisms. This adverse effect is represented by the oxidative stress (OS) that can arise in case of lack of antioxidant defense or by the increase of oxidative processes in the body. If OS becomes permanent it may cause a disease. Many different illnesses such as cardiovascular disease, cancer, neurological, and endocrinological disorders have been related to OS that can be either a cause or a consequence of the disease. In any case, no matter what determines its presence, the upregulation of OS is consistent with a pathological condition.

An appropriate equilibrium between oxidation and antioxidants is fundamental for life. Antioxidants and OS can be understood only through the knowledge of the mechanisms that generate oxidation and the activity of both endogenous antioxidants and those that are made available by food intake or its supplementation.

The author has no interests in any of the methods used to determine oxidative stress. The author is an executive manager of a company that develops antioxidants in the European market.

Oxygen, free radicals, and reactive species

The presence of O_2 in the atmosphere is a determinant for life since it makes available the energy necessary for living; 1 mole (M) of O_2 may generate 3 M of adenosine triphosphate (ATP).

The atomic oxygen (O) is formed by a nucleus containing eight protons (the positive charges), and 8, 9, or 10 neutrons (with no charge), which constitute the so-called nucleons. Three natural isomers of O exist, which may contain 16, 17, or 18 nucleons, and are represented, respectively, as ^{16}O, ^{17}O, and ^{18}O.

These three different types of natural isomers are present in the respective percentages of 99.76%, 0.04%, and 0.2%. Despite this difference in the number of nucleons, the number of electrons (e^-) rotating around the nucleus is always eight. The e^- rotates in five different orbitals represented as 1S, 2S, and $2P_z$ that each contain a couple of e^-, and as $2P_x$ and $2P_y$ that each contain one e^- only. Since every element that has a single e^- (unpaired) in an orbital is defined as a "free radical," O by definition is a biradical.

This is similar to the molecular oxygen O_2 (Fig. 1), since the combination of the two atoms does not allow a compensation of the two extreme "combined orbitals" and consequently O_2 also remains a biradical and should be represented as $\overset{\bullet\bullet}{O_2}$. However, the convention is to simply use the symbol O_2.

As such, O_2 is constantly in search of electrons to compensate the two unpaired orbital, and this is the essence of "oxidation." Starting as $\overset{\bullet\bullet}{O_2}$ the final aim will be to become H_2O, which can be achieved through many different steps, and each step will generate intermediates that are more oxidant than O_2 and are called ROS, as reported in Table 1.

It is known that O_2 is potentially toxic as was evident in premature infants where it caused retrolental fibroplasia (2) or in artificial ventilation where it caused pulmonary lesions (3) because of the formation of ROS.

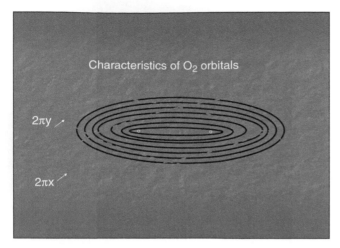

Figure 1
Oxygen with the unpaired orbital ($2\pi y$ and $2\pi x$) which determines the biradical nature.

However, the term oxidation has been used to define every process that ends up with a substrate that loses an e^- or a hydrogen atom (H), which contains one e^-, independently with or without the presence of O_2. Consequently, every substance that loses an e^- or an H is defined as "oxidized" and every substance that receives an e^- or an H is defined as "reduced."

The potential damage of O_2 is related to ROS, which are erroneously defined as "free radicals" and represent the tentative O_2 to compensate the orbitals that contain only one e-, with the aim of becoming H_2O—the real pacemaker of life.

The term "free radical" as a substance that is potentially toxic is incorrect, since most of the elements of the Mendeélev table are free radical elements (85 elements out of 103 are free radicals), however, the capability to oxidize a biological substrate is a greater determinant for toxicity.

The capacity to oxidize biological substrates is a common characteristic of a large group of substances (Table 1), which are defined as reactive species (RS).

They have been divided into ROS, reactive chlorine species (RCS), and reactive nitrogen species (RNS). There are many other RS that can be represented as $C^\bullet$, $L^\bullet$, or $R^\bullet$ depending on the nature of the compound, respectively, the carbon, lipidic, and generic radical. However, the entire body

Table 1   Some of the main reactive species divided according to the nature of the substance, free radical or nonradicals, and grouped by the element that determines the oxidation

Free radicals	Formula	Nonradicals	Formula
Reactive oxygen species			
Oxygen	$O_2^{\bullet a}$	Singlet oxygen	Δ or $\Sigma O_2^{\,b}$
Superoxide	$O_2^{\bullet -a}$	Hydrogen peroxide	H_2O_2
Hydroxyl	$OH^{\bullet a}$	Ozone	O_3
Hydroperoxyl	$HO_2^{\bullet a}$	Hypochlorus acid	$HOCl$
Peroxyl	$RO_2^{\bullet}$	Hypobromous acid	$HOBr$
Alcoxyl	$RO^{\bullet}$	Organic hydroperoxides	$ROOH$
Carbonate	$CO_3^{\bullet -}$	Peroxynitrite	$ONOO^-$
Carbon dioxide	$CO_2^{\bullet -}$	Peroxynitrous acid	$ONOOH$
Reactive chlorine species			
Atomic clorine	$Cl^{\bullet}$	Hypochloric acid	$HOCl$
		Nitryl chloride	NO_2Cl
		Chloramines RNHCl	
		Clorine gas	Cl_2
Reactive nitrogen species			
Nitric oxide	$NO^{\bullet}$	Nitrous acid	HNO_2
Nitrogen dioxide	$NO_2^{\bullet}$	Peroxynitrite	$ONOO^-$
		Peroxynitrous acid	$ONOOH$
		Alchyl peroxynitrite	$ROONO$
		Nitryl chloride	NO_2Cl

[a]Intermediate step of the transformation (quenching) of O_2 into H_2O.
[b]Generated by sun radiation (UV).

of RS in cells tends to be transformed, at least partially and by subsequent reaction, into ROS, which have to be considered the most important RS. The reason for this transformation of RS into an ROS is because the final product of the reaction of a ROS will be H_2O, which has an extremely low toxic value.

As shown in Table 1, the RS are divided into two categories: free radicals and nonradicals, which have in common the capacity to oxidize biological substrates. Some of the products belong to two different categories since very often they are regarded in one category or the other.

The presence of a large amount of RS in the body generates a condition defined as OS.

Oxidative stress

OS is caused by excess of oxidation and/or lack of antioxidant defense. Since it can damage all the constituents of the body (proteins, lipids, DNA, etc.), OS has to be a temporary condition, under strict control by the antioxidant defense network, which is represented by a variety of enzymatic and nonenzymatic systems.

There are schematically the following three different pathways to generate OS: energetic, reactive, and metabolic.

The energetic pathway

The energetic pathway is related to the production of ATP and is developed in mitochondria. The average caloric amount for human body functions is about 2100 Kcal/d.

A quantity of 300 M of ATP is produced (1 ATP = 7 Kcal) to fulfill the daily energetic needs, and a quantity of 100 M of O_2 is necessary to produce one ATP. At least 1% of O_2 escapes in the form of ROS, and tends to oxidize closer substrates (leakage). Since 100 M of O_2 are used to generate 300 M of ATP, at least 3M of ROS escape the cascade from the process of converting O_2 to H_2O, as reported in Scheme 1.

$$O_2\ddot{\ }+e^- \longrightarrow O_2^{\cdot}+e^-+2H^+ \longrightarrow H_2O_2+e^- \longrightarrow OH^{\cdot}+e^-+2H^+ \longrightarrow H_2O$$

oxygen   superoxide   hydrogen peroxide   hydroxy radical   water

Scheme 1
O_2 quenching.

Four e^- are involved in this process, and the ROS that are formed in each step can escape the process directed to the water formation. This event is known as "leakage" and is proportional to the production of ATP.

This cascade of reactions proceeds regularly and rapidly through a series of steps (enzymatic and non enzymatic) as reported in Scheme 2.

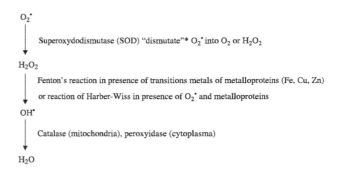

$O_2^{\cdot}$

Superoxydodismutase (SOD) "dismutate"* $O_2^{\cdot}$ into O_2 or H_2O_2

H_2O_2

Fenton's reaction in presence of transitions metals of metalloproteins (Fe, Cu, Zn) or reaction of Harber-Wiss in presence of $O_2^{\cdot}$ and metalloproteins

$OH^{\cdot}$

Catalase (mitochondria), peroxyidase (cytoplasma)

H_2O

* Dismutation is a biochemical process where an identical substrate is transformed into two different substances.

Scheme 2
Enzymes and reactions involved in O_2 quenching.

This cascade indicates that an increase of superoxydodismutase (SOD) activity brings to a concomitant increase of H_2O_2, which can diffuse through biological membranes. Since all the reactions of Scheme 2 have to proceed concomitantly, lack of coordination of the system may cause OS by leakage. An exhaustion of catalase and/or peroxydase do not consent the final quenching of $OH^{\cdot}$ into H_2O.

As an example, in Down syndrome SOD is very high because the gene for its code is on chromosome 21. These patients produce a large amount of hydrogen peroxide and are easily under OS since all of the H_2O_2 cannot be transformed efficiently into H_2O due to an alteration of the ratio in SOD/catalase + peroxidase (4).

In any cell producing energy, in case the quenching system is not efficient or even in case of excessive production of ATP, it is possible to generate OS by leakage. Since this happens within the matrix of the mitochondria, they are the first structures to be damaged, which results in the impairment of energy production. The cell will not produce the amount of ATP necessary for its normal activity and undergoes premature aging or apoptosis.

The reactive pathway

The reactive pathway is related to the so-called "oxidative burst."

In case of stimulation of a reactive cell (leukocytes, macrophages, etc.) by bacteria, virus, oxidized lipoproteins, or other substances, a large amount of $O_2^{\cdot}$ will be produced through the activation of nicotinamide adenine dinucleotide phosphate hydrogen (NADPH) oxidase, which is located on the cellular membrane of the cells. Following dismutation, H_2O_2 is immediately available and in the presence of the enzyme myeloperoxidase and chlorine (Cl^-) it is transformed into HClO. Furthermore, part of H_2O_2 becomes $OH^{\cdot}$ by Fenton's reaction (Scheme 1). HClO is a strong RS that oxidizes proteins and aminoacids, turning them into cloramines, which are also strong oxidants. The activation of the reactive cell also causes the production of $NO^{\bullet}$ via the induced nitrogen oxide synthase (iNOS). The concomitant presence of $NO^{\bullet}$ and $O^{\bullet}_2$ brings about the formation of $ONOO^-$, which in an acidic condition may generate $OH^{\bullet}$. This is one of the examples of how RS can be transformed into ROS.

In conclusion, the reactive modality ends up with a burst that produces a large amount of different RS, which together with proteases aggresses the environment.

Reactive pathway may follow the stimulation of angiotensin II receptors, which activate the NADPH oxidase (5). Hypertension may generate OS via this mechanism. A further reactive mechanism is related to the oxidized low-density lipoproteins (LDL) or even to the activity of free cholesterol on macrophages (6).

The metabolic pathway

There are many metabolic reactions that may generate $O^{\bullet}_2$. The most common is the transformation of arachidonic acid into a prostaglandin, or the production of norepinephrine from dopamine. In the cascade of production of uric acid from xantine, ROS are generated from hypoxantine to xantine and in the following step from xantine to uric acid, H_2O_2 and $O^{\bullet}_2$ are formed respectively, through the same enzyme—xantine oxidase.

These last reactions are considered the cause of the reperfusion damage (7–9). Both reactions need O_2 to be completed. Since during ischemia the availability of O_2 is extremely low, the tendency is to accumulate hypoxantine, locally. When suddenly the O_2 becomes available a massive OS is developed. Unfortunately, the antiproteases (anticoagulant enzymes) are much more sensitive to the oxidation than proteases (10,11) such as thrombin, and the consequence is the formation of a thrombus. OS facilitates the precipitation of acute ischemic episodes and antioxidants may limit the damage/incidence of an acute episode (165,167,168) for the prevention of acute episodes.

OS is also present in practically every woman under treatment with oral contraceptives, since a consistent OS has been shown (internal data of the author). The consequence can be the formation of superficial thrombus, which is one of the more frequent side effects of oral contraceptives.

The propagation of oxidative stress

One of the common issues in the production of RS is called "propagation," which may follow any pathway of RS formation. This is particularly effective in the case of fatty acids (L), which are located on the membrane phospholipids (in cells and lipoproteins), and proceeds according to the following steps:

1. The first oxidation (an H is taken out) transforms L into an alkyl radical ($L^{\bullet}$).
2. After an initial tentative of rearrangement (diene formation) a further reaction with O_2 generates a peroxy radical ($LOO^{\bullet}$).
3. At this moment the propagation reaction starts because $LOO^{\bullet}$ tears off an H from the closest L. The consequence is the formation of a hydroperoxide (LOOH) and $L^{\bullet}$.
4. LOOH undergoes the Fenton's reaction, which produces either an alkoxy radical ($LO^{\bullet}$) or an $LOO^{\bullet}$, both of which can oxidize the closest L and the reaction propagates.

In other terms, once an RS reacts with lipids, the propagation starts, which can be quenched only by the so-called "chain breakers" antioxidants (usually liposoluble antioxidants) such as vitamin E. This is one of the reasons for the presence of vitamin E in the cellular membranes.

The mechanism of propagation is very effective as a defense mechanism when it is oriented toward bacteria or virus membranes, but it may be very inappropriate once it is directed against the host membranes (lipoproteins, endothelial cells, internal membranes, etc.).

The most important pathway: the equilibrium

All the three pathways are important and it is useless to set up a classification in terms of quantity of RS produced endogenously. However, since oxidation is fundamental for life, it is necessary to maintain equilibrium between oxidation and antioxidant capacity in every compartment of the body. Usually, OS is a temporary condition; if it becomes constant, it may generate a disease. The real problem is to determine when an OS has to be counteracted to avoid the progression or the generation of a given disease.

OS can seriously damage molecules such as lipids, DNA, proteins, etc. following an imbalance between production/presence of RS and antioxidant defense. This consists of pool of nonenzymatic antioxidants and antioxidants enzymes, which have to be present and efficient in that part of the body where the oxidation is underway. Some examples may help clarify the concept.

Tropocollagen has to undergo oxidation to become mature collagen. By oxidation, lysine residuals of tropocollagen becomes allysine and forms a bridge between two different trimers of tropocollagen. In case of OS, more residuals of lysine are oxidized to allysine and many bridges are formed between tropocollagen trimers, and consequently the collagen becomes rigid, and inelastic. In this case antioxidants may control the reaction and allow an efficient production of collagen.

It may be that OS acts as a defense mechanism against bacteria or virus, and in this case OS is a protective "reactive" mechanism. In case of blocking this reaction with antioxidants a serious clinical problem can arise. Certain types of bacteria or even metastatic cells protect themselves with an efficient antioxidants system.

It is common knowledge that the activation of macrophages through the oxidative burst is a protective mechanism. However, it is potentially damaging to the sub-endothelium, and in case of inappropriate control of oxidation it can cause atherosclerosis.

This ambivalence has generated criticism against antioxidants because they may interfere with this protection derived from the oxidative processes. Antioxidant intakes have been analyzed during clinical/epidemiological studies, which focused usually on vitamin C and E, beta-carotene, and flavonoids, respectively. The results were a mixture of positive and negative outcomes.

However, for antioxidants, whatever prevails is the skepticism of doctors and the belief of consumers who tend to misuse them.

Only a comment can be addressed to this attitude:

"Antioxidants have to be used when there are conditions of OS that may generate or amplify chronic diseases."

OS has been implicated in many diseases. Diabetes, cancer, cardiovascular and neurodegenerative diseases are among the most common, but in many other diseases a particular emphasis is given to OS. With the increase of pollution, many other environmental sources such as O_3 and $CO_2^{\bullet-}$ are becoming very active partners for OS, and they are practically getting out of control.

Despite the threat to the equilibrium of oxidation/antioxidant defenses, OS was never measured in any of the epidemiological studies, but only in a few cases of acute or chronic diseases. Under these circumstances it is hard to draw any valid conclusions on the effect of antioxidants on health status.

Nobody would administer an antihypertensive drug to a patient with a normal blood pressure. At the same time, every doctor will use an antihypertensive drug in case of a hypertensive status. It makes no sense to give antihypertensive drugs to everybody and end up with the conclusion that sometimes they are working and sometimes they are toxic.

This raises the question of how to determine OS.

Evaluation of the oxidative stress

More than 100 different tests are used for the determination of OS. Most are experimental and some are clinically available.

To summarize, the following four categories of test are used to determine OS:

1. Determination of substances which have been oxidized by RS. These tests can be used in blood samples (whole blood, serum, plasma) and sometimes in urine. They are reported in Table 2 as C1.
2. Determination using "spin traps." These are products of different chemical structure capable of capturing RS. They are based on the determination of electron spin resonance, which is the paramagnetic signal derived from an unpaired electron. Spin traps have to be administered, and one of the main concerns is their potential toxicity. For this reason they are used only experimentally. These tests are reported in Table 2 as C2.
3. Determination through substances that become fluorescent or luminescent, when they get in contact with RS. These tests can be used ex vivo on biological samples and are reported in Table 2 as C3.
4. Determination of the antioxidant capability of blood. These test are reported in Table 2 as C4.

The prevalent methods are those regarding biomarkers of lipids, DNA, and protein oxidation or the antioxidant capacity of the body (12,13).

In general, those products that may be considered a mirror of the oxidation such as isoprostanes, hydroperoxides, or oxidized DNA are normally produced as a result of physiological processes. For this reason they can be found in the blood in relatively limited concentration, which increases under the condition of OS.

There are no comparative studies of different methods in humans or in experimental animals. Consequently, it is very difficult to decide which of the tests can be the ideal or the most reliable. The same problem arises for the comparison among tests for the determination of the total antioxidant capacity.

Up to now, there are no tests that are recognized as a standard test, and the suggestion is to use one or two tests (D-Roms, F2 isoprostanes) and learn how to interpret the results.

Particular attention is given to the D-Roms test (14), which is very simple and has been used also to evaluate the antioxidant activity of some products in patients and healthy subjects. The test is based on the determination of hydroperoxides that are derivatives of oxidized lipids and consequently indicate the OS at cellular level. The test is used for the epidemiological study on metabolic syndrome, in Italy by the European Society of Biological Nutrition.

The antioxidants network

Assuming that 1 M of ROS is the daily byproduct of ATP synthesis, and that hypothetically the quenching will derive

Table 2   Some of the most common tests under use for the determination of oxidative stress and the relative category from C1 to C4

Method	Type of substance that is determined	C	Reference
DNA	Deoxyribonucleic acid	1	(99)
SPC	Serum protein carbonyls	1	(100)
LHP	Lipids hydroperoxides D-Roms test	1	(101)
TBARS	Thiobarbituric acid reacting substances	1	(102)
LNO_2	Nitrolinoleate	1	(103)
MDA	Malondialdehyde	1	(104)
4-HNE	4-hydroxynonenal	1	(105)
IsoPs	$F_2/D_2/E_2$ isoprostanes	1	(106)
F neuroPs	F_3/F_4 isoprostanes	1	(107)
H_2O_2	Hydrogen peroxide	1	(108)
BH	Breath hydrocarbons	1	(109)
ONOO	Peroxynitrite	2	(110)
PTN	Alpha-phenyl-*N*-tert- butylnitrone	2	(111)
AHS	Aromatic hydroxylation of salicilate	2	(112)
TRAP	Total peroxyl radical scavenging antioxidant capacity	3	(113)
TOSCA	Total oxyradical scavenging capacity assay	4	(114)
UA	Uric acid	4	(14)
UAM	Uric acid metabolite allantoin	4	(115)
TEAC	Trolox equivalent antioxidant capacity	4	(116)
FRAP	Ferric reducing ability	4	(117)
ORAC	Oxygen radical absorbance capacity	4	(118)
DMPD	N,N-dimethyl-p-phenylenediamine	4	(119)
DPPH	1,1-diphenyl-2-picrylhydrazyl	4	(119)
TRX	Thioredoxine and glutaredoxine	4	(120,121)

from α-tocopherol (vitamin E) only, the total quantity of α-tocopherol needed would be 431 gm/day. Such a daily amount of vitamin E is unachievable. This indicates that to face the problem of oxidation more than one antioxidant is necessary, and that the complexity of the problem can be solved through an antioxidant network. Furthermore, antioxidants have to be present in many parts of the body, and because of this they have different structures and tissue affinities.

For these reasons, an antioxidant network becomes imperative.

Once an "antioxidant" has made available its e^- or H to another substance, it becomes an "oxidant," which is capable of subtracting from another substance the entity (e^- or H) that it has just given. In other terms, every antioxidant has to be regenerated and the paradigm is that:

Every antioxidant can become a pro-oxidant.

The combined processes of oxidation and reduction form couples of substances, which are called "redox" and may generate a cascade of reactions with other redox couples such that the final biological activity is determined by all the products formed during this cascade.

To understand the process it is necessary to underline that in biological systems many couples of products take part in the redox processes. Since this process is a cascade of reducing and oxidized products, it seems a never-ending story. Fortunately, an end exists which is represented in cells by the reduced glutathione (GSH) as such, or as the prosthetic reduced GSH of the reducing enzymes catalases, peroxidases, and tioredoxines. Enzymes usually do not act as strong oxidants and in case they are not regenerated they stop their activity.

Redox couples

Biochemical studies have made available (Table 3) the most common redox couples calculating the energy that is necessary to subtract an e^- from the reducing form to transform it into the oxidized form. By standardization the energy is expressed as E'o (volt at pH 7) and at 1 M concentration of each member of the couple.

The couple with the higher E'o value is capable of subtracting the e^- of any couple with a lower value. As an example oxidized glutathione (GSSG) can be regenerated to 2 GSH (reduced glutathion) with a redox potential of $E'_o = -0.23$ by

Table 3 Redox potential expressed as E'o (volt) indicates the difference of potential which is necessary to shift an e⁻ from the left to the right when the concentration of each member of the redox couple is 1 M at pH 7

Couple	E'o (volt)	e⁻	Site of the reaction
Acetate + CO_2/pyruvate	−0.70	2	Glycolysis/gluconeogenesis
Succinate + CO_2/α-ketoglutarate	−0.67	2	Krebs cycle
Acetate/acetaldehyde	−0.60	2	Piruvate dehydrogenase[a]
O_2/O_2^-	−0.45	1	Macrophages/neutrophils
$2H^+$/H_2	−0.42	2	(Potential at pH 7)
Acetoacetate/β-hydroxybutyrate	−0.35	2	Liver chetogenesys
NAD^+/NADH + H^+	−0.32	2	Ubiquitarian coenzyme
$NADP^+$/NAPH + H^+	−0.32	2	Ubiquitarian coenzyme
FMN/$FMNH_2$	−0.30	2	Riboflavine phosphate
2GSH/GSSG	−0.23	2	Intracellular antioxidant
FAD/$FADH_2$	−0.22	2	Mitochondrial complex II
Acetaldehyde/ethanol	−0.20	2	Ethanol metabolism
Pyruvate/lactate	−0.19	2	Anaerobic glycolysis
Oxaloacetate/malate	−0.17	2	Krebs cycle
α-chetoglutarate + NH_4^+/glutamate	−0.14	2	Glutamate synthesis/catabolism
Fumarate/succinate	0.03	2	Krebs cycle
CoQ_{10}/$CoQ_{10}H_2$	0.04	2	Mitochondrial complex II/III[b]
Dehydroascorbate/ascorbate	0.08	2	Ubiquitarian antioxidant
1/2 O_2 + H_2O/H_2O_2	0.30	2	Macrophages/neutrophils
Fe^{3+}/Fe^{2+}	0.77	1	Fenton's reaction (ubiquitarian)
1/2 O_2 + $2H^+$/H_2O	0.82	2	Mitochondria

Note: e⁻ represents the number of electrons that are transferred.
[a]Krebs cycle.
[b]Complexes of the oxidative phosphorylation.
Abbreviations: FAD, flavine adenine diphosphonucleotide; FMN, flavine mononucleotide; GSH, glutathione; NAD(P), nicotinamide adenine diphosphonucleotide (phosphate).
Source: From Ref. 122.

the NADPH, which will be transformed in the oxidized $NADP^+$ (E'_o = −0.32) or by any other couple having E'_o < −0.23.

However, the redox reactions reported in Table 3 are standardized to pH 7 and to 1 M concentration. When the pH and concentration change, the reaction can also change and it may happen such that a high concentration of an oxidized product (antioxidant which has given its e⁻) becomes pro-oxidant because the tendency to recuperate the lost e⁻ increases in parallel to its concentration as an oxidized product.

Furthermore, in the biological environment many couples may be localized in the same place where the oxidative process is underway, and consequently the final reaction belongs to the relative concentration of the different products. This means that although the in vitro activity of different compounds is defined quite precisely, in the in vivo situation they may behave very differently.

A wide number of molecules provide an antioxidant effect directly or indirectly. They are heterogeneous from the chemical point of view, and many different approaches were attempted in order to create a simple classification.

Table 4 reports a classification according to function and structure criteria (15,16).

Frequently omega 3 and omega 6 are represented as antioxidants. The problem is that they are polyunsaturated fatty acids (PUFA), which by definition are more sensitive to oxidation than saturated fatty acids. The administration of PUFA is one of the methods that clinical pharmacologists use to generate OS. When subjects treated with "fish oils" have a properly working antioxidant system, they can overcome this OS because the antioxidant system is well stimulated and generates an adequate compensation. In this case patients can take advantage of the use of these PUFA. On the other hand, when the antioxidant system is not working, the outcome will be an increase of the oxidative damage and relative consequences.

The literature has a lot of data concerning all the products listed in Table 4.

However, only those products with large clinical trials will be analyzed in more detail.

Appropriate clinical data are limited to five types of products and relative combinations. The products are vitamin E, β-carotene, vitamin C, polyphenols, and selenium (Se).

Table 4	Some of the compounds that are part of the antioxidant network in humans
Function/structure	*Type of product*
Vitamins	Retinol, vitamin E, vitamin C, nicotinamide, riboflavin, niacin
Fats and lipids	Omega 3, omega 6, squalene
Aminoacids and thiols	Taurine, *L*-arginine, histidine, glycine, cysteine; glutamine, methionine, *N*-acetyl cysteine, *S*-Adenosyl-*L*-methionine
Peptides	Carnosine, gamma-glutamyl cysteinyl glycine (GSH)
Proteins and enzymes	Albumin, thioredoxin, lactoferrin, transferrin, bilirubin, ceruloplasmin, superoxidodismutase, catalase, peroxidase
Plant-derived products	Polyphenols (derivatives of hydroxycinnamic acid, hydroxybenzoic acid, flavonols,[a] flavones,[a] anthocyanidins,[a] flavanols,[a] isoflavones,[a] flavanones,[a] stilbenes, lignans), glucosynolates, carotenoids (α-, β-, γ-, δ-carotene, lycopene, luthein, xeaxantin, canthaxantin), phytic acid, allicin
Minerals	Zinc, iron, copper, selenium, chromium
Metabolites	Uric acid, lipoic acid

[a]Within the class known also as flavonoids.
Abbreviation: GSH, glutathione.

Antioxidants: clinical definition

The evidence that a 24-hour fasting and tranquillity have both the ability for a strong antioxidant activity and may create some complexity in the definition of antioxidants. In many instances, subjects suffering from some diseases (hypertension, infection, inflammation) or under particular conditions such as menopause may also have OS, which can be considered as an epiphenomenon of that given condition. Once the disease (or the symptom and/or the condition) is controlled by a therapy, the OS may disappear. This means that a product can be considered as an antioxidant "indirectly." These aspects may further complicate the definition of an antioxidant.

At first a temporary definition could be:

> An antioxidant is a product that inhibits the oxidation in vitro and reduces the OS in vivo.

As we have previously shown, the determination of OS is made by many different tests. Most of these are experimental and those available for routine clinical use are capable of detecting some endogenous substances (DNA, lipids derivatives, proteins), which have been oxidized or have the total antioxidant capacity of body fluids. All these tests represent a derivatization of the OS and measure different type of substrates. The results that come out from each test cannot be comparable with the others, and it may turn out that the

products defined as an antioxidant in one test do not have similar activity in another test.

This modifies the temporary definition as follows:

> An antioxidant is a product that inhibits the oxidation in vitro and reduces the OS in vivo, no matter in which way OS is measured.

Typical compounds with these characteristics are some vitamins such as Vitamin C and E, which have a direct activity as scavengers and also some other indirect activities related to different mechanisms (17,18), which may have an impact on the OS.

All the studies conducted with vitamins or other compounds such as polyphenols cannot give precise information about any single product, even after supplementation, because foods provide the intake of many of them all together. The final activity belongs to the combination of a variety of antioxidants. As a consequence, sophisticated statistical analysis has to be applied to the data in order to isolate the effect of a given compound. Despite this effort, it is very hard to define the activity of a single product.

A certain amount of antioxidant is derived from food intake. Table 5 reports the data from the Division of Health and Nutrition Examination Survey concerning year 1999 and 2000 (19) in the U.S. population for some of the most common antioxidants.

From the data reported in Table 5, the difference between sexes is evident for Vitamin C, for which the intakes are higher in men—the only exception being β-carotene in young males. This may depend on the quantity of food intake—more food

Table 5 Dietary intakes of selected vitamins by sex and age mean values ± standard error: sample size from 641 to 1537 subjects

Type of vitamin	Male			Female		
	20–39 yr	40–59 yr	≥60 yr	20–39 yr	40–59 yr	≥60 yr
C mg	102 ± 4.5	107 ± 6.0	110 ± 7.5	85 ± 5.9	91 ± 5.3	99 ± 3.8
E mg[a]	10.4 ± 0.47	10.4 ± 0.44	9.2 ± 0.45	8.2 ± 0.32	9.1 ± 0.41	7.6 ± 0.24
β-carotene (RE)[b]	377 ± 36.4	537 ± 51.4	559 ± 47.3	522 ± 69.0	554 ± 47.3	507 ± 34.2
A (RE)[b]	878 ± 40.6	1115 ± 80.2	1117 ± 61.5	961 ± 74.4	945 ± 52.8	997 ± 58.5

Note: Systematic data on selenium (Se) and polyphenols (PP) are not available. However, for Se and PP the ranges of intake for U.S. population are approximately between 20 to 200 μg/day and 50 to 300 mg/day, respectively.
[a]Natural Vitamin E.
[b]Retinol equivalents (RE): 1 RE correspond to 1 μg of Vitamin A and 6 μg of β-carotene.
Abbreviation: RE, retinol equivalents.

usually gives more vitamins. The data concerning retinol equivalent (RE) suggests that certain types of vegetables and fruits do not fit young male tastes.

The dimension of standard error is such that many subjects are not reaching the Recommended Dietary Daily Allowance (RDA) and consequently they need to increase the vitamins, intake either with food or supplements. On the other hand, many subjects take a very high amount of vitamins with the food. In these last cases a further intake through supplements could generate the condition of a pro-oxidant effect.

In the following pages a single antioxidant will be considered on the basis of large epidemiological studies or long-term controlled clinical trials.

One particular characteristic of many studies reported is that more than one publication was issued based on different aspects of the trial. This is fully understandable because a large amount of data are available that may cover different aspects. However, in case of a bias, the error is spread out in all the data. Furthermore, to isolate the activity of the single class of product data are usually corrected by mathematical/statistical analysis that can contain some bias.

Vitamin E

Under the denomination of vitamin E are collected eight different isomers that are present in nature and particularly in oils commonly used as food. The synthetic vitamin E is the all racemic α-tocopherol (ART), whereas the natural vitamin E is the RRR α-tocopherol (RRRT).

Vitamin E directly scavenges most of the RS and may also upregulate antioxidant enzymes (20), reduces platelet aggregation and adhesion (21,22), and decreases smooth cell proliferation (23). It is considered as the most classical chain breaker antioxidant. The RDA of vitamin E is 10 mg/day.

The effect of vitamin E (as ART) on LDL oxidation was determined (24) following a treatment of eight weeks at different dosages from 60 to 1200 IU. Up to a dosage of 200 IU/day, vitamin E was found ineffective in reducing LDL oxidation.

In case LDL oxidation is considered as an important risk factor, the dosage of vitamin E may be important to determine a clinical effect. However, with respect to inhibition of protein kinase-C and the release of proinflammatory cytokines the intracellular transfer of RRRT (natural vitamin E) by the tocopherol-associated protein may be a crucial point. Consequently, natural vitamin E is considered more effective than the synthetic one. Since the activity on LDL oxidation was pointed out as important for the prevention of cardiovascular disease, most of the long-term trials with vitamin E were conducted at dosages >200 mg/day (about 200 IU/d). In a recent meta-analysis the association of plasma levels and mortality was studied in 1168 elderly European men and women (25). No association was found between the plasma concentration and all-cause or cause-specific mortality.

In Table 6 the most important clinical/epidemiological trials on vitamin E are reported with the main outcome (positive or negative).

The two largest studies, Nurse's Health Study (NHS) and Health Professional Follow-up Study (HPFS), were also examined together for the relationship of vitamin E and colon cancer but the findings do not provide consistent support of an inverse association between supplemental vitamin E and colon cancer risk (26).

Finnish Mobile Clinic Health Examination Survey is a typical study in which positive results were found both with the intake of vitamin E supplements and also with the dietary intake of vitamin C and carotenoids taken through fruits and vegetables. Despite the mathematical/statistical corrections it is very difficult to determine the effects of the interaction among the different antioxidants. Furthermore, fruits and vegetables contain polyphenols (PP), which were never considered in the old trials.

Table 6 Clinical/epidemiological studies with Vitamin E as all racemic α-tocopherol (ART), or as RRR-α tocopherol (RRRT)

Study	Daily dose	Period	N and sex	Outcome	Reference
NHS[a]	1–1000 IU (ART–RRRT)	5.6 yrs	121,700 F	Reduction of coronary heart disease comparing quintiles	123
HPFS	1–1000 IU (ART–RRRT)	3.5 yrs	39,910 M	Reduction of coronary heart disease comparing quintiles	124
FMC	1—1000 (ART–RRRT)	14 yrs	4697 M–F	Reduction of coronary heart disease comparing tertiles. Vegetables and fruits also reduce coronary heart disease due to the content of vitamin C and carotenoids.	125
ADCS	2000 IU (ART)	2 yrs	169	Slow progression of senile dementia	126
ATBC 1[b]	50 IU (ART)	6.1 yrs	11,635 M	No effect on major coronary events. Fewer cancers of the prostate and colorectum, more cancer in the stomach, no activity in lung cancer; reduction of cerebral infarction, increase of subarachnoid hemorrage mortality	41, 127–129
ATBC 2[c]	50 IU (ART)	6.1 yrs	904 M	Not recommended the use of α-tocopherol in men with previous myocardial infarction.	130
CHAOS	400/800 IU (RRRT)	510 day	2002 M–F	Reduction of composite cardiovascular death and fatal myocardial infarction	131
SPACE	800 IU (RRRT)	519 day	296 M–F	Reduction of composite cardiovascular disease	132
PPP	300 mg (ART)	3.6 yrs	4495 M–F	No activity on cardiovascular disease	133
HOPE	400 IU (RRRT)	4.5 yrs	9451 M–F	No activity on cardiovascular disease	134
GISSI	300 mg (ART)	3.5 yrs	5658 M–F	No activity on cardiovascular disease	135
VEAPS	400 IU (ART)	3 yrs	332 M–F	No activity on cardiovascular disease	136
DATATOP	2000 IU (ART)	8,2 yrs	800 M–F	No increase of life duration in Parkinson's disease patients	137
VECAT	500 IU (ART)	4 yrs	1193 M–F	No activity on prevention, development or slows the progression of age-related cataracts	138

[a]Data were corrected for the use of other vitamins.
[b]Four groups were randomized to receive α-tocopherol, β-carotene, or both, or placebo.
[c]Subjects of ABTC study with previous myocardial infarction.
Abbreviations: ADCS, Alzheimer's Disease Cooperative Study; ATBC, α-Tocopherol β-Carotene Cancer prevention; CHAOS, Cambridge Heart Antioxidant Study; DATATOP, Deprenyl and Tocopherol Antioxidative Therapy of Parkinsonism; FMC, Finnish Mobile Clinic Health Examination Survey; GISSI, Gruppo Italiano Studio Sopravvivenza Infarto; HOPE, Heart Outcome Prevention Evaluation; HPFS, Health Professional Follow-up Study; NHS, Nurses' Health Study; PPP, Primary Prevention Project; SPACE, Secondary Prevention with Antioxidants of Cardiovascular disease in End-stage renal disease; VEAPS, Vitamin E Atherosclerosis Prevention Study; VECAT, Vitamin E Cataract Age-related maculopathy Trial.

In the NHS study the reduced risk was only seen with vitamin E supplementation (at least 100 IU/day) and not with multivitamins. Although persons using vitamin E more commonly took other vitamins also, the effect was found to be independent from vitamin C and β-carotene.

In the HPFs, the maximal reduction in risk was seen among men consuming 100 to 249 IU/day with no further decrease at higher dosages, suggesting an inverse trend between the duration of vitamin E used and the risk of coronary disease.

The results coming out from these studies are such that they may confuse everybody.

It appears that the old trials end up with some positive results and the more recent do not show any real advantage in using vitamin E (26). The dosage of vitamin E and also the type of vitamin varied considerably. In the two studies with positive results, the natural vitamin E (RRRT) was more effective.

However, a meta-analysis of seven randomized trials of vitamin E (27) that involved 81,788 cases for a follow-up between 1.1 and 6.3 years and at a dosage range between 50 and 800 mg/day concluded, "Vitamin E did not provide benefit in mortality compared with the control group or significantly decrease risk of cardiovascular death or cerebrovascular accident."

Another meta-analysis has been conducted on 19 clinical trials with vitamin E supplementation and follow-up of a duration of more than one year. Nine trials were using vitamin E only without any other supplement and six of them were double-blind/placebo-controlled studies (28). The outcome of the analysis was that high dosages (>400 IU/d) may increase all-cause mortality and, therefore, should be avoided. Since in many studies other supplements were used concomitantly to vitamin E the authors concluded, "the use of any high-dose supplement should be discouraged until evidence of efficacy is documented from appropriately designed clinical trials."

The reason for this increase in mortality is considered to be due to the displacement of other fat-soluble antioxidant such as γ-tocopherol (29) and to the possible inhibition of the cytosolic glutathione S-transpherase, which is involved in the detoxification process of endogenous toxins (30). One of the oxidized metabolites of vitamin E, the vitamin E quinone, has a very strong activity as an inhibitor of vitamin K-dependent clotting mechanism (31).

In other words, the oxidation of vitamin E may generate problems.

There might be another crucial point as far as oxidized LDL is concerned. The presence of oxidized lipids in the gut allows the formation of oxidized chilomicrons followed by the production in the liver of oxidized lipoproteins. Once they are formed, vitamin E may reduce the propagation of the oxidation and becomes an α-tocopheryl radical (the major oxidation product of vitamin E). Once this radical is present at high concentration it is capable of oxidizing the apolipoprotein moiety of the LDL (32,33).

As a consequence, the effect of OS is binomial: one component of oxidation is generated by the cell (energy production, reactivity, and metabolism), while the other component is derived from food. This last is extremely variable and uncontrolled since it belongs to the eating habit/culture/environment.

Under OS vitamin E can generate pro-oxidant activity that is already in the gut and is directed against those structure such as chilomicrons, used to transport vitamin E.

One of the possibilities to counteract these tendencies to oxidate could be the concomitant use of products such as vitamin C or flavonoids, that are capable of regenerating vitamin E once it is oxidized.

β-Carotene

The other type of antioxidant that has been studied extensively is β-carotene. This is a peculiar type of antioxidant since it has a selectivity for the skin and it may be active even when the O_2 tension is lower than 150 mmHg (34). This last condition is typical of tissues. However, at higher oxygen pressure it may become pro-oxidant, particularly at high concentrations. Although carotenoids are more than 600 most of the attention was devoted to β-carotene, and only recently other carotenes such as α-carotene, lycopene, zeaxantin, and β-cryptoxantin are emerging as active compounds.

In the early 1980s, there were substantial epidemiological studies indicating association between high fruits and vegetables consumption, (high estimated β-carotene intake in the diet), high blood concentration of β-carotene, and lower incidences of cancer, particularly lung cancer. Twenty different studies coming from eight different countries were published at the end of 1970s (35,36) and much experimental evi-dence accumulated in favor of the cancer-preventing effect of β-carotene.

In a large trial (37) conducted in eight European countries—European Antioxidant Miocardial Infarction and Breast Cancer (EURAMIC) trial—the fatty acid composition, α-tocopherol, and β-carotene levels were determined in adipose tissue of patients with acute MI. The study supported the hypothesis that β-carotene protects against MI because it reduces the oxidation of PUFA. The concentration on adipose tissue was considered due to the dietary intake.

In another study (38) on coronary primary prevention, the placebo-controlled trial of colestyramine resin in coronary heart disease (CHD), the serum carotenoids levels were found inversely related to CHD events. In the same study, there was no evidence of activity of Se and α-tocopherol. The authors concluded that there was no proof of a cause-and-effect relation and that it was possible that another constituent of the diet could be present together with β-carotene in the same food products. Consequently, the final suggestion was to increase the consumption of yellow fruits and green leafy vegetables.

In a prospective nested case-control study on physicians diagnosed with MI who were part of the Physician Health Study (PHS) (39) in the United States, plasma levels of all carotenoids (α-carotene, β-carotene, β-cryptoxantin, lutein, and lycopene), retinol, and α- and γ-tocopherol were analyzed. No differences were noted by the physicians between the patients diagnosed with MI and the matched controls (40).

In a recent meta-analysis study on European men and women (25), high plasma concentrations of α- and β-carotene were associated both with lower mortality from all causes and cancer. For cardiovascular mortality the inverse association was confined to the elderly with body mass index <25.

A very different type of results came out from randomized long-term trials [The α-Tocopherol β-Carotene Cancer Prevention (ATBC), (41) in which β-carotene was given at very high dosages and ended up with an increase of first-ever non-fatal MI.

However, since β-carotene is a provitamin A, the combination of vitamin A and β-carotene have to be reported as μg RE such that 1 μg RE = 1 μg of vitamin A or to 6 μg of β-carotene. According to these equivalences, the RDA is 800 μg RE.

In the long-term clinical trials much higher dosages were used, since the lowest dosage was 3333 μg RE which is more than four times the RDA.

In Table 7 the most known studies published in the last 10 years on β-carotene are reported.

Selectivity for the skin of β-carotene is such that the palms of the hands of black people and Asian Indians have a yellowish color because of the β-carotene content. An environment rich in vegetables and fruits with high contents of carotenoids can protect natives from the high level of OS generated by solar radiation.

However, in the skin, vitamin D is also activated by oxidation, and an excess of quenching of this oxidation, due to high concentrations of β-carotene in the skin, may reduce the amount of vitamin D availability. This is not only important for bone construction, but also because vitamin D represents a powerful natural anticancer agent. This can be an explanation why an increase of lung cancer was found in Finland (country with relative lack of sun), where smoking people and subjects with asbestosis were treated with β-Carotene and Retinol Efficacy Trial. Concomitantly in ATBC, ischemic episodes were more severe due to the very high dosage of β-carotene, which can become pro-oxidant.

The relationship between dietary carotenoids and risk of lung cancer has been determined in a pooled analysis of seven cohort studies (studies with the asterisk in Table 7). The results (42) indicate that β-carotene was not associated with lung cancer, that smoking was the strongest risk factor for lung cancer, and β-cryptoxantin (contained in citrus fruit) may modestly reduce the risk.

In the same meta-analysis used for vitamin E (27), β-carotene was also analyzed in trials in which 138,113 cases

Table 7   Clinical/epidemiological studies using β-carotene. Dosage is reported also in terms of μg retinol equivalents (RE)

Study	Daily dose	Duration (yr)	N and sex	Outcome	Reference
ATBC 1[a]	20 mg (3333 μg RE[b])	6.1	11,609 M	Increase of first-ever nonfatal myocardial infarction	126,127
ATBC 2[c]	20 mg (3333 μg RE)	4.5	9451 M	No activity	134
ATBC 3[d,e]	Carotenoids and vitamin A	6.1	27,084 M	Lower risk of lung cancer in the highest quintile of carotenoids; same for highest quintile of consumption of fruit and vegetables; reduction of cerebral infarction	139,140
SCPSG	50 mg (8333 μg RE)	0.5	1383 M–F	No activity on nonmelanoma skin cancer	141
CARET	15–30 mg, vitamin A 25,000 IU (10,000–12,000 μg RE)	4	8889 M	May increase lung cancer	142
PHS	50 mg[f] (8333 μg RE)	12	22,071 M	Neither benefit nor harm in terms of the incidence of malignant neoplasms, cardiovascular disease, or death from all causes	39

(Continued)

Table 7 Clinical/epidemiological studies using β-carotene. Dosage is reported also in terms of μg retinol equivalents (RE) (*Continued*)

Study	Daily dose	Duration (yr)	N and sex	Outcome	Reference
PHS[g]	50 mg[f] (8333 μg RE)	12	1338 M	No activity on nonmelanoma skin cancer	143
Rotterdam	Case-cohort[h]	4	4802 M–F	High dietary intake of β-carotene may protect against cardiovascular disease; vitamin C and E seem ineffective	144
CNBSS[e]	Case-cohort[h]	13	5681 F	No association between dietary carotenoid intake and lung cancer risk	145
NYSC[e]	Case-cohort[h]	7	47.000 M–F	In men, vitamin C, folate, and carotenoids are inversely correlated lung cancer; no major role in women	145 146
IWHS[e]	Case-cohort[h]	4	2952 F	Intakes of fruits, vegetables, vitamin C, β-carotene in the uppermost quartile are related with a lower lung cancer risk	147
NCSDC[e]	Case-cohort[h]	6.3	2464 M	Protective effect on lung cancer incidence was found for folate and vitamin C, particularly, for current smokers; carotenoids do not show an evident protective activity	148
HPFS+NHS[e]	Case-cohort[h]	10	12.407 M-F	β-Carotenes do not significantly lower the lung cancer risk; α-Carotene and lycopene intakes were associated with a lower risk of lung cancer	149

[a]In smokers.
[b]Retinol equivalent (RE): 1 μg RE correspond to 1 μg vitamin A or 6 μg of β-carotene.
[c]Subjects with previous myocardial infarction.
[d]Analysis of dietary carotenoids.
[e]Trial used for pooled analysis of the data (41).
[f]Administration on alternative days.
[g]Nested case-control study within PHS for nonmelanoma skin cancer.
[h]Cases with a given disease under analysis were extracted from the entire cohort of subject and compared with noncases.
Abbreviations: ATBC, α-tocopherol β-carotene cancer prevention; CARET, β-carotene and retinol efficacy trial; CNBS, Canadian National Breast Screening Study; HPFS l NHS, Health Professional Follow-up Study l Nurses' Health Study; IWHS, Iowa Women's Health Study case-control with randomly selected noncases; NCSDC, Nederland Cohort Study on Diet and Cancer, a subcohort of subjects randomly sampled within the entire cohort; NYSC, New York State Cohort; PHS, Physician Health Study; SCP, Skin Cancer Prevention; SCPSG, Skin Cancer Prevention Study Group.

were studied, with a follow-up between 2.1 and 12 years, at dosages between 20 and 30 mg (or even 50 mg every other day). The outcome was that "β-carotene led to a small but significant increase in all cause of mortality and with a slight increase of cardiovascular death."

Among carotenoids, lycopene was analyzed for the risk of cardiovascular disease in women in a nested case-control group deriving from the Women's Health Study. Higher plasma lycopene concentrations (upper 3 quartiles; median > 16.5 μg/dL) were associated with a lower risk of cardiovascular disease (43). Additional adjustment for other carotenoids and retinol did not explain the association between plasma lycopene and cardiovascular disease (CVD).

In a similar study, the PHS (44) such a relation between lycopene and reduction of CVD in humans was not found. However, the average plasma levels of lycopene in women were about 60% higher than in men. Consequently the problem can be a matter of blood levels and not of gender.

In conclusion, as for vitamin E, old trials end up with positive results, whereas more controlled recent trials have an opposite outcome. However, once again, the dosages of β-carotene, which have been used in the more recent trials, are such that the pro-oxidant effects can prevail.

Vitamin C

The current RDA for vitamin C is 60 mg/day for a healthy non-smoking adult. Vitamin C is a cofactor for several enzymes involved in the biosynthesis of collagen, neurotransmitters, carnitine (45), hydroxylation of cholesterol (to form bile acids). It is also an important water-soluble antioxidant, which scavenges most of the RS and acts as a coantioxidant by regenerating α-tocopheryl radicals (46).

Ascorbate (AH⁻) can make two e⁻ available, and consequently both AH⁻ and its one e⁻ oxidation product, the ascorbyl radical (A•⁻), become antioxidants. The latter dismutates to form A•⁻ and dehydroascorbic acid (A), as shown in Scheme 3, or is reduced back by GSH or GSH-dependent enzymes (glutaredoxine, thioredoxin). Immediately, A is irreversibly hydrolized to 2,3-diketogluconic acid and then to oxalate, threonate, and many other metabolites. This last point is important because products derived from the hydrolysis of A may potentially damage proteins by glycation (47).

In vivo studies on the antioxidant activity of vitamin C were conducted on biomarkers of lipids, DNA, and proteins

$$A^{\bullet-} + A^{\bullet-} \longrightarrow AH^- + A$$

Scheme 3

oxidation, with conflicting results (45). However, a reduction of lipids oxidation after supplementation was shown, yet, the oxidation activity on DNA and proteins was not very clear. The dosage of vitamin C is also important because in case of high dosages (>200 mg/day) in subjects under OS the amount of metabolites that can be formed may damage proteins; in other words, there is a shift of compartment of OS from lipids to proteins. Again the moderation of the dosage together with a long period of time can be the keys to determine a beneficial clinical activity. Vitamin C maintains the intracellular concentration of GSH (48) and reduces nitrosation, thus preventing the formation of nitrosamines (49). This last activity is involved in the chemioprotection against mutagenicity induced by nitrosamines.

Numerous observational studies have found that vitamin C may decrease LDL cholesterol and elevate HDL (50). Some studies found an inverse association between serum vitamin C concentration and coagulation factor or coagulation activation markers (51).

A pooled analysis of nine prospective studies on 293,172 subjects for a follow-up of 10 years that included information on vitamin E, C, and carotenoids (52) was conducted the results suggest that high supplemental vitamin C intakes (>700 mg/day) reduced the incidence of major coronary heart disease. The risk reduction induced by vitamin E or carotenoids was very small.

According to the National Health and Nutrition Examination Survey (NHANES II), vitamin C status was related to mortality in U.S. adults (53) and data suggest that men with low serum ascorbate may have an increased risk of mortality because of an increased risk of cancer, whereas in women this relation was not found. However, the median level of serum ascorbate in women was much higher than in men, 64.2 μmol/L and 49.4 μg/mL, respectively (corresponding to 11.3 μg/mL and 8.7 μg/mL). In Europe similar plasma levels of 58.3 μmol/L for women and 47.2 μmol/L for men were found in a cohort of the European Prospective Investigation in Cancer and Nutrition study (EPIC-Norfolk). However, the conclusion was that both in men and women the plasma ascorbate concentration was inversely related to mortality from all causes, cardiovascular disease, and ischemic heart disease (54). Cancer mortality was inversely related in men but not in women. The suggestion that came out from this study was to increase fruit and vegetable intake of about one serving daily.

In some of the studies reported in Table 8 and in many other large studies vitamin C intake was analyzed for its possible activity against cancer.

Most of the studies reported no significant reduction in cancer risk, and those studies that reported a risk reduction (55–58) found an effect on subject with vitamin C intakes ≥80 to 110 mg/day.

Vitamin C results from long-term trials are also conflicting. However, high intake was never found to increase mortality, and moderate intake between 100 and 200 mg/day essentially shows some benefit either taken as a supplement or with a diet plus supplements, particularly in elderly. However, there is no benefit in using dosages higher than 400 mg/day.

Polyphenols

Polyphenols (PP) represent a very wide variety of about 6000 compounds divided into 11 different classes represented by hydroxybenzoic acids, hydroxycinnamic acid, anthocyanidins, flavonols, flavanones, flavanols (divided into monomeric catechins and polymeric proanthocyanidinsᵃ), flavones, isoflavones, stilbenes, and lignans (16).

They represent a sort of puzzle for "nonchemists" and to make the problem more complex the term "flavonoids" is sometimes erroneously used synonymously with PP.

Flavonoids consist of six out of 11 classes of polyphenols, precisely: anthocyanidins, flavonols, flavanones, flavonols,

---

ᵃThey are also named procyaniidins.

Table 8 Some of the most important clinical/epidemiological studies using vitamin C in cardiovascular disease

Study	Daily dose (mg)	Duration	N and sex	Outcome	Reference
MGH	200	6 mo	538 M–F	No activity on mortality in a geriatric hospital	(150)
SOP	50[a]	2 yr	297 M–F	No activity	(151)
VCS	200	6 mo	199 M–F	Moderate dose of vitamin C reduce the severity of the respiratory infections in geriatric patients	(152)
Almeda[b]	>250 <250	10 yr	3119 M–F	No activity	(153)
EVCS	<28 >45	20 yr	730 M–F	Reduction of stroke in the highest tertile No activity on coronary disease	(154)
Linxian[c]	180[c]	5 yr	29,584 M–F	No reduction of stroke	(155)
NHANES I	>50[d]	6.1 yr	11,348 M–F	Inverse correlation with all cause death, cancer, and cardiovascular disease	(54)
IWHS-D[e]	0>300[f]	15 yr	1923 F	>300 mg increase cardiovascular mortality in postmenopausal women with diabetes	(156)
PSCHD[g]	<93 >359	8 yr	87,245 F	Reduction of the risk of coronary heart disease in women	(157)
CPIHD	<37 >67	5 yr	2512 M	Trend of reduction of ischemic heart disease	(158)
MRCT	<70 >94	4.4 yr	1412 M–F	Low blood vitamin C concentration in the older British population are strongly predictive of mortality	(159)
CA	<56 >982	3 yr	4989 M	Reduction of intima thickness	(160)
CA	<64 >728	3 yr	6318 F	Reduction of intima thickness	(160)

[a]The initial dosage was 150 mg a day for 12 weeks followed by 50 mg/day.
[b]Alameda County, California, 250 mg of intake was taken as a cutoff.
[c]Linxian in China, association of vitamin C and molybdenum.
[d]Cutoff was .50 mg (by diet or supplement), vitamin E intake was not considered.
[e]Only women with diabetes were considered.
[f]Quintiles from 0 to .300 mg as supplements.
[g]In female nurses.
Abbreviations: CA, carotid atherosclerosis; CPIHD, Caerphilly Prospective Ischemic Heart Disease; EVCS, Elderly Vitamin C Status; IWHS-D, Lowa Women's Health Study; MGH, Mortality in a Geriatric Hospital; MRCT, Medical Research Council Trial; NAHNES I, National Health and Nutrition Examination Survey; PSCHD, Prospective Study of vitamin C in Coronary Heart Disease; SOP, Supplementation Old People; VCS, Vitamin C Supplementation.

flavones, and isoflavones, which have in common only a three-ring structure and are differentiated among them by the composition of the middle ring.

Plant foods contain a variety of PPs that are regarded as active agents and particularly as antioxidants. The chemical structures are quite complex and there are relatively small molecules such as hydrocinnamic acids (caffeic acid and ferulic acid) and also extremely large molecules like the proantho-cyanidins, which are known as condensed tannins (responsible for the astringent character of fruit).

Flavonoids are present in nature as glycosides, which means that different types of sugar are linked to the molecule, which during the metabolic/absorption processes are hydrolyzed generating the respective aglycone. Just for example, the difference between quercetin and rutin, which are among the most common flavonols, is the rutinose

Table 9   Different types of polyphenols and some of the relative sources

Class of polyphenol	Name of the product	Source
Hydroxy benzoic acid	Hydroxibenzoic acid Protochatecuic acid Gallic acid p-Hydroxibenzoic acid	Blackberry, raspberry, black currant, strawberry
Hydrocinnamic acid	Hydrocinnamic acid Caffeic acid Chlorogenic acid Cumaric acid Ferulic acid Sinapic acid	Blueberry, kiwi, cherry, plum, apple, pear, chicory, artichoke, aubergine
Anthocyanidins	Cyanidin Pelargonidin Peonidin Delphinidin Malvidin Petunidin	Blackberry, black currant, blueberry, black grape, cherry, rhubarb, red wine, tea, strawberries
Flavonols	Quercetin Rutin Kaempferol Myricetin	Yellow onions, curly kale, broccoli, blueberry, black tea, green tea
Flavones	Apigenin Luteolin Chrysin	Parsley, celery
Flavanones	Hesperidin Naringenin Eriodictyol Taxifolin Fisetin	Citrus fruit, orange juice, grapefruit juice, lemon
Isoflavones	Daidzein Genistein Glycitein	Soy flour, soybeans boiled, tofu, soy milk
Monomeric flavanols	Catechin Epicatechin	Chocolate, beans, apricot, green tea, black tea, red wine

(disaccharide containing glucose and ramnose) that is contained in rutin only. However, the most commonly known and tested PPs are included in the following eight classes: hydrocinnamic acids, hydrobenzoic acid, anthocyanidins, flavonols, flavanones, flavanols (cathechins and proanthocyanidins), and isoflavones.

The same fruit or vegetable may contain different types of PP and Table 9 gives an idea on how complex it can be to determine what kind of single polyphenol is responsible for a given "healthy" claim.

As a class, PPs are considered active as antioxidant, antithrombogenic, and anti-inflammatory compounds. Many of them show an in vitro activity as scavengers of a wide range of RS, and also show inhibition of cycloxygenase and lipoxygenase (59,60), xantine oxidase (61), metalloproteases (62), and angiotensin II converting enzyme (63). All these activities are compatible with a reduction of the cell reactivity. However, they are essentially xenobiotics, and the cytotoxic effects have been observed in vitro and in vivo. The antioxidant activity is due either to a direct scavenging activity or, at least for some of them, to the chelation of transition metals that can inhibit the Fenton's reaction (64,65). Furthermore, in vivo activity as antioxidants is very contradictory. There are studies where F2 isoprostanes are not modified by PP rich dietary intake (66–68), and others that show some activity (69). Other markers such as MDA and 8OHdG (70,71) were reduced using green tea as a source of PP. Clearly, the activity in vivo may depend on the type of food containing them and on the bioavailability of the compounds, and also on the biomarker used to determine the activity (66–71).

In some case, in vitro activity does not give a complete view of the activity of these products. In wine for instance, the process of fermentation generates esters of PP (72), which may allow an increase of the absorption of the compound in the gut. The subsequent hydrolysis will make the product available for the activity, whereas in vitro this activity can be masked.

> This is also true for fruit, vegetables, and tea because the maturation and fermentation processes may modify the bioavailability of the PP contained in the food or beverage.

Furthermore, metabolites generated either by the intestinal flora (73) or by the liver metabolism may have similar activity and longer half-life.

Several studies have shown the bioavailability of PP (16,74), which indicates that, in general, plasma concentration is relatively low, in the range of few μmol/L at the best, and the most well absorbed are isoflavones and gallic acid, followed by catechins, flavanones, and quercetin with a maximum concentration reached being between one and five hours, depending on the site of absorption. The tendency to accumulate is not evident for the parent compounds but could be the case of some metabolites.

PPs have been studied in many epidemiological studies conducted in Finland, United States, United Kingdom, and Netherlands, which addressed mainly the cardiovascular diseases and cancer.

The list of the studies is reported in Table 10.

In the Finnish Mobile Clinic examination there was an inverse relation between the dietary intake of some flavonoids and the incidence of several chronic diseases. The positive outcome was related to the consumption of apples. The authors concluded, "although our finding was independent of the intake of antioxidant vitamins, the potential

Table 10 Epidemiological studies on dietary polyphenols

Study	Type of polyphenol	Duration (yr)	N and sex	Outcome	Reference
FMC[a]	Flavonols Flavones Flavanones	24–26–28	9131 M–F	Reduction of total mortality, lung cancer, prostate cancer arthritis, asthma, coronary heart disease	(161–163)
Zuphten	Catechins Flavonols	10	806 M	Reduction of ischemic heart disease and stroke	(164–166)
ATBC	Flavones Flavonols	6.1	25,732 M	Reduction of fatal myocardial infarction, no reduction of stroke	(167,168)
ATBC[a]	Flavonols Flavones	6.1	27,110 M	Reduction of lung cancer	(169)
IWHS	Catechins Flavonols Flavones	13	32,857 F	Reduction of coronary heart disease, no reduction of stroke, reduction of rectal cancer	(170–173)
WHS	Flavanols Flavones	6.9	38,445 F	No association with reduction of cardiovascular disease	(174)
Caerphilly	Flavonols	14	1900 M	Increase of total mortality	(175)
Rotterdam	Flavonols	5.6	4807 M–F	Reduction of ischemic heart disease	(176)
HPFS	Flavonols Flavones	6	34,789 M	No activity in cardiovascular disease or cancer; activity on patients with established coronary disease is not excluded	(123,177)
FD	Flavanols	5	1376 M–F	Flavonoids intake is inversely related to the risk of dementia	(178)

[a]Studies characterized by analysis of different quality of flavonoids or conducted on a different number of eligible cases or with different follow-up.
Abbreviations: ATBC, α-Tocopherol β-Carotene Cancer prevention; Caerphilly, Welsh country study- Europe; FD, Flavonoids and Dementia; FMC, Finnish Mobile Clinical examination; HPFS, Health Professional Follow-up Study; IWHS, Iowa Women's Health Study; Rotterdam, Nederland-Europe; WHS, Women's Health Study—female health professional, postmenopausal, or not intending to become pregnant; Zuphten, was part of the Seven Country Study on the relationship between food and chronic diseases.

importance of other biological active compounds in fruit and vegetables on the relation cannot be excluded."

This last statement summarizes the entire story, in fact, going through all the data reported in the publications listed in Table 10, it is quite common to realize that those subjects consuming high quantities of flavonoids concomitantly were consuming less alcohol, and/or less saturated fats, and/or more vitamin E and C, and/or smoking was less frequent. In general, this denotes a more "healthy" way of living. The type of job and social/ economic conditions can be some times more important than coffee or apples. In a survey on Metabolic Syndrome (data on file) with a mobile unit, it was evident that scolarity has the same important of the diet scolarity.

From the data as a whole, it appears that flavonoids do not have a negative impact on health, and some positive outcome was found. However, it is very hard to state which flavonoid is responsible for positive effects. No epidemiological data on supplements are available. A long-term study on chronic venous insufficiency (CVI) showed that high dosages of an herbal medicine containing mainly quercetin were effective in the treatment of mild CVI (75).

There are many intervention studies in the literature that demonstrate significant biological effect of PP (76) such as improvement of plasma lipid profile, platelet aggregation, and blood pressure. However, they never have been tested as a therapy for a well-defined disease. A complete review of the most important epidemiological trials on PP is also available (77).

As for the other antioxidants, the suggestion is to avoid high dosages of PP. Particularly, for supplements the dosage should not exceed 25 to 50 mg/day for any type of PP, and those derived from common fruits and vegetables are recommended.

Selenium

Se is an essential trace element capable of exerting multiple actions in the body. At least 30 different selenoproteins are described (78) many of which have clearly defined functions such as glutathione peroxidase (GPXs) and thioredoxin reductase (TRs), which are among the most important antioxidant enzymes. One of the intriguing aspects of Se is why it has to be present in the prosthetic part of the enzymes or in GSH (glutation) forming, together with L-cystein—the selenocystein. In drosophila, the enzyme that is involved in similar types of reaction does not contain Se but the pH range of the optimal reaction is more restricted. Consequently, having Se in the molecule may constitute a genetic advantage.

One of the major roles of the Se-containing enzymes GPXs and TRs is to protect cells from the H_2O_2.

Se is involved in cell growth and control of the selenoprotein expression. A limited or insufficient supply of Se can be

the cause of several diseases and particular attention has be given to cancer. However, an upregulation of selenoproteins in case of a normal function of the antioxidant system may end up with a profound disregulation.

The first suggestion that Se might be anticarcinogenic was based on the inverse relationship of cancer mortality rates and forage crop content in the United States (79).

Since this first observation a large scientific body was generated, which indicates that Se may prevent cancer (80,81).

Mean serum levels in a survey in Finland were found to be around 60 ng/mL. Lower levels of blood Se were found in subjects with cancer (82–84) than in matched control, particularly in those cases on the lowest quintiles or deciles. In Northwest Washington State (85) and in men of Japanese ancestry in Hawaii (86) no relationship was found with cancer, and probably to be significant other concomitant factors have to be present.

A tentative trial to correlate toenail Se level and cancer was conducted in 62,461 women participating in the NHS and the results indicate that there was no inverse correlation between cancer and toenail level (87).

In a pooled analysis (88) of three studies (Wheat Bran Fiber Trial; Polyp Prevention Trial; Polyp Prevention Study) subjects with colorectal adenoma and Se levels in the highest quartile (median 150 ng/mL) had significant lower odds of developing new adenoma compared with those in the lowest quartile (median 113 ng/mL).

In the United States, the RDA for Se is 55 μg. Estimated intakes of Se by most of U.S. residents exceed that value, whereas in Europe the daily intake is sometimes lower than 30 μg, and in some rural regions of China it is <10 μg (84). The reduced dietary intake has to be considered together with a possible polymorphism that may result in a different requirement of Se or with the loss of chromosomes encoding selenoproteins, during the transformation of a premalignant cell to the cancer cell (89). Se baseline levels of the subjects participating in clinical studies were very different (84) and consequently a fixed supplementation may end up with different outcomes.

Some large trials have been conducted in China (179), where the ground does not contain sufficient amounts of Se and foods do not allow for a sufficient daily intake. It may be logical that results cannot be transferred to subjects who are accustomed to higher Se levels.

Table 11 reports the summary of some of the most known epidemiological studies on Se.

The Nutritional Prevention Cancer study generates many debates (90) that are still pending and data have been re-analyzed many times. The most robust effect was the reduction of prostate cancer, mostly among subjects who entered the trial with plasma Se levels at the bottom of the tertile of the cohort (<106.4 ng/mL), whereas subjects entering in the highest tertile (>123.2 ng/mL) showed no significant treatment effect.

The indication that may come out from these studies is the same for β-carotene. In both cases to improve antioxidant

Table 11 Epidemiological studies on selenium

Study	Daily dose (μg)	Period (yr)	N and sex	Outcome	Reference
Qidong (China)	200	8	20,847 M–F	35% Reduction of primary liver cancer	(179,180)
Linxian[a] (China)	50	6	3318 M–F	No effect on esophageal cancer	(181)
Linxian[b] (China)	50	5.2	29,584 M–F	No reduction of esophageal cancer, reduction of cancer mortality, reduction of cerebrovascular disease only in man	(182,183)
India[c]	50–100	1	298 M	Reduction of precancerous oral lesions	(184)
NPC	200		1312 M–F	Reduction of total cancer and increase, reduction of prostatic and colon rectum cancer; increase of squamous cell carcinoma and nonmelanoma skin cancer	(185,186)

[a]Vitamins and minerals were also added.
[b]β-carotene and vitamin E were added.
[c]100 μg for six months followed by 50 μg.
Abbreviation: NPC, Nutritional Prevention Cancer on subjects with confirmed history of nonmelanoma skin cancer within the year before enrollment.

activity it is not necessary to give supplements at dosages higher than RDA.

Antioxidant combinations

The link between high fruit/vegetables intake and reduced chronic disease may be related to the antioxidant protection.

However, a 24-hour fasting substantially reduces OS, indicating that food of any type generates a balance between oxidants/antioxidants. In other terms, caloric intake per se is increasing the oxidation, whether through fruits, vegetables, or fats.

> A pool of antioxidant taken for a week at very low dosages (very close to RDA or even less) and in fluid form was shown to reduce OS in healthy volunteers (91).

A higher dosage of antioxidants or an increase of the intake of antioxidant with food was not modifying substantially the oxidative markers, despite a significant increase of α-tocopherol, carotenoids, and vitamin C in serum (92,93).

Long-term administration (between 12 and 36 months) of vitamin C and E alone or in combination at respective daily dosages of 500 and 182 mg (as RRRA acetate) were not capable of modifying the antioxidant capacity of plasma (94),

measured through the total peroxyl radical trapping. However, the lipoprotein resistance to oxidation was improved in the group taking the association of the two vitamins.

The plasma antioxidant capacity after intake of fruits, vegetables, beverages, and some other foods (95) was determined using the Ferric reducing ability test. The antioxidant capacity was significantly correlated to carotenes and, surprisingly, the single greatest contributor to the total antioxidant intake was coffee, with 68% of the total capacity, whereas tea, wine, fruits, and vegetables were between 2% and 9% only (96).

The studies considering the intake of the antioxidant vitamins in foods can only be related to the combination of many components, which are also represented by PPs.

Some of these studies that analyzed antioxidant vitamins in food are reported in Table 12 with the relevant outcome.

A pooled analysis (52) of nine studies (NHS was divided into two studies) reached the following conclusion: "The results suggest a reduced incidence of major events at high supplemental vitamin C intakes. The risk reduction at high vitamin E or carotenoid intakes appear small."

A further pool analysis of eight perspective studies (97) concluded that the combination of vitamin A and C intakes from food alone were inversely associated to lung cancer risk and multivitamins or specific supplements did not add any advantage. Dosages of vitamin C that were found to start the

Table 12   Some of the most important clinical/epidemiological studies related to antioxidant combinations in food

Study	Duration	N and sex	Outcome	Reference
HPFS[a]	3.5 yr	39,910 M	Reduction of coronary heart disease comparing quintiles of vitamin E	(123)
ARIC[a]	11 yr	13,136 M–F	Reduction of cholesterol, increase HDL cholesterol control of hypertension can lower atherosclerosis progression	(187)
ATBC[+]	6.1 yr	29,133 M	No reduction of the incidence of lung cancer among smokers with supplementation of α-tocopherol or β-carotene	(188)
AHS[+]	6 yr	30,516 M–F	Fruit consumption protects from lung cancer	(189)
ATBC 4[a,b]	6.1 yr	4739 M	The highest quintile of fiber intake (median 34.8 g/d) is related to a reduction of major coronary events	(190)
CNBSS[c]	13 yr	56,837 F	No association between dietary carotenoids intake and lung cancer risk	(145)
FMC[a,d]	14 yr	4697 M–F	Reduction of coronary heart disease comparing tertiles	(124)
GPS[a]	11 yr	1824 M–F	Hostility may be associated to the risk of myocardial infarction	(191)
HPFS[a,c,e]	3.5 yr	19,687 M	Reduction of coronary heart disease comparing quintiles of vitamin E; no reduction of risk of stroke	(123)
NHS[a]	12 yr	70,089 F	Vitamin E supplement is associated with a reduced risk of coronary heart disease.	(122)
NHS[c]	6 yr	83,234 F	Consumption of fruit and vegetables high in carotenoids and vitamins may reduce postmenopausal breast cancer	(192)
NHScf	12 yr	14,968 F	The use of specific vitamin E supplements but not specific vitamin C supplement may be relate to modest cognitive benefits in older women	(193)
NHS II	8 yr	90,655 F	No evidence that higher intakes of vitamin C and E and folatel in early adult life reduce risk of breast cancer. Vitamin A including carotenoids was associated with a reduced risk of breast cancer among smokers.	(194)
VIP[a]	Case-control	16,517 M–F	This study is part of the WHO for the monitoring trends and determinants in cardiovascular disease. Suggestion of reduction of major coronary events	(195)
EPESE	6 yr	11,178 M–F	Simultaneous use of vitamin E and C is associated with a lower risk of total mortality; use of vitamin E reduces the risk of total mortality	(196)
WECS	24 yr	1556 M	Less coronary artery disease due to vitamin C > 113 mg	(197)
IWHS[+]	7 yr	34,486 F	Reduction of risk of death for coronary heart disease, the activity was determined by vitamin E not taken as a supplement; no activity was associated with vitamin A and C	(147,198)
CVCEE	10 yr	725 M–F	Reduction of cardiovascular disease	(199)
AHS[a]	5 yr	9364 M–F	Frequent consumption of nuts (containing vitamin E) protects against coronary heart disease	(200)
Rotterdam	6 yr	5395 M–F	High intakes of vitamin E and C are associated with a lower risk of Alzheimer disease; activity is more evident in smokers; high intakes of β-carotene may protect against cardiovascular disease	(201,202)
NECSSo	Case-control	2577 F	Higher intake of total vegetables and supplementation of vitamin E, B-complex vitamins and β-carotene protect from ovarian cancer	(203)
FMCHESd	23 yr	4304 M–F	Diabetes type 2 is reduced by the intake of vitamin E in the diet; no association was evident with vitamin C	(204)
SUVIMAX	7.5 yr	13,017 M–F	Antioxidant supplementation reduces the risk of cancer in man; no risk reduction in women. The baseline β-carotene and vitamin C status was lower in men than in women.	(205)

(Continued)

Table 12   Some of the most important clinical/epidemiological studies related to antioxidant combinations in food (*Continued*)

Study	Duration	N and sex	Outcome	Reference
SUVIMAX1	7.5 yr	1162 M–F	No activity on carotid atherosclerosis and arterial stiffness	(206)
ARCSd	6 yr	1353 M–F	No relation between diabetic retinopathy and intake of vitamin E and C from food and from food and supplements combined.	(207)
CCS	Case-control	4750 M–F	Use of vitamin E and C supplements in combination reduces the prevalence of Alzheimer's disease	(208)
CARETa	4 yr	14,120	Reduction of lung cancer for the higher versus lowest quintile of fruit consumption	(209)
NHNES III	Case-control	15,317 M–F	Antioxidant vitamins may prevent hypertension	(210)
NHNES IIIc	Case-control	8808 M–F	Participants with metabolic syndrome had lower circulating concentrations of vitamin C and E, carotenoids (except lycopene) and retinyl esters	(211)
NCSDC[c,f]	6.3 yr	3405; 3692; 1074 M–F	Dietary or supplemental intake of vitamin A, C, E, folates and carotenoids are not associated with bladder risk of cancer; inverse association were found between the intake of vitamins, carotenoids, and dietary fibers and risk of gastric carcinoma; inverse association with lung cancer is found both for vegetables and fruit intake.	(148,212) (213)
ASAP	6 yr	520 M–F	Supplementation with combination of vitamin and slow release vitamin C slow down atherosclerotic progression in hypercholesterolemic persons	(214)
MRC/BHF	5 yr	20,536 MF	Among the high-risk individuals antioxidant vitamin supplementation did not produce any significant reduction in mortality, vascular disease, or cancer	(215)
AREDS	6.3 yr	4757 M–F	High-dose formulation of vitamin C, vitamin E, and β-carotene had no apparent effect on the risk of development or progression of age-related lens opacity or visual acuity loss	(216)

[a]Studies that entered the pooled analysis (51).

[b]Subjects receiving vitamin E or β-carotene supplements were excluded.

[c]Studies that entered the pooled analysis (96).

[d]Same data were reported for the activity of vitamin E (which reduced both in man and women the risk of coronary mortality).

[e]Was related to vitamin E intake but subjects were also taking carotenoids and vitamin C.

[f]Cases are a subcohort with 6.3 years follow up deriving from a total of 120,852 cases; 3405 cases for gastric carcinoma; 3692 cases for bladder cancer; 1074 cases for lung cancer.

Abbreviations: AHS, Adventist Health Study; ARCSd, Atherosclerosis Risk in Communities Study in the cohort of cases suffering from diabetes type 2 II; AREDS, Age-Related Eye Disease Study; ARIC, Atherosclerosis Risk in Communities; ASAP, Antioxidant Supplementation in Atherosclerotic Prevention study; ATBC, α-Tocopherol β-Carotene Cancer prevention; CARETa, β-Carotene And Retinol Efficacy Trial, the placebo arm; CCS, Cache County Study (Utah); CNBSS, Canadian National Breast Screening Study; CVCEE, Carotenoids, Vitamin C and E in Elderly; EPESE, Established Population Epidemiological Study of the Elderly; FMC, Finnish Mobile Clinic examination; FMCHESd, Finnish Mobile Clinic Health Examination Survey for dietary antioxidant intake and risk of diabetes type 2; GPS, Glostrup Population Study (Denmark); HPFS, Health Professional Follow-up Study; HPS, Health Professional Study; IWHS, Iowa Women Health Study; MCR/BHF, Medical Research Council/British Heart Foundation Heart Protection Study—randomized placebo-controlled trial; NCSDC, Nederland Cohort Study Diet and Cancer; NECSSo, Canadian National Enhanced Cancer Surveillance System, part related to the ovarian cancer; NHNES III, National Health and Nutrition Examination Survey; NHNES IIIc, National Health and Nutrition Examination Survey for the part related to circulating concentration of vitamin A, C, and E—retinyl esters, carotenoids, and selenium; NHS, Nurse Health Study; NHScf, a cohort of Nurse's Health Study to study cognitive function; NHS II, related to breast cancer risk (Since NHS has been in progress for many years different set of data were available.); SUVIMAX, Supplementation of Vitamins and Mineral Antioxidant; SUVIMAX1, structure and function of large arteries; VIP, Västerbotten Intervention Program—Sweden part of WHO MONICA project (monitoring trends and determinants in vascular disease); WECS, Western Electric Company Study.

risk reduction were >140 mg/day for men and >180 mg/day for women, whereas for vitamin E the more evident effect is between 9 and 15 mg/day for both genders.

In the combination of NHS (77,283 women) and HPFS (47,778 men) studies of higher fruits and vegetables intakes were associated with lower risk of lung cancer in women but not in men, although fruits and vegetables were protective in both men and women who never smoked (98).

The Medical Research Council/British Heart Foundation study controlled the activity of antioxidants in the protection of a large group of patients (10,629) suffering from coronary disease who were treated daily with vitamin supplementation (vitamin E 600 mg, vitamin C 250 mg, and β-carotene 20 mg). Similar high dosages were used in Age-Related Eye Disease Study (vitamin E 400 UI, vitamin C 500 mg, and β-carotene 15 mg). In both studies the results were not positive. In these last two studies as in any of the studies reported in Table 9 the OS was measured to determine the real need of an antioxidant therapy.

> With high dosages of antioxidants, whether derived from diet and/or supplements, the pro-oxidant condition that could further compromise the clinical condition of some patient cannot be excluded.

Conclusions

In general, the old trials ended up with positive results with the use of supplements, whereas the new more controlled trials showed an opposite outcome. This can be explained partially by the increase of food intake and consequently of antioxidants. The lack of positive effects in the more recent trials may also derive from a more appropriate methodology in conducting clinical and epidemiological studies.

However, the daily intake of antioxidants can be a key to interpretation of the discrepancies between "old" and "new" trials.

On the light of this consideration, the most important concept to underline for the antioxidants belongs to the "Nutritional Paradigm."

This concept is reported in Figure 2 and it is valid for every Element (E), whether macro element (proteins, fats, carbohydrates, etc.) or microelement (vitamins, minerals, trace minerals) of nutrition.

Each E, when the intake is null or insufficient, generates a disease. Increasing its quantity up to the required daily allowance (DA), the disease disappears. However, when E is given in excess it reaches the toxicity limit (TL). In case of vitamins and some minerals RDA are well defined, whereas TL is sometimes less clear, and the tendency is to misuse both in megadoses.

Furthermore, each DA and TL can be different in healthy people and in patients suffering from a given disease. These areas of uncertainty have generated the tendency to

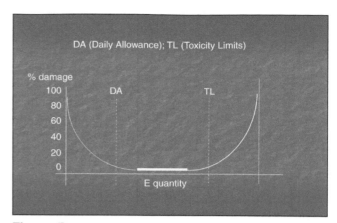

Figure 2
The nutritional paradigm.

increase dosages since the belief that "more is good" is prevailing, particularly in people who are oriented to self care.

Most of the epidemiological data presented in this chapter showed that high dosages of antioxidants are not active as preventive of chronic diseases, and the few positive results were found with moderation of the dosage and, particularly, by using a combination of products.

A single antioxidant given at high dosages may show some activity but not as antioxidant but for other reasons. For instance, high dosages of Vitamin E may increase fibrinolysis.

One of the major problems is the lack of a standard test to determine the OS. Despite the fact that they are not very precise, they still are the only possible tools to determine if an antioxidant treatment can be effective or not. Nobody would use an antihypertensive drug in case of a normal blood pressure. The same should be for antioxidant supplements, no matter which way they are combined.

The activity of fruits and vegetables for the prevention of cardiovascular disease and cancer indicates that only a combination of vitamins, minerals, and flavonoids taken in relatively low amounts can be considered active.

A few suggestions are emerging from all the data that have been analyzed in this chapter:

1. To counteract OS one should not use only one antioxidant at high dosages because the pro-oxidant activity may prevail over the antioxidant one.
2. It is better to use combinations of antioxidant and each product should be given in quantities close to the RDA or, in case the RDA is not determined, at dosages commonly taken with foods.
3. It is necessary to determine the OS in blood in order to avoid administering of antioxidants when is not necessary.
4. For the moment, the suggestion is to use more than one test to measure OS, because each test may address a different compartment of the oxidation. D-Roms test and F2 isoprostanes are recommended.

5. The increase of use of fruits and vegetables, or the moderate use of foods rich in antioxidants (such as extra virgin olive oil, tea, wine, coffee, black chocolate, etc.) can substitute for the use of supplement once OS is under control.

6. The change in eating habits reported in the previous point has to be monitored through the control of OS, particularly in patients suffering from chronic diseases.

7. The final sentence for antioxidants is very simple: . . . "take them if you need them."

Acknowledgment

The author is grateful to the American Journal of Clinical Nutrition who made available all the complete articles of the journal, free of charge and efficiently simply through the Internet connection.

References

1   Food and Nutrition Board, Institute of Medicine. Dietary Reference Intakes. Washington, DC: National Academy Press.

2   Comroe JH, Dripps RD, Dumke PR, Deming M. Oxygen toxicity. JAMA 1945; 128:707–710.

3   Nash G, Blennerhasset JB, Pontoppidan H. Pulmonary lesions associated with oxygen therapy and artificial ventilation. N Engl J Med 1967; 276:368–374.

4   Zitnanova I, Korytar P, Aruoma OI, et al. Uric acid and allantoin levels in Down syndrome: antioxidant and oxidative mechanism? Clin Chim Acta 2004; 341:139–146.

5   Das S, Engelman RM, Maulik N, Das DK. Angiotensin preconditioning of the heart evidence for redox signaling. Cell Biochem Biophys 2006; 44:103–110.

6   Hung YC, Hong MY, Huang GS. Cholesterol augments oxidative stress in macrophages. FEBS lett 2006; 580:849–861.

7   Cicco G, Panzera PC, Catalano G, Memeo V. Microcirculation and reperfusion injury in organ transplantation. Adv Exp Med Biol 2005; 566:563–573.

8   Campise M, Bamonti F, Novembrino C, et al. Oxidative stress in kidney transplantation. Transplantation 2003; 76:1474–1478.

9   Katz MA. The expanding role of oxygen free radicals in clinical medicine. West J Med 1986; 144:441–446.

10 Grisham MB. Oxidants and free radicals in inflammatory bowel disease. Lancet 1994; 344:859–861.

11 Stadtman ER, Oliver CN. Metal-catalyzed oxidation of proteins. J Biol Chem 1991; 266:2005–2008.

12 Halliwell B, Whiteman M. Measuring reactive species and oxidative damage in vivo and in cell culture: how should you do it and what do results mean? Br J Pharmac 2004; 142: 231–255.

13 Mayne ST. Antioxidant nutrients and chronic disease: use of biomarkers of exposure and oxidative stress status in epidemiological research. J Nutr 2003; 133:933S–940S.

14 Moison RM, de Baufort AJ, Haasnoot AA, et al. Uric acid and ascorbic acid redox ratio in plasma and tracheal aspirate of preterm babies with acute and chronic lung disease. Free Radic Biol Med 1997; 23:226–234.

15 Vertuani S, Angusti A, Manfredini S. The antioxidant and proantioxidant network. Curr Phamac Des 2004; 10:1677–1694.

16 Manach C, Scalbert A, Morand C, et al. Polyphenols: food sources and bioavailability. Am J Clin Nutr 2004; 79:727–747.

17 Carr AC, Zhu BZ, Frei B. Potential antiatherogenic mechanism of ascorbate (Vitamin C) and α-tocopherol (Vitamin E). Circ Res 2000; 87:349–354.

18 Diaz MN, Frei B, Vita JA, Keaney JF. Antioxidants and atherosclerotic heart disease. N Engl J Med 1997; 7:408–416.

19 Ervin RB, Wright JD, Wang CY, Kennedy-Stephenson J. Dietary intake of selected vitamins for the United States population: 1999–2000. Adv Data 2004: 339:1–8.

20 Masaki H, Okano Y, Ochiai Y, et al. Alpha-tocopherol increases the intracellular glutathione levels in HaCaT keratinocytes. Free Rad Res 2002; 36:705–709.

21 Colette C, Pare–Herbute N, Monnier LH, Cartry E. Platelet function in type 1 diabetes: effects of supplementation with large doses of vitamin E. Am J Clin Nutr 1998; 47:256–261.

22 Jandak J, Steiner M, Richardson PD. Alpha-tochopherol, an effective inhibitor of platelet adhesion. Blood 1989; 73:141–149.

23 Boskoboinik D, Szewozy KA, Hensey C, Azzi A. Inhibition of cell proliferation by alpha-tocopherol: role of protein kinase C. J Biol Chem 1991; 266:6188–6194.

24 Jialal I, Fuller CJ, Huet BA. The effect of α-tocopherol supplementation on LDL oxidation. Arteriosc Thromb Vasc Biol 1995; 15:190–198.

25 Bruijsse B, Feskens EJ, Schlettwein-Gsell D, et al. Plasma carotene and alpha-tocopherol in relation to 10-y all-cause and cause-specific mortality in European elderly: the Survey in Europe on Nutrition and Elderly, a Concerted Action (SENECA). Am J Clin Nutr 2005; 82:879–886.

26 Wu, K, Willet WC, Chan JM, et al. A prospective study on supplemental vitamin E intake and risk of colon cancer in women and man. Cancer Epidemiol Biomarkers Prev 2002; 11:1298–1304.

27 Vivekananthan DP, Penn MS, Saap KS, et al. Use of antioxidants vitamins for the prevention of cardiovascular disease: meta-analysis of randomized trials. Lancet 2003; 361:2017–2023.

28 Miller RE, Pastor-Barriuso R, Dalal D, et al. Meta-analysis: high-dosage vitamin E supplementation may increase all-cause mortality. Ann Intern Med 2005; 142:37–46.

29 Huang HY, Appel LJ. Supplementation of diets with alpha-tocopherol reduces serum concentration of γ- and δ-tocopherol in humans. J Nutr 2003; 133:3137–3140.

30 Van Haaften RI, Haenen GR, van Bladeren PJ, et al. Inhibition of various glutathione S-transpherase isoenzymes by RRR-alpha-tocopherol. Toxicol In Vitro 2003; 17:245–251.

31 Dowd P, Zheng ZB. On mechanism of the anticlotting action of vitamin E quinone. Proc Natl Acad Sci USA 1995; 92: 8171–8175.

32 Bowry VW, Stocker R. Tocopherol-mediated peroxidation: the prooxidant effect of vitamin E on the radical-initiated oxidation of human low density lipoprotein. 1993 J Am Chem Soc 1993; 115:6029–6044.

33 Neuzil J, Thomas SR, Stocker R. Requirement for, promotion, or inhibition by alpha-tocopherol of radical-induced initiation of plasma lipoprotein lipid peroxidation. Free Radic Biol Med 1997; 22:57–71.

34 Burton GW, Ingold KU. Beta-carotene: an unusual type of lipid antioxidant. Science 1984; 224:569–573.

35 Peto R, Doll R, Buckley JD Sporn MB. Can dietary β-carotene materially reduce human cancer rates? Nature 1981; 290: 201–208.

36 van Poppel G, Goldbohm RA. Epidemiological evidence for β-carotene and cancer prevention. Am J Clin Nutr 1995; 62:1393S–1402S.

37 Kardinaal AFM, Aro A, Kark JD, et al. Association between β-carotene and acute myocardial infarction depends on polyunsaturated fatty acid status. The EURAMIC study. Arteriosc Thromb Vasc Dis 1995; 15:726–732.

38 Morris D, Kritchevsky SB, Davis CE. Serum carotenoids and coronary heart disease. The Lipid Research Clinics Coronary Primary Prevention Trial and Follow-up Study. JAMA 1994; 272:1439–1441.

39 Hennekens CH, Buring JE, Manson JE, et al. Lack of effect of long-term supplementation with beta carotene on the incidence of malignant neoplasms and cardiovascular disease. N Engl J Med 1996; 334:1145–1149.

40 Hak AE, Stampfer MJ, Campos H, et al. Plasma carotenoids and tocopherol and risk of myocardial infarction in a low-risk population of US male physicians. Circulation 2003; 108:802–807.

41 Leppala JM, Virtamo J, Fogelholm R, et al. Controlled trial of alpha-tocopherol and beta-carotene supplements on stroke incidence and mortality in male smokers. Atherioscler Thromb Vasc Biol 2000; 20:250–235.

42 Männistö S, Smith-Warner SA, Spiegelman D, et al. Dietary carotenoids and risk of lung cancer in a pooled analysis of seven cohort studies. Cancer Epidemiol Biomarkers Prev 2004; 13:40–48.

43 Sesso H, Buring JE, Norkus EP, Gaziano JM. Plasma lycopene, other carotenoids, and retinol and the risk of cardiovascular disease in women. Am J Clin Nutr 2004; 79:47–53.

44 Sesso H, Buring JE, Norkus EP, Gaziano JM. Plasma lycopene, other carotenoids, and retinol and the risk of cardiovascular disease in man. Am J Clin Nutr 2005; 81:990–997.

45 Carr AC, Frei B. Towards a new recommended dietary allowance for vitamin C based on antioxidant and heath effects in humans. Am J Clin Nutr 1999; 69:1086–1107.

46 Bowry VW, Mohr D, Cleary J, Stocker R. Prevention of tocopherol-mediated peroxidation in ubiquinol-10-free human low density lipoprotein. J Biol Chem 1995; 270:5756–5763.

47 Ortwerth BJ, Chemoganskiy V, Mossine VV, Olesen PR. The effect of UVA light on the anaerobic oxidation of ascorbic acid and the glycation of proteins. Invest Ophthalmol Vis Sci 2003; 44:3094–3102.

48 Lenton KJ, Sané AT, Therriault H, et al. Vitamin C augments lymphocyte glutathione in subjects with ascorbate deficiency. Am J Clin Nutr 2003; 77:189–195.

49 Tannenbaum SR, Wishnok JS. Inhibition of nitrosamine formation by ascorbic acid. Ann NY Acad Sci 1987; 498:354–363.

50 Ness AR, Khaw KT, Bingham S, Day NE. Vitamin C status and serum lipids. Eur J Clin Nutr 1996; 50:724–729.

51 Khaw KT, Woodhose P. Interrelation of vitamin C, infection, hemostatic factors, and cardiovascular disease. BMJ 1995; 310:1559–1563.

52 Knekt P, Ritz J, Pereira MA, et al. Antioxidant vitamins and coronary heart disease risk: a pooled analysis of 9 cohort. Am J Clin Nutr 2004; 80:1508–1520.

53 Loria CM, Klag MJ, Caulfield LE, Whelton PK. Vitamin C status and mortality in US adults. Am J Clin Nutr 2000; 72:139–145.

54 Khaw K, Bingham S, Luben R, et al. Relation between plasma ascorbic acid and mortality in men and women in EPIC-Norfolk prospective study: a prospective population study. Lancet 2001; 357:657–663.

55 Ensrtom JE, Kanim LE, Klein MA. Vitamin C intake and mortality among a sample of United States population. Epidemiology 1992; 3:194–202.

56 Pandey DK, Shekelle R, Selwyn BJ, et al. Dietary vitamin C and β-carotene and risk of death in middle-aged men. Am J Epidemiol 1995; 142:1268–1278.

57 Kromhout D. Essential micronutrients in relation to carcinogenesis. Am J Clin Nutr 1987; 45:1361–1376.

58 Yong L, Brown CC, Schatzkin A, et al. Intake of vitamins E, C and A and risk of lung cancer. Am J Epidemiol 1997; 146:231–243.

59 Laughton MJ, Evans PJ, Moroney MA, et al. Inhibition of mammalian 5-lipoxygenase by flavonoids and phenolic dietary additives. Relationship to antioxidant activity and iron ion-reducing ability. Biochem Pharmacol 1991; 42:1673–1681.

60 Sadik, CD, Sies H, Schewe T. Inhibition of 15-lipoxigenase by flavonoids: structure-activity relation and mode of action. Biochem Pharmacol 2003; 65:773–781.

61 Van Hoorn DEC, Nijveldt RJ, Van Leewen PAM, et al. Accurate prediction of xantine oxidase inhibition based on the structure of flavonoids. Eur J Pharmacol 2002; 541:111–118.

62 Isemura M, Saeki K, Minami T, et al. Inhibition of matrix metalloproteinases by tea catechins and related polyphenols. Ann NY Acad Sci 1999; 878:629–631.

63 Actis-Goretta L, Ottaviani Ji, Keen CL, Fraga GC. Inhibition of angiotensin converting enzyme (ACE) activity by flavan-3-ols and procyanidins. FEBS Lett 2003; 555:597–600.

64 Silva MM, Santos MR, Caroco G, et al. Structure-antioxidant relationship of flavonoids: a reexamination. Free Radi Res 2002; 36:1219–1227.

65 Mira L, Fernandez MT, Santos M, et al. Interaction of flavonoids with iron and coppers ions: a mechanism for their antioxidant activity. Free Radic Res 2002; 36:1199–1208.

66 Abu-Amsha Caccetta R, Burke V, Mori TA, et al. Red wine polyphenols, in the absence of alcohol, reduce lipid peroxidative stress in smoking subjects. Free Radic Biol 2000; 30: 636–642.

67 Freese R, Basu S, Hietanen E, et al. Green tea extract decrease plasma malonilaldehyde concentration but does not affect other indicators of oxidative stress, nitric oxide production, or hemostatic factors during high-linolenic acid diet in healthy females. Eur J Nutr 1999; 38:149–157.

68 Hodgson JM, Croft KD, Mori TA, et al. Regular ingestion of tea does not inhibit in vivo lipid peroxidation in humans. J Nutr 2002; 131:55–58.

69 Wiseman H, O'Rilly JD, Aldercreutz H, et al. Isoflavone phytoestrogens consumed in soy decrease F(2)-isoprostane concentration and increase resistance of low-density lipoprotein to oxidation in humans. Am J Clin Nutr 2000; 72:395–400.

70 Klaunig JE, Xu Y, Han C, et al. The effect of tea consumption on oxidative stress in smokers and nonsmokers. Proc Soc Exp Biol Med 1999; 220:249–254.

71 Hakim IA, Harris RB, Brown S, et al. Effect of increased tea consumption on oxidative DNA damage among smokers: a randomized controlled study. J Nutr 2003; 133: 3303S–3309S.

72 Frega NG, Boselli E, Bendia E, et al. Ethyl caffeoate: liquid chromatography-tandem mass spectrometryc analysis in Verdicchio wine and effect on hepatic stellate cells and intracellular peroxidation. Analytica Chimica Acta 2006; 563:375–381.

73 Halliwell B, Rafer J, Jenner A. Health promotion by flavonoids, tocopherol, tocotrienols, and other phenols: direct or indirect effects? Antioxidant or not? Am J Clin Nutr 2005; 81:268S–276S.

74 Manach C, Williamson G, Morand C, et al. Bioavailability and bioefficacy of polyphenols in humans. I. Review on 97 bioavailability studies. Am J Clin Nutr 2005; 81:230S–242S.

75 Kiesewetter H, Koscienly J, Kalus U, et al. Efficacy of orally administered extract of red wine leaf as 195 (folia vitis viniferae) in chronic venous insufficiency (stages I-II). A randomized, double blind, placebo-controlled trial. Arzneimittelforshung 2000; 50:109–117.

76 Williamson G, Manach C. Bioavailability and efficacy of polyphenols in humans. II. Review of 93 intervention studies. Am J Clin Nutr 2005; 81:243S–255S.

77 Arts JCW, Hollman PCH. Polyphenols and disease risk in epidemiological studies. Am J Clin Nutr 2005; 81:317S–325S.

78 Beckett GI, Arthur JR. Selenium and endocrine system. J Endocrinol 2005; 184:455–456.

79 Shamberger R, Frost RJ. Possible protective effect of selenium against human cancer. Can Med Assoc 1969; 104:82–84.

80 Combs GF, Gray WP. Chemopreventive agents: selenium. Pharmacol Ther 1998; 79:179–192.

81 Whanger PD. Selenium and its relationship to cancer: an update dagger. Br J Nutr 2004; 91:11–28.

82 Knekt P, Aromaa A, Maatela J, et al. Serum selenium and subsequent risk of cancer among Finnish men and women. J Natl Cancer Inst 1990; 82:864–868.

83 Willet WC, Polk BF, Morris JS, et al. Prediagnostic serum selenium and risk of cancer. Lancet 1983; 2:130–134.

84 Xia J, Hill KE, Byrne DW, et al. Effectiveness of selenium supplements in a low-selenium area of China. Am J Clin Nutr 2005; 81:829–834.

85 Coates RJ, Weiss NS, Daling JR, et al. Serum levels of selenium and retinol and the subsequent risk of cancer. Am J Epidemiol 1988; 128:515–523.

86 Nomura A, Heilbrun LK, Morris JS, Stemmermann GN. Serum selenium and the risk of cancer, by specific sites: case-control analysis of prospective data. J Natl Cancer Inst 1987; 79:103–108.

87 Garland M, Morris JS, Stampfer MJ, et al. Prospective study of toenail selenium level and cancer among women. J Natl Cancer Inst 1995; 87:473–475.

88 Jacobs ET, Jiang R, Alberts DS, et al. Selenium and colorectal adenoma: results of a pooled analysis. J Natl Cancer Inst 2004; 96:1669–1675.

89 Diwadkar-Navsariwala V, Diamond AM. The link between selenium and chemioprevention: a case for selenoproteins. J Nutr 2004; 134:2899–2902.

90 Combs GF. Current evidence and research needs to support a Health claim for selenium and cancer prevention. J Nutr 2005; 135:343–347.

91 Cornelli U, Terranova R, Luca S, et al. Bioavailability and antioxidant activity of some food supplements in man and women using D-Roms test as a marker of oxidative stress. J Nutr 2001; 131:3208–3211.

92 Nelson J, Berstein PS, Schmidt MC, et al. Dietary modification and moderate antioxidant supplementation differentially affect serum carotenoids, antioxidant levels and markers of oxidative stress in older humans. J Nutr 2003; 3117–3123.

93 Jacob RA, Aiello GM, Stephensen CB, et al. Moderate antioxidant supplementation has no effect on biomarkers of oxidant damage in healthy men with low fruit and vegetable intakes. J Nutr 2003; 133:740–743.

94 Porkkala-Sarataho E, Salonen TJ, Nyyssönen K, et al. Long-term effects of vitamin E, vitamin C, and combined supplementation on urinary 7-hydro-8-Oxo-2'-deoxyguanosine, serum cholesterol oxidation products, and oxidation resistance of lipids in nondepleted men. Arterioscler Thromb Vasc Biol 2000; 20:2087–2093.

95 Halvorsen BL, Holte K, Mari CW, et al. A systematic screening of total antioxidant in dietary plants. J Nutr 2002; 132: 461–471.

96 Svilaas A, Sakhi AK, Frost Andersen L, et al. Intakes of antioxidant in coffee, wine, and vegetables are correlated with plasma carotenoids in humans. J Nutr 2004; 134:562–567.

97 Cho E, Hunter D, Spieglmann D, et al. Intakes of vitamin A, C and E and folate and miltivitamins and lung cancer: a pooled analysis of 8 prospective studies. Int J Cancer 2006; 118:970–978.

98 Feskanich D, Ziegler RG, Michaud DS, et al. Prospective study of fruit and vegetable consumption and risk of lung cancer among men and women. J Natl Can Inst 2000; 92:1812–1823.

99 Dizdaroglu M, Jaruga P, Birincioglu M, Rodriguex H. Free radical-induced damage to DNA: mechanism and measurement. Free Radic Biol Med 2002; 32:1102–1115.

100 Chevion M, Berenshtein E, Stadtman ER. Human studies related to protein oxidation: protein carbonyl content as a marker of damage. Free Rad Res 2000; 33:S99–S108.

101 Cesarone MR, Belcaro G, Carratelli M, et al. A simple test to monitor oxidative stress. Int Angiol 1999; 18:127–130.

102 Schimke I, Kahl PE, Romaniuk P, Papies B. Concentration of thiobarbituric acid reactive substances (TBARS) in serum following myocardial infarction. Klin Wochenschr 1986; 64:1237–1239.

103 Lima ES, Di Mascio P, Rubbo H, Abdalla DS. Characterization of linoleic acid nitration in human blood plasma by mass spectrometry. Biochemistry 2002; 41:10717–10722.

104 Liu J, Yeo HC, Doniger SJ, Ames BN. Assay of aldehydes from lipid peroxidation: gaschromatography–mass spectrometry compared to thiobarbituric acid. Annal Biochem 1997; 245:161–166.

105 Lang J, Celotto C, Esterbauer H. Quantitative determination of the lipid peroxidation product 4–hydroxynonenal by high performance liquid chromatography. Anal Biochem 1985; 150:369–378.

106 Montuschi P, Barnes PJ, Roberts LJ. Isoprostanes markers and mediators of oxidative stress. FASEB 2004; 18:1791–1800.

107 Montine TJ, Quinn JF, Milatovic D, et al. Peripheral F2-isoprostanes and F-4 isoprostanes are not increased in Alzheimer's disease. Annal Neurol 2003; 53:175–179.

108 Varma SD, Devamanoharan PS. Excretion of hydrogen peroxide in human urine. Free Radic Res Commun 1990; 8: 73–78.

109 Knutson MD, Handelman GJ, Viteri FE. Methods for measuring ethane and pentane in expired air from rats and humans. Free Radic Biol Med 2000; 28:514–519.

110 Radi R, Peluffo G, Alvarez MN, et al. Unraveling peroxynitrite formation in biological systems. Free Radic Biol Med 2001; 30:463–468.

111 Clermont G, Vergely C, Jazayeri S, et al. Systemic free radical activation is a major event involved in myocardial oxidative stress related to cardiopulmonary bypass. Anesthesiology 2002; 96:80–87.

112 Ingelman–Sundberg M, Kaur H, Terelius Y, et al. Hydroxylation of salicilate by microsomial fraction and cytochrome P-450. Lack of production of 2,3-dihydroxybenzoate unless hydroxyl radical formation is permitted. Biochem J 1991; 276: 753–757.

113 Aejmelaeus RT, Holm P, Kaukine U, et al. Age-related changes in the peroxyl radical scavenging capacity of human plasma. Free Radic Biol Med 1997; 23:69–75.

114 Winston GW, Regoli F, Dugas AJ, et al. A rapid gas chromatographic assay for determining oxyradical scavenging capacity of antioxidants and biological fluids. Free Radic Biol Med 1998; 24:480–493.

115 Mikami T, Tomita S, Qu GJ, et al. Is allantoin in serum and urine a useful indicator of exercise-induced oxidative stress in humans? Free Radic Res Med 2000; 32:235–244.

116 Miller NJ, Rice-Evans C, Davies MJ, et al. A novel method for measuring antioxidant capacity and its application on monitoring the antioxidant status in premature neonates. Clin Sci 1993; 84:407–412.

117 Benzie IF, Strain JJ. Ferric reducing ability of plasma (FRAP) as a measure of "antioxidant power": the FRAP assay. Anal Biochem 1996; 239:70–76.

118 Cao G, Prior RL. Measurement of oxygen radical absorbance capacity in biological samples. Methods Enzymol 1999; 299: 50–62.

119 Schleiser K, Harwat M, Bohm V, Bitsch R. Assessment of antioxidant activity by using different in vitro methods. Free Radic Res 2002; 36:177–187.

120 Nakamura H, Vaage J, Valev, et al. Measurement of plasma glutaredoxin and thioredoxin in healthy volunteers and during open heart surgery. Free Radic Biol Med 1998; 24: 1176–1186.

121 Hirai N, Kawano H, Yasue H, et al. Attenuation of nitrate tolerance and oxidative stress by an angiotensin II receptor blocker in patients with coronary spastic angina. Circulation 2003; 108: 1446–1450.

122 Mathews CK, van Hole KE. Biochimica Casa Editrice Ambrosiana. Milano: Seconda edizione, 2002:525.

123 Stampfer MJ, Hennekens CH, Manson JE, et al. Vitamin E consumption and the risk of coronary disease in women. N Engl J Med 1993; 328:1444–1449.

124 Rimm EB, Stampfer MJ, Ascherio A, et al. Vitamin E consumption and risk of coronary heart disease in men. N Engl J Med 1993; 328:1450–1456.

125 Knekt P, Reunanen A, Jarvine R, et al. Antioxidant vitamin intake and coronary mortality in a longitudinal population study. Am J Epidemiol 1994; 138:1180–1189.

126 Sano M, Ernesto C, Thomas RG, et al. A controlled trial of selegiline, alpha–tocopherol, or both as treatment for Alzheimer's disease. N Engl J Med 1997; 336:1216–1222.

127 Törnwall ME, Vitamo J, Korkonen PA, et al. Effect of α-tocopherol and β-carotene supplementation on coronary heart disease during 6-year post-trial follow up in the ATBC study. Europ Heart J 2004; 25:1171–1178.

128 Albanes D, Heinonen OP, Huttunen JK, et al. Effects of alpha-tocopherol and beta-carotene supplements on cancer incidence in the Alpha-tocopherol Beta-carotene Cancer Prevention Study. Am J Clin Nutr 1995; 62:1427S–1430S.

129 The effect of vitamin E and beta-carotene in the incidence of lung cancer and other cancers in male smokers. The Alpha-tocopherol Beta-carotene Cancer Prevention Study. N Engl J Med 1994; 330:1029–1035.

130 Rapla JM, Virtamo J, Ripatti S, et al. Randomized trial of α-tocopherol and β-carotene supplements on incidence of major coronary events in men with previous myocardial infarction. Lancet 1997; 349:1715–1720.

131 Stephens NG, Parsons A, Schofield PM, et al. Randomized controlled trial of vitamin E in patients with coronary disease: Cambridge Heart Antioxidant Study (CHAOS). Lancet 1996; 347:781–786.

132 Boaz M, Smetana S, Weinstein T, et al. Secondary prevention with antioxidants of cardiovascular disease in endstage renal disease (SPACE): randomised placebo-controlled trial. Lancet 2000; 356:1213–1218.

133 Collaborative Group of the Primary Prevention Project. Low-dose aspirin and vitamin E in people at cardiovascular risk: a randomized trial in general practice. Lancet 2001; 357:89–95.

134 Yusuf S, Dagenais G, Pogue J, et al. Vitamin E supplementation and cardiovascular events in high-risk patients. The Heart Outcomes Prevention Evaluation Study Investigators. N Engl J Med 2000; 342:154–160.

135 Dietary supplementation with n-3 polyunsaturated fatty acids and vitamin E after myocardial infarction: results of the GISSI-Prevenzione trial. Gruppo Italiano per lo studio della sopravvivenza nell'infarto miocardico. Lancet 2001; 357: 447–455.

136 Hodis HN, Mack WJ, LaBree L, et al. Alpha-tocopherol supplementation in healthy individuals reduces low-density lipoprotein oxidation but not atherosclerosis. The Vitamin E Atherosclerosis Prevention Study (VEAPS). Circulation 2002; 106:1453–1459.

137 Mortality in DATATOP: a multicenter trial in early Parkinson's disease. Parkinson's Study group. Ann Neurol 1999; 43: 318–325.

138 McNeil JJ, Robman L, Tikellis G, et al. Vitamin E supplementation and cataract: randomized controlled trial. Ophthalmology 2004; 111:75–84.

139 Hirvonen T, Virtamo J, Korhonen P, et al. Intake of flavonoids, carotenoids, Vitamin C and E, and risk of stroke in male smokers. Stroke 2000; 31:2301–2306.

140 Holick CN, Michaud DS, Stolzenberg-Solomon R, et al. Dietary carotenoids, serum beta-carotene, and retinol and risk of lung cancer in the alpha-tocopherol, beta-carotene cohort study. Am J Epidemiol 2002; 156:536–547.

141 Greenberg ER, Baron JA, Stukel TA, et al. A clinical trial of beta carotene to prevent basal-cell and squamous-cell cancers of the skin. The Skin Cancer Prevention Study Group. N Engl J Med 1990; 323:789–795.

142 Omenn GS, Goodman GE, Thornquist MK, et al. Effects of combination of beta carotene and vitamin A on lung cancer

and cardiovascular disease. N Engl J Med 1996; 334: 1150–1155.

143 Schaumberg DA, Frieling UM, Rifai N, Cook N. No effect of β-carotene supplementation on risk of nonmelanoma skin cancer among men with low baseline plasma β-carotene. Cancer Epidemiol Biomarkers Prev 2004; 13:1079–1080.

144 Grobusch KK, Geleijnse JM, den Breijen JH, et al. Dietary antioxidants and risk of myocardial infarction in the elderly: the Rotterdam study. Am J Clin Nutr 1999; 69:261–266.

145 Rohan TE, Jain M, Howe GR, Miller AB. A cohort study of dietary carotenoids and lung risk in women (Canada). Cancer Causes Control 2002; 13:231–237.

146 Bandera EN, Freudenheim JL, Marshall JR, et al. Diet and alcohol consumption and lung cancer risk in the New York State Cohort (United States). Cancer Causes Control 1997; 8:828–840.

147 Steinmetz KA, Potter JD, Folsom AR. Vegetables, fruit, and lung cancer in the Iowa Women's Health Study. Cancer Res 1993; 53:536–543.

148 Voorrips LE, Goldbohm RA, Brants HAM, et al. A prospective cohort study on antioxidant and folate intake and male lung cancer risk. Cancer Epidemiol Biomarkers Prev 2000; 9:357–365.

149 Michaud DS, Feskanich D, Rimm EB, et al. Intake of specific carotenoids and risk of lung cancer in 2 prospective US cohort. Am J Clin Nutr 2000; 72:990–997.

150 Wilson TS, Datta SB, Murrell JS, Andrews CT. Relation of vitamin C levels to mortality in a geriatric hospital: a study on the effect of vitamin C administration. Age Ageing 1973; 2:163–171.

151 Burr ML, Hurley RJ, Sweetnam PM. Vitamin C supplementation of old people with low blood levels. Gerontol Clin 1975; 17:236–243.

152 Hunt C, Chakravorty NK, Annan G. The clinical and biochemical effects of vitamin C supplementation in short-stay hospitalized geriatric patients. Int J Vitam Nutr Res 1984; 54: 65–74.

153 Emsrtom JE, Kanin LE, Breslow L. The relationship between vitamin C intake, general health practices, and mortality in Alameda County, California. Am J Public Health.

154 Gale CR, Martyn CN, Winter PD, Cooper C. Vitamin C and risk of death from stroke and coronary heart disease in cohort of elderly people. BMJ 1995; 310:1563–1566.

155 Mark SD, Wang W, Fraumeni JF, et al. Do nutritional supplements lower the risk of stroke or hypertension? Epidemiology 1998; 9:9–15.

156 Lee D, Folson AR, Harnak L, et al. Does supplemental vitamin C increase cardiovascular disease risk in women with diabetes? Am J Clin Nutr 2004; 80:1194–1200.

157 Osganian SK, Stampfer MJ, Rimm E, et al. Vitamin C risk of coronary heart disease in women. J Am Coll Cardiol 2003; 42:246–252.

158 Fehily AM, Yarnell JW, Sweetnam PM, Eldwood PC. Diet and incidence ischaemic heart disease: the Caerphilly Study. Br J Nutr 1993; 69:303–314.

159 Fletcher AE, Breeze E, Shetty PS. Antioxidant vitamins and mortality in older persons: finding from the nutrition add-on study to the Medical Research Council Trial of Assessment and Management of Older People in the Community. Am J Clin Nutr 2003; 78:999–1010.

161 Knekt P, Kumpulainen J, Järvinen R, et al. Flavonoid intake and risk of chronic disease. Am J Clin Nutr 2002; 76: 560–568.

162 Knekt P, Jarvinen R, Reunanen A, Maatela J. Flavonoid intake and coronary mortality in Finland: a cohort study. BMJ 1996; 312:478–481.

163 Knekt P, Jarvinen R, Seppanen R, et al. Dietary flavonoids and the risk of lung cancer and other malignant neoplasms. Am J Epidemiol 1997; 146:223–230.

164 Arts JCW, Feskens EJM, Bas Bueno de Mesquita H, Kromhout D. Catechin intake might explain the inverse relation between tea consumption and ischemic heart disease: the Zutphen Elderly Study. Am J Clin Nutr 2001; 74:227–232.

165 Hertog MG, Feskens EJ, Hollman PC, et al. Dietary antioxidant flavonoids and risk of coronary heart disease: the Zutphen Elderly Study. Lancet 1993; 42:1007–1011.

166 Arts IC, Hollman PC, Bueno de Mesquita H, et al. Dietary catechins and epithelial cancer incidence: the Zutphen elderly study. Int J Cancer 2001; 92:298–302.

167 Hirvonen T, Pietinen P, Virtanen M, et al. Intake of flavonols and flavones and risk of coronary heart disease in male smokers. Epidemiology 2001; 12:62–67.

168 Hirvonen T, Virtamo J, Korhonen P, et al. Intake of flavonoids, carotenoids, vitamin C and E, and risk of stroke in male smokers. Stroke 2000; 31:2301–2306.

169 Hirvonen T, Vitamo J, Korhonen P, et al. Flavonol and flavone intake and the risk of cancer in male smokers. Cancer Causes Control 2001; 12:789–796.

170 Arts IC, Jacobs DR, Harnack LJ, et al. Dietary catechins in relation to coronary heart disease death among postmenopausal women. Epidemiology 2001; 12:668–675.

171 Yochum L, Kushi LH, Meyer K, Folsom AR. Dietary flavonoid intake and risk of cardiovascular disease in postmenopausal women. Am J Epidemiol 1999; 149:943–949.

172 Kushi L, Folsom AR, Prineas RJ, et al. Dietary antioxidant vitamins and death from coronary heart disease in postmenopausal women. N Eng J Med 1996; 334: 1156–1162.

173 Arts IC, Jacobs DR, Gross M, et al. Dietary catechins and cancer incidence among postmenopausal women: the Iowa Women's Health Study (United States). Cancer Causes Control 2002; 13:373–382.

174 Sesso HD, Gaziano JM, Liu S, Buring JE. Flavonoid intake and the risk of cardiovascular disease in women. Am J Clin Nutr 2003; 77:1400–1408.

175 Hertog MG, Sweetnam PM, Fehily AM, et al. Antioxidant flavonols and ischemic heart disease in a welsh population of men: the Caerphilly Study. Am J Clin Nutr 1997; 65: 1489–1494.

176 Geleijnse JM, Launer LJ, van der Kuip DAM, et al. Inverse association of tea and flavonoid intakes with incident myocardial infarction: the Rotterdam Study. Am J Clin Nutr 2002; 75:880–886.

177 Rimm EB, Katan MB, Ascherio A, et al. Relation between intake of flavonoids and risk for coronary heart disease in male health professionals. Ann Inter Med 1996; 125:384–389.

178 Commenges D, Scote V, Renaud S, et al. Intake of flavonoids and risk of dementia. Eur J Epidemiol 2000; 16:357–363.

179 Yu SY, Li WG. Protective role of selenium against B virus and primary liver cancer in Qidong. Biol Trace Elemen Res 1997; 56:117–124.

180 Yu SY, Li WG, Huang QS, et al. A preliminary report on the intervention trials of primary liver cancer in high-risk population

with nutritional supplementation of selenium in China. Biol Trace Elem Res 1991; 29:289–294.

181 Li JY, Taylor PR, Li B, et al. Nutrition intervention trial in Linxian, China: multiple vitamin/mineral supplementation, cancer incidence, and disease specific mortality among adults with esophageal displasia. J Natl Cancer Inst 1993; 85:1492–1498.

182 Blot WJ, Li YW, Taylor PR, et al. Nutrition intervention in Linxian, china: supplementation with specific vitamin/mineral combinations, cancer incidence, and disease specific mortality in the general population. J Natl Cancer Inst 1993; 85: 1483–1492.

183 Blot WJ, Li JY, Taylor PR, et al. The Linxian trials: mortality rates by vitamin-mineral intervention group. Am J Clin Nutr 1995; 62:1424S–1426S.

184 Krishnaswamy K, Prasad MP, Krishna TP, et al. A case study of nutrient intervention of oral precancerous lesions in India. Eur J Cancer oral Oncol 1995; 31:41–48.

185 Combs GF. Status of selenium in prostate cancer prevention. Br J Cancer 2004; 91:195–199.

186 Reid ME, Duffield-Lillico AJ, Garland L, et al. Selenium supplementation and lung cancer incidence: an update of the Nutritional Prevention Cancer Trial. Cancer Epidemiol Biomark Prev 2002; 11:1285–1291.

187 Chambless LE, Folsom AR, Davis V, et al. Risk factors progression of common carotid atherosclerosis: the Atherosclerotic Risk in Communities Study, 1987–1998. Am J Epidemiol 2002;155:38–47.

188 Albanes D, Heinonen OP, Taylor PR, et al. Alpha-Tocopherol and beta-carotene supplements and lung cancer incidence in the alpha-tocopherol, beta-carotene cancer prevention study: effect of base-line characteristics and study compliance. J Natl Cancer Inst 1996; 88:1560–1570.

189 Fraser GE, Beeson WL, Phillips RL. Diet and lung cancer in California Seventh-day Adventists. Am J Epidemiol 1991; 133:683–693.

190 Pietinen P, Rimm EB, Korkonen P, et al. Intake of dietary fiber and risk of coronary heart disease in a cohort of Finnish men. The Alpha-Tocopherol, Beta-Carotene Cancer Prevention Study. Circulation 1996; 94:2720–2727.

191 Barefoot JC, Larsen S, von der Lieth L, Schroll M. Hostility, incidence of acute myocardial infarction, and mortality in a sample of older Danish men and women. Am J Epidemiol 1995; 42:477–484.

192 Zhang S, Hunter DJ, Forman MR, et al. Dietary carotenoids and vitamin A, C, and E and risk of breast cancer. J Natl Cancer Inst 1999; 9:547–556.

193 Grodstein F, Chen J, Wllet WC. High-dose antioxidant supplements and cognitive function in community-dwelling elderly women. Am J Clin Nutr 2003; 77:975–984.

194 Cho E, Spigenman D, Hunter DJ, et al. Premenopausal intakes of vitamin A, C, and E, folate, and carotenoids, and risk of breast cancer. Cancer Epidemiol Biomarkers Prev 2003; 12: 713–720.

195 The World Health Organization MONICA Project (monitoring trends and determinants in cardiovascular disease): a major international collaboration. WHO MONICA Project Principal Investigator. J Clin Epidemiol 1988; 41:105–114.

196 Losonczy KG, Harris TB, Havlik RJ. Vitamin E and vitamin C supplement use and risk of all-cause coronary heart disease

mortality in older persons: the Established Population for Epidemiologic Studies of the Elderly. Am J Cil Nutr 1996; 64: 190–196.

197 Pandet DK, Shekelle R, Selwyn BJ, et al. Dietary vitamin C and beta-carotene and risk of death in middle-aged men. The western Electric Study. Am J Epidemiol 1995; 142: 1269–1278.

198 Steinmetz KA, Potter JD, Folsom AR. Vegetables, fruits, and lung cancer in the Iowa Women's Health Study. Cancer Res 1993; 53:536–543.

199 Sahyoun NR, Jacques PF, Russell RM. Carotenoids, vitamin C and E, and mortality in a elderly population. Am J Epidemiol 1996; 144:501–511.

200 Fraser GE. Diet and coronary heart disease: beyond dietary fats and low-density-lipoprotein cholesterol. Am J Clin Nutr 1994; 59:1117S–1123S.

201 Klipstein-Grobush K, Gelejinse JM, den Breeijen JH, et al. Dietary antioxidants and risk of myocardial infarction in the elderly: the Rotterdam Study. Am J Clin Nutr 1999; 69:261–266.

202 Engelhart MJ, Geerlings MI, Ruitemberg A, et al. Dietary intake of antioxidants and risk of Alzheimer disease. JAMA 2002; 287: 3223–3229.

203 Pan SY, Ugnat AM, Mao Y, et al. A case-control study of diet and the risk of ovarian cancer. Cancer Epidemiol Biomarkers Prev 2004; 13:1521–1527.

204 Montonen J, Knekt P, Järvinen R, Reunanen A. Dietary antioxidant intake and risk of type II diabetes. Diabetes Care 2004; 27:362–366.

205 Hercberg S, Galan P, Preziosi S, et al. The SU.VI.MAX Study: a randomized, placebo-controlled trial of the health effects of antioxidant vitamins and minerals. Arch Intern Med 2004; 164: 2335–2342.

206 Zureik M, Galan P, Bertrais S, et al. Effect of long term daily low-dosage supplementation with antioxidants vitamins and minerals on structure and function of large arteries. Arterioscler Thromb Vasc Biol 2004; 24:1485–1491.

207 Millen AE, Klein R, Folsom AR, et al. Relation between intake of vitamin C and E and risk of diabetic retinopathy in the Atherosclerotic Risk in Communities Study. Am J Clin Nutr 2004; 79:865–873.

208 Zandi PP, Antony JC, Khachaturian AS, et al. Reduced risk of Alzheimer disease in users of antioxidant vitamin supplements: the Cache County Study. Arch Neurol 2004; 61: 82–88.

209 Neuhouser ML, Patterson RE, Thornquist MD, et al. Fruits and vegetables are associated with lower lung cancer risk only in the placebo arm of the beta-carotene and retinol efficacy trial (CARET). Cancer Epidemiol Biomarkers Prev 2003; 12:350–358.

210 Chen J, Hamm L, Batuman V, Whelton PK. Serum antioxidant vitamins and blood pressure in the United States population. Hypertension 2002; 40:810–816.

211 Ford ES, Mokdad AH, Giles WH, Brown DW. The metabolic syndrome and antioxidant concentrations. Finding from the third National Health and Nutrition Examination Survey. Diabetes 2003; 52:2346–2352.

212 Botterweck AA, van der Brandt PA, Goldbohm RA. Vitamins, carotenoids, dietary fiber, and the risk of gastric carcinoma: results from a prospective study after 6.3 years of follow-up. Cancer 2000; 88:743–748.

213 Zeegers MP, Goldbohm RA, van der Brandt PA. Are retinol, vitamin C, vitamin E, folate and carotene intake associated with bladder cancer risk? Result from Netherlands Cohort Study. Br J Cancer 2001; 85:977–983.

214 Salonen RM, Nyyssönen K, Kaikkonen J, et al. Six-years effect of combined vitamin C and E supplementation on atherosclerotic progression. The Antioxidant Supplementation on Atherosclerotic Progression. Circulation 2003; 107: 947–953.

215 MRC/BHF Heart Protection Study on antioxidant vitamin supplementation in 20536 high-risk individuals: a randomized placebo-controlled trial. Lancet 2002; 360: 23–33.

216 A randomized, placebo-controlled, clinical trial of high-dose supplementation with vitamins C and E and beta carotene for age related cataract and vision loss: AREDS report no. 9. Arch Ophthalmol 2001; 119:1439–1452.

20

Iron chelation: deferoxamine and beyond

Valeri S. Chekanov

Introduction

Investigations have shown that iron may contribute to endothelial cell function and increase the risk of cardiovascular disease. It is believed that strong metal chelators such as deferoxamine (DFO) can counteract iron cation formation. The primary targets of iron chelators used for treating iron overload are prevention of iron ingress into tissues and its intracellular scavenging.

Iron

Body iron stores

An average adult human absorbs and excretes (in iron balance) ~1 mg of iron each day. Even slight disturbances in this balance may lead to general or local iron overload or iron deficiency. Iron is essential for all cells for heme synthesis and obtained from extracellular transferrin. Mitochondrial and extramitochondrial cytochromes, oxygen-storage proteins, and hemoglobin and myoglobin are needed in heme iron. The liver is adapted to store and release iron when needed. Normally, all cells regulate the suitable level of catalytically active iron pool during iron uptake, synthesis of iron-containing proteins, and iron release. Excess iron can interact with oxygen to form very toxic superoxide and hydroxyl radicals. Several points are important to cardiovascular pharmacology in the case of iron overload: damage of endothelium as a base for development of atherosclerosis and tissue ischemia, existence in the iron pool of a weakly bound low-molecular-weight iron complex, and the possibility of the iron chelating drugs (DFO) interacting with this chelatable iron.

Iron and endothelial function

Nonprotein-bound iron may directly inactivate endothelium-derived nitric oxide (1), depress endothelial dysfunction, and be a potential mechanism for iron-related cardiovascular disease (2). Because the endothelium participates in the release of several paracrine factors, including nitric oxide, it is critical in regulating vasomotor tone, platelet activity, leukocyte adhesion, vascular smooth muscle proliferation, and endothelial activation (3). Large amounts of immunoreactive ferritin are focally detected in atherosclerotic lesions, specifically in endothelium. Endothelial dysfunction could potentially explain the association between iron and cardiovascular events, because endothelial dysfunction is commonly present in patients with atherosclerosis (2,4).

Iron and cardiovascular disease

Body iron level and iron depletion play an important role in the gender differences seen in death from cardiac disease. There is a better correlation with heart disease mortality in iron levels compared with levels of cholesterol (5). It was found that risk of coronary heart disease (6) and carotid atherosclerosis (7) is associated with increased iron stores. However, impaired endothelium-derived nitric oxide activity may be without overt atherosclerosis in patients with risk factors and may be associated with the presence of atherosclerosis (4). Thus, endothelial dysfunction related to iron activity not only may be an early marker for cardiovascular risk but also may contribute to the pathogenesis of atherosclerosis (2) by the stimulation of low-density lipoproteins (LDL) and membrane lipid peroxidation (1) and may be a key to the understanding of early mechanism in the development of atheroma (7,8). Nakayama et al. (9) showed the role of heme oxygenase induction in the modulation of macrophage activation in atherosclerosis. However, Howes et al. (10) concludes that at the moment, the available evidence on iron hypothesis remains circumstantial. Moreover, Kiechl et al. (7) showed that the adverse effect of iron is hypercholesterolemia. In patients referred for coronary angiography, higher ferritin concentration and transferrin saturation levels were not associated with an increased extent of coronary atherosclerosis (11). Results of Hetet et al. (12) do not support the hypothesis that reduced body iron stores lower coronary heart disease risk. Minqin et al. (13) and You et al. (14) confirm the role of iron in damage and progression of this disease. Stadler et al. (15) showed that cholesterol levels correlated positively with iron accumulation and that iron may contribute to disease progression. It is believed that myocardial iron deposition and the resultant cardiomyopathy only occurs in the presence of severe liver iron overload (16). A lower concentration of vitamin C and higher levels of labile iron pool may create an environment that promotes the development of atherosclerosis (17). A relationship between serum ferritin levels and carotid atherosclerosis in clinic was confirmed by Wolff et al. (18).

Pharmacology of deferoxamine

Structure and chemistry

DFO is an iron-chelating agent with a molecular weight of 657. Acetic acid, succinic acid, and 1-amino-5-hydroxylaminopentane are the three distinct moieties that compose DFO. They form an open-chain molecule with three amino groups and three hydroxamic acid groups. In each hydroxamic acid group, DFO has two coordination sites for iron (III) (six together). This hexadentate structure allows it to react with ferric ion, its chain structure entwining completely around the central ferric ion (19). As a result, the very stable (and protected from enzymatic degradation) DFO–iron complex (ferrioxamine) is formed. It is very important that other metal ions have no affinity to DFO and the treatment with DFO did not result in the depletion of other important metal ions from the body (19). For clinical treatment, DFO mesylate is used in sterile, lyophilized form (500 mg or 2 g in sterile, lyophilized form). DFO mesylate is a white powder, freely soluble in water. DFO mesylate is N-[5-[3-[(5-aminopentyl)hydroxycarbamoyl]propionamido]pentyl]-3-[[5-(N-hydroxyacetamido)pentyl]carbamoyl] pro-pionohydroxamic acid mono- methanesulfonate (salt), and its structured formula of deferoxamine mesylate is shown in Figure 1.

Clinical pharmacology

The mechanism of action of DFO is the formation of a stable complex with iron. It prevents the iron from entering into further chemical reactions. It is important that DFO chelates iron from hemosiderin and ferritin, but not from transferrin. It does not bind with the iron from hemoglobin and cytochromes. It is theorized that DFO is metabolized by plasma enzymes. The chelate is soluble in water and passed easily through the kidney (reddish color of urine).

Plasma pharmacokinetics

DFO may easily be absorbed from the gut and parenteral use is very efficient. If administered intravenously, DFO is eliminated from the systemic circulation very rapidly and in a biphasic manner (19). Both DFO and its major metabolites are cleared by the kidney and liver. However, ferrioxamine (DFO–iron complex) is cleared exclusively by the kidneys (19) and in the case of renal disease may accumulate in plasma and must be eliminated by dialysis.

Access to chelatable iron pools

The majority of body iron is not chelatable (iron from cytochromes and hemoglobin). There are two major pools of chelatable iron by DFO (19). The first is that delivered from the breakdown of red cells by macrophages. DFO competes with transferrin for iron released from macrophages. DFO will also compete with other plasma proteins for this iron, when transferrin becomes saturated in iron overload. The quantity of chelatable iron from this turnover is 20 mg/day in healthy individuals and iron chelated from this pool is excreted in the urine (19). The second major pool of iron available to DFO is derived from the breakdown of ferritin and hemosiderin. The ferritin is catabolized every 72 hours in hepatocytes, predominantly within lysosomes (1). DFO can chelate iron that remains within lysosomes shortly after ferritin catabolism or once this iron reaches a dynamic, transiently chelatable, cytosolic low-molecular-weight iron pool (20). Cellular iron status, the rate of uptake of exogenous iron, and the rate of ferritin catabolism are influent on the level of a labile iron pool (21). Excess ferritin and

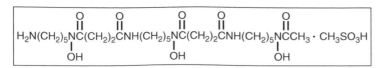

Figure 1
Structural formula of deferoxamine.

hemosiderin are turned over less often in myocytes than in the hepatocyte. This explains (16) why intensive chelation with DFO results in more rapid decrease in liver iron than in heart iron. Because of its hydrophilicity and relatively high molecular weight, DFO tends to move slowly across biomembranes. The rate of formation of intracellular iron chelate complexes is also slow (19). As a result, some nonheme-iron-containing enzymes (lipoxygenase) are not inhibited by DFO. Thus, the properties that limit DFO moving across biomembranes also limit access to metabolically important metal ion pools, thereby decreasing its potential toxicity (19).

Mechanism of action in myocardium

Anderson et al. (16) and Davis and Porter (19) believe that the more rapid chelation of the potentially toxic labile intracellular iron may explain the rapid reversal of cardiac dysarrhythmias and improvement in ventricular function with continuous DFO infusion, prior to achieving large decrements in myocardial iron. In experimental models, iron overload has been found to increase myocardial damage caused by anoxia and reperfusion, and the use of the iron chelator DFO resulted in a decrease in myocardial damage and protection of myocardial performance (22). Moreover, DFO significantly improved systolic function in both newborn and adults hearts exposed to 40 minutes of ischemia (23). The findings from the study of Nicholson et al. (24) indicated that there is protection against ischemia–reperfusion injury when DFO is added to the cardioplegic solution.

Indication, contraindication, and usage
General indication

DFO is generally indicated for treatment of acute iron intoxication and chronic iron overload due to transfusion depended anemias (including thalassemia). DFO is not recommended in primary hemochromatosis (PDR).

Contraindications

DFO is contraindicated in patients with severe renal disease or anuria as both DFO and the iron chelate are excreted primarily by the kidney. During pregnancy, DFO should be used only if clearly indicated (PDR).

Warnings

DFO causes a number of allergic reactions, including pruritus, wheals, rash, and anaphylaxis. Other adverse effects include dysuria, abdominal discomfort, diarrhea, fever, leg cramps, and tachycardia. Ocular disturbances may occur over prolonged periods of DFO use, or at high doses, or in patients with low ferritin levels. These include blurring of vision, cataracts, visual loss, visual defects, impaired peripheral, color and night vision, optic neuritis, corneal opacities, and retinal pigmentary abnormalities. Rapid development of severe toxic retinopathy associated with continuous intravenous DFO infusion was reported by Lai et al. (25). Auditory disturbances may occur after long-term use of DFO, including tinnitus, hearing loss, and especially high-frequency sensorineural hearing loss. In most cases, both ocular and auditory disturbances are reversible upon immediate cessation of treatment (26). A "pulmonary syndrome" (tachypnea, hypoxemia, fever, eosinophilia) was reported after high-dose (10–25 mg/kg/hr) DFO (27).

Precautions and drug interactions

Impairment of cardiac function may follow concomitant treatment with DFO and high doses of vitamin C (>500 mg/day). However, when vitamin C was discontinued, cardiac function was reversible. Patients with iron overload usually become vitamin C deficient (iron oxidizes the vitamin). Vitamin C increases availability of iron for chelation. Therefore, vitamin C should not be given to patients with cardiac failure and started only after an initial month of regular treatment with DFO. Clinical monitoring of cardiac function is advisable during such combined therapy (PDR). Hypotension and shock have occurred in a few patients when DFO was administered by rapid intravenous injection. Thus, DFO should be given intramuscularly or by slow subcutaneous or intravenous infusion (PDR). Concurrent treatment with prochlorperazine (a phenothiazine derivative) may lead to temporary impairment of consciousness (PDR). In some patients, the following adverse reactions have been observed at the injection site: irritation, pain, burning, swelling, indurations, infiltration, pruritus, erythema, crust, vesicles, and local edema (PDR). Some patients with hypersensitivity reaction may experience the following: hypotension, shock, abdominal discomfort, diarrhea, vomiting, blood dyscrasia, leg cramps, dizziness, neuropathy, paresthesias, dysuria, and impaired renal function (PDR).

Overdosage

Signs and symptoms: hypotension, tachycardia, transient loss of vision, aphasia, agitation, nausea, pallor, central nervous system depression (including coma), bradycardia, and acute renal failure (PDR). There is no specific antidote. DFO should be discontinued immediately.

Dosage and administration

DFO is preferably dissolved by adding 5 mL of sterile water for injection to each 500 mg vial or 20 mL of sterile water for injection to each 2 g vial. DFO reconstituted for injection is for single-use only.

Acute iron intoxication

Intramuscular administration is preferred and should be used for all patients not in shock. The intravenous route should be used only for patients in a state of cardiovascular collapse and then only by slow infusion. The rate of infusion should not exceed 15 mg/kg/hr for the first 1000 mg administered. Subsequent IV dosing, if needed, must be at a slower rate, not to exceed 125 mg/hr.

Chronic iron overload

A daily dose of 500 to 1000 mg should be administrated intra-muscularly; in addition, 2000 mg should be administrated intravenously with each unit of blood, but separately from the blood. The rate of IV transfusion must not exceed 15 mg/kg/hr. The total daily dose 1000 mg in the absence of a transfusion, but may be upto 6000 mg if three or more units of blood are transfused. For subcutaneous administration, a daily dose of 1000 to 2000 mg should be used (20–40 mg/kg/day) over 8 to 24 hours (PDR).

Special application in cardiology

Experimental data

Atherosclerosis

In animal models of atherosclerosis, vascular iron deposit is closely related to the progression of atherosclerosis and LDL oxidation, and restriction in dietary iron intake leads to significant inhibition of lesion formation (8). DFO forms a stable complex with ferric iron and decreases its availability for the production of reactive-oxygen species (28). Moreover, in high concentration (>0.5 mmol/L), DFO may also scavenge reactive-oxygen species (28). Matthews et al. (29) confirmed that iron chelators possess antioxidant activity in vitro and may reduce atherogenesis in vivo. Recently, Minqin et al. (13) showed that the iron chelator inhibits atherosclerotic lesion development and decreases lesion iron concentrations in the cholesterol-fed rabbit.

Muscle tissue ischemia

During ischemia, iron is released from erythrocytes. This increased iron level is cytotoxic to the vascular endothelium and acts as a catalyst for reactive-oxygen metabolism (30). DFO has been shown recently to activate the angiogenesis response (31). Some investigations also showed that DFO is effective in treatment of ischemic syndromes (32,33). DFO may attenuate the deleterious effects of iron on muscular tissue and has protected human endothelial cells in vitro from reoxygenation injury (34). DFO has recently been shown to be active in the treatment of acute ischemic syndrome (35,36). For local treatment of ischemia, a combination of DFO with fibrin sealant shows promising results: fibrin enhances angiogenesis and serves as a vehicle for delivering angiogenic growth factors (36). Local DFO application may be used to successfully promote neovascularization of ischemic tissue and is sufficient to revascularize an ischemic lower limb without damaging ischemic tissue. Fibrin sealant can activate migration of endothelial cells, macrophages, and myofibroblasts toward treated ischemic tissue, serving as a temporary matrix for gradual development of granulation tissue that is characterized by a high degree of vascularity, resulting in a new vessel formation within a loose collagenous interstitium (33,36). Studies (37) have shown that adding vascular endothelial growth factor (VEGF) and fibroblast growth factor (FGF) to the fibrin network increases angiogenesis in ischemic tissue and promotes sprout formation through enhancing the effect of the fibroblasts, vascular smooth muscle cells (VSMCs), and pericytes. Intracellular iron chelation indirectly stimulates endothelial cell growth by increasing VEGF release by VSMCs (38). Recently, Ulubayram et al. (39) confirmed that gelatin-based, controlled-release systems could be improved and could be good candidates for the production of long-term DFO-carrying systems. When DFO in fibrin sealant was applied in the case of acute limb ischemia (femoral artery excision), both angiogenesis and arteriogenesis were affected (Fig. 2) (36). Initial evidence based on arteriography and histological (immunostaining) studies indicated that angiogenesis improved to compensate for diminished blood flow in the ischemic limb (i.e., more capillaries occupied the same percentage of area as before surgery or, in some cases, even more of the area) as did arteriogenesis (i.e., more newly developed arterioles or remodeled pre-existing ones grew to become large collateral arteries).

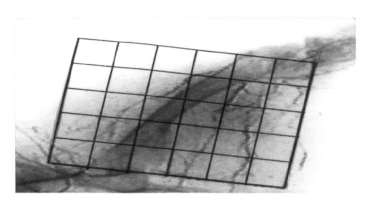

Figure 2

Angiogram one month after excision femoral artery and application deferoxamine in fibrin sealant. Many new collaterals formed to the distal part of femoral artery.

Protection from reperfusion injury

DFO is known to reduce the iron-dependent generation of toxic oxygen-derived radicals during reperfusion of ischemic tissue (40). It was shown experimentally that DFO reduces the early inflammatory reaction and improves myocardial microcirculation (41). Moreover, Dross et al. (42) showed that DFO's scavenging effect on superoxide anion could play a role in the cellular defense against oxygen radicals during cardiac operation.

Clinical evidence of cardioprotective effect

Reversal of established heart disease

In most cases, the reversal of symptomatic myocardiopathy has been achieved without drug toxicity (19,43). Davis and Porter (19) and Tsironi et al. (44) confirmed clinically the laboratory data of Link et al. (45) that DFO therapy reverses cardiac arrhythmias in some patients previously unresponsive to medical treatment. This may be attributed to removal of a toxic labile iron pool. They also mentioned improvement of left ventricular ejection fraction in seven of nine patients. It is important to note that oral chelators are less effective than DFO and are unable to prevent cardiac mortality in patients with established heart disease (46).

Coronary artery atherosclerosis

Duffy et al. (2) showed that DFO improved endothelium-dependent vasodilatation in patients with coronary artery disease. In his review of 68 references regarding iron-mediated cardiovascular injury, Horwitz and Rosenthal (47) concluded that iron chelation may prevent restenosis and atherogenesis in coronary arteries. Paraskevaidis et al. (48)

demonstrated that in patients undergoing elective coronary artery bypass grafting for the first time, the infusion of the free-radical scavenger DFO, for eight hours, starting immediately after the induction of anesthesia, improves the postischemic recovery of the left ventricle, mainly in those patients with the poorest pre-operative cardiac function. Of particular interest, this benefit remains for 12 months of follow-up.

Future chelation therapy

For 30 years, DFO has been the only approved iron chelator. Recently, several oral iron chelators and variations of DFO to prolong the half-life have been developed. The best conclusion for the future of chelation therapy in cardiology was done by Hershko et al. in 2005 (49): "Prevention of cardiac mortality is the most important beneficial effect of iron chelation therapy. Unfortunately, compliance with the rigorous requirements of daily subcutaneous DFO infusions is still a serious limiting factor in treatment success. The development of orally effective iron chelators such as deferiprone and ICL670 (deferasirox) is intended to improve compliance. Although total iron excretion with deferiprone is somewhat less than that with DFO, deferiprone may have a better cardioprotective effect than DFO due to deferiprone's ability to penetrate cell membranes. For the patient with transfusional iron overload in whom results of DFO treatment are unsatisfactory, several orally effective agents are now available to avoid serious organ damage. Finally, combined chelation treatment is emerging as a reasonable alternative to chelator monotherapy. Combining a weak chelator that has a better ability to penetrate cells with a stronger chelator that penetrates cells poorly but has a more efficient urinary excretion may result in improved therapeutic effect through iron shuttling between the two compounds. The efficacy of combined chelation treatment is additive and offers an increased likelihood of success in patients previously failing DFO or deferiprone monotherapy."

References

1 Cooper CE. Nitric oxide and iron proteins. Biochim Biophys Acta 1999; 340:115–126.

2 Duffy SJ, Biegelsen ES, Holbrook M, et al. Iron chelation improves endothelial function in patients with coronary artery disease. Circulation 2001; 103:2799–2804.

3 Zhang WJ, Frei B. Intracellular metal ion chelators inhibit TNFalpha-induced SP-1 activation and adhesion molecule expression in human aortic endothelial cells. Free Radic Biol Med 2003; 34(6):674–682.

4 Celermajer DS, Sorensen KE, Gooch VM, et al. Non-invasive detection of endothelial dysfunction in children and adults at risk of atherosclerosis. Lancet 1992; 340:1111–1115.

5 Lauffer RB. Iron stores and the international variation in mortality from coronary artery disease. Med Hypoth 1991; 35:96–102.

6 de Valk B, Marx JJ. Iron, atherosclerosis, and ischemic heart disease. Arch Intern Med 1999; 159:1542–1548.

7 Kiechl S, Willeit J, Egger G, et al. Body iron stores and the risk of carotid atherosclerosis: prospective results from the Bruneck study. Circulation 1997; 96:3300–3307.

8 Lee TS, Shiao MS, Pan CC, et al. Iron-deficient diet reduces atherosclerotic lesions in apoE-deficient mice. Circulation 1999; 99:1222–1229.

9 Nakayama M, Takahashi K, Komura T, et al. Increased expression of heme oxygenase-1 and bilirubin accumulation in foam cells of rabbit atherosclerotic lesions. Arterioscler Thromb Vasc Biol 2001; 21(8):1373–1377.

10 Howes PS, Zacharski LR, Sullivan J, Chow B. Role of stored iron in atherosclerosis. J Vasc Nurs 2000; 18(4):109–114.

11 Auer J, Rammer M, Berent R, et al. Body iron stores and coronary atherosclerosis assessed by coronary angiography. Nutr Metab Cardiovasc Dis 2002; 12(5):285–290.

12 Hetet G, Elbaz A, Gariepy J, et al. Associated studies between haemochromatosis gene mutations and the risk of cardiovascular disease. Eur J Clin Invest 2001; 31(5):382–388.

13 Minqin R, Watt F, Huat BT, Halliwell B. Correlation of iron and zinc levels with lesion depth in newly formed atherosclerotic lesions. Free Radic Biol Med 2003; 34(6):746–752.

14 You SA, Archacki SR, Angheloiu G, et al. Proteomic approach to coronary atherosclerosis show ferritin light chain as a significant marker: evidence consistent with iron hypothesis in atherosclerosis. Physiol Genomics 2003; 13(1):25–30.

15 Stadler N, Lindner RA, Davies MJ. Direct detection and quantification of transition metal ions in human atherosclerotic plaques: evidence for the presence of elevated levels of iron and copper. Arterioscler Thromb Vasc Biol 2004; 24(5): 949–954.

16 Anderson LJ, Westwood MA, Prescott E, et al. Development of thalassaemic iron overload cardiomyopathy despite low liver iron levels and meticulous compliance to desferrioxamine. Acta Haematol 2006; 115(1–2):106–108.

17 Gackowski D, Kruszewski M, Jawien A, et al. Further evidence that oxidative stress may be a risk factor responsible for the development of atherosclerosis. Free Radic Biol Med 2001; 31(4):542–547.

18 Wolff B, Volzke H, Ludermann J, et al. Association between high serum ferritin levels and carotid atherosclerosis in the study of health in Pomerania (SHIP). Stroke 2004; 35(2):453–457.

19 Davis BA, Porter JB. Results of long term iron chelation treatment with deferoxamine. In: Hershko C, ed. Advances in Experimental Medicine and Biology. Vol. 509. New York: Kluwer Academic/Plenum Publisher, 2002.

20 Konijn AM, Glickstein H, Vaisman B, et al. The cellular labile iron pool and intracellular ferritin in K562 cells. Blood 1999; 94:2128–2134.

21 Epsztejn S, Kakhlon O, Glickstein H, et al. Fluorescence analysis of the labile iron pool of mammalian cells. Anal Biochem 1997; 248:31–40.

22 Araujo A, Kosaryan M, MacDowell A, et al. A novel delivery system for continuous desferrioxamine infusion in transfusional iron overload. Br J Haematol 1996; 93:835–837.

23 Nakamura H, del Nido PJ, Jimenez E, et al. Age-related differences in cardiac susceptibility to ischemia/reperfusion injury. Response to deferoxamine. J Thorac Cardiovasc Surg 1992; 104(1):165–172.

24 Nicholson SC, Squier M, Ferguson DJ, et al. Effect of desferrioxamine cardioplegia on ischemia-reperfusion injury in isolated rat heart. Ann Thorac Surg 1997; 63(4): 1003–1011.

25 Lai TY, Lee GK, Chan WM, Lam DS. Rapid development of severe toxic retinopathy associated with continuous intravenous deferoxamine infusion. Br J Ophthalmol 2006; 90(2): 243–244.

26 Chen SH, Liang DC, Lin HC, et al. Auditory and visual toxicity during deferoxamine therapy in transfusion-dependent patients. J Pediatr Hematol Oncol 2005; 27(12): 651–653.

27 Freedman MH, Grisaru D, Olivieri N, et al. Pulmonary syndrome in patients with thalassemia major receiving intravenous deferoxamine infusions. Am J Dis Child 1990; 144:565–569.

28 Halliwell B. Use of desferrioxamine as a probe for iron-dependent formation of hydroxyl radicals. Evidence for a direct reaction between desferal and the superoxide radical. Biochem Pharmacol 1985; 34(2):229–233.

29 Matthews AJ, Vercellotti GM, Menchaca HJ, et al. Iron and Atherosclerosis: inhibition by the iron chelator deferiprone. J Surg Res 1997; 73:35–40.

30 Muntane J, Mitjavila MT, Rodriquez MC, et al. Dietary lipid and iron status modulate lipid peroxidation in rats with induced adjuvant arthritis. J Nutr 1995; 125(7):1930–1937.

31 Chawla PS, Keelan MN, Kipshidze N. Angiogenesis for treatment of vascular diseases. Int Angiol 1999; 18 (3): 185–192.

32 Baffour R, Garb JL, Kaufman J, et al. Angiogenic therapy for the chronically ischemic lower limb in a rabbit model. J Surg Res 2000; 93(2):219–229.

33 Chekanov VS, Nikolaychik VV. Iron contributes to endothelial dysfunction in acute ischemic syndrome. Circulation 2002; 105(4):E35.

34 Hickey MJ, Knight KR, Lepore DA, et al. Influence of postischemic administration of oxyradical antagonists on ischemic injury to rabbit skeletal muscle. Microsurgery 1996; 17(9):517–523.

35 Beerepoot LV, Shima DT, Kuroki M, et al. Up-regulation of vascular endothelial growth factor production by iron chelator. Cancer Res 1996; 56(16):3747–3751.

36 Chekanov VS, Zargarian M, Baibekov IM, et al. Deferoxamine-fibrin accelerates angiogenesis in a rabbit model of peripheral ischemia. Vasc Med 2003; 8(3):157–162.

37 Pandit AS, Feldman DS, Caulfield J, Thompson A. Stimulation of angiogenesis by FGF-1 delivered through a modified fibrin scaffold. Growth Factors 1998; 15(2):113–123.

38 Hodges YK, Reese SM, Pahl PM, Horwitz LD. Paradoxical effects of iron chelation on growth of vascular endothelial cells. J Cardiovasc Pharmacol. 2005; 45(6): 539–544.

39 Ulubayram K, Kiziltay A, Yilmaz E, Hasirei H. Desferrioxamine release from gelatin-based systems. Biotechnol Appl Biochem 2005; 42(Pt 3):237–245.

40 Spencer KT, Lindower PD, Buettner GR, Kerber RE. Transition metal chelators reduce directly measured myocardial free radical production during reperfusion. J Cardiovas Pharmacol 1998; 32(3):343–348.

41 Dulchavsky SA, Davidson SB, Cullen WJ, et al. Effects of deferoxamine on H_2O_2-induced oxidative stress in isolated rat heart. Basic Res Cardiol 1996; 91(6):418–424.

42 Dross G, Lazou A, Panagopoulos P, et al. Deferoxamine cardioplegia reduces superoxide radical production in human myocardium. Ann Thorac Surg 1995; 59(1):169–172.

43 Hershko C, Link G, Konijn AM. Cardioprotective effect of iron chelators. In: Hershko C, ed. Advances in Experimental Medicine and Biology. Vol. 509. New York: Kluwer Academic/Plenum Publisher, 2002.

44 Tsironi M, Deffereos S, Andriopoulos P, et al. Reversal of heart failure in thalassemia major by combined chelation therapy: a case report. Eur J Haematol 2005; 74(1):84–85.

45 Link G, Saada A, Pinson A, et al. Mitochondrial respiratory enzymes are a major target of iron toxicity in rat heart cells. J Lab Clin Med 1998; 131:466–474.

46 Hoffbrand AV, Al-Refaie F, Davis B, et al. Long-term trial of deferiprone in 51 transfusion-dependent iron overloaded patients. Blood 1998; 91:295–300.

47 Horwitz LD, Rosenthal SA. Iron-mediated cardiovascular injury. Vasc Med 1999; 4(2):93–99.

48 Paraskevaidis IA, Iliodromitis EK, Vlahakos D, et al. Deferoxamine infusion during coronary artery bypass grafting ameliorates lipid peroxidation and protects the myocardium against reperfusion injury: immediate and long-term significance. Eur Heart J 2005; 26(3):263–270.

49 Hershko C, Link G, Konijn AM, Cabantchik ZI. Objectives and mechanism of iron chelation therapy. Ann N Y Acad Sci 2005; 1054:124–135.

21

Stent-mediated local drug delivery

Yanming Huang, Lan Wang, and Ivan De Scheerder

Coronary stent implantation prevents vessel elastic recoil and reduces restenosis in some subsets of lesions compared to balloon angioplasty alone. However, because of inducing a foreign body reaction and causing deep vessel injury during stent deployment, sub(acute) thrombosis and increased neointimal hyperplasia have limited their efficacy. Systemic drug administration has been limited by side effects and insufficient drug concentration at the target sites. Stent, uncoated or coated with polymer matrix, has been proposed as a platform for local drug delivery. Stent mediated local drug delivery could achieve a high local drug concentration and sustained drug release. Until now, different stents, polymer coatings, and drugs have been explored to reduce stent-related thrombosis and to suppress the cascade of neointimal formation.

Thromboresistant stents

Optimal stent implantation and new antiplatelet therapy have reduced the thrombotic complication after stent implantation, dramatically. However, thrombosis remains a challenge in some lesions and patient subgroups. As an initial and unavoidable event during stent implantation, thrombosis and platelet activation are also involved in the development of neointimal hyperplasia. Stents coated with heparin and other antithrombotic drugs have been demonstrated to decrease thrombotic complications, although their effect on neointimal hyperplasia remains uncertain. As heparin is attached to the stent surface, we divide thromboresistant stents as heparin-coated stents and drug-eluting thromboresistant stents.

Heparin-coated stents

Heparin is an antithrombin III factor. It can be attached to a metallic surface either chemically or physically. Endpoint covalent attachment of heparin to a polymer-coated surface is a stable and efficient method. By this bond, the immobilized heparin interacts with circulating antithrombin III. In vitro experimental work showed that heparin-coated stents could decrease the platelet aggregation and thrombus weight (Table 1). Furthermore, most in vivo studies demonstrated that heparin-coated stents could reduce stent thrombogenicity. For the effects on neointimal hyperplasia, controversial results have been published. Most studies showed that heparin-coated stents have a limited effect on neointimal hyperplasia. Even in one study, histomorphometric analysis after four weeks showed a significant increase in neointimal thickness with the highest heparin activity, although no significant difference was observed at 12 weeks follow-up (1). Heparin also has interactions with several growth factors and other glycoproteins (GPs). By this way, the heparin coating could hamper endothelial cell coverage of the coated stents. However, two recent studies in pigs have found that heparin-coated stents could decrease neointimal hyperplasia compared to bare control stents (2,3).

Heparin-coated Palmaz-Schatz, Wiktor, Jostent, BX Velocity, and beStent have been investigated in clinical studies. All studies showed that heparin-coated stents are safe, even in high-risk lesions. When compared with balloon angioplasty, heparin-coated stents could significantly reduce the rate of subacute stent thrombosis and the late restenosis. However, no significant difference of restenosis was observed between the heparin-coated stent and the bare stent control.

Drug-eluting thromboresistant stents

Drug-eluting stents to reduce thrombotic complication have also been evaluated (Table 2). It is known that a final common pathway for platelet aggregation exists. Platelet aggregation is

Table 1 Heparin-coated stents

First author (reference)	Year	Type of stent	Polymer	Model	Control	Thrombosis reduction	Neointima reduction
In vitro studies							
Kocsis (39)	1996	P-S	Carmeda	In vitro	Bare stent	Yes	—
Chronos (40)	1996	P-S	Carmeda	Baboon A-V	Bare stent	Yes	—
Blezer (41)	1998	Tantalum	NA	In vitro	Bare stent	Yes	—
Christensen (42)	1998	Stent-graft	PTFE	In vitro	Bare stent	Yes	—
Beythien (43)	1999	NA	NA	Pulsed floating	Bare stent	Yes	—
Bickel (44)	2001	NA	NA	In vitro	Bare stent Carbon-coated stent	Yes	—
Brockmann (45)	2002	NA	NA	Pulsed floating	Bare stent	Yes	—
Hietala (46)	2003	NA	PCL95/ L-LA5-PLA	In vitro	Bare	Yes	—
In vivo studies							
Bonan (47)	1991	Zig-zag	NA	Dog coronary art	Bare stent	No	No
Zidar (48,49)	1992	Cordis	NA	Dog coronary art	Bare stent	No	No
Baily (50)	1992	P-S	NA	Rabbit iliac art	Bare stent	Yes	—
Stratienko (51)	1993	P-S	NA	Rabbit iliac art	Bare stent	Yes	—
van der Giessen (52)	1994	P-S	NA	Pig coronary art	Bare stent	Yes	No
Jeong (53)	1995	Wallstent	NA	Pig carotid art	Bare stent	Yes	—
Sheth (54)	1995	Harts	SPUU-PEO	Rabbit carotid art	Bare stent	Yes	—
Chronos (55)	1995	Cordis	Hepamed	Baboon carotid	Bare stent	Yes	Yes
Wilczek (56)	1996	Copper	PUR	Pig coronary art	Bare stent	Yes	No
Gao (57)	1996	Biodegradable	CL + LA	Pig carotid art	—	—	—
Hardhammar (1)	1996	P-S	Carmeda	Pig coronary art	Bare stent	Yes	No
De Scheerder (58)	1997	Self-designed	Duraflo II	Rat A-V shunt pig coronary art	Bare stent	Yes	No
Schurmann (59)	1997	Cragg	Dacron	Sheep iliac art	Bare stent	—	No
Ahn (60)	1999	Wiktor	Hepamed	Pig coronary art	Bare stent	Yes	Yes
Armstrong (61)	1999	Cordis	Hepamed	Baboon carotid art	Cordis CCS	Yes	Yes
Goodwin (62)	2000	Collagen stent-graft	Collagen	Pig peripheral art	—	No	No
Matsumoto (2)	2002	NA	NA	Pig coronary art	Bare stent	—	Yes
Lin (3)	2003	P-S	NA	Baboon iliac art	Bare stent	—	Yes
Clinical studies							
Serruys (63)	1996	P-S	Carmeda	Human coronary art	—	Yes	—

(Continued)

Table 1   Heparin-coated stents (*Continued*)

First author (reference)	Year	Type of stent	Polymer	Model	Control	Thrombosis reduction	Neointima reduction
Vrolix(64)	1997	Wiktor	Hepamed	Human coronary art	—	—	—
Serruys (63)	1998	P-S	Carmeda	Human coronary art	PTCA	Yes	Yes
Wöhrle (65)	1999	Jomed	Corline	Human coronary art	Bare stent	No	No
Vrolix (66)	2000	Wiktor	Hepamed	Human coronary art	—	Yes	—
Van Langenhove (67)	2000	Wiktor	Hepamed	Human coronary saphenous vein bypass	—	—	Yes
Degertekin (68)	2000	Jomed	Corline	Human coronary art	Bare stent	—	No
Degertekin (69)	2000	Jomed	Corline	Human coronary art (CTO)	PTCA	—	Yes
Shin(70)	2000	Jomed	Corline	Human coronary art (AMI)	—	Yes	—
Wohrle (71)	2001	Jostent	Corline	Human coronary art	Jostent	—	No
Kedev (72)	2002	NA	NA	Human coronary art	P-S	Yes	—
Moer (73) (SISCA)	2002	beStent	Hepamed	Human coronary art	PTCA	—	Yes
Semiz (74)	2003	Jostent	NA	Human coronary art	NIR stent	No	No
Gurbel (75)	2003	NA	NA	Human coronary art	Bare	Yes	—
Mehran(76) (HOPE)	2003	BX Velocity	Carmeda	Human coronary art	—	Yes	—
Haude (77)	2003	JOSTENT	Corline	Human coronary art	Angioplasty	—	Yes
		Flex			Bare stent	—	No
Jaster (78)	2003	Coiled wire stent	NA	Human coronary art (AMI)	PTCA	Yes	—
Gupta (79)	2004	BX Velocity	Hepacoat	Human coronary art	Bare stent	Yes	—
Madduri (80)	2004	HC BX Velocity	Hepacoat	Human coronary art	—	—	—

Abbreviations: AMI, acute myocardial infarction; Art, artery; A-V, arteriovenous; CL, caprolactone; CTO, chronic total occlusion; LA, D,L-lactide; NA, not available; PTCA, percutaneous transluminal coronary angioplasty; PTFE, polytetrafluoroethylene; P-S, Palmaz-Schatz; PUR, polyurethane; SPUU-PEO, segmented polyurethaneurea-polyethylene oxide.

Table 2 Thromboresistant drug-eluting stents

First author (reference)	Year	Type of stent	Polymer	Model	Drug	Amount	Control stent	Thr-R	Neo-R
In vitro studies									
Baron (81)	1997	NA	NA	In vitro	C7E3 Fab	466 ng/cm wire	—	—	—
Schmidmaier (7,8)	1997	NA	PLLA	In vitro	5% PEG-hirudin 1% PGI_2	10 μg 2 μg	—	—	—
Schmidmaier (82)	1997	NA	PLLA	Human stasis	5% PEG-hirudin 1% PGI_2	NA	Bare	Yes	—
Foo (12)	1998	NA	NA	In Vitro	Activated protein C	NA	Bare polymer	Yes Yes	— —
Herrmann (9)	1999	In-Flow	PLLA	Human stasis ex vivo	5% PEG-hirudin 1% iloprost	10 μg 2 μg	Bare	Yes	—
Baron (83,84)	2000	Cook GR II	CHC	In vitro	C7E3 Fab	1146 ng/cm wire	Bare	Yes	—
Lahann (85)	2001	Nitinol	paracyclo phanes	In vitro	γ-hirudin	NA	Bare	Yes	—
In vivo studies									
Lambert (13)	1994	Harts	PUR	Rabbit carotid art	Forskolin	1.58 mg	—	Yes	—
Dev (86)	1995	Nitinol	PUR	Rabbit carotid art	Forskolin Etedrinate	1.5 mg 2.8 mg	—	—	—
Tanguay (87)	1996	NA	NA	Dog coronary art	GPIIb/IIIa inhibitor	NA	Bare	Yes	—
Aggarwal (88)	1996	Cook	CEL	Rabbit iliac art	GPIIb/IIIa inhibitor	1.15 μg	CEL	Yes	No
Aggarwal (89)	1997	NA	CEL	Rabbit iliac art	GPIIb/IIIa inhibitor + UK	—	CEL	Yes	—
Alt (10)	1997	P-S	PLLA	Sheep coronary art	PEG-hirudin PGI_2	10 μg 2 μg	Bare	—	Yes
Santos (90)	1998	NA	NA	Dog coronary art	L703,081	40w%	Bare	Yes	—
Kruse (91)	1999	NA	NA	Pig coronary art	Argatroban	NA	Bare	Yes	
Foo (14,15)	1999 2000	Cook	CEL	In vitro rabbit iliac art	Activated protein C	67.5 μg	Bare CEL Albumin loaded	Yes Yes Yes	— — —
Jeong (11)	2000	ReoPro	NA	Pig coronary art	GPIIb/IIIa inhibitor	NA	Bare	Yes	Yes
Alt (92)	2000	P-S	PLLA	Pig coronary art	5% r-PEG-hirudin	NA	Bare	—	Yes
				Sheep coronary art	1% iloprost	NA			
Fontaine (4)	2001	Wallstents	NA	Dog iliac art	Abciximab	21.53 μg	Bare	—	Yes

(Continued)

Table 2   Thromboresistant drug-eluting stents (*Continued*)

First author (reference)	Year	Type of stent	Polymer	Model	Drug	Amount	Control stent	Thr-R	Neo-R
Clinical studies									
Kim (5)	2004	NA	NA	Human coronary	Abciximab	NA	Bare	—	Yes
Hong (6)	2004	NA	NA	Human coronary	Abciximab	NA	Bare	—	Yes

Abbreviations: CEL, cellulose; CHC, chlorohydrocarbon; GP, glycoprotein; GR, gianturco-roubin; NA, not available; Neo-R, neointima reduction; PEG, polyethyleneglycol; PGI$_2$, prostaglandin I$_2$; PLLA(PLA), poly-L-lactic acid; P-S, Palmaz-Schatz; PUR, polyurethane; Thr-R, thrombosis reduction.

mediated through GPIIb/IIIa receptors on the platelet membrane. Stents loaded with different kinds of GPIIb/IIIa inhibitors have been investigated. Results showed that GPIIb/IIIa inhibitor-loaded stents could significantly decrease the thrombus formation in different models, even compared to polymer-coated control. Furthermore, in recent preclinical and clinical studies, abciximab, a GPIIb/IIIa inhibitor, coated on stents could significantly suppress neointimal hyperplasia compared to bare stents (4–6).

Hirudin, a specific and direct thrombin inhibitor, does not require a cofactor to antagonize the thrombin activity. It, however, has no direct effects on platelets. Prostacyclin is a potent inhibitor of platelet aggregation. Stent coatings impregnated with hirudin and prostacyclin analogs have been investigated. Incorporation of a polyethyleneglycol (PEG)-hirudin and a prostaglandin I$_2$ (PGI$_2$) analog in a polylactic acid stent coating showed initial exponential release characteristic of PEG-hirudin and a slow release of PGI$_2$ (7–9). These release properties resulted in a fast and prolonged antithrombotic effect after stent implantation. PEG-hirudin and PGI$_2$ analog loaded stent coatings demonstrated a significant inhibitive effect on both platelet activation and blood coagulation in a human shunt model. Furthermore, in a sheep and pig coronary artery model, favorable effects on neointimal formation were observed (10,11).

Other antithrombotic agent loaded stents, such as activated protein C and forskolin, have also been studied (12–15).

Drug-eluting stents to decrease neointimal hyperplasia

Neointimal formation is a multifactorial process, that consists of thrombotic formation, inflammatory response, and smooth muscle cells differentiation, migration, and proliferation (Table 3). Mural thrombi may serve as a scaffold for subsequent cell proliferation and undergo organization. However, early thrombus formation alone is not responsible for the development of neointimal hyperplasia. As discussed earlier, controversial results on neointimal hyperplasia with thromboresistant stents have been reported.

Inflammatory response after stent implantation plays an important role in the cascade of neointimal formation. A positive correlation between inflammatory reaction and restenosis has been observed (16). Perivasculitis caused by stent deployment also participates in the neointimal formation (17). Corticosteroids, as an anti-inflammatory agent, have been evaluated. Methylprednisolone (MP)-loaded stents with different doses showed a positive dose-related effect on neointimal hyperplasia (18). Furthermore, MP-coated stents showed decreased macrophages at the stented sites (19). In clinic, dexamethasone-coated stents showed an inhibitive effect on neointimal hyperplasia in selected patients (20), although no beneficial effect was observed in a randomized trial compared to bare stents (21). For other type of drugs with anti-inflammatory characteristics, such as ibuprofen, colchicine, atorvastatin, and probucol, no favorable effects on neointimal hyperplasia were observed (18,22,23).

Histological analysis of in-stent restenosis showed that smooth muscle cells and activated smooth muscle cells comprised 59% and 25% of all cells, respectively (24). Interference with smooth muscle cell differentiation, migration, and proliferation could inhibit neointimal formation. Paclitaxel- and sirolimus-coated stents could significantly reduce restenosis, even in complex coronary lesions, such as small vessels, chronic total occlusions, in-stent restenosis, and in diabetic patients. Consistent effects on neointimal formation have been reported in long-term follow-up studies up to four years (25). Apart from paclitaxel and sirolimus, other drugs such as angiopeptin, RGD, ST638, actinomycin D, 7-hexanoyltaxol, and tacrolimus have all been evaluated. Cytotoxic effects of actinomycin D and 7-hexanoyltaxol induced thrombosis and neointimal growth (26,27).

Table 3   Drug-eluting stents to decrease neointimal hyperplasia

First author (reference)	Year	Type of stent	Polymer	Model	Drug	Amount	Control stent	Neo-R
In vitro studies								
Swanson (93)	2000	BiodivYsio	PC	In vitro	Paclitaxel	127 µg	—	—
In vivo studies								
Cox (94)	1992	Cook	CEL	Pig coronary art	Heparin; methotrexate; heparin+ methotrexate	NA	Bare	No
Eccleston (95)	1995	Tantalum	PLLA	Pig coronary art	Colchicine	3.96 mg 0.99 mg	—	No
De Scheerder (96)	1996	Wiktor	POP	Pig coronary art	MP	300 µg	POP	Yes
Baker (97)	1996	PEAK	FIB	Rabbit iliac art	RGD	NA	Bare	Yes
De Scheerder (98)	1996	Wiktor	POP	Pig coronary art	Angiopeptin	250 µg	POP	Yes
Lincoff (99)	1997	Wiktor	PLLA	Pig coronary art	DXM	0.8 mg	PLLA Bare	No No
Strecker (100)	1998	Strecker	dL-PLA or PLA-co-TMC	Dog femoral art	DXM	8 mg	Bare	Yes
Drachman (101)	1998	NA	NA	Rabbit iliac art	Paclitaxel	NA	Bare polymer	Yes
Yamawaki (102)	1998	PLLA biodegradable	PLLA	Pig coronary art	ST638	0.8 mg	PLLA	Yes
Amstrong (103)	1999	BiodivYsio	PC	Pig coronary art	Angiopeptin	8.3 µg	—	—
De Scheerder (18)	2000	Self-designed	PFM-P75	Pig coronary art	MP	Dipcoating: 10–15 µg in 5% (g/g) 20–25 µg in 10% (g/g) Spraycoating 100–150 µg in 9% (g/g) 400–450 µg in 33% (g/g) 700–1000 µg in 50% (g/g)	PFM-P75 PFM-P75	Yes Yes
De Scheerder (18)	2000	Self-designed	PFM-P75	Pig coronary art	Ibuprofen Valsartan	10–15 µg in 5% (g/g) 20–25 µg in 10% (g/g)	PFM-P75 PFM-P75	No No
De Scheerder (18)	2000	Self-designed	PFM-P75	Pig coronary art	Trapidil	92 µg in 10% (g/g)	PFM-P75	No
Rogers (104)	2000	NIR	NA	Pig coronary art	Paclitaxel	NA	Bare	Yes
Carter (105)	2000	NA	NA	Pig coronary art	Sirolimus	NA	Bare polymer	Yes Yes

(Continued)

Table 3 Drug-eluting stents to decrease neointimal hyperplasia (*Continued*)

First author (reference)	Year	Type of stent	Polymer	Model	Drug	Amount	Control stent	Neo-R
Klugherz (106)	2000	BX Velocity	NA	Rabbit iliac art	Sirolimus	64 mg 196 mg	Bare Polymer	Yes Yes
Klugherz (107)	2000	BX Velocity	NA	Pig coronary art	Sirolimus	NA	—	—
Hong (108)	2001	Gianturco-Roubin II	NA	Pig coronary art	Paclitaxel	175–200 μg/stent	Bare	Yes
Suzuki (109)	2001	NA	Nonerodable	Pig coronary art	Sirolimus DXM Sirolimus +DXM	185 μg/stent 350 μg/stent 185 + 350 μg/stent	Bare	Yes No Yes
Heldman (110)	2001	P-S	—	Pig coronary art	Paclitaxe l	0.2, 15 μg/stent 187 μg/stent	Bare	No Yes
New (111)	2002	BiodivYsio	PC	Pig coronary art	17beta-estradiol	67 μg/stent 240 μg/stent	Bare	Yes
Klugherz (112)	2002	BX Velocity	NA	Rabbit iliac art	Sirolimus	Low dose High dose	Bare Coated	Yes
Armstrong (113)	2002	BiodivYsio	PC	Pig coronary art	Angiopeptin	126 μg/stent	Bare Coated	No
Yoon (114)	2002	Coil	PU	Pig coronary art	SNP	Low dose High dose	Bare	No
Finkelstein (115)	2003	Conor	Biodegradable	Pig coronary art	Paclitaxel	95 μg/stent	Bare	Yes
Wu (116)	2003	NA	PC	Pig coronary art	TIMP-3	NA	Bare	Yes
Scheller (117)	2003	BiodivYsio	PC	Pig coronary art	Atorvastatin	56 μg	Bare	No
Salu (22)	2003	NA	Biological oil	Pig coronary art	Cytochalasin D	93 μg	Bare	Yes
Wieneke (118)	2003	NA	Aluminum oxide	Rabbit carotid art	Tacrolimus	60,120 μg	Bare Coated	Yes
Huang (119)	2003	BiodivYsio	PC	Pig coronary art	MP	269 μg	Coated	Yes
Banai (120)	2004	NA	PLGA Polylactic/glycolic	Pig coronary art	AGL-2043	180 mcg	Coated	Yes
Carter (121)	2004	NA	NA	Pig coronary art	Sirolimus	140 μg/cm^2	Bare	30 days yes; 90, 180 days, No
Huang (122)	2004	Jostent	Biolog	Pig coronary art	Methotrexate	150 μg/stent	Coated	Yes
Chen (123)	2004	NA	Jelly	Rabbit iliac art	EIPA	NA	Coated	Yes

(*Continued*)

Table 3 Drug-eluting stents to decrease neointimal hyperplasia (*Continued*)

First author (reference)	Year	Type of stent	Polymer	Model	Drug	Amount	Control stent	Neo-R
Jaschke (124)	2005	NA	NA	Rat carotid art	Cerivastatin	NA	Bare	Yes
Qiu (125)	2005	NA	Polyolefin	Pig coronary art	Mytrolimus	160 μg/stent	Bare coated	Yes
Uurto (126)	2005	Wallstent	PLA: PCL	Pig iliac art	DXM Simvastatin	NA	Coated	Yes No
Collingwood (127)	2005	BiodivYsio	PC	Pig coronary art	ABT-578	10 μg/mm	Coated	Yes
Kim (128)	2005	BiodivYsio	PC	Pig coronary art	Carvedilol Probucol	7 μg/stent 52 μg/stent	Coated	Yes No
Huang (23)	2005	Jostent	Biolog	Pig coronary art	Tacrolimus	200 μg/stent	Coated	Yes
Wang (129)	2005	Jostent	Biolog	Pig coronary art	MP	530 μg/stent	Coated	Yes
Clinical studies								
Sousa (19)	2000	BX Velocity	NA	Human coronary art	Sirolimus	NA	—	—
Grube (130)	2000	Q-DL	NA	Human coronary art	Microtubuler inhibitor	NA	Q-M	Yes
Rensing (131)	2001	BX Velocity	NA	Human coronary art	Sirolimus	1.4 μg/mm^2	—	—
Morice (132) (RAVEL)	2002	BX Velocity	Polyethyl methacrylate	Human coronary art	Sirolimus	1.4 μg/mm^2	Bare	Yes
Liu (133) (STRIDE)	2003	BiodivYsio	PC	Human coronary art	DXM	0.5 μg/mm^2	—	Yes
Lemos (20) (RSEARCH)	2003	BX Velocity	Polyethyl methacrylate	Human coronary art (Acute coronary syndromes)	Sirolimus	1.4 μg/mm^2	Bare	No
Park (134) (ASPECT)	2003	Supra G	—	Human coronary art	Paclitaxel	1.3, 3.1 μg/mm^2	Bare	Yes
Schofer (135) (E-SIRIUS)	2003	BX Velocity	Polyethyl methacrylate	Human coronary art (Small art)	Rapamycin	1.4 μg/mm^2	Bare	Yes
De Scheerder (136)	2003	BiodivYsio	PC	Human coronary art	Batimatstat	0.30 μg/mm^2	Coated	No
Grube (137) (TAXUS I)	2003	NIRx	Translute	Human coronary art	Paclitaxel	1 μg/mm^2	Bare	Yes
Bullesfeld (138) (TAXUS I)	2003	NIRx	Translute	Human coronary art	Paclitaxel	1 μg/mm^2	Bare	Yes
Colombo (139) (TAXUS II)	2003	NIR	Translute	Human coronary art	Paclitaxel	1 μg/mm^2	Bare	Yes

(Continued)

Table 3   Drug-eluting stents to decrease neointimal hyperplasia (*Continued*)

First author (reference)	Year	Type of stent	Polymer	Model	Drug	Amount	Control stent	Neo-R
Tanabe (140) (TAXUS III)	2003	NIRx	Translute	Human coronary art (in-stent restenosis)	Paclitaxel	1 µg/mm^2	Bare	Yes
Moses (141) (SIRIUS)	2003	BX Velocity	Polyethyl methacrylate	Human coronary art	Sirolimus	1.4 µg/mm^2	Bare	Yes
Schampaert (142) (C-SIRIUS)	2004	BX Velocity	Polyethyl methacrylate	Human coronary art (long lesion, small art)	Sirolimus	1.4 µg/mm^2	Bare	Yes
Grube (143) (SCORE)	2004	QuaDDS	Acrylate polymer sheeves	Human coronary art	7-hexanoyl taxol	800 µg	Bare	Yes
Serruys (26) (ACTION)	2004	Multilink-Tetra	NA	Human coronary art	Actinomycin D	2.5 or 10 µg/cm^2	Bare	No
Grube (144) (FUTURE I)	2004	S-Stent	Poly (D.L-lactide)	Human coronary art	Everolimus	NA	Bare	Yes
Lansky (145) (DELIVER)	2004	Multi-link PENTA	NA	Human coronary art	Paclitaxel	3 µg/mm^2	Bare	Yes
Gershlick (146) (ELUTES)	2004	V-flex Plus	NA	Human coronary art	Paclitaxel	0.2, 0.7, 1.4, 2.7 µg/mm^2	Bare	Yes with 2.7 µg/mm^2
Ardissino (147)	2004	BX Velocity	Translute	Human coronary art (small art)	Sirolimus	1.4 µg/mm^2	Bare	Yes
Hoye (148)	2004	BX Velocity	Translute	Human coronary art (chronic total occlusion)	Sirolimus	1.4 µg/mm^2	Bare	Yes
Stone (149 (TAXUS-IV)	2004	EXPRESS	Translute	Human coronary art	Paclitaxel	1 µg/mm^2	Bare	Yes
Kwok (150)	2005	BiodivYsio	PC	Human coronary art	Angiopeptin	22 µg: 126 µg/stent	—	—
Nakamura (151)	2005	BX Velocity	Polyethyl methacrylate	Human coronary art	Sirolimus	1 µg/mm^2	—	—
Airoldi (152)	2005	BiodivYsio	PC	Human coronary art	17beta-estradiol	2.5 µg/mm^2	PC coated	No
Hausleiter (153)	2005	NA	—	Human coronary art	Sirolimus	—	Bare	Yes
Sabaté (154) (DIABETES)	2005	BX Velocity	Polyethyl methacrylate	Human coronary art (Diabetic patients)	Sirolimus	1.4 µg/mm^2	Bare	Yes
Commeau (155) (ISR II study)	2005	BX Velocity	Polyethyl methacrylate	Human coronary art (In-stent restenosis)	Sirolimus	1.4 µg/mm^2	—	—

(*Continued*)

Table 3 Drug-eluting stents to decrease neointimal hyperplasia (*Continued*)

First author (reference)	Year	Type of stent	Polymer	Model	Drug	Amount	Control stent	Neo-R
Voudris (156) (ONASSIS)	2005	BX Velocity	Polyethyl methacrylate	Human coronary art	Sirolimus	$1.4\,\mu g/mm^2$	Bare	Yes
Hofma (157)	2005	BX Velocity	Polyethyl methacrylate	Human coronary art	Sirolimus	$1.4\,\mu g/mm^2$	Paclitaxel (Taxus)	No
Ge (158)	2005	BX Velocity	Polyethyl methacrylate	Human coronary art (chronic total occlusion)	Sirolimus	$1.4\,\mu g/mm^2$	Bare	Yes
Goy (159) (TAXi)	2005	BX Velocity	Polyethyl methacrylate	Human coronary art	Sirolimus	$1.4\,\mu g/mm^2$	Paclitaxel coated	No
Serruys (160) (PISCES)	2005	Conor	Erodable	Human coronary art	Paclitaxel	10, 30 μg	Bare	Yes
Stone (161) (TAXUS V)	2005	Express	Translute	Human coronary art (complex lesions)	Paclitaxel	$1\,\mu g/mm^2$	Bare	Yes

Abbreviations: CEL, cellulose; DXM, dexamethasone; EIPA, ethylisopropylamiloride; FIB, fibrin; MP, methylprednisolone; NA, not available; Neo-R, neointima reduction; PC, phosphorylcholine; PCL, polycaprolactone; PFM-P75, polyfluoroalkoxyphosphazene; PLLA(PLA), poly-L-lactic acid; POP, polyorganophosphazene; PU, polyurethane; Q-DL, Quanam drug eluting stent; Q-M, Quanam metal stent; SNP, sodium nitroprusside; TIMP, tissue inhibitors of metalloproteinase.

Endothelial cell seeding and gene transfer

Endothelial regeneration after stent implantation can influence the vascular thrombogenecity and neointimal hyperplasia. Endothelial cell seeding on stents or locally delivered endothelium-derived relaxing factors have been proposed for inhibiting the restenosis process (Table 4). Genetically modified endothelial cells can be seeded on stents. Recently, a first study by using an endothelial progenitor cell (EPC) capture stent has been performed in patients (28). This technology has been demonstrated to be safe and feasible for the treatment of de novo coronary artery disease. Furthermore, it has been demonstrated that vascular endothelial growth factor (VEGF)-loaded stents can significantly decrease thrombus formation and neointimal hyperplasia (29,30). Nitric oxide (NO)-loaded stents showed decreased thrombosis, although controversial results on neointimal formation were observed (31–35).

Gene therapy has been proposed to transfer a desired gene from the stent coating to the cells of the arterial wall. Naked DNA, viral vector containing DNA, and antisense oligonucleotides have been evaluated. Using DNA-coated stents as gene carriers, transgene expression was observed.

As shown in the tables, both biodegradable and nonbiodegradable polymers have been used as matrix for local drug delivery. The most important consideration in the selection of polymers for drug-eluting stents is the long-term biocompatibility. Increased thrombogenicity and inflammatory reaction induced by the polymer coating can counteract the beneficial effects of the local stent-mediated drug delivery. As most synthetic polymer coatings induce an inflammatory response, biological polymers as fibrin and phosphorylcholine (PC) have been evaluated to coat stents for local drug delivery. The biological polymers have the theoretical advantage of low thrombogenicity and minimizing the inflammatory response. Studies have demonstrated that PC coating did not provoke increased arterial neointimal hyperplasia in rabbit iliac and porcine coronary artery model, although the coating could not reduce restenosis (36,37).

Recently, also biological oil-based stent coatings were introduced to deliver drugs. Advantages of these coatings are that they are metabolized by the vascular smooth muscle cells without activating inflammatory cells.

Although drug-loaded stents have shown beneficial effects on restenosis and thrombosis compared to bare stents in clinical trials and real-world practice, there are still concerns about their long-term safety and efficacy. It has been reported that clinical trials of drug-eluting stents were stopped because of increased (sub)acute thrombosis and neointimal growth or insufficient efficacy. Furthermore, increased late thrombosis has been reported, especially with cytotoxic drug-coated

Table 4   Endothelial cell seeding and gene therapy

First author (reference)	Year	Type of stent	Polymer	Model	Drug	Amount	Control stent	Thr-R	Neo-R
In vitro studies									
Dichek (162)	1989	Johnson–Johnson	Fibronectin	In vitro	Sheep EC seeding	—	—	—	—
Flugeman (163)	1992	Johnson—Johnson	Fibronectin	Pulsatile flow	Sheep EC seeding	—	—	—	—
Amstrong (164)	2000	BiodivYsio	PC	Pig carotid art ex vivo	AS-ODN-c-myc	500 µg	—	—	—
Leclerc (165)	2000	BiodivYsio	PC		DNA oligonucleotide				
Shirota (166)	2003	NA	Gelatin: SPU film	In vitro	EPC	—	—	—	—
In vivo studies									
Scott (167)	1995	Cordis	—	In vitro pig coronary art	Human EC seeding	—	—	—	—
Folts (31,32)	1995	P-S	PSNO-BSA	Pig carotid art	NO	NA	Bare	Yes	Yes
Landau (168)	1995	PLLA/PCL biodegradable	PLLA/PCL	Rabbit carotid art	Recombinant adenovirus vectors	NA	—	—	—
Labhasetwar (169)	1998	DNA-polymer-coated suture	NA	Rat skeletal muscle Dog atrial myocardium	Plasmid DNA	777.2 µg	—	—	—
Mir-Akbari (29)	1999	Cook	NA	Rabbit iliac art	phVEGF	—	Bare	—	Yes
Klugherz (170)	1999	Crown	NA	Pig coronary art	Plasmid DNA	NA	—	—	—
Buergler (33)	2000	Cordis	PCL	Pig coronary art	NO	1 mg	PCL	—	No
Yuan (171)	2001	NA	Gelatin	Pig coronary art	Ad-beta gal	—	—	—	—
Panetta (172)	2002	Mesh-stent	Fibronectin	Pig coronary art	Autologous porcine SMC	—	—	—	—
Swanson (173)	2003	NA	NA	Rabbit iliac art	VEGF	18.5 µg	Bare	Yes	No
Takahashi (174)	2003	NA	Polyurethane	Rabbit iliac art	Plasmid DNA	NA	—	—	—
Walter (30)	2004	BiodivYsio	PC	Rabbit iliac art	PhVEGF-2	100 or 200 µg	—	—	Yes
Fleser (34)	2004	Polyurethane vascular graft	NA	Sheep arteriovenous bridge graft	NO-donor		Sham-coated; uncoated	Yes	—
Radke (175)	2005	BiodivYsio	PC	Rabbit aorta	ODNs	41 µg	—	—	—

(Continued)

Table 4 Endothelial cell seeding and gene therapy (*Continued*)

First author (reference)	Year	Type of stent	Polymer	Model	Drug	Amount	Control stent	Thr-R	Neo-R
Johnson (176)	2005	NA	NA	Pig coronary art	RAdTIMP-3	—	Bare	—	Yes
Hou (35)	2005	aSpire	ePTFE covered	Pig carotid art	SNP	54.5 μg/stent	Bare	Yes	
Clinical Studies									
Aoki (28)	2005	NA	NA	Human coronary art	EPC	—	—	—	—

Abbreviations: Ad-beta gal, beta-galactosidase; AS-ODN, antisense oligonucleotides; EC, endothelial cell; EPC, endothelial progenitor cell; NA, not available; Neo-R, neointima reduction; NO, Nitric oxide; PC, phosphorylcholine; PLLA(PLA), poly-L-lactic acid; PSNO, polyntrosated nitric oxide albumin; P-S, Palmaz-Schatz; RAdTIMP-3, recombinant adenovirus metalloproteinase-3; SMC, smooth muscle cell; SPU, segmented polyurethane; Thr-R, thrombosis reduction; VEGF, vascular endothelial growth factor.

stents. Intravascular ultrasound revealed that drug-eluting stents presented more incomplete stent apposition than the bare control (38). In a porcine coronary stent model, sirolimus-coated stents could effectively inhibit neointimal hyperplasia at 30 days follow-up; however, no effect was observed at 90 or 180 days (18). Although a very limited neointimal formation of sirolimus-coated stents was demonstrated up to four years in a small trial, long-term efficacy of drug-eluting stents is still a major concern.

References

1   Hardhammar P, Van Beusekom H, Emanuelsson H, et al. Reduction in thrombotic events with heparin-coated Palmaz-Schatz stents in normal coronary arteries. Circulation 1996; 93:423–430.

2   Matsumoto Y, Shimokawa H, Morishige K, et al. Reduction in neointimal formation with a stent coated with multiple layers of releasable heparin in porcine coronary arteries. J Cardiovasc Pharmacol 2002; 39(4):513–522.

3   Lin PH, Chronos NA, Marijianowski MM, et al. Carotid stenting using heparin-coated balloon-expandable stent reduces intimal hyperplasia in a baboon model. J Surg Res 2003; 112(1):84–90.

4   Fontaine AB, Borsa JJ, Dos Passos S, et al. Evaluation of local abciximab delivery from the surface of a polymer-coated covered stent: in vivo canine studies. J Vasc Interv Radiol 2001; 12(4):487–492.

5   Kim W, Jeong MH, Hong YJ, et al. The long-term clinical results of a platelet glycoprotein IIb/IIIa receptor blocker (Abciximab: Reopro) coated stent in patients with coronary artery disease. Korean J Intern Med 2004; 19(4):220–229.

6   Hong YJ, Jeong MH, Kim W, et al. Effect of abciximab-coated stent on in-stent intimal hyperplasia in human coronary arteries. Am J Cardiol 2004; 94(8):1050–1054.

7   Schmidmaier G, Stemberger A, Alt E, Gawaz M, Schömig A. Time release characteristics of a biodegradable stent coating with polylactic acid releasing PEG-hirudin and PGI$_2$-analog [abstr]. J Am Coll Cardiol 1997; 29:94A.

8   Schmidmaier G, Stemberger A, Alt E, et al. Non-liner time release characteristics of a biodegradable polylactic acid coating releasing PEG hirudin and a PGI$_2$ analog [abstr]. Eur Heart J 1997; 18(suppl):571.

9   Herrmann R, Schmidmaier G, Markl B, et al. Antithrombogenic coating of stents using a biodegradable drug delivery technology. Thromb Haemost 1999; 82(1):51–57.

10   Alt E, Beilharz C, Preter G, et al. Biodegradable stent coating with polylactic acid, hirudin and prostacyclin reduces restenosis [abstr]. J Am Coll Cardiol 1997; 29:238A.

11   Jeong M, Ahn Y, Kang K, et al. ReoPro® coated stent inhibits porcine coronary stent thrombus and restenosis [abstr]. Circulation 2000; 102(18):II-666.

12   Foo RS, Hogrefe K, Baron JH, et al. Activated protein C adsorbed on a stent reduces its thrombogenicity [abstr]. Circulation 1998; 17(suppl):I855.

13   Lambert T, Dev V, Rechavia E, Forrester J, Litvak F, Eigler N. Localized arterial wall drug delivery from a polymer-coated removable metallic stent: kinetics, distribution, and bioactivity of forskolin. Circulation 1994; 90:1003–1011.

14   Foo RS, Hogrefe K, Baron JH, et al. Activated protein C eluting stent inhibits platelet deposition in an in vivo model [abstr]. Eur Heart J 1999; 20(suppl):367.

15   Foo RS, Gershlick AH, Hogrefe K, et al. Inhibition of platelet thrombosis using an activated protein C-loaded stent: in vitro and in vivo results. Thromb haemost 2000; 83(3):496–502.

16   Kornowski R, Hong MK, Tio FO, et al. In-stent restenosis: contributions of inflammatory response and arterial injury to neointimal hyperplasia. J AM Coll Cardiol 1998; 31:224–230.

17   De Scheerder I, Szilard M, Huang Y, et al. Evaluation of the effect of oversizing on vascular injury, thrombogenicity and neointimal hyperplasia using the Magic Wallstent™ in a porcine coronary model [abstr]. JACC 2000; 35(2):70A.

18   De Scheerder I, Huang Y, Schacht E. Now concepts for drug eluting stents. 6th Local Drug Delivery Meeting and Cardiovascular Course on Radiation and Molecular Strategies, Geneva, Switzerland, Jan 27–29, 2000.

19 Sousa JE, Abizaid AAC, Abizaid ACLS, et al. First human experience with sirolimus coated BX Velocity stent: clinical, angiographic and ultrasound late results [abstr]. Circulation 2000; 102(18):II-815.

20 Lemos PA, Lee CH, Degertekin M, et al. Early outcome after sirolimus-eluting stent implantation in patients with acute coronary syndromes: insights from the Rapamycin-Eluting Stent Evaluated At Rotterdam Cardiology Hospital (RESEARCH) registry. J Am Coll Cardiol 2003; 41(11):2093–2099.

21 Hoffmann R, Langenberg R, Radke P, et al. Evaluation of a high-dose dexamethasone-eluting stent. Am J Cardiol 2004; 94(2):193–195.

22 Salu KJ, Huang Y, Bosmans JM, et al. Addition of cytochalasin D to a biocompatible oil stent coating inhibits intimal hyperplasia in a porcine coronary model. Coron Artery Dis 2003; 14(8):545–555.

23 Huang Y, Salu K, Wang L, et al. Use of a tacrolimus-eluting stent to inhibit neointimal hyperplasia in a porcine coronary model. J Invasive Cardiol 2005; 17(3):142–148.

24 Newby AC. Biological/pharmacological treatment and prevention. XXIInd Congress of the European Society of Cardiology, Amsterdam, Netherlands, Aug 27–30, 2000.

25 Sousa JE, Costa MA, Farb A, et al. Images in cardiovascular medicine. Vascular healing 4 years after the implantation of sirolimus-eluting stent in humans: a histopathological examination. Circulation 2004; 110(1):e5–e6.

26 Serruys PW, Ormiston JA, Sianos G, et al. Actinomycin-eluting stent for coronary revascularization: a randomized feasibility and safety study: the ACTION trial. J Am Coll Cardiol 2004; 44(7):1363–1367.

27 Liistro F, Colombo A. Late acute thrombosis after paclitaxel eluting stent implantation. Heart 2001; 86:262–264.

28 Aoki J, Serruys PW, van Beusekom H, et al. Endothelial progenitor cell capture by stents coated with antibody against CD34: the HEALING-FIM (Healthy Endothelial Accelerated Lining Inhibits Neointimal Growth-First In Man) Registry. J Am Coll Cardiol 2005; 45(10):1574–1579.

29 Mir-Akbari H, Sylven C, Lindvall B, et al. phVEGF coated stent reduces restenosis intimal hyperplasia [abstr]. Eur heart J 1999; 20(suppl):275.

30 Walter DH, Cejna M, Diaz-Sandoval L, et al. Local gene transfer of phVEGF-2 plasmid by gene-eluting stents: an alternative strategy for inhibition of restenosis. Circulation 2004; 110(1):36–45.

31 Folts J, Maalej N, Keaney J, Loscalzo J. Coating Palmaz-Schatz stents with a unique NO donor renders them much less thrombogenic when placed in pig carotid arteries [abstr]. Circulation 1995; 92:I-670.

32 Folts J, Maalej N, Keaney J, Loscalzo J. Palmaz-Schatz stents coated with a NO donor reduces reocclusion when placed in pig carotid arteries for 28 days [abstr]. J Am Coll Cardiol 1996; 27:86A.

33 Buergler JM, Tio FO, Schulz DG, et al. Use of nitric-oxide-eluting polymer-coated coronary stents for prevention of restenosis in pigs. Coron Artery Dis 2000; 11(4):351–357.

34 Fleser PS, Nuthakki VK, Malinzak LE, et al. Nitric oxide-releasing biopolymers inhibit thrombus formation in a sheep model of arteriovenous bridge grafts. J Vasc Surg 2004; 40(4):803–811.

35 Hou D, Narciso H, Kamdar K, et al. Stent-based nitric oxide delivery reducing neointimal proliferation in a porcine carotid overstretch injury model. Cardiovasc Intervent Radiol 2005; 28(1):60–65.

36 Kuiper KK, Robinson KA, Chronos NA, et al. Phosphorylcholine-coated metallic stents in rabbit iliac and porcine coronary arteries. Scand Cardiovasc J 1998; 32(5):261–268.

37 Whelan DM, van der Giessen WJ, Krabbendam SC, et al. Biocompatibility of phosphorylcholine coated stents in normal porcine coronary arteries. Heart 2000; 83(3):338–345.

38 Serruys PW, Degertekin M, Tanabe K, et al. Intravascular ultrasound findings in the multicenter, randomized, double-blind RAVEL (RAndomized study with the sirolimus-eluting VElocity balloon-expandable stent in the treatment of patients with de novo native coronary artery Lesions) trial. Circulation 2002; 106(7):798–803.

39 Kocsis JF, Lunn AC, Mohammad SF. Incomplete expansion of coronary stents: risk of thrombogenesis and protection provided by a heparin coating [abstr]. J Am Coll Cardiol 1996; 27(suppl A):84A.

40 Chronos N, Robinson K, White D, et al. Heparin coating dramatically reduces platelet deposition on incompletely deployed Plamaz-Schatz in the baboon A-V shunt [abstr]. J Am Coll Cardiol 1996; 27:84A.

41 Blezer R, Cahalan I, Cahalan PT, et al. Heparin coating of tantalum coronary stents reduces surface thrombin generation but not factor Ixa generation. Blood Coagul Fibrinolysis 1998; 9(5):435–440.

42 Christensen K, Larsson A, Emanuelsson H, et al. The stent graft: modulation of platelet and coagulation activation with heparin coating [abstr]. Eur Heart J 1998; 19 (suppl):498.

43 Beythien C, Gutensohn K, Bau J, et al. Influence of stent length and heparin coating on platelet activation: a flow cytometric analysis in a pulsed floating model. Thromb Res 1999; 94(2):79–86.

44 Bickel C, Rupprecht HJ, Darius H, et al. Substantial reduction of platelet adhesion by heparin-coated stents. J Interv Cardiol 2001; 14(4):407–413.

45 Brockmann MA, Gutensohn K, Bau J, et al. Influence of heparin coating of coronary stents and ex vivo efficacy of different doses of acetylsalicylic acid and ticlopidine in a pulsed floating model of recirculating human plasma. Platelets 2002; 13(8):443–449.

46 Hietala EM, Maasilta P, Valimaa T, et al. Platelet responses and coagulation activation on polylactide and heparin-polycaprolactone-L-lactide-coated polylactide stent struts. J Biomed Mater Res A2003; 67(3):785–791.

47 Bonan R, Bhat K, Lefevre T, et al. Coronary artery stenting after angioplasty with self-expanding parallel wire metallic stents. Am Heart J 1991; 121:1522–1530.

48 Zidar I, Jackman J, Gmmon R, et al. Serial assessment of heparin coating on vascular response to a new tantalum stent [abstr]. Circulation 1992; 89:I-185.

49 Zidar I, Virmani R, Culp S, et al. Quantitative histopathologic analysis of the vascular response to heparin coating of the Cordis stent [abstr]. J Am Coll Cardiol 1993; 12:336A.

50 Baily SR, Paige S, Lunn A, et al. Heparin coating of endovascular stents decreases subacute thrombosis in a rabbit model. Circulation 1992; 86(suppl):I186.

51 Stratienko A, Zhu D, Lambert C, et al. Improved thromboresistance of heparin coated Palmaz-Schatz coronary stents in an animal model [abstr]. Circulation 1993; 88:I-596.

52   van der Giessen WJ, Hardhammar PA, van Beusekom HMM, et al. Prevention of (sub)acute thrombosis using heparin-coated stents. Circulation 1994; 90(suppl):I–650.

53   Jeong M, Owen W, Staab M, et al. Does heparin release coating of the Wallstent limit thrombosis and platelet deposition? Results in a porcine carotid injury model [abstr]. Circulation 1995; 92:I–37.

54   Sheth S, Dev V, Jacobs H, et al. Prevention of subacute stent thrombosis by polymer-polyethylene oxide-heparin coating in rabbit carotid artery [abstr]. J Am Coll Cardiol 1995; 25:348A.

55   Chronos N, Robinson K, Kelly A, et al. Thrombogenicity of tantalum stents is decreased by surface heparin bonding: scintigraphy of ¹¹¹In-platelet deposition in baboon carotid arteries. Circulation 1995; 92:I–490.

56   Wilczek KL, De Scheerder IK, Wang K, et al. Implantation of balloon expandable copper stents in porcine coronary arteries. A model for testing the efficacy of stent coating in decreasing stent thrombogenicity [abstr]. Eur Heart J 1996; 17(suppl):455.

57   Gao R, Shi R, Qiao S, et al. A novel polymeric local heparin delivery stent: initial experimental study [abstr]. J Am Coll Cardiol 1996; 27:85A.

58   De Scheerder I, Wang K, Wilczek K, et al. Experimental study of thrombogenicity and foreign body reaction induced by heparin-coated coronary stents. Circulation 1997; 95: 1549–1553.

59   Schurmann K, Vorwerk D, Uppenkamp R, et al. Iliac arteries: plain and heparin-coated Dacron-covered stent-grafts compared with noncovered metal stents–an experimental study. Radiology 1997; 203(1):55–63.

60   Ahn YK, Jeong MH, Kim JW, et al. Preventive effects of the heparin-coated stent on restenosis in the porcine model. Catheter Cardiovasc Interv 1999; 48(3):324–330.

61   Armstrong

62   Goodwin SC, Yoon HC, Wong GC, et al. Percutaneous delivery of a heparin-impregnated collagen stent-graft in a porcine model of atherosclerotic disease. Invest Radiol 2000; 35(7):420–425

63   Serruys P, Emanuelsson H, Van der Giessen W, et al. Heparin-coated Palmaz-Schatz stents in human coronary arteries: early outcome of the Benestent-II pilot study. Circulation 1996; 93:412–422.

64   Vrolix M, Grollier G, Legrand V, et al. Heparin-coated wire coil (Wiktor) for elective stent placement-The MENTOR trial (abstract). Eur Heart J 1997; 18:155.

65   Wöhrle J, Grotzinger U, Al-Kayer I, et al. Comparison of the heparin-coated and the uncoated version of the JOMED stent with regards to stent thrombosis and restenosis rates [abstr]. Eur Heart J 1999; 20(suppl):271.

66   Vrolix M, Legrand V, Reiber JH, et al. Heparin-coated wiktor stents in human coronary arteries. Am J Cardiol 2000; 86(4):385–389.

67   Van Langenhove G, Vermeersch P, Serrano P, et al. Saphenous vein graft disease treated with the Wiktor Hepamed stent: procedural outcome, in-hospital complications and six-month angiographic follow-up. Can J Cardiol 2000; 16(4):473–480.

68   Degertekin M, Gencbay M, Sonmez K, et al. Comparison of heparin-coated jomed stents with uncoated stents in patients with coronary artery disease. 3rd International Congress on Coronary Artery Disease, Lyon, France, Oct 2–5, 2000:128.

69   Degertekin M, Sonmez K, Gencbay M, et al. Heparin-coated stent implantation in chronic total occlusion. 3rd International Congress on Coronary Artery Disease, Lyon, France, Oct 2–5, 2000:67.

70   Shin EK, Sohn S, Son JW, et al. Efficacy of heparin coated stent in the early setting of acute myocardial infarction. 3rd International Congress on Coronary Artery Disease, Lyon, France, Oct 2–5, 2000:152.

71   Wohrle J, Al-Khayer E, Grotzinger U, et al. Comparison of the heparin coated vs the uncoated Jostent–no influence on restenosis or clinical outcome. Eur Heart J 2001; 22(19):1808–1816.

72   Kedev S, Guagliumi G, Valsechi O, Tespili M. Heparin-coated versus uncoated Palmaz-Schatz stent in native coronary circulation. A randomized study with blind angioscopic assessment. Int J Artif Organs 2002; 25(5):461–469.

73   Moer R, Myreng Y, Molstad P, et al. Clinical benefit of small vessel stenting: one-year follow-up of the SISCA trial. Scand Cardiovasc J 2002; 36(2):86–90.

74   Semiz E, Ermis C, Yalcinkaya S, et al. Comparison of initial efficacy and long-term follow-up of heparin-coated Jostent with conventional NIR stent. Jpn Heart J 2003; 44(6):889–898.

75   Gurbel PA, Bliden KP. Platelet activation after stenting with heparin-coated versus noncoated stents. Am Heart J 2003; 146(4):E10.

76   Mehran R, Aymong ED, Ashby DT, et al. Safety of an aspirin-alone regimen after intracoronary stenting with a heparin-coated stent: final results of the HOPE (HEPACOAT and an Antithrombotic Regimen of Aspirin Alone) study. Circulation 2003; 108(9):1078–1083.

77   Haude M, Konorza TF, Kalnins U, et al. Heparin-coated stent placement for the treatment of stenoses in small coronary arteries of symptomatic patients. Circulation 2003; 107(9):1265–1270.

78   Jaster M, Schwimmbeck P, Spencker S, et al. Randomized comparison of platelet-leukocyte aggregates and platelet activation in blood: heparin-coated coiled wire stent implantation versus balloon angioplasty in acute myocardial infarction. Thromb Res 2003; 112(5–6):285–289.

79   Gupta V, Aravamuthan BR, Baskerville S, et al. Reduction of subacute stent thrombosis (SAT) using heparin-coated stents in a large-scale, real world registry. J Invasive Cardiol 2004; 16(6):304–310.

80   Madduri J, Assali A, Solodky A, et al. Acute and intermediate-term clinical outcomes following Heparin coated BX coronary stent implantation in patients with thrombus containing lesions. Int J Cardiovasc Intervent 2004; 6(2):77–81.

81   Baron JH, Aggrawal R, de Bono D, Gershlick AH. Adsorption and elution of c7E3 Fab from polymer-coated stents in-vitro [abstr]. Eur Heart J 1997; 18(suppl):503.

82   Schmidmaier G, Stemberger A, Alt E, Gawaz M, Neumann F, Schömig A. A new biodegradable polylactic acid coronary stent-coating, releasing PEG-Hirudin and a prostacycline analog, reduces both platelet activation and plasmatic coagulation [abstr]. J Am Coll Cardiol 1997; 29:354A.

83   Baron JH, Gershlick AH, Hogrefe K, et al. In vitro evaluation of c7E3-Fab (ReoPro) eluting polymer-coated coronary stents. Cardiovasc Res 2000; 46(3):585–594.

84   Baron JH, Aggrwal RK, Azrin MA, et al. Development of c7E3 Fab (abciximab) eluting stents for local drug delivery: effect of

sterilization and storage [abstr]. Circulation 1998; 98(17 suppl):I855.

85 Lahann J, Klee D, Pluester W, Hoecker H. Bioactive immobilization of r-hirudin on CVD-coated metallic implant devices. Biomaterials 2001; 22(8):817–826.

86 Dev V, Eigler N, Sheth S, et al. Kinetics of drug delivery to the arterial wall via polyurethane-coated removable nitinol stent: comparative study of two drugs. Cathet Cardiovasc Diagn 1995; 34:272–278.

87 Tanguay JF, Santos RM, Kruse KR, et al. Local delivery of a potent GPIIb/IIIa inhibitor using a composite polymeric stent reduces platelet deposition [abstr]. Eur Heart J 1996; 17(suppl):454.

88 Aggarwal R, Ireland D, Azrin M, Ezekowitz M, De Bono D, Gershlick A. Antithrombotic potential of polymer-coated stents eluting platelet glycoprotein IIb/IIIa receptor antibody. Circulation 1996; 94:3311–3317.

89 Aggarwal R, Ireland D, Azrin M, de Bono D, Gershlik A. Reduction in thrombogenicity of cellulose polymer-coated stents by immobilisation of platelet-targeted urokinase [abstr]. J Am Coll Cardiol 1997; 29:353A.

90 Santos RM, Tanguay JF, Crowley JJ, et al. Local administration of L-703,081 using a composite polymeric stent reduces platelet deposition in canine coronary arteries. Am J Cardiol 1998; 82(5):673–675,A8.

91 Kruse KR, Crowley JJ, Tanguay JF, et al. Local drug delivery of argatroban from a polymeric-metallic composite stent reduces platelet deposition in a swine coronary model. Catheter Cardiovasc Interv 1999; 46(4):503–507.

92 Alt E, Haehnel I, Beilharz C, et al. Inhibition of neointima formation after experimental coronary artery stenting: a new biodegradable stent coating releasing hirudin and the prostacyclin analogue iloprost. Circulation 2000; 101(12):1453–1458.

93 Swanson N, Hogrefe K, Javed Q, et al. Drug-eluting stents—could drugs tailored to the patient be loaded in the cather lab [abstr]? Eur Heart J 2000; 21(suppl):285.

94 Cox D, Anderson P, Roubin G, Chou C, Agrawal S, Cavender J. Effects of local delivery of heparin and methotrexate on neointimal proliferation in stented porcine coronary arteries. Coron Artery Dis 1992; 3:237–248.

95 Eccleston D, Lincoff A, Furst J. Administration of colchicine using a novel prolonged delivery stent produces a marked local biological effect within the porcine coronary artery(abstract). Circulation 1995; 92:I–87.

96 De Scheerder I, Wang K, Wilczek K, et al. Local methylprednisolone inhibition of foreign body response to coated intracoronary stents. Coronary Artery Dis 1996; 7:161–166.

97 Baker J, Nikolaychik V, Zulich A, et al. Fibrin coated stents as depot to deliver RGD peptide inhibit vascular reaction in atherosclerosis rabbit model [abstr]. J Am Coll Cardiol 1996; 27:197A.

98 De Scheerder I, Wilczek K, Van Dorpe J, et al. Local angiopeptin delivery using coated stents reduces neointimal proliferation in overstretched porcine coronary arteries. J Inves Cardiol 1996; 8:215–222.

99 Lincoff A, Furst J, Ellis S, Tuch R, Topol E. Sustained local delivery of dexamethasone by a novel intravascular eluting stent to prevent restenosis in the porcine coronary injury model. J Am Coll Cardiol 1997; 29:808–816.

100 Strecker EP, Gabelmann A, Boos I, et al. Effect on intimal hyperplasia of dexamethasone released from coated metal stents compared with non-coated stents in canine femoral arteries. Cardiovasc Intervent Radiol 1998; 21:487–496.

101 Drachman DE, Edelman ER, Kamath KR, et al. Sustained stent-based delivery of paclitaxel arrests neointimal thickening and cell proliferation [abstr]. Circulation 1998; 17(suppl):I740.

102 Yamawaki T, Shimokawa H, Kozai T, et al. Intramural delivery of a specific tyrosine kinase inhibitor with biodegradable stent suppresses the restenotic change of the coronary artery in pigs in vivo. J Am Coll Cardiol 1998; 32:780–786.

103 Armstrong J, Gunn J, Holt CM, et al. Local angiopeptin delivery from coronary stents in porcine coronary arteries [abstr]. European Heart J 1999; 20(suppl):336.

104 Rogers C, Groothuis A, Toegel G, et al. Paclitaxel release from inert polymer material-coated stents curtails coronary in-stent restenosis in pigs [abstr]. Circulation 2000; 102(18):II-1566.

105 Carter AJ, Bailey LR, Llanos G, et al. Stent based sirolimus delivery reduces neointimal proliferation in a porcine coronary model of restenosis [abstr]. J Am Coll Cardiol 2000; 35(suppl A):13.

106 Klugherz BD, Lianos G, Lieuallen W, et al. Dose-dependent inhibition of neointimal formation using a sirolimus-eluting stent [abstr]. Eur Heart J 2000; 21(suppl):283.

107 Klugherz BD, Lianos G, Lieuallen W, et al. Intramural kinetics of sirolimus eluting from an intracoronary stent [abstr]. Circulation 2000; 102(18):II-733.

108 Hong MK, Kornowski R, Bramwell O, et al. Paclitaxel-coated gianturco-roubin II (GR II) stents reduce neointimal hyperplasia in a porcine coronary in-stent restenosis model. Coron Artery Dis 2001; 12(6):513–515.

109 Suzuki T, Kopia G, Hayashi S, et al. Stent-based delivery of sirolimus reduces neointimal formation in a porcine coronary model. Circulation 2001; 104(10):1188–1193.

110 Heldman AW, Cheng L, Jenkins GM, et al. Paclitaxel stent coating inhibits neointimal hyperplasia at 4 weeks in a porcine model of coronary restenosis. Circulation 2001; 103(18):2289–2295.

111 New G, Moses JW, Roubin GS, et al. Estrogen-eluting, phosphorylcholine-coated stent implantation is associated with reduced neointimal formation but no delay in vascular repair in a porcine coronary model. Catheter Cardiovasc Interv 2002; 57(2):266–271.

112 Klugherz BD, Llanos G, Lieuallen W, et al. Twenty-eight-day efficacy and pharmacokinetics of the sirolimus-eluting stent. Coron Artery Dis 2002; 13(3):183–188.

113 Armstrong J, Gunn J, Arnold N, et al. Angiopeptin-eluting stents: observations in human vessels and pig coronary arteries. J Invasive Cardiol 2002; 14(5):230–238.

114 Yoon JH, Wu CJ, Homme J, et al. Local delivery of nitric oxide from an eluting stent to inhibit neointimal thickening in a porcine coronary injury model. Yonsei Med J 2002; 43(2):242–251.

115 Finkelstein A, McClean D, Kar S, et al. Local drug delivery via a coronary stent with programmable release pharmacokinetics. Circulation 2003; 107(5):777–784.

116 Wu YX, Johnson T, Herdeg C, et al. Stent-based local delivery of therapeutic adenovirus effectively reduces neointimal proliferation in porcine coronaries. Di Yi Jun Yi Da Xue Xue Bao 2003; 23(12):1263–1265.

117 Scheller B, Schmitt A, Bohm M, Nickenig G. Atorvastatin stent coating does not reduce neointimal proliferation after coronary stenting. Z Kardiol 2003; 92(12):1025–1028.

118 Wieneke H, Dirsch O, Sawitowski T, et al. Synergistic effects of a novel nanoporous stent coating and tacrolimus on intima proliferation in rabbits. Catheter Cardiovasc Interv 2003; 60(3):399–407.

119 Huang Y, Liu X, Wang L, et al. Local methylprednisolone delivery using a BiodivYsio phosphorylcholine-coated drug-delivery stent reduces inflammation and neointimal hyperplasia in a porcine coronary stent model. Int J Cardiovasc Intervent 2003; 5(3):166–171.

120 Banai S, Gertz SD, Gavish L, et al. Tyrphostin AGL-2043 eluting stent reduces neointima formation in porcine coronary arteries. Cardiovasc Res 2004; 64(1):165–171.

121 Carter AJ, Aggarwal M, Kopia GA, et al. Long-term effects of polymer-based, slow-release, sirolimus-eluting stents in a porcine coronary model. Cardiovasc Res 2004; 63(4):617–624.

122 Huang Y, Salu K, Liu X, et al. Methotrexate loaded SAE coated coronary stents reduce neointimal hyperplasia in a porcine coronary model. Heart 2004; 90(2):195–199.

123 Chen YX, Ma X, Whitman S, O'brien ER. Novel antiinflammatory vascular benefits of systemic and stent-based delivery of ethylisopropylamiloride. Circulation 2004; 110(24):3721–3726.

124 Jaschke B, Michaelis C, Milz S, et al. Local statin therapy differentially interferes with smooth muscle and endothelial cell proliferation and reduces neointima on a drug-eluting stent platform. Cardiovasc Res 2005; 68(3):483–492.

125 Qiu H, Gao RL, Tang ZR, et al. Experimental study of Mytrolimus-eluting stents on preventing restenosis in porcine coronary model. Zhonghua Xin Xue Guan Bing Za Zhi 2005; 33(6):561–564.

126 Uurto I, Mikkonen J, Parkkinen J, et al. Drug-eluting biodegradable poly-D/L-lactic acid vascular stents: an experimental pilot study. J Endovasc Ther 2005; 12(3):371–379.

127 Collingwood R, Gibson L, Sedlik S, et al. Stent-based delivery of ABT-578 via a phosphorylcholine surface coating reduces neointimal formation in the porcine coronary model. Catheter Cardiovasc Interv 2005; 65(2):227–232.

128 Kim W, Jeong MH, Cha KS, et al. Effect of anti-oxidant (carvedilol and probucol) loaded stents in a porcine coronary restenosis model. Circ J 2005; 69(1):101–106.

129 Wang L, Salu K, Verbeken E, et al. Stent-mediated methyl-prednisolone delivery reduces macrophage contents and in-stent neointimal formation. Coron Artery Dis 2005; 16(4):237–243.

130 GrubeE, Gerckens U, Rowold S, et al. Inhibition of in-stent restenosis by a drug eluting polymer stent: pilot trail with 18 month follow-up [abstr]. Circulation 2000; 102(18):II-554.

131 Rensing BJ, Vos J, Smits PC, et al. Coronary restenosis elimination with a sirolimus eluting stent: first European human experience with 6-month angiographic and intravascular ultrasonic follow-up. Eur Heart J 2001; 22(22):2125–2130.

132 Morice MC, Serruys PW, Sousa JE, et al. A randomized comparison of a sirolimus-eluting stent with a standard stent for coronary revascularization. N Engl J Med 2002; 346(23):1773–1780.

133 Liu X, Huang Y, Hanet C, et al. Study of antirestenosis with the BiodivYsio dexamethasone-eluting stent (STRIDE): a first-in-human multicenter pilot trial. Catheter Cardiovasc Interv 2003; 60(2):172–178.

134 Park SJ, Shim WH, Ho DS, et al. A paclitaxel-eluting stent for the prevention of coronary restenosis. N Engl J Med 2003; 348(16):1537–1545.

135 Schofer J, Schluter M, Gershlick AH, et al. Sirolimus-eluting stents for treatment of patients with long atherosclerotic lesions in small coronary arteries: double-blind, randomised controlled trial (E-SIRIUS). Lancet 2003; 362(9390):1093–1099.

136 De Scheerder I, Xianshun Liu, Chevalier B, LeClerc G, Colias A. Batimastat: mode of action, preclinical and clinical studies. In: Camenzind E, De Scheerder I, eds. Local Drug Delivery for Coronary Artery Disease. London and New York: Taylor & Francis, 2005:483–498.

137 Grube E, Silber S, Hauptmann KE, et al. TAXUS I: six- and twelve-month results from a randomized, double-blind trial on a slow-release paclitaxel-eluting stent for de novo coronary lesions. Circulation 2003; 107(1):38–42.

138 Bullesfeld L, Gerckens U, Muller R, Grube E. Long-term evaluation of paclitaxel-coated stents for treatment of native coronary lesions. First results of both the clinical and angiographic 18 month follow-up of TAXUS I. Z Kardiol 2003; 92(10):825–832.

139 Colombo A, Drzewiecki J, Banning A, et al. Randomized study to assess the effectiveness of slow- and moderate-release polymer-based paclitaxel-eluting stents for coronary artery lesions. Circulation 2003; 108(7):788–794.

140 Tanabe K, Serruys PW, Grube E, et al. TAXUS III Trial: in-stent restenosis treated with stent-based delivery of paclitaxel incorporated in a slow-release polymer formulation. Circulation 2003; 107(4):559–564.

141 Moses JW, Leon MB, Popma JJ, et al. Sirolimus-eluting stents versus standard stents in patients with stenosis in a native coronary artery. N Eng J Med 2003; 349:1315–1323.

142 Schampaert E, Cohen EA, Schluter M, et al. The Canadian study of the sirolimus-eluting stent in the treatment of patients with long de novo lesions in small native coronary arteries (C-SIRIUS). J Am Coll Cardiol 2004; 43(6):1110–1115.

143 Grube E, Lansky A, Hauptmann KE, et al. High-dose 7-hexanoyltaxol-eluting stent with polymer sleeves for coronary revascularization: one-year results from the SCORE randomized trial. J Am Coll Cardiol 2004; 44(7):1368–1372.

144 Grube E, Sonoda S, Ikeno F, et al. Six- and twelve-month results from first human experience using everolimus-eluting stents with bioabsorbable polymer. Circulation 2004; 109(18):2168–2171.

145 Lansky AJ, Costa RA, Mintz GS, et al. Non-polymer-based paclitaxel-coated coronary stents for the treatment of patients with de novo coronary lesions: angiographic follow-up of the DELIVER clinical trial. Circulation 2004; 109(16):1948–1954.

146 Gershlick A, De Scheerder I, Chevalier B, et al. Inhibition of restenosis with a paclitaxel-eluting, polymer-free coronary stent: the European evaLUation of pacliTaxel Eluting Stent (ELUTES) trial. Circulation 2004; 109(4):487–493.

147 Ardissino D, Cavallini C, Bramucci E, et al. Sirolimus-eluting vs uncoated stents for prevention of restenosis in small coronary arteries: a randomized trial. JAMA 2004; 292(22):2727–2734.

148 Hoye A, Tanabe K, Lemos PA, et al. Significant reduction in restenosis after the use of sirolimus-eluting stents in the treatment of chronic total occlusions. J Am Coll Cardiol 2004; 43(11):1954–1958.

149 Stone GW, Ellis SG, Cox DA, et al. One-year clinical results with the slow-release, polymer-based, paclitaxel-eluting TAXUS stent: the TAXUS-IV trial. Circulation 2004; 109(16):1942–1947.

150 Kwok OH, Chow WH, Law TC, et al. First human experience with angiopeptin-eluting stent: a quantitative coronary angiography and three-dimensional intravascular ultrasound study. Catheter Cardiovasc Interv 2005; 66(4):541–546.

151 Nakamura M, Wada M, Hara H, et al. Angiographic and clinical outcomes of a pharmacokinetic study of sirolimus-eluting stents: lesson from restenosis cases. Circ J 2005; 69(10): 1196–1201.

152 Airoldi F, Di Mario C, Ribichini F, et al. 17-beta-estradiol eluting stent versus phosphorylcholine-coated stent for the treatment of native coronary artery disease. Am J Cardiol 2005; 96(5):664–667.

153 Hausleiter J, Kastrati A, Wessely R, et al. Prevention of restenosis by a novel drug-eluting stent system with a dose-adjustable, polymer-free, on-site stent coating. Eur Heart J 2005; 26(15):1475–1481.

154 Sabate M, Jimenez-Quevedo P, Angiolillo DJ, et al. Randomized comparison of sirolimus-eluting stent versus standard stent for percutaneous coronary revascularization in diabetic patients: the diabetes and sirolimus-eluting stent (DIABETES) trial. Circulation 2005; 112(14): 2175–2183.

155 Commeau P, Barragan PT, Roquebert PO, Simeoni JB. ISR II study: a long-term evaluation of sirolimus-eluting stent in the treatment of patients with in-stent restenotic native coronary artery lesions. Catheter Cardiovasc Interv 2005; 66(2): 158–162.

156 Voudris V, Alexopoulos E, Karyofillis P, et al. Prospective native coronary artery stenosis treated with sirolimus-eluting stent (ONASSIS) registry—acute results and mid-term outcomes: a single-center experience. J Invasive Cardiol 2005; 17(8):401–405.

157 Hofma SH, Ong AT, Aoki J, et al. One year clinical follow up of paclitaxel eluting stents for acute myocardial infarction compared with sirolimus eluting stents. Heart 2005; 91(9):1176–1180.

158 Ge L, Iakovou I, Cosgrave J, et al. Immediate and mid-term outcomes of sirolimus-eluting stent implantation for chronic total occlusions. Eur Heart J 2005; 26(11):1056–1062.

159 Goy JJ, Stauffer JC, Siegenthaler M, et al. A prospective randomized comparison between paclitaxel and sirolimus stents in the real world of interventional cardiology: the TAXi trial. J Am Coll Cardiol 2005; 45(2):308–311.

160 Serruys PW, Sianos G, Abizaid A, et al. The effect of variable dose and release kinetics on neointimal hyperplasia using a novel paclitaxel-eluting stent platform: the Paclitaxel In-Stent Controlled Elution Study (PISCES). J Am Coll Cardiol 2005; 46(2):253–260.

161 Stone GW, Ellis SG, Cannon L, et al. Comparison of a polymer-based paclitaxel-eluting stent with a bare metal stent in patients with complex coronary artery disease: a randomized controlled trial. JAMA 2005; 294(10):1215–1223.

162 Dichek DA, Neville RF, Zwiebel JA, et al. Seeding of intravascular stents with genetically engineered endothelial cells. Circulation 1989; 80:1347–1353.

163 Flugelman MY, Virmani R, Leon MB, et al. Genetically engineered endothelial cells remain adherent and viable after stent deployment and exposure to flow in vitro. Circulation Res 1992; 70:348–354.

164 Amstrong J, Chan KH, Gunn J, et al. Antisense delivery from phosphorycholine (PC) coated stents [abstr]. Eur Heart J 2000; 21(suppl):285.

165 Leclerc G, Martel R, Vicks T, et al. Optimalization of parameters affecting DNA oligonucleotide loading onto phosphorylcholone (PC) coated Biodiv Ysio drug delivery stent. 6th Local Drug Delivery Meeting and Cardiovascular Course on Radiation and Molecular Strategies, Geneva, Switzerland, Jan 27–29. 2000.

166 Shirota T, Yasui H, Shimokawa H, Matsuda T. Fabrication of endothelial progenitor cell (EPC)-seeded intravascular stent devices and in vitro endothelialization on hybrid vascular tissue. Biomaterials 2003; 24(13):2295–2302.

167 Scott NA, Candal FJ, Robinson KA, et al. Seeding of intracoronary stents with immortalized human microvascular endothelial cells. Am Heart J 1995; 129:860–866.

168 Landau C, Willard JE, Clagett GP, et al. Biodegradable stents function as vehicles for vascular delivery of recombinant adenovirus vectors [abstr]. Circulation 1995; 92(8):I-670.

169 Labhasetwar V, Bonadio J, Goldstein S, et al. A DNA controlled-release coating for gene transfer: transfection in skeletal and cardiac muscle. J Pharm Sci 1998; 87(11): 1347–1350.

170 Klugherz BD, Chen w, Jones PL, et al. Successful gene transfer to the arterial wall using a DNA-eluting polymer-coated intracoronary stent in swine [abstr]. Eur Heart J 1999; 20:367.

171 Yuan J, Gao R, Shi R, et al. Intravascular local gene transfer mediated by protein-coated metallic stent. Chin Med J (Engl) 2001; 114(10):1043–1045.

172 Panetta CJ, Miyauchi K, Berry D, et al. A tissue-engineered stent for cell-based vascular gene transfer. Hum Gene Ther 2002; 13(3):433–441.

173 Swanson N, Hogrefe K, Javed Q, et al. Vascular endothelial growth factor (VEGF)-eluting stents: in vivo effects on thrombosis, endothelialization and intimal hyperplasia. J Invasive Cardiol 2003; 15(12):688–692.

174 Takahashi A, Palmer-Opolski M, Smith RC, Walsh K. Transgene delivery of plasmid DNA to smooth muscle cells and macrophages from a biostable polymer-coated stent. Gene Ther 2003; 10(17):1471–1478.

175 Radke PW, Griesenbach U, Kivela A, et al. Vascular oligonucleotide transfer facilitated by a polymer-coated stent. Hum Gene Ther 2005; 16(6):734–740.

176 Johnson TW, Wu YX, Herdeg C, et al. Stent-based delivery of tissue inhibitor of metalloproteinase-3 adenovirus inhibits neointimal formation in porcine coronary arteries. Arterioscler Thromb Vasc Biol 2005; 25(4):754–759.

22

The application of controlled drug delivery principles to the development of drug-eluting stents

Kalpana R. Kamath, Kathleen M. Miller, and James J. Barry

Background

Drug delivery systems that can precisely control drug release rates or target drugs to a specific body site have had an enormous medical and economic impact (1). The controlled-release drug delivery market is expanding rapidly, paralleled by active and aggressive research in the field (2). Conceptually, the ideal controlled drug delivery (CDD) system should fulfill two prerequisites: First, to deliver the drug at a rate dictated by the needs of the body over a period of treatment and second, to achieve spatial targeting to specific sites (3). A number of technological advancements with regard to regulating the rate of drug delivery, sustaining the duration of therapeutic action, and/or targeting the drug to a specific site or tissue have been made over recent years. The ability of CDD systems to release the drug in an amount sufficient to maintain the therapeutic levels over an extended time period provides significant improvements over traditional pharmaceutical formulations, such as tablets, capsules, or intravenous injections (4,5), as shown in Figure 1. The use of drug-eluting stents (DES)—now hailed as the pioneering technology in the interventional cardiology community—was the first successful application of CDD principles for the localized delivery of pharmacologic agents in the management of coronary artery disease.

Stent-based drug delivery as a treatment modality for occlusive coronary artery disease

In the setting of percutaneous coronary intervention (PCI), the use of bare-metal stents (BMS) enabled direct mechanical treatment of occluded vessels. BMS were successful in improving the outcomes of the procedure by alleviating the acute elastic recoil associated with balloon angioplasty and by reducing the angiographic restenosis rates in simple lesions, such as vessels >3.0 mm and focal lesions (6). However, in complex lesion subsets (i.e., small vessels <3.0 mm diameter), bifurcations, diffuse lesions, and in complex patients, such as diabetics, the use of BMS was still associated with restenosis in 30% to 60% of the stented patient population (7,8). An exuberant neointimal hyperplastic response post-stenting was considered to be the primary culprit leading to restenosis and late lumen loss associated with BMS use (9). Revascularization strategies prior to the introduction of DES centered on mechanical approaches, such as repeat angioplasty, restenting, cutting balloon, directional coronary atherectomy (DCA), phototherapy, and brachytherapy, among others. Most of these approaches met with limited clinical success in the management of restenosis.

The mid-to-late 1990s also experienced a plethora of studies that examined systemic pharmacotherapy to address the issue of restenosis post-PCI (10–12), although with minimal or no success, which could be attributed to many components. First, the systemic administration of a drug may not be effective in sustaining drug concentrations within the therapeutic window at the target site and, therefore, may induce untoward side effects due to high systemic drug concentrations. In addition, long-term, repeat-dose, and systemic therapy may be difficult due to the potential issues of patient noncompliance.

Given the numerous drawbacks associated with the approaches discussed earlier and the obvious advantage offered by the stent as a drug delivery platform, CDD via DES offers the potential to circumvent these problems by providing localized, sustained release of drug within the required therapeutic window. The delivery of drugs directly to the tissues affected by PCI minimizes the impact on nontarget tissues.

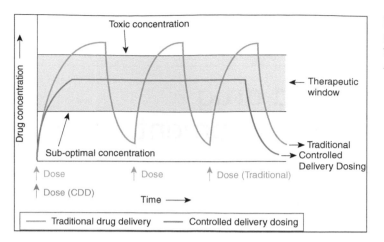

Figure 1
(*See color plate.*) Drug levels in the blood with traditional drug delivery and controlled-delivery dosing. *Abbreviation*: CDD, controlled drug delivery.

A multidisciplinary approach has been adopted to define the best DES design for use as a CDD system. This chapter discusses the principles of CDD and considers its application to the development of polymer-based DES using the TAXUS® paclitaxel-eluting stent (Boston Scientific Corporation, Natick, Massachusetts, U.S.A.) as an example of this technology.

Types of controlled drug delivery

Several types of CDD systems have been designed based on various mechanisms of drug release (Table 1). These mechanisms are dependent on the required site of drug delivery, the physicochemical properties of the drug and also of the delivery vehicle (13). Modes of administration can be oral, sublingual, transdermal, rectal, intrauterine, ocular, or parenteral (intramuscular, peritoneal, and subcutaneous routes of injection).

Drug release from CDD systems can be controlled by physical and/or chemical methods. Physical mechanisms rely on the properties of the drug delivery system, that is, the drug and the polymer carrier; drug release, in this case, is governed by diffusion of drug molecules through a polymer matrix, degradation of the polymer matrix, osmotic pressure, or ion exchange. Chemical mechanisms of drug release, on the other hand, involve the breaking of covalent bonds connecting the drug to the delivery vehicle by chemical or enzymatic degradation, as in prodrugs. Disadvantages associated with chemical mechanisms of drug release include the chemical modification of the drug molecules in order that they can be grafted to the delivery vehicle. Additionally, chemical modification of approved drug molecules results in the creation of new chemical entities (NCEs), which require new regulatory approvals. Given the simplicity and effectiveness of physical mechanisms in achieving precise control over drug-release kinetics, these mechanisms have dominated the CDD field (13).

Diffusion-controlled release can be achieved through reservoir or matrix designs. Typically, reservoir systems employ rate-controlling membranes to control drug release, as in transdermal patches. A diffusion-controlled matrix system, in contrast, typically has the drug dispersed within a polymer and the drug is released without the use of a rate-controlling barrier layer. A combination of matrix and reservoir systems can also be used as a means of controlling drug-release kinetics. Very recently, Implanon® (Organon International, Roseland, New Jersey, U.S.A.), a small rod implant made of an ethylene-vinyl acetate (EVA) core and etonorgestrel covered by an outer EVA membrane, was approved by the Food and Drug Administration. In addition, reservoir and matrix systems can be based on degradation-controlled drug release mechanisms. Such mechanisms would involve the dissolution or degradation of either the polymer that encapsulates the drug reservoir or of the polymer matrix in which the drug is dispersed.

Many commercial controlled-release products are based on both diffusion and degradation mechanisms (14). Such

Table 1   Mechanisms of controlled drug release

Diffusion-controlled
  Reservoir system
  Matrix system
Degradation-controlled
  Reservoir system
  Matrix system
Ion exchange
Osmosis
Prodrug

Source: From Ref. 13.

systems have the benefit of being injectable (if delivered as microspheres), implantable (thin rods), and/or resorbable (no retrieval surgery required). A few examples of commercially available CDD products based on degradable polymers include Lupron Depot® (TAP Pharmaceuticals Inc., Deerfield, Illinois, U.S.A.), ZOLADEX® (AstraZeneca Pharmaceuticals LP, Wilmington, Delaware, U.S.A.), Sandostatin LAR® Depot (Novartis Pharmaceutical Corp., East Hanover, New Jersey, U.S.A.), Risperdal® Consta™ (Janssen Pharmaceutical Products, Titusville, New Jersey, U.S.A.), and Vivitrol™ (Alkermes, Inc., Cambridge, Massachusetts, U.S.A.).

In some CDD systems, osmotic pressure acts as the driving force to generate a constant release of drug. The advantage of such a system is that it requires only osmotic pressure to be effective and is essentially independent of the environment (13,15).

Ion exchange can be an effective method for the controlled release of ionizable drugs that are coupled with the oppositely charged ionic groups on a polymer matrix, as in ion-exchange resins used in gastrointestinal (GI) applications. The drug release from such a system depends on the ionic environment, that is, pH and electrolyte concentration within the GI tract, as well as the properties of the resin (5).

Regardless of the drug release mechanism, utilizing polymers as a drug delivery vehicle enables controlled and sustained release of the drug. Moreover, for a DES, this has the added benefit of localized delivery to a specific target, that is, the stented artery area.

Controlled drug delivery— considerations for the vascular setting

As described earlier, selection of the appropriate CDD mechanism depends on the application and the nature of the drug to be delivered. The development of DES was centered on addressing the issue of restenosis occurring secondary to neointimal hyperplasia, which was the major limiting factor after BMS implantation (16–20).

The pathophysiology of restenosis

PCI, be it stent deployment, balloon angioplasty, or both, inevitably leads to injury to the vessel wall and damage to the endothelium. This vessel damage provokes the activation of platelets and the development of mural thrombi (21–26). Combined with the presence of a metallic foreign body, these events further trigger the activation of circulating neutrophils and tissue macrophages (23,25–27). The resulting biologic response often leads to uncontrolled proliferation of intimal and medial smooth muscle cells (SMCs), migration of SMCs from

the media into the vessel intima, and the deposition of extracellular matrix material. This leads to significant luminal narrowing three to six months after the procedure and is known as in-stent restenosis (ISR) (28). As other approaches proved to be ineffective in preventing ISR (29), local drug delivery was considered as a means to control hyperplastic responses in the section of the coronary vessel affected by the PCI.

Developing the optimal controlled drug delivery system for the prevention of restenosis

Catheter-based drug delivery devices were initially investigated for the local delivery of potential antirestenotic agents, but these met with limited success (30–33). Such catheter-based systems typically delivered the drug over a few minutes in forms that included liquids, gels, and microspheres. Ultimately, the use of this approach was found to be clinically ineffective in the prevention of restenosis. The reasons for this lack of efficacy could be the rapid washout of the drug downstream into the coronary circulation, poor tissue bioavailability, short duration of local drug residence, and/or selection of drugs that are ineffective in targeting restenosis (34).

In parallel to catheter-based delivery, stent-based approaches, such as passive stent coatings (diamond-like carbon, phosphorylcholine, and silicon carbide coatings) and immobilized drug coatings (heparin-coated stents), were evaluated for their ability to inhibit restenosis. Although animal studies demonstrated some promise, none of these technologies were clinically successful for restenosis prevention. The failure of these surface modification technologies further added to the need for the development of DES based on the principles of sustained CDD.

As a result of the significant collaborative efforts among polymer scientists, pharmacologists, engineers, chemists, and medical researchers, CDD systems suitable for the prevention of restenosis have been developed and shown to be clinically effective (35).

Controlled drug delivery via drug-eluting stents

Polymers—the optimal system for controlled drug-eluting stents

It is imperative that the kinetics of drug release are aligned with the kinetics of the restenotic cascade, as well as the pharmacologic mechanism of the drug being released (7,36). Rate-controlling systems, such as polymers, are ideal for this

Table 2 Some desired characteristics of polymers suitable for a drug-eluting stent
Good coating integrity through manufacturing, sterilization and deployment Vascular compatibility Compatibility with drug Ability to provide uniform drug distribution along the stent Ability to retain the drug on the stent during stent deployment Ability to control drug release Stable shelf life
Source: From Ref. 55.

application since they ensure drug retention during stent deployment, as well as modulation of drug-release kinetics.

Ideally, DES polymers should have the characteristics listed in Table 2, namely, the ability to maintain mechanical integrity on stent expansion (i.e., it must not crack, flake, or delaminate) and to withstand sterilization. The polymer should demonstrate vascular compatibility in order to avoid inflammatory reactions. In addition, the polymer should enable consistent and predictable dosing and release kinetics (37).

Figure 2A–C demonstrate the negative impact of sterilization, stent expansion, and inappropriate drug loading on various polymer carriers investigated in early DES studies, indicating the importance of formulation and process parameters on the coat integrity. This also emphasizes the need to subject the drug–polymer coating to rigorous testing at various stages of DES manufacturing, as it goes through coating, crimping, sterilization, and expansion.

Investigation of polymers for use in drug-eluting stents

Various synthetic and natural polymers in biostable and biodegradable classes were investigated over the last decade to assess their potential as DES coatings or coverings. The types of polymers included polyurethanes (38–40), silicone (41), polyorganophosphazenes (42), and fibrin (43,44) to name but a few. A multicenter preclinical study published by van der Giessen et al. (45) described the inflammatory sequelae in a porcine coronary artery model in response to the implantation of polymers with a wide range of chemistries. Polyglycolic acid/polylactic acid (PLGA), polycaprolactone (PCL), polyhydroxybutyrate valerate (PHBV), polyorthoester (POE), polyethylene oxide/polybutylene terephthalate (PEO/PBTP), polyurethane, silicone, and polyethylene terephthalate (PETP) were investigated in the form of strips cast onto stents, providing partial asymmetric stent coverings. The aggravated inflammatory and proliferative response of stented vessels at four weeks was ascribed to the asymmetric geometry of the implant, the lack of terminal sterilization of the implanted stents, or the inadequate surface and bulk physicochemical characterization of the polymers investigated.

In addition to the polymer-only studies, combined drug–polymer coatings were examined in animal models. These early DES coatings showed little or no difference in the inhibition of neointimal proliferation versus BMS. Some of these studies are listed in Table 3. The lack of success of these early studies could be attributed to many reasons, including suboptimal manufacturing processes, lack of desirable

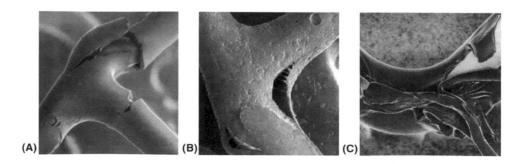

(A) (B) (C)

Figure 2

The effect of formulation and process parameters on early polymeric drug-eluting stent systems investigated. (A) Cracking of a polylactide (PLA)/polycaprolactone (PCL)-based coating with high paclitaxel loading, (B) disruption of a PLA/PCL-based coating post ethylene oxide sterilization, and (C) delamination of an ethylene-vinyl acetate-based coating post expansion.

Table 3 Some examples of early drug–polymer coating investigations

Polymer	Drug	Animal model	References
Polyurethane	Forskolin	Rabbit carotid	(74)
	Forskolin, etretinate	Rabbit carotid	(75)
Poly(organo) phosphazene	Methylprednisone	Porcine coronary	(76)
Poly-L-lactic acid	Dexamethasone	Porcine coronary	(34,77)
	Colchicine	Porcine coronary	(78)
Cellulose ester	Platelet glycoprotein IIb—IIIa inhibitors	Rabbit iliac	(79)
	Heparin/methotrexate	Porcine coronary	(80)
Poly-lactic acid/poly caprolocatone	Paclitaxel	Rabbit iliac	(81,82)

mechanical and physicochemical properties of the coating, vascular incompatibility of the polymers, nonuniform drug loading, inappropriate release kinetics, and/or use of ineffective antirestenotic drugs. Therefore, polymers with the desirable mechanical and biologic properties, as well as potentially more effective antirestenotic agents, were subsequently investigated.

The importance of preclinical models in the selection of polymer carriers

Studies conducted over the course of the last decade suggest that the outcomes of preclinical studies for DES are impacted significantly by the choice of the animal model. A consensus document assembled by clinical, academic, and industrial investigators engaged in preclinical interventional device evaluations provided an integrated view of the requirements for evaluating DES in preclinical models (46). The suggested requirements encompass study design, experimental performance, and histopathologic evaluations, emphasizing safety and efficacy at multiple points in time. The porcine coronary artery model has been the most widely used model of ISR since porcine coronary arteries have a structure and physiology similar to human coronary arteries (28,46–48), are generally of a similar diameter (49,50), and show similar responses to overstretch injury (28,47,48). Furthermore, the amount of neointimal hyperplasia induced in this animal model is closely linked to the degree of injury sustained by the vessel wall, enabling a straightforward comparison between the experimental and control groups. Another animal model of ISR is the rabbit iliac artery model, in which endothelial injury is induced using an angioplasty balloon, provoking pathological changes similar to those observed in human coronary arteries after stent implantation (28,51). However, the elasticity of the rabbit iliac artery can lead to difficulties in

the induction of the vascular damage that is required for these studies. Canine models are also commonly used in stent evaluation; although a more modest level of neointimal induction compared with that observed in the porcine model makes canine models less suitable for restenosis investigations (52). Figure 3 demonstrates the differential response to the same polymer in two different animal models. As seen from the histology data, a polyurethane coating appeared comparable with the BMS when examined in a rat subcutaneous model, but resulted in severe vessel wall damage and an exuberant hyperplastic response in the porcine coronary model. This example indicates the importance of conducting the evaluation of the stent coatings in the appropriate animal model in order to assess the impact of the DES components, individually and in combination.

Marketed drug-eluting stents employing controlled drug delivery systems

At present, a number of DES are marketed in the United States and Europe. The most widely used DES are the CYPHER® sirolimus-eluting stent (SES; Cordis Corp., Miami Lakes, Florida, U.S.A.) and the TAXUS paclitaxel-eluting stent. Sirolimus and paclitaxel are immunosuppressive and anticancer agents, respectively, and have known biological mechanisms of actions for these indications. As an anticancer agent, paclitaxel binds to microtubules, antagonizing their disassembly and preventing their depolymerization, thereby causing cells to arrest in the G2/M phase of the cell cycle (53). However, as an antirestenotic agent, paclitaxel was found to inhibit SMC proliferation and migration in a concentration-dependent manner (54–56) and caused G1 arrest in the cell cycle of SMCs. The mechanism of action of paclitaxel as an antirestenotic agent in a DES system is described in more detail in Chapter 10. As an immunosuppressive agent, one of

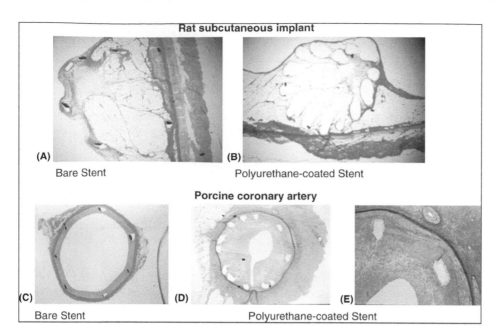

Figure 3
(*See color plate.*) Effect of animal model and implant site on biologic response to polyurethane-coated stents. Comparable biologic responses to a bare-metal stent (A) and a polyurethane-coated stent (B) in the rat subcutaneous model at 28 days. Dramatically different biological response to a bare-metal stent (C) and polyurethane-coated stent (D: low magnification image) and (E: high magnification image) in the porcine coronary artery model at 28 days.

the mechanisms of action of sirolimus is that it binds to the immunophilin FK506-binding protein 12, inhibits mammalian target of rapamycin (mTOR) activity and the subsequent activity of mitogen-activated kinases associated with cell proliferation, leading to cell-cycle arrest at the G1/S transition point (57,58). Additional information on the antirestenotic effects of sirolimus can be found in Chapter 10.

Clinical experience with the CYPHER® sirolimus-eluting stent

The pivotal Sirolimus-coated BX VELOCITY® Balloon-Expandable Stent in Treatment of Patients with De Novo Coronary Artery Lesions (SIRIUS) study of the CYPHER SES demonstrated a low rate of reintervention compared with

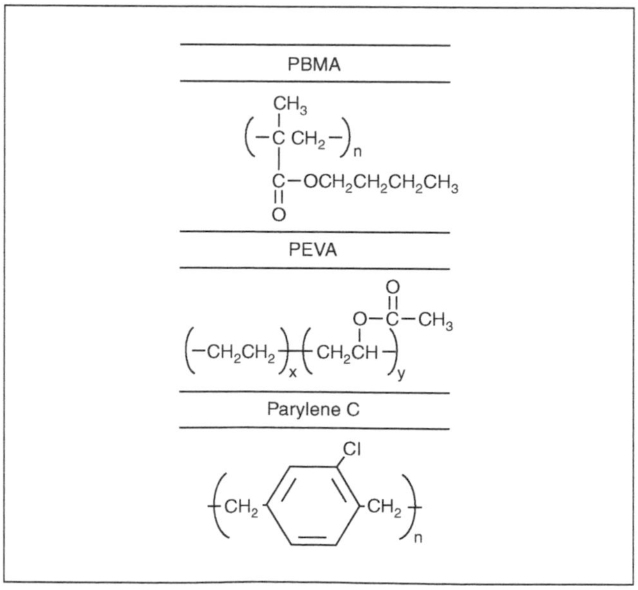

Polymers used in the CYPHER® sirolimus-eluting stent

The CYPHER stent employs two nonerodible polymers: polyethylene-co-vinyl acetate (PEVA) and poly-*n*-butyl methacrylate (PBMA). The combination of sirolimus and these two polymers constitutes the basecoat formulation that is applied to a stent treated with parylene C. In addition, a drug-free topcoat of PBMA polymer is applied to control the release kinetics of sirolimus (59), making this a diffusion-controlled reservoir device. The chemical structure of the polymers used in the CYPHER stent is shown in Figure 4.

The biocompatibility of the PBMA/PEVA was assessed in porcine as well as canine models (60). The results of these studies indicated a greater inflammatory response in the porcine coronary model compared with the canine model, pointing to the differences in the animal model governing the biologic response. The low coat weight of 750 μg polymer coating was well tolerated in both models at two months after implantation. However, a more severe strut-associated inflammation for the higher coat weight (1300 μg polymer-coated stents) was observed in the porcine model, but not in the canine model (Fig. 5).

Figure 4
Polymers used in the CYPHER™ sirolimus-eluting stent. *Abbreviations*: PBMA, poly-*n*-butyl methacrylate; PEVA, polyethylene-co-vinyl acetate.

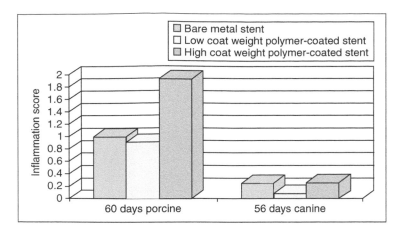

Figure 5
(*See color plate.*) Strut-associated inflammation in response to the polyethylene-co-vinyl acetate—poly-*n*-butyl methacrylate polymers in porcine and canine models at two months. *Source*: Adapted from Ref. 60.

BMS in over 1000 patients (61). These and other studies provided evidence for the clinical utility of the CYPHER stent for the prevention of ISR and are discussed in Chapter 10.

SIBS-coated stents (no paclitaxel) and BMS in the porcine coronary artery model indicate that SIBS has a biologic response comparable with BMS with no adverse impact on vessel biology (Fig. 8).

The Taxus® paclitaxel-eluting controlled drug delivery system

The TAXUS DES utilizes the Translute™ polymer—a matrix-controlled system made of a soft elastomeric triblock co-polymer, poly(styrene-*b*-isobutylene-*b*-styrene) (SIBS) (37). The chemical structure of SIBS is shown in Figure 6.

The TAXUS stent coating is a smooth, conformal coating with uniform stent coverage and good mechanical integrity. Figure 7A and B shows representative low and high magnification scanning electron micrograph (SEM) images of the TAXUS stent that underwent ethylene oxide sterilization, followed by stent expansion under aqueous conditions.

Vascular compatibility of poly (styrene-b-isobutylene-b-styrene)

The short- and long-term vascular compatibility of SIBS was examined in the porcine coronary model in an extensive portfolio of studies. Histomorphometric comparisons for the

In vitro characterization of the paclitaxel–poly(styrene-b-isobutylene-b-styrene) coatings

The paclitaxel–SIBS coatings were also characterized to assess drug distribution within the polymer matrix, drug–polymer interactions, and in vitro release kinetics (37). Various instrumentation techniques and methods were used to provide an in-depth evaluation of these crucial parameters in order to understand the factors governing the functional performance of the TAXUS stent. Transmission electron microscopy (TEM), nuclear magnetic resonance (NMR), differential scanning calorimetry (DSC), and atomic force microscopy (AFM) evaluations of the TAXUS coating indicated no measurable solubility of paclitaxel within the SIBS matrix, as well as a lack of chemical interactions between the drug and the polymer (55). The AFM images demonstrated that paclitaxel exists as discreet particles on the surface and in the bulk of the SIBS matrix (Fig. 9A). In addition, as the drug-to-polymer ratio increases from 8.8% to 25% and to 35% paclitaxel in the SIBS polymer, the size of the subsurface drug domain increases.

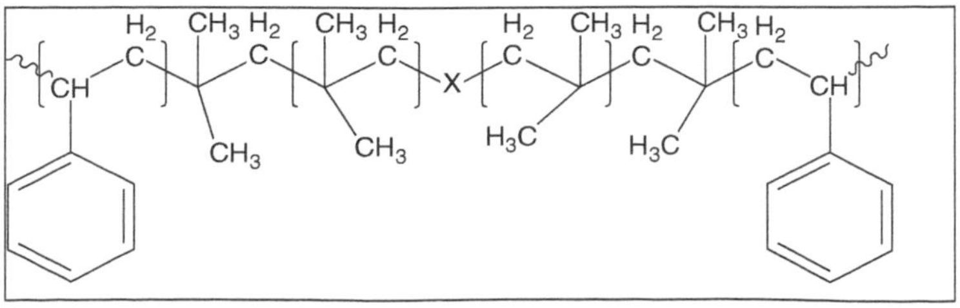

Figure 6
The chemical structure of poly(styrene-*b*-isobutylene-*b*-styrene).

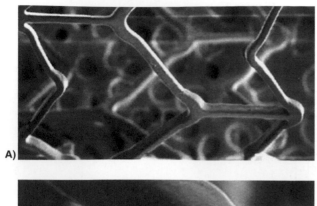

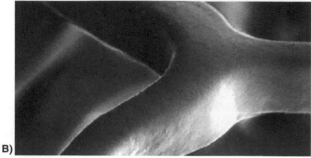

Figure 7
Scanning electron micrographs of the TAXUS stent poststerilization and expansion. (A) Low magnification, (B) high magnification. *Source*: From Ref. 55.

This increase in the domain size of the drug correlates well with the in vitro drug release behavior of these three formulations when examined in a physiologically relevant release medium [phosphate-buffered saline (PBS) with Tween 20; Fig. 9B]. As seen in the figure, increasing the drug loading from 8.8% to 35% weight by weight (w/w) had a notable effect on the cumulative amounts of the drug released. The 35% formulation, which has the largest drug domain size,

showed a high initial burst with more than half of the drug released within two days. The 8.8% formulation, with the smallest drug domain size, on other hand, showed a low level, sustained release. Based on the release kinetics, these formulations were termed slow release (8.8% w/w paclitaxel), moderate release (25% w/w paclitaxel), and fast release (35% w/w paclitaxel).

Furthermore, there is a direct correlation between the paclitaxel dose delivered to the artery and the vascular response when examined in the porcine coronary artery model. The slow-release formulation demonstrated patent lumen, struts covered by stable intima and re-endothelialization with minimal fibrin, whereas the fast-release formulation resulted in noticeable fibrin accumulation, an indication of higher level of drug exposure to the arteries (Fig. 10). It should be noted that the 8.8% slow-release formulation is currently marketed as TAXUS SR and has demonstrated efficacy in clinical studies; this is discussed in the next section.

Clinical experience with nonpolymeric paclitaxel drug-eluting stent systems

Paclitaxel has been tested in three studies that used a nonpolymeric delivery of paclitaxel from a stent (62,63). In the Asian Paclitaxel-Eluting Stent Clinical Trial (ASPECT) trial, patients were randomized to controls (BMS) or one of two doses of paclitaxel (1.3 or 3.1 μg/mm^2) on a Supra G^{TM} stent (Cook Incorporated, Bloomington, Indiana, U.S.A.) (63). The European EvaLuation of pacliTaxel ElUting Stent (ELUTES) trial in de novo lesions investigated the safety and efficacy of V-Flex Plus coronary stents (Cook Incorporated,

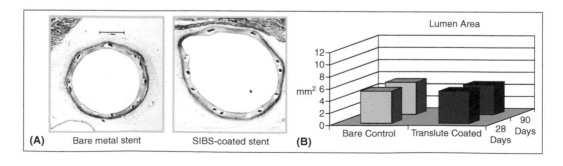

Figure 8
(*See color plate.*) Vascular compatibility of poly(styrene-*b*-isobutylene-*b*-styrene) (SIBS) as examined in the porcine coronary model. (A) Histology in the porcine coronary artery for the control bare metal versus SIBS-coated stents at 180 days. (B) Comparative vessel lumen area for the control bare metal versus SIBS-coated stents at 28 and 90 days. *Abbreviation*: SIBS, poly(styrene-*b*-isobutylene-*b*-styrene). *Source*: From Ref. 55.

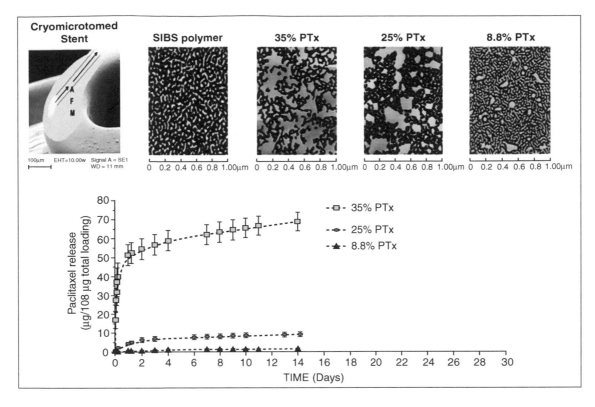

Figure 9

(*See color plate.*) Atomic force microscopy images and drug release kinetics of the paclitaxel-poly(styrene-*b*-isobutylene-*b*-styrene) polymer combination. *Abbreviations*: PTx, paclitaxel; SIBS, poly(styrene-*b*-isobutylene-*b*-styrene).

Bloomington, Indiana, U.S.A.) coated with escalating doses of paclitaxel (0.2, 0.7, 1.4, and 2.7 μg/mm² of stent surface area) applied directly to stent surface. In both trials, there was a dose-dependent effect on the angiographic parameters of restenosis (64). However, clinical outcomes at 6 and 12 months were not improved in these studies (65). The subsequent Drug ELuting coronary stent systems in the treatment of patients with de noVo nativE coronaRy lesions

I (DELIVER I) pivotal trial, undertaken in the United States, examined the nonpolymeric delivery of paclitaxel at the dose density of 3.0 μg/mm² in a much larger patient population by using target vessel failure (TVF) as a primary endpoint, a clinical rather than angiographic measurement. This study showed similar disappointing clinical outcomes to those seen in the earlier ASPECT and ELUTES studies (65).

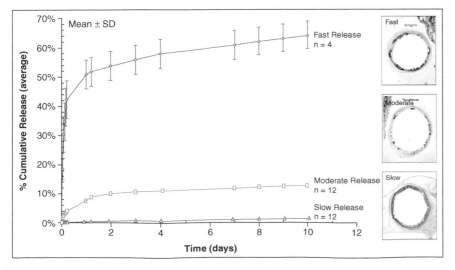

Figure 10

(*See color plate.*) Vascular response to slow-, moderate-, and fast-release formulations of paclitaxel in the porcine coronary artery model. Vascular response to 1 μg/mm² slow-, moderate-, and fast-release formulations in the porcine coronary artery model. *Source*: From Ref. 55.

Overall, key takeaways from the nonpolymeric paclitaxel delivery studies were that despite their improvement of angiographic parameters, paclitaxel-eluting stents without a polymer carrier did not demonstrate a positive effect on clinical outcomes, as seen with polymer-based paclitaxel elution (65), discussed in the next section. Potential reasons for the failure of such an approach could be loss of drug to the systemic circulation prior to reaching the target site during the stent deployment procedure, variability associated with the dose delivered to the lesion, and lack of control over drug-release kinetics due to the absence of a polymer carrier.

Clinical experience with Taxus® paclitaxel-eluting stent

The TAXUS paclitaxel-eluting stent clinical trial program comprised the largest dataset of randomized clinical trials (RCTs) and registries of DES to date, with over 6200 patients enrolled across six RCTs and multiple registries. The program included treatment of de novo lesions, as well as higher-risk lesion and patient populations (66–73). The data from the RCTs suggest that the TAXUS DES provides consistent and durable benefits across multiple lesion and patient types, even in patients with high risk factors and complex lesions (67). Evidence from peri and postapproval registries, where patient populations are more heterogeneous than those eligible and included in the RCTs, corroborate these findings, with overall low rates of cardiac events, including re-interventions. Extended follow-up after implantation of the polymer-based, paclitaxel-eluting TAXUS SR stent in de novo native coronary lesions confirmed the safety of this approach, with low overall major adverse cardiac events rates at three years and no late stent thrombosis between two and three years.

Conclusions

The development of localized CDD systems for vascular applications, specifically, for the prevention of restenosis, has presented significant challenges. The use of polymer-based systems as DES coatings to obtain precise control over the drug-release kinetics has allowed the delivery of potent antirestenotic agents directly into the tissues affected by the procedure. The clinical benefits of the paclitaxel- and SESs in randomized trials and registries suggest that this development marks a new era in the treatment of obstructive coronary artery diseases. Continued understanding of vascular biology and disease pathophysiology coupled with the knowledge of CDD principles will be crucial in future multidisciplinary efforts.

Acknowledgments

The authors would like to thank Cecilia Schott, PharmD for her assistance in the preparation of this chapter.

References

1 Langer R. Foreword. In: Mathiowitz EE, ed. Encyclopedia of Controlled Drug Delivery. Vol. 1. New York: John Wiley & Sons, Inc., 1999:xi.

2 Varma MVS, Kaushal AM, Garg A, Garg S. Factor affecting mechanism and kinetics of drug release from matrix-based oral controlled drug delivery systems. Am J Drug Deliv 2004; 2(1):43–67.

3 Chien YW. Controlled- and modulated-release drug-delivery systems. In: Swarbrick J, Baylan JC, eds. Encyclopedia of Pharmaceutical Technology. New York: Dekker, 1999: 281–313.

4 Khan GM. Controlled release oral dosage forms: some recent advances in matrix type drug delivery systems. Sciences 2001; 1(5):350–354.

5 Longer MA, Robinson JR. Sustained-release drug delivery systems. In: Gennaro AR, ed. Remington's Pharmaceutical Sciences. Easton, PA: Mack Publishing Company, 1990: 1676–1693.

6 Mitsuuchi Y, Johnson SW, Selvakumaran M, Williams SJ, Hamilton TC, Testa JR. The phosphatidylinositol 3-kinase/AKT signal transduction pathway plays a critical role in the expression of p21WAF1/CIP1/SDI1 induced by cisplatin and paclitaxel. Cancer Res 2000; 60(19):5390–5394.

7 Hiatt BL, Ikeno F, Yeung AC, Carter AJ. Drug-eluting stents for the prevention of restenosis: in quest for the Holy Grail. Catheter Cardiovasc Interv 2002; 55(3):409–417.

8 Mehran R, Dangas G, Abizaid AS, et al. Angiographic patterns of in-stent restenosis: classification and implications for long-term outcome. Circulation 1999; 100(18):1872–1878.

9 The Bypass Angioplasty Revascularization Investigation (BARI) Investigators. Comparison of coronary bypass surgery with angioplasty in patients with multivessel disease. N Engl J Med 1996; 335(4):217–225.

10 Bailey SR. Coronary restenosis: a review of current insights and therapies. Catheter Cardiovasc Interv 2002; 55(2): 265–271.

11 Eccleston D, Topol EJ. Clinical trials of restenosis. In: Feuerstein GZ, ed. Coronary Restenosis—From Genetics to Therapeutics. New York: Marcel Dekker, Inc., 1997:333–370.

12 Lau K-W, Sigwart U. Restenosis—an accelerated arteriopathy: pathophysiology, preventive strategies and research horizons. In: Edelman ER, Levy RJ, eds. Molecular Interventions and Local Drug Delivery. London: W. B. Saunders Co. Ltd., 1995:1–28.

13 Acharya G, Park K. Mechanisms of controlled drug release from drug-eluting stents. Adv Drug Deliv Rev 2006; 58(3):387–401.

14 Okada H, Toguchi H. Biodegradable microspheres in drug delivery. Crit Rev Ther Drug Carrier Syst 1995; 12(1):1–99.

15 Langer M, Leong J. Optimization of beam weights under dose-volume restrictions. Int J Radiat Oncol Biol Phys 1987; 13(8):1255–1260.

16 Farb A, Sangiorgi G, Carter AJ, et al. Pathology of acute and chronic coronary stenting in humans. Circulation 1999; 99(1):44–52.

17 Farb A, Weber DK, Kolodgie FD, Burke AP, Virmani R. Morphological predictors of restenosis after coronary stenting in humans. Circulation 2002; 105(25):2974–2980.

18 Hoffmann R, Mintz GS, Dussaillant GR, et al. Patterns and mechanisms of in-stent restenosis. A serial intravascular ultrasound study. Circulation 1996; 94(6):1247–1254.

19 Virmani R, Farb A. Pathology of in-stent restenosis. Curr Opin Lipidol 1999; 10(6):499–506.

20 Wahlgren CM, Frebelius S, Swedenborg J. Inhibition of neointimal hyperplasia by a specific thrombin inhibitor. Scand Cardiovasc J 2004; 38(1):16–21.

21 Alfonso F, Goicolea J, Hernandez R, et al. Angioscopic findings during coronary angioplasty of coronary occlusions. J Am Coll Cardiol 1995; 26(1):135–141.

22 Bauters C, Lablanche JM, Renaud N, McFadden EP, Hamon M, Bertrand ME. Morphological changes after percutaneous transluminal coronary angioplasty of unstable plaques. Insights from serial angioscopic follow-up. Eur Heart J 1996; 17(10):1554–1559.

23 Komatsu R, Ueda M, Naruko T, Kojima A, Becker AE. Neointimal tissue response at sites of coronary stenting in humans: macroscopic, histological, and immunohistochemical analyses. Circulation 1998; 98(3):224–233.

24 Liu MW, Hearn JA, Luo JF, et al. Reduction of thrombus formation without inhibiting coagulation factors does not inhibit intimal hyperplasia after balloon injury in pig coronary arteries. Coron Artery Dis 1996; 7(9):667–671.

25 Ott I, Neumann FJ, Kenngott S, Gawaz M, Schomig A. Procoagulant inflammatory responses of monocytes after direct balloon angioplasty in acute myocardial infarction. Am J Cardiol 1998; 82(8):938–942.

26 Smith-Norowitz TA, Shani J, Weiser W, et al. Lymphocyte activation in angina pectoris. Clin Immunol 1999; 93(2):168–175.

27 Kornowski R, Hong MK, Tio FO, Bramwell O, Wu H, Leon MB. In-stent restenosis: contributions of inflammatory responses and arterial injury to neointimal hyperplasia. J Am Coll Cardiol 1998; 31(1):224–230.

28 Babapulle MN, Eisenberg MJ. Coated stents for the prevention of restenosis: Part I. Circulation 2002; 106(21):2734–2740.

29 Sousa JE, Serruys PW, Costa MA. New frontiers in cardiology: drug-eluting stents: Part II. Circulation 2003; 107(18):2383–2389.

30 Bailey SR. Local drug delivery: current applications. Prog Cardiovasc Dis 1997; 40(2):183–204.

31 Camenzind E, Kint PP, Di Mario C, et al. Intracoronary heparin delivery in humans. Acute feasibility and long-term results. Circulation 1995; 92(9):2463–2472.

32 Mitchel JF, McKay RG. Treatment of acute stent thrombosis with local urokinase therapy using catheter-based, drug delivery systems: a case report. Cathet Cardiovasc Diagn 1995; 34(2):149–154.

33 Tahlil O, Brami M, Feldman LJ, Branellec D, Steg PG. The Dispatch catheter as a delivery tool for arterial gene transfer. Cardiovasc Res 1997; 33(1):181–187.

34 Lincoff AM, Topol EJ, Ellis SG. Local drug delivery for the prevention of restenosis. Fact, fancy, and future. Circulation 1994; 90(4):2070–2084.

35 Hunter WL. Drug-eluting stents: beyond the hyperbole. Adv Drug Deliv Rev 2006; 58(3):347–349.

36 Jenkins NP, Prendergast BD, Thomas M. Drug eluting coronary stents. BMJ 2002; 325(7376):1315–1316.

37 Ranade SV, Miller KM, Richard RE, Chan AK, Allen MJ, Helmus MN. Physical characterization of controlled release of paclitaxel from the TAXUS Express2 drug-eluting stent. J Biomed Mater Res A 2004; 71(4):625–634.

38 Fontaine AB, Dos Passos S, Spigos D, Cearlock J, Urbaneja A. Use of polyetherurethane to improve the biocompatibility of vascular stents. J Endovasc Surg 1995; 2(3):255–265.

39 Fontaine AB, Koelling K, Passos SD, Cearlock J, Hoffman R, Spigos DG. Polymeric surface modifications of tantalum stents. J Endovasc Surg 1996; 3(3):276–283.

40 Rechavia E, Litvack F, Fishbien MC, Nakamura M, Eigler N. Biocompatibility of polyurethane-coated stents: tissue and vascular aspects. Catheter Cardiovasc Diagn 1998; 45(2):202–207.

41 Widenhouse CW, Seeger JM, Baptist N, Martin PJ, Goldberg EP. Polydimethylsiloxane (PDMS) coatings for stainless steel endovascular stents: uniform, stable, highly adherent coatings for reduced thrombogenicity and drug delivery. 24th Annual Meeting of the Society for Biomaterials.

42 de Scheerder IK, Wilczek KL, Verbeken EV, et al. Biocompatibility of polymer-coated oversized metallic stents implanted in normal porcine coronary arteries. Atherosclerosis 1995; 114(1):105–114.

43 Holmes DR, Camrud AR, Jorgenson MA, Edwards WD, Schwartz RS. Polymeric stenting in the porcine coronary artery model: differential outcome of exogenous fibrin sleeves versus polyurethane-coated stents. J Am Coll Cardiol 1994; 24(2):525–531.

44 McKenna CJ, Camrud AR, Sangiorgi G, et al. Fibrin-film stenting in a porcine coronary injury model: efficacy and safety compared with uncoated stents. J Am Coll Cardiol 1998; 31(6):1434–1438.

45 van der Giessen WJ, Lincoff AM, Schwartz RS, et al. Marked inflammatory sequelae to implantation of biodegradable and nonbiodegradable polymers in porcine coronary arteries. Circulation 1996; 94(7):1690–1697.

46 Schwartz RS, Edelman ER, Carter A, et al. Drug-eluting stents in preclinical studies: recommended evaluation from a consensus group. Circulation 2002; 106(14):1867–1873.

47 Badimon JJ, Ortiz AF, Meyer B, et al. Different response to balloon angioplasty of carotid and coronary arteries: effects on acute platelet deposition and intimal thickening. Atherosclerosis 1998; 140(2):307–314.

48 Karas SP, Gravanis MB, Santoian EC, Robinson KA, Anderberg KA, King SB III. Coronary intimal proliferation after balloon injury and stenting in swine: an animal model of restenosis. J Am Coll Cardiol 1992; 20(2):467–474.

49 Hughes HC. Swine in cardiovascular research. Lab Anim Sci 1986; 36(4):348–350.

50 Lowe HC, Schwartz RS, Mac Neill BD, et al. The porcine coronary model of in-stent restenosis: current status in the era of drug-eluting stents. Catheter Cardiovasc Interv 2003; 60(4):515–523.

51 Carter AJ, Farb A, Gould KE, Taylor AJ, Virmani R. The degree of neointimal formation after stent placement in atherosclerotic rabbit iliac arteries is dependent on the underlying plaque. Cardiovasc Pathol 1999; 8(2):73–80.

52 Kantor B, Ashai K, Holmes DR Jr, Schwartz RS. The experimental animal models for assessing treatment of restenosis. Cardiovasc Radiat Med 1999; 1(1):48–54.

53 Rowinsky EK, Wright M, Monsarrat B, Lesser GJ, Donehower RC. Taxol: pharmacology, metabolism and clinical implications. Cancer Surv 1993; 17:283–304.

54 Axel DI, Kunert W, Goggelmann C, et al. Paclitaxel inhibits arterial smooth muscle cell proliferation and migration in vitro and in vivo using local drug delivery. Circulation 1997; 96(2):636–645.

55 Kamath KR, Barry JJ, Miller KM. The Taxus drug-eluting stent: a new paradigm in controlled drug delivery. Adv Drug Deliv Rev 2006; 58(3):412–436.

56 Signore PE, Machan LS, Jackson JK, et al. Complete inhibition of intimal hyperplasia by perivascular delivery of paclitaxel in balloon-injured rat carotid arteries. J Vasc Interv Radiol 2001; 12(1):79–88.

57 Formica RN Jr, Lorber KM, Friedman AL, et al. Sirolimus-based immunosuppression with reduce dose cyclosporine or tacrolimus after renal transplantation. Transplant Proc 2003; 35(3 suppl):95S–98S.

58 Marx SO, Jayaraman T, Go LO, Marks AR. Rapamycin-FKBP inhibits cell cycle regulators of proliferation in vascular smooth muscle cells. Circ Res 1995; 76(3):412–417.

59 Cypher Instructions for Use. Cypher sirolimus-eluting coronary stent on Raptor over-the-wire delivery system. http://www.fda.gov/cdrh/PDF2/p020026c.pdf Accessed Aug 8, 2006.

60 Suzuki T, Kopia G, Hayashi S, et al. Stent-based delivery of sirolimus reduces neointimal formation in a porcine coronary model. Circulation 2001; 104(10):1188–1193.

61 Moses JW, Leon MB, Popma JJ, et al. Sirolimus-eluting stents versus standard stents in patients with stenosis in a native coronary artery. N Engl J Med 2003; 349(14):1315–1323.

62 Gershlick A, de Scheerder I, Chevalier B, et al. Inhibition of restenosis with a paclitaxel-eluting, polymer-free coronary stent: the European evaLUation of pacliTaxel Eluting Stent (ELUTES) trial. Circulation 2004; 109(4):487–493.

63 Hong MK, Mintz GS, Lee CW, et al. Paclitaxel coating reduces in-stent intimal hyperplasia in human coronary arteries: a serial volumetric intravascular ultrasound analysis from the Asian Paclitaxel-Eluting Stent Clinical Trial (ASPECT). Circulation 2003; 107(4):517–520.

64 Grube E, Buellesfeld L. Paclitaxel-eluting stents: current clinical experience. Am J Cardiovasc Drugs 2004; 4(6):355–360.

65 Silber S. Paclitaxel-eluting stents: are they all equal? An analysis of six randomized controlled trials in de novo lesions of 3,319 patients. J Interv Cardiol 2003; 16(6):485–490.

66 Colombo A, Drzewiecki J, Banning A, et al. Randomized study to assess the effectiveness of slow- and moderate-release polymer-based paclitaxel-eluting stents for coronary artery lesions. Circulation 2003; 108(7):788–794.

67 Dawkins KD, Grube E, Guagliumi G, et al. Clinical efficacy of polymer-based paclitaxel-eluting stents in the treatment of complex, long coronary artery lesions from a multicenter, randomized trial: support for the use of drug-eluting stents in contemporary clinical practice. Circulation 2005; 112(21):3306–3313.

68 Dawkins KD, Stone GW, Colombo A, et al. Integrated analysis of medically treated diabetic patients in the TAXUS® program: benefits across stent platforms, paclitaxel release formulations, and diabetic treatments. Eurointervention 2006; 2:61–68.

69 Grube E, Silber S, Hauptmann KE, et al. Two-year-plus follow-up of a paclitaxel-eluting stent in de novo coronary narrowings (TAXUS I). Am J Cardiol 2005; 96(1):79–82.

70 Grube E, Silber S, Hauptmann KE, et al. TAXUS I: six- and twelve-month results from a randomized, double-blind trial on a slow-release paclitaxel-eluting stent for de novo coronary lesions. Circulation 2003; 107(1):38–42.

71 Stone GW, Ellis SG, Cannon L, et al. Comparison of a polymer-based paclitaxel-eluting stent with a bare metal stent in patients with complex coronary artery disease: a randomized controlled trial. JAMA 2005; 294(10):1215–1223.

72 Stone GW, Ellis SG, Cox DA, et al. One-year clinical results with the slow-release, polymer-based, paclitaxel-eluting TAXUS stent: the TAXUS-IV trial. Circulation 2004; 109(16):1942–1947.

73 Tanabe K, Serruys PW, Grube E, et al. TAXUS III Trial: in-stent restenosis treated with stent-based delivery of paclitaxel incorporated in a slow-release polymer formulation. Circulation 2003; 107(4):559–564.

74 Lambert TL, Dev V, Rechavia E, Forrester JS, Litvack F, Eigler NL. Localized arterial wall drug delivery from a polymer-coated removable metallic stent. Kinetics, distribution, and bioactivity of forskolin. Circulation 1994; 90(2):1003–1011.

75 Dev V, Eigler N, Sheth S, Lambert T, Forrester J, Litvack F. Kinetics of drug delivery to the arterial wall via polyurethane-coated removable nitinol stent: comparative study of two drugs. Catheter Cardiovasc Diagn 1995; 34(3):272–278.

76 de Scheerder I, Wang K, Wilczek K, et al. Local methylprednisolone inhibition of foreign body response to coated intracoronary stents. Coron Artery Dis 1996; 7(2):161–166.

77 Lincoff AM, Furst JG, Ellis SG, Tuch RJ, Topol EJ. Sustained local delivery of dexamethasone by a novel intravascular eluting stent to prevent restenosis in the porcine coronary injury model. J Am Coll Cardiol 1997; 29(4):808–816.

78 Eccleston D, Lincoff A, Furst J. Administration of colchicine using a novel prolonged delivery stent produces a marked local biological effect within the porcine coronary artery [abstract]. Circulation 1995; 92:1–67.

79 Aggarwal RK, Ireland DC, Azrin MA, Ezekowitz MD, de Bono DP, Gershlick AH. Antithrombotic potential of polymer-coated stents eluting platelet glycoprotein IIb/IIIa receptor antibody. Circulation 1996; 94(12):3311–3317.

80 Cox DA, Anderson P, Roubin G, Chou C, Agrawal S, Cavender J. Effects on the local delivery of heparin and methotrexate on neotimal proliferation in stented porcine coronary arteries. Coron Artery Dis 1992; 3:237–248.

81 Drachman DE, Edelman ER, Kamath KR, et al. Sustained stent-based delivery of paclitaxel arrests neointimal thickening and cell proliferation. Abstracts from the 71st Scientific Sessions, AHA, 1998.

82 Drachman DE, Edelman ER, Seifert P, et al. Neointimal thickening after stent delivery of paclitaxel: change in composition and arrest of growth over six months. J Am Coll Cardiol 2000; 36(7):2325–2332.

23

Brachytherapy

Ravi K. Ramana, Ferdinand Leya, and Bruce E. Lewis

Introduction

Following introduction into clinical practice, the long-term success of percutaneous coronary intervention (PCI) has been most limited by restenosis of the target-vessel segment. Initially, restenosis rates following percutaneous coronary angioplasty (PTCA) exceeded 50% (1,2), and attempts to reduce the frequency of restenosis and possible repeat revascularization included the use of bare-metal stents (BMS). Long-term studies using BMS revealed improved, yet still significant, rates of restenosis (~17%–20%) (3–5). Therefore, in the late 1990s, newer therapies including intracoronary brachytherapy (ICB) were developed in attempts to treat in-stent restenosis (ISR). Initial studies using ICB were promising, but limited by predictable complications such as edge restenosis and late thrombosis. More recently, the introduction of drug-eluting stents (DES) into the practice of interventional cardiology has nearly eliminated the use of ICB. This chapter attempts to summarize the theoretical basis, clinical trials, limitations, and possible therapeutic role of ICB in the drug-eluting stent era.

General physics

Today, there are two radiation delivery systems approved for the treatment of ISR in the United States: one the gamma-radiation device using 192Ir (Cordis Checkmate, no longer commercially available) and the other beta-radiation device using 32P, 90Sr/90Y (Novoste Beta-Cath, Fig. 1). The ICB procedure involves transient placement of gamma- or beta-emitting radiation seeds or wires (delivered within an indwelling coronary-artery catheter) into the coronary vasculature. The given radiation therapy penetrates the coronary arterial endothelium and breaks the bonds of single-stranded DNA in rapidly dividing cells. Theoretically, this results in attenuation and/or cessation of smooth-muscle and fibroblast proliferation, decreased collagen synthesis, and ensuing target-lesion restenosis (6,7).

Electrons (produced by beta emitters) produce their ionizing energy directly on nuclear DNA; photons (produced by gamma emitters) produce their ionizing effects indirectly by producing fast-moving electrons. For the same energy, beta emitters result in a smaller field of radiation and less penetration to surrounding parts of the body (than do gamma emitters) (8). Therefore, limitations specific to gamma radiation include the need for longer treatment times and higher generalized radiation exposure (9).

The optimal dosing of ICB for the treatment of ISR provides sufficient radiation to the targeted vessel wall in order to block cell proliferation and neointimal hyperplasia. Previous dose-finding randomized trials using the beta-radiation source recommend 18.4 Gy at 2 mm from the source center (if the target-vessel diameter is 2.7–3.35 mm) or 23 Gy (if the target-vessel diameter is 3.35–4.0 mm). At these radiation doses, there was a reported 4% restenosis rate at six months (10). Also, it is imperative that radiation therapy be directed at the entire segment injured by balloon inflation and/or stent deployment including a 5-mm margin on each side of the stent (11).

Background and previous research

Restenosis is caused by an exaggerated healing response involving smooth-muscle migration, neointimal hyperplasia, and a lack of compensatory vessel wall dilation, which result in a reduced vessel luminal diameter at the site of previous endothelial trauma or injury (12–14). Therefore, ICB attempts to attenuate this process and reduce target-vessel restenosis and repeat revascularization.

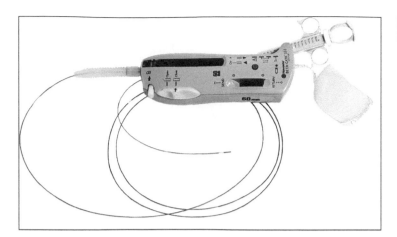

Figure 1
Novoste beta-cath system. *Source*: From Ref. 74.

In 1994, Liermann et al. (15) pioneered clinical application of vascular brachytherapy by showing feasibility, safety, and short-term efficacy of intraluminal radiation in patients undergoing percutenous angioplasty of restenosed femoral or popliteal arteries. In that same year, ICB was first introduced as an effective modality to reduce the restenosis process following balloon angioplasty of coronary arteries in animal models (16). These investigators showed that ICB reduced the bulk of the neointimal lesion by 71% and percent area stenosis by 63% compared with control animals. There was no evidence of radiation vasculopathy or myocardial damage immediately following the procedure and at six-month follow-up (17). Further studies validated these findings and provided a dose–response curve relationship between radiation dose and inhibition of neointimal proliferation (18,19).

In 1997, Condado et al. was the first to investigate the effectiveness of ICB after PTCA in human coronary arteries. Twenty-one patients who underwent PTCA for unstable angina received ICB (gamma radiation) for prevention of restenosis. Immediate and six-month follow-up revealed improved freedom from major adverse cardiac event (MACE) defined as death, myocardial infarction or target lesion revascularization compared with several previously completed balloon angioplasty trials (20). More importantly, this trial demonstrated that ICB was a feasible technique for the prevention of restenosis without any unexpected acute complications in humans.

In addition, attempts to deliver radiation therapy to symptomatic de novo or restenotic native coronary-artery lesions included the deployment of very low activity 32P radioactive stents. Preliminary data for clinical endpoints (e.g., subacute stent thrombosis, TLR, and death at 30 days) appeared promising, but the long-term angiographic follow-up revealed an unacceptable restenosis rate at or beyond the stent edges (21,22). Consequently, further studies to evaluate this technique were abandoned.

Since these original studies, there have been numerous clinical randomized trials and prospective registries detailing the efficacy of ICB as an adjunctive therapy for de novo native coronary or sapheneous vein graft lesions treated with balloon angioplasty and/or stent implantation (Table 1). The majority of these studies revealed that there was no additional benefit, but possible harm, of ICB therapy for patients who undergo PCI for de novo stenosis (10,23–25).

Also, studies investigating the use of ICB with patients with SVG ISR had a significantly reduced need for repeat target-lesion revascularization, but not target-vessel revascularization (TVR) or combined TVR–MACE endpoints (28,29).

Current clinical application

Although ICB has been studied in various clinical conditions, the Food and Drug Administration (FDA) has approved ICB only when delivered in combination with standard PCI for the treatment of ISR. Therefore, there is no current FDA approval for the use of ICB in the prevention of ISR during treatment of de novo lesions. Similarly, the American College of Cardiology has deemed ICB a "safe and effective treatment for ISR" (Class IIa, Level of Evidence A: conditions for which there is conflicting evidence and/or a divergence of opinion about the usefulness/efficacy of a procedure or treatment, but the weight of evidence/opinion is in favor of usefulness/efficacy). These data were derived from multiple randomized clinical trials or meta-analyses (30). These recommendations are based on several randomized control trials that suggested a reduced restenosis and target-lesion revascularization rates when ICB is used immediately following standard PCI for ISR (Table 2) (24,31–35). Although many of these trials' results initially appeared promising, more recent studies suggested that ICB following standard PCI treatment of ISR only delays the restenotic process rather than preventing it (36).

Brachytherapy in the drug-eluting stent ERA

The introduction of DES for the treatment of symptomatic coronary-artery disease has significantly reduced the previous

Table 1 Selected randomized clinical trials of intracoronary brachytherapy as adjunctive therapy during PCI

Trial	Year	Source	F/U	N	Inclusion	Randomization	Restenosis	TLR	MI	Death
Condado (20)	1997	G	12	21	De novo PCI	None: all ICB	19%	19%	9.5%	0%
GENEVA (27) (Pilot study)	1997	B	6	15	De novo POBA	None: ICB w/POBA/BMS	33%	33%	6.7%	6.7%
BERT (66)	1998	B	6	21	De novo POBA	None: ICB p POBA	14.2%	N/A	N/A	N/A
ARREST (67) (Pilot study)	1998	G	6	25	De novo/ISR	PCI/BMS + ICB vs. PCI/BMS	47%	16%	NA	0%
BERT 1.5 (68)	1998	B	6	31	De novo PCI	None: all ICB p PCI	24%	23%	NA	N/A
PREVENT (25)	2000	B	12	105	De novo PCI	PCI + ICB vs. PCI + Placebo	8/39	6/24	10/4	1/0
							$P = 0.012$	$P < 0.05$	NS	NS
Beta-Cath (69)	2001	B	8	1100	De novo PCI/PCBA	PCI + ICB vs. PCI	21/33	13.7/15.4	MACE	N/A
							$P < 0.05$	NS	18.7/20.6	NS
Dose-Finding Trial (22)	2001	B	6	181	De novo PCI	Various doses of ICB	N/A	11.1%	2.8%	0.6%
BRIE (26)	2002	B	12	149	De novo PCI	None: PCI + ICB	N/A	20.6%	10.1%	2%
BRIDGE (23)	2004	B	12	112	De novo stent	BMS + ICB vs. BMS	N/A	20.4/11.1	11.2/5.2	0/0
								NS	NS	NS

Abbreviations: BMS, bare-metal stents; ICB, intracoronary brachytherapy; N/A, results not published; NS, not statistically significant ($P > 0.05$); PCI, percutaneous coronary intervention; PTCA, percutaneous transluminal coronary angioplasty; POBA, plain old balloon angioplasty.

Table 2   Selected randomized clinical trials of intracoronary brachytherapy for in-stent restenosis

Trial	Year	Source	F/U	N	Inclusion	Randomization	Restenosis (%)	TVR (%)	MI (%) / MACE	Death (%)
ARTISTIC (67)	1998	G	6	26	ISR	PTCA/BMS/RA + ICB vs. PTCA/BMS/RA	20%	3.8	15 / MACE	7.7
WRIST (31) (Waksman)	2000	G	60	65/65	ISR	PCI + ICB vs. PCI	NA	39/66 $P = 0.008$	19/19 NS	15/15 NS
GAMMA-ONE (32) (Leon)	2001	G	9	131/121	ISR	PCI + ICB vs. PCI	55/32 $P = 0.01$	42/24 $P < 0.01$	4.1/9.9 $P = 0.09$	0.8/3.1 $P = 0.17$
SCRIPPS (44) (Grise)	2002	G	72	29/26	Restenotic area (±ISR)	BMS + ICB vs. BMS	N/A	48/23 $P = 0.05$	10/4 NS	31/19 NS
Long WRIST (70) (Waksman)	2003	G	12	60/60	ISR + Lesion >36 mm	PCI + ICB vs. PCI	45/73 $P < 0.05$	39/62 $P < 0.05$	23.7/18.3 NS	1.7/6.8 NS
Cha et al. (71)	2003	G/B	6	1275	ISR	BMS + ICB vs. ICB	N/A	18.9/12.6 $P = 0.002$	16.8/11.5 $P < 0.05$	1.0/1.3 NS
Chu et al. (72)	2005	G/B	10	54/34	Previous ICB with Re-ISR	DES + ICB vs. ICB	N/A	4/20.6 $P = 0.02$	0/0 NS	2/0 NS
Beta WRIST (25) (Waksman)	2000	B	6	50/50	De novo PCI	PCI + ICB vs. PCI	NA	17/36 $P = 0.001$	7/5 NS	0/4 $P = 0.11$
INHIBIT (34)	2002	B	9	166/166	ISR	PCI + ICB vs. PCI	16/48 $P < 0.0001$	8/26 $P < 0.0001$	5/3 NS	3/2 NS
START (35) (Popma)	2002	B	8	244/232	ISR	PTCA* + ICB vs. PTCA*	0.8/0.4 NS	57/76 $P = 0.027$	10/13 NS	7/11 NS
SISR (40) (Holmes)	2006	B	9	259/125	ISR	SES vs. ICB	N/A	10.8/21.6 $P = 0.008$	2.7/0 NS	0/0 NS
TAXUS V ISR (39) (Stone)	2006	B	9	194/199	ISR	PES vs. ICB	N/A	6.3/13.9 $P = 0.01$	3.7/4.6 NS	0/0.5 NS

Abbreviations: BMS, bare-metal stents; DES, drug-eluting stent; ICB, intracoronary brachytherapy; N/A, results not published; NS, not statistically significant ($P > 0.05$); PCI, percutaneous coronary intervention; PES, paclitaxel-eluting stent; PTCA, percutaneous transluminal coronary angioplasty; PTCA*, balloon angioplasty ± rotational atherectomy, directional atherectomy, or excimer laser angioplasty; SES, sirolimus-eluting stent.

limitation of restenosis with BMS (~25% vs. ~4%) or repeat revascularizations (~20% vs. ~4%) (36,37). Based on these data, it seemed plausible that DES may be as effective, if not more effective, therapy for the treatment of BMS ISR as that of ICB.

Therefore, prospective randomized trials have compared the use of DES with angioplasty versus DES combined with ICB for the treatment of BMS ISR. After six- and nine-month follow-up, it was evident that patients who had received DES (paclitaxal- and sirolimus-eluting) alone (and not ICB) had a >50% reduction in angiographic restenosis, ischemic target-lesion revascularization, and major cardiac events. There was no significant difference in rates of myocardial infarction or death between the two groups (38,39). A current trial, the TROPICAL study, is a multicenter nonrandomized trial evaluating the efficacy of sirolimus-eluting stent in the treatment with an ISR lesion attempting to validate these results (40).

Similar studies have used intravascular ultrasound (IVUS) at six-month follow-up to evaluate differences in target-lesion healing and have found less intimal hyperplasia and late lumen loss due to increased plaque burden in patients who had received DES without ICB for the treatment of BMS ISR (41). On the other hand, other IVUS-guided studies have described a significant "black-hole phenomenon" in patients who have undergone ICB. The "black hole," a homogeneous, echolucent intraluminal entity depicted on IVUS, is felt to be a result of an impaired response to endothelial injury and an altered molecular proliferative response (Fig. 2). This intraluminal tissue, which accounted for ~50% of the neo-intimal growth in areas of restenosis after radioactive stent implantation (42), leads to a hypocellular matrix with abundant proteoglycans but no elastin or mature collagen. This ultrasound "phenomenon" was not consistently seen in patients who had only received DES or BMS.

Limitations and complications

Although ICB has proven to improve clinical outcomes in patients with ISR, ICB is extremely logistically demanding, since it requires a radiation oncologist, interventional cardiologist, and medical radiation physicist to be available simultaneously at all times (i.e., emergent, on-call cardiac catheterization cases). Also, there remain several predictable complications with the use of ICB, including injury to normal vessels, edge stenosis, delayed healing of dissections, coronary-artery spasm, thrombosis, and late occlusion as described subsequently.

Injury to normal vessels

Initial concern of possible deleterious effects of ICB on adjacent normal coronary-artery endothelium was refuted with studies showing three- and five-year follow-up results of patients randomized to PCI with IRB or PCI with placebo

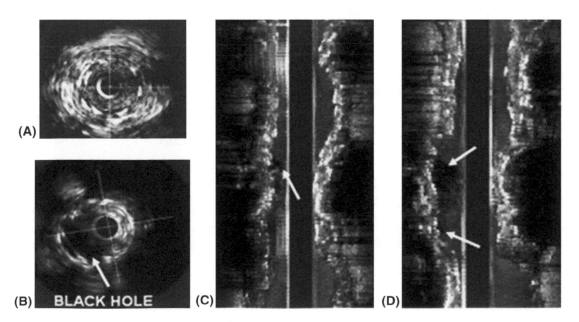

Figure 2
Black-hole phenomenon. IVUS image of black-hole formation after drug-eluting stents. (A) Cross-sectional IVUS image of typical appearance of neointimal hyperplasia after bare-metal stents implantation, (B) cross-sectional IVUS image of echolucent intraluminal tissue (*black hole, white arrow*) that is intraluminal, juxtaposed to stent strut, and (**C,D**) longitudinal IVUS image reconstructions of stented segment with black hole (*white arrows*). *Abbreviation*: IVUS, intravascular ultrasound. *Source*: From Ref. 43.

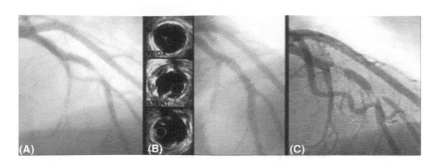

Figure 3
Edge restenosis: representative angiographic images of a candy-wrapper edge restensosis effect four months after radioactive ^{32}P β-emitting stent implantation. Baseline angiography (A) demonstrates a significant stenosis in the left anterior coronary artery. After implantation (B) of a ^{32}P β-emitting stent, IVUS images show minimal plaque burden. At four-month follow-up (C), there is little in-stent late loss, but severe stenosis at both stent edges. *Source*: From Ref. 22.

"sham" therapy. Data analysis of these studies revealed no significant change in IVUS appearance of the adjacent normal coronary-artery endothelium and no increased rates of non-TVR (43,44).

Edge stenosis

Earlier clinical application of ICB was complicated by a pattern of recurrent edge restenosis. This pattern of restenosis, referred to as a "candy-wrapper effect" (Fig. 3), was first described in trials investigating radioactive stent efficacy (21,22) and has been attributed to lower-dose radiation stimulating proliferation at the edges of the prior treatment zones (i.e., a "geographical miss" describing inadequate coverage of the diseased/injured segment) (44,45), neointimal proliferation, negative remodeling (21,22,46,49), and longitudinal plaque displacement (47,48). Continued research proved that this pattern of restenosis can be avoided by distribution of the radiation treatment to the entire site of injured endothelium with extension of the radiation margins to 5 to 14.5 mm beyond each end of the stent. Also, a higher dose of radiation is essential to eliminate further increases in neointimal hyperplasia at the overlapped segments of multiple stents (50,51).

Delayed dissection healing and pseudoaneursym formation

There are data suggesting that the same mechanisms which ICB impairs the exaggerated healing process leading to lesion restenosis also may cause reduced healing of coronary-artery dissections following high-pressure ballon inflation and/or stent deployment. An IVUS-guided study which compared immediate postangioplasty and six-month follow-up findings in patients who underwent balloon angioplasty with and without subsequent ICB, found no difference in clinical endpoints at six months, but did find a significant increase in residual dissection (and possible early aneurysm formation) in patients who underwent ICB (Fig. 4) (52). Related research has

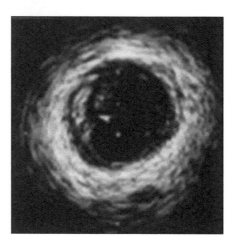

Figure 4
Delayed dissection healing. A clear dissection plane noted six months' postangioplasty and irradiation, demonstrating nonresolution of the dissection. *Source*: From Ref. 52.

provided further evidence that ICB can induce arterial dilatation and pseudoaneursym formation (20).

Coronary-artery spasm and thrombosis

Although deemed a "safe and effective therapy," there are considerable reports of angina and ischemic electrocardiographic (ECG) changes during the ICB therapy. Further investigation has revealed that the use of high-dose beta-radiation following de novo coronary-artery stent deployment resulted in a higher incidence of coronary-artery spasm proximal and distal to the stent as measured by qualitative coronary angiography when compared with placebo "sham" therapy (67% vs. 9%). Although only a minority of these spasm episodes were classified as severe (>90% diameter stenosis) with significant ECG changes or hemodynamic instability, these severe episodes resolved only after repetitive doses of intra-coronary vasodilator injection (53). Additionally, ICB can induce endothelial damage with subsequent significant vasomotor dysfunction (54) via severely impairing endothelium-dependent

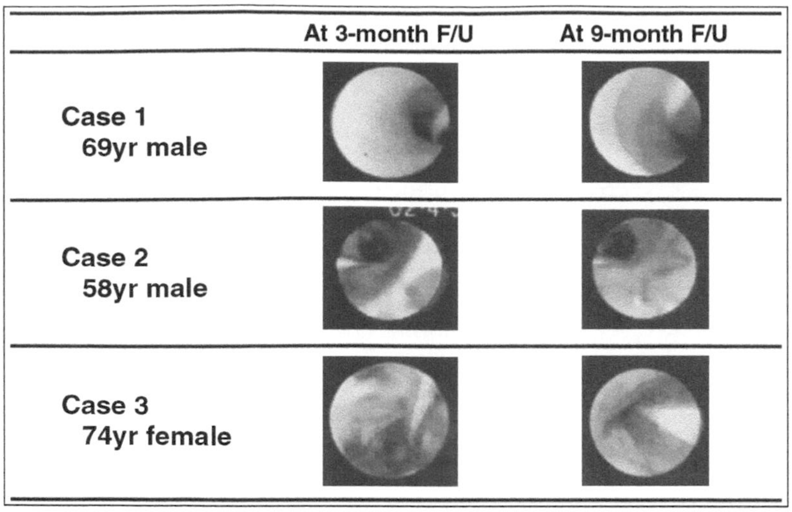

Figure 5
Delayed endothelial healing. In case 1, a smooth, white lesion was detected at three and nine months. In case 2, erosion with a superficial thrombus was seen at three months. At nine months, the erosion had disappeared, although an uncovered stent was observed. In case 3, severe, circumferential erosion with superficial thrombus was detected at three months, with erosion still evident but partly improved at nine months. These results suggest that the healing process was not completed nine months after brachytherapy. *Source*: From Ref. 73.

smooth-muscle relaxation (53,54). Furthermore, studies have reported that ICB can stimulate a dose-dependent increase in platelet recruitment release of vasoconstrictive mediators, leading to coronary arterial spasm (55,56).

Late thrombosis and occlusion/need for dual antiplatelet

Early evaluation of patients receiving ICB following PCI revealed a sudden thrombotic event rate of 6% to 9% confirmed by angiography 2 to 15 months following balloon angioplasty and/or stent deployment (57,58). This late thrombosis is possibly due to pronounced delay in endothelialization (Fig. 5), poor healing dissections at the edges of the recently deployed stents, and regression or erosion of tissue outside the stent that occurs after exposure to ICB (58). This pathophysiology leads to a continued thrombogenic coronary surface that requires longer dual-antiplatelet therapy with aspirin and clopidogrel for at least 6 to 12 months (30,59,60).

Future considerations

Initial clinical investigations suggested that ICB used in combination with PCI could be most beneficial in those patients with high-risk ISR lesions (24,61). But, as previously stated, long-term follow-up has been less promising. However, there may remain a small subset of patients with ISR in which ICB may prove useful. More specifically, definitive statements cannot be made addressing the optimal treatment strategy (DES vs. ICB) in the treatment of ISR in bifurcation (62), diffuse (>50 mm) (63,64), or heavily calcified lesions, smaller target vessels (<2.25 mm) (65), or patients with renal

dysfunction (7) due to persistent high restenosis rates or lack of comparative research in these patient populations.

From a clinical standpoint, there remain no randomized controlled trials evaluating the optimal treatment strategy for ISR of DES (DES vs. ICB). For now, it seems reasonable to consider DES therapy alone in any initial restenosis of previously deployed DES, and only consider ICB or surgical revascularization in situations of recurrent restenosis of DES.

References

1 Chaitman BR, Rosen AD, Williams DO, et al. Myocardial infarction and cardiac mortality in the Bypass Angioplasty Revascularization Investigation (BARI) randomized trial. Circulation 1997; 96(7):2162–2170.
2 King SB, Barnhart HX, Kosinski AS, et al. Angioplasty or surgery for multivessel coronary artery disease: comparison of eligible registry and randomized patients in the EAST trial and influence of treatment selection on outcomes. Emory Angioplasty versus Surgery Trial Investigators. Am J Cardiol 1997; 79(11):1453–1459.
3 SoS Investigators. Coronary artery bypass surgery versus percutaneous coronary intervention with stent implantation in patients with multivessel coronary artery disease (the Stent or Surgery trial): a randomised controlled trial. Lancet 2002; 360(9338):965–970.
4 Serruys PW, Ong AT, van Herwerden LA, et al. Five-year outcomes after coronary stenting versus bypass surgery for the treatment of multivessel disease: the final analysis of the Arterial Revascularization Therapies Study (ARTS) randomized trial. J Am Coll Cardiol 2005; 46(4):575–581.
5 Rodriguez A, Mele E, Peyregne E, et al. Three-year follow-up of the argentine randomized trial of percutaneous transluminal coronary angioplasty versus coronary artery bypass surgery in multivessel disease (ERACI). J Am Coll Cardiol 1996; 27(5):1178–1184.
6 Fischer-Dzoga K, Dimitrievich GS, Schaffner T. Effect of hyperpliemic serum and irradiation wound healing in primary

quiescent cultures of vascular cells. Exp Mol Pathol 1989; 52: 1–12.

7   Mukherjee M, Moliterno DJ. Brachytherapy for in-stent restenosis: a distant second choice to drug-eluting stent placement. JAMA 2006; 295:1307–1309.

8   Stack R, Roubin GS, O'Neill WW. Interventional Cardiovascular Medicine. 2nd ed. Philadelphia, Pennsylvania: Churchill Livingstone, 2002.

9   Waksman R. Vascular brachytherapy: applications in the era of drug-eluting stents. Rev Cardiovasc Med 2002; 3(S5):S23–S30.

10 Verin V, Popowski Y, de Bruyne B, et al. Endoluminal beta-radiation therapy for the prevention of coronary restenosis after balloon angioplasty. N Engl J Med 2001; 344(4): 243–249.

11 User's Manual, Beta-Cath System, Novoste Corporation, 2002.

12 Gertz SD, Gimple LW, Banai S, et al. Geometric remodeling is not the principal pathogenetic process in restenosis after balloon angioplasty. Evidence from correlative angiographic – histomorphometric studies of atherosclerotic arteries in rabbits. Circulation 1994; 90:3001–3008.

13 Lafont A, Guzman LA, Whitlow PL, Goormastic M, Cornhill JF, Chisholm GM. Restenosis after experimental angioplasty. Intimal, medial and adventitial changes associated with constrictive remodeling. Circ Res 1995; 76:996–1002.

14 Post MJ, Borst C, Kuntz RE. The relative importance of arterial remodeling compared with intimal hyperplasia in lumen narrowing after balloon angioplasty. Circulation 1994; 89:2816–2821.

15 Liermann DD, Bauernsachs R. Schopohl B, et al. Five year follow-up after brachytherapy for restenosis in peripheral arteries. Sem Interv Cardiol 1997; 2(2):133–137.

16 Wiedermann JG, Marboe C, Amols H, Schwartz A, Weinberger J. Intracoronary irradiation markedly reduces restenosis after balloon angioplasty in a porcine model. J Am Coll Cardiol 1994; 23(6):1491–1498.

17 Wiedermann JG, Marboe C, Amols H, et al. Intracoronary irradiation markedly reduces neointimal proliferation after balloon angioplasty in swine: persistent benefit at 6-month follow-up. J Am Coll Cardiol 1995; 25(6):1451–1456.

18 Waksman R, Robinson KA, Crocker IR, et al. Endovascular low-dose irradiation inhibits neointima formation after coronary artery balloon injury in swine: a possible role for radiation therapy in restenosis prevention. Circulation 1995; 91:1533–1539.

19 Verin V, Popowski Y, Urban P, et al. Intra-arterial beta irradiation prevents neointimal hyperplasia in a hypercholesterolemic rabbit restenosis model. Circulation 1995; 92: 2284–2290.

20 Condado JA, Waksman R, Gurdiel O, et al. Long-term angiographic and clinical outcome after percutaneous transluminal coronary angioplasty and intracoronary radiation therapy in humans. Circulation 1997; 96:727–732.

21 Albiero R, Nishida T, Adamian M, et al. Edge restenosis after implantation of high activity ^{32}P radioactive β-emitting stents. Circulation 2000; 101:2454–2457.

22 Albiero R, Adamian M, Kobayashi N, et al. Short- and intermediate-term results of ^{32}P radioactive β-emitting stent implantation in patients with coronary artery disease: the Milan Dose-Response Study. Circulation 2000; 101:18–26.

23 Serruys PW, Wijns W, Sianos G, et al. Direct stenting versus direct stenting followed by centered beta-radiation with intravascular ultrasound-guided dosimetry and long term platelet treatment: results of a randomized trial BRIDGE. J Am Coll Cardiol 2004; 44(3):228–537.

24 Teirstein PS, Massullo V, Jani S, et al. Catheter-based radiotherapy to inhibit restenosis after coronary stenting. N Engl J Med 1997; 336:1697–1703.

25 Raizner AE, Oesterle SN, Waksman R, et al. Inhibition of restenosis with beta-emitting radiotherapy: report of the Proliferation Reduction with Vascular Energy Trial (PREVENT). Circulation 2000; 102:951.

26 Serruys PW, Sianos G, van der Giessen, et al. Intracoronary beta-radiation to reduce restenosis after balloon angioplasty and stenting; the Beta Radiation In Europe (BRIE) study. Eur Heart J 2002; 23(17):1351–1359.

27 Verin V, Urban P, Popowski Y, et al. Feasibility of intracoronary β-irradiation to reduce restenosis after balloon angioplasty: a clinical pilot study (GENEVA). Circulation 1997; 95:1138–1144.

28 Waksman R, Ajani AE, White RL, et al. Intravascular gamma radiation for in-stent restenosis in saphenous-vein bypass grafts. N Engl J Med 2002; 346:1194–1199.

29 Castagna MT, Mintz GS, Waksman R, et al. Comparitive efficacy of gamma-irradition for treatment of in-stent restenosis in sapheneous vein graft versus native coronary artery in-stent restenosis. Circulation 2001; 104:3020–3022.

30 Smith, SC, Feldman TE, Morrison DA, et al. Percutaneous coronary intervention: ACC/AHA/SCAI 2005 guideline update for (Update of the 2001 PCI Guidelines). J Am Coll Cardiol 2006; 47:216–235.

31 Waksman R, White RL, Chan RC, et al. Intracoronary gamma-radiation therapy after angioplasty inhibits recurrence in patients with in-stent restenosis. Circulation 2000; 101:2165–2171.

32 Leon MB, Teirstein PS, Moses JW, et al. Localized intracoronary gamma-radiation therapy to inhibit the recurrence of restenosis after stenting. N Engl J Med 2001; 344:250–256.

33 Waksman R, Bhargava B, White L, et al. Intracoronary beta-radiation therapy inhibits recurrence of in-stent restenosis. Circulation 2000; 101:1895–1898.

34 Waksman R, Raizner AE, Yeung AC, et al. Use of localised intracoronary beta radiation in treatment of in-stent restenosis the INHIBIT randomized controlled trial. Lancet 2002; 359:551–557.

35 Popma JJ, Suntharalingam M, Lanksy AJ, et al. Randomized trial of 90Sr/90Y beta-radiation versus placebo control for treatment of in-stent restenosis. Circulation 2002. 106: 1090–1096.

36 Baierl V, Baumgartner S, Pollinger B, et al. Three-year clinical follow-up after strontium/yttrium beta-irradiation for the treatment of in-stent coronary restenosis. Am J Cardiol 2005; 96: 1399–1403.

37 Morice MC, Serruys PW, Sousa JE, et al. A randomized comparison of a sirolimus-eluting stent with a standard stent for coronary revascularization. The RAVEL trial. N Engl J Med 2002; 346:1773–1780.

38 Holmes DR, Leon MB, Moses JW, et al. SIRIUS analysis of 1-year clinical outcomes in the SIRIUS trial. A randomized trial of a sirolimus-eluting stent versus a standard stent in patients at high risk for coronary restenosis. Circulation 2004; 109: 634–640.

39 Stone G, Ellis S, O'Shaughnessy, et al. Paclitaxel-eluting stents vs vascular brachytherapy for in-stent restenosis within bare-metal

stents: the TAXUS V ISR randomized trial; for the TAXUS V ISR investigators. JAMA 2006; 295:1253–1263.

40　Holmes DR, Teirstein P, Satlet L, et al. Sirolimus-eluting stents vs vascular brachytherapy for in-stent restenosis within bare-metal stents: the SISR randomized trial. JAMA 2006; 295: 1264–1273.

41　Cordis Corporation. A Multi-Center, Non-Randomised Study of the CYPHER™ Sirolimus-Eluting Stent in the Treatment of Patient With an in-Stent Restenotic Native Coronary Artery Lesion (TROPICAL Study), 2006.

42　Schiele TM, Konig A, Rieber J, et al. Sirolimus-eluting stent implantation and beta-irradiation for the treatment of in-stent restenotic lesions: comparison of underlying mechanisms of acute gain and late loss as assessed by volumetric intravascular ultrasound. Am Heart J 2005; 150(2):351–357.

43　Costa MA, Sabate M, Angiolillo DJ, et al. Intravascular ultrasound characterization of the "black hole" phenomenon after drug-eluting stent implantation. Am J Cardiol 2006; 97(2): 203–206.

44　Grise MA, Massullo V, Jani S, et al. Five-year clinical follow-up after intracoronary radiation: results of a randomized clinical trial. Circulation 2002; 105:2737–2740.

45　Ahmed JM, Mintz GS, Waksman R, et al. Safety of intracoronary γ-radiation on uninjured reference segments during the first 6 months after treatment of in-stent restenosis: a serial intravascular ultrasound study. Circulation 2000; 101: 2227–2230.

46　Kim H, Waksman R, Cottin Y, et al. Edge stenosis and geographical miss following intracoronary gamma radiation for in-stent restenosis. J Am Coll Cardiol 2001; 37:1026–1030.

47　Sabate M, Serruys PW, van der Giessen WJ, et al. Geometric vascular remodeling after balloon angioplasty and β-radiation therapy: a three-dimensional intravascular ultrasound study. Circulation 1999; 100:1182–1188.

48　Ahmed JM, Mintz GS, Weissman NJ, et al. Mechanism of lumen enlargement during intracoronary stent implantation: an intravascular ultrasound study. Circulation 2000; 102:7–10.

49　Limpjankit T, Waksman R, Yock PG, et al. Intravascular ultrasound volumetric assessment of intimal hyperplasia in stents treated with intracoronary radiation. Am J Cardiol 1999; 84: 850–854.

50　User's Manual. Beta-Cath System. Atlanta, GA: Novoste Corporation; 2002.

51　Cheneau E, Waksman R, Yazdi H, et al. How to fix the edge effect of catheter-based radiation therapy in stented arteries. Circulation 2002; 106(17):2271–2277.

52　Meerkin D, Tardif JC, Bertrand OF, et al. The effects of intracoronary brachytherapy on the natural history of postangioplasty dissections. J Am Coll Cardiol 2000; 36(1):59–64.

53　Scheinert D, Strand V, Muller R, et al. High-dose beta-radiation after de novo stent implantation induces coronary artery spasm. Circulation 2002; 105:1420–1423.

54　Wiedermann JG, Leavy JA, Amolls H, et al. Effects of high-dose intracoronary radiation on vasomotor function and smooth muscle histopathology. Am J Physiol 1994; 267: H125–H132.

55　Salame MY, Verheye S, Mulkey SP, et al. The effect of endovascular radiation on platelet recruitment at sites of balloon angioplasty in pig coronary arteries. Circulation 2000; 101:1087–1090.

56　Vodovotz Y, Waksman R, Kim WH, et al. Effects of intracoronary radiation on thrombosis after balloon overstretch injury in the porcine model. Circulation 1999; 100:2527–2533.

57　Costa MA, Sabaté M, van der Giessen JM, et al. Late coronary occlusion after intracoronary brachytherapy. Circulation 1999; 100(8):789–792.

58　Waksman R, Bhargava B, Mintz G, et al. Late total occlusion after intracoronary brachytherapy for patients with in-stent restenosis. J Am Coll Cardiol 2000; 36(1):65–68.

59　Food and Drug Administration. FDA approval of coronary artery brachytherapy. N Engl J Med 2001; 344(4):297–299.

60　Waksman R, Ajani AE, Pinnow E, et al. Twelve versus six months of clopidogrel to reduce major cardiac events in patients undergoing gamma-radiation therapy for in-stent restenosis: Washington Radiation for In-Stent restenosis Trial (WRIST) 12 versus WRIST PLUS. Circulation 2002; 106(7):776–778.

61　Mehran, R, Dangas G, Abizaid AS, et al. Angiographic patterns of instent restenosis: classification and implications for long term outcome. Circulation 1999; 100:1872–1878.

62　Colombo A, Moses JW, Morice MC, et al. Randomized study to evaluate sirolimus-eluting stents implanted at coronary bifurcation lesions. Circulation 2004; 109:1244–1249.

63　Ajani AE, Waksman R, Cha D, et al. The impact of lesion length and reference vessel diameter on angiographic restenosis and target vessel revascularization in treating in-stent restenosis with radiation. J Am Coll Cardiol 2002; 39:1290–1296.

64　Kaluza GL, Raizner AE. Brachytherapy for restenosis after stenting for coronary artery disease: its role in the drug-eluting stent era. Curr Opin Cardiol 2004; 19(6):601–607.

65　Lemos PA, Chourmouzios AA, Saia F, et al. Treatment of very small vessels with 2.25-mm diameter sirolimus-eluting stents (RESEARCH registry). Am J Cardiol 2004; 93(5): 633–636.

66　King SB III, Williams DO, Chougule P, et al. Endovascular b-radiation to reduce restenosis after coronary balloon angioplasty: results of the β Energy Restenosis Trial (BERT). Circulation 1998; 97:2025–2030.

67　Durairaj A, Faxon DP. The ARTISTIC and ARREST trials. J Invasive Cardiol 2000; 12(1):44–49.

68　Coen VL, Knook AH, Wardeh AJ, et al. Endovascular brachytherapy in coronary arteries: the Rotterdam experience. Cardiovasc Radiat Med 2000; 2(1):42–50.

69　Knutz R. Beta-Cath Trial. Annual Scientific Session of the American College of Cardiology, 2001.

70　Waksman R, Cheneau E, Ajani AE, et al. Intracoronary radiation therapy improves the clinical and angiographic outcomes of diffuse in-stent restenotic lesions: results of the Washington Radiation for In-Stent Restenosis Trial for Long Lesions (Long WRIST) Studies. Circulation 2003; 107:1744.

71　Cha DH, Ajane AE, Cheneua E, et al. Clinical trials of intracoronary gamma radiation therapy for in-stent restenosis. J Invasive Cardiol 2002; 14(7):432–437.

72　Chu WW, Toguson R, Pichard AD, et al. Drug-eluting stents versus repeat vascular brachytherapy for patients with recurrent in-stent restenosis after failed intracoronary radiation. J Invasive Cardiol 2005; 17(12):659–662.

73　Okada M, Tamai H, Kyo E, et al. Serial angioscopic findings after successful intracoronary brachytherapy for in-stent restenosis. Am J Cardiol 2006; 97(1):21–25.

74　Beta-Cath 3.5F System. Best Vascular Inc. Novoste Company Website www.novoste.com

24

Polymers and drug-eluting stents

Robert Falotico and Jonathon Zhao

Introduction

Stents are fenestrated hollow metal tubes that are used to scaffold arteries following balloon angioplasty. Both balloon-expandable and self-expanding stent designs have been used in the coronary circulation. Stenting of de novo lesions with balloon-expandable stents has been shown to produce a significant reduction in restenosis rates when compared with balloon angioplasty in randomized trials (1,2). However, restenosis rates after bare metal stenting still remained at 15% to 20% in patients with simple lesions and over 30% in patients with complex lesions (3).

The pathophysiology of in-stent restenosis is fundamentally a wound-healing response in which inflammation, cell proliferation, migration, and extracellular matrix production are key steps. Studies using intravascular radiation demonstrated that blocking smooth muscle cell proliferation could ameliorate the problem of the restenosis (4) and raised the possibility that pharmacological therapy could produce similar benefits. However, it was not clear what was the right drug or how to deliver it to the vessel wall and for what length of time.

Stent-based drug delivery soon emerged as the most promising and practical approach to treating restenosis since the stent could serve the dual role of a lumenal scaffold and a platform for local drug delivery. An important requirement for the success of this strategy would be to find an effective drug and a drug carrier. A study of interaction of various polymers with porcine coronary arteries suggested that such efforts would be challenging due to polymer-induced inflammatory reactions (5). However, persistent efforts that included identification of a potent antirestenotic drug and a biocompatible polymer matrix, as well as effective coating technology led to the first successful trial of a drug-eluting stent (DES) in December 1999 (6) and commercialization of the first DES (Cypher®) in 2002. There are two commercially available DES in the United States at this time. They are the Cypher sirolimus-eluting stent manufactured by Cordis, a division of Johnson & Johnson and the Taxus® paclitaxel-eluting stent manufactured by Boston Scientific.

Rationale for drug-eluting stent

DES represent the integration of a medical device, pharmaceutical, and polymer technologies and they have revolutionized the practice of interventional cardiology (7). DES are superior to bare metal stents because they not only treat the mechanical problem of restenosis (i.e., acute vessel recoil and chronic negative remodeling), but also treat the biological problem of neointimal hyperplasia by eluting a drug into the vessel wall. The sustained presence of a therapeutic agent in an effective concentration at the site of vascular injury is key to preventing neointimal hyperplasia. In addition, because DES has a local site-specific action, they minimize systemic drug exposure and the potential for drug toxicity and expand the option to use more powerful therapeutic agents.

Components of a drug-eluting stent

Antirestenotic drug

There are currently two successful drugs that are used in commercial DES. They are sirolimus (also known as rapamycin) and paclitaxel. Both drugs are highly potent and lipophilic cell cycle inhibitors. Sirolimus and its analogs inhibit a protein kinase involved in growth factor signaling called the mammalian target of rapamycin that leads to inhibition of smooth muscle cell proliferation by blocking the G1/S phase of the cell cycle (8). These agents also have potent immunosuppressive and anti-inflammatory activity. Paclitaxel inhibits microtubular disassembly and exerts its inhibitory effect on smooth muscle cell proliferation at the G2/M phase of the cell cycle (9). Paclitaxel also has potent antimigratory activity and is used as a chemotherapeutic agent. Drugs used in DES must remain stable to device sterilization procedures. That is why small molecules have a potential advantage over proteins and genes as therapeutic agents for DES.

Stent platform

Balloon-expandable coronary stents are fabricated from stainless steel, cobalt chromium, and other metal alloys and composites. Important attributes of a stent platform include high radial strength, low recoil, minimal foreshortening, uniform scaffolding, and radiopacity (10–13). As drug delivery platforms, stent surface area, and cell pattern (open-cell or closed-cell designs) are important factors in determining the amount of drug that can be loaded and the uniformity of drug delivery to the vessel wall (14,15).

Polymer carrier

Various methods have been proposed to deliver the drugs from a stent, including nonpolymeric drug coatings (16,17), covalent drug attachment to the stent surface through linkers, drug-infused polymer sleeves (18,19), nonabsorbable polymer carriers, and bioabsorbable polymer carriers. Polymer carriers have to demonstrate tissue compatibility, physical/chemical compatibility with the drug, resistance to cracking and pealing, conformability during stent expansion (elasticity), and the ability to sustain drug release over prolonged intervals. The polymer formulation must be matched to the drug to achieve optimal performance.

Requirements for a polymer carrier

Physical stability

The polymer carrier should remain stable and durable during coating, crimping, sterilization, packaging, shelf-storage, and implantation. Physical stability of the polymer is necessary to maintain the integrity of the stent coating, the uniform distribution of drug in the coating, and the shelf life of the product. The important parameters to be considered are the glass transition temperature (Tg) and its mechanical strength of the polymer. Common ways to adjust the stability are through copolymerization or polymer blending.

Compatibility of incorporated drug

This is an important aspect as many drugs and polymeric materials contain functional groups that may chemically interact with each other, potentially leading to denaturing of the drug. Such interactions often negatively affect the intended pharmacological activity of the drug as well as the shelf life of a drug eluting stent.

Compatible with sterilization

The most commonly used method for DES sterilization is ethylene oxide (EO), which may interact with active functional groups such as amine, sulphydryl, and unsaturated bonds in a drug molecule. A polymer carrier can help to shield the drug from the effects of EO. Similarly, the polymer material itself may be affected by the sterilization process, causing the re-arrangement of the drug in the polymer matrix and ultimately affecting the shelf life and release kinetics of the drug. Likewise, e-beam and gamma irradiation are generally not compatible with most drugs because their high energy can disrupt a molecular structure of a drug.

Control of drug elution

Effective DES are able to control drug elution from the polymer. Clinical experience has demonstrated that excessively rapid drug elution often fails to achieve desired clinical efficacy. Rapid drug elution can also produce vascular toxicity by exceeding the safety threshold for the drug. The ideal situation is to have a sustained release of drug for at least 30 days, as this is the critical time window for the resolution of local tissue inflammation and the suppression of neointimal proliferation.

Compatibility with vascular tissue

All polymeric materials used in a DES must be extensively screened using standard in vitro and in vivo preclinical biocompatibility tests. These tests examine the potential of polymer-coated stents to induce inflammation and vessel injury over periods ranging from one to six months or longer. Extrapolation of animal data to human biocompatibility should be done cautiously as it is known that certain species such as the porcine coronary model are more prone to inflammation after implantation of foreign materials than other species. Long-term compatibility in humans generally requires years to ascertain safety.

Polymers that degrade in the body over time present a special biocompatibility challenge. Bioabsorbable polymers have been shown to induce an inflammatory response in acute animal studies (5) as they undergo matrix degradation. This response may be reduced by the therapeutic agent that elutes during degradation of the matrix. Since bioabsorbable materials have different degradation rates, it is necessary to evaluate these materials after drug loading and during the entire degradation phase to assess biocompatibility. A challenge of using bioabsorbable polymers is to control drug release through matrix degradation.

Compatibility with processing techniques

Selection of a suitable application technology is another important aspect of DES development. Spray coating, dip coating, ink-jet coating, and microdroplet coating are among the methods used in DES processing. For the same drug/polymer combination, different processing methods may lead to drastically different coating morphologies, drug distribution in the polymer matrix, drug release rates, and long-term efficacy.

Polymers used in drug-eluting stent

Biostable polymers

Biostable polymers have been chosen for use in the majority of DES that are marketed or in clinical development. The main attractiveness of biostable polymers is their physical stability, inertness toward the drug, and predictable drug kinetics. In Cypher, a blend of poly(ethylene-co-butyl methacrylate) (PEVAc/PBMA) is used as the drug carrier. This hydrophobic polymer, along with additional polymer process steps, effectively controls the release of sirolimus, eluting 80% of the drug over 30 days after implantation. In the case of Taxus, a tri-block copolymer of styrene-isobutylene-styrene (SIBS) is used as the hydrophobic polymer matrix that releases ~10% of incorporated paclitaxel in the first 30 days (20).

Phosphorylcholine (PC) is a class of biostable methacrylate-based copolymers that contain a PC monomer to mimic the charged phospholipid component of the plasma membrane of cells (21). The rational for using PC as a drug delivery matrix is to have a biomimetic material that can serve as a biocompatible drug delivery matrix. In practice, the charged moieties in the PC polymer make it relatively hydrophilic and require extensive cross-linking to slow drug efflux. Despite this modification, the Endeavor® zotarolimus-eluting stent (Medtronic) that uses a PC coating has reported rapid drug release (60–70%) after only one day of implantation (22). The ZoMaxx® zotarolimus-eluting stent (Abbott) uses a PC coating reportedly with a topcoat over the drug layer to slow drug elution (23).

Bioabsorbable polymers

Bioabsorbable polymers were among the first materials to be used as coatings for DES. Early attempts to develop bioabsorbable stent coatings recognized the problem of inflammatory responses generated by polymer degradation products. Material properties and degradation rates are dependent upon the molecular weight of the polymer and the ratio of monomers in the copolymer. The most commonly used bioabsorbable polymers and their key properties are listed in Table 1. Currently, there are several DES in development using a bioabsorbable polymer. The most advanced is the CoStar® paclitaxel-eluting stent from ConorMed, which uses a $PLGA_{85/15}$ polymer matrix to release paclitaxel over a period of 30 days (24).

Natural biopolymers

Proteins such as albumin, collagen, gelatin, and fibrin or polysaccharides such as hyaluronic acid and dextran have been used as natural polymeric materials for DES coatings (26,27). These attempts have not been successful for a variety of reasons. The hydrophilic nature of these materials usually produces a matrix with poor physical integrity and poor ability to control drug elution. In the case of cross-linked gelatin encapsulating paclitaxel, the drug load is completely exhausted in two weeks after implantation (28). Mitigating strategies such as cross-linking often lead to unwanted damage to the drug incorporated. Potential immunogenicity of these biological materials (especially after cross-linking) also raises additional safety concerns.

Control of drug elution

There are a number of excellent reviews on the subject of controlled drug elution from polymers (29–32). The general

Table 1 Properties of common biodegradable polymers

Polymer	Melting point (°C)	Glass-transition temperature (°C)	Modulus (Gpa)[a]	Degradation time (mo)[b]
PGA	225–230	35–40	7.0	6–12
LPLA	173–178	60–65	2.7	>24
DLPLA	Amorphous	55–60	1.9	12–16
PCL	58–63	−65 to −60	0.4	>24
PDO	N/A	−10 to 0	1.5	6–12
PGA-TMC	N/A	N/A	2.4	6–12
85/15 DLPLG	Amorphous	50–55	2.0	5–6
75/25 DLPLG	Amorphous	50–55	2.0	4–5
65/35 DLPLG	Amorphous	45–50	2.0	3–4
50/50 DLPLG	Amorphous	45–50	2.0	1–2

[a]Tensile or flexural modulus.

[b]Time to complete mass loss. Rate also depends on part geometry.

Abbreviations: DLPLA. poly (D, L-lactide); DLPLG. poly (D, L-lactide-co-glycolide); LPLA. poly (L-lactide); PCL. poly (caprolactone); PDO. poly (dioxanone); PGA. poly (glycolide); PGA-TMC. poly (glycolide-co-trimethylene carbonate).

Source: From Ref. 25.

mechanisms that govern drug elution from a polymer matrix are listed in Table 2. They can be broadly divided into physical and chemical/enzymatic mechanisms. Physical mechanisms govern water permeation into the polymer and drug diffusion out of the matrix, degradation of the polymer matrix to allow drug release, osmotic pressure gradients for drug release, and an ion exchange mechanism for ionized entities. The main advantages of physical mechanisms are that drug release kine-stics may be controlled by the polymer matrix itself with minimal influence of external factors. Drug elution kinetics may be roughly controlled by varying system parameters such as physical dimension of the matrix, surface to volume ratio of the system, and the drug loading percentage. In contrast, a chemical mechanism relies on cleavage of covalent bonds between a drug and a carrier through either a hydrolytic or enzymatic reaction, which may vary among individuals and disease states. A very limited number of drugs are suitable for conjugation or grafting with a polymer matrix and a wide array of cleaved products may be generated during the release phase. It is important to remember that these mechanisms describe ideal situations for a particular polymer/drug design.

Diffusion control

This is the most common mechanism of drug elution in which water permeates through water-insoluble polymer membrane and causes drug molecules to dissolve and diffuse through the polymer matrix. A schematic depicting diffusion controlled drug release is shown in Figure 1. Both Cypher and Taxus rely on this mechanism for drug elution. In vivo drug release from the polymeric coating is influenced by several factors, such as the hydrophobicity of the polymer, the water solubility of the drug, the percentage of drug loaded in the coating, and the use of a diffusion barrier. Most diffusion-controlled drug elution follows first-order kinetics for non-swelling polymer matrices. Matrices that swell, such as PC, lead to relatively fast drug elution in vivo, as in the case of Endeavor that releases ~60% of its drug load in the first day (33). On the other hand, a highly hydrophobic coating such as SIBS used in the Taxus stent coupled with a low drug loading level limits the amount of drug that is released in vivo.

Table 2 Mechanisms of drug elution from drug-eluting stent

Diffusion control
    Reservoir system
    Monolithic matrix
Matrix degradation
    Surface erosion
    Bulk erosion
Osmosis
Ion exchange
Enzymatic cleavage
Hydrolytic degradation

Matrix degradation

This mechanism is applied to bioabsorbable polymer matrices in which drug elution is a function of both the matrix degradation

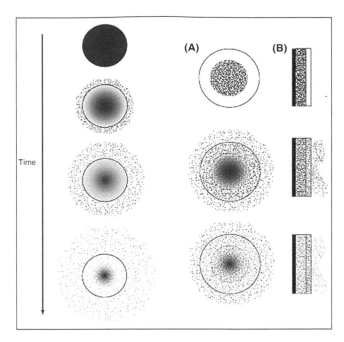

Figure 1
Diffusion controlled drug elution. Left panel shows a matrix diffusion type, the right panel shows a reservoir type diffusion control. *Source*: From Ref. 34.

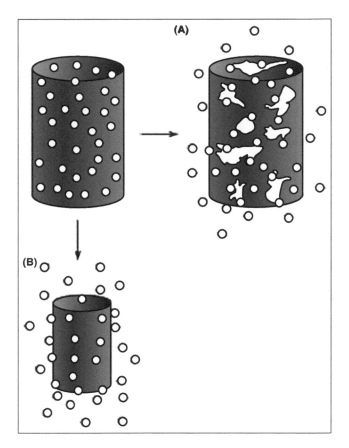

Figure 2
Matrix degradation for controlled drug release: (A) bulk erosion of a matrix, (B) surface erosion of a matrix. *Source*: From Ref. 34.

and drug diffusion in the degrading matrix. The schematic of matrix degradation for control of drug delivery in shown in Figure 2.

The exact drug release mechanism is dependent upon multiple factors including the nature of the polymer matrix (bulk degradation or surface erosion), the percentage of drug loaded in the matrix, and distribution of the drug within the polymer matrix. For a bulk degradation polymer matrix, initial burst release of drug is mainly caused by the dissolution and elution of the drug located at or near the surface of the matrix. Subsequent drug release from the bulk of the matrix requires both water diffusion into the matrix and the degradation of the polymer. A majority of the bioabsorbable polymers used for DES are in this category, such as polylactide (PLA), poly(lactide-co-glycolide) (PLGA), and polyphosphoester. For a surface erosion polymer matrix, drug located on or near the surface of the coating is released initially. Due to the inherent hydrophobicity of the polymer, water cannot diffuse into the bulk of the matrix to release the drug. Additional drug is eluted in a near zero-order fashion when the surface of polymer is degraded in an onion-peel fashion. Prominent examples of these polymers include poly(anhydride), poly(orthoester), poly(phosphazene), and poly(carbonate) (PC) that are constructed from hydrophobic monomers. In reality, some drug elution occurs via rearrangement of drug in the polymer matrix and diffusion

through the polymer matrix, creating elution kinetics that are somewhere between zero- and first-order kinetics.

Polymeric coating designs in drug-eluting stent

Thin layer coating

This is the most prevalent form of polymer carrier and most DES on the market or in development use this as a drug carrier. The appealing feature of thin layer coatings is that they can form a conformal drug layer on the surface of a stent, utilizing the whole stent surface for maximal drug release. Another advantage is that a wide array of coating processes, such as ultrasonic-spray coating, dip-coating, spin-coating, vapor deposition, piezoelectric inkjet coating, and micro-droplet atomization, are available for this application. Several of these techniques such as spray coating and ink-jet coating are all capable of providing thin and uniform drug coatings.

Protective or diffusion barrier polymer layer

This type of polymer barrier is mainly used to provide additional protective layer or further regulate drug release kinetics. For instance, the top layer in the Infinnium® paclitaxel-eluting stent utilizes a drug-free layer that both protects the drug and decreases the drug release (35). Abbott's ZoMaxx zotarolimus-releasing stent uses a topcoat to reduce the fast drug elution of drug from the underlying PC coating (36).

Hydrogel matrix

This type of matrix has been evaluated with limited success. The chief drawbacks include poor control of drug release, particularly for drugs that are water-soluble, and poor biocompatibility due to matrix swelling in preclinical animal studies. Hydrogels comprising heparin (37) or poly(EO) (38,39) in the very top layer of DES coating may have local antithrombotic activity.

Polymer matrix covalently linked to drug molecules

This is an extension of the polymeric drug concept in which the drug can be conjugated to a polymeric matrix and released over time via hydrolytic and/or enzymatic cleaving. The potential stumbling blocks to this approach are that such conjugates are not achieved quantitatively, the degradation is not homogeneous, and the local enzyme levels are influenced by the disease state and may vary from person to person.

Drug-eluting stent incorporating a polymer component

A comparison of polymer coating and drug delivery technologies in leading DES is shown in Table 3.

Cypher

The Cypher sirolimus-eluting stent from Cordis uses a blend of poly(ethylene-co-vinyl acetate) (PEVA) and poly(n-butyl methacrylate) (PBMA) as the polymeric matrix for sirolimus release. Both PEVA and PBMA have individually been used as implants in humans and demonstrated excellent biocompatibility. The blend of PEVA and PBMA is physically mixed with sirolimus in a weight ratio of 2:1. In vivo studies have shown that the majority of the drug is released in a sustained fashion in 30 days with complete drug release in 90 days as

Table 3 Leading drug eluting stents on the market or in late development that incorporate a polymer component

Features	CYPHER™ (6)	TAXUS™ (20)	Endeavor (22)	ZoMaxx (23)	CoStar (24)
Stent Platform	316L Close cell	316L Open cell	CoCr alloy Open cell	SS/Ta/SS Sandwich	L605 Holes in strut
Polymer matrix	PEVAc/PBMA blend	SIBS Block	PC-Copolymer	PC Copolymer topcoat	PLGA
Coating wt (16–18 mm)	550 μg				347 μg
Drug dose (16–18 mm)	140 μg/cm^2 180 μg	100 μg/cm^2 100 μg	10 μg/mm 160 μg	10 μg/mm 160 μg	3–30 μg/17 mm
Drug elution kinetics	80%/30 days 100%/90 days	10% in 30 days	70%/first day	75%/10 days 100%/30 days	100%/30 days
Unique features		Single layer	Asymmetric single layer	Asymmetric topcoat	Asymmetric multiple layers
Thickness	10 μm	16–18 μm			

Abbreviations: PBMA, poly (ethylene-co-butyl methacrylate); PC, phosphoryl choline; PEVAc, poly (ethylene-co-vinyl autate); PLGA, poly (lactide-co-glycolide); SIBS, styrene-isobutylene-styrene; SS, ____.

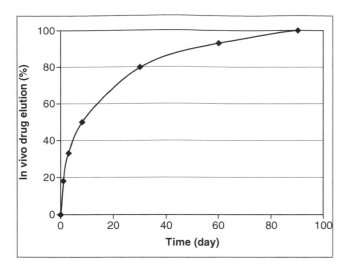

Figure 3
In vivo sirolimus release profile from the Cypher sirolimus eluting stent.

shown in Figure 3. Four-year clinical follow-up data have unequivocally demonstrated the long-term efficacy and safety of this device (40).

Taxus

The Taxus stent by Boston Scientific uses a tri-block copolymer [poly(styrene-*b*-isobutylene-*b*-styrene)] for sustained delivery of paclitaxel. This new polymer is specifically designed for this use and has a trade name of Translute™. Paclitaxel can be released at a fast or a slow rate by varying the drug loading in the polymer matrix as shown in Figure 4.

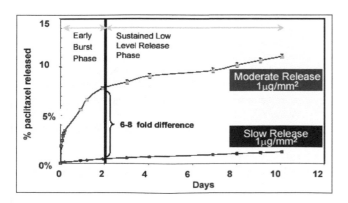

Figure 4
Schematic of paclitaxel release from TAXUS with a moderate and a slow release profile (41).

Endeavor and ZoMaxx

Endeavor and ZoMaxx are being developed by Medtronic and Abbott Vascular, respectively. The common components shared by these two DES are the PC copolymers and the drug Zotarolimus (previously known as ABT-578). The difference is that Endeavor uses a thin single-layer coating which results in fast in vivo release of the drug (22), whereas ZoMaxx employs additional PC topcoat to reduce in vivo drug elution kinetics (23).

CoStar

The CoStar paclitaxel-eluting stent made by Conor MedSystems is distinct in that the polymer and drug are not bonded to the stent structure through a coating (42). Instead, multiple holes are drilled through the structure of the stent and filled with bioabsorbable polymer/drug mixture to serve as local drug release depots. Various loading configurations can be employed to control drug elution direction toward arterial side alone or toward both the blood stream and arterial wall. They are developing a paclitaxel-eluting stent in a bioabsorbable $PLGA_{85/15}$ matrix that completely elutes the drug over 30 days.

Future trends
Totally bioabsorbable stents

A totally bioabsorbable stent is pursued by several companies (Guidant, Boston Scientific). Unlike early bioabsorbable stents, such as the Igaki-Tamai stent (43), the new generation of bioabsorbable stents incorporates a pharmacological component. Another difference lies in the way a drug is incorporated: either in the bulk of the stent or on the stent surface. Another important aspect is the choice of polymeric materials. poly (L, L-lactide) (PLLA), PLGA blends, polycarbonate, and poly (ester-amide) are among the leading candidates. The attractive feature is that the drug is released as the polymer degrades, eventually eliminating both the stent scaffold and the drug from the stent implant site once the pathological processes accompanying the angioplasty and stenting procedures are fully resolved. Whether polymers have the mechanical properties to replace metallic scaffolds remains to be demonstrated. Guidant has recently initiated a clinical trial with a totally bioabsorbable balloon-expandable stent that consists of a PLLA core and an everolimus containing bio- absorbable drug coating (44).

Poly(ester-amide)

This class of material is being evaluated by MediVas and its licensees including Guidant, Boston Scientific, and Microport

(45). Surmodics also recently licensed similar technology from Intralytix. The potential attractiveness of this material is a wide range of physical and chemical properties through utilizing different combinations of monomers, including natural amino acids such as lysine, glycine, etc. This new class of polymer may also allow incorporation of additional functional moieties for enzymatic degradation in vivo. In contrast, traditional monomers such as lactic acid, glycolic acid, and caprolactone afford comparatively limited options.

Polymers designed to carry biomolecules

Recent advances in the biopharmaceutical industry have made available a large array of biological molecules that are potentially useful for treating vascular diseases. The choices include monoclonal antibodies, DNA, RNA, and single-stranded RNA. The main challenges to implementing this approach lies in maintaining the biological activity of these molecules through manufacturing and controlling release of these molecules which are generally water soluble. A recent attempt to incorporate plasmid DNA in a PLGA coating demonstrated the feasibility of loading and releasing a gene from a stent coating (46). The PC coating was recently used to incorporate a naked plasmid DNA (5283-bp) encoding a human vascular endothelial growth factor gene (phVEGF-2) (47). The loading is achieved through the ionic interaction between the negative charges of the plasmid and the positive charges of a PC head group. The bound plasmids were slowly eluted from the coating after being displaced by negative ions in the surrounding tissue.

Tailored polymers and constructs

With the inherent versatility in choosing the monomers and comonomers, the different repeating sequences in the polymer chain (random and alternative blocks), introduction of functional and ionic groups through side chains, and the different polymerization methods, polymer can be tailor-made to posses additional special properties as well. For instance, layer-by-layer strategy may be used to coat stent surface with alternating layers of charge carrying polyelectrolytes and opposite charged drug molecules to achieve specific properties (48–51).

In addition, a monomer having an inherent pharmacological activity can be used to build a polymer for use in DES. This approach is analogous to the prodrug concept in the pharmaceutical industry that relies on chemical or enzymatic degradation to affect the drug release. Drug release kinetics, however, is likely to be influenced by local pH and the enzyme concentration locally, which may not be entirely controlled by the system. Additional excipients such as pH buffering agents may bring about improved control. The

coming years will likely witness experiments with these special-purpose polymers for applications in DES.

Concluding remarks

The past decade has witnessed a breakthrough in medical technology. The success of DES has expanded the reach of interventional cardiologists and will continue to generate new DES for peripheral, neurovascular, and urological applications. These devices will have their own challenges and may include the need to deliver multiple drugs, proteins, or genes. Novel polymers are expected to play an important role in these future developments.

References

1 Erbel R, Haude M, Hopp HW, et al. Coronary-artery stenting compared with balloon angioplasty for restenosis after initial balloon angioplasty. Restenosis Stent Study Group. New Engl J Med 1998; 339:1672–1678.

2 Serruys PW, de Jaegere P, Kiemeneij F, et al. A comparison of balloon-expandable-stent implantation with balloon angioplasty in patients with coronary artery disease. Benestent Study Group. New Engl J Med 1994; 331:489–495.

3 Fattori R, Piva T. Drug eluting stents in vascular intervention. Lancet 2003; 361:247–249.

4 King SB III, Williams DO, Chougule P, et al. Endovascular beta-radiation to reduce restenosis after coronary balloon angioplasty: results of the beta energy restenosis trial (BERT). Circulation 1998; 97(20):2025–2030.

5 Ven der Giessen W, Lincoff AM, Schwartz RS, et al. Marked inflammatory sequelae to implantation of biodegradable and nonbiodegradable polymers in porcine coronary arteries. Circulation 1996; 94:1690–1697.

6 Morice MC, Serruys PW, Sousa JE, et al. A randomized comparison of a sirolimus-eluting stent with a standard stent for coronary revascularization. New Engl J Med 2002; 346(23):1773–1780.

7 van der Hoeven BL, Pires NMM, Warda HM, et al. Drug eluting stents: results, promises and problems. Int J Cardiol 2005; 99:9–17.

8 Parry TJ, Brosius R, Thyagarajan R, et al. Drug-eluting stents: sirolimus and paclitaxel differentially affect cultured cells and injured arteries. Eur J Pharm 2005; 524(1–3):19–29.

9 Wessely R, Schomig A, Kastrati A. Sirolimus and Paclitaxel on polymer-based drug-eluting stents: similar but different. J Am Coll Cardiol 2006; 47(4):708–714.

10 Lally C, Dolan F, Prendergast PJ. Cardiovascular stent design and vessel stresses: a finite element analysis. J Biomech 2005; 38:1574–1581.

11 Walke W, Paszenda Z, Filipiak J. Experimental and numerical biomechanical analysis of vascular stent. J Mater Process Technol 2005; 164/165:1263–1268.

12 Mori K, Saito T. Effects of stent structure on stent flexibility measurements. Ann Biomed Eng 2005; 33:733–742.

13 McClean DR, Eigler NL. Stent design: implications for restenosis. Rev Cardiovasc Med 2002; 3(suppl 5):S16–S22.

14 Hwang CW, Wu D, Edelman ER. Physiological transport forces govern drug distribution for stent-based delivery. Circulation 2001; 104(5):600–605.

15 Rogers CDK. Drug-eluting stents: role of stent design, delivery vehicle, and drug selection. Rev Cardiovasc Med 2002; 3: S10–S15.

16 Heldman AW, Cheng L, Jenkins GM, et al. Paclitaxel stent coating inhibits neointimal hyperplasia at 4 weeks in a porcine model of coronary restenosis. Circulation 2001; 103: 2289–2295.

17 Lansky AJ, Costa RA, Mintz GS, et al. Non-polymer-based paclitaxel-coated coronary stents for the treatment of patients with de novo coronary lesions. Circulation 2004; 109: 1948–1954.

18 Hiatt BL, Carter AJ, Yeung AC. The drug-eluting stent: is it the Holy Grail? Rev Cardiovasc Med 2001; 2:190–196.

19 Nakayama Y, Nishi S, Ueda-Ishibashi H, et al. Fabrication of micropored elastomeric film-covered stents and acute-phase performances. J Biomed Mater Res 2003; 64A:52–61.

20 TAXUS II, http://www.tctmd.com/csportal/appmanager/ tctmd/main?_nfpb=true&_pageLabel=TCTMDContent&hdCon=895183.

21 Rose SF, Lewis AL, Hanlon GW, et al. Biological responses to cationically charged phosphorylcholine-based materials in vitro. Biomaterials 2004; 25:5125–5135.

22 Medtronic Endeavor ABT-578 Program update http://www.tctmd.com/csportal/appmanager/tctmd/main?_nfpb=true&_pageLabel=TCTMDContent&hdCon=822596.

23 Nowak SA, Sabaj KM, Zielinski DA, et al. The effects of adding a polymer topcoat on the elution rate from drug-eluting stents (abstr). Cardiovascular Revascularization Therapeutics 2005; 503–505.

24 Conor Medsystems website: http://www.conormed.com/tech/stent.html.

25 Middleton JC, Tipton AJ. Synthetic Biodegradable Polymers as Medical Devices. Medical Device and Diagnosis Industry. Los Angeles, CA: A Canon Communications LLC, 1998.

26 Chen MC, Liang HF, Chiu YL, et al. A novel drug-eluting stent spray coated with multi-layers of collagen and sirolimus. J Control Release 2005; 108:178–189.

27 Holmes DR, Camrud AR, Jorgenson MA, et al. Polymeric stenting in the porcine coronary artery model: differential outcome of exogenous fibrin sleeves versus polyurethane-coated stents. J Am Coll Cardiol 1994; 24:524–531.

28 Farb A, Heller PF, Shroff S, et al. Pathological analysis of local delivery of paclitaxel via a polymer-coated stent. Circulation 2001; 104:473–479.

29 Robinson JR. Sustained and Controlled Release Drug Delivery Systems, Drugs and Pharmaceutical Sciences. Vol. 6. New York, NY: Marcell Dekker, 1978.

30 Chien YW. Novel Drug Delivery Systems, Drugs and the Pharmaceutical Sciences. Vol. 126. New York, NY: Marcel Dekker, 1992.

31 Ansel HC, Popovich NG, Allen LV. Pharmaceutical Dosage Forms and Drug Delivery Systems. Baltimore: Williams and Wilkins, 1995.

32 Saltzman WM. Drug Delivery. Engineering Principles for Drug Therapy. New York, NY: Oxford University Press, 2001.

33 Meredith I. Medtronic Endeavor ABT-578 program: http://www.tctmd.com/csportal/appmanager/tctmd/main?_nfpb=true&_pageLabel=TCTMDContent&hdCon=822596.

34 Brannon-Pepas L. Polymers in Controlled Drug Delivery. Medical Device and Diagnosis Industry. Los Angeles, CA: A Canon Communications LLC, 1998.

35 Vaishnav R, Kothwala D, Chand R. The Millennium Matrix Coronary Stent. In: Surreys P, ed. Handbook of Drug Eluting Stent. London and New York: Taylor and Francis, 2005:215–226.

36 ABT-578 Drug-eluting Stent II: The Abbott Zomaxx Stent http://www.tctmd.com/csportal/appmanager/tctmd/main?_nfpb=true&_pageLabel=TCTMDContent&hdCon=766016.

37 Hardhammar PA, Beusekom HM, Emanuelsson HU, et al. Reduction in thrombotic events with heparin-coated Palmaz–Schatz stents in normal porcine coronary arteries. Circulation 1996; 90:423–430.

38 Park K, Shim HS, Dewanjee MK, et al. In vitro and in vivo studies of PEO-grafted blood-contacting cardiovascular prostheses. J Biomater Sci Polym Ed 2000; 11:1121–1134.

39 Mcpherson TB, Shim HS, Park K. Grafting of PEO to glass, nitinol, and pyrolytic carbon surfaces by gamma irradiation. J Biomed Mater Res Appl Biomater 1997; 38:289–302.

40 Sousa E, et al. Four-year angiographic and intravascular ultrasonic follow-up of patients treated with sirolimus-eluting stents, circulation. Circulation 2005; 111:2326–2329.

41 Russell ME. The BSC drug-eluting stent systems: polymer characteristics and drug delivery: http://www.tctmd.com/ csportal/appmanager/tctmd/main?_nfpb=true&_pageLabel=TCTMDContent&hdCon=864064.

42 Finkelstein A, Mcclean D, Kar S, et al. Local drug delivery via a coronary stent with programmable release pharmacokinetics. Circulation 2003; 107:777–784.

43 Tamai H. Igaki-Tamai bioerodable stent (not drug-loaded): four-year follow-up in patients and future design iterations, http://www.tctmd.com/csportal/appmanager/tctmd/main?_nfpb=true&_pageLabel=TCTMDContent&hdCon=771400.

44 The Future of Polymer Based Bioabsorbable Drug Eluting Stents http://www.tctmd.com/csportal/appmanager/tctmd/main?_nfpb=true&_pageLabel=TCTMDContent &hd Con=1270085.

45 A New Generation Bioabsorbable Drug Delivery Platform, http://www.tctmd.com/csportal/appmanager/tctmd/main?_nfpb=true&_pageLabel=TCTMDContent&hdCon=820634.

46 Klugherz BD, Jones PL, Cui X, et al. Gene delivery from a DNA controlled-release stent in porcine coronary arteries. Nat Biotechnol 2000; 18:1181–1184.

47 Walter DH, Cejna M, Diaz-Sandoval L, et al. Local gene transfer of phVEGF-2 plasmid by gene-eluting stents. Circulation 2004; 110:36–45.

48 Decher G. Fuzzy nano-assemblies: toward layered polymeric multicomposites. Science 1997; 277:1232–1237.

49 Kotov NA. Layer-by-layer assembly of nanoparticles and nanocolloids: intermolecular interactions, structure and materials perspectives. In: Decher G, Schlenoff JB, eds. Multilayer Thin Films. Sequential Assembly of Nanocomposite Materials. Germany: Wiley-VCH, 2003:207–243.

50 Thierry B, Winnik FM, Merhi Y, et al. Bioactive coatings of endovascular stents based on polyelectrolyte multilayers. Biomacromolecules 2003; 4:1564–1571.

51 Tan Q, Ji J, Barbosa MA, et al. Constructing thromboresistant surface on biomedical stainless steel via layer-by-layer deposition anticoagulant. Biomaterials 2003; 24: 4699–4705.

25

Utilization of antiproliferative and antimigratory compounds for the prevention of restenosis

Kalpana R. Kamath and James J. Barry

Background

The advent of drug-eluting stents (DES) and their clinical success has brought about a paradigm shift in the treatment of occlusive coronary artery disease. Prior to the introduction of DES, the restenosis rate in patients who had undergone coronary stenting or balloon angioplasty varied between 20% and 50%, depending on the complexity of the lesion and the patient subset being treated (1–3). The use of DES has offered an elegant and effective de novo therapeutic approach to addressing the major components of postangioplasty restenosis, negative remodeling, and neointimal hyperplasia, while potentially minimizing the risk of systemic toxicity by potent therapeutic agents (4). This chapter provides an overview of the restenotic cascade—the arch enemy of percutaneous coronary intervention (PCI)—a summary of pharmacologic therapies investigated for the prevention of restenosis both prior to and during the DES era, and a discussion of antiproliferative and antimigratory compounds used as part of DES systems, using the TAXUS® DES (Boston Scientific Corporation, Natick, Massachusetts, U.S.A.) as an example.

Pathophysiology of restenosis

The introduction of bare-metal stents (BMS) alleviated the problem of elastic recoil associated with balloon angioplasty, the predecessor of coronary stenting. However, neointimal hyperplasia leading to restenosis and luminal narrowing continued to be a major limitation of BMS (5–9). The angiographic late lumen loss attributed to in-stent neointimal hyperplasia ranges from 0.8 to 1.0 mm, leading to a 56% to 75% cross-sectional area loss (4). Understanding restenosis,

a process with an iatrogenic etiology involving multiple biologic pathways, has been an ongoing area of research since the arrival of PCI. The salient features of the restenotic cascade are shown in Figure 1 (10,11).

The initial consequence of stent placement is endothelial denudation, followed by adhesion of platelets and fibrinogen at the site of injury. This prothrombotic layer recruits leukocytes, which adhere and transmigrate drawn by the chemokines secreted by smooth muscle cells (SMCs) and resident macrophages (10,11). The release of growth factors and cytokines by the cellular milieu, composed of platelets, leukocytes, and SMCs, stimulates the migration of medial SMCs into the neointima and the proliferation of medial and intimal SMCs. The secretion of extracellular matrix and subsequent remodeling completes the process of vascular repair (12–15), resulting in a hyperplasic neointimal mass that compromises the coronary lumen. Given the biochemical, cellular, and molecular complexities involved in the cascade of restenosis, delivery of a therapeutic entity that could target one or more of the events of this cascade is probably the most attractive—although challenging—approach to addressing the problem of restenosis (16).

Systemic therapy of antirestenotic agents

Several drugs from various pharmacologic classes, including antithrombotics, vasomotor tone modulators, antiproliferatives, anti-inflammatories, and lipid modulators, were examined via systemic approach preceding and during the era of BMS (Table 1) (17). Unfortunately, the systemic therapies investigated to prevent in-stent restenosis (ISR) have shown

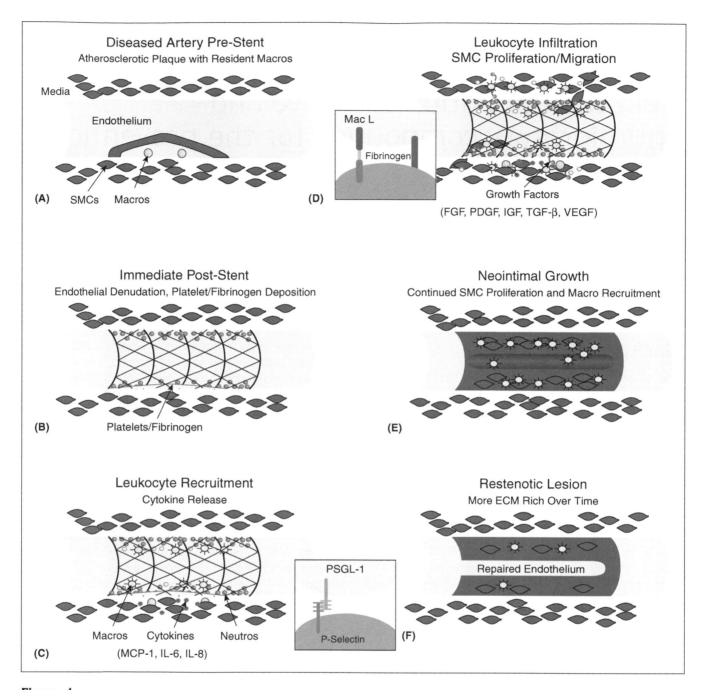

Figure 1

(*See color plate.*) Pathophysiology of restenosis: (A) atherosclerotic vessel before intervention. (B) immediate result of stent placement with endothelial denudation and platelet/fibrinogen deposition. (C) and (D) leukocyte recruitment, infiltration, and SMC proliferation and migration in the days after injury. (E) neointimal thickening in the weeks after injury, with continued SMC proliferation and monocyte recruitment. (F) long-term (weeks to months) change from a predominantly cellular to a less cellular and more ECM-rich plaque. *Abbreviations*: ECM, extracellular matrix; FGF, fibroblast growth factor; IGF, insulin-like growth factor; IL, interleukin; MCP, monocyte chemoattractant protein; PDGF, platelet-derived growth factor; PSGL, P-selectin glycoprotein ligand; SMC, smooth muscle cell; TGF, transforming growth factor; VEGF, vascular endothelial growth factor. *Source*: From Ref. 11.

disappointing results, despite most having shown promise in animal models (18). Their failure in the clinical setting could be attributed to many reasons, namely, differences between animal and human responses, systemic intolerance of doses successful in animal studies, and selection of an inappropriate pharmacologic agent, to name but a few (18,19). Therefore, the focus of investigation shifted to alternate agents as well as alternate methods of delivery.

Table 1 Clinical studies of systemic therapies investigated for the treatment of restenosis

Agent (dose)	Rate of restenosis (%)	Postulated mechanism	References
Nifedipine (40 mg/day)	28.0	Vasodilation	(77)
Diltiazem (270 mg/day)	15.0		(78)
Verapamil (48.3 mg/day)	48.3		(79)
Aspirin (990 mg/day) plus dipyrimadole (225 mg/day)	37.7	Inhibition of platelet aggregation and thrombus formation	(80)
Ticlopidine (750 mg/day)	49.6		(81)
Trapidil (600 mg/day)	19.0	Blocks PDGF	(82)
GR32191B (80 mg/day)	21.0	Inhibits platelet aggregation and vasodilation	(83)
Prostacyclin (5 μg/kg/min IV) plus aspirin plus dipyrimadole	27.0	Platelet inhibition and vasodilation Inhibition of thrombus formation	(84)
Therapeutic warfarin plus verapamil	29.0		(85)
Therapeutic heparin (IV)	41.0		(86)
Methylprednisone (im) plus prednisolone (60 mg/day)	42.0	Anti-inflammatory and antiproliferative	(87)
Methylprednisolone (1 g IV before PTCA)	43.0		(88)
Cilazapril (10 mg/day)	28.0	Antiproliferative and	(89)
Fosinopril (40 mg/day)	39.4	vasodilation	(90)
Colchicine (1.2 mg/day)	41.0	Antiproliferative, antifibrotic and anti-inflammatory	(91)
Angiopeptin (190 μg/day; 750 μg/day; 3000 μg/day)	38.0; 35.6; 38.6	Inhibits growth hormone and antiproliferative	(92)
Angiopeptin (750 μg/day continuous infusion)	7.5		(93)
Ketanserin (40 mg/day)	32	Inhibits SMC proliferation and platelet aggregation	(94)
Lovastatin (20–40 mg/day)	12	Reduces serum lipids and inhibits SMC proliferation	(95)
Omega-3 fatty acids (3.2–6 mg/day)	19–36	Inhibits platelet aggregation and SMC proliferation	(96–100)

Abbreviations: IM, intramuscular; IV, intravenous; PDGF, platelet-derived growth factor; SMC, smooth muscle cells.
Source: From Ref. 17.

Catheter-based drug delivery for restenosis management

Given the obvious issues associated with the systemic delivery of agents to address the local pathology of restenosis, other local delivery modalities were investigated prior to the DES era. Catheter-based delivery, which combines drug delivery and balloon angioplasty, received significant attention (20). Types of catheters used for local drug delivery included those utilizing passive diffusion, active or pressure-driven devices, and mechanical devices (Fig. 2) (21); this type of technology required a catheter providing acceptable delivery efficiency as well as a pharmacologic agent effective in decreasing restenosis at the dose delivered. Delivery of several agents using catheter-based delivery was investigated in animal models and in humans, including heparin (22–24).

Unfortunately, the clinical successes of this approach to address restenosis were limited, for many reasons, including, but not limited to, short duration of delivery, rapid downstream

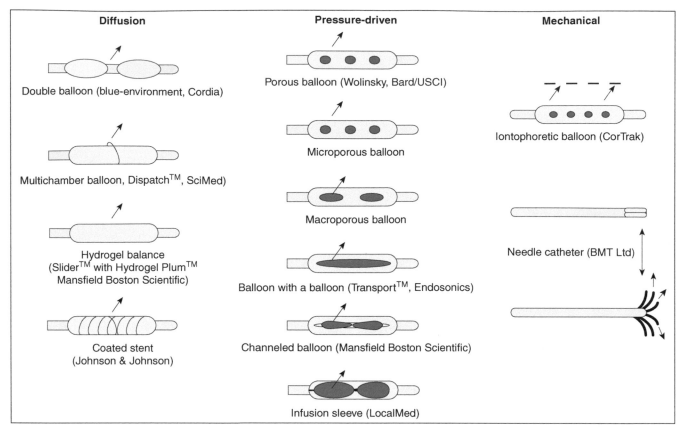

Figure 2
(*See color plate*.) Types of catheter-based local delivery devices. *Source*: From Ref. 21.

drug washout, selection of inappropriate drug and dose, and inadequate sample size (25,26).

Restenosis and fibroproliferative conditions: Similarities and differences

With advances in the field of vascular biology and a deeper understanding of restenosis pathology, it was recognized that restenosis had a significant fibroproliferative component. Animal and human pathology studies have demonstrated that SMC proliferation is critical to neointimal formation following mechanical injury (27–29). Using proliferation markers, peak proliferation rates of up to 20% of total medial cells have been observed five to seven days after injury (30,31). The inevitable comparison of restenosis with other fibroproliferative conditions, such as cancer, rheumatoid arthritis, psoriasis, and transplant rejection (32,33), narrowed the focus of investigation of antirestenotic therapies to agents also used for the treatment of fibroproliferative conditions.

Antiproliferative and antimigratory agents in restenosis

Several antiproliferative and antimigratory agents used in the treatment of cancer and other fibroproliferative conditions have been evaluated for their ability to prevent restenosis, with mixed results. Table 2 lists the outcomes of preclinical studies for some of these agents in various animal models, ranging from rat, rabbit to porcine.

Promising data from these studies stimulated subsequent examination of these agents in clinical trials via stent-based delivery.

Antirestenotic agents incorporated into drug-eluting stents

Several of the agents that showed promise in preclinical studies were evaluated as part of a DES system. The

Table 2 Preclinical studies of antimigratory and antiproliferative agents for their ability to prevent restenosis

Drug	Postulated mechanism of action	Model	Delivery method	Key findings	References
Methotrexate	Antiproliferative: inhibits folate metabolism, purine synthesis and cell proliferation	Porcine coronary artery	Local application by balloon catheter	Did not prevent neointimal thickening	(101)
Colchicine	Inhibits microtubule assembly and cell division	Rabbit femoral artery	Local infusion of drug-containing biodegradable microparticles	Did not reduce restenosis Induced toxicity to adjacent musculature	(102)
Batimastat	Inhibits matrix metalloproteinase	Rat carotid artery	Intraperitoneal administration	Inhibited neointimal hyperplasia	(103)
		Atherosclerotic porcine femoral artery		No significant decrease in neointimal thickness	(104)
Actinomycin D	Inhibits DNA directed RNA synthesis and DNA synthesis at higher concentrations	Rat carotid artery	Periadventitial application	Significant reduction in neointimal hyperplasia	(105)
Sirolimus	Inhibits mammalian target of rapamycin and cell cycle progression	Porcine coronary artery	Drug-eluting stent	Significant reduction in neointimal hyperplasia	(106)
Paclitaxel	Stabilizes microtubules, inhibiting cell-cycle progression	Rat carotid artery	Intraperitoneal administration	Prevented medial SMC migration and neointimal SMC proliferation	(47)
		Rabbit iliac artery	Drug-eluting stent	Prevented intimal thickening	(56)
		Porcine coronary artery		Inhibited neointimal hyperplasia and luminal encroachment	(57)

Abbreviation: SMC, smooth muscle cell.

development of DES allowed local sustained delivery of an appropriate drug directly to the affected tissue, avoiding the high doses and undesirable systemic effects associated with systemic delivery as well as the issues associated with catheter-based delivery. The Batimastat (BB-94) antiRestenosis trIaL utiLizIng the BiodivYsio® (Biocompatibles Ltd., Farnham, U.K.) local drug delivery PC steNT(BRIL-LIANT 1) clinical study of the antimigratory matrix metalloproteinase inhibitor, batimastat, coated on a stent, did not show the benefit that was evident in the preclinical studies and further investigation was suspended. In addition, the ACTinomycin-eluting stent Improves Outcomes by reduction of Neointimal hyperplasia clinical study of an actinomycin-eluting stent, which also was initiated on the basis of encouraging preclinical data, demonstrated an unacceptably high rate of major adverse cardiac events [MACE; a composite of death, Q-wave myocardial infarction (MI), non-Q-wave MI or target lesion revascularization (TLR) (PCI or coronary artery bypass grafting)] in the treatment arms (18.3% in the $2.5 \,\mu g/cm^2$ group and 28.1% in the $10 \,\mu g/cm^2$ group) versus the control group (10.2%) and was, therefore, halted prematurely. Figure 3 shows the event free survival at six months in this study (34).

The first two DES to be commercialized incorporated sirolimus (rapamycin; Rapamune®, Wyeth Pharmaceuticals, Inc., Collegeville, Pennsylvania, U.S.A.), an immunosuppressive agent used for the prevention of transplanted organ rejection, or paclitaxel (Taxol®, Bristol-Myers Squibb, Princeton, New Jersey, U.S.A.) an agent with an extensive history as an anti-cancer therapy.

Sirolimus

Sirolimus, a macrolide antibiotic, in one mode of action, binds to FK506-binding protein (FKBP12), inhibiting the activation of mammalian target of rapamycin (mTOR), which, in turn, blocks the cellular transition from G_1 to the S phase of the cell cycle (35). Sirolimus was approved by the Food and Drug Administration (FDA) in 1999 for the prevention of renal

transplant rejection. Interestingly, due to the antiangiogenic properties of sirolimus, it is also now being evaluated as an anticancer agent in preclinical studies (36). The use of sirolimus as an antirestenotic agent delivered from a DES is discussed further in Chapter 10.

Paclitaxel

Originally developed as part of a large-scale effort headed by the United States National Cancer Institute to investigate chemotherapeutic agents from natural sources, paclitaxel was approved by the FDA in 1992 as an antineoplastic agent to treat metastatic ovarian cancer after failure of first-line or subsequent chemotherapy (37). Further studies demonstrated efficacy in other solid tumors (38). In addition, paclitaxel was shown to inhibit T- and B-cell proliferation when tested for transplant-rejection application (39,40) and has demonstrated inhibition of matrix-metalloproteinase synthesis in studies conducted to test its utility for rheumatoid arthritis (41).

Cellular and molecular mechanism of paclitaxel as an antirestenotic agent

Paclitaxel is a well-established antiproliferative agent with a microtubule-targeting pharmacologic activity (37,42,43). As an anticancer agent, paclitaxel causes polymerization and stabilization of microtubules (43–45). The stabilization of microtubule dynamics by paclitaxel can interrupt many cellular processes, including cell division, migration, activation, maintenance of cytoskeletal framework, and intracellular as well as transmembrane protein transport (42,46,47).

It is widely assumed in the oncology therapeutic area that paclitaxel is cytotoxic to cancer cells and induces apoptosis, a rapid, programmed cell death associated with the activation of caspases (48) and mediated via the mitotic arrest of cells.

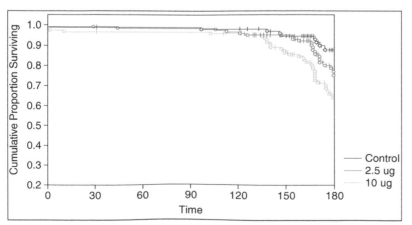

Figure 3
(*See color plate.*) Event free survival at six months in the ACTinomycin-eluting stent Improves Outcomes by reduction of Neointimal hyperplasia trial of the actinomycin-eluting stent. *Source*: From Ref. 34.

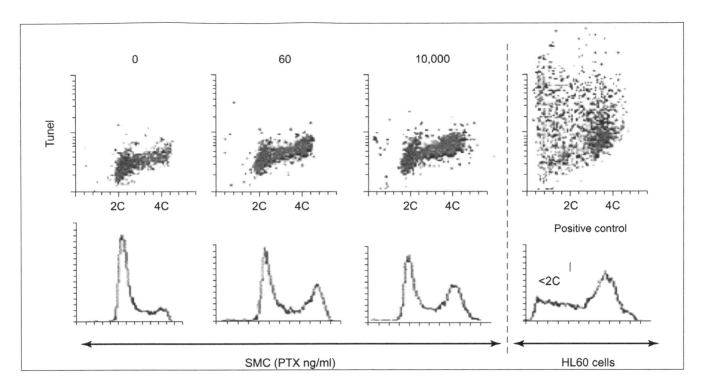

Figure 4
Terminal deoxynucleotidyl transferase biotin-dUTP nick end labeling assay examining apoptosis in smooth muscle cells and HL60 leukemia cells treated with paclitaxel. *Abbreviations*: HL60, human leukemia 60. PTX, paclitaxel; SMC, smooth muscle cells; Tunel, terminal deoxynucleotidyl transferase biotin-dUTP nick end labeling. *Source*: From Ref. 49.

However, this effect of paclitaxel was found to be dependent on the drug dose and cell type (49,50). A number of studies have demonstrated that paclitaxel has several biologic attributes that are critical to the cascade of events involved in preventing restenosis. Paclitaxel was shown to inhibit SMC proliferation over a broad concentration range (0.01 – 10,000 ng/mL) without causing cell death or apoptosis (49,51). A comparison of human coronary artery SMCs and HL60 leukemia cells showed that paclitaxel did not induce apoptosis in SMCs at concentrations as high as 10,000 ng/mL (Fig. 4) (49).

Unlike the mitotic arrest seen in cancer cells, in coronary artery SMCs, paclitaxel induced a primary and postmitotic G1 arrest (49,52). Coronary artery SMCs arrested in G1 remained metabolically active, becoming senescent over time (52). Furthermore, coronary artery SMCs exposed to paclitaxel maintained normal cellular and nuclear morphology (Fig. 5).

This cytostatic mechanism of action of paclitaxel in SMCs differentiates its antirestenotic activities from the antineoplastic activities in cancer cells. Paclitaxel has also been shown to be a potent inhibitor of SMC migration and chemotaxis (3,16,47,51). As shown in Figure 6, paclitaxel inhibited the migration of SMCs in a cell-culture wound assay at very low concentrations (16).

Studies by Axel et al. examined the effect of paclitaxel on the distribution of the contractile filament SMC α-actin and the intermediate filament vimentin in arterial SMCs (51). At a concentration of 1 μm/L, paclitaxel induced partial circumferential orientation of the actin filaments and disarrangement of actin bundles but without remarkable effects on vimentin assembly

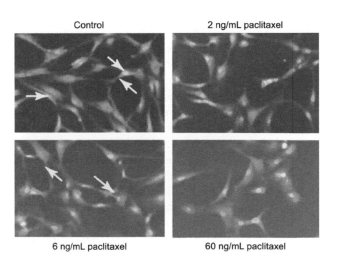

Figure 5
(*See color plate.*) Effect of paclitaxel on smooth muscle cell morphology. Normal interphase nuclei (*arrowheads*) and typical smooth muscle cell morphology with extended cellular processes (*arrow*) seen in the absence as well as presence of paclitaxel. *Source*: From Ref. 16.

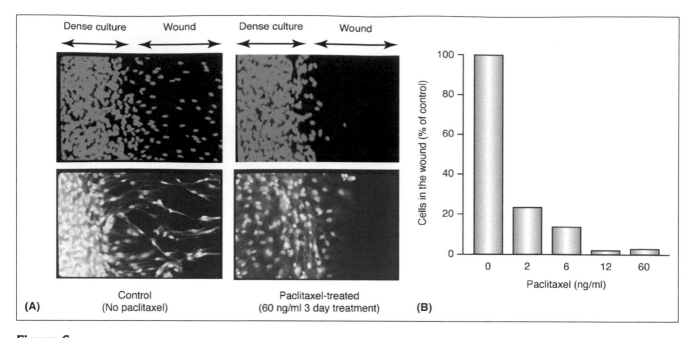

Figure 6

(*See color plate.*) The effects of paclitaxel on smooth muscle cell migration. (A) Inhibition of smooth muscle cell (SMC) migration by paclitaxel in a culture wound assay model and (B) paclitaxel dose–response relationship for SMC migration inhibition. (In collaboration with Dr. M. Blagosklonny.) *Source*: From Ref. 16.

(Fig. 7). Therefore, the investigators attributed the antimigratory activity of paclitaxel to its effect on the actin bundles.

In other studies, paclitaxel was found to inhibit the secretion of extracellular matrix proteins (3,53) and neovascularization-mediated intima progression (54), pointing to the multimodal activities of paclitaxel in various pathways relevant to the cascade of restenosis.

Studies under challenged conditions, such as in the cell culture models of insulin resistance, published recently by Patterson et al., have examined the antimigratory activity of DES agents. A comparison of the effects of paclitaxel and sirolimus on SMC migration and survival under conditions of high glucose and subsequent insulin resistance (as in diabetes), showed that the migratory effect of paclitaxel was maintained even under conditions of high glucose. Conversely, under these conditions, the antimigratory effects of sirolimus were reduced in comparison to those seen in normal glucose conditions (Fig. 8) (55). These data demonstrate the need to examine the effects of the drugs used in DES under a variety of conditions that simulate the potential "real-life" biologic environment.

In addition to the in vitro evidence of the antirestenotic effects of paclitaxel, various in vivo models of restenosis have demonstrated its ability to reduce neointimal hyperplasia and inhibit the restenotic cascade (47,56–60). Intraperitoneal administration of paclitaxel following rat carotid artery injury showed a significant (70%) reduction in neointimal proliferation at blood concentrations 100 times lower than antineoplastic levels (Fig. 9) (47).

The effect of intrapericardial administration of paclitaxel on neointimal proliferation was examined after balloon over-stretch of porcine coronary arteries (58). The study found that a single intrapericardial dose of 50 mg/25 mL of paclitaxel significantly reduced vessel narrowing in this model at 28 days, albeit at much higher doses than that delivered via DES-based delivery. The effect was found to be mediated by a reduction of neointimal mass, as well as by positive vascular remodeling. In a separate study, nonpolymeric, stent-based delivery of paclitaxel was examined in the porcine coronary model using various doses of paclitaxel (0, 0.2, 15, or 187 µg/stent) (57). At four weeks after stent implantation, there was a corresponding reduction in mean luminal diameter with increasing paclitaxel dose. In the rabbit iliac artery model, Farb et al. demonstrated that local delivery of paclitaxel from a polymer-coated (chondroitin sulfate and gelatin) stent induced a similar dose-dependent inhibition of neointimal hyperplasia at 28 days (Fig. 10) (61).

Another study of stent-based paclitaxel delivery, which also used a degradable polymer [poly(lactide-co-$\widetilde{\Sigma}$caprolactone)] to control the drug-release kinetics, demonstrated sustained reduction in neointimal hyperplasia in the rabbit iliac model (Fig. 11) (56).

The concept of using polymeric coatings for prolonged, localized stent-based delivery of antirestenotic agents has been an important advance in interventional cardiology (62,63). The combination of the right drug, dose, and release kinetics with a vascular compatible polymer that has the right mechanical, chemical, and biologic features, is crucial in achieving the desirable biologic benefit. A description of the characteristics of the polymer used in the marketed TAXUS paclitaxel DES can be found in Chapter 22 of this book.

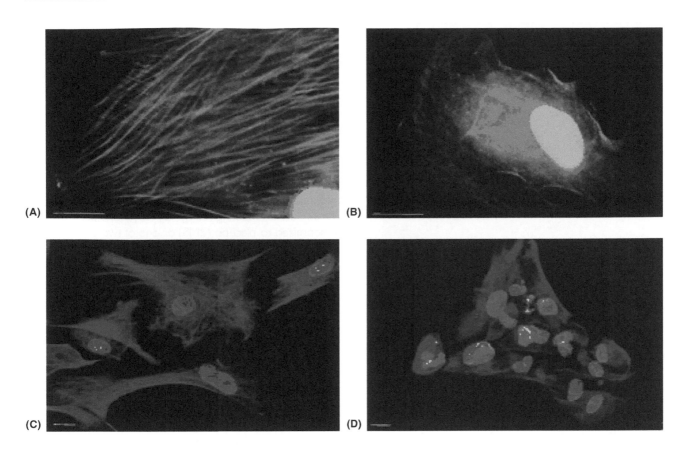

Figure 7

(*See color plate.*) Immunofluorescence micrographs demonstrating the effect of 1.0 μmol/L paclitaxel on the distribution of the contractile filament smooth muscle α-actin and the intermediate filament vimentin in haSMCs. (A) Smooth muscle α-actin staining of control cultures showing typical, straight α-actin filaments predominantly orientated along the cell axis; (B) paclitaxel causes a disarrangement of α-actin bundles with a partial circumferential orientation of the filaments; (C) the vimentin network of untreated control cells is expanded over the entire cytoplasm; and (D) paclitaxel treatment has no remarkable effects on vimentin assembly. Only the arrangement within the cytoplasm is altered according to the changes of cell shape and size. Scale bars represent 5 μm. *Source*: From Ref. 51.

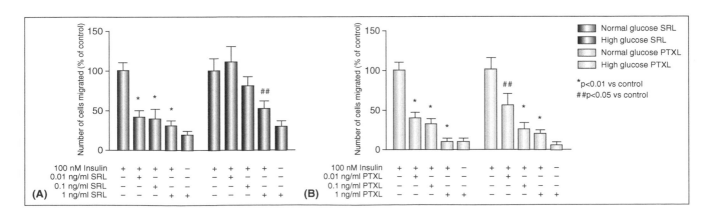

Figure 8

(*See color plate.*) The effects of sirolimus and paclitaxel on smooth muscle cell migration under conditions of normal and high glucose. Insulin-dependent smooth muscle cell migration was measured using modified Boyden chamber assays in insulin-stimulated cells grown under low-glucose or high-glucose conditions in the presence of escalating doses of sirolimus (A) and paclitaxel (B). Migrating cells were counted and expressed as a percentage of control. *Abbreviations*: PTXL, paclitaxel; SRL, sirolimus (rapamycin). *Source*: From Ref. 55.

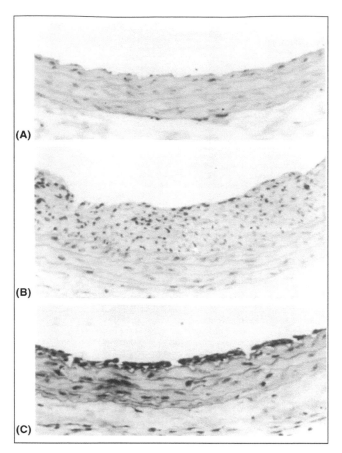

Figure 9

Inhibition of restenosis by paclitaxel in the rat carotid artery injury model. Paclitaxel inhibits the accumulation of smooth muscle cells 11 days after balloon catheter injury of rat carotid artery. Animals were treated with 2 mg/kg body weigh paclitaxel in vehicle (control animals were treated with vehicle alone) two hours after injury and daily for the next four days. Representative hematoxylin- and eosin-stained cross sections from (A) uninjured, (B) vehicle-treated, and (C) paclitaxel-treated, injured rat carotid arteries. X240. *Source*: From Ref. 47.

Clinical trials investigating stent-based delivery of paclitaxel

A number of randomized clinical trials (RCTs) have investigated stent-based delivery of paclitaxel. These studies utilized a number of different delivery methods, including polymeric sleeves, nonpolymeric drug delivery and from drug-polymer coatings on stents.

The Study to COmpare REstenosis rate between QueSt and QuaDDS-QP2 trial was designed to control neointimal proliferation through prolonged high-dose (800 μg) delivery of the paclitaxel derivative 7-hexanoyltaxol (QP2) via acrylate polymer membranes on the QuaDDS stent (Quanam Medical, Santa Clara, California, U.S.A.) (64). Despite a potential antirestenotic effect, enrollment in the trial was terminated early, due to an unacceptable safety profile, as

seen by high rates of early stent thrombosis and MI. The very high doses of paclitaxel used in this study and the unknown vascular compatibility of the polymeric sleeve used for delivery could be a few of the many reasons responsible for failure of the study.

Data from the European EvaLuation of pacliTaxel ElUting Stent clinical trial, in which a Cook V-Flex Plus DES (Cook Incorporated, Bloomington, Indiana, U.S.A.) was coated with escalating doses of paclitaxel (0.2, 0.7, 1.4, and 2.7 μg/mm^2) applied directly to the abluminal surface of the stent, showed a binary restenosis rate of 3.1% in the paclitaxel-eluting stent group compared with 20.6% in the BMS group (65). In the Asian Paclitaxel-Eluting Stent Clinical Trial, patients were randomized to placebo (BMS) or one of two doses of paclitaxel (1.3 or 3.1 μg/mm^2) on a Supra G™ stent (Cook Incorporated, Bloomington, Indiana, U.S.A.) (66). These studies demonstrated a positive result using angiographic endpoints and were used as the basis for the larger Drug ELuting coronary stent systems in the treatment of patients with de noVo nativE coronaRy lesions (DELIVER I) study. However, no significant reduction in angiographic restenosis rate or target vessel failure (TVF) was seen in the DELIVER-I trial (67). Therefore, despite the improvement seen in angiographic parameters in the earlier clinical trials, delivery of paclitaxel via a nonpolymeric approach did not demonstrate a positive clinical benefit. This failure may have several causes, such as the loss of the drug to the systemic circulation before its deployment at the target site, as well as variability of the drug-release kinetics and dose delivered. The use of polymers to control the release of a drug is discussed in Chapter 22, "The Application of Controlled Drug Delivery Principles to the Development of Drug-Eluting Stents."

The TAXUS DES, which utilizes a polymeric delivery approach for paclitaxel, has been examined across multiple patient and lesion types in various clinical trials with successful results demonstrating its antirestenotic potential. These clinical data are described next.

Clinical studies using the TAXUS Express® paclitaxel-eluting stent

The first study of the TAXUS paclitaxel-eluting stent in humans, TAXUS I, reported major adverse cardiac events at one-year follow-up at 3.2% for the TAXUS DES group versus 10.0% for the BMS control group (p = NS) (68). TAXUS I, now has data through four years and these benefits were maintained for the TAXUS group (Fig. 12).

These data formed the basis of the most comprehensive RCT program of a DES to date, evolving to encompass higher patient numbers and higher-risk lesions and patients. Over 6200 patients have been enrolled in the clinical trial

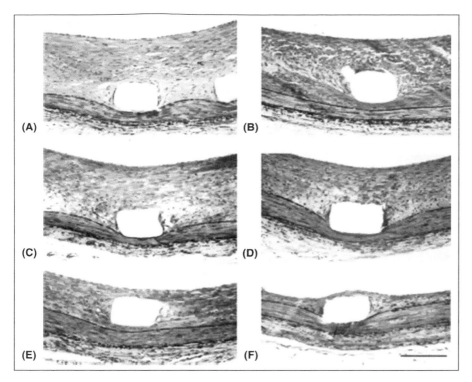

Figure 10

(*See color plate.*) Inhibition of restenosis by paclitaxel inhibits in a porcine coronary model. Photomicrographs demonstrating neointimal thickness in arteries 28 days after stent deployment. (**A**) Uncoated (bare) stent without paclitaxel; (**B**) chondroitin sulphate and gelatin-coated stent with paclitaxel; (**C**) chondroitin-sulphate and gelatin stent containing 1.5 μg of paclitaxel; (**D**) chondroitin-sulphate and gelatin stent containing 8.6 μg of paclitaxel; (**E**) chondroitin-sulphate and gelatin stent containing 20.2 μg of paclitaxel; and (**F**) chondroitin-sulphate and gelatin stent containing 42.0 μg of paclitaxel. Movat pentochrome stain; Scale bar represents 0.12 mm. *Source*: From Ref. 61.

program and a number of peri- and post-approval registries have also been completed.

The TAXUS II study compared slow-release (SR) and moderate-release (MR) formulations of the PES with BMS in patients with relatively noncomplex lesions (69,75). At three years, the TLR rate was 5.4% for the SR group and 3.7% for the MR group, compared with 15.7% for the combined control groups (p = 0.0001) (Fig. 12). TAXUS III was a single-arm, pilot study assessing the feasibility of implanting up to two PES for the treatment of ISR (70). The TAXUS IV pivotal study

in the United States is the largest ongoing PES RCT designed to assess the safety and efficacy of the SR TAXUS Express™ DES for the treatment of de novo, coronary artery lesions (62, 63). In this study, TLR rates at three years were significantly lower with the TAXUS DES group than the BMS control group [6.9% vs. 18.6%, respectively ($P \leq 0.0001$); Fig. 12].

The remaining trials, TAXUS V and VI, incorporated higher-risk patients or patients with higher-risk lesions. TAXUS V expanded on the TAXUS IV pivotal study by including a higher proportion of diabetic patients (31%) as well as those with

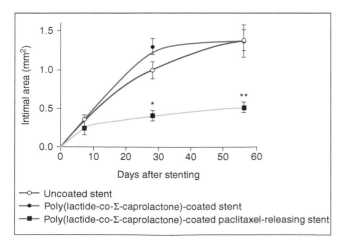

Figure 11

(*See color plate.*) Sustained reduction in neointimal hyperplasia in the rabbit iliac model. *Source*: From Ref. 107.

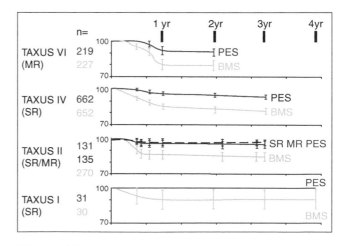

Figure 12

(*See color plate.*) Sustained freedom from target lesion revascularization in TAXUS clinical trials. *Abbreviations*: BMS, bare-metal stent; MR, moderate-release; PES, paclitaxel-eluting stent; SR, slow-release. *Source*: From Ref. 73.

small or large vessels, and patients with long lesions requiring multiple overlapping stents (71). In this study, PES reduced the nine-month TLR rate from 15.7% for BMS-treated patients to 8.6% for TAXUS DES-treated patients (p = 0.0003). The TAXUS VI moderate release paclitaxel-eluting stent study comprised the longest mean lesion lengths and highest-risk patient population of any DES study to date, and currently has data for three years of follow-up. A total of 28% of the patients had long lesions with overlapping stents; the small vessel subpopulation was also 28% of the total patient population. Diabetic patients represented 20% of the study population. Even in this more challenging study population, two-year TLR rates were low in the PES group (9.7%) compared with the BMS control group (21.0%) (p = 0.0013) (68).

Similar findings to those demonstrated in RCTs have been seen in postapproval registries (72,73), corroborating the findings of RCTs with "real-world" data. In addition, recent studies have demonstrated significant benefit by DES when used for the treatment of ISR, comparable with that seen with intracoronary radiation (71,74). These findings point to the potential utility of DES platforms in scenarios other than de novo lesions, emphasizing the need to continue to understand and assess this technology for unmet clinical needs.

Conclusions

Stent-based delivery of antirestenotic agents, now considered a major technological advance in the interventional cardiology area, was the first successful application of controlled drug delivery technology in the management of occlusive coronary artery disease. The success of DES in preventing coronary restenosis has opened doors to other potential indications suitable for local and regional drug delivery. Various pharmacotherapeutic options and delivery modalities are being considered for a number of pathologies, such as vulnerable plaque, stroke, valvular heart disease, and congestive heart failure (76). A thorough understanding of disease biology, drug pharmacology, and a delivery technology appropriate for the intended clinical application would be critical elements of a successful therapeutic strategy.

Acknowledgments

The authors would like to thank Cecilia Schott, PharmD, and Michael Eppihimer, PhD, for their assistance in the preparation of this chapter.

References

1   Investigators TBARIB. Comparison of coronary bypass surgery with angioplasty in patients with multivessel disease. The Bypass Angioplasty Revascularization Investigation (BARI) Investigators. N Engl J Med 1996; 335(4):217–225.

2   Serruys PW, Unger F, Sousa JE, et al. Comparison of coronary-artery bypass surgery and stenting for the treatment of multivessel disease. N Engl J Med 2001; 344(15):1117–1124.

3   Wiskirchen J, Schober W, Schart N, et al. The effects of paclitaxel on the three phases of restenosis: smooth muscle cell proliferation, migration, and matrix formation: an in vitro study. Invest Radiol 2004; 39(9):565–571.

4   Hiatt BL, Ikeno F, Yeung AC, Carter AJ. Drug-eluting stents for the prevention of restenosis: in quest for the Holy Grail. Catheter Cardiovasc Interv 2002; 55(3):409–417.

5   Farb A, Sangiorgi G, Carter AJ, et al. Pathology of acute and chronic coronary stenting in humans. Circulation 1999; 99(1):44–52.

6   Farb A, Weber DK, Kolodgie FD, Burke AP, Virmani R. Morphological predictors of restenosis after coronary stenting in humans. Circulation 2002; 105(25):2974–2980.

7   Hoffmann R, Mintz GS, Dussaillant GR, et al. Patterns and mechanisms of in-stent restenosis. A serial intravascular ultrasound study. Circulation 1996; 94(6):1247–1254.

8   Virmani R, Farb A. Pathology of in-stent restenosis. Curr Opin Lipidol 1999; 10(6):499–506.

9   Wahlgren CM, Frebelius S, Swedenborg J. Inhibition of neointimal hyperplasia by a specific thrombin inhibitor. Scand Cardiovasc J 2004; 38(1):16–21.

10 Costa MA, Simon DI. Molecular basis of restenosis and drug-eluting stents. Circulation 2005; 111(17):2257–2273.

11 Welt FG, Rogers C. Inflammation and restenosis in the stent era. Arterioscler Thromb Vasc Biol 2002; 22(11):1769–1776.

12 Chesebro JH, Lam JY, Badimon L, Fuster V. Restenosis after arterial angioplasty: a hemorrheologic response to injury. Am J Cardiol 1987; 60(3):10B–16B.

13 Ferns GA, Raines EW, Sprugel KH, Motani AS, Reidy MA, Ross R. Inhibition of neointimal smooth muscle accumulation after angioplasty by an antibody to PDGF. Science 1991; 253(5024):1129–1132.

14 Ip JH, Fuster V, Israel D, Badimon L, Badimon J, Chesebro JH. The role of platelets, thrombin and hyperplasia in restenosis after coronary angioplasty. J Am Coll Cardiol 1991; 17(6 suppl B):77B–88B.

15 Willerson JT, Yao SK, McNatt J, et al. Frequency and severity of cyclic flow alternations and platelet aggregation predict the severity of neointimal proliferation following experimental coronary stenosis and endothelial injury. Proc Natl Acad Sci USA 1991; 88(23):10624–10628.

16 Kamath KR, Barry JJ, Miller KM. The Taxus drug-eluting stent: a new paradigm in controlled drug delivery. Adv Drug Deliv Rev 2006; 58(3):412–436.

17 Lau K-W, Sigwart U. Restenosis—an accelerated arteriopathy: pathophysiology, preventive strategies and research horizons. In: Edelman ER, Levy RJ, eds. Molecular Interventions and Local Drug Delivery. London: W. B. Saunders Co. Ltd, 1995:1–28.

18 Chorny M, Fishbein I, Golomb G. Drug delivery systems for the treatment of restenosis. Crit Rev Ther Drug Carrier Syst 2000; 17(3):249–284.

19 Lincoff AM, Topol EJ, Ellis SG. Local drug delivery for the prevention of restenosis. Fact, fancy, and future. Circulation 1994; 90(4):2070–2084.

20 Kavanagh CA, Rochev YA, Gallagher WM, Dawson KA, Keenan AK. Local drug delivery in restenosis injury: thermo-responsive co-polymers as potential drug delivery systems. Pharmacol Ther 2004; 102(1):1–15.

21 Bailey SR. Local drug delivery: current applications. Prog Cardiovasc Dis 1997; 40(2):183–204.

22 Camenzind E, Kint PP, Di Mario C, et al. Intracoronary heparin delivery in humans. Acute feasibility and long-term results. Circulation 1995; 92(9):2463–2472.

23 Mitchel JF, McKay RG. Treatment of acute stent thrombosis with local urokinase therapy using catheter-based, drug delivery systems: a case report. Cathet Cardiovasc Diagn 1995; 34(2):149–54.

24 Tahlil O, Brami M, Feldman LJ, Branellec D, Steg PG. The Dispatch catheter as a delivery tool for arterial gene transfer. Cardiovasc Res 1997; 33(1):181–187.

25 Bailey SR. Coronary restenosis: a review of current insights and therapies. Catheter Cardiovasc Interv 2002; 55(2):265–271.

26 Lambert CR, Leone JE, Rowland SM. Local drug delivery catheters: functional comparison of porous and microporous designs. Coron Artery Dis 1993; 4(5):469–475.

27 Hanke H, Strohschneider T, Oberhoff M, Betz E, Karsch KR. Time course of smooth muscle cell proliferation in the intima and media of arteries following experimental angioplasty. Circ Res 1990; 67(3):651–659.

28 Holmes DR Jr, Simpson JB, Berdan LG, et al. Abrupt closure: the CAVEAT I experience. Coronary angioplasty versus excisional atherectomy trial. J Am Coll Cardiol 1995; 26(6): 1494–1500.

29 Linde J, Strauss BH. Pharmacological treatment for prevention of restenosis. Expert Opin Emerg Drugs 2001; 6(2): 281–302.

30 Rogers C, Edelman ER, Simon DI. A mAb to the beta2-leukocyte integrin Mac-1 (CD11b/CD18) reduces intimal thickening after angioplasty or stent implantation in rabbits. Proc Natl Acad Sci U S A 1998; 95(17):10134–10139.

31 Simon DI, Dhen Z, Seifert P, Edelman ER, Ballantyne CM, Rogers C. Decreased neointimal formation in Mac-1(−/−) mice reveals a role for inflammation in vascular repair after angioplasty. J Clin Invest 2000; 105(3):293–300.

32 Fidler J. Clinical Oncology. New York: Churchill Livingstone, 2000.

33 Li JJ, Gao RL. Should atherosclerosis be considered a cancer of the vascular wall? Med Hypotheses 2005; 64(4):694–698.

34 Serruys PW, Ormiston JA, Sianos G, et al. Actinomycin-eluting stent for coronary revascularization: a randomized feasibility and safety study: the ACTION trial. J Am Coll Cardiol 2004; 44(7):1363–1367.

35 Marx SO, Jayaraman T, Go LO, Marks AR. Rapamycin-FKBP inhibits cell cycle regulators of proliferation in vascular smooth muscle cells. Circ Res 1995; 76(3):412–417.

36 Bruns CJ, Koehl GE, Guba M, et al. Rapamycin-induced endothelial cell death and tumor vessel thrombosis potentiate cytotoxic therapy against pancreatic cancer. Clin Cancer Res 2004; 10(6):2109–2119.

37 Adams JD, Flora KP, Goldspiel BR, Wilson JW, Arbuck SG, Finley R. Taxol: a history of pharmaceutical development and current pharmaceutical concerns. J Natl Cancer Inst Monogr 1993; 15:141–147.

38 Ramaswamy B, Puhalla S. Docetaxel: a tubulin-stabilizing agent approved for the management of several solid tumors. Drugs Today (Barc) 2006; 42(4):265–279.

39 Mullins DW, Koci MD, Burger CJ, Elgert KD. Interleukin-12 overcomes paclitaxel-mediated suppression of T-cell proliferation. Immunopharmacol Immunotoxicol 1998; 20(4):473–492.

40 Tange S, Scherer MN, Graeb C, et al. The antineoplastic drug paclitaxel has immunosuppressive properties that can effectively promote allograft survival in a rat heart transplant model. Transplantation 2002; 73(2):216–223.

41 Hui A, Min WX, Tang J, Cruz TF. Inhibition of activator protein 1 activity by paclitaxel suppresses interleukin-1-induced collagenase and stromelysin expression by bovine chondrocytes. Arthritis Rheum 1998; 41(5):869–876.

42 Rowinsky EK, Donehower RC. Paclitaxel (taxol). N Engl J Med 1995; 332(15):1004–1014.

43 Schiff PB, Fant J, Horwitz SB. Promotion of microtubule assembly in vitro by taxol. Nature 1979; 277(5698):665–667.

44 Jordan MA, Thrower D, Wilson L. Mechanism of inhibition of cell proliferation by Vinca alkaloids. Cancer Res 1991; 51(8):2212–2222.

45 Schiff PB, Horwitz SB. Taxol stabilizes microtubules in mouse fibroblast cells. Proc Natl Acad Sci U S A 1980; 77(3):1561–1565.

46 Jordan MA, Toso RJ, Thrower D, Wilson L. Mechanism of mitotic block and inhibition of cell proliferation by taxol at low concentrations. Proc Natl Acad Sci U S A 1993; 90(20):9552–9556.

47 Sollott SJ, Cheng L, Pauly RR, et al. Taxol inhibits neointimal smooth muscle cell accumulation after angioplasty in the rat. J Clin Invest 1995; 95(4):1869–1876.

48 Ganansia-Leymarie V, Bischoff P, Bergerat JP, Holl V. Signal transduction pathways of taxanes-induced apoptosis. Curr Med Chem Anti-canc Agents 2003; 3(4):291–306.

49 Blagosklonny MV, Darzynkiewicz Z, Halicka HD, et al. Paclitaxel induces primary and postmitotic G1 arrest in human arterial smooth muscle cells. Cell Cycle 2004; 3(8):1050–1056.

50 Giannakakou P, Robey R, Fojo T, Blagosklonny MV. Low concentrations of paclitaxel induce cell type-dependent p53, p21 and G1/G2 arrest instead of mitotic arrest: molecular determinants of paclitaxel-induced cytotoxicity. Oncogene 2001; 20(29):3806–3813.

51 Axel DI, Kunert W, Goggelmann C, et al. Paclitaxel inhibits arterial smooth muscle cell proliferation and migration in vitro and in vivo using local drug delivery. Circulation 1997; 96(2):636–645.

52 Blagosklonny MV, Demidenko ZN, Giovino M, et al. Cytostatic activity of paclitaxel in coronary artery smooth muscle cells is mediated through transient mitotic arrest followed by permanent post-mitotic arrest: comparison with cancer cells. Cell Cycle 2006; 5(14):1574–1579.

53 Oberhoff M, Herdeg C, Al Ghobainy R, et al. Local delivery of paclitaxel using the double-balloon perfusion catheter before stenting in the porcine coronary artery. Catheter Cardiovasc Interv 2001; 53(4):562–568.

54 Celletti FL, Waugh JM, Amabile PG, Kao EY, Boroumand S, Dake MD. Inhibition of vascular endothelial growth factor-mediated neointima progression with angiostatin or paclitaxel. J Vasc Interv Radiol 2002; 13(7):703–707.

55 Patterson C, Mapera S, Li HH, et al. Comparative effects of paclitaxel and rapamycin on smooth muscle migration and survival. Role of Akt-dependent signaling. Arterioscler Thromb Vasc Biol 2006; 26(7):1479–1480.

56 Drachman DE, Edelman ER, Seifert P, et al. Neointimal thickening after stent delivery of paclitaxel: change in composition and arrest of growth over six months. J Am Coll Cardiol 2000; 36(7):2325–2332.

57 Heldman AW, Cheng L, Jenkins GM, et al. Paclitaxel stent coating inhibits neointimal hyperplasia at 4 weeks in a porcine model of coronary restenosis. Circulation 2001; 103(18):2289–2295.

58 Hou D, Rogers PI, Toleikis PM, Hunter W, March KL. Intrapericardial paclitaxel delivery inhibits neointimal proliferation and promotes arterial enlargement after porcine coronary overstretch. Circulation 2000; 102(13):1575–1581.

59 Kolodgie FD, John M, Khurana C, et al. Sustained reduction of in-stent neointimal growth with the use of a novel systemic nanoparticle paclitaxel. Circulation 2002; 106(10):1195–1198.

60 Signore PE, Machan LS, Jackson JK, et al. Complete inhibition of intimal hyperplasia by perivascular delivery of paclitaxel in balloon-injured rat carotid arteries. J Vasc Interv Radiol 2001; 12(1):79–88.

61 Farb A, Heller PF, Shroff S, et al. Pathological analysis of local delivery of paclitaxel via a polymer-coated stent. Circulation 2001; 104(4):473–479.

62 Stone GW, Ellis SG, Cox DA, et al. A polymer-based, paclitaxel-eluting stent in patients with coronary artery disease. N Engl J Med 2004a; 350(3):221–231.

63 Stone G, Ellis S, Cox D, et al. One-year clinical results with the slow-release, polymer-based, paclitaxel-eluting TAXUS stent: the TAXUS-IV trial. Circulation 2004b; 109(16):1942–1947.

64 Grube E, Lansky A, Hauptmann KE, et al. High-dose 7-hexanoyltaxol-eluting stent with polymer sleeves for coronary revascularization: one-year results from the SCORE randomized trial. J Am Coll Cardiol 2004; 44(7):1368–1372.

65 Gershlick A, De Scheerder I, Chevalier B, et al. Inhibition of restenosis with a paclitaxel-eluting, polymer-free coronary stent: the European evaLUation of pacliTaxel Eluting Stent (ELUTES) trial. Circulation 2004; 109(4):487–493.

66 Hong MK, Mintz GS, Lee CW, et al. Paclitaxel coating reduces in-stent intimal hyperplasia in human coronary arteries: a serial volumetric intravascular ultrasound analysis from the Asian Paclitaxel-Eluting Stent Clinical Trial (ASPECT). Circulation 2003; 107(4):517–520.

67 Silber S. Paclitaxel-eluting stents: are they all equal? An analysis of six randomized controlled trials in de novo lesions of 3,319 patients. J Interv Cardiol 2003; 16(6):485–490.

68 Grube E, Silber S, Hauptmann KE, et al. TAXUS I: six- and twelve-month results from a randomized, double-blind trial on a slow-release paclitaxel-eluting stent for de novo coronary lesions. Circulation 2003; 107(1):38–42.

69 Colombo A, Drzewiecki J, Banning A, et al. Randomized study to assess the effectiveness of slow- and moderate-release polymer-based paclitaxel-eluting stents for coronary artery lesions. Circulation 2003; 108(7):788–794.

70 Tanabe K, Serruys PW, Grube E, et al. TAXUS III Trial: in-stent restenosis treated with stent-based delivery of paclitaxel incorporated in a slow-release polymer formulation. Circulation 2003; 107(4):559–564.

71 Stone GW, Ellis SG, Cannon L, et al. Comparison of a polymer-based paclitaxel-eluting stent with a bare metal stent in patients with complex coronary artery disease: a randomized controlled trial. JAMA 2005; 294(10):1215–1223.

72 Abizaid A, Chan C, Lim Y-T, et al. Twelve-month outcomes with a paclitaxel-eluting stent transitioning from controlled trials to clinical practice: the WISDOM registry. Am J Cardiol 2006; 98:1028–1032.

73 Lasala JM, Stone GW, Dawkins KD, et al. An overview of the TAXUS® EXPRESS® paclitaxel-eluting stent clinical trial program. J Interv Cardiol 2006; 19:422–431.

74 Saia F, Lemos PA, Hoye A, et al. Clinical outcomes for sirolimus-eluting stent implantation and vascular brachytherapy for the treatment of in-stent restenosis. Catheter Cardiovasc Interv 2004; 62(3):283–288.

75 Tanabe K, Serruys PW, Degertekin M, et al. Chronic arterial responses to polymer-controlled paclitaxel-eluting stents: comparison with bare metal stents by serial intravascular ultrasound analyses: data from the randomized TAXUS-II trial. Circulation 2004; 109(2):196–200.

76 Sousa JE, Serruys PW, Costa MA. New frontiers in cardiology: drug-eluting stents: Part II. Circulation 2003; 107(18): 2383–2389.

77 Whitworth HB, Roubin GS, Hollman J, et al. Effect of nifedipine on recurrent stenosis after percutaneous transluminal coronary angioplasty. J Am Coll Cardiol 1986; 8(6): 1271–1276.

78 Corcos T, David PR, Val PG, et al. Failure of diltiazem to prevent restenosis after percutaneous transluminal coronary angioplasty. Am Heart J 1985; 109(5 Pt 1):926–931.

79 Hoberg E, Dietz R, Frees U, et al. Verapamil treatment after coronary angioplasty in patients at high risk of recurrent stenosis. Br Heart J 1994; 71(3):254–260.

80 Schwartz L, Bourassa MG, Lesperance J, et al. Aspirin and dipyridamole in the prevention of restenosis after percutaneous transluminal coronary angioplasty. N Engl J Med 1988; 318(26):1714–1719.

81 Bertrand ME, Allain H, Lablanche JM. Results of a randomized trial of ticlopidine vs placebo for prevention of acute closure and restenosis after coronary angioplasty. The TACT study. Circulation 1990; 82(suppl 3):190.

82 Okamoto S, Inden M, Setsuda M, Konishi T, Nakano T. Effects of trapidil (triazolopyrimidine), a platelet-derived growth factor antagonist, in preventing restenosis after percutaneous transluminal coronary angioplasty. Am Heart J 1992; 123(6): 1439–1444.

83 Serruys PW, Rutsch W, Heyndrickx GR, et al. Prevention of restenosis after percutaneous transluminal coronary angioplasty with thromboxane A2-receptor blockade. A randomized, double-blind, placebo-controlled trial. Coronary Artery Restenosis Prevention on Repeated Thromboxane-Antagonism Study (CARPORT). Circulation 1991; 84(4):1568–1580.

84 Knudtson ML, Flintoft VF, Roth DL, Hansen JL, Duff HJ. Effect of short-term prostacyclin administration on restenosis after percutaneous transluminal coronary angioplasty. J Am Coll Cardiol 1990; 15(3):691–697.

85 Urban P, Buller N, Fox K, Shapiro L, Bayliss J, Rickards A. Lack of effect of warfarin on the restenosis rate or on clinical outcome after balloon coronary angioplasty. Br Heart J 1988; 60(6):485–488.

86 Ellis SG, Roubin GS, Wilentz J, Douglas JS Jr, King SB III. Effect of 18- to 24-hour heparin administration for prevention of restenosis after uncomplicated coronary angioplasty. Am Heart J 1989; 117(4):777–782.

87 Stone GW, Rutherford BD, McConahay DR, et al. A randomized trial of corticosteroids for the prevention of restenosis in 102 patients undergoing repeat coronary angioplasty. Cathet Cardiovasc Diagn 1989; 18(4):227–231.

88 Pepine CJ, Hirshfeld JW, Macdonald RG, et al. A controlled trial of corticosteroids to prevent restenosis after coronary angioplasty. M-HEART Group. Circulation 1990; 81(6): 1753–1761.

89 Multicenter European Research Trial with Cilazapril after Angioplasty to Prevent Transluminal Coronary Obstruction and Restenosis (MERCATOR) Study Group. Does the new angiotensin converting enzyme inhibitor cilazapril prevent restenosis after percutaneous transluminal coronary angioplasty? Results of the MERCATOR study: a multicenter, randomized, double-blind placebo-controlled trial. Circulation 1992; 86(1):100–110.

90 Desmet W, Vrolix M, De Scheerder I, Van Lierde J, Willems JL, Piessens J. Angiotensin-converting enzyme inhibition with fosinopril sodium in the prevention of restenosis after coronary angioplasty. Circulation 1994; 89(1):385–392.

91 O'Keefe JH Jr, McCallister BD, Bateman TM, Kuhnlein DL, Ligon RW, Hartzler GO. Ineffectiveness of colchicine for the prevention of restenosis after coronary angioplasty. J Am Coll Cardiol 1992; 19(7):1597–1600.

92 Kent KN, Williams DO, Cassagneau B, et al. Double-blind, controlled trial of the effect of angiopeptin on coronary restenosis following coronary angioplasty. Circulation 1993; 88(suppl 1):5063.

93 Eriksen UH, Amtorp O, Bagger JP, et al. Continuous angiopeptin infusion reduces coronary restenosis following balloon angioplasty. Circulation 1993; 88(suppl 1):594.

94 Serruys PW, Klein W, Tijssen JP, et al. Evaluation of ketanserin in the prevention of restenosis after percutaneous transluminal coronary angioplasty. A multicenter randomized double-blind placebo-controlled trial. Circulation 1993; 88(4 Pt 1): 1588–1601.

95 Sahni R, Maniet AR, Voci G, Banka VS. Prevention of restenosis by lovastatin after successful coronary angioplasty. Am Heart J 1991; 121(6 Pt 1):1600–1608.

96 Bairati I, Roy L, Meyer F. Double-blind, randomized, controlled trial of fish oil supplements in prevention of recurrence of stenosis after coronary angioplasty. Circulation 1992; 85(3):950–956.

97 Dehmer GJ, Popma JJ, van den Berg EK, et al. Reduction in the rate of early restenosis after coronary angioplasty by a diet supplemented with n-3 fatty acids. N Engl J Med 1988; 319(12):733–740.

98 Grigg LE, Kay TW, Valentine PA, et al. Determinants of restenosis and lack of effect of dietary supplementation with eicosapentaenoic acid on the incidence of coronary artery restenosis after angioplasty. J Am Coll Cardiol 1989; 13(3):665–672.

99 Nye ER, Ablett MB, Robertson MC, Ilsley CD, Sutherland WH. Effect of eicosapentaenoic acid on restenosis rate, clinical course and blood lipids in patients after percutaneous transluminal coronary angioplasty. Aust N Z J Med 1990; 20(4):549–552.

100 Reis GJ, Boucher TM, Sipperly ME, et al. Randomised trial of fish oil for prevention of restenosis after coronary angioplasty. Lancet 1989; 2(8656):177–181.

101 Muller DW, Topol EJ, Abrams GD, Gallagher KP, Ellis SG. Intramural methotrexate therapy for the prevention of neointimal thickening after balloon angioplasty. J Am Coll Cardiol 1992; 20(2):460–466.

102 Gradus-Pizlo I, Wilensky RL, March KL, et al. Local delivery of biodegradable microparticles containing colchicine or a colchicine analogue: effects on restenosis and implications for catheter-based drug delivery. J Am Coll Cardiol 1995; 26(6): 1549–1557.

103 Margolin L, Fishbein I, Banai S, et al. Metalloproteinase inhibitor attenuates neointima formation and constrictive remodeling after angioplasty in rats: augmentative effect of alpha(v)beta(3) receptor blockade. Atherosclerosis 2002; 163(2):269–277.

104 van Beusekom HM, Post MJ, Whelan DM, de Smet BJ, Duncker DJ, van der Giessen WJ. Metalloproteinase inhibition by batimastat does not reduce neointimal thickening in stented atherosclerotic porcine femoral arteries. Cardiovasc Radiat Med 2003; 4(4):186–191.

105 Wu CH, Pan JS, Chang WC, Hung JS, Mao SJ. The molecular mechanism of actinomycin D in preventing neointimal formation in rat carotid arteries after balloon injury. J Biomed Sci 2005; 12(3):503–512.

106 Suzuki T, Kopia G, Hayashi S, et al. Stent-based delivery of sirolimus reduces neointimal formation in a porcine coronary model. Circulation 2001; 104(10):1188–1193.

26

Anti-inflammatory drugs, sirolimus, and inhibition of target of rapamycin and its effect on vascular diseases

Steven J. Adelman

Introduction

The role of immune cells and inflammatory mediators in cardiovascular disease has been well documented. Atherosclerosis has been described as a chronic inflammatory syndrome, a systemic disorder characterized by focal lesions throughout the vasculature (1,2). Immune cells such as T-cells and macrophages are recruited to the vascular wall where they and their signaling molecules play important roles at all stages of lesion development including plaque initiation, progression, and rupture leading to thrombotic events (3,4). Compositionally, varying sections of the plaque may be engorged with soft, pliable lipid (cholesterol ester) and immune components such as foam-cell-like macrophages, typical of either newly formed or shoulder regions of mature lesions versus regions with more stable transformations comprised of proliferated smooth muscle cells (SMCs), fibroblasts, and matrix (5–7). With growth and maturation, remodeling occurs with thickening and breakdown of the architecture and function of the vascular wall, ultimately impinging on the size of the lumen and reducing blood flow. It is these larger lesions, those more easily identified by angiography, that are typically treated with interventional procedures.

Attempts at treating stenotic vessels due to vascular plaque have included surgical interventions such as bypass and, since the late 1970s, angioplasty. Unfortunately, in nearly 30% to 40% of patients, these procedures failed leading to re-occlusion of the vessel within 6 to 12 months (8). Pathologically, this failure has been ascribed to either an acute closure from stretching and recoil of the vessel or a more chronic biologically mediated lumen loss. This longer-term failure, or restenosis, is due to a response to the mechanical disruption and endothelial denudation from the procedure and results from a cellular response to repair the injury. The major component of restenotic plaque is neointima, primarily misaligned, proliferated/migrated SMCs and fibroblasts, and matrix material appearing somewhat in disarray. Early attempts to treat restenosis focused on the local proliferative process, primarily SMC expansion, with numerous therapeutic agents and approaches investigated over more than two decades (9).

Recently, a breakthrough has been achieved leading to a significant shift in therapeutic paradigm, initially by use of the Cypher sirolimus drug-eluting stent (DES). Sirolimus, an immune suppressant approved for use in patients undergoing kidney transplant, has pleotropic effects on cellular metabolism. Specifically, the compound appears to act as an inhibitor of cell cycle progression, and based on this, may combine the activities required on the numerous mechanisms and cell types purported to participate in the restenotic process. Utilizing this approach, a clear improvement has occurred in outcomes, despite the reality that we really still do not completely understand the restenotic participants or mechanisms.

This chapter focuses on percutaneous transluminal coronary angioplasty (PTCA), provides a summary of the underlying immune activities of the diseased vasculature, and focuses in part on the role of immune and inflammatory mediators in the restenotic process. In addition, the mechanism of action of sirolimus, the drug used in the first successful DES for reduction of restenosis will be highlighted. Finally, the potential role for immune mediators on the overall processes of atherosclerosis will be explored.

Percutaneous transluminal coronary angioplasty

Today, standard therapy for myocardial infarction or luminal narrowing includes thrombolytics, anticoagulants, and often interventional procedures such as PTCA. With its introduction in the late 1970s, improvement was seen in the treatment of luminal narrowing from obstructive coronary artery disease or blockage due to myocardial infarction. The procedure involves placing a balloon-tipped catheter at the site of occlusion and disrupting and expanding the occluded vessel by inflating the balloon. Although initially successful at removal of the blockage and achieving luminal enlargement, the process also damages the blood vessel wall extensively including the loss of the endothelial lining. The ensuing response to this severe injury is often enhanced expression of cytokines and growth factors and, subsequently, a rapid reclosure or recoil, and/or a slow progressive re-occlusion or restenosis of the vessel. With the introduction of stents, metal-based cage/tube-like structures placed into the vessel lumen, a step toward improving outcomes was achieved. Coronary stents provide luminal scaffolding, eliminating elastic recoil which can occur rapidly following an interventional procedure. Unfortunately, although acute reclosure was reduced, neointimal hyperplasia was not, and in fact, the procedure lead to an increase in the proliferative comportment of restenosis (10).

As a consequence of PTCA, a neointima is formed within the vascular wall, typically including myointimal hyperplasia, proliferation and migration of SMCs and fibroblasts, connective tissue matrix remodeling, and formation of thrombus. Restenosis, referring to the renarrowing of the vascular lumen following an intervention such as balloon angioplasty, is defined clinically as >50% loss of the initial luminal diameter gain following the interventional procedure and has affected anywhere from 30% to 40% of treated vessels.

Restenosis: role of inflammation

Initial attempts at treating or preventing restenosis focused primarily on inhibition of the proliferation of vascular SMCs (VSMCs). A series of agents successful at inhibition of SMC proliferation in vitro as well as in vivo in animal models such as carotid injury models in the rat failed to demonstrate benefit in the clinic. More recently, it has been shown in addition to effects on SMCs, that mechanical intervention also activates the recruitment and activation of immune cells. Cell signaling through cytokines, chemokines, and adhesion molecule expression results in the recruitment to the vascular wall of cells of many types, as well as their proliferation, migration, and/or maturation.

As with atherosclerosis itself, recruitment of inflammatory cells is now recognized as an essential step in the pathogenesis of neointima formation in humans (11,12). In various animal models, reduction of leukocyte recruitment by selective blockade of adhesion molecules significantly reduced neointima formation and restenosis (13–16). Recent studies also concluded a role of pre-existing inflammation within the treated lesion itself and also, a correlation with systemic markers of inflammation. Interestingly and in addition, there are also current data suggesting a mobilization of hematopoeitic progenitor cells (HPC) contributing to restenosis, both from studies in mice and in humans (17).

Activation of inflammation

Following PTCA, responses within the vascular wall are typical of a response to injury. Numerous studies in animals demonstrate that the inflammatory response is strongly related to degree of arterial injury, with balloon dilation damaging the endothelial lining and stimulating cytokine and adhesion molecule expression (12,18). A layer of platelets and fibrin forms at the injured site and circulating cells are recruited. P-selectin mediates the adhesion of activated platelets with monocytes and neutrophils and the rolling of leukocytes on the endothelium (14,15). This is the main pathophysiological process linking inflammation with thrombosis after arterial wall injury.

Leukocytes are recruited to the site of injury and NFkB is activated. Recent findings support a role for nuclear factor-kappa B (NFkB) as a key player in restenosis. NFkB, a central mediator of expression of inflammatory genes including cytokines and interleukins (ILs), is activated by degradation of its inhibitor IkB through the ubiquitin–proteasome system. This system regulates mediators of proliferation, inflammation, and apoptosis that are fundamental mechanisms for the development of restenosis. In animal studies, blocking the proteasome system reduced intimal hyperplasia (19,20) showing that inflammation contributes significantly. Activation of cytokines enhances the migration of leukocytes across the platelet–fibrin layer into the tissue. Growth factors are released from platelets and leukocytes, and SMCs and fibroblasts proliferate and undergo a transformation to myofibroblasts 3 to 14 days after the intervention (11). With the release of growth factors, the initiation of the first phase (G1) of the cell cycle is activated, regulated by the assembly and phosphorylation of cyclin/cyclin-dependent kinase (CDK) complexes. Growth factors trigger signaling pathways that activate these CDK complexes.

Studies using human arterial segments strongly support a role for inflammation in restenosis. Immediately following stent implantation, studies by Grewe et al. (21) demonstrate that a mural thrombus is formed, followed by invasion of SMCs, T-lymphocytes, and macrophages. Additional studies in atherectomy specimens following PTCA demonstrate an increase of monocyte chemoattractant protein-1 and specimens from restenotic lesions show an increased number of macrophages (22). These results indicate that local expression of macrophage activity may be associated with the mechanisms of intimal hyperplasia. A correlation was found between stent strut penetration with inflammatory cell density and neointimal thickness (23). Neointimal inflammatory cell content was 2.4-fold greater in segments with restenosis, and inflammation was associated with neoangiogenesis. Coronary stenting that is accompanied by medial damage or penetration of the stent into the lipid core induces increased arterial inflammation, which is associated with increased neointimal growth.

Circulating markers of inflammation

Similar to a growing body of evidence in studies of atherosclerosis and cardiovascular disease, assessment of markers from blood samples has provided information regarding the role of inflammation after PTCA. Included among markers for atherosclerosis are C-reactive protein (CRP), IL-6, serum amyloid A (SAA), and even white blood cell (WBC) count. With respect to PTCA, many of these same markers provide insight. In studies by Serrano et al. (24) coronary sinus blood samples taken 15 minutes after angioplasty showed evidence of leukocyte and platelet activation with increased adhesion molecule expression on the surface of neutrophils and monocytes. Late lumen loss was correlated with the changes in IL-6 concentrations post-PTCA and MAC-1 activation in coronary sinus blood (25,26). Recent studies demonstrated that stent deployment is associated with an increase in CRP (27). Interestingly, CRP plasma levels were significantly higher and more prolonged in patients with restenosis compared with patients without restenosis. Similar findings were reported in a series of patients with stable angina who underwent PTCA (28). The association between the extent of vascular inflammatory response with long-term outcome was even observed in patients with stable angina undergoing stent implantation (29). Finally, a recent study showed that the inflammatory response after stent implantation can be assessed by measuring the circulating monocytes in the peripheral blood. The maximum monocyte count after stent implantation showed a significant positive correlation with in-stent neointimal volume at six-month follow-up. In contrast, other fractions of WBCs were not correlated with in-stent neointima volume (30). These findings demonstrate that there is an inflammatory stimulus following PTCA, which needs to be assessed for the risk stratification for restenosis.

Pre-existing inflammation

The studies discussed earlier demonstrate that vascular injury caused by PTCA triggers inflammation. Importantly, however, at the time of stent implantation, the overall inflammatory status is not equivalent in all patients and, critically, in all atherosclerotic

plaques. Therefore, PTCA in an already inflamed plaque may have significant impact on clinical and angiographic outcome. Studies in patients with unstable angina and elevated baseline CRP, SAA, and IL-6 values showed an enhanced inflammatory response to angioplasty. Pretreatment CRP level is an independent predictor for one-year major adverse cardiac events (MACE), including the need for re-intervention in patients not receiving statins. CRP levels were significantly higher in patients with recurrent angina compared with asymptomatic patients (31,32). Walter et al. (33) found that tertiles of CRP levels were independently associated with a higher risk of MACE and angiographic restenosis after stenting, and Buffon et al. (34) found that baseline CRP and SAA levels were independent predictors of clinical restenosis. Additionally, Patti et al. (35) found that preprocedural IL-1 receptor antagonist (IL-1Ra) plasma levels were an independent predictor of MACE during the follow-up period. Furthermore, the overall activation status of the immune system, estimated by the amount of IL-1β produced by monocytes, had positive correlation with late lumen loss, while the expression of CD66 by granulocytes has shown to prevent luminal renarrowing (36). Finally, the concentration of macrophages was also reported to be an independent predictor for restenosis (23).

The role of pre-existing inflammation in clinical outcome after stenting was also studied by measuring the temperature of the culprit lesion (37), a marker of inflammation. Patients with MACE had increased plaque temperature before the intervention. During a clinical follow-up of 18 months, the incidence of MACE in patients with increased temperature was higher compared with those without increased thermal heterogeneity. The adverse cardiac events were mainly due to restenosis at the culprit lesions.

It appears that the overall and local inflammatory status at the time of PTCA plays a significant role in the development of restenosis. The current evidence arises from studies combining data from the clinical syndrome and peripheral markers of inflammation. For patients with unstable clinical syndromes and with increased levels of monocytes and CRP, there is strong evidence for increased risk of restenosis. The measurement of other inflammatory indices, such as SAA, IL-6, IL-1β, IL-1Ra plasma levels, Lp(a), and fibrinogen, seems to provide additional information.

Thus, overall, there is considerable evidence for an important role for inflammation contributing to the restenotic process.

Sirolimus: molecular mechanism of action

Sirolimus (rapamycin, Rapamune) is a naturally occurring macrocyclic lactone produced by *Streptomyces hygroscopicus*, a streptomycete isolated from a soil sample collected from

Easter Island (Rapa Nui) first discovered and characterized by Sehgal in 1975 (38). Initially identified as an antifungal agent, the compound was subsequently found to posses potent immunosuppressive activities, initially demonstrated through its ability to prevent adjuvant-induced arthritis and experimental allergic encephalomyelitis in rodent models. As a potent immunosuppressive agent, sirolimus has been developed and marketed by Wyeth Pharmaceuticals for the prevention of renal transplant rejection (Rapamune®) (39).

Sirolimus has pleotropic effects on a wide variety of cell types with relevance to restenosis. The underlying mechanism of action of the compound is as an inhibitor of the cell cycle, with its principal effect on the G1 to S transition (40). Importantly, sirolimus affects the numerous cell types thought to be involved in the restenotic process including cells typically resident to the vascular wall, such as SMCs, as well as those recruited from the circulation at times of injury such as immune constituents. As the complete delineation of the steps and mechanisms of restenosis remain to be determined, the benefit of sirolimus may be due to its ability to affect the multiple cell types involved.

Although the mechanism of action of sirolimus is unique, it belongs to a class of immunosuppressive agents whose cellular activity depends on their complexing to specific cytosolic binding proteins called immunophilins. Cyclosporin A and tacrolimus (FK506) are also members of this class. Specific to cyclosporin A and tacrolimus, when complexed to their respective immunophilins, the phosphatase calcineurin is inhibited, thus blocking its ability to dephosphorylate the cytoplasmic subunit of NF-AT, a transcription factor contributing to cytokine production (41–43). Without dephosphorylatin, translocation to the nucleus is blocked, resulting in reduced transcription of cytokines (44,45). In contrast, although sirolimus binds to the same immunophilin, FKBP12, as does tacrolimus (46), but rather than affecting calcineurin, puts the complex into a conformation that interacts with and blocks activation of target of rapamycin (TOR), a kinase critical to cell cycle progression from G1 to S (47). Consequently, rather than proliferative, cells generally are driven to a more quiescent or differentiated state.

This critical nuclear protein TOR [also known as FKBP12 rapamycin-associated protein (FRAP), rapamycin and FKBP12 target 1 (RAFT 1), sirolimus effector protein (SEP), and regulatory associated protein of mTOR (RAPT)] is a 289 kDa protein highly conserved across species with similarities to several PI kinases and is thought to be an important mediator of cellular proliferation/differentiation processes (48–50). Through its complex formation, sirolimus inhibits the activation of the kinase, p70S6k, an enzyme involved in the phosphorylation of the S6 ribosomal protein, regulating the translocation of critical cell-cycle regulating proteins (51–53). In addition, through its effects on TOR, sirolimus diminishes the kinase activity of the CDK-4/cyclin D and CDK2/cyclin E complexes that peak in mid-to-late G1 in the cell cycle (54,55). Normally, this activation involves a change in

stoichiometry with the CDK inhibitors p21 and p27kip1 (56). Sirolimus blocks the elimination of kip1 and the activation of CDK/cyclin complexes. Consequently, downstream events including hyperphosphohorylation of retinoblastoma proteins and dissociation of Rb:E2F complexes are inhibited resulting in decreased synthesis of cell cycle proteins cdc2, cyclin A, and TTK, a serine threonine tyrosine kinase. Sirolimus does not affect early response genes c-fos/c-jun and c-myc, but inhibits transcription of bcl-2, a proto-oncogene induced by IL-2 critical for cell cycle progression (57,58).

Based on the activities described earlier, sirolimus had been found to have effects on several cells of the immune response. Similar to other immunosuppressive drugs, sirolimus inhibits T-cell proliferation (59). In contrast to cyclosporin A and tacrolimus which inhibit calcineurin and subsequent IL-2 production, however, the antiproliferative effect of sirolimus results from the inhibition of the kinase TOR and regulation of the CDK inhibitor p27kip1 (60–62). The T-cell proliferative effects of sirolimus are not limited to inhibition of IL-2 or IL-4 mediated growth as it has also been found to inhibit intermediate or late-acting IL-12, IL-7, and IL-15, driven proliferation of activated T-cells, demonstrated by the findings that it blocks lymphocyte proliferation even when added up to 12 hours after stimulation. In addition to effects on T-cell activity, sirolimus has been found to inhibit IL-2-dependent and -independent proliferation of B-cells in the mid-G1-phase of the cell cycle and to prevent cytokine-induced B-cell differentiation into antibody-producing cells, thereby decreasing IgM, IgG, and IgA production.

The role and benefit of sirolimus on the restenotic process may be due to its ability to affect the many cell types and many mechanisms involved. As well summarized by Marks (63), in addition to immune cells, sirolimus also has inhibitory effects on SMC proliferation and migration through pathways that are similar or identical to those observed in the immune cells. Inhibition of TOR by sirolimus results in the upregulation of p27kip1 and p21cip, leading to growth arrest of cultured VSMCs. In addition, recent evidence by Martin et al. (64) also suggests an effect of sirolimus on SMC differentiation. Upon injury of the arterial wall, VSMC de-differentiate into a synthetic, proliferative phenotype and these studies suggest that sirolimus may play a new role as differentiator of vascular smooth muscle (SM) phenotype, with a focus on the TOR/p70 S6K1 pathway regulating differentiation. TOR inhibition promotes the coordinated regulation of not only cell cycle progression but also the expression of contractile proteins to induce the differentiated phenotype. Sirolimus treatment of primary human, porcine, or rat VSMC caused a marked increase in expression of SM-myosin heavy chain, SM-actin, and calponin. Interestingly, overexpression of the TOR target p70 S6 kinase (S6K1) reversed the effects on contractile protein and p21cip expression. Although regulation of PI3-K/Akt (upstream activators of TOR) signaling has been shown to change platelet-derived growth factor-induced proliferative response of VSMC toward enhanced contractile protein expression (65), the study by Martin et al. provides the first evidence that S6K1 actively opposes VSMC differentiation. Moreover, because VSMC dedifferentiation (characterized by decreased contractile protein expression) is a prerequisite for the transformation of VSMC into a migratory, proliferative phenotype, these novel results add new mechanistic insight for the prevention of restenosis. It is possible that the drug may promote the maintenance of functional, quiescent VSMC at the site of injury. Finally, Nuhrenberg et al. (17) has demonstrated both the recruitment of HPCs to the vascular wall with restenosis and the inhibition of their recruitment in the presence of sirolimus.

Effects of sirolimus on percutaneous transluminal coronary angioplasty: animal models

In vivo, studies have demonstrated efficacy of sirolimus on vascular disease from a diverse array of animal models thought to mimic aspects of human vascular disorders.

Initially, Gregory et al. (66) and Morris et al. (67) demonstrated that sirolimus was a potent inhibitor of the intimal thickening that occurs following balloon injury of the carotid artery in the rat. In these studies, short-term (~3–13 days) treatment with sirolimus combined with mycophenolic acid reduced arterial intimal thickening when studied out to 44 days following mechanical injury. Endothelial replacement was also observed. Subsequent studies by Gallo et al. (68) reported that sirolimus significantly reduced the arterial proliferative response after PTCA in the pig. Administration was associated with a significant inhibition in coronary stenosis in treated (36% stenosis) versus control (63%; $p < 0.001$) animals, resulting in a concomitant increase in luminal area (3.3 vs. 1.7 mm^2; $p < 0.001$) after PTCA. Drug administration significantly reduced the arterial proliferative response after PTCA in the pig by increasing the level of the CDKI p27kip1 and inhibition of pRb phosphorylation within the vessel wall. These studies demonstrating efficacy on induced vascular injury in the pig ultimately led to the investigation and development of the Cypher® stent, the first drug (sirolimus)-eluting coronary stent as discussed further below.

Clinical observations

With the recent development of angioplasty combined with DES such as the Cypher-Coronary Stent marketed by Cordis/J&J Pharmaceuticals, treatment of the culprit vessel in myocardial infarction has had a significant and meaningful advance (69,70). By engineering the device to elute sirolimus

over ~14 days (71), the intimal thickening and restenosis formally associated with angioplasty is now reduced to near zero over the long-term, and utilization of these DES has brought about a new era in the practice of interventional cardiology. Importantly, its use has greatly reduced the burden of follow-up procedures. Sirolimus, the agent utilized in this first successful DES is an immune mediator shown to quiet the local immune activation and also to reduce or eliminate cellular proliferation. Locally, the DESs have been shown to be of substantial benefit to the culprit lesion, effectively reducing the restenotic process and maintaining the patency of the treated vessel over the long term. Their use has changed the practice of interventional cardiology.

As shown in a human organ culture model (17), sirolimus combines antiproliferative and anti-inflammatory properties and reduces neointima formation after angioplasty in patients. Vascular wall inflammation is attenuated as are progenitor cell promoters as assessed by gene expression during neointima formation.

In the RAVEL trial (69), as studied by intravascular ultrasound (IVUS), the difference in neointimal hyperplasia (2 vs. 37 mm^3) and percent of volume obstruction (1% vs. 29%) at six months between the two groups were highly significant ($p < 0.001$), emphasizing the nearly complete abolition of the proliferative process inside the DES. In an update by Kipshidze et al. (72), it is quoted that the introduction of DES to interventional cardiology practice has resulted in a significant improvement in the long-term efficacy of percutaneous coronary interventions. DES successfully combines mechanical benefits of bare-metal stents in stabilizing the lumen, with direct delivery and the controlled elution of a pharmacological agent to the injured vessel wall to suppress further neointimal proliferation. The dramatic reduction in restenosis has resulted in the implementation of DES in clinical practice and has rapidly expanded the spectrum of successfully treatable coronary conditions, particularly in high-risk patients and complex lesions.

In long-term follow-up of the RAVEL trial (73), clinical benefit with sirolimus-eluting coronary stents has been maintained. Using cumulative one to three-year event-free survival rates, treatment with sirolimus-eluting stents was associated with a sustained clinical benefit and very low rates of target lesion revascularization up to three years after device implantation. As recently shown by both Kastrati and coworkers (74) and Windecker et al. (75), the Cypher stent eluting sirolimus is highly effective and may have clinical benefit beyond alternative DES products.

Cardiovascular disease and immune mechanisms

Despite the success of the DESs, the incidence of atherosclerosis and accompanying acute coronary syndromes remain significant issues. With an estimated 180 million individuals affected at various stages of the disease process, clinically symptomatic disease accounts for ~34 million patients worldwide (76). It has recently been recognized that myocardial infarctions often occur in patients with plaques with only mild to moderate obstruction, more often than not, in vessels with <50% stenosis (77–79). These most dangerous lesions are typically not detected with routine imaging techniques such as angiography and, thus, are not treated. Recently, the concept of a vulnerable plaque has emerged, characterized by a lipid core, an excessive inflammatory cell component, and a thin fibrous cap (80–82). The presence of increased macrophage and activated T-cell infiltration may be critical, as these appear to be the lesions that are more likely to rupture and are responsible for many of the acute coronary thrombosis leading to myocardial infarction (83). Mortality here remains high and, short of death, rupture of plaques is associated with significant morbidities including stable and unstable angina as well as non-ST elevation myocardial infarction and ST elevation myocardial infarction (84,85). Consequently, vulnerable plaques and vulnerable patients, those having a high systemic total plaque burden, remain of substantial concern.

Although treatment of the culprit lesion is now possible with DES and the overall event rate including the need for re-intervention is reduced, the more serious events such as a second myocardial infarction have not changed significantly. In addressing this issue, it has been found in patients undergoing angioplasty due to an event with plaque rupture, that there was clear evidence of additional ruptures at sites distal to the culprit or treated lesion. By utilizing IVUS in patients undergoing angioplasty for an infarcted artery, Rioufol et al. (86) observed distal ruptures in at least 80% of patients examined. These ruptures occurred in plaques that were <50% stenosed and thus their detection likely would have been missed by angiography. This finding suggests that treating the culprit lesion alone as is accomplished with stent therapy is not sufficient and that intervention at multiple active lesion sites will be required to reduce secondary events and mortality.

Finally, in addition to the issues of costs and secondary events, treatment is also lacking for many more at-risk patients who cannot undergo successful angioplasty. These patients, who may have either diffuse, nonstentable, bifurcated lesions, or multivessel disease (i.e., diabetics), are not benefiting as much from DES, and improved treatments here also remain a clear clinical need. Often there is a systemic and local activation of the immune response, followed by a consequent local vascular incident. The role of the systemic immune response in these individuals, as well as in cardiovascular patients in general, is evidenced by the numerous reports of correlation of disease with increases in plasma markers such as CRP, tumor necrosis factor, and even circulating white cell counts (87–89).

The understanding of atherosclerosis as a chronic inflammatory process represents an interesting paradigmatic shift.

Plasma concentrations of immune markers such as CRP, SAA, IL-6, and WBC count may reflect the intensity of occult plaque inflammation and the vulnerability to rupture. Monocyte chemoattractant protein-1 and IL-8 play a crucial role in initiating atherosclerosis by recruiting monocytes/macrophages to the vessel wall (90), which promotes atherosclerotic lesions and plaque vulnerability. In addition, circulating levels of these proinflammatory cytokines increase in patients with acute myocardial infarction and unstable angina, but not in those with stable angina. Based on the above information, there is clearly a need for new therapies to quiet the inflammation within areas of disease of the vascular wall. Such therapy would be of importance for secondary intervention following an initial event as described above, where there is documentation of multiple sites of rupture, for patients with nonstentable diffuse or multivessel disease and potentially for use as primary prevention in those patients with documented atherosclerotic disease and elevated immune markers.

Potential for immune/ inflammation intervention in atherosclerotic vascular disease

In addition to induced injury models, recent studies suggest that drugs such as sirolimus may have benefit beyond PTCA and may include atherosclerosis itself. In a series of studies in the apoprotein E deficient mouse model of atherosclerosis (91,92), it has been found that sirolimus can eliminate the development of lesion formation. This was observed despite an excessively high circulating lipid load, with total cholesterol exceeding 1300 mg/dL in these animals. Based on morphological evidence, as well as on vascular cholesterol/cholesteryl ester content, sirolimus-treated animals developed no lesions at doses ranging from 2 to 8 mg/kg q.o.d. Spleen expression of T-cell markers for TH-1 (IL-12 p40, interferon γ) and TH-2 (IL-10) was reduced and TGFβ expression was increased. Atherogenic lipids such as total cholesterol, triglycerides, and LDL cholesterol were either not effected or, in some instances, were increased from control. Waksman et al. (93) and Naoum et al. (94) also demonstrated inhibitory effects on lesion development in similar models with sirolimus administration and also on vascular expression, at the transcriptional level, of a variety of genes thought to be involved in vascular disorders.

More recently, studies of sirolimus in a vascular allograft rejection model in nonhuman primates by Ikonen et al. (95), a severe immune-mediated vascular disorder, have shown lesion inhibition and possibly regression. Finally, clinical studies by Mancini et al. (96) and Eisen et al. (97) with a sirolimus analog on vasculopathy and also by Keogh et al. (98) on coronary artery disease in subjects who have undergone heart transplantation have demonstrated that sirolimus (or analogs) has the ability to maintain patency and potentially reverse stenosis of coronary vessels in patients.

Thus, the TOR pathway and sirolimus in particular has been shown to be a promising approach to the treatment of a variety of vascular disorders, both mechanistically at the preclinical level and verified in the clinic. Clearly, there are serious liabilities and toxicities with this approach if it were to be used in a chronic systemic fashion. Immune modulation with such a powerful agent would not be an acceptable approach for treatment of cardiovascular disease. However, results here do point to pathways for study and opens possible further understanding of the potential for intervention in this serious condition affecting millions of patients.

References

1 Ross R. Atherosclerosis—an inflammatory disease. N Engl J Med 1999; 340:115–126.

2 Libby P. Inflammation in atherosclerosis. Nature 2002; 420:868–874.

3 Hansson GK. Inflammation, atherosclerosis, and coronary artery disease. N Engl J Med 2005; 352:1685–1695.

4 Tousoulis D, Davies G, Stefanadis C, Toutouzas P, Ambrose JA. Inflammatory and thrombotic mechanisms in coronary atherosclerosis. Heart 2003; 89:993–997.

5 Choudhury RP, Fuster V, Badimon JJ, Fisher EA, Fayad ZA. MRI and characterization of atherosclerotic plaque: emerging applications and molecular imaging. Arterioscler Thromb Vasc Biol 2002;:22:1065–1074.

6 Schroeder AP, Falk E. Pathophysiology and inflammatory aspects of plaque rupture. Cardiol Clin 1996; 14:211–220.

7 Fuster V, Stein B, Ambrose JA, Badimon L, Badimon JJ, Chesebro JH. Atherosclerotic plaque rupture and thrombosis. Evolving concepts. Circulation 1990; 82(suppl 3):II47–II59.

8 Mintz GS, Hoffmann R, Mehran R, et al. In-stent restenosis: the Washington Hospital Center experience. Am J Cardiol 1998; 81(7A):7E–13E.

9 Kester M, Waybill P, Kozak M. New strategies to prevent restenosis. Am J Cardiovasc Drugs 2001; 1(2):77–83.

10 Edelman ER, Rogers C. Hoop dreams. Stents without restenosis. Circulation 1996; 94(6):1199–1202.

11 Toutouzas K, Colombo A, Stefanadis C. Inflammation and restenosis after percutaneous coronary interventions. Eur Heart J 2004; 25(19):1679–1687.

12 Kornowski R, Hong MK, Tio FO, et al. In-stent restenosis: contributions of inflammatory responses and arterial injury to neointimal hyperplasia. J Am Coll Cardiol 1998; 31:224–230.

13 Welt FG, Tso C, Edelman ER, et al. Leukocyte recruitment and expression of chemokines following different forms of vascular injury. Vasc Med 2003; 8(1):1–7.

14 Wang K, Zhou Z, Zhou X, et al. Prevention of intimal hyperplasia with recombinant soluble P-selectin glycoprotein ligand-immunoglobulin in the porcine coronary artery balloon injury model. J Am Coll Cardiol 2001; 38:577–582.

15 Hayashi S, Watanabe N, Nakazawa K, et al. Roles of P-selectin in inflammation, neointimal formation, and vascular remodeling in balloon-injured rat carotid arteries. Circulation 2000; 102:1710–1717.

16 Conde ID, Kleiman NS. Arterial thrombosis for the interventional cardiologist: from adhesion molecules and coagulation factors to clinical therapeutics. Catheter Cardiovasc Interv 2003; 60:236–246.

17 Nuhrenberg TG, Voisard R, Fahlisch F, et al. Rapamycin attenuates vascular wall inflammation and progenitor cell promoters after angioplasty. FASEB J 2005;19(2):246–248.

18 Schwartz RS, Holmes DR Jr, Topol EJ. The restenosis paradigm revisited: an alternative proposal for cellular mechanisms. J Am Coll Cardiol 1992; 20:1284–1293.

19 Breuss JM, Cejna M, Bergmeister H, et al. Activation of nuclear factor-kappa B significantly contributes to lumen loss in a rabbit iliac artery balloon angioplasty model. Circulation 2002; 105:633–638.

20 Meiners S, Laule M, Rother W, et al. Ubiquitin–proteasome pathway as a new target for the prevention of restenosis. Circulation 2002; 105:483–489.

21 Grewe PH, Deneke T, Machraoui A, et al. Acute and chronic tissue response to coronary stent implantation: pathologic findings in human specimen. J Am Coll Cardiol 2000; 35:157–163.

22 Hokimoto S, Oike Y, Saito T, et al. Increased expression of monocyte chemoattractant protein-1 in atherectomy specimens from patients with restenosis after percutaneous transluminal coronary angioplasty. Circ J 2002; 66:114–116.

23 Moreno PR, Bernardi VH, Lopez-Cuellar J, et al. Macrophage infiltration predicts restenosis after coronary intervention in patients with unstable angina. Circulation 1996; 94:3098–3102.

24 Serrano CV Jr, Ramires JA, Venturinellie M, et al. Coronary angioplasty results in leukocyte and platelet activation with adhesion molecule expression. Evidence of inflammatory responses in coronary angioplasty. J Am Coll Cardiol 1997; 29:1276–1283.

25 Hojo Y, Ikeda U, Katsuki T, et al. Interleukin 6 expression in coronary circulation after coronary angioplasty as a risk factor for restenosis. Heart 2000; 84:83–87.

26 Inoue T, Uchida T, Yaguchi I, et al. Stent-induced expression and activation of the leukocyte integrin Mac-1 is associated with neointimal thickening and restenosis. Circulation 2003; 107:1757–1763.

27 Gottsauner-Wolf M, Zasmeta G, Hornykewycz S, et al. Plasma levels of C-reactive protein after coronary stent implantation. Eur Heart J 2000; 21:1152–1158.

28 Almagor M, Keren A, Banai S. Increased C-reactive protein level after coronary stent implantation in patients with stable coronary artery disease. Am Heart J 2003; 145:248–253.

29 Gaspardone A, Crea F, Versaci F, et al. Predictive value of C-reactive protein after successful coronary-artery stenting in patients with stable angina. Am J Cardiol 1998; 82:515–518.

30 Fukuda D, Shimada K, Tanaka A, et al. Circulating monocytes and in-stent neointima after coronary stent implantation. J Am Coll Cardiol 2004; 43:18–23.

31 Chan AW, Bhatt DL, Chew DP, et al. Relation of inflammation and benefit of statins after percutaneous coronary interventions. Circulation 2003; 107:1750–1756.

32 Rahel BM, Visseren FL, Suttorp MJ, et al. Preprocedural serum levels of acute-phase reactants and prognosis after percutaneous coronary intervention. Cardiovasc Res 2003; 60:136–140.

33 Walter DH, Fichtlscherer S, Sellwig M, et al. Preprocedural C-reactive protein levels and cardiovascular events after coronary stent implantation. J Am Coll Cardiol 2001; 37:839–846.

34 Buffon A, Liuzzo G, Biasucci LM, et al. Preprocedural serum levels of C-reactive protein predict early complications and late restenosis after coronary angioplasty. J Am Coll Cardiol 1999; 34:1512–1521.

35 Patti G, Di Sciascio G, D'Ambrosio A, et al. Prognostic value of interleukin-1 receptor antagonist in patients undergoing percutaneous coronary intervention. Am J Cardiol 2002; 89:372–376.

36 Pietersma A, Kofflard M, de Wit LE, et al. Late lumen loss after coronary angioplasty is associated with the activation status of circulating phagocytes before treatment. Circulation 1995; 91:1320–1325.

37 Stefanadis C, Toutouzas K, Tsiamis E, et al. Increased local temperature in human coronary atherosclerotic plaques: an independent predictor of clinical outcome in patients undergoing a percutaneous coronary intervention. J Am Coll Cardiol 2001; 37:1277–1283.

38 Vezina C, Kudelski A, Sehgal SN. Rapamycin (AY-22,989), a new antifungal antibiotic. I. Taxonomy of the producing streptomycete and isolation of the active principle. J Antibiot (Tokyo) 1975; 10:721–726.

39 Sehgal SN. Sirolimus: its discovery, biological properties, and mechanism of action. Transplant Proc 2003; 35(suppl 3):7S–14S. Prog Cell Cycle Res 1995; 1:53–71.

40 Wiederrecht GJ, Sabers CJ, Brunn GJ, Martin MM, Dumont FJ, Abraham RT. Mechanism of action of rapamycin: new insights into the regulation of G1-phase progression in eukaryotic cells. Prog Cell Cycle Res 1995; 1:53–71.

41 Liu J, Farmer JD Jr, Lane WS, Friedman J, Weissman I, Schreiber SL. Calcineurin is a common target of cyclophilin–cyclosporin A and FKBP-FK506 complexes. Cell 1991; 66(4):807–815.

42 Liu J, Albers MW, Wandless TJ, et al. Inhibition of T cell signaling by immunophilin-ligand complexes correlates with loss of calcineurin phosphatase activity. Biochemistry 1992; 31(16):3896–3901.

43 Parsons JN, Wiederrecht GJ, Salowe S, et al. Regulation of calcineurin phosphatase activity and interaction with the FK-506.FK-506 binding protein complex. J Biol Chem 1994; 269(30):19610–19616.

44 Flanagan WM, Corthesy B, Bram RJ, Crabtree GR. Nuclear association of a T-cell transcription factor blocked by FK506 and cyclosporin A. Nature 1992; 352:803–807.

45 McCaffrey PG, Perrino BA, Soderling TR, Rao A. NF-ATp, a T lymphocyte DNA-binding protein that is a target for calcineurin and immunosuppressive drugs. J Biol Chem 1993; 268(5):3747–3752.

46 Fruman DA, Wood MA, Gjertson CK, Katz HR, Burakoff SJ, Bierer BE. FK506 binding protein 12 mediates sensitivity to both FK506 and rapamycin in murine mast cells. Eur J Immunol 1995; 25(2):563–571.

47 Cardenas ME, Zhu D, Heitman J. Molecular mechanisms of immunosuppression by cyclosporine, FK506, and rapamycin. Curr Opin Nephrol Hypertens 1995; 4(6):472–477.

48 Sarbassov Dos D, Ali SM, Sabatini DM. Growing roles for the mTOR pathway. Curr Opin Cell Biol 2005; 17(6):596–603.

49 Wullschleger S, Loewith R, Hall MN. TOR signaling in growth and metabolism. Cell 2006 10; 124(3):471–484.

50 Dann SG, Thomas G. The amino acid sensitive TOR pathway from yeast to mammals. FEBS Lett 2006 22; 580(12):2821–2829.

51 Chung J, Kuo CJ, Crabtree GR, Blenis J. Rapamycin-FKBP specifically blocks growth-dependent activation of and signaling by the 70 kda S6 protein kinases. Cell 1992; 69(7):1227–1236.

52 Kuo CJ, Chung J, Fiorentino DF, Flanagan WM, Blenis J, Crabtree GR. Rapamycin selectively inhibits interleukin-2 activation of p70 S6 kinase. Nature 1992; 358(6381):70–73.

53 Price DJ, Grove JR, Calvo V, Avruch J, Bierer BE. Rapamycin-induced inhibition of the 70-kilodalton S6 protein kinase. Science 1992 14; 257(5072):973–977.

54 Sehgal SN, Molnar-Kimber K, Ocain TD, Weichman BM. Rapamycin: a novel immunosuppressive macrolide. Med Res Rev 1994; 14(1):1–22.

55 Wood MA, Bierer BE. Rapamycin: biological and therapeutic effects, binding by immunophilins and molecular targets of action. Perspect Drug Discov Design 1994; 2:163–184.

56 Nourse J, Firpo E, Flanagan WM, et al. Interleukin-2-mediated elimination of the p27Kip1 cyclin-dependent kinase inhibitor prevented by rapamycin. Nature 1994; 372:570–573.

57 Flanagan WM, Crabtree GR. Rapamycin inhibits p34cdc2 expression and arrests T lymphocyte proliferation at the G1/S transition. Ann N Y Acad Sci 1993; 696:31–37.

58 Miyazaki T, Liu ZJ, Kawahara A, et al. Three distinct IL-2 signaling pathways mediated by bcl-2, c-myc, and lck cooperate in hematopoietic cell proliferation. Cell 1995; 81:223–231.

59 Dumont FJ, Staruch MJ, Koprak SL, Melino MR, Sigal NH. Distinct mechanisms of suppression of murine T cell activation by the related macrolides FK-506 and rapamycin. J Immunol 1990; 144:251–258.

60 Aagaard-Tillery KM, Jelinek DF. Inhibition of human B lymphocyte cell cycle progression and differentiation by rapamycin. Cell Immunol 1994; 156(2):493–507.

61 Kim HS, Raskova J, Degiannis D, Raska K Jr. Effects of cyclosporine and rapamycin on immunoglobulin production by preactivated human B cells. Clin Exp Immunol 1994; 96:508–512.

62 Ferraresso M, Tian L, Ghobrial R, Stepkowski SM, Kahan BD. Rapamycin inhibits production of cytotoxic but not noncytotoxic antibodies and preferentially activates T helper 2 cells that mediate long-term survival of heart allografts in rats. J Immunol 1994 1; 153(7):3307–3318.

63 Marks AR. Rapamycin: signaling in vascular smooth muscle. Transplant Proc 2003; 35(suppl 3):231S–233S.

64 Martin KA, Rzucidlo EM, Merenick BL, et al. The mTOR/p70 S6K1 pathway regulates vascular smooth muscle cell differentiation. Am J Physiol Cell Physiol 2004; 286(3):C507–C517.

65 Hegner B, Weber M, Dragun D, Schulze-Lohoff E. Differential regulation of smooth muscle markers in human bone marrow-derived mesenchymal stem cells. J Hypertens 2005; 23(6):1191–202.

66 Gregory CR, Huang X, Pratt RE, et al. Treatment with rapamycin and mycophenolic acid reduces arterial intimal thickening produced by mechanical injury and allows endothelial replacement. Transplantation 1995; 59:655–661.

67 Morris RE, Cao W, Huang X, et al. Rapamycin (Sirolimus) inhibits vascular smooth muscle DNA synthesis in vitro and

suppresses narrowing in arterial allografts and in balloon-injured carotid arteries: evidence that rapamycin antagonizes growth factor action on immune and nonimmune cells. Transplant Proc 1995; 27(1):430–431.

68 Gallo R, Padurean A, Jayaraman T, et al. Inhibition of intimal thickening after balloon angioplasty in porcine coronary arteries by targeting regulators of the cell cycle. Circulation 1999; 99:2164–2170.

69 Morice MC, Serruys PW, Sousa JE, et al. A randomized comparison of a sirolimus-eluting stent with a standard stent for coronary revascularization. N Engl J Med 2002; 346:1773–1780.

70 Moses JW, Leon MB, Popma JJ, et al. Sirolimus-eluting stents versus standard stents in patients with stenosis in a native coronary artery. N Engl J Med 2003; 349:1315–1323.

71 Klugherz BD, Llanos G, Lieuallen W, et al. Twenty-eight-day efficacy and pharmacokinetics of the sirolimus-eluting stent. Coron Artery Dis 2002; 13(3):183–188.

72 Kipshidze NN, Tsapenko MV, Leon MB, Stone GW, Moses JW. Update on drug-eluting coronary stents. Expert Rev Cardiovasc Ther 2005; 3:953–968.

73 Fajadet J, Morice MC, Bode C, et al. Maintenance of long-term clinical benefit with sirolimus-eluting coronary stents: three-year results of the RAVEL trial. Circulation 2005; 111(8):1040–1044.

74 Dibra A, Kastrati A, Mehilli J, et al. Paclitaxel-eluting or sirolimus-eluting stents to prevent restenosis in diabetic patients. N Engl J Med 2005; 353(7):663–670.

75 Windecker S, Remondino A, Eberli FR, et al. Sirolimus-eluting and paclitaxel-eluting stents for coronary revascularization. N Engl J Med 2005; 18:353(7):653–662.

76 Rosamond W, Flegal K, Friday G, et al. Heart disease and stroke statistics—2007 update. A Report from the American Heart Association Statistics Committee and Stroke Statistics Subcommittee. Circulation 2006; 115:e69–171e.

77 Hausmann D, Johnson JA, Sudhir K, et al. Angiographically silent atherosclerosis detected by intravascular ultrasound in patients with familial hypercholesterolemia and familial combined hyperlipidemia: correlation with high density lipoproteins. J Am Coll Cardiol 1996; 27:1562–1570.

78 Schoenhagen P, Nissen SE. Assessing coronary plaque burden and plaque vulnerability: atherosclerosis imaging with IVUS and emerging noninvasive modalities. Am Heart Hosp J 2003; 1(2):164–169.

79 Schoenhagen P, McErlean ES, Nissen SE. The vulnerable coronary plaque. J Cardiovasc Nurs 2000; 15:1–12.

80 Schroeder AP, Falk E. Vulnerable and dangerous coronary plaques. Atherosclerosis 1995; 118 (suppl):S141—S149.

81 Naghavi M, Libby P, Falk E, et al. From vulnerable plaque to vulnerable patient: a call for new definitions and risk assessment strategies: Part I. Circulation 20037; 108(14):1664–1672.

82 Vink A, Schoneveld AH, Richard W, et al. Plaque burden, arterial remodeling and plaque vulnerability: determined by systemic factors? J Am Coll Cardiol 2001; 38(3):718–723.

83 Corti R, Hutter R, Badimon JJ, Fuster V. Evolving concepts in the triad of atherosclerosis, inflammation and thrombosis. J Thromb Thrombolysis 2004; 17(1):35–44.

84 Virmani R, Burke AP, Farb A, Kolodgie FD. Pathology of the vulnerable plaque. J Am Coll Cardiol 2006; 47(suppl 8): C13–C18.

85 Klein LW. Clinical implications and mechanisms of plaque rupture in the acute coronary syndromes. Am Heart Hosp J 2005; 3(4):249–255.

86 Rioufol G, Finet G, Ginon I, et al. Multiple atherosclerotic plaque rupture in acute coronary syndrome: a three-vessel intravascular ultrasound study. Circulation 2002; 106: 804–808.

87 Jialal I, Devaraj S. Inflammation and atherosclerosis: the value of the high-sensitivity C-reactive protein assay as a risk marker. Am J Clin Pathol 2001; 116(suppl):S108–S115.

88 Ridker PM, Brown NJ, Vaughan DE, Harrison DG, Mehta JL. Established and emerging plasma biomarkers in the prediction of first atherothrombotic events. Circulation 2004; 109(25 suppl 1):IV6–IV19.

89 Ridker PM. C-reactive protein in 2005. J Am Coll Cardiol 2005; 46(1):CS2–CS5.

90 Gerszten RE, Garcia-Zepeda EA, Lim YC, et al. MCP-1 and IL-8 trigger firm adhesion of monocytes to vascular endothelium under flow conditions. Nature 1999; 398:718–723.

91 Elloso MM, Azrolan N, Sehgal SN, et al. Protective effect of the immunosuppressant sirolimus against aortic atherosclerosis in apo E-deficient mice. Am J Transplant 2003; 3:562–569.

92 Basso MD, Nambi P, Adelman SJ. Effect of sirolimus on the cholesterol content of aortic arch in ApoE knockout mice. Transplant Proc 2003; 35(8):3136–3138.

93 Waksman R, Pakala R, Burnett MS, et al. Oral rapamycin inhibits growth of atherosclerotic plaque in apoE knock-out mice. Cardiovasc Radiat Med 2003; 4(1):34–38.

94 Naoum JJ, Woodside KJ, Zhang S, Rychahou PG, Hunter GC. Effects of rapamycin on the arterial inflammatory response in atherosclerotic plaques in Apo-E knockout mice. Transplant Proc 2005; 37(4):1880–1884.

95 Ikonen TS, Gummert JF, Hayase M, et al. Sirolimus (rapamycin) halts and reverses progression of allograft vascular disease in non-human primates. Transplantation 2000; 70(6):969–975.

96 Mancini D, Pinney S, Burkhoff D, et al. Use of rapamycin slows progression of cardiac transplantation vasculopathy. Circulation 2003; 108(1):48–53.

97 Eisen HJ, Tuzcu EM, Dorent R, et al. Everolimus for the prevention of allograft rejection and vasculopathy in cardiac-transplant recipients. N Engl J Med 2003; 349:847–858.

98 Keogh A, Richardson M, Ruygrok P, et al. Sirolimus in de novo heart transplant recipients reduces acute rejection and prevents coronary artery disease at 2 years: a randomized clinical trial. Circulation 2004; 110(17):2694–2700.

27

Anti-migratory drugs and mechanisms of action

Ivan De Scheerder, Xiaoshun Liu, and Yanming Huang

Cell migration: a target for the control of restenosis

It has long been considered that restenosis following balloon angioplasty is the result of the formation of excessive neointima. More recently, both animal and human studies have shown that constrictive arterial remodeling is the major determinant of restenosis after balloon angioplasty, and it is responsible for up to 70% of late lumen loss. Arterial remodeling in this context means a structural change of the vessel wall, where re-organization of cells and matrix at sites of injury leads to decreased lumen diameter. At the heart of this remodeling process is the degradation of the extra cellular matrix by a group of enzymes known as matrix metalloproteinases (MMPs), secreted predominantly by vascular smooth muscle cells (VSMCs) and also by macrophages and monocytes.

The matrix metalloproteinases

The MMPs are a family of zinc-dependent neutral endopeptidases that share structural domains but differ in substrate specificity, cellular sources, and inductivity (Table 1). All the MMPs are important for remodeling of the extra cellular matrix and share the following functional features: (*i*) they degrade extracellular matrix components, including fibronectin, collagen, elastin, proteoglycans, and laminin, (*ii*) they are secreted in a latent proform and require activation for proteolytic activity, (*iii*) they contain zinc at their active site and need calcium for stability, (*iv*) they function at neutral pH, and (*v*) they are inhibited by specific tissue inhibitors of metalloproteinases (TIMPs).

The activity of the MMPs is controlled at the transcriptional level by activation of the latent proenzymes and by their endogenous inhibitors, the TIMPs. Although low-level expression of most MMPs is generally found in normal adult tissue, it is upregulated during certain physiological and pathological remodeling processes. Induction or stimulation at transcriptional level is mediated by a variety of inflammatory cytokines, hormones, and growth factors, such as IL-1, IL-6, tumor necrosis factor-α, epidermal growth factor, platelet-derived growth factor, basic fibroblast growth factor, and CD40. Binding of these stimulatory ligands to their receptors triggers a cascade of intracellular reactions that are mediated through at least three different classes of mitogen-activated protein (MAP) kinases: extracellular signal-regulated kinase, stress activated protein kinase/Jun N-terminal kinases, and p38. Activation of these kinases culminates in the activation of a nuclear AP-1 transcription factor, which binds to the AP-1 *cis* element and activates the transcription of corresponding MMP gene. Other factors such as corticosteroids, retinoic acid, heparin, and IL-4 have been demonstrated to inhibit MMP gene expression (1).

The role of matrix metalloproteinases in restenosis

Although the precise role of MMPs in inducing VSMC migration is not fully understood, there are multiple proposed mechanisms of action, which include the removal of physical restraints by the severing of cell-matrix contacts via integrins or cell–cell contacts via adherins. Additionally, contact with interstitial matrix components may be facilitated and migration may be stimulated through exposure of cryptic extracellular

Table 1 Matrix metalloproteinase family

Enzyme	MMP classification	Substrate(s)
Collagenases		
Interstitial collagenase	MMP-1	Collagen types I, II, III, VII, and X, gelatin, entactin, aggrecan
Neutrophil collagenase	MMP-8	Collagen types I–III, aggrecan
Collagenase-3	MMP-13	Collagen types I–III, gelatin, fibronectin, laminins, tenascin
Collagenase-4	MMP-18	Not known
Gelatinases		
Gelatinase A	MMP-2	Collagen types I, IV, V, and X, fibronectin, laminins, aggrecan, tenascin-C, vitronectin
Gelatinase B	MMP-9	Collagen types IV, V, XIV, aggrecan, elastin, entactin, vitronectin
Stromelysins		
Stromelysin 1	MMP-3	Collagen types III, IV, IX, and X, gelatin, fibronectin, laminins, tenascin-C, vitronectin
Stromelysin 2	MMP-10	Collagen IV, fibronectin, aggrecan
Stromelysin 3	MMP-11	Collagen IV, fibronectin, aggrecan, laminins, gelatin
Membrane-type (MT-MMPs)		
MT1-MMP	MMP-14	Collagen types I–III, fibronectin, laminins, vitronectin, proteoglycans; activates proMMP-2
MT2-MMP	MMP-15	Activates proMMP-2
MT3-MMP	MMP-16	Activates proMMP-2
MT4-MMP	MMP-17	Not known
MT5-MMP	MMP-24	Activates proMMP-2
MT6-MMP	MMP-25	Not known
Nonclassified MMPs		
Matrilysins	MMP-7	Gelatin, fibronectin, laminins, elastin, collagen IV, vitronectin, tenascin-C, aggrecan,
Metalloelastase	MMP-12	Elastin
Unnamed	MMP-19	Not known
Enamelysin	MMP-20	Aggrecan
	MMP-23	Not known
Endometase	MMP-26	Not known

Abbreviations: MMP, matrix metalloproteinase; MT-MMP, membrane-type matrix metalloproteinase.
Source: From Ref. 16.

matrix sites, production of extracellular matrix fragments, and the release of matrix or cell-bound growth factors (2). Other recent studies also demonstrate that MMP activity is required for lymphocyte transmigration across endothelial venules into lymph nodes, providing some evidence for the concept that MMPs are important players in transendothelial migration (3).

Coronary angioplasty inevitably produces a mechanical injury to the vessel. Damage to the endothelia is thought to trigger phenotypic modulation of medial VSMCs, changing them from a normal contractile (differentiated) phenotype to a synthetic (proliferative) state. To enable VSMC migration, remodeling of the basement membrane and the interstitial collagenous matrix that maintains VSMCs in a quiescent state must occur. Intimal thickening ensues because of the migration of medial VSMCs to the intima, where they proliferate and secrete extracellular matrix proteins. This is supported by studies on aortic explants (4), in rat carotid arteries (5), and in human saphenous vein (2) which have shown that mechanical injury stimulates the production of MMPs. More specifically, remodeling following injury in the rat carotid artery model has been shown to be associated with increased expression of the gelatinases, MMP-9 and MMP-2, and subsequently with increased migration and proliferation of VSMCs (6). Furthermore, the response to arterial balloon injury involves MMP-dependent VSMC migration and can be attenuated by TIMP-1 expression. In vivo arterial gene transfer of TIMP-1 attenuates neointimal hyperplasia after vascular injury, with a marked reduction in VSMC migration but without altering proliferation (7). These results confirm that the balance of MMPs/TIMPs is important and support the supposition that targeting can be a powerful approach to control the migratory capabilities of the cells and, consequently, to control restenosis following balloon angioplasty and stenting.

Batimastat: mode of action

Batimastat, (4-N-Hydroxyamino)-2R-isobutyl-3s-(thiopen-2-ylthiomethyl)-succinyl-l-phenylalanin-n-methylamide, was originally developed by British Biotech Pharmaceuticals Limited as a broad-spectrum matrix metalloproteinase inhibitor (MMPI). It is a low-molecular-weight (478) peptide mimetic comprising the peptide residues found on one side of a principal cleavage site in type I collagen, containing a hydroxamate group (Fig. 1). This group chelates a zinc atom in the active site of the MMP, inhibiting the enzyme reversibly.

The three classes of MMP (collagenases, stromelysins, and gelatinases) are potently inhibited by batimastat, with an IC_{50} in the low-nanomolar range. It shows no activity against unrelated metalloproteinases such as enkephalinase or angiotensin converting enzyme. These enzymes are critical in matrix degradation and invasion by cancer cells (development of cancer metastasis), in the process of arterial remodeling after injury, in cytokine receptor shedding and in the development of restenosis after coronary angioplasty.

Batimastat has been shown to suppress injury-induced phosphorylation of MAP kinase ERK1/ERK2, which is an important signaling pathway of the injury-induced activation of the cells, both restraining the phenotypic modulation and suppressing injury induced-DNA synthesis and migration in VSMC cultures (8). In an in vitro model of baboon aortic medial explants, batimastat was able to inhibit basal cell migration (9), and more specifically in a rat carotid model, it inhibited intimal thickening after balloon injury by decreasing VSMC migration and proliferation (10). A study in Yucatan mini-pigs showed batimastat significantly reduced late lumen loss after balloon angioplasty by inhibition of constrictive arterial remodeling (11). In studies with other MMPIs, marimastat was also shown to affect the arterial wall following balloon angioplasty in favor of neutral and expansive remodeling (12), whereas in a double balloon injury model in rabbits, the broad spectrum

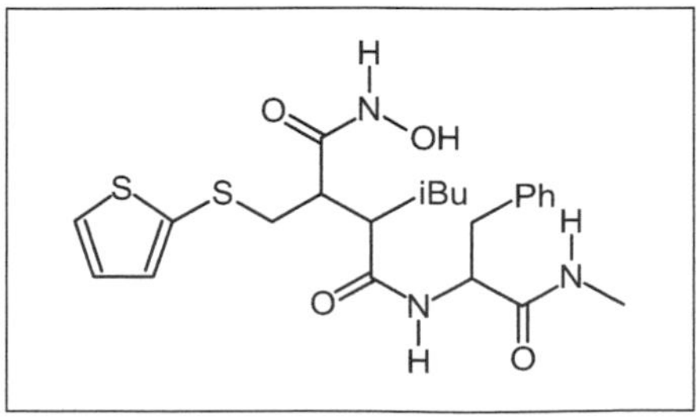

Figure 1
Chemical structure of batimastat.

MMPI GM6001 was shown to reduce intimal cross-sectional area and collagen content by 40% in stented arteries (13). These data help support the rationale for the use of a batimastat-loaded stent to help reduce the restenotic response of the artery after stenting.

Preclinical assessment of the biodivysio batimastat stent

A total of five animal studies, ranging from five days to three months implantation, have been conducted with the batimastat-loaded BiodivYsio Stent (Fig. 2). A summary of the preclinical studies is shown in Table 2. In all the animal studies, batimastat was loaded on either the BiodivYsio AS or OC stents since these stents are more applicable to the vessel size of the selected animal models.

In all cases, stent implantation over-sizing (i.e., balloon/artery ratio >1) was performed to cause an injury to the artery wall, which would result in neointimal formation resembling that occurring in stented human coronary arteries. Angiographic data were obtained before and just after implantation of the stent and were compared to those obtained at the end of each study. In some studies, the performance of the batimastat doses was evaluated by histological measurement of neointimal hyperplasia formation and lumen area changes and compared with the performance of the nondrug loaded stents as a control. Appropriate antiplatelet therapy was administered according to the type of study performed.

Short-term studies

The five-day farm swine study evaluated the sub-acute safety and re-endothelialization of two doses of batimastat $0.30 \pm 0.13 \, \mu g/mm^2$ [clinical trial dose (CTD)] and $1.43 \pm 0.20 \, \mu g/mm^2$ (>CTD) delivered from the 15mm BiodivYsio Batimastat OC Stent compared with BiodivYsio PC coated OC stents without batimastat (control). All stents were implanted without problems and there were no deaths during the five-day follow-up period. All animals were sacrificed at five days. The SEM analysis was performed on all arteries from a total of three animals selected randomly. The rate and extent of endothelialization of the stent struts and the presence of any cellular/biological debris within the stented segment were assessed, and the results showed that batimastat did not interfere with the process of stent endothelialization, the degree of cell coverage being similar to that of the control stent. A continuous and confluent layer of endothelial cells was observed on the inner surface of the stented vessel segments for all stents including control stents. The high degree of endothelial cell coverage over the inner

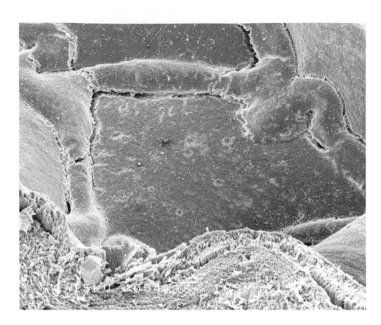

Figure 2
Scanning electron micrograph showing continuous endothelial cell coverage of the stent struts after five-day implantation (preclinical study of clinical trial dose BiodivYsio Batimastat Stent).

surface of the vessel in each of these cases is consistent with previous observations made by Whelan et al. (14). Some white cells and mural thrombus were also observed. It can be concluded that batimastat loaded onto the Bio*divYsio* stent at the CTD or >CTD dose does not affect the in vivo endothelialization process at five days in comparison to the control.

Off-line qualitative coronary angiography (QCA) analysis of all stented vessel segments was also performed and indicated that there were no stent thromboses nor significant differences in percent stenosis between the control group (3.8%) versus CTD (4.8%) and >CTD (4.4%). The fact that both the controls and the batimastat-loaded stents showed a low-stenosis rate demonstrates that the processes

Table 2   Preclinical study summary

Study	Implantation period	Stent	Total dose/μg batimastat per mm² of stent (number of stents implanted)				Animals
			Control	<CTD[a]	CTD[b]	>CTD[c]	
Short-term	5 days	Preloaded 15 mm OC stent	0 (6)		0.30 (7)	1.39 (7)	10 farm swine
	1 month	Nonpreloaded OC stent	0 (8)		0.30 (8)	1.09 (8)	12 farm swine
	1 month	Preloaded AS stent	0 (10)		0.30 (10)		10 farm swine
Short- and Long-term	1 and 3 months	Preloaded AS stent	0 (15)	0.03 (17)	0.30 (30)		26 Yucatan mini-pigs
Pharmaco-kinetic	24 hrs and 1 month	Preloaded OC stent	0.37 (12)	(1 μCi radio-labeled batimastat ¹⁴C per stent)			9 New Zealand white rabbits

Note: CTD specification established for larger vessel clinical trials (i.e., BRILLIANT-EU) and the actual measured dose for the animal study dose is within this CTD range.
[a]These samples were produced using a less concentrated drug solution to achieve a dose lower than clinical trial dose.
[b]The manufacturing range during the preparation of these stents was 0.30 μg batimastat per mm² of stent surface area.
[c]These samples were prepared as for CTD stents; additional batimastat was added by pipette to increase the dose.
Abbreviations: AS, added support; BRILLIANT-EU, batimastat (BB94) anti-restenosis trial utilizing the Bio*divYsio* local drug delivery PC-stent; CTD, clinical trial dose; OC, open cell.

of migration, proliferation, and remodeling were in their early stages (15) (Fig. 3).

The one-month farm swine studies evaluated safety following implantation of two doses of batimastat loaded on the 18 mm Bio*divYsio* stent in comparison to control stent without batimastat. Two batimastat doses were evaluated as described in Table 2. No deaths occurred during the implantation procedure and no sub-acute death or stent thrombosis was observed during the follow-up period. Histological examination confirmed that all the vessels were patent, without the presence of thrombus in the vessel lumen. All sections showed stent struts to be completely covered, leading to a smooth endoluminal surface. There was no excessive inflammatory response at stent struts in Bio*divYsio*-Batimastat-treated sections compared with the control sections. Medial and adventitial layers appeared similar in all three groups. The perivascular nerve fibers, the adipose tissue, and adjacent myocardium appeared normal in control and Bio*divYsio*-Batimastat-treated sections. Therefore, these studies demonstrated that the Bio*divYsio* Batimastat stent at CTD and >CTD was well tolerated up to 28 days.

The study of the pharmacokinetics of release of batimastat from the Bio*divYsio* Batimastat stent was initiated to investigate the deposition of the drug from the stent in the arterial wall and major organs. These studies used the well-established New Zealand white rabbit model where ^{14}C batimastat loaded Bio*divYsio* OC stents, at a dose of 0.37 μg/mm^2, were placed in the left and right iliac arteries and levels of batimastat deposited in the iliac arteries and solid organs were measured 28 days after stent implantation. A total of 18 Bio*divYsio* Batimastat OC stents were implanted in nine rabbits. Three of the nine rabbits were implanted for only one day whereas the remaining six rabbits were implanted for 28 days. The study demonstrated the reproducible release and deposition of drug from the Bio*divYsio* Batimastat stent. Release was reproducible at all time points and was of first-order. Within the first 24 hours, 72.9 ± 4.0% was released and the bulk of loaded drug (94%) was eluted 28 days postimplantation. Drug released from each stent is primarily localized to the 15 mm long-stented region and to a lesser degree the adjacent adventitia and regions immediately proximal and distal to the stent. The data follow the expected patterns of release and deposition and indicate that there is unlikely to be a long-term issue of residual drug within the artery wall after the release has terminated. Very little of the drug was found in the distal organs (brain, liver, kidney, spleen, carotid artery, gonad, heart, lung, and intestine); the amount obtained being so low, it could be considered as undetectable.

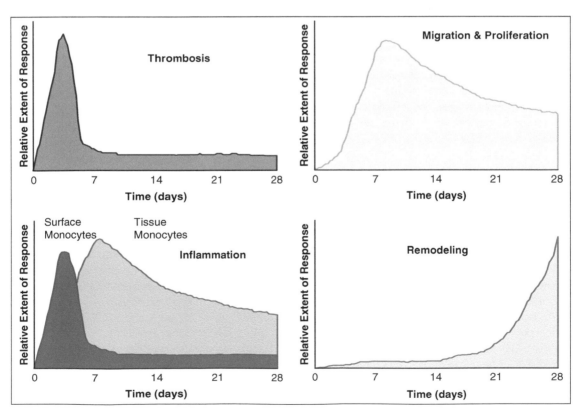

Figure 3
(*See color plate.*) The phases and their timing in the restenosis process.

Table 3 Three month qualitative coronary angiography and histological analysis

	Control	<CTD	CTD
Injury score	1.6	1.5	1.3
In-stent stenosis (%)	34.10	27.20	22.50
Vessel area (mm^2)	9.4	9.9	9.4
Lumen area (mm^2)	3.2	3.3	3.6
Neointimal area (mm^2)	3.9	3.9	3.3
Intimal/medial ratio	0.74	0.72	0.74
Thrombus present	No	No	No

Abbreviation: CTD, clinical trial dose.

Long-term studies

The long-term (three months) safety study was carried out on Yucatan mini-pigs using two doses of batimastat loaded on the 15 mm BiodivYsio stent in comparison to a control stent without batimastat, as outlined in Table 2. The evaluation criteria included vessel lumen area, neointimal thickness and area, absence/presence of thrombus, angiographic percent stenosis, and lumen loss. The QCA and histological analysis at three months follow-up are presented in Table 3.

At three-months, the stenosis was reduced by 20 and 34% in the <CTD and CTD dose, respectively. These data show a trend in favor of the treatment groups. Histopathology evaluation showed that there were no adverse effects of the drug-loaded stent compared to the controls, and no deleterious phenomenon could be attributed to the drug tested. The intensity of fibrosis, hemorrhages, and inflammatory cell infiltration was not significantly different from the control group at three months.

Clinical studies with the bio*divysio* batimastat stent

One clinical registry has been performed to evaluate the safety of the BiodivYsio Batimastat stent in countries outside the U.S.

The Batimastat (BB94) anti-restenosis trial utilizing the BiodivYsio local drug delivery PC-stent (BRILLIANT-EU) was a multi-center, prospective, noncontrolled, European-based single pilot trial performed at eight interventional cardiovascular sites in Belgium, 10 sites in France, and two sites in the Netherlands (Fig. 4). The primary purpose of this multi-center, prospective registry was to evaluate the acute safety and effectiveness of the BiodivYsio Batimastat OC stent (2.0 μg batimastat per mm^2 of stent surface area) in patients with a single, de novo lesion ≤25.0 mm in length, requiring endovascular stenting following percutaneous transluminal coronary angioplasty

(PTCA). The primary objective was to evaluate the occurrence of major adverse cardiac events (MACE) [death, recurrent myocardial infarction (MI), or clinically driven target lesion revascularization] 30 days postprocedure. The secondary objectives were to evaluate the binary restenosis, incidence of (sub)acute stent thrombosis at 30 days follow-up, MACE at 6 and 12 months and the QCA endpoints at 6 months. This study was designed to allow a comparison with the patient population and the results of a larger randomized DISTINCT (BiodivYsio stent in controlled clinical trial) study previously conducted in the U.S.

Study design

One hundred and seventy-three patients (134 males and 39 females), symptomatic patients with stable angina pectoris (Canadian Cardiovascular Society 1, 2, 3, or 4) or unstable angina pectoris with documented ischaemia (Braunwald Class IB-C, IIB-C, or IIIB-C) or documented ischemia with a single de novo lesion in a coronary artery suitable for treatment with a single BiodivYsio DD OC-coated coronary stent preloaded with Batimastat of 11, 15, 18, 22, or 28 mm length by 3.0, 3.5, or 4.0-mm diameter were included in the study, providing they met the selection criteria.

All patients were required to agree to a six-month clinical and angiographic follow-up and had to be over 18 years old. The reference vessel diameter (RVD) of the treated lesion was visually estimated >2.75 and <3.5 mm in diameter, target lesion stenosis >50% and <100%. Noncalcified lesions, de novo lesions within a native coronary artery, ≤25 mm long, requiring one appropriately sized BiodivYsio Batimastat OC stent were included.

The following patient categories were excluded from the study: patients with ostial and bifurcation lesions, left ventricular ejection fraction <30%, known hypersensitivity or contraindication to aspirin or stainless steel, or a sensitivity to contrast dye, allergy to heparin or ticlopidine.

BATMAN-Pilot	
BATiMastat (BB94) Anti-restenosis trial utilizing the Bio*divY sio* local drug delivery PC-steNt	
Purpose	To evaluate the acute safety and effectiveness of the Bio*divYsio* Batimastat Stent
Structure	Single center, prospective, non-controlled study
Study devices	11 mm, 15 mm and 18 mm Bio*divYsio* Batimastat OC stents in diameters of 3.0 mm, 3.5 mm and 4.0 mm
Batimastat dose	0.30 µg batimastat per mm^2
Enrollment	35 patients
Clinical sites	Single center in Brazil
Clinical follow-up	Patients will undergo clinical follow-up at 30 days, 4 and 9 months post procedure
Angiographic follow-up	All patients will undergo angio graphic follow-up 4 months post procedure.
Primary endpoint	MACE (death, recurrent myocardial infarction or clinically driven target vessel revascularisation) at 30 day follow-up
Secondary endpoints	Binary restenosis at 4 months follow-up (defined as ≥ 50% diameter stenosis by QCA) Quantitative coronary angiography endpoints including late loss, loss index, late absolute MLD at 4 months Incidence of (sub)acute stent thrombosis (SAT) to 30 day follow-up, MACE at 4 and 9 months
PI	Dr Mangione – Real e Benemerita Soc. Port de Beneficia, Sao Paulo

BATMAN	
BATiMastat(BB94) Anti-restenosis trial utilizing the Bio*divYsio* local drug delivery PC-steNt	
Purpose	To evaluate safety and efficacy of the Bio*divYsio* Batimastat SV stent versus balloon angioplasty in small coronary arteries
Structure	Multi-center, prospective, randomized study
Study devices	7, 10, 15 and 18 mm Bio*divYsio* Batimastat SV stents in diameters of 2.0, 2.25 & 2.5 mm
Batimastat dose	0.20 µg batimastat per mm^2
Enrollment	600 patients
Clinical sites	45 centers in the US and Canada
Clinical follow-up	Patients will undergo clinical follow-up at 30 days, 6, 8, 9, 12, 24, 36, 48 and 60 months
Angiographic follow-up	All patients will undergo angiographic follow-up at 8 months post procedure
Primary endpoint	Binary restenosis at 8 months follow-up, including late loss, absolute MLD
Secondary endpoints	MACE at 30 days + 1 year, vascular complications, TLR, TVF, TVR
PIs	Dr C Buller (Canada) Dr J Zidar (USA)

Figure 4

Structure of BRILLIANT EU. *Abbreviations*: IVUS, intravascular ultrasound; MACE, major adverse cardiac events; MLA, minimal luminal area; MLD, minimal luminal diameter; QCA, qualitative coronary angiography; SAT, subacute stent thrombosis; TLR, target lesion revascularization; TVF, target vessel failure; TVR, target vessel revascularization.

BRILLIANT - EU	
Batimastat(BB94)anti-**R**estenosis tr**Ia**L uti**L**iz**I**ng the Bio*divYsio* loc**A**l drug Delivery PC-ste**NT**	
Purpose	To evaluate the acute safety and effectiveness of the Bio*divYsio* Batimastat stent
Structure	Multi-center, prospective, non-controlled study
Study devices	11 mm, 15 mm, 18 mm, 22 mm and 28 mm Bio*divYsio* Batimastat stents in diameters of 3.0 mm, 3.5 mm and 4.0 mm
Batimastat dose	0.30 µg batimastat per mm^2
Enrollment	European study of 150 patients
Clinical sites	22 sites in France, Belgium and Holland.
Clinical follow-up	All patients will undergo clinical follow-up at 30 days, 6 and 12 months post procedure
Angiographic follow-up	Patients will undergo angiographic follow-up at 6 months post procedure
Primary endpoint	MACE (death, recurrent myocardial infarction or clinically driven target lesion revascularisation) at 30 days.
Secondary endpoints	Binary restenosis at 6 months follow-up (defined as ≥ 50% diameter stenosis by QCA)Quantitative coronary angiography endpoints including late loss, loss index, late absolute MLD at 6 months Incidence of (sub)acute stent thrombosis (SAT) to 30 day follow-up MACE at 6 months and 12 months
PIs	Dr de Scheerder – UH Gasthuisberg, Leuven Dr Chevalier - Centre Cardiologique du Nord, Paris

BRILLIANT – II Randomized		
Batimastat(BB94)anti-**R**estenosis tr**Ia**L uti**L**iz**I**ng the Bio*divYsio* loc**A**l drug Delivery PC-ste**NT**-II		
Purpose	To evaluate the acute safety and effectiveness of the Bio*divYsio* Batimastat stent compared to the standard BiodivYsio stent	
Structure	Multi-center, prospective, randomized study	
Study devices	11 mm, 15 mm, 18 mm, 22 mm and 28 mm Bio*divYsio* Batimastat and standard Bio*divYsio* OC stents in diameters of 3.0 mm, 3.5 mm and 4.0 mm	
Batimastat dose	0.30 µg batimastat per mm^2	
Enrollment	450 subjects	
Clinical sites	Approximately 30 sites in Europe	
Clinical follow-up	Patients will undergo clinical follow-up at 30 days and 6 months post procedure	
Angiographic follow-up	Angiographic and IVUS follow-up on 100 patients (50 in each arm) at 6 months post procedure	
Primary endpoint	MACE (death, recurrent myocardial infarction or clinically driven target lesion revascularisation) at 6 months.	
Secondary endpoints	Incidence of (sub)acute stent thrombosis (SAT) to 30 days, MACE at 30 day follow-up TVR, TVF at 6 month follow-up, IVUS endpoints including neo intimal hyperplasia, mean lumen area (MLA) at 6 months in 100 patients (50 from each arm of the study) in addition to angiographic endpoints including late loss, loss index, and late absolute MLD	
PIs	Dr de Scheerder – UH Gasthuisberg, Leuven Dr Chevalier - Centre Cardiologique du Nord, Paris	

Figure 4
(*Continued*)

The ethics committee at each center approved the protocol. The consent form or modification based on local independent ethics committee recommendations was completed by all enrolled subjects and signed by the operating physician.

Medication

All patients were premedicated with acetyl salicylic acid (160 mg/day) orally. Oral clopidogrel 300 mg or ticlopidine 500 mg was given before PTCA. Heparin (100 U/kg) after insertion of the arterial sheath was weight-adjusted and administered as needed to maintain an activated clotting time (ACT) of ~250 to 300 seconds. (If a GB IIb/IIIa blocker is used, an ACT of 150–200 sec suffices.) Intracoronary nitroglycerin 50 to 200 μg was administered immediately prior to baseline angiography, poststent deployment, and after final postdilatation angiography. Aspirin was continued indefinitely and clopidogrel 75 mg or ticlopidine (250 mg/day) was prescribed for 28 days in all cases.

Quantitative coronary angiographic analysis

Preprocedural, postprocedural, and at six-month follow-up angiography was performed in at least two orthogonal projections after intracoronary injection of nitrates. Quantitative analyses were performed by an independent core laboratory (Brigham and Women's, Boston, MA, U.S). RVD, minimal luminal diameter (MLD), and degree of stenosis (as percentage of diameter) were measured before dilatation, at the end of the procedure, and at a six-month follow-up. Restenosis was defined as >50% diameter stenosis at follow-up. Late loss was defined as MLD after the procedure minus MLD at follow-up.

Clinical follow-up

All patients were asked to return to the investigative site for a clinical visit four weeks ± one-week postprocedure to repeat clinical labs and monitor acute clinical events. All patients were contacted by telephone by the investigative site at three months ± one week for a safety evaluation. All subjects were required to return to the investigative site for a repeat coronary angiography whether they were experiencing symptoms or not. If a patient had a positive exercise stress test at any time up to and including his required follow-up, a repeat angiogram was performed.

Definitions and statistics

Safety analysis patient set was defined as all patients who received the Bio*divYsio* Batimastat OC stent. per-protocol analysis patient set was defined as all patients in the Safety analysis set who did not deviate from the protocol. Categorical variables were summarized using counts and percentages. Continuous variables were summarized using mean, standard deviation, minimum and maximum, and median for variable not showing a normal distribution. For comparison of subgroups, the unpaired two-tailed student's t-test was used. Results were considered statistically significant at $P < 0.05$.

Results

Demographic characteristics, procedural, and in-hospital outcomes

The baseline clinical and angiographic characteristics are summarized in Table 4. In total, 173 patients were enrolled in the study and had at least one study stent implanted. Nine patients (5%) were excluded from the per-protocol analysis, among which six violated the inclusion/exclusion criteria for the study and four (one violated the inclusion/exclusion) had a second stent placed in the study vessel. The mean age was 61 with a range from 34 to 83 years old. Hypercholesterolemia (62%), hypertension (46%), and family coronary history (43%) were the most frequently reported risk factors. The majority of patients (69%) had one diseased vessel and the mean left ventricular ejection fraction was 67%. Fifty-nine patients (34%) had experienced a previous MI, 22 patients (13%) had undergone previous PTCA, and four patients (2%) had undergone previous coronary artery bypass graft (CABG). At preprocedural evaluation, 100 patients (58%) had unstable angina pectoris (including class 4), 56 patients (32%) had stable angina (classes 1–3), and 17 patients (10%) had silent ischemia.

The most frequent locations of the target lesion were the mid-left anterior descending vessel (39 patients, 23%), proximal left descending vessel (37 patients, 21%), and mid-right coronary artery (35 patients, 20%). Mean lesion length was 11.5 ± 5.0 mm (range from 4 to 25 mm). The most commonly recorded target lesion classification was type B1 (86 patients, 50%).

The majority of patients received either a 15 mm stent (71 patients, 41%), a 18 mm stent (38 patients, 22%), or an 11 mm stent (32 patients, 18%). Mean balloon diameter and length were 3.3 and 16.6 mm, respectively. Mean maximum balloon inflation pressure was 13.3 atm. Delivery balloon rupture occurred in four patients (2%) during the stent placement. The

Table 4 Baseline clinical characteristics

	BRILLIANT-EU N = 173 (N,%)
Male	134(77)
Mean age (yr)	60.6 ± 10.6(34–83)
Risk factors	
Family history CHD	74(43)
Hypercholesterolaemia	108(62)
Hypertension	79(46)
Peripheral vascular disease	19(11)
Previous stroke	10(6)
Diabetes	23(13)
Current smokers	55(32)
Ex smokers	67(39)
History of	
Previous MI	59(34)
Previous PTCA	22(13)
Previous CABG	4(2)
Left ventricular ejection fraction	67.0 ± 11.6(30–93)
Angina status	
Stable angina	62(36)
Unstable angina	94(54)
Silent ischemia	17(10)
Number of diseased vessels	
One vessel	119(69)
Two vessels	36(21)
Three vessels or more	18(10)
Target vessels	
LAD	77(45)
RCA	60(35)
LCX	32(18)
Ramus	4(2)
AHA/ACC classification[a]	
A	32(19)
B1	86(50)
B2	44(25)
C	11(6)
Lesion length (mm)	11.5 ± 5.0 (4–25)

Note: Values are mean ± SD or *N* (%).

[a]According to AHA/ACC classification.

Abbreviations: BRILLIANT-EU, batimastat (BB94) antirestenosis trial utilizing the Bio*divYsio* local drug delivery PC-stent; CABG, coronary artery bypass graft; CHD, coronary heart disease; LAD, left anterior descending artery; LCX, left circumflex artery; PTCA, percutaneous transluminal coronary angioplasty; RCA, right coronary artery.

stent was adequately positioned in 170 patients (98%). Three patients (2%) experienced a residual dissection after stent placement. Two patients (1%) experienced three postprocedural in the hospital complications. One experienced a pseudoaneurysm or arteriovenous fistula at arterial access site requiring surgery and blood loss requiring transfusion. One patient experienced hypotension.

There were no MACE resulting from the angioplasty or stenting procedure. Two non-Q-wave MI occurred postprocedural during hospitalization. Technical device success,

defined as intended stent successfully implanted as the first stent, was achieved in 170 patients (98%). Clinical device success, defined as technical device success in the absence of MACE, was achieved in 168 patients (97%). Procedural success, defined as ≥20% reduction in percent stenosis of the target lesion from immediately prior to intervention to immediately after stent deployment and ≤50% diameter stenosis immediately after stent deployment, using the assigned treatment alone was achieved in 162 patients (94%).

Clinical results

Short-term (up to 30 days) results

At the 30-day (±7 days) follow up, one cardiac death was reported. There were no significant changes in blood parameters either immediately postprocedure or at 30 day follow-up. There were no reports of Q-wave MI, CABG, or repeated angioplasty up to 30 days postprocedure. In addition, there were no reported cases of (sub)acute thrombosis. The MACE free rate at 30 days was 98%.

The six-month follow-up

Between 30 days and six months postprocedure, 32 MACE were reported (18%), one patient experienced cardiac death (ventricular fibrillation), two patients had non-Q-wave MI, and one experienced CABG, and 28 patients underwent TLR (Table 5).

Angiographic outcome

Angiographic data were available from 146 patients (Table 7). Mean reference vessel diameter (defined as the average of normal segments within 10 mm proximal and distal to the target lesion from two views using QCA) was similar at pre PTCA, poststent implantation and at six months postprocedure (2.91, 2.99, and 3.12 mm, respectively). PrePTCA, mean MLD in the target lesion was 1.01 ± 0.34

and mean DS of the lesion was 65.20 ± 10.70%. At six months, mean MLD was 1.81 ± 0.63 mm and mean DS was 37.65 ± 20.20%. Mean acute gain was 1.81 ± 0.38 mm, mean late loss was 0.88 ± 0.63 and mean loss index was 0.50 ± 0.39. Thirty-seven patients (23%) had a significant restenosis at six-month follow-up angiographic assessment.

Summary

The data suggest that the Bio*divYsio* Batimastat OC Stent is safe during the period of drug elution from the stent (pharmacokinetic studies have shown that 94% of the batimastat will have eluted from the PC coating after one month). The final 30 days results suggest that the presence of the batimastat in the coating is not associated with an increased occurrence of MACE or serious adverse events, therefore, the Bio*divYsio* Batimastat OC Stent is safe in the short term for use in patients. However, the long-term (six months) data demonstrate that the Bio*divYsio* Batimastat OC Stent has no additional beneficial effect on restenosis (Table 6).

This study was set up to allow a comparison of the patient population and the results with the larger randomized DISTINCT study previously conducted in the U.S.A. The Bio*divYsio* Batimastat OC Stent showed no improvement in the overall unadjudicated MACE (18%) and restenosis (23%) rate at six months when compared to the nondrug-coated BiodivYsio stent used in the DISTINCT study, where the reported adjudicated MACE and restenosis rate were 17% and 19.7%, respectively. This six-month follow-up data suggest that the Bio*divYsio* Batimastat OC Stent did not offer the additional benefit over the standard BiodivYsio stent (Table 7).

Table 5   Ranked major adverse cardiac events by descending severity and number of events during six-month follow-up

| MACE | BRILLIANT-EU N = 173 (%) | | | | | |
	In hospital N (%) patients	Number events	Up to 30 day follow-up N (%) of patients	Number of events	Up to 6-month follow-up N (%) patients	Number of events
Cardiac death	0(0)	0	1(1)	1	2(1)	2
Q-wave MI	0(0)	0	0(0)	0	0(0)	0
Non-Q-wave	2(1)	2	2(1)	2	4(2)	4
CABG	0(0)	0	0(0)	0	1(1)	1
TLR	0(0)	0	0(0)	0	24(14)	28
Total MACE	2(1)	2	3(2)	3	31(18)	35

Abbreviations: BRILLIANT-EU, Batimastat (BB94) anti-restenosis trial utilizing the Bio*divYsio* local drug delivery PC-stent; CABG, coronary artery bypass graft; MACE, major adverse cardiac events; MI, myocardial infarction; TLR, target lesion revascularization.

Table 6 Six-month clinical follow-up: comparison between BRILLIANT-EU and DISTINCT

	BRILLIANT-EU N = 173 (%)	DISTINCT N = 313 (%)	P-value
Cardiac death	1	1	NS
Q-wave MI	0	1	NS
Non-Q-Wave	2	1	NS
TLR	14	11	NS
CABG	1	3	NS
Total MACE	18	17	NS

Abbreviations: BRILLIANT-EU, batimastat (BB94) anti-restenosis trial utilizing the Bio*divYsio* local drug delivery PC-stent; CABG, coronary artery bypass graft surgery; DISTINCT, Bio*DIvYsio* stent in randomized control trial; MACE, major adverse cardiac events; MI, myocardial infarction; NS, no significant difference; TLR, target lesion revascularization.

Table 7 Qualitative coronary angiography data: comparison between BRILLIANT-EU and DISTINCT

	BRILLIANT-EU	DISTINCT	P-value
Before procedure	N = 163	N = 313	
RVD (mm)	2.91 ± 0.41	2.95 ± 0.48	0.366
MLD (mm)	1.01 ± 0.34	0.81 ± 0.37	$P < 0.001$
%DS	65.20 ± 10.70	72.27 ± 11.92	$P < 0.001$
After procedure	N = 163	N = 146	
RVD (mm)	2.99 ± 0.39	2.92 ± 0.47	0.154
MLD (mm)	2.50 ± 0.45	2.87 ± 0.43	$P < 0.001$
%DS	16.54 ± 8.39	2.87 ± 12.08	$P < 0.001$
Acute gain (mm)	1.81 ± 0.38	2.03 ± 0.49	$P < 0.001$
Follow-up	N = 146	N = 143	
RVD (mm)	3.12 ± 2.96	2.90 ± 0.45	0.380
MLD (mm)	1.81 ± 0.63	1.94 ± 0.67	0.090
%DS	37.65 ± 20.20	33.27 ± 20.67	0.070
Late loss (mm)	0.88 ± 0.63	0.94 ± 0.61	0.412
Loss index	0.50 ± 0.39	0.48 ± 0.33	0.639
Binary restenosis rate (%)	23	19.7	NS

Abbreviations: BRILLIANT-EU, batimastat (BB94) antirestenosis trial utilizing the BiodivYsio local drug delivery PC-stent; DISTINCT, *BioDIvYsio* stent in randomized control trial; DS, diameter stenosis; MLD, minimal luminal diameter; NS, no significant difference; RVD, reference vessel diameter.

Conclusions

The five-day, one-, and three-month preclinical data are available for PC-stents loaded with the CTD of batimastat. Histological analysis showed that the degree of fibrosis, hemorrhages, and inflammatory cell infiltration was not significantly different between the control and CTD stents at all three time points. Five-day and one-month data are available for stents containing greater than three times the CTD. Taken together, these studies demonstrate that the Bio*divYsio* Batimastat Stent is well tolerated in appropriate animal models for the evaluation of restenosis after stent implantation in coronary arteries. The pharmacokinetics release data for the Bio*divYsio* Batimastat Stent follow the expected patterns of release and deposition and indicate that there is unlikely to be a long-term issue of residual drug within the artery wall after release has terminated. The preclinical data at three months with the Bio*divYsio* Batimastat stent showed a change in the rate of stenosis, where a reduction of 20% and 34% in the <CTD and CTD dose, respectively, as measured by QCA was observed. These data showed a trend in favor of the treatment groups.

In addition to the preclinical studies, the clinical studies demonstrate that stent-based delivery of batimastat in coronary artery using the Bio*divYsio* DD stents is a feasible and safe procedure. Results from the BRILLIANT study however did not show a positive effect of the BiodivYsio Batimastat OC stent on TLR, late loss, and binary restenosis.

References

1   Hidalgo M, Eckhardt SG. Development of matrix metalloproteinase inhibitors in cancer therapy. J Natl Cancer Inst. 2001; 93(3):178–193.

2   Jason LJ, Guillaume JJM, Van Eyes GD, et al. Injury induces dedifferentiation of smooth muscle cells and increased matrix-degrading metalloproteinase activity in human saphenous vein. Arterioscler Thromb Vasc Biol 2001; 21(7):1146–1151.

3   Faveeuw C, Preece G, Ager A. Transendothelial migration of lymphocytes across high endothelial venules into lymph nodes is affected by metalloproteinases. Immunobiology 2001; 98(3):688–695.

4   James TW, Wagner R, White LA, et al. Induction of collagenase and stromyelysin gene expression by mechanical injury in a vascular smooth muscle-derived cell line. J Cell Physiol 1993; 157(2):426–437.

5   Jenkins GM, Crow MT, Bilato C, et al. Increased expression of membrane-type matrix metalloproteinase and preferential localitation of matrix metalloproteinase-2 to the neointima of balloon-injured rat carotid arteries. Circulation 1998; 97:82–90.

6   Bendeck MP, Zempo N, Clowes, AW, et al. Smooth muscle cell migration and matrix metalloproteinase expression after arterial injury in the rat. Circ Res 1994; 75:539–545.

7   Dollery CM, Humphries SE, McClelland A, et al. Expression of tissue inhibitor of matrix metalloproteinases 1 by use of an adenoviral vector inhibits smooth muscle cell migration and reduces neointimal hyperplasia in the rat model of vascular balloon injury. Circulation 1999; 99:3199–3205.

8   Lovdahl D, Thyberg J, Hultgardh-Nilsson A. The synthetic metalloproteinase inhibitor batimastat suppresses injury-induced phosphorylation of MAP kinase ERK1/ERK2 and phenotypic modification of arterial smooth muscle cells in vitro. J Vasc Res 2000; 37(5):345–354.

9   Kenagy RD, Vergel S, Mattsson E, et al. The role of plasminogen, plasminogen activators, and matrix metalloproteinases in primate arterial smooth muscle cell migration. Arterioscler Thromb Vasc Biol 1996; 16(11):1373–1382.

10 Zempo N, Koyama N, Kenagy RD, et al. Regulation of vascular smooth muscle cell migration and proliferation in vitro and in injured rat arteries by a synthetic matrix metalloproteinase inhibitor. J Vasc Biol 1996; 16(1):28–33.

11 De Smet BJG, De Kleijn D, Hanemaaijer R, et al. Metalloproteinase inhibition reduces constrictive arterial remodeling after balloon angioplasty: a study in the atherosclerotic yucatan micropig. Circulation 2000; 101:2962–2967.

12 Sierevogel MJ, Pasterkamp G, Velema E, et al. Oral matrix metalloproteinase inhibition and arterial remodeling after balloon dilation—an intravascular ultrasound study in the pig. Circulation 2001; 103:302–307.

13 Li CW, Cantor WJ, Robinson R, et al. Matrix metalloproteinase inhibitor GM6001 selectively reduces intimal hyperplasia and intima collagen in stented but not balloon treated arteries. Can J Cardiol 2000; 16(suppl F):143F.

14 Whelan DM, van der Giessen WJ, Krabbendam SC, et al. Biocompatibility of phosphorylcholine coated stents in normal porcine coronary arteries. Heart 2000; 83(3):338–345.

15 Edelman ER, Rogers C. Pathobiologic responses to stenting. Am J Cardiol 1998; 81(7A):4E–6E.

16 Creemers EE, Cleutjens JP, Smits JF, Daemen MJ. Matrix metalloproteinase inhibition after myocardial infarction: a new approach to prevent heart failure? Circ Res 2001; 89(3):201–210.

28

Antioangiogenetic drugs—mechanisms of action

Christodoulos Stefanadis and Konstantinos Toutouzas

Introduction

Angiogenesis, the growth of new blood vessels, is essential during fetal development, female reproductive cycle, and tissue repair. In contrast, uncontrolled angiogenesis promotes the neoplastic disease and retinopathies, whereas inadequate angiogenesis can lead to coronary artery disease. Although unregulated angiogenesis is seen in several pathological conditions including psoriasis, nephropathy, cancer, and retinopathy, it is essential for embryonic development, menstrual cycle, and wound repair (1–7). The deregulated and excessive vessel growth can have a significant impact on health and contribute to various diseases, such as rheumatoid arthritis, obesity, and infectious diseases. However, it can also be therapeutic in the treatment of some diseases.

More than a dozen endogenous proteins that act as positive regulators or activators of tumor angiogenesis have been identified. These include vascular endothelial growth factor (VEGF), basic fibroblast growth factor (bFGF), tumor necrosis factor-alpha, angiopoietin-1 and -2, interleukin-8 (IL-8), and platelet-derived growth factor-beta (PDGF-b) (6,8). There are also endogenous angiogenic inhibitors, which include angiostatin, endostatin, and interferon-a and -b (6). Thrombospondin (TSP), a 450 kDa matricellular protein, was the first antiangiogenic factor discovered in early 1990s. Gupta and Zhang (5) found that TSP prevented VEGF-induced angiogenesis by directly binding to it and by interfering with its binding to cell surface heparan sulfates (9). Because of the large size (450 kDa), poor bioavailability, and proteolytic breakdown, the clinical use of TSP is limited. However, ABT-510, a mimetic peptide sequence of TSP possessing antiangiogenic activity is in phase II clinical trials (5,9). Pigment epithelium-derived growth factor (PEDF) is a secreted glycoprotein with a molecular weight of 50 kDa. It is a member of the serpin superfamily of serine protease inhibitors and is the most recently discovered antiangiogenesis factor (10). PEDF can promote neuronal cell survival, but acts as a potent inhibitor of angiogenesis (11). Wang et al. (12) reported that adenovirus-mediated gene transfer of PEDF could significantly reduce tumor neoangiogenesis and tumor growth in animal models with hepatocellular carcinoma and Lewis lung carcinoma. The factor that determines whether the angiogenic switch is on or off is the balance of angiogenic activators and inhibitors (13). It also depends on the presence or the absence of receptors.

Angiogenesis and atheromatosis

The development of vasa vasorum in the vascular bed is believed to be critical for atheromatosis. The concept that neovascularization provokes atherosclerotic plaques destabilization, mainly expressed clinically as acute coronary syndrome, is currently being explored. Although safe conclusions cannot still be drawn, several studies demonstrated a correlation between the extent of atherosclerosis and plaque neovascularization in the human pathological samples (14–17) and in the coronary arteries of hypercholesterolemic primates (18). In those specimens with chronic inflammatory cell infiltration by macrophages and lymphocytes, increased number of microvessels are observed (19). These newly formed plaque vessels mainly originate from adventitial vasa vasorum and develop a reach net within the intima, media, and adventitia of the vessel wall. Moreover, their density is increased in the shoulder of atheromatic plaques (20), where the plaque rupture occurs more often. Human ex vivo studies in aorta specimens demonstrated a correlation between the extent of neovascularization in atheromatic plaques and plaque vulnerability, as well as plaque rupture.

The most important stimuli for vessel formation within the vessel wall are the reduction in oxygen supply. The lack of oxygen in a tissue promotes the production of proangiogenic factors, leading to increased neovascularization by migration and hyperplasia of vascular endothelial cells. In the vessel wall, the most prominent proangiogenic factors are VEGF, FGF, and tissue growth factor (TGF).

The importance of neovascularization in atherosclerotic plaques has been demonstrated in several studies (19,21–27). As part of a cellular inflammatory reaction in the presence of damage, small vessels contribute to the healing process. In pathological states, neovascularization differs from a periodic compromise in healing (cocciomatosis in trauma tissue) to a permanent compromise in tissue regeneration. Neovessels are then accompanied by giant cells similar to osteoclastes (with cholesterol crystals inside), immunological cells, and macrophages in a enhanced reaction similar to cocciomatosis, which characterizes the further atherosclerosis of the arterial wall (28). Recently, the inhibition of neovascularization by endostatin reduced the plaque burden by 70% to 85%, implying the significant role of neovascularization in the disease progression (29).

Atherosclerotic neovascularization was studied by Kumamoto et al. (19), who showed that the vasa vasorum have close impact with the external coronary vessel wall in 97% of human coronary atherosclerotic plaques. The possible relationship between microvessels, inflammation, and lipid core enlargement in atherosclerosis is studied. Microvessels facilitate inflammatory cells to penetrate the vessel wall by provoking the macrophages infiltration. Furthermore, inflammation enhances microangiogenesis, causing even greater macrophages infiltration (30). This study showed the synergetic role of neovascularization and inflammation. Another mechanism for plaque neovascularization has also been suggested. The density of microvessels is greater in larger plaques. Therefore, the increased number of microvessels in ruptured plaques may be due to their size. Nevertheless, the number of microvessels was independently related with the plaque rupture. Furthermore, the density of microvessels was smaller in great fibrous-calcified plaques (11). More accurate imaging techniques [magnetic resonance imaging (MRI) or contrast ultrasound] may enlighten the precise mechanisms involved in plaque rupture (31,32).

Angiogenic and antiangiogenic agents

Various angiogenic agents are in clinical trials for treating ischemic heart disease. Hypoxia is a strong stimulus for angiogenesis in numerous disorders, and it can switch on the expression of several angiogenic factors including VEGF, nitric oxide synthase, and PDGF by activating hypoxia inducible transcription factors (HIFs) (Table 1). HIF-1 is an ab-heterodimer that was first recognized as a DNA binding factor. Both HIF-a and -b subunits exist as a series of isoforms encoded by distinct genetic loci. Among three isoforms of HIF-a, HIF-1a and HIF-2a are more closely related with hypoxia response elements to induce transcriptional activity (7). Several strategies have been carried out in the experimental treatment on the basis of HIF-a. However, the most exciting possibility is the use of small molecule inhibitors of the HIF hydroxylases. For example, favorable response to one such compound, FG0041, in a rat model of myocardial infarction was seen even in the face of little detectable fibrosis in control animals (33).

However, one growth factor may not be sufficient by itself, but may require additional growth promoting cytokines. VEGF and placental growth factor (PlGF) have been shown to stimulate angiogenesis and collateral growth with comparable efficiency in the ischemic heart and limb (34). Many studies showed that additional mechanisms including the recruitment of myeloid progenitors and hematopoietic precursors are also required in addition to angiogenic agents to stimulate the growth of new vessels in the ischemic tissue (5,35). The formation of new vessels by tissue engineering holds promise to regenerate vessels for cardiac collateralization and in vascular healing (36).

Besides tissue healing, main interest is currently shown in adopting strategies to reduce in-stent restenosis (37–39). Stent-based approaches include the attachment of anticoagulants, such as heparin (40), or the use of radioactive stents (41) to reduce local cell proliferation. Simply coating stents with biocompatible polymers to mask the underlying thrombotic metal surface is another approach.

Table 1 Antiangiogenic factors

Angiostatin
Antithrombin III
Endostatin
Fibronectin fragment
Heparinases
Human chorionic gonadotropin
Interferon
PEDF
Platelet factor 4
Retinoits
Thrombospodin-S
Tissue inhibitors of metalloporteinases
TGF
Vasostatin

Abbreviations: PEDF, pigment epithelium-derived growth factor; TGF, tissue growth factor.

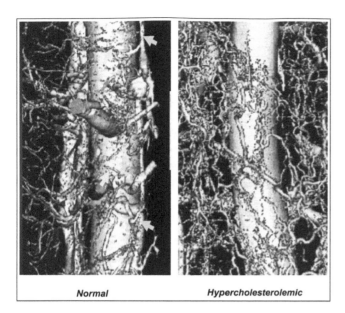

Figure 1

(*See color plate.*) The development of neovascularization in a hypercholesterolemic model is shown in the right panel. The density of vasa vasorum in the aortic wall is clearly increased after administration of hypercholesterolemic diet, compared with the control group (*left panel*). *Arrows* indicate the vasa vasorum. *Source*: From Ref. 72.

Local delivery with stents

Earlier studies on stents coated with a variety of biodegradable and biostable polymers showed marked inflammatory responses and subsequent neointimal thickening (42). Recently, it has been reported that rapamycin-eluting stents can significantly improve patency rates when compared with conventional stents (43). Virmani et al. (44) reported the possibility that the hypersensitivity to the polymer of rapamycin-eluting stent can cause late coronary thrombosis. Ganaha et al. (45) examined the efficacy of the local stent-based release of angiostatin, to inhibit neovascularization and to limit subsequent in-stent plaque progression. Consistent with its primary action as an angiogenesis inhibitor, this study found that local stent-based release of angiostatin significantly limited plaque microvessel formation versus the control group.

Same beneficial results were obtained from SOPHOS? and studies in lesions <15 mm long (46). Four hundred and twenty-five patients from 24 centers were enrolled. In patients of SOPHOS A study ($n = 200$), a second angiography was performed in six months and the whole study population was followed-up for one year. The endpoint was death, acute myocardial infarction (AMI), or need for angioplasty and was observed in 13.4%. Two deaths, five AMIs, and 32 revascularizations were observed. Angiographical restenosis was 17.7% with a lumen loss of 0.8 mm. Recently, the results of the SV stent study showed in 150 patients with reference vessel diameter of 2 to 2.75 mm in 19 centers in

Europe and Israel that in six months of follow-up, one death was recorded, four patients suffered from non-Q AMI, and 24 patients underwent revascularization. Lumen loss was 0.55 mm and restenosis occurred in 32% (47).

Except decreasing platelet adhesion, phosphorylcholine (PC) may be used for transporting other substances and releasing them within the vessel wall. Therefore, experimental studies for the evaluation of angiopeptin-, eostradiol-, or dexamethazone-coated BiodivYsio stents have been performed. After angiopeptin coated stent implantation, the substance was detected in porcine arterial wall (48) for only 28 days and no further than the site of implantation. The study proved this stent-based release to be safe and successful. In the clinical study of 13 patients, no side effects and no cardiac events were observed for one year. Angiographical results were equally positive. No restenosis was detected, whereas lumen loss was 0.46 mm and lumen area loss estimated by intravascular ultrasound was 18.4% (49).

Local corticoids release was also successfully performed by BiodivYsio stents. Methylprednisolone-coated BiodivYsio stents reduced the inflammatory reaction and intimal wall hyperplasia in porcine coronary arteries (50). The clinical multicenter pilot STRIDE study was designed for the evaluation of safety and efficacy of dexamethasone ($0.5 \, \mu g/mm^2$)—releasing BiodivYsio stents. Seventy-one patients, 42% suffering from unstable angina, were enrolled. Angiographic restenosis was 13.3% and lumen loss was 0.45 mm. Especially in the subgroup of patients with unstable angina known to have greater inflammatory activation, lumen loss was 0.32 mm and angiographic restenosis was 6% (51).

Later studies from Japan showed beneficial effect of antioxidants-releasing BiodivYsio stent. Carvedilole and prombucole were induced in porcine coronary arteries.

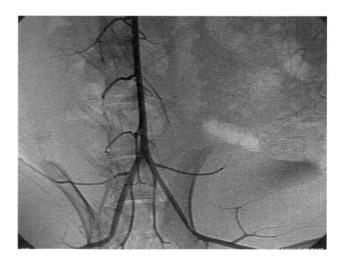

Figure 2

Four weeks after the implantation of bevacizumab-eluting stent in the right iliac artery of a hypercholesterolemic rabbit. Angiographically, there is no detectable intimal hyperplasia. *Source*: From Ref. 71.

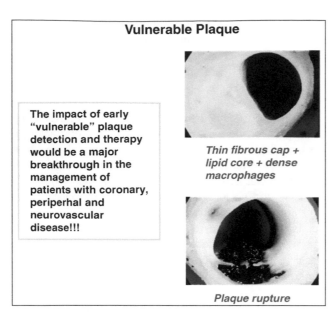

Vulnerable Plaque

The impact of early "vulnerable" plaque detection and therapy would be a major breakthrough in the management of patients with coronary, periperhal and neurovascular disease!!!

Thin fibrous cap + lipid core + dense macrophages

Plaque rupture

Figure 3

In the upper panel, a "vulnerable plaque" is demonstrated with thin fibrous cap, large lipidcore, and increased density of microphages. In the lower panel, a plaque rupture with accompanying thrombi is shown.

Carvedilol-releasing BiodivYsio stents minimized the hyperplasia by 42% and maximized the lumen area by 20% compared with simple BiodivYsio stents. No positive effect was observed in the Probucole group (52).

Bevacizumab

Bevacizumab (Avastin, Roche) is the first approved anticancer agent developed on angiogenesis-based treatment. Bevacizumab is a recombinant humanized monoclonal antibody directed against VEGF. Several studies with anti-VEGF factors have been performed. First in 1997 (53), on a phase I study, 25 patients with solid tumors received intravenously different doses (0.1, 0.3, 1.0, 3.0, of $\kappa\alpha$? 10mg/kg bevacizumab for 90 minutes on 0th, 28th, 35th, and 42nd day. In a later phase Ib study, bevacizumab was combined with other cytotoxic drugs such as doxorubicin, carboplatin, and paclitaxel. Bevacizumab was intravenously delivered in 3 mg/kg weekly doses for eight weeks and no further deterioration of known cytotoxic-related side effects was shown (54). Five more studies were performed in different forms of cancers, with the most promising results obtained in kidney and colon cancer (54–56). Then, phase III studies were performed, which showed that bevacizumab added to the conventional therapy of patients with metastatic colon cancer an increase in median survival by 15.6 to 20.3 months (57).

No deterioration of the therapy toxicity was shown. However, a moderate blood pressure elevation, without proteinuria, was observed and also thrombotic and bleeding events were encountered (58).

It was significantly effective when used in combination with fluorouracil-based chemotherapy and led to the improvement of overall response rates, time to progression, and survival of patients with metastatic colon cancer (55,57,58). Bevacizumab and irinotecan, fluorouracil, leucovorin (IFL) chemotherapy regimen showed an increase in median survival by 4.7 months, in progression free survival by 4.36 months, and in overall response rates (complete and partial responses) by 10.2% when compared with IFL plus placebo.

In February 2004, the Food and Drug Administration (FDA) approved the use of bevacizumab in patients with metastatic colon cancer in United States. In an additional phase III study, with 462 participating patients suffering from breast cancer, capecitabine with or without bevacizumab was delivered and better results were observed in the group with the combined therapy, although there was no significant change in the median survival (59). In a late stage study, paclitaxel combined with bevacizumab in patients with metastatic breast cancer is investigated. Bevacizumab is also evaluated in phase II studies for the treatment of sarcomas and pancreatic cancer.

Bevacizumab

Local delivery of bevacizumab at the vessel wall can be performed by dedicated stents coated with PC. The PC polymer mimics the chemical structure of the PC headgroup, which makes up 90% of phospholipids in the outer membrane of a red blood cell. PC has been shown to decrease protein absorption and platelet adhesion; thereby we can expect that the PC coating reduces the thrombus formation of the stainless steel stent, allowing the prevention of subacute thrombosis. Both in vitro and in vivo researches have demonstrated that PC-based polymers are effective in improving the biocompatibility of inert materials (60–62).

Galli et al. (63,64) demonstrated that primary stenting of AMI with PC-coated stent leads to excellent short- and mid-term clinical outcomes and a low restenosis, despite a reduced heparin therapy. As in other studies, the reported restenosis rate using the BiodivYsio stent in the small vessels is lower than that using any other metallic stents (46,47, 49,64–68).

Several attempts in the past have been made to achieve local gene delivery via coated balloon catheters or infusion catheters using both naked plasmid DNA and adenoviral vectors for the transfer of VEGF-1 or -2 (69,70). Walter et al. (69) demonstrated that local VEGF-2 plasmid gene delivery of a therapeutic gene via coated stents appears feasible, safe, and effective.

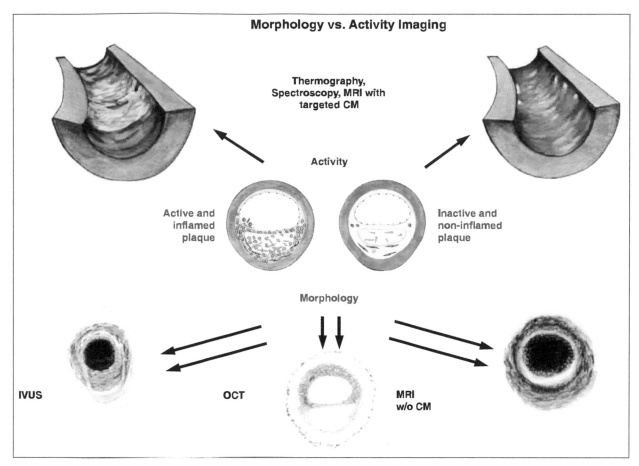

Figure 4
Methods for recognizing morphological and functional characteristics include intracoronary thermography, spectroscopy, intravascular ultrasound (IVUS), optical coherence tomography (OCT), and intravascular magnetic resonance imaging (MRI).

Bevacizumab-eluting stents

For local inhibition of vasa vasorum development, we hypothesized that delivery of bevacizumab by stent would inhibit the neovascularization in an atheromatic rabbit model. In a recent study, we used 10 New Zealand atheromatic rabbits. BiodivYsio stents were immersed in a solution of 4 mL bevacizumab according to previous studies. Both eluting stents and noneluting BiodivYsio stents were implanted in the middle segment of the two iliac arteries of the animals, with the same procedural characteristics. There was no acute or subacute thrombosis. The angiographic follow-up at 28 days demonstrated that there was no restenosis. Gross pathological analysis did not show any evidence of vascular necrosis. On the basis of these results, we currently performed the first-in-man study to evaluate the safety of bevacizumab-eluting stents in patients with coronary artery disease (71,72).

Conclusion

In conclusion, neovascularization seems to play an important role in the development of atheromatic plaques, especially in the process of destabilization. Inhibitors of plaque neovascularization are under animal and clinical investigation. In the following years, we can obtain safe results for the novel treatment of high-risk plaques.

References

1   Kim KJ, Li B, Winer J, et al. Inhibition of vascular endothelial growth factor-induced angiogenesis suppresses tumour growth in vivo. Nature 1993; 362:841–844.

2   Majack RA, Clowes AW. Inhibition of vascular smooth muscle cell migration by heparin-like glycosaminoglycans. J Cell Physiol 1984; 118:253–256.

3 Carmeliet P. Angiogenesis in health and disease. Nat Med 2003; 9:653–660.

4 Folkman J. Angiogenesis in cancer, vascular, rheumatoid and other disease. Nat Med 1995; 1:27–31.

5 Gupta K, Zhang J. Angiogenesis: a curse or cure? Postgrad Med J 2005; 81:236–242.

6 Westphal JR, Van't Hullenaar R, Peek R, et al. Angiogenic balance in human melanoma: expression of VEGF, bFGF, IL-8, PDGF and angiostatin in relation to vascular density of xenografts in vivo. Int J Cancer 2000; 86:768–776.

7 Pugh CW, Ratcliffe PJ. Regulation of angiogenesis by hypoxia: role of the HIF system. Nat Med 2003; 9:677–684.

8 Poon RT, Fan ST, Wong J. Clinical implications of circulating angiogenic factors in cancer patients. J Clin Oncol 2001; 19: 1207–1225.

9 Gupta K, Gupta P, Wild R, Ramakrishnan S, Hebbel RP. Binding and displacement of vascular endothelial growth factor (VEGF) by thrombospondin: effect on human microvascular endothelial cell proliferation and angiogenesis. Angiogenesis 1999; 3:147–158.

10 Becerra SP, Sagasti A, Spinella P, Notario V. Pigment epithelium-derived factor behaves like a noninhibitory serpin. Neurotrophic activity does not require the serpin reactive loop. J Biol Chem 1995; 270:25992–25999.

11 Doll JA, Stellmach VM, Bouck NP, et al. Pigment epithelium-derived factor regulates the vasculature and mass of the prostate and pancreas. Nat Med 2003; 9:774–780.

12 Wang L, Schmitz V, Perez-Mediavilla A, Izal I, Prieto J, Qian C. Suppression of angiogenesis and tumor growth by adenoviral-mediated gene transfer of pigment epithelium-derived factor. Mol Ther 2003; 8:72–79.

13 Hanahan D, Folkman J. Patterns and emerging mechanisms of the angiogenic switch during tumorigenesis. Cell 1996; 86: 353–364.

14 Kamat BR, Galli SJ, Barger AC, Lainey LL, Silverman KJ. Neovascularization and coronary atherosclerotic plaque: cinematographic localization and quantitative histologic analysis. Hum Pathol 1987; 18:1036–1042.

15 Zamir M, Silver MD. Vasculature in the walls of human coronary arteries. Arch Pathol Lab Med 1985; 109:659–662.

16 Zhang Y, Cliff WJ, Schoefl GI, Higgins G. Immunohistochemical study of intimal microvessels in coronary atherosclerosis. Am J Pathol 1993; 143:164–172.

17 Sueishi K, Yonemitsu Y, Nakagawa K, Kaneda Y, Kumamoto M, Nakashima Y. Atherosclerosis and angiogenesis. Its pathophysiological significance in humans as well as in an animal model induced by the gene transfer of vascular endothelial growth factor. Ann N Y Acad Sci 1997; 811:311–322, 322–324.

18 Williams JK, Armstrong ML, Heistad DD. Vasa vasorum in atherosclerotic coronary arteries: responses to vasoactive stimuli and regression of atherosclerosis. Circ Res 1988; 62:515–523.

19 Kumamoto M, Nakashima Y, Sueishi K. Intimal neovascularization in human coronary atherosclerosis. Hum Pathol 1995; 26:450–456.

20 O'Brien ER, Garvin MR, Dev R, et al. Angiogenesis in human coronary atherosclerotic plaques. Am J Pathol 1994; 145: 883–894.

21 Fuster V, Moreno PR, Fayad ZA, Corti R, Badimon JJ. Athero-thrombosis and high-risk plaque: part I: evolving concepts. J Am Coll Cardiol 2005; 46:937–954.

22 Arbustini E, Morbini P, D'Armini AM, et al. Plaque composition in plexogenic and thromboembolic pulmonary hypertension: the critical role of thrombotic material in pultaceous core formation. Heart 2002; 88:177–182.

23 Fleiner M, Kummer M, Mirlacher M, et al. Arterial neovascularization and inflammation in vulnerable patients: early and late signs of symptomatic atherosclerosis. Circulation 2004; 110:2843–2850.

24 Hayden MR, Tyagi SC. Vasa vasorum in plaque angiogenesis, metabolic syndrome, type 2 diabetes mellitus, and atheroscleropathy: a malignant transformation. Cardiovasc Diabetol 2004; 3:1.

25 Jeziorska M, Woolley DE. Local neovascularization and cellular composition within vulnerable regions of atherosclerotic plaques of human carotid arteries. J Pathol 1999; 188: 189–196.

26 Mofidi R, Crotty TB, McCarthy P, Sheehan SJ, Mehigan D, Keaveny TV. Association between plaque instability, angiogenesis and symptomatic carotid occlusive disease. Br J Surg 2001; 88:945–950.

27 Nakata Y, Maeda N. Vulnerable atherosclerotic plaque morphology in apolipoprotein E-deficient mice unable to make ascorbic Acid. Circulation 2002; 105:1485–1490.

28 Raines E, Rosenfeld M, Ross R. The Role of Macrophages. Atherosclerosis and Coronary Artery Disease. Philadelphia: Lippincott-Raven Publishers, 1996:539–555.

29 Moulton KS, Heller E, Konerding MA, Flynn E, Palinski W, Folkman J. Angiogenesis inhibitors endostatin or TNP-470 reduce intimal neovascularization and plaque growth in apolipoprotein E-deficient mice. Circulation 1999; 99: 1726–1732.

30 Polverini PJ, Cotran PS, Gimbrone MA Jr, Unanue ER. Activated macrophages induce vascular proliferation. Nature 1977; 269:804–806.

31 Leong-Poi H, Christiansen J, Klibanov AL, Kaul S, Lindner JR. Noninvasive assessment of angiogenesis by ultrasound and microbubbles targeted to alpha(v)-integrins. Circulation 2003; 107:455–460.

32 Casscells W, Hassan K, Vaseghi MF, et al. Plaque blush, branch location, and calcification are angiographic predictors of progression of mild to moderate coronary stenoses. Am Heart J 2003; 145:813–820.

33 Nwogu JI, Geenen D, Bean M, Brenner MC, Huang X, Buttrick PM. Inhibition of collagen synthesis with prolyl 4-hydroxylase inhibitor improves left ventricular function and alters the pattern of left ventricular dilatation after myocardial infarction. Circulation 2001; 104:2216–2221.

34 Luttun A, Tjwa M, Moons L, et al. Revascularization of ischemic tissues by PlGF treatment, and inhibition of tumor angiogenesis, arthritis and atherosclerosis by anti-Flt1. Nat Med 2002; 8:831–840.

35 Avecilla ST, Hattori K, Heissig B, et al. Chemokine-mediated interaction of hematopoietic progenitors with the bone marrow vascular niche is required for thrombopoiesis. Nat Med 2004; 10:64–71.

36 Koike N, Fukumura D, Gralla O, Au P, Schechner JS, Jain RK. Tissue engineering: creation of long-lasting blood vessels. Nature 2004; 428:138–139.

37 Gershlick AH, Baron J. Dealing with in-stent restenosis. Heart 1998; 79:319–323.

38 Kim KI, Bae J, Kang HJ, et al. Three-year clinical follow-up results of intracoronary radiation therapy using a rhenium-188-diethylene-triamine-penta-acetic-acid-filled balloon system. Circ J 2004; 68:532–537.

39 Suzuki J, Ito H, Gotoh R, Morishita R, Egashira K, Isobe M. Initial clinical cases of the use of a NF- B decoy at the site of coronary stenting for the prevention of restenosis. Circ J 2004; 68:270–271.

40 Hardhammar PA, van Beusekom HM, Emanuelsson HU, et al. Reduction in thrombotic events with heparin-coated Palmaz-Schatz stents in normal porcine coronary arteries. Circulation 1996; 93:423–430.

41 Fischell TA, Carter AJ, Laird JR. The beta-particle-emitting radioisotope stent (isostent): animal studies and planned clinical trials. Am J Cardiol 1996; 78:45–50.

42 van der Giessen WJ, Lincoff AM, Schwartz RS, et al. Marked inflammatory sequelae to implantation of biodegradable and nonbiodegradable polymers in porcine coronary arteries. Circulation 1996; 94:1690–1697.

43 Moses JW, Leon MB, Popma JJ, et al. Sirolimus-eluting stents versus standard stents in patients with stenosis in a native coronary artery. N Engl J Med 2003; 349:1315–1323.

44 Virmani R, Guagliumi G, Farb A, et al. Localized hypersensitivity and late coronary thrombosis secondary to a sirolimus-eluting stent: should we be cautious? Circulation 2004; 109:701–705.

45 Ganaha F, Kao EY, Wong H, et al. Stent-based controlled release of intravascular angiostatin to limit plaque progression and in-stent restenosis. J Vasc Interv Radiol 2004; 15: 601–608.

46 Boland JL, Corbeij HA, Van Der Giessen W, et al. Multicenter evaluation of the phosphorylcholine-coated biodivYsio stent in short de novo coronary lesions: The SOPHOS study. Int J Cardiovasc Intervent 2000; 3:215–225.

47 Bakhai A, Booth J, Delahunty N, et al. The SV stent study: a prospective, multicentre, angiographic evaluation of the BiodivYsio phosphorylcholine coated small vessel stent in small coronary vessels. Int J Cardiol 2005; 102:95–102.

48 Armstrong J, Gunn J, Arnold N, et al. Angiopeptin-eluting stents: observations in human vessels and pig coronary arteries. J Invasive Cardiol 2002; 14:230–238.

49 Kwok OH, Chow WH, Law TC, et al. First human experience with angiopeptin-eluting stent: a quantitative coronary angiography and three-dimensional intravascular ultrasound study. Catheter Cardiovasc Interv 2005; 66:541–546.

50 Huang Y, Liu X, Wang L, Verbeken E, Li S, De Scheerder I. Local methylprednisolone delivery using a BiodivYsio phosphorylcholine-coated drug-delivery stent reduces inflammation and neointimal hyperplasia in a porcine coronary stent model. Int J Cardiovasc Intervent 2003; 5:166–171.

51 Liu X, Huang Y, Hanet C, et al. Study of antirestenosis with the BiodivYsio dexamethasone-eluting stent (STRIDE): a first-in-human multicenter pilot trial. Catheter Cardiovasc Interv 2003; 60:172–178; discussion 179.

52 Kim W, Jeong MH, Cha KS, et al. Effect of anti-oxidant (carvedilol and probucol) loaded stents in a porcine coronary restenosis model. Circ J 2005; 69:101–106.

53 Gordon M, Margolin K, Talpaz M. Phase I safety and pharmacokinetic study of recombinant human anti-vascular endothelial growth factor in patients with advanced cancer. J Clin Oncol 2001; 19:843–850.

54 Margolin K, Gordon M, Holmgren E. Phase Ib trial of intravenous recombinant humanised monoclonal antibody to vascular endothelial growth factor in combination with chemotherapy in patients advanced cancer: Pharmacologic and long term results. J Clin Oncol 2001; 19:851–859.

55 Kabbinavar F, Hurwitz HI, Fehrenbacher L, et al. Phase II, randomized trial comparing bevacizumab plus fluorouracil (FU)/leucovorin (LV) with FU/LV alone in patients with metastatic colorectal cancer. J Clin Oncol 2003; 21:60–65.

56 Yang J, Hawworth L, Sherry R. A randomised trial of bevacizumab, an antivascular endothelial growth antibody for metastatic renal cancer. N Engl J Med 2003; 349: 427–434.

57 Hurwitz H, Fehrenbacher L, Novotny W, et al. Bevacizumab plus irinotecan, fluorouracil, and leucovorin for metastatic colorectal cancer. N Engl J Med 2004; 350:2335–2342.

58 Zondor SD, Medina PJ. Bevacizumab: an angiogenesis inhibitor with efficacy in colorectal and other malignancies. Ann Pharmacother 2004; 38:1258–1264.

59 Midgley R, Kerr D. Bevacizumab-current status and future directions. Ann Oncol 2005; 16:999–1004.

60 Kuiper K, Robinson K, Chronos N, Nordrehaug J. Biocompatibility of phosphorylcholine coated stents in a procine coronary moedl. Circulation 1998; 96:I-289.

61 Malik N, Gunn J, Shepherd L, Crossman DC, Cumberland DC, Holt CM. Phosphorylcholine-coated stents in porcine coronary arteries: in vivo assessment of biocompatibility. J Invasive Cardiol 2001; 13:193–201.

62 Lewis AL, Vick TA, Collias AC, et al. Phosphorylcholine-based polymer coatings for stent drug delivery. J Mater Sci Mater Med 2001; 12:865–870.

63 Galli M, Sommariva L, Prati F, et al. Acute and mid-term results of phosphorylcholine-coated stents in primary coronary stenting for acute myocardial infarction. Catheter Cardiovasc Interv 2001; 53:182–187.

64 Galli M, Bartorelli A, Bedogni F, et al. Italian BiodivYsio open registry (BiodivYsio PC-coated stent): study of clinical outcomes of the implant of a PC-coated coronary stent. J Invasive Cardiol 2000; 12:452–458.

65 Moreno R, Fernandez C, Alfonso F, et al. Coronary stenting versus balloon angioplasty in small vessels: a meta-analysis from 11 randomized studies. J Am Coll Cardiol 2004; 43: 1964–1972.

66 Shinozaki N, Yokoi H, Iwabuchi M, et al. Initial and follow-up results of the BiodivYsio phosphorylcholine coated stent for treatment of coronary artery disease. Circ J 2005; 69:295–300.

67 Grenadier E, Roguin A, Hertz I, et al. Stenting very small coronary narrowings (<2mm) using the biocompatible phosphorylcholine-coated coronary stent. Catheter Cardiovasc Interv 2002; 55:303–308.

68 Beaudry Y, Sze S, Fagih B, Constance C, Kwee R. Six-month results of small vessel stenting (2.0–2.8 mm) with the Biodivysio SV stent. J Invasive Cardiol 2001; 13:628–631.

69 Walter DH, Cejna M, Diaz-Sandoval L, et al. Local gene transfer of phVEGF-2 plasmid by gene-eluting stents: an alternative

strategy for inhibition of restenosis. Circulation 2004; 110:36–45.

70 Asahara T, Chen D, Tsurumi Y, et al. Accelerated restitution of endothelial integrity and endothelium-dependent function after phVEGF165 gene transfer. Circulation 1996; 94:3291–3302.

71 Stefanadis C, Toutouzas K, Stefanadi E, Kolodgie F, Virmani R, Kipshidze N. First experimental application of bevacizumab-eluting

PC coated stent for inhibition of vasa vasorum of atherosclerotic plaque: angiographic results in a rabbit atheromatic model. Hellenic J Cardiol 2006; 47:7–10.

72 Stephanidis C, Toutouzas K, Stefanadi E, et al. Inhibition of plague neovascularization and intimal hyperplasia by specific targeting vascular endothelial growth factor with bevacizumab–eluting stent: an experimental study. Atherosclerosis 2007; in press.

29

Vasculoprotective approach for restenosis

Nicholas Kipshidze, Jean-François Tanguay,
Alexandre C. Abizaid, and Antonio Colombo

Introduction

Coronary stent implantation has been proven superior to conventional balloon angioplasty for the treatment of coronary de novo lesions (1–4) and by extension has transformed the field of percutaneous coronary intervention (PCI). However, despite the advent of stents, restenosis continues to limit the long-term success of PCI. Stenting may evoke an exuberant proliferative healing response compared to balloon angioplasty. The favorable effect of stents in countering constrictive remodeling is therefore, in some cases, offset by the increased neointimal hyperplasia associated with stenting, causing difficult-to-treat in-stent restenosis.

As discussed elsewhere, drug-eluting stents (DESs) will revolutionize PCI to a greater extent in the near future. Recently, the utilization of antiproliferative agents, sirolimus and paclitaxel, delivered locally via DES has dramatically reduced neointimal growth in various animal models. In human trials, this has translated clinically to a reduction in the incidence of restenosis (5–7) to the single digits. These early clinical results appear to be maintained at longer term follow-up. However, as in the case of vascular brachytherapy, in the last several months, concerns arise from delayed healing of the arterial wall, occurrence of late thrombosis in high-risk subsets, and potentially unknown long-term effects of the cell-cycle inhibitors on the vasculature.

Because the endothelium has important inhibitory effects on platelet aggregation, monocyte adhesion, and smooth muscle cell (SMC) proliferation, strategies to improve vascular healing after spontaneous or induced injury may improve clinical outcomes in the long-term (Fig. 1).

Endothelium and restenosis

The endothelium acts as a selective permeability barrier and participates in vascular tone regulation via production of vasodilators such as endothelium-derived relaxing factor, nitric oxide (NO), and prostacyclin. The endothelium also produces vasoconstrictors (endothelin), which influence the local coagulation homeostasis via antithrombotic (thrombomodulin, tissue plasminogen activator, prostacyclin, NO, heparin sulfate) or prothrombotic substances (von Willebrand factor, tissue factor, plasminogen activator inhibitor) and produces cytokines interleukin (IL) [(IL-1, IL-6, IL-8)], growth factors [platelet-derived growth factor (PDGF), fibroblast growth factor (bFGF), transforming growth factor (TGF-β)], adhesion molecules (selectins, vascular cell adhesion molecule, intracellular adhesion molecule), and extracellular matrix components (laminin, collagen, proteoglycans) (8–10).

Following vascular injury, the loss of the endothelial cell (EC) is critical in favoring thrombosis, platelet–leukocyte adhesion, vasospasm, and SMC activation and proliferation. Endothelium regeneration may take several weeks under the influence of vascular endothelial growth factor and bFGF. Re-endothelialization and recovery of endothelial nitric-oxide synthase (eNOS) activity may influence restenosis (11–12). Indeed, administration of L-arginine (13) and eNOS gene therapy (14) has been shown to reduce intimal thickening and restenosis after balloon injury.

Endothelial denudation is considered a primary injury event following balloon angioplasty and/or stent implantation. Although ECs are firmly attached to each other and to their basement membrane forming a monolayer throughout the vascular tree, balloon injury denudes these cells from the

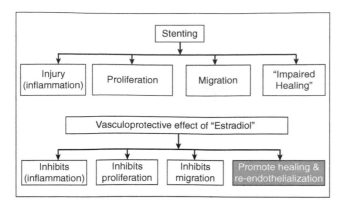

Figure 1
Vasculoprotective approach to prevent restenosis.

vessel wall. ECs, when in confluent monolayer, cease replication. Disruption of cell contact inhibition results in rapid EC replication from the proximal and distal untraumatized segments. Overlying ECs likely play an important role in controlling SMC proliferation via secretion of heparin and other growth-inhibitory factors, with some evidence that neointimal proliferation ceases when ECs regenerate. ECs might themselves maintain the mitogenic quiescence of SMCs by the growth inhibitory effect of NO (15).

Besides modulating local hemostasis and thrombolysis, producing vasoactive compounds, and providing a nonpermeable barrier protecting SMCs against circulating growth-promoting factors, ECs themselves synthesize several growth factors including FGF, PDGF, and TGF-β, which are important in SMC proliferation. ECs also produce a significant number of the components of EC basement membrane: types IV and V collagen, laminin, proteoglycans, and extracellular matrix (fibronectin). EC denudation thus leads not only to endothelial dysfunction but also to exposure of the thrombogenic and adhesive subendothelial layer to platelets and leukocytes with concomitant release of growth factors (16). This wound-healing response elicited by endothelial denudation often leads to luminal narrowing and restenosis.

Using scanning electron microscopy, Grewe et al. (17) studied the pathomorphological findings of the vessel wall after stent insertion. On the basis of the results, they divided the stent integration process with intra-individual differences into three phases: In the acute phase (<six weeks), the border between the vascular lumen and arterial wall is constituted by a thin, multilayered thrombus. During the time course of integration, increasing amounts of SMC and extracellular matrix can be detected. No ECs can be found in the implantation zone. In the intermediate phase (6–12 weeks), the neointima consists of extracellular matrix and increasing numbers of SMC. The borderline between lumen and neointima is generated by SMC and extracellular matrix. Increasing amounts of ECs are found on the luminal surface of the stent neointima. Complete re-endothelialization is first noted in the chronic phase, three months after stenting. Matrix structures

increase, whereas the amount of SMC decreases. In all the phases of stent incorporation, the alloplastic stent material is covered by a thin (few nanometers) proteinaceous layer.

Time-course analysis in a rabbit iliac artery model disclosed <20% stent re-endothelialization at four days, <40% at seven days, and near-complete endothelialization at 28 days following stent implantation (18). The re-endothelialization process has been studied in several other animal models using different types of injuries with very controversial results, suggesting, in part, a diversity in the response and capacity of vascular healing.

Furthermore, the regenerating endothelium can demonstrate long-term (more than three months) dysfunction with a decreased vascular integrity and an increased permeability, which is more pronounced after stenting than after percutaneous transluminal coronary angioplasty (19). This dysfunction is also characterized by impaired endothelium-dependent vasodilatation (20). Influences that lead to an increased intracellular cyclic adenosine monophosphate (cAMP) may promote re-endothelialization, reduce endothelial permeability, and attenuate fibromuscular proliferation (21). Intima affected by atherosclerosis also has ECs with lowered cAMP content, which points at similarities in the development of both pathological conditions: restenosis and atherosclerosis. Thus, re-endothelialization of an injured atherosclerotic vessel may take a longer period of time that could become a substantial factor in restenosis formation. In theory, early confluent re-endothelialization by EC seeding may reduce SMC proliferation, migration, or both.

Estradiol and endothelium

An alternative approach for the prevention of in-stent restenosis involves the use of a naturally occurring vasculoprotective hormone such as 17β-estradiol (Fig. 2). Estradiol is the most potent naturally occurring female hormone (Fig. 3). It is well known that premenopausal women have a low

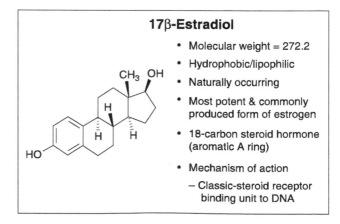

Figure 2
Chemistry of 17β-estradiol.

17β-Estradiol: Low Toxicity
• Circulates free / bound to plasma proteins
• Metabolized in liver
• Excreted in urine/bile
• Half-life 12-14 hours
• Low acute toxicity
– oral, intraperitoneal, intra-coronary, sublingual, subcutaneous & intravenous

Figure 3
Pharmacology of 17β-estradiol.

incidence of coronary heart disease (22). Estradiol is known to have pleomorphic properties. It has antiatherogenic, anti-inflammatory, and antioxidant properties as well as a wide therapeutic window.

Many experimental studies have demonstrated that estradiol has a vasculoprotective effect that is mediated via a number of cellular mechanisms (23). In particular, estradiol can inhibit SMC proliferation and migration (24),accelerate re-endothelialization (25), and restore normal endothelial function following balloon arterial injury (26,27). Inhibition of neointimal proliferation and accelerated re-endothelialization and function, with the local injection of 17β-estradiol following balloon angioplasty in a porcine model was initially reported (26). In another study, no vasoconstrictive response to acetylcholine was detected in injured arteries treated with 17β-estradiol compared to the control (27). Recent animal data suggest that local delivery of 17β-estradiol, either via an infusioncatheter or an impregnated one on a stent, inhibits neointimal proliferation without affecting endothelial repair and function (26–29). In addition, for a similar injury score, it has been shown that 17β-estradiol decreased the neointimal thickness in a stented artery. To date, the safety and efficacy of the 17β-estradiol eluting stent system on neointimal proliferation in human coronaries has not been reported. 17β-estradiol has a low molecular weight, is hydrophobic, and lipophilic making it pharmacokinetically suitable for loading on a stent delivery system.

Estradiol may improve vascular healing, reduce SMC migration and proliferation, and promote local angiogenesis. Indeed, several animal and human studies have demonstrated the protective effect of estrogen on coronary circulation (30–32). Estrogen not only appears to have a beneficial effect on lipids, but also stimulates NO production by ECs, as well as inhibits expression of the proto-oncogene, c-*myc*, the activity of which is implicated in the development of intimal hyperplasia (31,32).

Some of the mechanisms for the rapid effects of 17β-estradiol on vascular cells were recently elucidated (33,34). It was observed that 17β-estradiol rapidly increases proliferation of ECs and their migration through rapid upregulation of mitogen-activated protein kinases while decreasing the same events in SMC. These regulatory effects were abrogated by the use of estrogen receptor (ER) antagonists, tamoxifen (Tam), 4-OH-tamoxifen, or Raloxifen (Ral) (33). More recently, it was demonstrated using an antisense strategy that these effects of 17β-estradiol on EC were mediated through ERα, whereas the effects on SMC were mediated via ERβ (34).

Based on these data, we conducted a study to determine the effects of a 17β-estradiol-eluting stent on neointimal formation in a high-injury porcine coronary model (29). Our study showed that 17β-estradiol-eluting PC-coated stents (Abbott/ Biocompatibles) were associated with a 40% reduction in neointimal formation without affecting endothelial regeneration. This approach could have a potential clinical benefit in the prevention and treatment of in-stent restenosis.

Human clinical experiences

First in-human study: the estrogen and stents to eliminate restenosis-1 trial

The first human experience with a 17β-estradiol-eluting stent was recently published (35). The Estrogen and Stents to Eliminate Restenosis (EASTER) trial was a single-center feasibility study testing 17β-estradiol-eluting BiodivYsio stents in 30 patients with de novo coronary lesions. The purpose of the EASTER study was to evaluate the feasibility of 17β-estradiol-eluting stents to inhibit restenosis in humans.

This was a prospective trial of patients who were scheduled to undergo elective percutaneous intervention for single, short (<18 mm in length), de novo lesions in native coronary arteries of 2.5 to 3.5 mm in diameter. All patients received aspirin (325 mg) at least 12 hours before the procedure (and 325 mg/day, indefinitely), and clopidogrel (300 mg at least six hours prior to stent implantation and 75 mg daily continued for 60 days). All patients underwent angiographic and intravascular ultrasound (IVUS) follow-up at six months. The patients returned for clinical visits at 30 days and 6 and 12 months in which physicians were blinded to the angiographic and ultrasonographic data. All patients were enrolled after protocol approval by the Medical Ethics Committee of the Institute Dante Pazzanese of Cardiology in Sao Paulo, Brazil.

The mean age of the patients was 61 ± 12 years. A total of 21 patients (70%) were males. Systemic hypertension was the most frequent coronary risk factor, involving 15 patients (49%), followed by smoking in 10 patients (33%), and dyslipidemia in 8 (27%), whereas only three patients (10%) were diabetics. Eleven patients (37%) had a prior history of myocardial infarction (MI). The procedure was successful in all patients. There were no in-hospital events and no elevation

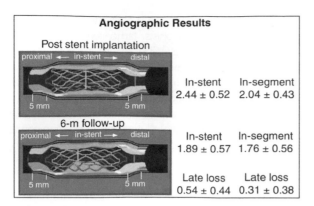

Angiographic Results

Post stent implantation

proximal ← in-stent → distal

5 mm   5 mm

	In-stent	In-segment
	2.44 ± 0.52	2.04 ± 0.43

6-m follow-up

proximal ← in-stent → distal

5 mm   5 mm

	In-stent	In-segment
	1.89 ± 0.57	1.76 ± 0.56
	Late loss	Late loss
	0.54 ± 0.44	0.31 ± 0.38

Figure 4
Clinical follow-up.

of cardiac enzymes postprocedure. One patient underwent target lesion revascularization at six-month follow-up due to symptomatic angiographic restenosis. All other patients were asymptomatic at six-month angiographic follow-up. There were no stent thromboses or other major cardiovascular events [including death, MI, stroke, or target vessel revascularization (TVR)] up to 12 months clinical follow-up (Fig. 4). The angiographic results are presented in the table (Fig. 5). Mean lesion length was 9.1 ± 2.4 mm. Two patients developed in-stent restenosis (>50% diameter stenosis). One patient with a 60% lesion was asymptomatic with a negative noninvasive stress test and did not undergo repeat revascularization. There was no restenosis at the stent edge segments, and the in-segment late loss was 0.34 mm.

By IVUS, the neointimal hyperplasia volume amounted to 32.3 ± 16.4 mm³ with the stent volume of 143.7 ± 43.7 mm³, resulting in a mean neointimal volume obstruction of 23.5 ± 12.5%. None of the patients had ≥50% volume obstruction by IVUS (Fig. 6). There was no evidence of stent malapposition or echolucent images ("black hole").

This study represents the first human experience with 17β-estradiol-eluting stents for the prevention of restenosis. The clinical outcome that was maintained up to one-year follow-up suggests that the use of 17β-estradiol-eluting, PC-coated stents is safe and feasible, with a low incidence of restenosis and without associated local or systemic toxicity. The angiographic and IVUS follow-up results at six months demonstrated a low amount of intimal hyperplasia and late-loss, which compared favorably with previous studies testing the same PC-coated

Vessel (mm³)	268 ± 66
Stent (mm³)	147 ± 43.6
Lumen (mm³)	115 ± 41.9
Intimal hyperplasia (mm³)	32.6 ± 14.7
% obstruction	23 ± 11%

Figure 5
Quantitative coronary angiography at six months.

	n = 30
Death	0%
Q wave MI	0%
TLR	3.3%
Non-TLR (other vessel)	3.3%
Event-free survival	93.4%

Figure 6
Intravascular ultrasound results at six months. *Abbreviations*: MI, myocardial infarction; TLR, target lesion revascularization.

BiodivYsio stents without estradiol (Figs. 7 and 8). Only 3.3% (1 of 30) patients required TVR. In addition, there was minimal in-segment late-loss and no edge restenosis. These early results may reflect an improved vessel healing after stenting, which would be clinically very desirable.

Nevertheless, neointimal proliferation was not completely abolished by estradiol-eluting stents. It is possible that drug dosing, absorption, and elution kinetics, may have influenced our results and partially limited the antiproliferative effects of estradiol. Estradiol elution from "hand"-loaded PC-coated stents is only carried out within the first 24-hour interval. Nonetheless, the amount of intimal hyperplasia detected by IVUS in the present study compares favorably with bare metal stents (36), suggesting an antirestenotic effect of estradiol in spite of the suboptimal stent elution.

The loading of the 17β-estradiol onto the stent was performed in the catheterization laboratory just prior to stent insertion. Although a strict loading protocol was utilized, this process was still a manual method, and a lack of good reproducibility by this technique could result in varying doses of the hormone being loaded on the stent. Using this "manual" loading process is also not practical and preloaded stents would eliminate this problem. Theoretically, preloaded stents with different pharmacokinetics, higher-drug doses, and more homogeneous and programmed drug release may further improve the results observed in this study. A second phase of EASTER using a preloaded 17β-estradiol-eluting stents was recently completed in Italy and the results are pending.

Randomized clinical study: the estradiol to cure restenosis trial

The Estradiol to Cure Restenosis (ESTRACURE) trial is a randomized clinical trial of 360 patients undergoing stent implantation evaluating the efficacy and safety of local 17β-estradiol delivery prior to stent implantation to reduce angiographic late luminal loss and restenosis. The hypothesis of this prospective, randomized, multicenter trial is that a single local administration of 17β-estradiol will improve vascular healing and reduce late

EASTER

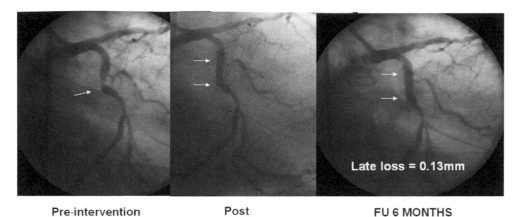

Pre-intervention   Post   FU 6 MONTHS

Figure 7
Six month angiography after 17β-estradiol-eluting stent implantation in circumflex artery demonstrates late loss of only 0.13 mm.
Abbreviations: EASTER, estrogen and stents to eliminate restenosis; FU, follow-up.

loss after stenting. The study will randomize patients undergoing stent implantation to control low or high 17β-estradiol doses delivered locally, using the REMEDY™ catheter (Boston Scientific, Natick, Massachusetts, U.S.A.). Clinical follow-up and a six-month angiographic evaluation will be obtained. This ongoing study will confirm the feasibility of a prohealing approach to vascular stenting and, if proven successful, may lead to a new paradigm in the field of DESs.

Future studies

The clinical utility of this approach will depend on the results of these initial clinical trials evaluating 17β-estradiol and the outcomes of current DESs in higher-risk patients. Speculations about the clinical results are that an improved healing and re-endothelialization, although not completely abolishing neointima formation, will allow a controlled

regrowth and more importantly a better stent passivation with a reduced risk of late thrombosis or vascular toxicity. Very recently, long DESs were associated with a 70-fold increase in the occurrence of intraprocedural stent thrombosis (37). This very rare event with bare metal stents ($<$0.01%) occurred during elective implantation of a sirolimus-eluting stent in 0.7% (5 of 670) patients. Stent length was the only variable by univariate analysis to be associated with intraprocedural stent thrombosis. More data will be required to confirm this observation and the potential clinical impact of this association. Meanwhile, particular attention is recommended when using long DESs.

The possibilities for a prohealing approach using 17β-estradiol remains of clinical relevance either as monotherapy or as adjunctive therapy. The combination therapy approach could be an effective way to decrease the dose or potential negative effects of a given antiproliferative compound and combine the beneficial effects of 17β-estradiol to optimize vascular healing.

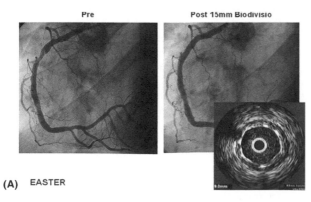

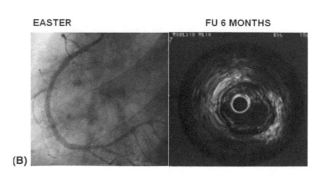

Figure 8
(A and B) Angiographic and intravascular ultrasound follow-up at six months after stent in proximal portion of right coronary artery.
Abbreviation: FU, follow-up.

The growing clinical interest of detection and treatment of the vulnerable plaques or patients opens a new area of investigation. The promise of using 17β-estradiol on a DES platform as a prohealing strategy could potentially improve the clinical outcome in such high-risk populations. Because of the beneficial effects of 17β-estradiol on vascular cells, this approach could offer patients a safer method of plaque stabilization.

Conclusion

We are still in the early phases of investigating the use of DES as a platform for local delivery of prohealing compounds. Because 17β-estradiol is a naturally occurring substance, ERs are present in human endothelial and SMC and numerous beneficial effects on vasculature have already been demonstrated. Thus, utilization of this local therapeutic approach remains one of the most promising and clinically relevant approaches at this time. Current investigations will provide important data about the safety and potential of this technology to prevent restenosis. Whether results similar to the EASTER trial will be reproduced in a larger population with more complex lesion morphology in a randomized trial remains to be tested. The ESTRACURE trial will add important information about dosing and long-term late loss in a randomized population. These ongoing investigations and future experimental work will confirm whether vasculoprotective agents such as 17β-estradiol can provide an alternative approach to antiproliferative agents in the prevention of restenosis and vessel passivation.

References

1 Serruys PW, de Jaegere P, Kiemeneij F, et al. A comparison of balloon-expandable-stent implantation with balloon angioplasty in patients with coronary artery disease. Benestent Study Group. N Engl J Med 1994; 331:489–495.

2 Erbel R, Haude M, Hopp HW, et al. Coronary-artery stenting compared with balloon angioplasty for restenosis after initial balloon angioplasty. Restenosis Stent Study Group. N Engl J Med 1998; 339:1672–1678.

3 Fischman DL, Leon MB, Baim DS, et al. A randomized comparison of coronary-stent placement and balloon angioplasty in the treatment of coronary artery disease. Stent Restenosis Study Investigators. N Engl J Med 1994; 331:496–501.

4 Savage MP, Fischman DL, Schatz RA, et al. Coronary intervention in the diabetic patient: improved outcome following stent implantation compared with balloon angioplasty. Clin Cardiol 2002; 25:213–217.

5 Sousa JE, Costa MA, Sousa AG, et al. Two-year angiographic and intravascular ultrasound follow-up after implantation of sirolimus-eluting stents in human coronary arteries. Circulation 2003; 107:381–383.

6 Grube E, Silber S, Hauptmann KE, et al. TAXUS I: six- and twelve-month results from a randomized, double-blind trial on a slow-release paclitaxel-eluting stent for de novo coronary lesions. Circulation 2003; 107:38–42.

7 Tanabe K, Degertekin M, Regar E, Ligthart JM, van der Giessen WJ, Serruys PW. No delayed restenosis at 18 months after implantation of sirolimus-eluting stent. Catheter Cardiovasc Interv 2002; 57:65–68.

8 Ross R. The pathogenesis of atherosclerosis: A perspective for the 1990s. Nature 1993; 362:801–809.

9 Lijnen HR, Collen D. Endothelium in hemostasis and thrombosis. Prog Cardiovasc Dis 1997; 39:343–350.

10 Vanhoutte PM, Mombouli JV. Vascular endothelium: Vasoactive mediators. Prog Cardiovasc Dis 1996; 39:229–238.

11 Van Belle E, Christophe B, Takayaki A, Isner JM. Endothelial regrowth after arterial injury: From vascular repair to therapeutics. Cardiovasc Res 1998; 38:54–68.

12 Myers PR, Webel R, Thondapu V, et al. Restenosis is associated with decreased coronary artery nitric oxide synthase. Int J Cardiol 1996; 55:183–191.

13 Hamon M, Vallet B, Bauters C, et al. Long-term oral administration of L-arginine reduces intimal thickening and enhances neoendothelium-dependent acetylcholine-induced relaxation after arterial injury. Circulation 1994; 90:1357–1362.

14 Janssens S, Flaherty D, Nong Z, et al. Human endothelial nitric oxide synthase gene transfer inhibits vascular smooth muscle cell proliferation and neointima formation after balloon injury in rats. Circulation 1998; 97:1274–1281.

15 Garg UC, Hasssid A. Nitric oxide-generating vasodilators and 8-bromo-cyclic-guanosine monophosphate inhibit mitogenesis and proliferation of cultured rat vascular smooth muscle cells. J Clin Invest 1989; 83:1774–1777.

16 McBride W, Lange RA, Hillis LD. Restenosis after successful coronary angioplasty. Pathophysology and prevention. N Engl J Med 1988; 318:1734–1737.

17 Grewe PH, Deneke T, Holt SK, et al. Scanning electron microscopic analysis of vessel wall reactions after coronary stenting. Z Kardiol 2000; 89(1):21–27.

18 Asahara TC, Tsurumi Y, Kearney M, et al. Accelerated restitution of endothelial integrity and endothelium dependent function following rh VEGF$_{165}$ gene transfer. Circulation 1996; 94:3291–3302.

19 van Beusekom HM, Whelan DM, Hofma SH, et al. Long-term endothelial dysfunction is more pronounced after stenting than after balloon angioplasty in porcine coronary arteries. J Am Coll Cardiol 1998; 32(4):1109–1117.

20 Meurice T, Vallet B, Bauters C, et al. Role of endothelial cells in restenosis after coronary angioplasty. Fundam Clin Pharm 1996; 10:234–242.

21 Fantidis P, Fernandez-Ortiz A, Aragoncillo P, et al. Effect of cAMP on the function of endothelial cells and fibromuscular proliferation after the injury of the carotid and coronary arteries in a porcine model. Rev Esp Cardiol 2001; 54(8): 981–989.

22 Lerner DJ, Kannel WB. Patterns of coronary heart disease morbidity and mortality in the sexes: a 26-year follow-up of the Framingham population. Am Heart J 1986; 111:383–390.

23 White MM, Zamudio S, Stevens T, et al. Estrogen, progesterone, and vascular ractivity: potential cellular mechanisms. Endocr Rev 1995; 16:739–751.

24 Dai-Do D, Espinosa E, Liu G, et al. 17 beta-estradiol inhibits roliferation and migration of human ciated with reduced neointimal formation but no delay in vascular repair in a porcine coronary model. Catheter Cardiovasc Interv 2002; 57:266–271.

25 Brouchet L, Krust A, Dupont S, Chambon P, Bayard F, Arnal JF. Stradiolaccelerates reendothelialization in mouse carotid artery through estrogen receptor-alpha but not estrogen receptor-beta. Circulation 2001; 103:423–428.

26 Chandrasekhar B, Tanguay JF. Local delivery of 17-beta-estradiol decreases neointimal hyperplasia after coronary angioplasty in a porcine model. J Am Coll Cardiol 2000; 36:1972–1978.

27 Chandrasekar B, Nattel S, Tanguay JF. Coronary artery endothelial protection after local delivery of 17beta-estradiol during balloon angioplasty in a porcine model: a potential new pharmacologic approach to improve endothelial function. J Am Coll Cardiol 2001; 38:1570–1576.

28 Krasinski K, Spyridopoulos I, Asahara T, van der Zee R, Isner JM, Losordo DW. Estradiol accelerates functional endothelial recovery after arterial injury. Circulation 1997; 95:1768–1772.

29 New G, Moses JW, Roubin GS, et al. Estrogen-eluting, phosphorylcholine-coated stent implantation is associated with reduced neointimal formation but no delay in vascular repair in a porcine coronary model, Cathet Cardiovasc Intervent 2002; 57:266–271.

30 Herrington DM, Reboussin DM, Brosnihan KB, et al. Effects of estrogen replacement on the progression of coronary-artery atherosclerosis. N Engl J Med 2000; 343: 522–529.

31 Kishnankutty S, Chiu T, Mullen W, et al. Mechanisms of estrogen-induced vasodilation: in vivo studies in canine coronary conductance and resistance arteries. J Am Coll Cardiol 1995; 26:807–814.

32 White CR, Shelton J, Chen SJ, et al. Estrogen restores endothelial cell function in an experimental model of vascular injury. Circulation 1997; 96:1624–1630.

33 Geraldes P, Sirois MG, Bernatchez PN, Tanguay JF. Estrogen regulation of endothelial and smooth muscle cell migration and proliferation: role of p38 and p42/44 mitogen-activated protein kinase. Arterioscler Thromb Vasc Biol 2002; 22: 1585–1590.

34 Geraldes P, Sirois MG, Tanguay JF. Specific contribution of estrogen receptors on mitogen-activated protein kinase pathways and vascular cell activation. Circ Res 2003; 93:399–405.

35 Abizaid A, Albertal M, Costa MA, et al. First human experience with the 17β-E stradiol-eluting stent: The Estrogen And Stents To Eliminate Restenosis (EASTER) Trial J Am Coll Cardiol 2004; 43:1118–1121.

36 Costa MA, Sabate M, Kay IP, et al. Three-dimensional intravascular ultrasonic volumetric quantification of stent recoil and neointimal formation of two new generation tubular stents. Am J Cardiol 2000; 85:135–139.

37 Chieffo A, Bonizzoni E, Orlic D, et al. Intraprocedural stent thrombosis during implantation of sirolimus-eluting stents. Circulation 2004; 109:2732–2736.

30

Vascular endothelial growth factor

Neil Swanson and Anthony Gershlick

Introduction

Vascular endothelial growth factor (VEGF) is a much-studied cytokine active in the growth and maintenance of blood vessels. This occurs in fetal development and normal growth. In clinical terms, it is of interest with regards to its key role in supporting the neoangiogenesis, which is necessary for the growth of solid tumors. Extensive research has been directed in understanding this role and attempting to block the actions of VEGF in cancers. VEGF research interest has also been active with regard to rheumatoid arthritis and proliferative diabetic retinopathy. This chapter will not deal further with such other aspects of VEGF's properties.

In the cardiovascular area, it has been studied for its potential to enhance neovascularization of ischemic tissue, including the myocardium, particularly when delivered locally. By virtue of promoting endothelial cell growth, it is also involved in the recovery of a normal, functional endothelium at the site of vascular injury, for example, after percutaneous coronary intervention. Finally, VEGF appears to have a role in the microvasculature of the atherosclerotic plaque.

Structure and regulation of vascular endothelial growth factor

VEGF is a heparin-binding, homodimeric peptide found in vivo as a glycoprotein. It comprises a family of peptides (VEGF-A to -E) of which VEGF-A is the most thoroughly studied. VEGF-A (more often called just VEGF) occurs in five isoforms of 121, 145, 165, 189, and 206 amino acids. VEGF-C is also known as VEGF-2. VEGF is almost exclusively bound by endothelial cells, although receptors for VEGF have also been found in human atherosclerotic artery tissue (1). This suggests that VEGF is not solely active on the endothelial cell and may have effects on other cells within the vascular wall.

VEGF promotes endothelial cell growth and stimulates endothelial cell production of factors such as nitric oxide and prostacycline. VEGF is a chemotactic factor and increases vascular permeability, causing edema. VEGF inhibits apoptosis by the upregulation of apoptosis inhibitors. All of these properties, which are illustrated in Figure 1, are mediated by nitric oxide-dependent pathways.

The release of VEGF from cells is under the influence of a number of humoral, chemical, and physical factors. Cytokines and hormones including interleukin (IL)-6, insulin-like growth factor (IGF)-1, endothelin-1, fibroblast growth factor (FGF)-4, transforming growth factor β (TGFβ), platelet-derived growth factor (PDGF), angiotensin-II, basic FGF (bFGF), and tumor necrosis factor (TNF)-α have all been shown to regulate the expression of VEGF or its receptors.

Chemical conditions have shown effects on VEGF production in cardiac myocytes. Principally, hypoxia stimulates VEGF production. VEGF is often found in the relatively ischemic and hypoxic microenvironment of the interior of a solid tumour. A transcription promoter for the VEGF gene has been identified that upregulates VEGF synthesis in response to hypoxia-inducible factor (HIF-1) (2). HIF-1 is also responsible for the upregulation of erythropoietin, emphasizing the close functional similarities between the angiogenic and hematopoietic growth factors.

Reactive oxygen species and oxidized-low density cholesterol (LDL), which promote the progression of atherosclerotic plaques, potentiate the production of VEGF.

Electrical stimulation of skeletal muscle, either directly or via chronic motor nerve stimulation demonstrate increased VEGF production that leads to angiogenesis in vivo.

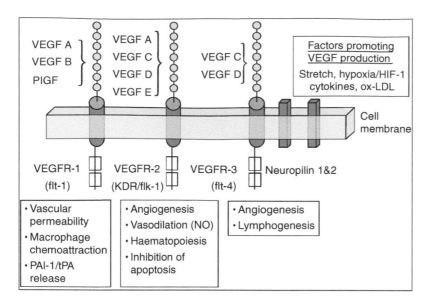

Figure 1

Diagrammatic representation of actions of VEGF and receptors. *Abbreviations:* HIF-1, hypoxia-inducible factor; LPA, lysophosphatidic acid; ox-LDL, oxidized low-density; PAI, plasminogen activation inhibitor; PlGF, placental growth factor; VEGF, vascular endothelial growth factor.

The effects of VEGF that have led to most research interest in the field of cardiovascular disease can be broadly divided in two categories: re-endothelialization and angiogenesis.

Vascular endothelial growth factor delivery to promote re-endothelialization

Percutaneous coronary intervention (PCI) inevitably causes extensive denudation of the vascular endothelium at the stenosis site. In animal models of stent placement, re-endothelialization begins to occur in the first two to seven days postplacement. Full re-endothelialization of the stent takes three or four weeks. This process has been called stent passivation. It is thought that a similar or longer time course occurs in humans, although this has been difficult to quantify from the rarity of available autopsy specimens from patients' poststent insertion (3). In animals, endothelial dysfunction is seen up to three months poststenting (4).

The loss of the protective endothelial lining of the artery is a stimulus to the cell proliferation that is typical of the restenotic lesion. Correspondingly, it may be that accelerated recovery of the endothelium might reduce the complications that result from endothelial loss or dysfunction. The use of a number of locally delivered agents to test this hypothesis have been reported positively including prostacyclin synthase, hepatocyte growth factor, estrogen, and thrombospondin blockade. VEGF has also been widely investigated for this potential. Endogenous VEGF and VEGFR-2 receptors begin to be expressed in increasing amounts within 48 hours of an angioplasty injury. The effects of VEGF on the restenosis process are complex, involving the clotting process, as well as re-endothelialization.

In endothelial cell cultures, vascular endothelial growth factor (VEGF) produces nitric oxide and PGI_2, wherein both inhibit platelet aggregation and smooth muscle cell growth. VEGF may therefore have antithrombotic properties. VEGF increases the expression and activation of urokinase and tissue-type plasminogen activator, promoting the generation of the thrombolytic enzyme, plasmin (5). In vivo, reduced clot formation has been seen on stents implanted in rabbit iliac arteries when washed with VEGF by a channel balloon system (6).

Late thrombosis following intervention and the role of the endothelium

An intact endothelium acts as a physical barrier to platelets adhesion. As well as causing vessel thrombosis, platelets produce factors that stimulate smooth muscle cells, leading to restenosis.

The relatively high incidence (up to 11% of patients) of late stent thrombosis (i.e., more than 30 days postprocedure) in patients receiving vascular brachytherapy has been attributed to delayed re-endothelialization. This technique is rarely used now in the era of drug-eluting stents, but the experience of such high complication rates related to impaired endothelial function has fueled ongoing anxieties about the long-term safety of the use of drug-eluting stent (DES).

Late stent thrombosis (LST) after the use of DES is a rare complication. The SIRTAX (7) trial has shown LST rates of 0.5% to 0.9% using DES. A case series (8) of four patients with LST who had stopped taking aspirin many months after DES implant has been reported. Registry data of DES use (9) reported a 0.7% late thrombosis rate, half of which patients died as a consequence.

Several meta-analyses of DES trials have examined this further with conflicting results. Indolfi et al. (10) have reported a nonsignificant trend in favor of using DES in terms of lower stent thrombosis. Bavry et al. (11), looking only at trials of paclitaxel-eluting stents (PES), found no difference in the incidence of thrombosis, while Katritsis et al. (12) found a nonsignificant trend favoring base metal stent (BMS) in lowering stent thrombosis rates. The Reality trial (13) comparing the two main DES platforms found LST rates of 0.3% for sirolimus-eluting stents (SES), 0.9% for PES, $P = 0.3$, suggesting that there may be a differential risk in the development of LST from one DES to another.

The reasons for any increase in the occurrence of LST in other DES trials compared with bare metal stent (BMS) are unclear. The strongest predictor found by Iakovou et al. (9) in their study for the development of LST was premature discontinuation of antiplatelet medications. The requirement for prolonged potent antiplatelet treatment is because of the possible inhibition of re-endothelialization after DES use as a result of direct inhibition of endothelial cell growth by the antirestenotic agents delivered by the stent.

Re-endothelialization

To promote re-endothelialization, VEGF has been administered in animal studies by a variety of means, using varying isoforms of the VEGF family either in protein form or as a plasmid.

Local infusion

Locally delivered VEGF infusion appeared to accelerate re-endothelialization of damaged arteries in the rat carotid artery (14). A 30-minute infusion of VEGF into the carotid artery at the site of balloon injury caused superior re-endothelialization and reduced intimal hyperplasia. Antibodies against VEGF inhibited this effect on re-endothelialization (15).

These reported findings have not been confirmed by other groups. Six-hour, two- and six-week infusions of VEGF into the aortic arch of rats with denuded endothelium in the carotid artery or aorta showed no evidence of endothelial regrowth, nor indeed the presence of any VEGFR-2 receptors in large vessels (16). These include the carotid vessel that Asahara et al. (14) had reported as demonstrating endothelial recovery. Furthermore, in the porcine restenosis model bolus, delivery of 1 mg of VEGF as a five-minute local infusion into the coronary arteries failed to demonstrate any inhibition of restenosis (17).

Balloon-delivered vascular endothelial growth factor

Locally delivered VEGF-A protein was used in a rabbit hindlimb stent model. A clear increase in the rate of re-endothelialization was shown (18). In further studies, naked plasmid coding for VEGF-A was administered locally using a hydrogel-coated balloon. Passivation of the stent occurred quickly and completely in the rabbits given VEGF DNA, associated with a decreased incidence of both intimal hyperplasia and thrombus formation on the stent. Not only was endothelial integrity restored, but also the regenerated endothelium was functional, restoring vasomotor responsiveness and thromboresistance (19).

Hiltunen et al. (20) have reported balloon catheter delivery of VEGF-C plasmid after angioplasty injury in vivo. They found a significant reduction in intima–media ratio of the vessels compared with controls. They also studied the effects of VEGF-A plasmid in the same model, but found no benefit. VEGF-D plasmid has also been infused into balloon-injured rabbit aortae. A nitric oxide-dependent significant reduction in intima/media ratio was observed at 14 days (21).

Stent-based delivery of vascular endothelial growth factor

A study deployed phVEGF-2 (VEGF-C) plasmid-coated, polymer stents and uncoated stents in iliac arteries of normocholesterolemic and hypercholesterolemic rabbits. Re-endothelialization in phVEGF stents at 10 days was significantly greater than in control stents (98.7 ± 1% vs. 79.0 ± 6%, $P < 0.01$). At three months, cross-sectional area was significantly greater in the VEGF. Transfected areas showed a 2.4-fold increase in nitric oxide production, suggesting functional recovery of the endothelium (22).

VEGF protein can be absorbed into the polymer coating of a stent. About 18.5 ± 4.1 μg of VEGF has been shown to be passively absorbed into a polymer-coated stent (23). Elution of VEGF from these stents follows a biexponential release pattern with 20% of initial VEGF load persisting on the stent for nine days. In an ex vivo model, using stented internal mammary artery tissue in a perfusion circuit, 11 ± 6.8% of the initial VEGF loaded onto the stents was seen in the tissue after 24 hours perfusion. About 12.3 ± 1.7% remained on the stents. VEGF-loaded stents were effective in significantly promoting endothelial cell growth.

These VEGF-eluting stents were tested in vivo in a rabbit iliac artery model. After seven days, median clot demonstrated was 12.5 mg in control stents versus 0 mg [$P = 0.0142$; 95% confidence interval (CI) 8.49, 55.99] in VEGF stents. Quantifiable re-endothelialization was poor in both groups (Fig. 2), with no significant differences between them. Neointimal cross-sectional area at 28 days showed no statistically significant differences (Table 1) (24).

The VEGF-eluting stent did not lead to the expected rapid re-endothelialization, which may well explain the lack of effect in reducing restenosis. The reduction in thrombosis may be because of the antithrombotic effects of VEGF discussed

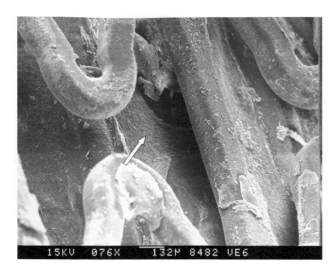

Figure 2

Scanning electron micrograph of a vascular endothelial growth factor (VEGF)-eluting stent in situ in rabbit iliac artery. The artery and stent have been split longitudinally and gently prised open. Endothelialization between stent struts is noted (*arrowed*).

Vascular endothelial growth factor delivery to promote angiogenesis

Vascular endothelial growth factor has mitogenic effects on the vascular endothelium via the VEGFR-2 receptor. VEGF in normal arteries is not expressed in detectable quantities. In angioplastied vessels, it is expressed and correlates with the adventitial angiogenesis that causes the growth of *vasa vasorum* (26). These new vessels may be of importance in the repair of the damaged vessel. It is also detectable in coronary sinus blood samples from patients with complete coronary artery occlusions. VEGF levels in patients with severe stenosis are much lower. It is felt that this may represent the natural angiogenic response to an ischemic stimulus in the total occlusion group (27). Similarly, VEGF may have a role in the neovascularization of atherosclerotic plaques (28).

Exogenous VEGF may stimulate the growth of new collateral vessels in ischemic areas of the myocardium. A single, intra-arterial bolus of VEGF promoted collateral growth in rabbit hindlimb ischemia (29). Other workers have tried to replicate these results but have found that while VEGF plasmid injection was correlated with increased angiogenesis, no actual VEGF could be detected in the tissues (30).

In pigs, high dose of VEGF delivered extraluminally after coronary occlusion caused higher blood flow in the ischemic territory (31). In a canine model of chronic coronary ischemia, VEGF showed enhanced collateral vessel density and blood flow when delivered as a local infusion, although not when administered systemically (32).

VEGF has been delivered by injecting it directly into the ischemic muscle and showed a dose-dependent improvement of collateral growth in the rabbit model (33). Intramuscular injections of VEGF plasmid showed synthesis of VEGF up to two weeks following the procedure despite only 2% of cells having incorporated the plasmid (34). Conflicting with these results is the finding that injection of an entirely unrelated gene into the myocardium of pigs also shows an upregulation of VEGF expression (35). It may be that merely

before. Such an effect might make these stents less thrombogenic than the current clinically used ones. VEGF may be a suitable agent for local delivery by stent in patients in whom a high risk of stent thrombosis may be anticipated, including patients with small vessel stenoses.

Genetically modified, VEGF-producing, immortalized endothelial cells (ECs) have been coated onto a stent (25), although the efficacy of this has not been reported. Cell seeding has several disadvantages. It requires delicate handling and would require harvesting and culturing ECs from the patient prior to stent placement. The use of cultured cells raises the possibility of introducing infection into the coronary circulation. It is unclear to what extent ECs will remain on a stent in vivo or how long they will remain viable. The long-term effects of genetically altered cells are unknown. The use of cell seeding is not currently practical in human trials.

Table 1 Digital morphometry of cross-sections of stented iliac arteries at 28 days using vascular endothelial growth factor and control polymer-coated stents

	Area (mm²)		Thickness (μm)	
Intima-VEGF	2.4 ± 1.8	P = 0.81	163 ± 50	P = 0.26
-control	2.2 ± 0.9		189 ± 39	
Media-VEGF	0.9 ± 0.3	P = 0.07	93 ± 28	P = 0.1
-control	1.2 ± 0.3		117 ± 27	

Note: Results are mean ± SD. No significant differences are seen between the two groups, including the intima/media ratio.

Abbreviation: VEGF, vascular endothelial growth factor.

Source: From Ref. 24.

the trauma of injection is itself a stimulus for VEGF production, undermining the scientific rationale for performing the treatment. VEGF appears to stimulate the activity of circulating endothelial progenitor cells (EPCs). In the mouse hindlimb-ischemia model, EPCs transfected with the VEGF gene were administered and showed an improvement in neovascularization (36).

Clinical trials of vascular endothelial growth factor

Clinical trials of VEGF use (Table 2) have looked at its potential to promote angiogenesis, both peripherally and in the ischemic myocardium. The clinical point in using VEGF has been to try and treat patients with refractory, severe ischemic heart disease not amenable to intervention or surgery to produce new collaterals perfusing the ischemic myocardium. VEGF has also been used in a limited fashion to test the potential to reduce restenosis by virtue of accelerating re-endothelialization.

A small study of plasmid-derived VEGF showed collateral vessel growth and improved outcome in patients with critical limb ischemia (37). In the regional angiogenesis with VEGF (RAVE) study, AdVEGF-121 was injected into the skeletal muscle of the lower extremity and safety and efficacy were compared with placebo control in patients with unilateral, severe, disabling intermittent claudication. No symptomatic or objective evidence of clinical benefit were reported at 26-week follow-up (38).

The VIVA (VEGF in Ischemia for Vascular Angiogenesis) trial gave patients with untreatable severe ischemia VEGF-165, most of it by systemic delivery, the rest by intracoronary bolus delivery. No benefit was seen in the functional status (exercise time or reduction of angina) of the treated patients over controls despite some signs of improved perfusion (39). A strong, sustained placebo effect was seen. The route of administration may have meant that a poor local concentration of the drug was achieved. The amounts of drug administered were significantly less than the doses per kilogram found to be effective in animal models.

Conversely, direct application of VEGF DNA through a mini left anterior thoracotomy did show functional improvement in a very small group of treated patients (40). An adenovirus vector to deliver VEGF-121 cDNA was administered by direct intramyocardial injection during surgery in patients with severe coronary artery disease. This phase I trial suggested a subjective benefit for the treatment although no statistically significant improvement in symptoms related to augmented angiogenesis occurred (41). A study using VEGF-165 plasmid delivery into the myocardium of inoperable coronary disease patients showed objective improvements in perfusion as well as subjective improvement in anginal symptoms in a small group of nonrandomized patients (42). A randomized, double-blind, placebo-controlled study has been reported in a small group of patients using percutaneous delivery to the ischemic myocardium of the VEGF plasmid. This study showed a reduction in anginal class in the VEGF group (43).

The phase II Randomized Evaluation of VEGF for Angiogenesis in Severe Coronary disease (REVASC) trial randomized 71 patients unsuitable for conventional

Table 2 Clinical trials of the use of vascular endothelial growth factor in cardiovascular disease. Of these trials, VIVA, RAVE, euroinject, and KAT were randomized, blinded studies

Trial	Method	Endpoint	Results
VIVA (39) (n = 178)	Systemic and i.c. bolus of VEGF-165	Anginal class, perfusion at four months	No improvement in perfusion
REVASC (44) (n = 71)	Direct intramyocardial injection of adVEGF-121	ST depression at six months	Significant reduction in ST depression and improved anginal class
Losordo et al. (43) (n = 19)	VEGF-C plasmid percutaneous intramyocardial	Exercise ability, anginal class	Reduction in angina, trend to improved exercise
Euroinject (45) (n = 80)	Intramyocardial VEGF plasmid via NOGA	Myocardial perfusion, wall motion at three months	No improvement in perfusion, but improved wall motion
KAT (47) (n = 103)	adVEGF locally	Restenosis at six months, myocardial perfusion	No reduction in restenosis, improved perfusion
Laitinen et al. (46) (n = 10)	Local coronary infusion of VEGF plasmid	Restenosis at six months	No benefit
RAVE (38) (n = 105)	adVEGF-121 direct intramuscular injection	Claudication, quality of life at six months	No benefit

Abbreviations: adVEGF, adenoviral delivered VEGF; KAT, kuopio angiogenesis trial; RAVE, regional angiogenesis with VEGF; REVASC, randomized evaluation of VEGF for angiogenesis in severe coronary; VEGF, vascular endothelial growth factor; VIVA, VEGF in ischemia for vascular angiogenesis.

revascularization to medical therapy or direct intramyocardial administration of AdVEGF-121 (adenoviral delivered VEGF plasmid) via left lateral thoracotomy. Time to 1 mm ST depression on exercise, the primary end point, and anginal class were significantly improved in the treatment group at 26 weeks. Four adverse events were associated with minithoracotomy. This study gives some objective evidence of benefit of VEGF therapy (44). The trial, inevitably, was not blinded, thus risking significant bias due to placebo effects from surgery.

In the Euroinject One phase II randomized, double-blind trial, 0.5 mg of phVEGF-165 was delivered directly into the ischemic myocardium of 80 inoperable patients, using the NOGA-MyoStar delivery system, At three months, myocardial stress perfusion defects did not differ significantly between groups. Compared with placebo, VEGF gene transfer did improve local wall motion abnormalities, assessed by contrast ventriculography ($P = 0.03$). Improvements in functional class classification of angina did not differ significantly between the groups. NOGA procedure-related adverse events occurred in five patients (45).

Local delivery of VEGF plasmid into human angioplastied coronaries has been reported by Laitinen et al. At six months, no improvement in restenosis was seen (46). This study was not performed in stented patients. It also used a local delivery balloon, which may cause intimal hyperplasia and so obscure any beneficial response from the drug.

The kuopio angiogenesis trial (KAT), a phase II clinical trial involving 103 patients, used adenovirus gene transfer for VEGF, mainly in stented patients. At six months, no detectable difference was seen in restenosis rates compared with controls, but there was a significant improvement in myocardial perfusion (47).

Adverse effects of locally delivered vascular endothelial growth factor

There are obstacles to be overcome before local VEGF delivery could be used in mainstream clinical practice. These obstacles include concerns over the safety of VEGF administration in humans.

The aspect of most concern to any future use of VEGF in clinical trials is the risk of death consequent to the therapy. Use of VEGF in clinical trials was temporarily halted in 2000 after the death of a young man in an angiogenesis trial. In this case, large amounts of the adenoviral vector used to deliver DNA coding for VEGF was accidentally injected into the patient's hepatic artery with fatal consequences (48). Ultimately, it was felt that this case was not directly because of the use of VEGF, but rather of the viral vector. No other deaths have yet been associated with VEGF use in humans,

but the total number of patients who have been treated with VEGF in any form is still significantly less than 1000.

VEGF is a potential carcinogen. Use of VEGF may have unwanted neoplastic effects either in the heart or at distal sites, although this has not yet been demonstrated in human subjects. Myoblasts genetically engineered to synthesise VEGF have been implanted into the heart in a mouse model. Most animals treated with VEGF either died or developed large tumors, usually of vascular origin (49). In cell culture, VEGF receptors have been demonstrated in uterine smooth muscle cells. VEGF receptors have also been demonstrated in human cell tumor lines including glioma, melanoma, and squamous cell carcinoma of the neck.

Species differences in response to VEGF may be significant. VEGF has been shown to reduce restenosis in a rabbit model. However, in a porcine model, workers have not shown a reduction in restenosis. Results in rats have been variable. If interspecies differences can be so great in the animal models, there is therefore no guarantee that VEGF will exert a positive effect in humans, regardless of any encouraging initial studies in animals. As discussed, the VIVA and KAT studies failed to show any clinically significant beneficial effects.

VEGF is not purely an endothelial cell growth factor. One group has reported the detection of KDR (VEGR-2) receptors on human smooth muscle cells in specimens of atherosclerotic arteries (1). The authors suggest that the atherosclerotic process itself is the stimulus for the production of VEGF receptors in the smooth muscle cells. It is not known whether these receptors have a significant effect in vivo. VEGF mRNA and VEGF receptors have been demonstrated in atherosclerotic, but not normal, human coronary arteries (28). VEGF may have the potential to accelerate atherosclerosis/destabilize plaques. The additional effects of VEGF (vascular permeability, chemoattraction for macrophages) may destabilize existing plaques leading to increased risk of plaque rupture and resulting acute coronary syndromes. There is some question of the appropriateness of using VEGF as an agent to reduce restenosis in atherosclerotic vessels like the diseased coronary. It is possible that, in the presence of atherosclerosis, VEGF promotes smooth muscle cell replication and might in fact exacerbate the growth of neointima.

Summary

Vascular endothelial growth factor in cardiovascular disease has a complex range of actions. It stimulates growth and function of endothelial cells, including the generation of new blood vessels. There are perceived advantages in promoting such an angiogenic potential in ischemic tissues and hypothetical benefits in terms of passivation of the site of percutaneous interventions.

There have been mixed results when these hypotheses have been tested in preclinical studies. In clinical trials of locally delivered VEGF, few clinically meaningful benefits have been demonstrated in many of these areas. Concerns regarding the safety of this mitogenic agent remain, including the potential to cause plaque destabilization.

VEGF has an undoubted important role in cardiovascular (dys)function. Despite the disappointments of the current clinical studies, it seems likely that its actions in cardiac pathology will still need to be understood and manipulated as part of the overall management of cardiovascular disease.

References

1. Belgore F, Blann A, Neil D, Ahmed AS, Lip GYH. Localisation of members of the vascular endothelial growth factor (VEGF) family and their receptors in human atherosclerotic arteries. J Clin Pathol 2004; 57(3):266–272.

2. Forsythe JA, Jiang BH, Iyer NV, et al. Activation of vascular endothelial growth factor gene transcription by hypoxia-inducible factor 1. Mol Cell Biol 1996; 16(9):4604–4613.

3. Grewe PH, Deneke T, Machraoui A, Barmeyer J, Muller KM. Acute and chronic tissue response to coronary stent implantation: pathologic findings in human specimen. J Am Coll Cardiol 2000; 35(1):157–163.

4. van Beusekom HM, Whelan DM, Hofma SH, et al. Long-term endothelial dysfunction is more pronounced after stenting than after balloon angioplasty in porcine coronary arteries. J Am Coll Cardiol 1998; 32(4):1109–1117.

5. Zachary I, Mathur A, Yla-Herttuala S, Martin J. Vascular protection: a novel nonangiogenic cardiovascular role for vascular endothelial growth factor. Arterioscler, Thromb Vasc Biol 2000; 20(6):1512–1520.

6. Van Belle E, Tio FO, Chen D, Maillard L, Kearney M, Isner JM. Passivation of metallic stents after arterial gene transfer of phVEGF165 inhibits thrombus formation and intimal thickening. J Am Coll Cardiol 1997; 29(6):1371–1379.

7. Windecker S, Remondino A, Eberli FR, et al. Sirolimus-eluting and paclitaxel-eluting stents for coronary revascularization. N Engl J Med 2005; 353(7):653–662.

8. McFadden E, Stabile E, Regar E, et al. Late thrombosis in drug-eluting coronary stents after discontinuation of antiplatelet therapy. Lancet 2004; 364(9444):1466–1467.

9. Iakovou I, Schmidt T, Bonizzoni E, et al. Incidence, predictors, and outcome of thrombosis after successful implantation of drug-eluting stents. JAMA 2005; 293(17):2126–2130.

10. Indolfi CF, Pavia MF, Angelillo IF. Drug-eluting stents versus bare metal stents in percutaneous coronary interventions (a meta-analysis). Am J Cardiol 2005; 95(10):1146–1152.

11. Bavry AA, Kumbhani DJ, Helton TJ, Bhatt DL. What is the risk of stent thrombosis associated with the use of paclitaxel-eluting stents for percutaneous coronary intervention? A meta-analysis. J Am Coll Cardiol 2005; 45(6):941–946.

12. Katritsis DG FAU—Karvouni E, Karvouni E FAU—Ioannidis J, Ioannidis JP. Meta-analysis comparing drug-eluting stents with bare metal stents. Am J Cardiol 2005; 95(5):640–643.

13. Morice MC. Reality 8 month results. Conference presentation at the American College of Cardiology Scientific Sessions 2005.

14. Asahara T, Bauters C, Pastore C, et al. Local delivery of vascular endothelial growth factor accelerates reendothelialization and attenuates intimal hyperplasia in balloon-injured rat carotid artery. Circulation 1995; 91(11):2793–2801.

15. Qi F, Sugihara T, Hattori Y, Yamamoto Y, Kanno M, Abe K. Functional and morphological damage of endothelium in rabbit ear artery following irradiation with cobalt-60. Br J Pharmacol 1998; 123(4):653–660.

16. Lindner V, Reidy MA. Expression of VEGF receptors in arteries after endothelial injury and lack of increased endothelial regrowth in response to VEGF. Arterioscler, Thromb Vasc Biol 1996; 16(11):1399–1405.

17. Belli G, Eccleston MC, Horrigan JG. Locally delivered vascular endothelial growth factor (VEGF) does not inhibit neointimal proliferation in the porcine restenosis model. J Am Coll Cardiol 1997; Abstracts:52A.

18. Van Belle E, Tio FO, Couffinhal T, Maillard L, Passeri J, Isner JM. Stent endothelialization. Time course, impact of local catheter delivery, feasibility of recombinant protein administration, and response to cytokine expedition. Circulation 1997; 95(2):438–448.

19. Asahara T, Chen D, Tsurumi Y, et al. Accelerated restitution of endothelial integrity and endothelium-dependent function after phVEGF165 gene transfer. Circulation 1996; 94(12):3291–3302.

20. Hiltunen MO, Laitinen M, Turunen MP, et al. Intravascular adenovirus-mediated VEGF-C gene transfer reduces neointima formation in balloon-denuded rabbit aorta. Circulation 2000; 102(18):2262–2268.

21. Rutanen JF, Turunen AM FAU, Teittinen MF, et al. Gene transfer using the mature form of VEGF-D reduces neointimal thickening through nitric oxide-dependent mechanism. Gene Ther 2005; 12(12):980–987.

22. Walter DH, Cejna M, Diaz-Sandoval L, et al. Local gene transfer of phVEGF-2 plasmid by gene-eluting stents: an alternative strategy for inhibition of restenosis. Circulation 2004; 110(1):36–45.

23. Swanson N, Hogrefe K, Javed Q, Gershlick A. In vitro evaluation of vascular endothelial growth factor (VEGF) eluting stents. Int J Cardiol 2003; 92:2–3.

24. Swanson N, Hogrefe K, Javed Q, Malik N, Gershlick A. Vascular endothelial growth factor (VEGF) eluting stents. In vivo effects on thrombosis, endothelialisation and intimal hyperplasia. J Invas Cardiol 2003; 15(12):688–692.

25. Flugelman MY, Weisz A, Koren B, Fischer L, Lewis BS. Stent-based gene therapy: from transfection efficiency to biological effect. Sixth International LDD&R Local Drug delivery meeting and Cardiovascular Course on Radiation & Molecular strategies—Abstract book. (abstr 26). January 28, 2000.

26. Pels K, Labinaz M, Hoffert C, O'Brien ER. Adventitial angiogenesis early after coronary angioplasty: correlation with arterial remodeling. Arterioscler Thromb Vasc Biol 1999; 19(2):229–238.

27. El Gendi H, Violaris AG, Foale R, Sharma HS, Sheridan DJ. Endogenous, local, vascular endothelial growth factor production in patients with chronic total coronary artery occlusions: further evidence for its role in angiogenesis. Heart 2002; 87(2):158–159.

28. Inoue M, Itoh H, Ueda M, et al. Vascular endothelial growth factor (VEGF) expression in human coronary atherosclerotic lesions: possible pathophysiological significance of VEGF in progression of atherosclerosis. Circulation 1998; 98(20):2108–2116.

29 Takeshita S, Zheng LP, Brogi E, et al. Therapeutic angiogenesis. A single intraarterial bolus of vascular endothelial growth factor augments revascularization in a rabbit ischemic hind limb model. J Clin Invest 1994; 93(2):662–670.

30 Dulak J, Partyka L, Jozkowicz A, et al. Gene transfer of naked VEGF plasmid induces the formation of microvessels but not mature collaterals in ischaemic limb muscles. Eur Surg—Acta Chirurgica Austriaca 2002; 34(2):105–110.

31 Pearlman JD, Hibberd MG, Chuang ML, et al. Magnetic resonance mapping demonstrates benefits of VEGF-induced myocardial angiogenesis. Nat Med 1995; 1(10):1085–1089.

32 Lazarous DF, Shou M, Scheinowitz M, et al. Comparative effects of basic fibroblast growth factor and vascular endothelial growth factor on coronary collateral development and the arterial response to injury. Circulation 1996; 94(5):1074–1082.

33 Takeshita S, Pu LQ, Stein LA, et al. Intramuscular administration of vascular endothelial growth factor induces dose-dependent collateral artery augmentation in a rabbit model of chronic limb ischemia. Circulation 1994; 90(5 Pt 2):II228–II234.

34 Tsurumi Y, Takeshita S, Chen D, et al. Direct intramuscular gene transfer of naked DNA encoding vascular endothelial growth factor augments collateral development and tissue perfusion. Circulation 1996; 94(12):3281–3290.

35 Glennon PE, Clarke SC, Kume SM, Wright MJ, Charnock-Jones DS, Rotavatn S, Nordrehaug JE, Weissberg PL, Schofield P. Catheter-based endomyocardial injection of viral or plasmid DNA in vivo stimulates local VEGF production irrespective of the gene delivered. Eur Heart J 2000; 21(Suppl):58.

36 Iwaguro H, Yamaguchi J, Kalka C, et al. Endothelial progenitor cell vascular endothelial growth factor gene transfer for vascular regeneration. Circulation 2002; 105(6):732–738.

37 Baumgartner I, Pieczek A, Manor O, et al. Constitutive expression of phVEGF165 after intramuscular gene transfer promotes collateral vessel development in patients with critical limb ischemia. Circulation 1998; 97(12):1114–1123.

38 Callow AD. Does vascular endothelial growth factor (VEGF) work for lower extremity ischemia: results of a randomized controlled evaluation. Conference presentation at the Veithsymposium 2003:2.1–2.2.

39 Henry TD FAU—Annex B, Annex BH FAU—McKendall G, McKendall GR FAU —Azrin M, Azrin MA FAU—Lopez J, Lopez JJ FAU—Giordano F, Giordano FJ FAU, et al. The VIVA trial: vascular endothelial growth factor in ischemia for vascular angiogenesis. Circulation 2003; 107(10):1359–1365.

40 Losordo DW, Vale PR, Symes JF, et al. Gene therapy for myocardial angiogenesis: initial clinical results with direct myocardial injection of phVEGF165 as sole therapy for myocardial ischemia. Circulation 1998; 98(25):2800–2804.

41 Rosengart TK, Lee LY, Patel SR. Angiogenesis gene therapy: phase I assessment of direct intramyocardial administration of an adenovirus vector expressing VEGF121 cDNA to individuals with clinically significant severe coronary artery disease. Circulation 1999; 100:468–474.

42 Symes JF, Losordo DW, Vale PR, et al. Gene therapy with vascular endothelial growth factor for inoperable coronary artery disease. Ann Thorac Surg 1999; 68(3):830–836.

43 Losordo DW, Vale PR, Hendel RC, et al. Phase 1/2 placebo-controlled, double-blind, dose-escalating trial of myocardial vascular endothelial growth factor 2 gene transfer by catheter delivery in patients with chronic myocardial ischemia. Circulation 2002; 105(17):2012–2018.

44 Stewart DJ, on behalf of the REVASC investigators. Late-breaking clinical trial abstracts. Circulation 2002; 106(23): 2986-a.

45 Kastrup JF, Jorgensen E FAU—Ruck A, Ruck AF, Tagil KF, Glogar DF, Ruzyllo WF, et al. Direct intramyocardial plasmid vascular endothelial growth factor-A165 gene therapy in patients with stable severe angina pectoris A randomized double-blind placebo-controlled study: the Euroinject One trial. J Am Coll Cardiol 2005; 45(7):982–988.

46 Laitinen M, Hartikainen J, Hiltunen MO, et al. Catheter-mediated vascular endothelial growth factor gene transfer to human coronary arteries after angioplasty. HumGene Ther 2000; 11(2):263–270.

47 Hedman M, Hartikainen J, Syvanne M, et al. Safety and feasibility of catheter-based local intracoronary vascular endothelial growth factor gene transfer in the prevention of postangioplasty and in-stent restenosis and in the treatment of chronic myocardial ischemia. Circulation 2003; 107:2677–2683.

48 Epstein SE, Kornowski R, Fuchs S, Dvorak HF. Angiogenesis therapy. Circulation 2001; 104(1):115–119.

49 Harada K, Friedman M, Lopez JJ, et al. Vascular endothelial growth factor administration in chronic myocardial ischemia. Am J Physiol 1996; 270(5 Pt 2):H1791–H1802.

31

Gene therapy: role in myocardial protection

Alok S. Pachori, Luis G. Melo, and Victor J. Dzau

Introduction

Despite significant advances in the clinical management of cardiovascular disease (CVD), acute myocardial infarction (MI) and heart failure (HF) as a result of coronary artery disease (CAD), cardiomyopathy and systemic vascular disease remain the prevalent causes of premature death across all ages and racial groups (1). The complexity of the pathological processes leading to heart disease and the lack of specific predictive markers has been a major impediment to the development of effective preventive therapies, despite the identification of various risk factors and sensitive risk assessment technologies (2–4). Consequently, the focus has been on the design of "rescue" treatments for overt symptoms of the disease, such as hyperlipidemia, myocardial ischemia, left ventricular pump failure, and hemodynamic overload (5). Although these therapies have improved the clinical outlook for patients affected by MI and HF, morbidity and mortality associated with these diseases remain high, indicating the need for more effective treatments.

The current availability of efficient vector systems such as adeno-associated virus (AAV) (6,7), and the recent identification of several gene targets associated with heart disease (8,9) offer opportunities for the design of gene therapies for myocardial protection and rescue. The ability of AAV to confer long-term and stable protein expression with a single administration of the therapeutic gene (10) renders them ideally suited for delivery of therapeutic genes.

In this chapter, we review the major advances in gene-based therapies for heart disease, with emphasis on strategies for protection and rescue of the failing heart, their clinical feasibility, and a perspective on future developments in the field. We will highlight the breakthroughs, the challenges in making the transition from preclinical studies to clinical application, and the opportunities ahead in this exciting and growing field.

Mechanism of action: tools and strategies for genetic manipulation of the cardiovascular system

The major hindrance to the development of effective gene therapies for CVD has been the unavailability of efficient vectors and delivery tools for genetic manipulation of the heart and blood vessels. The main types of vectors used in cardiovascular gene therapy are summarized in Table 1. Most of the current vectors lack tissue specificity and express transgenes only transiently (11,12), rendering them unsuitable for use in chronic CVD. Nonviral vectors usually yield low and transient gene transfer efficiency as a result of lack of genomic integration and rapid degradation (12). Therefore, recombinant viruses have become the preferred vectors for cardiovascular gene transfer (Table 1). These replication-deficient viral particles deliver genetic material with higher efficiency than nonviral vectors (11). Some viral vectors, such as AAV and lentivirus are capable of sustained expression of the therapeutic gene (11), rendering them suitable for use in chronic myocardial and vascular diseases.

The most common somatic gene therapy strategy for CVD involves the exogenous overexpression of a full length or partial complementary DNA (cDNA) encoding a gene whose endogenous activity may be absent or attenuated as a result of the disease. The goal is to restore normal function or reverse disease progression (13). The therapeutic gene may encode an intracellular protein, in which case the therapeutic effect is predominantly autocrine. Alternatively, the therapeutic protein may be secreted and can exert physiological effects in a paracrine or endocrine fashion. Such "gain-of-function" strategies have been employed for the overexpression of cytoprotective and proangiogenic genes in animal models and in patients with vascular and myocardial disease (13,14). In

Table 1 Vectors used for transfer and manipulation of genetic material in cardiovascular tissues

Vector	Transfer efficiency in vivo	Sustainability of therapeutic effect	Level of expression	Target cells	Potential risks	Host immune response
Nonviral						
Cationic liposomes	+	Short	+	Quiescent and dividing	Cytotoxicity	+
HVJ-liposomes	+++	Short	++	Quiescent and dividing	Cytotoxicity	+
Naked plasmid	+	Short	+	Quiescent and dividing	Cytotoxicity	+
Viral						
Retrovirus	++	Life-long	++	Dividing	Cytotoxicity Oncogenesis	+
Lentivirus	+++	Life-long	+++	Quiescent and dividing	Cytotoxicity Viral mutation	+
Adenovirus	+++++	Moderate	+++++	Quiescent and dividing	Cytotoxicity Inflammation	++++
Adeno-associated virus	+++	Life-long	+++	Quiescent and dividing	Oncogenesis Viral mutation	+
Herpes simplex virus	+++	Long	+++	Quiescent and dividing	Cytotoxicity Viral mutation	+++

Abbreviation: HVJ, hemaglutannin-virus of Japan.

other instances, the short-term silencing of (loss-of-function) pathogenic genes may be desirable and sufficient to halt disease progression. Toward this goal, acute inhibition of transcription and translation can be achieved by treatment with short single-stranded antisense oligodeoxynucleotides, ribozymes, and more recently, using RNA interference technology (15,16). These molecules inhibit translation by hybridizing in a sequence-specific manner to the target mRNA. As an alternative strategy, double-stranded "decoy" oligonucleotides bearing DNA consensus binding sequences (cis-elements) have been used to inhibit the transactivating activity of target transcription factors (15). The decoy is usually delivered in molar excess, effectively sequestering the target transcription factor and rendering it incapable of binding to the promoter region of the target gene(s).

Indications (1): pathogenesis of heart disease and targets for gene therapy

Myocardial ischemia associated with CAD is the primary cause of myocardial failure (17). Acute ischemic events, if sufficiently prolonged will lead to irreversible damage and infarction, underlined by alterations in membrane fluidity, intracellular hydrogen ion concentration, and metabolic activity and eventual cell death, resulting in arrhythmia and impaired pump function (18). Paradoxically, reoxygenation of the ischemic myocardium induces a robust increase in reactive oxygen species (ROS), which triggers a profound inflammatory response and may exacerbate the damage initiated during ischemia (18,19). In time the left ventricle undergoes a process of remodeling characterized by myocyte hypertrophy, interstitial fibrosis, chamber dilatation, and increased propensity for contractile dysfunction that ultimately leads to ventricular failure (20). The remodeling process is complex and highly dependent on the activity of matrix metalloproteinases (MMPs), a group of zinc-dependent proteases that are involved in extracellular matrix degradation (21). Chronic ischemic heart disease is also characterized by heightened inflammatory state and oxidative stress (22). The increased levels of proinflammatory cytokines suppress myocardial contractility and activate neurohormonal systems such as the renin–angiotensin system, which promote ventricular fibrosis and remodeling. Taken together, the pathophysiology of ischemic heart disease offers several exciting targets for intervention with gene therapy which may provide benefits to HF patients.

Indications (2): protection against myocardial ischemia

The vascular endothelium usually remains in a quiescent, nonproliferative state, and with the exception of the female reproductive tract and neoplastic disease, postnatal neovascularization is rare (23). However, injury, inflammation, and oxidative stress activate the endothelium, resulting in cell proliferation, migration, and formation of new vascular networks by angiogenesis (23). In patients and animal models with ischemic heart disease, the progressive occlusion of the coronary artery leads to a chronic imbalance in myocardial oxygen supply and demand, which stimulates the development of collateral vessels aimed and maintaining tissue perfusion and oxygenation (24). This native adaptive response of the myocardium, however, does not provide adequate compensation in face of severe ischemia, and depression of cardiac function ensues, which in time leads to HF.

Evidence of enhanced neovascularization and functional recovery of ischemic myocardium has been reported in animal and human studies after exogenous supplementation of proangiogenic cytokines by gene transfer (25–30). This novel strategy, commonly known as therapeutic angiogenesis, offers a potentially efficacious method for treatment of CAD in clinical cases where percutaneous angioplasty or surgical revascularization has been excluded. In all cases, improvement in tissue perfusion was accompanied by morphological and angiographic evidence of new vessel formation, thus establishing a relationship between improved tissue viability and neovascularization. For example, Mack et al. (26) demonstrated improvement in regional myocardial perfusion and left ventricular function in response to stress in an ameroid constrictor model of chronic myocardial ischemia in pigs following intramyocardial delivery of vascular endothelial growth factor (VEGF)-121 by adneovirus. Using intracoronary injection of an adenovirus vector encoding human fibroblast growth factor (FGF)-5, Giordano et al. (27) also showed a significant improvement in blood flow and a reduction in stress-induced functional abnormalities as early as two weeks after ameroid placement around the proximal left circumflex coronary artery in pigs, in association with an increase in capillary to fiber ratios.

Indications (3): protection from ischemia and reperfusion injury

The continuum of myocardial injury that is initiated by a coronary ischemic event and perpetuated by reperfusion [ischemia/reperfusion (I/R) injury] may be clinically manifested in patients undergoing thrombolytic therapy following an acute coronary episode. The increase in ROS formation during reperfusion of the ischemic myocardium may eventually deplete the buffering capabilities of endogenous antioxidant systems, thereby exacerbating the cytotoxic effects of these reactive species (31). The development of gene therapies for acute MI has been difficult because the time required for transcription and translation of therapeutic genes with the current generation of vectors exceeds the time window for successful intervention. An alternative gene therapy for myocardial protection is to "prevent" I/R by the transfer of cytoprotective genes into the myocardium of high-risk patients prior to ischemia, using a gene delivery method that could confer long-term therapeutic gene expression. This novel concept of "preventive" gene therapy would protect the heart from future I/R injury, thereby minimizing the need for acute intervention. Given the prominent role of oxidative stress in I/R injury, a therapeutic approach aimed at increasing endogenous antioxidant reserves should, in principle, be a useful strategy for prevention/protection in patients at risk of acute MI. This strategy would potentiate the native protective response of the myocardium (32), rendering it resistant to future ischemic insults.

We have evaluated the feasibility of antioxidant enzyme gene transfer as a long-term first line of defence against I/R-induced oxidative injury, using an rAAV vector for intramyocardial delivery of heme oxygenase-1 (HO-1) gene in a rat model of myocardial I/R injury (33). Our findings show that HO-1 gene delivery to the left ventricular risk area several weeks in advance of MI results in approximately 80% reduction in infarct size. The reduction in myocardial injury in the treated animals is accompanied by decreases in oxidative stress, inflammation, and interstitial fibrosis. Consistent with the histopathology, echocardiographic assessment showed postinfarction recovery of left ventricular function in the HO-1-treated animals, whereas the untreated control animals presented evidence of ventricular enlargement and significantly depressed fractional shortening and ejection fraction. Thus, these findings suggest that AAV-mediated delivery of HO-1 may be a viable therapeutic option for long-term myocardial protection from I/R injury in patients with CAD. Comparable findings were found with extracellular superoxide dismutase (ecSOD) gene transfer (34,35). This secreted metalloenzyme plays an essential role in maintenance of redox homeostasis by dismutating the oxygen-free radical superoxide.

The inhibition of proinflammatory genes involved in the pathogenesis of I/R injury offers another option for cardioprotection. Morishita et al. (36) showed that pretreatment with a decoy oligonucleotide capable of inhibiting the transactivating activity of the proinflammatory transcription factor NF-κB reduces MI after coronary artery ligation in rats. Similarly, intravenous administration of antisense oligonucleotide against angiotensin-converting enzyme mRNA (37) significantly reduces myocardial dysfunction and injury following ischemia and reperfusion. Although the rapid in vivo degradation of oligonucleotides would preclude their use in long-term myocardial protection, they may be useful in treatment of acute myocardial ischemia and cardiac transplantation (38) by providing a tool for inhibition of pro-oxidant, proinflammatory, and immunomodulatory genes activated by ischemia and reperfusion. For example, treatment with antisense oligonucleotide directed against intercellular adhesion molecule-1 (ICAM-1) was shown to prolong cardiac allograft tolerance and long-term survival when administered ex vivo prior to transplantation into the host (39). Such an approach could be beneficial in the preparation of donor hearts for transplantation. For example, oligonucleotide-mediated inhibition of anti-inflammatory genes and adhesion molecules in donor organs in advance of transplantation could be used to suppress the acute inflammatory response that ensues upon reperfusion of the transplanted organ in the recipient.

Indications (4): myocardial hypertrophy and remodeling

The progression of HF as a result of hemodynamic overload, chronic myocardial ischemia, or acute MI is invariably accompanied by hypertrophy and remodeling of the left ventricle (40). This process, which usually begins as an adaptive physiological mechanism aimed at normalizing wall stress in response to the increased load or myocyte death from infarction eventually becomes maladaptive, resulting in alteration in ventricular geometry, mechanical decompensation, and contractile failure. Following MI, the left ventricle undergoes an early healing phase during which the infarcted area expands, resulting in wall thinning and ventricular dilation that leads to increased wall stress. This is followed by long-term dilation of the noninfarcted region and myocyte hypertrophy and interstitial fibrosis, leading to ventricular chamber distortion and enlargement (40).

Inhibition of ventricular remodeling is a prime target in the treatment of HF, and the long-term survival benefits of therapies such as acetylcholinesterase (ACE) inbition and β-blockade in patients suffering from MI or HF are attributed, at least in part, to a decrease in left ventricular (LV) remodeling. Pharmacological inhibition of these pathways attenuates the hypertrophic and remodeling process and delays the progression of the disease (5). More recently, treatment with MMP inhibitors was shown to effectively attenuate postinfarction LV dilation (41), indicating that this could be a potential therapeutic strategy for the treatment of HF. Genetic manipulation of these targets may prove to be an effective alternate therapy to current pharmacological approaches for treatment of HF. Gene therapies aimed at inhibiting hypertrophic and profibrotic pathways should be useful in limiting the extent of remodeling. For example, inhibition of AT_1-R signaling by antisense reduces cardiac hypertrophy in a renin-overexpressing transgenic rat, independently of systemic effects (42), suggesting a role of local

angiotensin II (ANG II) in inducing the hypertrophic phenotype. A similar approach could be used for inhibition of cardiotrophic factors such as calcineurin and protein kinases (43). Antisense inhibition of myocardial tumor growth factor (TGF)-β1 factor signaling and metalloproteinase activity could be employed as strategies to reduce fibrosis and remodeling. Conversely, myocardial overexpression of antihypertrophic factors may be used as a strategy to reverse hypertrophy in failing hearts. Li et al. (44) demonstrated that cardiac-specific overexpression of insulin-like growth factor-1 in mice prevented myocyte death in the viable myocardium and attenuated ventricular dilation and hypertrophy after MI. Similarly, cardiac overexpression of glycogen synthase-3β, an endogenous antagonist of calcineurin action, was reported to inhibit hypertrophy in response to chronic β-adrenergic stimulation and pressure overload (45).

Complications

One disadvantage of using viral vectors for gene therapy is that some viral proteins may trigger a robust immune reaction which may reduce the duration of transgene expression (11); however, recent developments have led to the production of vectors with attenuated immunogenicity (46). Furthermore, there is a risk, albeit remote, that these vectors may revert to their wild-type phenotype, raising concerns about biological hazards such as oncogenesis and insertional mutagenesis (11). The impetus at the current time is to develop vectors with enhanced tissue specificity that are capable of directing expression of the therapeutic transgene in response to pathophysiological stimuli such as hypoxia and oxidative stress.

Vector delivery to cardiovascular tissues is problematic. The selectivity of endothelium and the presence of the basement membrane restrict the diffusion of some vectors. A variety of specialized balloon catheters have been developed for intravascular delivery, but the efficiency of vector delivery is moderate, at best (47). A novel approach for local vascular gene delivery uses stents coated with genetically engineered cells or with plasmid or adenoviral vectors expressing therapeutic genes [for review, see Ref. (48)]. Specific modifications of the vector backbone or capsid proteins have also been reported to increase the efficiency of vector uptake by the endothelium. Catheters have also been used for intracoronary gene delivery to the myocardium, but efficiency is low (14). Intramyocardial injection is routinely used as a strategy for local transgene delivery in the myocardium, but transgene expression is restricted to the vicinity of the injection site (14). New catheters are now available which allow more precise intramyocardial gene injection with the assistance of transesophageal echocardiographic and mapping techniques (49).

As discussed before, gene therapy can be used to target transcription factors which control downstream signaling systems. However, this strategy lacks specificity because several genes may be under the control of the targeted transcription factor, and the target gene may be under the influence of multiple transcription factors (15). New strategies are currently being developed to improve the specificity of gene knockdown. For example, nucleic acid and peptide aptamers have been used to inhibit protein function without altering the genetic complement of the host (50).

Combination and synergistic use of gene therapy

As discussed before, induction of blood vessel formation or "angiogenesis" has been a popular target of gene therapy as several studies have used agents like VEGF and FGF to enhance collateral blood vessel formation following myocardial ischemia (51). Recent studies have demonstrated the therapeutic potential of administering various angiogenic growth factors to augment revascularization in the ischemic limb (51) as well as myocardium (26,27). However, it has been demonstrated that although VEGF is a strong angiogenic factor, it also increases the permeability of capillaries. Indeed, the presence of severe edema has been reported following VEGF delivery (52,53). Therefore, several studies have explored the possibility of a "synergistic" therapy with combined use of VEGF and FGF for induction of functional capillary formation (51). It has been demonstrated that such a combination approach may be a better one than using a single factor alone. The mechanisms of such an effect are not clear. However, it can be speculated that as leakage of the fluid component and worsening of edema might decrease the efficiency of tissue perfusion, there is a possibility that the net blood flow conduction in capillaries formed by VEGF would be considerably less than the expected blood flow matching the gross volume of the capillary bed. In contrast, basic FGF (bFGF) does not only promote the proliferation of endothelial cells, but also induces development of the medial layer and adventitia (54), which could sustain and support the endothelial layer from the outside. Therefore, bFGF possibly increases the function of VEGF-induced capillaries by preventing leakage of the fluid, resulting in synergistic angiogenic effects after combined gene delivery of VEGF and bFGF.

Clinical gene therapy: applications to interventional cardiology

Despite the compelling preclinical evidence about the feasibility and efficacy of gene therapy in the treatment of CVDs, only a few small-scale trials have been carried out (55). Of the 918 trials that have been finished or currently under way worldwide, only 8.3% are CVDs. The majority of these trials evaluated the therapeutic efficacy of angiogenic gene transfer

in treatment of coronary and peripheral ischemia [for review see Refs. (14,56)]. Although the trials generally support the feasibility and safety of angiogenic gene transfer, the clinical findings have been inconclusive with regard to the efficacy of angiogenesis gene therapy. In a phase I study in five male patients aged 53–71 years of age with CAD that did not respond to conventional antiangina therapy, intramyocardial delivery of naked plasmid encoding VEGF-165 into the ischemic myocardium led to reduction of anginal symptoms and improvement, albeit modest, in left ventricular function concomitant with reduced ischemia (57). Vale et al. (58) reported significant reductions in weekly anginal attacks for as long as one year after catheter-based delivery of naked VEGF-2 (VEGF-C) assisted by electromechanical NOGA mapping of the left ventricle in patients with chronic myocardial ischemia. The recently published results of the Angiogenic GENe Therapy (AGENT) double-blinded, randomized, placebo-controlled trial using dose-escalating adenovirus-mediated intracoronary delivery of FGF-4 in 79 patients with angina showed a general trend toward an increase in exercise tolerance and improved stress echocardiograms at 4 and 12 weeks after gene transfer in the patients treated with FGF-4 gene therapy compared with the patients receiving placebo, in association with angiographic evidence of neovascularization (59). However, the trial was not sufficiently powered to detect statistically significant differences between the treated and placebo groups in the treadmill exercise time to fatigue.

Some early phase trials have also been undertaken to evaluate the effect of cell cycle inhibition on neointima proliferation and vein graft failure. We carried out a phase I prospective, randomized double-blind trial of human saphenous vein graft treatment with E2F decoy (Project in Ex-Vivo Vein Graft Engineering via Transfection, PREVENT-I) in a high-risk patient suffering form peripheral arterial occlusive disease (60). Using nondistending pressure to deliver the E2F decoy oligonucleotide ex vivo prior to arterial interpositional grafting, we demonstrated that E2F decoy treatment was safe and feasible. Although the results were preliminary, the study provided evidence that cytostatic gene therapy is feasible for clinical application. More recently, the PREVENT-II has largely confirmed the finding of the PREVENT-I trial. The PREVENT-II is a randomized double-blinded, placebo-controlled phase II trial designed to evaluate the effect of E2F decoy treatment on coronary artery bypass graft surgery (CABG) failure [unpublished findings, Grube et al., American Heart Association meeting, Nov. 2001, for commentary see Ref. (61)]. The interim results confirmed the feasibility and safety of using E2F-1 decoy. Analysis of the secondary endpoints using quantitative coronary angiography and three-dimensional intravascular ultrasound demonstrated increased patency and adaptive vessel remodeling characterized by reduction in neointimal size and volume in the treated group one year after treatment, leading to 40% reduction in critical stenosis. These results will now need to be confirmed in adequately sampled and powered phase III studies in patients with coronary and peripheral vessel disease in order to further validate the therapeutic value of this approach. Another phase I trial (Restenosis Gene Therapy Trial, REGENT-I) is currently underway to evaluate the efficacy of catheter-based inducible nitric oxide synthase (iNOS) gene delivery to prevent restenosis of coronary arteries treated by percutaneous transluminal coronary angioplasty (PTCA).

The success of clinical gene therapy will ultimately be determined by our ability to resolve the outstanding issues regarding safety and efficacy. Larger and more adequately controlled multicenter trials are warranted. Stringent criteria need to be applied in the selection of patients. For example, candidates for therapeutic angiogenesis often have an impaired angiogenic response because of underlying endothelial dysfunction (56). In addition, objective endpoints for assessing efficacy need to be standardized and implemented, as well as measures to assess and overcome potential short- and long-term complications, such as edema, hypotension, retinopathy, and neovascularization of occult neoplasms. The use of gene therapy for vasculoproliferative diseases also has to overcome efficacy issues. The complexity of the pathological process involved in restenosis suggests that genetic manipulation of multiple targets may be necessary for effective and sustained therapeutic benefit. Strategies to accelerate endothelial recovery should also be considered, as endothelial damage plays a pivotal role in the subsequent development of restenosis and graft atherosclerosis.

Perspectives and future directions

Several molecular mechanisms underlying many of the most common CVDs have recently been identified. This has led to the development of an array of gene-based strategies with potential therapeutic value for treatment of these diseases. Some of these strategies have already made the transition from the preclinical phase into clinical trial and are now being considered for use in human patients, while several others are currently undergoing safety and feasibility evaluation in early phase trials. Notwithstanding these significant advances, there is still need for further developments in several aspects of cardiovascular gene therapy. Progress in vector and delivery technologies have not kept pace with the identification of novel therapeutic targets. All vectors currently in use for transfer of genetic material do not meet the criteria of the "ideal" vector. Emphasis needs to be put on the development of vectors that are amenable to endogenous regulation and with the capability of conferring tissue specificity of transgene expression. Such a degree of spatial and temporal control over transgene expression will enhance the safety of human gene therapy protocols and potentially overcome many of the potential ethical issues that can arise as a result of nonspe-

cific transgene expression, such as germ cell line transmission. Much of this development can be carried out using current vector platforms. Rigorous systematic evaluation of the safety and efficacy of delivery strategies and improvement of delivery devices are also essential prerequisites for human gene therapy protocols.

The optimal genetic therapy for complex diseases such as CAD and MI may require a combination of cell transplantation and proangiogenic gene therapy for long-term sustenance of the regenerated myocardium. Such potentially synergistic combinatorial approaches have seldom been considered in the design of cardiovascular gene therapy strategies, which have traditionally been developed around a single therapeutic target. Genomic profiling and screening is being employed for molecular phenotyping of patients and will permit the detection of disease-causing polymorphisms and the design of individualized therapies. The convergence of gene transfer technology and genomic technology will facilitate the elucidation of novel genes and may help uncover new roles for previously known genes, thereby leading to the discovery of novel therapeutic targets and approaches for myocardial protection.

Summary

Heart failure associated with CAD is a major cause of morbidity and mortality. Recent developments in the understanding of the molecular mechanisms of HF have led to the identification of novel therapeutic targets which combined with the availability of efficient gene delivery vectors offer the opportunity for the design of gene therapies for protection of the myocardium. Viral-based therapies have been developed to treat polygenic and complex diseases such as myocardial ischemia, hypertension, atherosclerosis, and restenosis. Some of these experimental therapies are now undergoing clinical evaluation in patients with CVDs. In this review, we will focus on the latest advances in the field of gene therapy for treatment of HF and their clinical application.

References

1 Kannel WB, Belanger AJ. Epidemiology of heart failure. Am Heart J 1991; 12:951–957.
2 Stein EA. Identification and treatment of individuals at high risk of coronary artery disease. Am J Med 2002; 112(8A).
3 Wilson PWF, D'Agostino RB, Levy D, Belanger AJ, Silbershatz H, Kannel WB. Prediction of coronary heart disease using risk factor categories. Circulation 1998; 97:1837–1847.
4 D'Agostino RB, Russel MW, Huse DM, et al. Primary and subsequent coronary risk appraisal: new results from the Framingham study. Am Heart J 2000; 139:272–281.

5 McMurray JC, Pfeffer MA. New therapeutic options in congestive heart failure. Circulation 2002; 105:2099–2106.

6 Robbins PD, Ghivizzani SC. Viral vectors for gene therapy. Pharmacol Ther 1998; 80:35–47.

7 Monahan PE, Samulski RJ. Adeno-associated virus vectors for gene therapy: more pros than cons? Mol Med Today 2000; 6:433–440.

8 Colucci WS. Molecular and cellular mechanisms of myocardial failure. Am J Cardiol 1997; 80(11A):15L–25L.

9 Givertz MM, Colucci WS. New targets for heart failure therapy: endothelin, inflammatory cytokines, and oxidative stress. Lancet 1998; 352(suppl 1):S134–S138.

10 Kaplitt MG, Xiao X, Samulski RJ, et al. Long term gene transfer in porcine myocardium after coronary infusion of and adeno-associated virus vector. Ann Thorac Surg 2000; 62:1669–1676.

11 Mah C, Byrne BJ, Flotte TR. Virus-based gene delivery systems. Clin Pharmacokinet 2002; 41:901–911.

12 Niidome T, Huang L. Gene therapy progress and prospects: non-viral vectors. Gene Ther 2002; 9:1647–1652.

13 Melo LG, Pachori AS, Kong D, Gnecchi M. Gene and cell-based therapies for heart disease. FASEB J 2004; 18:648–663.

14 Isner JM. Myocardial gene therapy. Nature 2002; 415:234–239.

15 Mann MJ, Dzau VJ. Therapeutic applications of transcription factor decoy oligonucleotides. J Clin Invest 2000; 106:1071–1075.

16 Stein CA. The experimental use of antisense oligonucleotides: a guide for the perplexed. J Clin Invest 2001; 108:641–644.

17 Funk M, Krumholz HM. Epidemiologic and economic impact of advanced heart failure. J Cardiovasc Nurs 1996; 10(2):1–10.

18 Carden DL, Granger DN. Pathophysiology of ischemia-reperfusion injury. Am J Pathol 2000; 190:255–266.

19 Yellon DM, Baxter GF. Reperfusion injury revisited. Is there a role for growth factor signalling in limiting lethal reperfusion injury? Trends Cardiovasc Med 2000; 9:245–249.

20 Pfeffer JM, Pfeffer MA, Fletcher PJ, Braunwald E. Progressive ventricular remodelling in rat myocardial infarction. Am J Physiol 1991; 260:H14106–H1414.

21 Peterson JT, Li H, Dillon L, Bryant JW. Evolution of metalloprotease and tissue inhibitor expression during heart failure progression in the infarcted heart. Cardiovasc Res 2000; 46:307–315.

22 Mehta JL, Li DY. Inflammation in ischemic heart disease: response to tissue injury or a pathogenic villain? Cardiovasc Res 1999; 43:291–299.

23 Carmeliet P. Mechanisms of angiogenesis and arteriogenesis. Nat Med 2000; 6:389–395.

24 Ware JH, Simons M. Angiogenesis in ischemic heart disease. Nat Med 1997; 3:158–164.

25 Tio RA, Tkebuchava T, Scheurermann TH, et al. Intramyocardial gene therapy with naked DNA encoding vascular endothelial growth factor improves collateral blood flow to ischemic myocardium. Hum Gene Ther 1999; 10:2953–2960.

26 Mack CA, Patel SA, Schwarz EA, et al. Biological bypass with the use of adenovirus-mediated transfer of the complementary deoxyribonucleic acid for vascular endothelial growth factor 121 improves myocardial perfusion and function in the ischemic porcine heart. J Thorac Cardiovasc Surg 1998; 115:168–177.

27 Giordano FJ, Ping P, McKirnan MD, et al. Intracoronary gene transfer of fibroblast growth factor-5 increases blood flow and contractile function in an ischemic region of the heart. Nat Med 1996; 2:534–539.

28 Ueno H, Li JJ, Masuda S, Qi Z, Yamamoto H, Takeshita A. Adenovirus-mediated expression of the secreted form of basic fibroblast growth factor (FGF-2) induces cellular proliferation and angiogenesis in vivo. Arterioscler Thromb Vasc Biol 1997; 17: 2453–2460.

29 Ueda H, Sawa Y, Matsumoto K, et al. Gene transfection of hepatocyte growth factor attenuates reperfusion injury in the heart. Ann Thorac Surg 1999; 67:1726–1731.

30 Symes JF, Losordo DW, Vale PR, et al. Gene therapy with vascular endothelial growth factor for inoperable coronary artery disease. Ann Thorac Surg 1999; 68:830–837.

31 Park JL, Lucchesi BR. Mechanisms of myocardial reperfusion injury. Ann Thorac Surg 1999; 68:1905–1912.

32 Williams RS, Benjamin IJ. Protective responses of the ischemic myocardium. J Clin Invest 2000; 106:813–818.

33 Melo LG, Agrawal R, Zhang L, et al. Gene therapy strategy for long-term myocardial protection using adeno-associated virus-mediated delivery of heme oxygenase gene. Circulation 2002; 105:602–607.

34 Li Q, Bolli R, Qiu Y, Tang X-L, Guo Y, French BA. Gene therapy with extracellular superoxide dismutase protects conscious rabbits against myocardial infarction. Circulation 2001; 103:1893–1898.

35 Chen EP, Bittner HB, Davis RD, Van Trigt P, Folz RJ. Physiological effects of extracellular superoxide dismutase transgene overexpression on myocardial function after ischemia and reperfusion injury. J Thorac Cardiovasc Surg 1998; 115:450–458.

36 Morishita R, Sugimoto T, Aoki M, et al. In vivo transfection of cis element "decoy" against nuclear factor factor κB binding sites prevents myocardial infarction. Nat Med 1997; 3:894–899.

37 Chen H, Mohuczy D, Li D, et al. Protection against ischemia/reperfusion injury and myocardial dysfunction by antisense-oligodeoxynucleotide directed at angiotensin-converting enzyme mRNA. Gene Ther 2001; 8:804–810.

38 Stepkowski SM. Development of antisense oligodeoxynucleotides for transplantation. Curr Opin Mol Ther 2000; 2:304–317.

39 Poston RS, Mann MJ, Hoyt EG, Ennen M, Dzau VJ, Robbins RC. Antisense oligodeoxynucleotides prevent acute cardiac allograft rejection via a novel, non-toxic, highly efficient transfection method. Transplantation 1999; 68:825–832.

40 St. John Sutton MG, Sharpe N. Left ventricular remodeling after myocardial infarction. Pathophysiology and therapy. Circulation 2000; 101:2981–2988.

41 Asakura M, Kitakaze M, Taskashima S, et al. Cardiac hypertrophy is inhibited by antagonism of ADAM12 processing of HB-EGF: metalloproteinase inhibitors as a new therapy. Nat Med 2002; 8:35–40.

42 Pachori AS, Numan MT, Ferrario CM, Diz DM, Raizada MK, Katovich MJ. Blood pressure-independent attenuation of cardiac hypertrophy by AT(1)R-AS gene therapy. Hypertension 2002; 20:969–975.

43 Taigen T, Windt LJ, Lim HW, Molkentin JD. Targeted inhibition of calcineurin prevents agonist-induced cardiomyocyte hypertrophy. Proc Natl Acad Sci USA 2000; 97:1196–1201.

44 Li Q, Li B, Wang X, et al. Overexpression of insulin-like growth factor-I in mice protects from myocyte death after infarction, attenuating ventricular dilation, wall stress, and cardiac hypertrophy. J Clin Invest 1997; 100:1991–1999.

45 Antos CL, McKinsey TA, Frey N,. Activated glycogen synthase kinase 3-β suppresses cardiac hypertrophy in vivo. Proc Natl Acad Sci USA 2002; 99:907–912.

46 Chirmule N, Kutschke W, McAnally J, Shelton J. Immune responses to adenovirus and adeno-associated virus in humans. Gene Ther 1999; 6: 1574–1583.

47 Feldman LJ, Steg G. Optimal techniques for arterial gene transfer. Cardiovasc Res 1997; 35:391–404.

48 Sharif F, Daly K, Crowley J, O'Brien T. Current status of catheter- and stent-based gene therapy. Cardiovasc Res 2004; 64:208–216.

49 Sylvein C, Sarkar N, Insulander P, Kennenback G, Blomberg P, Islam K. Catheter-based transendocardial myocardial gene transfer. J Interv Cardiol 2002; 15:7–13.

50 White RR, Sullenger BA, Rusconi CP. Developing aptamers into therapeutics. J Clin Invest 2000; 106:929–934.

51 Asahara T, Bauters C, Zheng LP, et al. Synergistic effect of vascular endothelial growth factor and basic fibroblast growth factor on angiogenesis in vivo. Circulation 1995; 92(9 suppl):II365–II371.

52 Masaki I, Yonemitsu Y, Yamashita A, et al. Angiogenic gene therapy for experimental critical limb ischemia: acceleration of limb loss by overexpression of vascular endothelial growth factor 165 but not of fibroblast growth factor-2. Circ Res 2002; 90(9):966–973.

53 Vajanto I, Rissanen TT, Rutanen J, et al. Evaluation of angiogenesis and side effects in ischemic rabbit hindlimbs after intramuscular injection of adenoviral vectors encoding VEGF and LacZ. J Gene Med 2002; 4(4):371–380.

54 Klagsbrun M. The fibroblast growth factor family: structural and biological properties. Prog Growth Factor Res 1989; 1(4): 207–235.

55 Edelstein ML, Abedi MR, Wixon J, Edelstein RM. Gene therapy clinical trials worldwide 1989–2002—an overview. J Genet Med 2004; 6: 597–602.

56 Herttuala SY, Alitalo K. Gene transfer as a tool to induce therapeutic vascular growth. Nat Med 2003; 9:694–700.

57 Losordo DW, Vale PR, Symes JF, Dunnington CH, et al. Gene therapy for myocardial angiogenesis. Initial clinical results with direct myocardial injection of phVEGF$_{165}$ as sole therapy for myocardial ischemia. Circulation 1998; 98:2800–2804.

58 Vale PR, Losordo DW, Milliken CE, McDonald MC, Gravelin LM, Curry CM, et al. Randomized, single-blind, placebo-controlled pilot study of catheter-based myocardial gene transfer for therapeutic angiogenesis using left ventricular electromechanical mapping in patients with chronic myocardial ischemia. Circulation 2001; 103:2138–2143.

59 Grines CL, Watkins MW, Helmer G, Penny W, Brinker J, Marmur JD. Angiogenic gene therapy (AGENT) trial in patients with stable angina pectoris. Circulation 2002; 105:1291–1297.

60 Mann MJ, Whittemore AD, Donaldson MC, Belkin M, Conte MS, Polak JF. Ex-vivo gene therapy of human vascular bypass grafts with E2F decoy: The PREVENT single-centre, randomized, controlled trial. Lancet 1999; 354:1493–1498.

61 McCarthy M. Molecular decoy may keep bypass grafts open. Lancet 2001; 358:1703.

32

Antisense approach

Patrick Iversen and Martin B. Leon

Introduction

Medical therapy of coronary artery disease (CAD) has changed considerably in recent years. It is characterized by expanding the use of percutaneous coronary intervention (PCI) and continued conversion to minimally invasive percutaneous transluminal coronary angioplasty (PTCA) and stent therapy despite significant advances in pharmacological treatment and implementation of novel surgical techniques in treatment of the CAD (1). Introduction of stents showed a significant decrease in vessel remodeling and elastic recoil at the site of intervention and clearly demonstrated the superiority of stent implantation over PTCA alone with respect to restenosis in de novo coronary lesions. Extensive use of coronary stents to prevent restenosis has produced a new disease, in-stent restenosis. Unfortunately, this complication continues to be difficult to prevent; regardless of the treatment strategy, the rate of in-stent restenosis (20% to 60% after bare metal stent implantation) is still unacceptably high, depending on vessel and patient bias (2–5). This is particularly true in patients with diabetes and in some lesion sublets, such as bifurcated lesions, long diffuse lesions, and/or small vessels (5). However, it was also evident that neointimal proliferation is not affected by stenting technique (6). Thus, despite significant advances in the treatment of cardiovascular disease, intimal hyperplasia remains the most common cause of early failure after revascularization.

In addition to mechanical procedures, current treatment strategy on intimal hyperplasia includes two main approaches: (i) inhibiting vascular smooth muscle cell (VSMC) proliferation and growth, and stimulating the pathways that lead to VSMC apoptosis, as well as (ii) promoting re-endothelialization and augmenting endothelial functions. New trend toward stent-based drug delivery explored the potential of antiproliferative drugs in treatment and prevention of the intimal hyperplasia. Several completed studies on sirolimus and paclitaxel eluting stents showed great capability of this approach in the prevention and/or treatment of in-stent restenosis. However, recent advances in vascular gene transfer have shown potential new treatment modalities for cardiovascular disease, particularly in the treatment of vascular restenosis.

Antisense oligonucleotides

Until recently, the clinical applicability of antisense technology to the problem of restenosis has been limited because of a relative lack of target specificity, slow uptake across the cell membranes, and rapid intracellular degradation of the antisense oligonucleotides (4). The only randomized study in humans with c-myc antisense demonstrated no reduction in restenosis after stent implantation when arteries were pretreated with the drug (6). However, the recently introduced AVI-4126 (Resten-NG) belongs to a new family of molecules known as the phosphorodiamidate morpholino oligomers (PMO). In general, PMO are capable of binding to ribonucleic acid (RNA) in a sequence-specific fashion with sufficient avidity to be useful for the inhibition of the translation of mRNA into protein in vivo, a result commonly referred to as an "antisense" effect.

Chemistry

The oligomers are comprised of (dimethylamino)phosphinylideneoxy-linked morpholino backbone moieties (Fig. 1). These morpholino moieties contain a heterocyclic base recognition moiety of DNA (A, C, G, T) attached to a substituted morpholine ring system. When linked to each other via the (dimethylamino)phosphinylideneoxy function, the functional

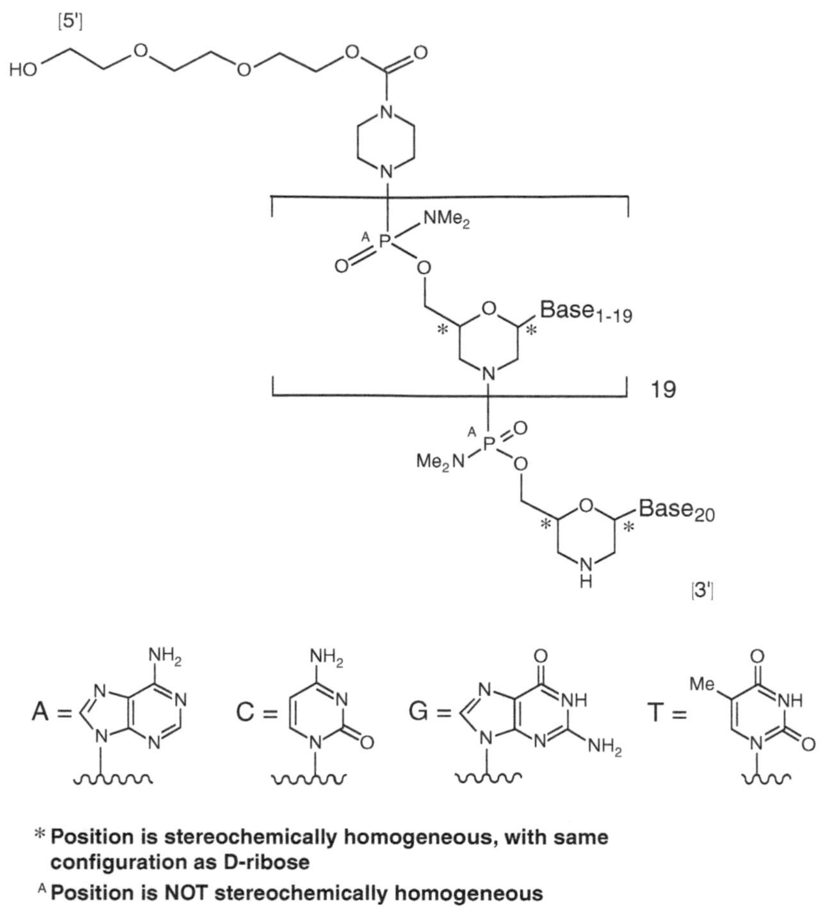

Figure 1
Phosphorodiamidate morpholino oligomers.

group formed by the intersubunit linkage is commonly referred to as a phosphorodiamidate.

Mechanism of action

Genetic information is accessed by a process known as transcription, in which the double-stranded DNA splits and the genetic code is transcribed onto a single-strand messenger RNA (mRNA). The mRNA is comprised of the same bases as the DNA, arranged in the same sequence, but in a complementary fashion. The mRNA migrates out of the nucleus and into the cytoplasm, where it attaches to ribosomes. The ribosomes assemble amino acids to form protein molecules through a process known as translation.

The mRNA is known as the "sense" strand because it is the portion of the DNA that is ultimately translated by the cell into proteins. An "antisense" strand is the other, complementary strand in DNA's double helix structure—or any nucleic acid that is complementary to, and can pair exactly with, at least part of a sense strand.

Antisense oligonucleotides are designed as mirror images to specific mRNA sequences that trigger production of disease-causing proteins. They are generally 15 to 20 bases in length. Their base sequence is complementary to a segment of the target gene that confers specificity to a single site in the genome. This complementary sequence allows the oligonucleotide to bind specifically to the corresponding segment of mRNA that is transcribed from the gene during expression. By recognizing and binding to these sense strands, antisense compounds block the translation of their genetically encoded messages, prevent formation of unwanted proteins, and interrupt the disease at its inception. In contrast, traditional therapeutic agents act to alter the function of unwanted proteins after disease initiation is under way.

Contraindications

The very specific activity of PMOs makes them inherently less toxic than other antisense agents. In addition, the neutral morpholino backbone reduces the opportunity for nonspecific interactions with charged entities such as α-adrenergic blood pressure receptors that can lead to catastrophic loss of blood pressure.

Moreover, the morpholino backbone's immunity to enzymatic attack avoids the potential for nonspecific interactions associated with degradation by-products. In contrast, modified nucleosides or nucleotides resulting from degradation of other antisense compounds might be toxic or might be incorporated into cellular genetic material and thereby lead to mutations or other undesired biologic effects.

Complications

The neutral character combined with no metabolism avoids most types of deleterious drug interactions. Further, clinical monitoring of over a dozen clinical trials has yet to identify a drug-related serious adverse event. No complications have been identified.

Rationale for using antisense oligonucleotides in the treatment of intimal hyperplasia

Gene therapy of intimal hyperplasia

Gene therapy, which has been defined as the transfer of nucleic acids (either functional genes or oligonucleotides) to the somatic cells of an individual with a resulting therapeutic effect (7), targets particular genes and thus appears to be more selective and suited to a site-specific treatment approach, as in the case of intimal hyperplasia, than conventional drug therapy. Moreover, vascular gene transfer can be used not only to overexpress or block therapeutically important proteins and correct genetic defects, but also study various genes and experimentally test their role in the development of particular pathologic conditions.

Neointimal hyperplasia involves a complex interaction between multiple growth factors that promotes VSMC migration and proliferation (8–10). Platelet aggregation and simultaneous activation of SMCs in the media immediately follow injury to the vessel wall. Within 24 hours, DNA replication in the medial SMCs can be observed; in approximately four days, migration of SMC from the media to the intima becomes apparent. In the intima, proliferation of SMC occurs for several days and stops in about four weeks, even

in the absence of endothelial regeneration. Furthermore, synthesis and deposition of the extravascular matrix leads to intimal hyperplasia (11,12).

Multiple factors are implicated in the development of intimal hyperplasia. Many of them have been identified and studied. They involve the release of a host of cytokines and growth factors by platelets, leukocytes, and SMCs, which can induce the synthesis of gene products that stimulate VSMC migration and proliferation, thereby contributing to excessive intimal growth. These appear to be feasible targets for future therapy and prevention of the intimal hyperplasia. Gene transfer studies (e.g., eNOS, p53, kallikrein gene, herpes simplex virus (HSV) with ganciclovir therapy, cytosine deaminase with 5-FC therapy, tissue factor pathway inhibitor, adrenomedullin, and c-myc antisense) have shown the potential advantages of gene therapy in the prevention of intimal hyperplasia (13–22). However, several hurdles must be overcome before gene-based stent therapy can be applied successfully in clinical trials. This includes: (*i*) increasing the efficiency of gene delivery through atherosclerotic plaque; (*ii*) increasing intramural retention times; preventing the inflammatory reaction that stents coated with biodegradable polymers can elicit; (*iii*) overcoming the risk of systemic gene delivery; and (*iv*) accessing the adventitia via a percutaneous approach (23).

Antisense approach to inhibit gene expression

The first successful experience that used oligonucleotides to inhibit gene expression and virus replication was presented by Zamecnik and Stephenson in 1978 (24). They synthesized a 13-mer oligodeoxynucleotide complementary to the 5′ and 3′ reiterated terminal sequences of the Rous sarcoma virus 35S RNA and showed that exposure of infected fibroblasts to this oligomer led to a 99% decrease in reverse transcriptase activity in the medium, which also correlated with a decrease in cellular transformation. This study showed that such compounds may have a therapeutic advantage by specifically targeting genetic sequences that are critical to disease processes.

Three major classes of oligonucleotides exist: (*i*) antisense sequences (commonly called antisense oligonucleotides, or ODN); (*ii*) antigen sequences; (*iii*) ribozymes and *cis*-element double-stranded decoy ODN. Antisense sequences are derivatives of nucleic acids (DNA or RNA sequences) that hybridize cytosolic mRNA strands through hydrogen bonding to complementary nucleic acid bases. Antigene sequences hybridize double-stranded DNA in the nucleus, forming triple helixes. Instead of inhibiting protein synthesis simply by binding to a single targeted mRNA, ribozymes combine enzymatic processes with the specificity of base pairing, creating a molecule that can incapacitate multiple targeted mRNAs (25). Transfection of decoy ODN will result in attenuation of authentic cis–trans interaction, leading to the removal of trans-factors from the endogenous cis-elements, with subsequent modulation of gene expression (26).

The antisense approach to inhibit gene expression involves introducing oligonucleotides complementary to mRNA into cells to block any one of the following processes: uncoiling of DNA, transcription of DNA, export of RNA, DNA splicing, RNA stability, or RNA translation involved in the synthesis of proteins in cellular proliferation (27). It includes the use of antisense oligonucleotides, antisense mRNA, autocatalytic ribozymes, and the insertion of a section of DNA to form a triple helix. The inhibition of gene expression thus achieved is believed to be highly specific and is dependent on formation of the antiparallel duplex by complementary base pairing between the antisense DNA and the target mRNA, in which adenosine and thymidine or guanosine and cytidine interact through hydrogen bonding. This elegant specificity of the Watson-Crick base pairing between the ODN and the target mRNA may form the basis for a highly effective and specific therapeutic modality and might be used to eliminate the expression of any cellular protein (28).

Oligonucleotides that are complementary or antisense to individual mRNA sequences bind to the particular sequence and prevent translation (29). Once inside the cell, ODN binds to its target mRNA in the cytoplasm, nucleus, or both. This hybridization with the mRNA explains two main mechanisms of action of the oligonucleotides (30,31). First, oligonucleotides have been suggested to exert steric interference (32) to ribosome binding and translation, or splice excision. Evidence for steric interference came from studies in which antisense to the 5′ cap of mRNA was found to be most effective in inhibiting rabbit B-globin protein synthesis (33); the 5′ cap is the site where a number of initiation factors bind for ribosome assembly; the unwinding of DNA; and ribosome translocation along the mRNA (34).

Second, the effect of antisense oligonucleotides is because of induction of cleavage of mRNA by the nuclease RNAse H that specifically recognizes DNA–RNA duplexes (35–37). Antisense oligonucleotides can also enter the nucleus where they may inhibit splicing (38), preventing the process of pre-mRNA or mRNA, or block transport of the mRNA out of the nucleus. Introduction of oligonucleotides thus results in a reduction of specific mRNA and protein levels if mediated by RNAse H, or a reduction in specific protein levels if mediated by steric interference.

It was also found that SMC proliferation could be inhibited by antisense oligomers via nonantisense mechanisms (39). In this case, the presence of four contiguous guanosine residues (G-4 tract) within the oligonucleotide sequence caused a sequence-specific, but not antisense-dependent, antiproliferative effect.

Efficacy of antisense oligonucleotides in the prevention of restenosis

Inhibition of several cellular proto-oncogenes including DNA binding protein c-myb (40,41), nonmuscle myosin heavy chain, proliferating-cell nuclear antigen (PCNA) (42,43), platelet-derived growth factor (PDGF) (44), basic fibroblast growth factor (bFGF) (45), c-raf (46), and c-myc (47,48) have been shown to inhibit SMC proliferation in vitro; the efficacy of these oligomers has been confined in in vivo studies as well (49–51). Most recent data showed great efficacy of antisense oligonucleotides in study of FGF–receptor interaction and revealing possible new sites targeted for restenosis prevention (52). Another study found in vivo that downregulation of N-cadherin expression by antisense transfection significantly altered cell–cell adhesion, decreased SMC migration, and prevented restenosis (53). These in vitro and in vivo studies not only demonstrated efficacy of the ODN in the inhibition of SMC migration, proliferation, and intimal hyperplasia, but also revealed key points in the development of antisense therapy of arterial restenosis.

The combination of two different oligonucleotides has demonstrated an inhibitory effect on arterial intimal hyperplasia following balloon injury (54). Even after single intraluminal delivery, the antisense oligomer combination directed against PCNA and cell division cycle 2 kinase (cdc2) was effective in suppressing neointima formation in the rat model of carotid artery balloon injury (50). Another combination of ODNs, antisense cdc2, and cdk2 oligonucleotides, was successfully used by Abe et al. (55) to suppress neointimal SMC accumulation in vivo in the rat carotid artery. At the same time, Robinson et al. (56) demonstrated that single endoluminal delivery of PCNA/cdc2 antisense oligonucleotides by porous balloon catheter does not affect neointima formation or vessel size in the pig coronary artery model of postangioplasty restenosis.

The time frame of antisense ODN introduction to injured vessel may play an important role in the prevention of restenosis. Schmidt et al. (57) showed that rat carotid artery SMC proliferation begins one to two days after balloon catheter-induced injury, and entry of cells into the growth phase was completed within three days of injury. At the same time, minimally modified b-FGF-specific antisense ODN exerted its antiproliferative activity within this time frame. This strategy has also been successfully applied in the inhibition of various targets, such as c-cbl and c-src (58), HSV-1 (59), and c-myc (47).

Different structural types of antisense ODN demonstrate different efficacies and specificities in inhibiting targeted mRNA. Stein et al. (60) carried out cell-free translation studies to compare the efficacy and specificity of four antisense structural types: DNA, phosphorothioate DNA, 2′-O-methyl RNA, and morpholino oligonucleotides, a novel antisense oligonucleotide. It was shown that at low concentrations of antisense oligomer, all four types provide high specificity, but the morpholino oligos and 2'-O-methyl RNA afford better efficacy. At high oligomer concentrations, all four types provide high efficacy, but the morpholino oligos and 2'-O-methyl RNA provide substantially better specificity than the DNA and S-DNA. It was also shown that mRNA could discriminate between oligonucleotides that differ only by one or two bases (30,60,61). Changes in a c-myc antisense ODN sequence of only two bases resulted in almost complete loss of its activity (61).

Frequent nonspecific effects may follow the use of antisense oligonucleotides. Some of these effects are sequence-specific, as described for 4-guanosine residue, which causes an aptamer effect leading to nonantisense-dependent inhibition (39). Although in vitro studies have clearly established that antisense oligomers can inhibit target genes without producing gross toxic effects on cultured cells, in vivo studies in *Xenopus* oocytes reveal that it is not possible to obtain specific cleavage of an intended target RNA without also causing at least the partial destruction of many nontargeted RNA (42).

Limitations of antisense therapy

Despite the apparent success of antisense oligonucleotide therapy, several limitations of this technology have been manifested. First, the ODN must effectively cross the cell membrane to reach the cytoplasm or nucleus (permeation). Once inside the cell, the ODN must be resistant to degradation (stability). Finally, the ODN must be able to bind specifically and with a high affinity to the RNA target to inhibit the desired gene (affinity and specificity) (28,30).

Oligonucleotides are strongly negatively charged, which prevent them from passing the cell surface passively. Uptake of ODN appears to occur by receptor-mediated endocytosis and is determined by various factors including the length of the ODN, the total charge of the molecule, its lipid solubility, and the nucleotide concentration (62,63).

Naturally occurring nucleotide oligomers are easily and rapidly degraded by exo- and endonucleases, which can significantly limit their utilization in antisense technology (64,65). Previous studies have confirmed that the presence of simple 3' or 3' plus 5' modifications may provide protection from degradation by exonucleases (66,67). However, the action of intracellular endonucleases is sufficient to degrade the end-modified oligomers; uniform modification throughout the oligomers has been suggested. Interestingly, previous studies (41) have shown that unmodified ODN is more efficacious in vivo and in vitro than modified ODN.

The affinity of the oligonucleotides depends on their length and base composition. An increase in ODN length also increases its affinity; however, after a particular oligonucleotide length has been reached, its affinity decreases. The affinity also increases as the number of guanosine–cytidine pairs increase (68). The effect of ODN is believed to be highly specific because of complementary base pairing between the antisense DNA and the target mRNA, but it does not prevent frequent nonspecific effects described earlier (42).

Clinical implications and first experience of antisense therapy in the treatment of vascular proliferative disease

Delivery systems for antisense oligonucleotides

One of the most important technical problems in the clinical applicability of antisense technology is the development of an efficient and suited delivery system for oligonucleotides. Local drug delivery was designed to bring the antisense agent to the coronary artery during the period of time corresponding to peak-injury response. The earliest attempts to deliver antisense agents to prevent restenosis involved a rat carotid artery model using adventitial (49) or surgical application (50). The initial clinically applicable devices were catheter-based and provided local delivery as a bolus injection, at which time the catheter was withdrawn. The combination of antisense targeting to c-myc with catheter-based delivery to coronary arteries of pigs for prevention of restenosis began with phosphorothioate oligonucleotides (29). The bolus injection of phosphorothioate oligomers produced a reduction in heart rate, blood pressure, and cardiac output in primate models that was sometimes lethal (69–72).

Modified angioplasty balloons have been designed and developed for local delivery of genes or drugs into the vascular wall (73). Some examples of modified angioplasty balloons are the double balloon catheter, in which the agent is infused into a closed compartment between the balloons and can diffuse with minimal pressure onto the vessel wall; perforated balloon, in which the agent is infused under pressure through pores in the balloon wall and onto the vessel tissue; and the hydrogel-coated balloon, in which the agent is mixed in hydrogel, which dissolves in the blood stream when the balloon is inflated and pressed against the vessel wall (the agent can then diffuse into the luminal cells). The limitation of these devices is pressure-driven delivery that causes additional vessel damage and low efficacy. Viral vectors or different lipid carriers may increase the efficacy of delivery. Fibrin meshwork is an alternative vehicle for sustained release of antisense, a factor that may be important in the case of stent implantation.

Polymer-coated stents have been used successfully to deliver micromolar concentrations of c-myc antisense PMO into the vessel wall (74) (Fig. 2). Zhang et al. (75) reported effective local delivery of c-myc antisense ODN by gelatin-coated platinum–ipidium stents in rabbits. These experiences showed that ultimate success will require polymers that are capable of rapid elution of the oligonucleotide with minimal capacity to inflame or otherwise cause additional injury to the vessel wall.

Perfluorobutane gas microbubbles with a coating of dextrose and albumin efficiently bind antisense oligomers (76). These 0.3- to 10-μm particles bind to sites of vascular injury. Furthermore, perfluorobutane gas is an effective cell membrane fluidizer. The potential advantages of microbubble carrier delivery include minimal additional vessel injury from delivery; no resident polymer to degrade, leading to eventual inflammation; rapid bolus delivery; and the high likelihood of repeated delivery. In addition, the potential for perfluorocarbon gas microbubble carriers (PGMC) to deliver to vessel regions both proximal and distal to stents in vessels suggests this mode of delivery will serve as an excellent adjuvant to a variety of catheter and coated-stent delivery techniques.

First clinical experience of antisense therapy in the treatment of restenosis

The clinical applicability of antisense technology remains limited by a relative lack of specificity, slow uptake across the cell membrane, and rapid degradation of oligonucleotides.

Promising results emerged from the PREVENT trial (77), which showed efficacy of ex vivo gene therapy of human vascular bypass grafts with an antisense oligonucleotide to E2F transcription factor, which is essential for VSMC proliferation in lowering the incidence of venous bypass graft failure. Recently reported results of another clinical trial (ITALICS) in Rotterdam (78) that examined the effectiveness of antisense compound directed against c-myc, however, were disappointing. The authors considered several reasons for the observed lack of effect of the antisense compound. Among them, the local concentration of antisense compound achieved may not have been high enough to show a significant effect. Also, the single administration of the antisense compound might not be effective in suppressive c-myc, which showed biphasic response to the vessel injury. The authors also used a self-expanding stent, which can cause chronic injury of stented arteries. Under these circumstances, a single injection of antisense may not be adequate to reduce myointimal response.

Optimistic results have been obtained with the newly introduced AVI-4126, which belongs to a family of molecules known as the PMOs (28). These oligomers are comprised of (dimethylamino)phosphinylideneoxy-linked morpholino subunits, which contain a heterocyclic base recognition moiety of DNA attached to a substituted morpholine ring system. In general, PMOs are capable of binding to RNA in a sequence-specific fashion with sufficient avidity to be useful for the inhibition of the translation of mRNA into protein in vivo.

Although PMOs share many similarities with other substances that are capable of producing antisense effects [e.g., DNA, RNA, and their analogous oligonucleotide analogs such as the phosphorothioates (PSOs)], there are several critical differences. Most importantly, PMOs are uncharged and resistant to degradation under biological conditions, exceptionally stable at temperature extremes, and resistant to degradation in plasma and to the nucleases found in serum and liver extracts (79). They also exhibit a high degree of specificity and efficacy, both in vitro and in cell culture (80), which averts a variety of potentially significant limitations observed in PSO chemistry. The antisense mechanism of action appears to be through the PMO hybrid duplex with mRNA to inhibit translation. Finally, PMOs have

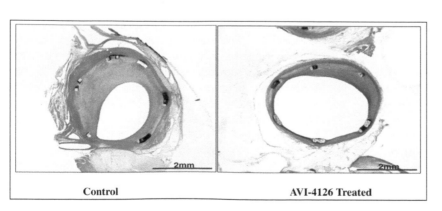

Control   AVI-4126 Treated

Figure 2
(*See color plate.*) Polymer-coated stent delivery of c-myc antisense phosphorodiamidate morpholino oligomers into swine vessels.

demonstrated antisense activity against c-myc pre-mRNA in living human cells (81). The combined efficacy, potency, and lack of nonspecific activities of PMO chemistry have compelled us to re-examine the approach to antisense c-myc in the prevention of restenosis following balloon angioplasty.

PMOs have been evaluated for adverse effects after intravenous bolus injections in both primates (GLP studies by Sierra Biomedical) and man (GCP studies at MDS Harris). No alterations in heart rate, blood pressure, or cardiac output were observed. In summary, bolus injections of PMO by local catheter-based delivery devices are feasible.

Our studies with endoluminal delivery of advanced c-myc antisense PMO into the area of PTCA (Transport Catheter™; rabbit iliac artery model) (82) and into coronary arteries following stent implantation (Infiltrator™ delivery system; pig model) (83) demonstrated complete inhibition of c-myc expression and a significant reduction of the neointimal formation in the treated vessels in a dose-dependent fashion while allowing for complete vascular healing. Similar results were obtained after implantation of advanced c-myc antisense PMO-eluting phosphorylcholine-coated stents in the porcine coronary restenosis model (74). We also observed less inflammation after implantation of the antisense-loaded stent. This favorable influence on hyperplasia (a 40% reduction of intima) in the absence of endothelial toxicity may represent an advantage of antisense PMO over more destructive methods such as brachytherapy (84) or cytotoxic inhibitors (85). We also tested novel perfluorocarbon gas microbubble carriers (PGMS) for site specific delivery of AVI-4126 to the injured vessel wall and obtained encouraging results (86).

The most robust of observations to date by multiple investigators is the finding that AVI-4126 is safe and effective in vascular application in a number of species. Different methods for local delivery have also been tested, but these observations fall short of proof that AVI-4126 will be effective in the treatment of human restenosis. Efficacy in animal models has also been encouraging. Furthermore, all these studies with AVI-4126 indicated that the agent is safe.

The last remaining question is if AVI-4126 will find a place in future therapeutic regimens for the prevention of restenosis; this answer might be found in the results of phase II clinical studies currently being conducted, such as AVAIL. Our recent data on six-month follow-up on the patients enrolled in the AVAIL study (87) showed that AVI-4126 is effective in reducing neointimal formation, particularly when locally delivered in high dose. We also concluded that local delivery of antisense is safe and feasible. The results indicate that antisense (AVI-4126) can be as effective in prevention of the restenosis as most of the well-known antiproliferative agents do, but in contrast to other chemotherapeutics (paclitaxel, actinomycin D) c-myc antisense inhibits cell cycle in the G-1 phase, which make its effect less toxic and comparable with that of rapamycin.

Conclusion

Proof of principle has been established that inhibition of several cellular proto-oncogenes including DNA-binding protein c-myb, nonmuscle myosin heavy chain, proliferating-cell nuclear antigen, PDGF, bFGF, and c-myc inhibit SMC proliferation in vitro and in several animal models. The first clinical study demonstrated the safety and feasibility of local delivery of antisense in treatment and prevention of restenosis; another randomized clinical trial (AVAIL) with local delivery of c-myc morpholino compound in patients with CAD demonstrated its long-term effect in reducing neointimal formation as well as its safety. These preliminary findings from the small cohort of patients require confirmation in a larger trial utilizing more sophisticated drug eluting technologies.

Further identification of new transcriptional factors and signaling mediators would be an important step in the development of new potential targets for therapy of vascular restenosis.

References

1 Simonsen M. Changing role for cardiac surgery as use of stents continues growth. Cardiovasc Device Update 2003; 9:1–7.
2 Topol EJ, Serruys PW. Frontiers in interventional cardiology. Circulation 1998; 98:1802–1820.
3 Serruys PW, Foley DP, Suttorp M-J, et al. A randomized comparison of the value of additional stenting after optimal balloon angioplasty for long coronary lesions. J Am Coll Cardiol 2002; 39:393–399.
4 van den Brand M, Rensing J, Morel MM, et al. The effect of completeness of revascularization on event-free survival at one-year in the ARTS trial. J Am Coll Cardiol 2002; 39:559–564.
6 Nakatani M, Takeyama Y, Shibata M, et al. Mechanisms of restenosis after coronary intervention. Difference between plain old balloon angioplasty and stenting. Cardiovasc Pathol 2003; 12:40–48.
5 Goldberg SL, Loussararian A, De Gregorio J, Di Mario C, Albierro R, Colombo A. Predictors of diffuse and aggressive intrastent restenosis. J Am Coll Cardiol 2001; 37:1019–1025.
7 Yla-Herttuala S, Martin JF. Cardiovascular gene therapy. Lancet 2000; 355:213–222.
8 Libby P, Schwartz D, Bogi E, Tanaka H, Clinton SK. A cascade model for restenosis: special case of atherosclerosis progression. Circulation 1992; 86:47–52.
9 Clowes AW, Clowes MM, Fingerle J, Reidy MA. Regulation of smooth muscle cell growth in injured artery. J Cardiovasc Pharmacol 1989; 14:S12–S15.
10 Fingerle J, Johnson R, Clowes AW, Majesky MW, Reidy MA. Roles of platelets in smooth muscle cell proliferation and migration after vascular injury in rat carotid artery. Proc Natl Acad Sci USA 1989; 86:8412–8416.
11 Nikkari ST, Clowes AW. Restenosis after vascular reconstruction. Ann Med 1994; 26:95–100.

12 Schwartz SM, De Blois D, O'Brien RM. The intima – soil for restenosis and atherosclerosis. Circ Res 1997; 77:445–465.

13 Agata J, Zhang JJ, Chao L. Adrenomedullin gene delivery inhibits neointima formation in rat artery after ballon angioplasty. Regul Rep 2003; 112:115–120.

14 Kipshidze N, Moses J, Shankar LR, et al. Perspectives on antisense therapy for the prevention of restenosis. Curr Opin Mol Ther 2001; 3:265–277.

15 Kipshidze N, Iversen P, Keane E, et al. Complete vascular healing and sustained suppression of neointimal thickening after local delivery of advanced c-myc antisense at six months follow-up in a rabbit balloon injury model. Cardiovasc Radiat Med 2002; 3:26–30.

16 George SJ, Andelini GD, Capogrossi MC, et al. Wild-type p53 gene transfer inhibits neointima formation in human saphenous vein by modulation of smooth muscle cell migration and induction of apoptosis. Gene Ther 2001; 8:668–676.

17 Murakami H., Yayama K, Miao RQ, et al. Kallikrein gene delivery inhibits vascular smooth muscle cell growth and neointima formation in the rat artery after balloon angioplasty. Hypertension 1999; 34:164–170.

18 Steg GP, Tahlil O, Aubailly N, et al. Reduction of restenosis after angioplasty in an atheromatous rabbit model by suicide gene therapy. Circulation 1997; 96:408–411.

19 Harell RL, Rajanayagam S, Doanes AM, et al. Inhibition of vascular smooth muscle cell proliferation and neointimal accumulation by adenovirus-mediated gene transfer of cytosine deaminase. Circulation 1997; 96:621–627.

20 Zoldheliy P, McNatt J, Shelat H, et al. Thromboresistance of balloon-injured porcine carotid arteries after local gene transfer of human tissue factor pathway inhibitor. Circulation 2000; 101:289–295.

21 Van Belle E, Tio Fo, Chen D, et al. Passivation of metallic stents after arterial gene transfer of phVEGF 165 inhibits thrombus formation and intimal thickening. J Am Coll Cardiol 1997; 29:1371–1379.

22 Yoon J, Wu CJ, Homme J, et al. Local delivery of nitric oxide from an eluting stent to inhibit neointimal thickening in a porcine coronary injury model. Yonsei Med J 2002; 43:242–251.

23 Feldman MD, Bo Sun, Koci B, et al. Stent-based gene therapy. J Long-Term Eff Med Implants 2000; 10:47–68.

24 Zamecnik P, Stephenson M. Inhibition of Rous sarcoma virus replication and cell transformation by a specific deoxyoligonucleotide. Proc Natl Acad Sci USA 1978; 75:280–284.

25 Wang A, Creasy A, Lardner M, et al. Molecular cloning of the complementary DNA for human tumor necrosis factor. Science 1985; 228:149–154.

26 Morishita R, Kaneda Y, Ogihara T. Therapeutic potential of oligonucleotide-based therapy in cardiovascular disease. Bio Drugs 2003; 17(6):383–389.

27 Helene C, Toulme JJ. Specific regulation of gene expression by antisense, sense and antigene nucleic acids. Biochem Biophys Acta 1990; 1049:99–125.

28 Stein CA, Cheng YC. Antisense oligonucleotides as therapeutic agents—is the bullet really magical? Science 1993; 261: 1004–1012.

29 Shi Y, Fad A, Galleon A, et al. Transcatheter delivery of c-myc antisense oligomers reduced neointimal formation in a porcine model of coronary artery balloon injury. Circulation 1994; 90: 944–951.

30 Bennett MR, Schwartz SM. Antisense therapy for angioplasty restenosis: some critical considerations. Circulation 1995; 92: 1981–1993.

31 Stein CA, Tokinson JL, Yakubov L. Phosphorothioate oligodeoxynucleotides antisense inhibitors of gene expression? Pharmacol Ther 1991; 52:365–384.

32 Bolziau C, Kurfist R, Cazenave C, Roig V, Thoung NT, Toulme JJ. Inhibition of translation initiation by antisense oligonucleotides via an RNAase independent mechanism. Nucleic Acid Res 1991; 19:1113–1119.

33 Goodchild J. Inhibition of gene expression by oligonucleotides. In: Cohen J, ed. Oligonucleotides: Antisense Inhibitors of Gene Expression. London, UK: MacMillan press, 1989: 53–77.

34 Kozak M. Influences of mRNA secondary structure on inhibition by eucaryotic ribosome. Proc Natl Acad Sci USA 1996; 83:2850–2854.

35 Wagner R, Nishikura K. Cell cycle expression of RNA duplex unwinding activity in cells. Mol Cell Biol 1988; 8:770–777.

36 Dash P, Lotan L, Knapp M, Kandel ER, Goelet P. Selective elimination of mRNA in vivo: complementary oligodeoxynucleotides promote RNA degradation by RNAse-H like activity. Proc Natl Acad Sci 1987; 84:7896–7900.

37 Dagle JM, Walder JA, Weeks DL. Target degradation of mRNA in Xenopus oocytes and embryos directed by modified oligonucleotides: studies of An2 and cyclin in embryogenesis. Nucleic Acid Res 1990; 18:4751–4757.

38 McMannaway ME, Neckers LM, Loke SL, et al. Tumor-specific inhibition of lymphoma growth by an antisense oligodeoxynucleotide. Lancet 1990; 335:808–811.

39 Burgess TL, Fisher EF, Ross SL, et al. The antiproliferative effect of c-myb and c-myc antisense oligonucleotides in smooth muscle cells is caused by a non antisense mechanism. Proc Natl Acad Sci USA 1995; 92(9):4051–4055.

40 Simons M, Rosenburg RD. Antisense non-muscle, myosin, heavy chain and c-myb oligonucleotides suppress smooth muscle cell proliferation in vitro. Circ Res 1992; 70: 835–843.

41 Gunn J, Holt CM, Francis SE, et al. The effect of oligonucleotides to c-myb on vascular smooth muscle cell proliferation and neointima formation after porcine coronary angioplasty. Circ Res 1997; 80:520–531.

42 Speir E, Epstein SE. Inhibition of smooth muscle cell proliferation by an antisense deoxyoligonucleotide targeting the mRNA coding proliferating cell nuclear antigen. Circulation 1992; 86: 538–547.

43 Simons M, Edelman ER, Rosenberg RD. Antisense PCNA oligonucleotides inhibit neointimal hyperplasia in a rat carotid artery injury model. J Clin Invest 1994; 93: 2351–2356.

44 Sugiki H. Suppression of vascular smooth muscle cell proliferation by an antisense oligonucleotide against PDGF receptor. Hokkaido Igaku Zasshi 1995; 70(3):485–495.

45 Hanna AK, Fox JC, Necklis DG, et al. Antisense basic fibroblast growth factor gene transfer reduces neointimal thickening after arterial injury. J Vasc Surg 1997; 25(2):320–325.

46 Mandiyan S, Schumacher C, Cioffi C, et al. Molecular and cellular characterization of baboon C-Raf as target for antiproliferative effects of antisense oligonucleotides. Antisense Nucleic Acid Drug Dev 1997; 7(6):539–548.

47 Biro S, Fu YM, Yu ZX, Epstein SE. Inhibitory effects of oligodeoxynucleotides targeting c-myc RNA on smooth muscle cell proliferation and migration. Proct Natl Acad Sci USA 1993; 90:654–658.

48 Daum T, Engels JW, Mag M, et al. Antisense deoxynucleotide: inhibitor of splicing of mRNA of human immunodeficiency virus. Intern Virol 1992; 89:7031–7035.

49 Simons M, Edelman ER, Dekeyser JL, Langer R, Rosenberg RD. Antisense c-myb oligonucleotides inhibits intimal arterial smooth muscle cell accumulation in vivo. Nature 1992; 359:67–70.

50 Morishita R, Gibbons GH, Ellison KE, et al. Single intraluminal delivery of antisense cdc kinase PCNA results in chronic inhibition of neointimal hyperplasia. Proc Natl Acad Sci USA 1993; 90:8474–8478.

51 Bayever E, Iversen PL, Bishop MR, et al. Systemic administration of a phosphorothioate oligonucleotide with a sequence complementary to p53 for acute myelogenous leukemia and myelodysplastic syndrome: initial results of a phase I trial. Antisense Res Dev 1993; 4(4):383–390.

52 Agrotis A, Kanellakis P, Kostolias G, et al. Proliferation of neointimal smooth muscle cells after arterial injury: dependency on interaction between fibroblast growth factor receptor-2 and fibroblast growth factor-9. J Biol Chem 2004 [EPub ahead of print].

53 Blindt R, Bosserhoff AK, Dammers J, et al. Downregulation of N-cadherin in the neointima stimulates migration of smooth muscle cells by RhoA deactivation. Cardiovasc Res 2004; 62(1):212–222.

54 Summerton J, Stein D, Huang B, Matthews P, Weller D, Partridge M. Morpholino and phosphorothioate antisense oligomers compared in cell-free and in-cell systems. Antisense Nucleic Acid Drug Dev 1997; 7:63–70.

55 Abe J, Zhou W, Taguchi J. Suppression of neointimal smooth muscle cell accumulation in vivo by antisense cdc2 and cdk2 oligonucleotides in rat carotid artery. Biochem Biophys Commun 1994; 198:16–24.

56 Robinson KA, Chronos NAF, Schieffer E, et al. Endoluminal local delivery of PCNA/cdc2 antisense oligonucleotides by porous balloon catheter does not affect neointima formation or vessel size in the pig coronary artery model of post angioplasty restenosis. Catheter Cardiovasc Diagn 1997; 41: 348–353.

57 Schmidt A, Sindermann J, Peyman A, et al. Sequence specific antiproliferative effects of antisense and end-capping modified antisense oligodeoxynucleotides targeted against the 5′-terminus of basic-fibroblast growth factor mRNA in coronary smooth muscle cells. Eur J Biochem 1997; 248(2):543–549.

58 Tanaka S, Amling M, Neff L, et al. c-cbl downstream of c-src in a signaling pathway necessary for bone resorption. Nature 1996; 383:528–531.

59 Peyman A, Helsberg M, Kretzschmar G, Mag M, Ryte A, Uhlmann E. Nuclease stability as dominant factor in the antiviral activity of oligonucleotides directed against HSV-1 IE 1 10. Antiviral Res 1997; 33:135–139.

60 Stein D, Foster E, Huang SB, Weller D, Summerton J. A specificity comparison of four antisense types: morpholino, 2′-O methyl RNA, DNA and phosphorothioate DNA. Antisense Nucleic Acid Drug Dev 1997; 7:151–157.

61 Holt JT, Render RL, Nelhus AW. An oligomer complementary to c-myc RNA inhibits proliferation of HL-60 promyelocytic cells and induces differentiation. Mol Cell Biol 1988; 8:963–973.

62 Villa AE, Guzman LA, Poptic EJ, et al. Effects of antisense c-myb oligonucleotides on vascular smooth muscle cell proliferation and response to vessel wall injury. Circ Res 1995; 76:505–513.

63 Muller DM. The role of proto-oncogenes in coronary restenosis. Pro Cardiovasc Ids 1997; 40(2):117–128.

64 Wickstrom E. Antisense c-myc inhibition of lymphoma growth. Antisense Nucleic Acid Drug Dev 1997; 7(3):225–228.

65 Cazenave C, Loreau N, Thuong NT, Toulme JJ. Enzymatic amplification of translation inhibition of rabbit beta-globin mRNA mediated by anti-messenger oligodeoxynucleotides covalently linked to intercalating agents. Nucleic Acid Res 1995; 15(12):4717–4736.

66 Shaw JP, Kent K, Bird J, Fishback J, Froehler BF. Modified deoxyoligonucleotide stable to exonuclease degradation in serum. Nucleic Acid Res 1991; 19:747–750.

67 Ott J, Eckstein F. Protection of oligonucleotide primers against degradation by DNA polymerase I. Biochemistry 1987; 26(25):8237–8241.

68 Hoke GD, Draper K, Freier SM, et al. Effect of phosphorothioate capping on antisense oligonucleotide stability, hybridization and antiviral efficacy versus herpes simplex virus infection. Nucleic Acid Res 1991; 20:5743–5748.

69 Cornish KG, Iversen PL, Smith L, Arneson M, Bayever E. Cardiovascular effects of a phosphorothioate oligonucleotide with sequence antisense to p53 in the conscious rhesus monkey. Pharmacol Commun 1993; 3:239–247.

70 Galbraith WM, Hobson WC, Giclas PC, Schechter PJ, Agrawal S. Complement activation and hemodynamic changes following intravenous administration of phosphorothioate oligonucleotides in the monkey. Antisense Res Dev 1994; 4:201–206.

71 Henry SP, Bolte H, Auletta C, Kornburst DJ. Evaluation of the toxicity of ISIS 2302, a phosphorothioate oligonucleotide, in a four week study in cynomolgus monkeys. Toxicology 1997; 120:145–155.

72 Iversen PL, Cornish KG, Iversen LJ, Mata JE, Bylund DB. Bolus intravenous injection of phosphorothioate oligonucleotides causes hypotension by acting as a 1-adrenergic receptor antagonists. Toxicol Appl Pharmacol 1999; 160:289–296.

73 Hedin U, Wahlberg E. Gene therapy and vascular disease: potential applications in vascular surgery. Eur J Vasc Endovasc Surg 1997; 13:101–111.

74 Kipshidze NN, Iversen P, Kim HS, et al. Advanced c-myc antisense (AVI-4126)-eluting phosphorylcholine-coated stent implantation is associated with complete vascular healing and reduced neointimal formation in the porcine coronary restenosis model. Catheter Cardiovasc Interv 2004; 61(4):518–527.

75 Zhang XX, Cui CC, Xu XG, Hu XS, Fang WH, Kuang BJ. In vivo distribution of c-myc antisense oligonucleotides local delivered by gelatin-coated platinum-iridium stent in rabbits and its effect on apoptosis. Chin Med J (Engl) 2004; 117(2): 258–263.

76 Porter TR, Iversen PL, Li S, Xie F. Interaction of diagnostic ultrasound with synthetic oligonucleotide-labeled perfluorocarbon-exposed sonicated dextrose albumin microbubbles. J Ultrasound Med 1996; 15:577–584.

77 Mann MJ, Whittemore AD, Donaldson MC, et al. Ex-vivo gene therapy of human vascular bypass grafts with E2F decoy:

the PREVENT single-centre, randomised, controlled trial. Lancet 1999; 354(9189):1493–1498.

78   Kutryk MJ, Foley DP, van den Brand M, et al. Local intracoronary administration of antisense oligonucleotide against c-myc for the prevention of in-stent restenosis: results of the randomized investigation by the Thoraxcenter of antisense DNA using local delivery and IVUS after coronary stenting (ITALICS) trial. J Am Coll Cardiol 2002; 39(2):281–287.

79   Hudziak RM, Barofsky E, Barofsky DF, et al. Resistance of morpholino phosphorodiamidate oligomers to enzymatic degradation. Antisense Nucleic Acid Drug Dev 1996 6: 267–272.

80   Hudziak RM, Summerton J, Weller DD, Iversen PL. Antiproliferative effects of steric blocking phosphorodiamidate morpholino antisense agents directed against c-myc. Antisense Nucleic Acid Drug Dev 2000; 10:163–176.

81   Dani C, Blanchard JM, Piechaczyk M, El Sabouty S, Marty L, Jeanteur P. Extreme instability of myc mRNA in normal and transformed human cells. Proc Natl Acad Sci USA 1984; 81:7046–7050.

82   Kipshidze N, Keane E, Stein D, et al. Local delivery of c-myc neutrally charged antisense oligonucleotides with transport catheter inhibits myointimal hyperplasia and positively affects vascular remodeling in the rabbit balloon injury model. Catheter Cardiovasc Interv 2001; 54:247–256.

83   Kipshidze NN, Kim H-S, Iversen P et al. Intramural delivery of advanced antisense oligonucleotides with infiltrator catheter inhibits c-myc expression and intimal hyperplasia in the porcine. J Am Coll Cardiol 2002; 39(10):1686–1691.

84   Sheppard R, Eisenberg MJ. Intracoronary radiotherapy for restenosis. N Engl J Med 2001; 344 (4):295–297.

85   Herdeg C, Oberhoff M, Baumbach A, et al. Local paclitaxel delivery for the prevention of restenosis: biological effects and efficacy in vivo. J Am Coll Cardiol 2000; 35(7): 1969–1976.

86   Kipshidze NN, Porter TR, Dangas G, et al. Systemic targeted delivery of antisense with perflourobutane gas microbubble carrier reduced neointimal formation in the porcine coronary restenosis model. Cardiovasc Radiat Med 2003; 4(3): 152–159.

87   Kipshidze N, Iversen P, Overlie P, et al. First human experience with local delivery of novel antisense AVI-4126 with infiltrator catheter in de novo native and restenotic coronary arteries: six-month clinical and angiographic follow-up from AVAIL study. Cardiovasc Revasc Med 2007 (in press).

33

Principles of photodynamic treatment

Thomas L. Wenger and Nicholas H. G. Yeo

Introduction

Phototherapy, the therapeutic application of light in the treatment of diseases has evolved over thousands of years from its origins in Asia. The earliest understanding that photonic energy in visible light could be harnessed through the presence of a photoreactive substance to promote a biological effect in an oxygenated tissue is attributed to the work of Professor von Tappeiner on xanthene derivatives, first published in 1900 (1). This work led to the realization that the destructive skin lesions observed in porphyrias could be attributable to a photodynamic effect.

Early photodynamic agents were naturally derived porphyrins such as hematoporphyrin and typically were mixtures of many porphyrins leading to inconsistent biological results. A purified form, hematoporphyrin derivative (HpD), was shown through red fluorescence under ultraviolet light to localize in tumors (2). Thus, the synthesis of first-generation photoreactive agents was directed toward their use in disease diagnosis. It was not until the observation by Diamond et al. in 1972 that the photodynamic effect caused selective necrosis of a glioma implant in a rat (3), that the term photodynamic treatment (PDT) was coined.

The 1980s saw the advent of second-generation photoreactive agents characterized by greater purity, favorable pharmacokinetics, and stronger absorption of light in the far red part of the spectrum that is least attenuated on transmission through tissue. PDT development programs have resulted in marketing approval of several photoreactive agents by the Food and Drug Administration (FDA) and other regulatory agencies including Photofrin® (esophageal/bronchial cancer), Levulan® (actinic keratosis), and Visudyne® (age-related macular degeneration). The use of PDT in interventional cardiovascular therapy is experimental. However, the unique combination of site-specific, endovascu-lar activity and potential application for focal or regional intervention makes PDT an attractive concept for primary treatment of atherosclerosis or as an adjunct to inhibit restenosis. The following sections provide an overview of the principles of photodynamic effect and highlight potential application of PDT to structural targets underlying certain cardiovascular diseases.

Mechanisms of photodynamic effect and modes of cell death in photodynamic treatment

At the core of the photodynamic effect is a photoreactive agent with a stable electronic configuration that exists as a singlet in the ground state—(Fig. 1). Upon excitation by the absorption of photonic energy from light of a specific wavelength ($h\nu_{exc}$) the photoreactive molecule is elevated to a higher though short-lived first excited energy state, which is also a singlet. The molecule either relaxes to its ground singlet state releasing energy as a photon through fluorescence ($h\nu_F$), or may convert to a triplet state by intersystem crossing (ISX). The photoreactive triplet has greater longevity than its parent singlet, in the order of milliseconds, increasing the probability of interaction with the surrounding oxygen molecules.

Higher intersystem crossing probabilities and higher triplet quantum yields are inherent in those photoreactive agents selected for clinical development, as these parameters indicate the quantity of cytotoxic species produced. Energy in the photoreactive triplet state molecule provides the basis for biomolecular interactions in photodynamic treatment. The predominant mechanism involves generation of singlet oxygen ($^1O_2$).

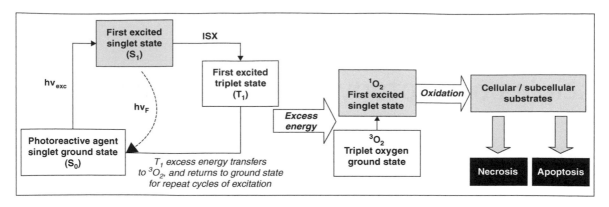

Figure 1
Summary of the photodynamic effect.

The diffusion distance of $^1O_2$ is around 0.01–0.02 μ before being quenched (4) and so the photoreactive drug must be associated intimately with the target substrate for maximal impact. Biomolecules present in cellular membranes react rapidly with $^1O_2$ and are prime targets for PDT. Membranous intracellular organelles such as mitochondria, lysosomes, and nuclei are also potential targets for attack by $^1O_2$.

Photodynamic cytotoxicity is initiated through various signaling pathways. Both apoptotic and necrotic modes of cell death have been described (5). Modulating the components of PDT dosimetry (e.g., administered doses of photoreactive agent and light, and the time interval between these) together with the specific binding characteristics of the photoreactive agent, can alter the balance between apoptosis and necrosis (6–9). Endovascular PDT of injury-induced hyperplastic arteries has been shown to induce neointimal and medial apoptosis in vivo (10). PDT-mediated translocation of a pro-apoptotic mitochondrial protein (apoptosis-inducing factor) from the mitochondria to the nucleus appears to play a role in smooth muscle cell (SMC) apoptosis (11). Cytotoxic free radicals formed during PDT also inactivate cell-associated basic fibroblast growth factor and inhibit the stimulation of SMC mitogenesis after tissue injury (12).

Managing photodynamic treatment at the threshold

The principles of photodynamic effect require that each of the elements (e.g., photoreactive molecules, photons of the appropriate wavelength, and molecular oxygen) is present at the site of the intended treatment effect coincidently and in such numbers that the yield of $^1O_2$ is sufficient to overcome the target's ability to sustain itself against the oxidative stress being inflicted. The corollary is also important, namely that where any one or more of the elements is present below the threshold the target may tolerate the resultant oxidative stress. It is self-evident then that dosimetry is critical. The challenge is thus to establish dosimetry parameters that provide a working surface of safety and efficacy that accommodates the biologic and pathologic variability present in patients undergoing treatment.

Figure 2 highlights the required intersection of the three elements of PDT necessary to generate $^1O_2$. The principal criteria influencing each element's contribution to the photodynamic effect are also listed.

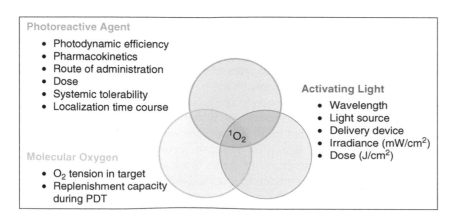

Figure 2
(*See color plate.*) Summary of the interaction of the three elements required for photodynamic effect. *Abbreviation*: PDT, photodynamic treatment.

Configuring photodynamic therapy for endovascular intervention

Photoreactive agents

Table I provides a summary of the principal photoreactive agents that have been investigated clinically or are currently undergoing industry-sponsored development for endovascular use. A small number of other photoreactive agents (including various porphyrin and phthalocyanine derivatives) have been investigated in basic cardiovascular research studies or in in vivo models of cardiovascular disease.

Certain photophysical and pharmacokinetic characteristics are of particular importance in determining the potential utility of photoreactive agents in endovascular treatment of cardiovascular disease. Agents having a high triplet state quantum yield are more efficient generators of $^1O_2$ and this productivity advantage can translate to less photosensitivity burden on the patient and a lower energy requirement for effective activation. In the cath lab, more efficient photoreactive agents requiring shorter activation times may minimize procedure times for endovascular PDT.

Selection of photoreactive agents has been largely directed toward those having strong absorption in the far red part of the visible spectrum, offering the deeper tissue effect that goes with longer wavelength activation (see section on Light Activation). This characteristic has been a long-held holy grail of PDT researchers seeking to enlarge the volume of tissue ablation to treat advanced cancers. Most of the photoreactive agents under investigation today have evolved from this selection process.

Another important characteristic of photoreactive agents is their apparent affinity for certain targets that are of special interest for interventional vascular therapists. As most photosensitizers fluoresce, the kinetics of their distribution in vascular tissue can be investigated both at macroscopic and microscopic levels using fluorescence imaging techniques (Fig. 3). Numerous studies on porphyrin, chlorin, texaphryin, pheophorbide and phthalocyanine photosensitizers in various animal models have documented selective localization in

Table 1 Principal photoreactive agents with cardiovascular development experience

Drug ID (cardiovascular sponsor)	Code/generic name	Cardiovascular development status		Sponsor-defined clinical development target (from company publication)	Other information
		Preclinical	Clinical phase (P)		
Antrin® (*Pharmacyclics*)	Motexafin lutetium	✔	Coronary P1 Peripheral P2	Vulnerable plaque	
Photofrin®	Porfimer sodium	✔	Coronary P1 (pilot study)	—	Marketed internationally as Photofrin for PDT of cancer
ALA	Aminolevulinic acid/ALA-induced protoporphrin-IX	✔	Peripheral P1 (pilot study)	—	Can be administered orally
LS11 (*Vascular Reconditioning*™)	Talaporfin, NPe6 Mono-L-aspartyl chlorin e6, MACE	✔	—	SFA restenosis and vulnerable plaque	Marketed in Japan as Laserphyrin® for PDT of cancer
PhotoPoint®(*Miravant*)	MV0633	✔	—	Vulnerable plaque and coronary restenosis	
	MV2101	✔	—	Vascular access failure in hemodialysis patients	

Abbreviations: ALA, 5-aminolevulinic acid; PDT, photodynamic treatment; SFA, superficial femoral artery.

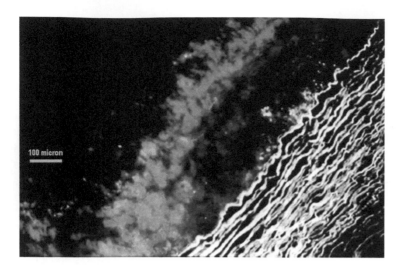

Figure 3
(*See color plate*.) Microscopy with 405 nm excitation reveals red fluorescence from talaporfin (LS11/NPe6) in macrophages within atheromatous plaque on abdominal aorta in hyper- cholesterolemic rabbit, 24 hours after 5 mg/kg intra- venous administration. Note green autofluorescence from elastic fibers in adventitia with no detected LS11. *Source*: Courtesy of Prof. K Aizawa, Tokyo Medical University, Tokyo, Japan.

atheromatous plaque and sites of endothelial injury (13–26). Despite differences in the molecular configurations and physicochemical properties of these photoreactive agents their affinities follow a remarkably consistent pattern of uptake. In normal uninjured and nonatheromatous control arteries there is little accumulation except in the endothelium. In atheromatous lesions there is typically strong accumulation in the intima, weak accumulation in the media, and rare presence in the adventitia. In balloon-injured, but nonatheromatous arteries, there is strong uptake into the media, less in the intima, and no uptake in the adventitia. Balloon-injured, atheromatous lesions show both intimal and medial accumulation. Uptake into diffuse atherosclerotic lesions in a model of vein graft disease has also been demonstrated (27).

Factors such as the structure, charge, and lipophilicity of a photoreactive agent will determine serum protein binding, cellular uptake, subcellular localization and ultimately the biological effect at the time of light activation. The mechanism of photoreactive agent accumulation in plaque has not been fully elucidated but may relate to a tendency to bind to low-density lipoproteins (LDL). During the development of atherosclerosis, scavenger receptors present on the surface of accumulating macrophages mediate the uptake of modified (oxidized) lipoproteins transforming the cells into foam cells (28). The level of expression of scavenger receptors on macrophage-derived foam cells increases dramatically as the disease progresses (29). This may increase the cellular uptake of photoreactive agents that are carried on LDL particles. For example, electron microscopy has revealed the presence of the gold salt of talaporfin (LS11/NPe6) in macrophages within an atherosclerotic plaque (30). Furthermore, the uptake of LDL by another key interventional cardiovascular target— arterial smooth muscle cells (SMC)—is reported to be significantly increased by hypoxia exclusive of LDL

receptor activity (31). LDL transport may thus provide receptor-mediated and direct modes of entry of photoreactive agents into macrophages and SMCs within a thickening intima as atherosclerosis progresses. Perhaps these processes also explain the uptake of photoreactive agents in the media of vessels injured by angioplasty. Time-dependent accumulation of motexafin lutetium within murine macrophages and human SMCs has been shown by real-time monitoring of the agent's fluorescence emission at 750 nm (32).

Some photoreactive agents, especially those that are hydrophobic or amphiphilic, may also be transported in complexes loosely or tightly formed with serum albumin. It is believed that albumin-binding proteins on the surface of endothelial cells create a specific pathway for gp60-mediated transcytosis of the albumin-photoreactive agent complex across the endothelial cell monolayer (33).

Drug to light activation interval

Although there may be a number of similarities in the process of uptake of photoreactive agents into sites of atherosclerosis and vascular injury, there may be substantial differences in the time during which this occurs. The ideal time to undertake light activation is when the photoreactive agent is present in the pathologic target and absent elsewhere. Thus, careful selection of the drug to light activation interval (DLI) is an important parameter in maximizing the benefit versus the risk in this treatment. The real attraction of endovascular PDT as a regional intervention for diffuse atherosclerotic disease is based on the opportunity to combine an agent that self-localizes in pathologic foci, coupled with regionally distributed light energy that itself has no affect on the tissue in absence of the photoreactive agent. This also provides a basis to mitigate geographic miss during adjunctive use through extending light activation beyond the edge of the lesion.

The presence of photoreactive agent in blood within the light activation field may mask the activation site by absorbing the activating light's energy before it reaches the intended target. However, delaying activation while the photoreactive agent clears from the blood may require many hours. Preadministering a photoreactive agent hours or days in anticipation of an intended intervention, so as to achieve an accumulation threshold in a cellular target but not in blood, may be inconvenient. The ideal is a photoreactive agent that can be administered *during* an interventional procedure, which rapidly accumulates within the target and can be efficiently activated by light with only a marginal increment in the overall procedure time.

Light activation

Longer wavelengths of light at the far red end of the visible light spectrum penetrate tissues more deeply than shorter wavelengths near the blue part of the spectrum. When light passes into tissue, the optical properties of the tissue determine the extent to which it is reflected, transmitted, scattered, or absorbed. The optical properties of tissue are defined by the presence of chromophores that absorb energy in the light, and structures within the tissue (e.g., cells and subcellular organelles) that scatter light. Scattering becomes more significant as wavelength decreases toward the blue-violet (i.e., 390–420 nm) and ultraviolet (i.e., <380 nm) parts of the spectrum limiting the depth that light penetrates. As wavelength increases toward the infrared (i.e., beyond 1000 nm) the depth of light penetration is reduced by water absorption. Between these regions in the visible part of the spectrum, and with specific reference to the photodynamic treatment of arterial disease, the major light-absorbing chromophores are oxyhemoglobin, which absorbs strongly in the blue-green regions (420 and 540–580 nm), and yellow chromophores in carotenoids contained in the atheroma that strongly absorb blue-green light at 420–530 nm (34) with a peak absorption around 470 nm.

Thus, blue light will not penetrate deeply into tissue and yellow light will be variably attenuated. While blue light may be a viable choice for a subendothelial treatment field, red light can activate photoreactive drugs more deeply into the tissue and is perhaps a better choice for targeting SMCs in the media, for example, after angioplasty.

Atherosclerotic plaque evolves to be an optically complex lesion ranging from diffuse intimal thickening through lipid-rich regions and the presence of calcification, neovascularization, and intraplaque hemorrhage. In this setting, red light above 650 nm wavelength may be the most effective activation strategy. Alternatively, as photoreactive agents typically have several wavelengths at which they activate strongly within the

blue to red color range (although the $^1O_2$ yields may be very different) contemporaneous light activation with multiple activating wavelengths may potentially enable "through the lesion" treatment.

Light transmission through blood to the arterial wall must contend with scattering by blood elements, absorption by oxyhemoglobin, and absorption by the photoreactive drug present in the blood. It is claimed that motexafin lutetium which absorbs around 730 nm does not require blood exclusion from the vascular treatment field during light activation. Other photoreactive agents under cardiovascular development with activation wavelengths in the region 630 to 670 nm are believed to require blood exclusion. It is unclear whether these perceived distinctions are real. With oxyhemoglobin, the absorption nadir is between 660 and 710 nm, whereas with de-oxyhemoglobin the absorption graph declines across the range 580–800 nm with two inflections around 750 nm. However, hemoglobin in arterial blood is greater than 90% saturated with oxygen; thus, the absorption of light by oxyhemoglobin carries greater weight in considering appropriate wavelengths for efficient light transmission through arterial blood. In this regard, there appears to be little to differentiate between photoreactive agents that are activated across the range 650 to 730 nm (Fig. 4). Light transmission may depend on hematocrit, hemoglobin concentration, light catheter diameter to vessel diameter distance relationships, drug pharmacokinetics and DLI, and other factors. Various strategies have been used to eliminate blood from the lumen including balloon occlusion of blood flow at the light delivery site and saline flush [hemodilution technique (35)]. Ultimately, whether complete blood exclusion is needed is uncertain.

The duration of light delivery can be defined by the total optical energy required (i.e., light dose or fluence measured in J/cm^2 across the endovascular surface being treated) and the optical power (i.e., irradiance, measured in mW/cm^2) applied to the endovascular surface, according to the formula:

$$Time (sec) = Joules (J) / Watts (W)$$

Long durations of light exposure, where occlusion is required, may require light delivery to be fractionated with one or more reperfusion intervals, especially in coronary applications. Light activation protocols based on intense energy delivery may appear attractive in terms of shortened light exposure but may lead to photobleaching (destruction of the photoreactive agent), and, in the presence of hypoxia or restricted re-oxygenation capacity, may be ineffective.

Light for endovascular PDT has typically been generated by pumped-dye or solid-state diode lasers and delivered to the site of treatment through a fiberoptic with a diffusing segment at the distal end of the device that provides radial distribution of the light. Where blood flow occlusion is required, the fiberoptic may be delivered to the treatment site through the guidewire channel of an angioplasty catheter with the diffusing segment positioned within the translucent balloon (36,37). Laser light is coherent, collimated, and

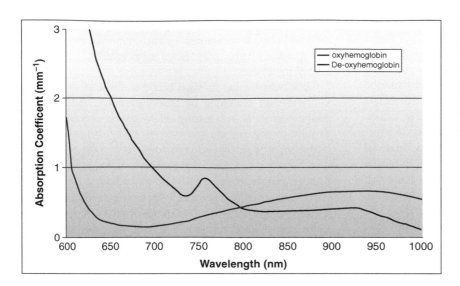

Figure 4
(*See color plate.*) Absorption coefficient of oxyhemoglobin and de-oxyhemoglobin as a function of wavelength. *Source:* Based on data consolidated by Scott Prahl (Oregon Medical Laser Center) from various sources that are available at: http://omlc.ogi.edu/spectra/hemoglobin/index.html.

monochromatic. Of these characteristics, the only one that is important for endovascular PDT is that it is monochromatic and can be matched to the specific peak absorption wavelength of the photoreactive agent. A noncoherent light source such as a light-emitting diode (LED) is also able to provide a spectral output matching a specific peak absorption wavelength of the photoreactive agent. Highly efficient LEDs fabricated into single-use, percutaneous catheter devices have been used clinically for the light activation of talaporfin in patients with refractory solid tumors (38) and their use in endovascular PDT avoids the procedural and economic disadvantages associated with lasers.

Oxygen

The importance of the unrestricted availability of molecular oxygen at the site of, and throughout, the photodynamic process will be clear from earlier discussion on the formation of $^1O_2$. Namely hypoxic tissue may not provide sufficient oxygen for the photodynamic process to occur. In an environment of limited oxygen availability, longer light exposure at lower intensity may provide an effective photodynamic effect, provided that the yield of $^1O_2$ exceeds the tissue's ability to quench.

In one report, the benefit of PDT with 5-aminolevulinic acid (ALA) in preventing intimal hyperplasia after endovascular balloon injury in a rabbit model was present when light activation took place before stenting and was lost when activation followed stenting (39). The authors proposed that this result was because of hypoxia caused by compression of the arterial wall by the expanded stent. On the other hand, in-stent restenosis was not evident in a pilot clinical study involving porfimer sodium where light activation was applied after coronary stenting (35). These potentially discrepant observations may have resulted from the experimental conditions using different drugs.

Biological activities and therapeutic goals

Much animal research on potential cardiovascular applications of PDT has focused on medial smooth muscle cell depletion as a means to reduce neointimal hyperplasia and thus restenosis. Light activation studies on several photoreactive agents using various models of balloon-injured artery in rats, rabbits, or pigs have demonstrated medial SMC depletion and prevention of neointimal hyperplasia (23,25,26,36,39,40–44). In one study in rabbits (40), 30 minutes after intravenous talaporfin (LS11— Table 1) administration, drug fluorescence was found only in the balloon-injured region of the carotid artery. Light activation was applied at that time. At three days, no SMCs were seen in the media of the talaporfin PDT-treated arterial segments. Intimal hyperplasia developed progressively in the untreated balloon-injured segments. However, in the segments treated with PDT intimal hyperplasia was markedly suppressed through to the end of the study at 25 weeks by which time the media had been repopulated by SMCs but no macrophages were present.

At therapeutic dosimetries in vivo, the main photodynamic mechanism for vascular SMC depletion is apoptosis (10). Re-endothelialization appears to be accelerated after PDT and may contribute to the sustained inhibition of neointimal formation (26,45–47). If so, this would be an important advantage over other restenosis prevention strategies such as brachytherapy or certain drug-eluting stents.

In the high cholesterol-fed rabbit atherosclerosis model there is further evidence for macrophage depletion (40) and loss of cholesterol from the plaque (48), suggesting that PDT might actually reduce plaque volume ("atherolysis") (49). PDT mitigates cytokine activity and enhances collagen cross-linking (50) potentially stabilizing the arterial wall. Indeed, burst pressure studies in PDT-treated arterial segments do not indicate that an artery becomes predisposed to rupture through the application of PDT, unless high-energy PDT is used (51,52).

As atherosclerotic plaque progresses the arterial wall vasa vasora contribute branches to support its maintenance (53). Eventually, however, the formation of this fragile, leaky neovascular nest beneath the plaque correlates more closely with inflammatory elements and cytokine production, than with wall thickening per se (54–56). This subintimal neovasculature may contribute to the pathological process, including microvascular hemorrhage, cholesterol deposition, and inflammatory cell delivery (57). Inflammation stimulates neovascular formation, and neovascularization supports the inflammatory process; this pathological positive feedback drives atherosclerotic progression. Thus, subintimal neovascularization might well be a therapeutic target to reduce plaque expansion and to prevent plaque rupture. Antiangiogenic drugs might also be a reasonable approach to attenuate this process (56) presumably by preventing further growth rather than closing existing neovascularization. PDT is able to ablate neovessels clinically both in human cancers and in wet macular degeneration of the eye, so it is reasonable to pursue its potential for targeting neovascularization of the arterial wall as a way to stabilize or reduce atherosclerotic plaque in man. There may be a role here for activation by blue light, which can be highly efficient for many of these drugs but penetrates much less deeply than red light. Work in these areas is at its inception.

Based on these mechanisms of activity, it is obvious that PDT has a potential role preventing neointimal hyperplasia and, therefore, restenosis following angioplasty or stenting of either coronary or peripheral atherosclerotic arteries. It might be useful adjunctively with angioplasty or stents to reduce restenosis, or perhaps as a primary treatment in de novo disease. Long lesions, narrow vessels, diffuse disease, branch or bifurcation disease, in-stent restenosis, and so-called "stent-free zones" all would seem good targets for PDT, as would "vulnerable plaque" stabilization. Re-treatment as needed should be feasible with this technology.

Although the success of drug-eluting stents has curtailed the development of alternative therapeutic strategies in obstructive coronary and carotid artery stenosis, superficial femoral artery and other leg vessels may be a particularly attractive target for PDT because the disease is typically multifocal and/or diffuse, no hardware is left behind that would be subject to wall stresses common in these sites, or that would interfere with future surgical options for care. Some preclinical work and clinical observations suggests PDT might also be useful as an adjunct to angioplasty in vascular access graft dysfunction in hemodialysis patients.

Another exciting potential application of PDT in cardiovascular disease is as a treatment for nonobstructive coronary artery lesions. As PDT has potential atherolytic effects and might reduce pathological neovascularization in highly active plaques, it might be possible to reduce plaque processes that lead to progression and/or plaque rupture. As the low power

of light needed to activate photodynamic drugs will not adversely affect areas of the vessel wall without the drug, and the drug is expected to be inert in the absence of light activation, treatment can theoretically be administered regionally with increased effect in the most diseased areas and little to no effect in normal areas of vessel wall. Thus, it seems ideally suited for regional treatment of arterial segments likely to contain the so-called vulnerable plaques to prevent acute coronary syndromes.

Furthermore, photodynamic drugs fluoresce and can theoretically also diagnose and localize atherosclerotic lesions, with a more intense signal in areas of more intense disease or disease closer to the endothelial surface, for example, thin-cap fibroatheroma or superficial inflammatory erosive disease. Coupled with a sophisticated light catheter an intervention could theoretically be designed to diagnose, localize, and treat atherosclerosis in regions of risk throughout the cardiovascular system (58). Obviously these are areas for future research, not proven uses of photoreactive agents in the cardiovascular system.

Clinical experience

The largest cardiovascular clinical trial experience with PDT has been with motexafin lutetium. These studies were as adjunctive therapy to bare metal stenting in coronary disease and as de novo therapy ("photoangioplasty") in peripheral arterial disease. Light activation in all cases was provided by a light source without blood occlusion following a drug light interval of 18–24 hours (see discussion on Drug to Light Interval and Light Activation). In a phase I study in 79 patients undergoing coronary intervention and stenting (59), motexafin lutetium administration was generally safe. However, there was a dose-related incidence of mild-to-moderate side effects including peripheral paresthesias and skin rashes that were not related to cutaneous photosensitivity. Patients had been instructed to avoid direct, intense sunlight for one week after drug administration and skin photosensitivity reactions were not reported. Analysis of a subgroup of patients who underwent intravascular ultrasound (IVUS) evaluation at baseline and six months suggested a beneficial dose-associated effect on restenosis [transcatheter cardiovascular therapeutics (TCT) 2004]. A similar safety profile was reported in a phase I photoangioplasty study in 47 patients with symptomatic claudication arising from ilio-femoral disease (60). These authors also reported secondary efficacy measures suggesting a beneficial effect.

Another drug, ALA, has been used to treat restenosis of the superficial femoral artery. These have been small, uncontrolled studies. In one report, ALA was given orally in a clinical study of adjuvant PDT in patients undergoing femoral angioplasty (61). Patients left the hospital after an overnight stay and there were no reports of skin photosensitivity. The authors suggested a benefit and no evident safety concerns, leading them to recommend that this therapeutic modality be pursued (37).

Potential complications

The most obvious potential complication of PDT is cutaneous photosensitivity. Careful avoidance of intense, direct light was required for weeks after treatment with first-generation photoactive agents. This risk has been greatly reduced in incidence and severity with the latest generation of photosensitizers, which clear more rapidly from the skin. Nevertheless, minor photosensitivity may remain a factor. Typically, depending on the drug characteristics and dose, patients can leave the treatment facility on the same day but may need to wear dark glasses and avoid bright light for a few days. Skin should be protected from bright lights in the procedure room or from other sources, such as pulse oximeters, as these may emit wavelengths capable of activating photoreactive drugs.

Photosensitivity might possibly be eliminated with intra-arterial drug delivery, enabling the use of much lower doses to achieve similar target tissue concentrations. Various passive (43) or pressure-driven (13) endovascular balloon catheters have been used for this purpose. For example, porfimer sodium was administered through a Dispatch™ catheter (Boston Scientific, Maple Grove, MN, USA) to the site of coronary stenting prior to light activation in a pilot clinical safety investigation in five patients. The intervention was well tolerated and there were no clinical sequelae at 18-month follow-up (62). Apart from cutaneous or ocular photosensitivity, photoreactive agents hold the theoretical prospect of being biologically inert away from the site of light activation.

One of the important theoretical advantages of PDT is that the treatment field is limited by drug, light, and oxygen co-localization. However, inappropriate dosimetry has the potential to create contiguous tissue toxicity or inadequate photodynamic effect. Also, numerous non-PDT drugs have mild photosensitization properties that might augment activity if given concomitantly. Conversely, free radical scavengers may attenuate activity. Drugs or foods that are chromophores might attenuate light delivery, depending on their wavelengths.

In summary, the main beneficial features of PDT that suggest its utility in cardiovascular disease are the localization of photoreactive compounds to injured, and especially to atherosclerotic, arterial wall; the ability to treat a specific site through drug and light co-localization; targeted destruction of medial SMCs, plaque macrophages, and possibly sub-endothelial neovessels by an apparently apoptotic process, with preservation of structural wall elements, rapid re-endothelialization, and SMC repopulation. In addition, there may be a specific effect to reduce plaque cholesterol. Unlike brachytherapy, PDT does not deliver ionizing radiation that is toxic to healthy as well as diseased vessel wall within its

range of penetration. There is no hardware left within the vessel wall, which may be of benefit especially in peripheral vascular disease where long, multifocal lesions occur in vessels that bend and stretch during ambulation. Furthermore, specialists in vascular therapy can perform PDT without the need for separate specialists to manage radiation risks. At least some PDT agents should be able to be used conveniently in the interventional vascular therapy setting without undue constraints to standard practice, and should be able to be repeated if necessary.

Clinical development issues

Photodynamic treatment involves both a photoreactive agent and a light source. Photoreactive agents are energy transducers, helping light to activate oxygen, rather than a "drug"; that is, the treatment effect is a result of the interaction of $^1O_2$ with tissues, not a direct effect of the photoreactive agent. PDT is regulated as a combination product by FDA and as separate drug and medical device entities in Europe.

Combining a drug with a device creates development issues that are factorial in complexity. Within the field of drug development, establishing the best dose range remains an area of underachievement (authors' opinion). Most devices do not have doses, but light-generating devices are an exception. Furthermore, the energy for light activation can be adjusted by changes in power and time of exposure to give an overall dose. As such, establishing the best drug dose in combination with the best light dose is more complicated than simply establishing a drug dose alone. While this issue can be managed by thoughtful development it does not readily fit into the rapid time-to-market mode of most medical devices.

Photosensitizers self-localize to areas of atherosclerosis and vascular wall injury so it makes sense to deliver these agents by intravenous administration. This route offers the flexibility of a single administration regardless of how many sites are treated. On the other hand, high local wall concentrations can be achieved with minimal total body exposure if the agent is administered at the treatment site. Local or regional administration may be particularly useful in applications such as saphenous vein graft disease or arteriovenous grafts dysfunction in hemodialysis patients. Adding an arterial drug delivery device would introduce additional complications to the development process.

After the photosensitizer is administered intravenously it accumulates in areas of the disease and is eliminated from the circulation over a time course that varies from compound to compound. So, in addition to choice of the drug dose and light dose, another important variable is the time from drug administration to light activation. This time is called the DLI (discussed in an earlier section). With drugs that accumulate slowly in plaque and/or have a long half-life of elimination from blood, it makes sense to use a long DLI, typically 4 to 24 hours, between drug administration and light activation. With a long DLI either the drug must be administered before the treatment intervention or else the patient must be brought back to the catheterization laboratory. Depending on the drug, or perhaps the treatment target, a DLI of 30 minutes or less seems feasible. Verteporfin for example, an approved photodynamic treatment that ablates neovascularization to treat age-related wet macular degeneration, uses a DLI of 15 minutes. Drug accumulation in areas of vascular disease is much faster after regional delivery than intravenous infusion, and might be a way to shorten the DLI.

Light can be administered in a variety of forms. There may be interesting opportunities to activate superficial arteries such as the carotid artery, superficial femoral artery (SFA), or an arteriovenous graft from outside the vessel lumen. This approach is limited by potential skin irritation and by loss of irradiance as the light traverses the near side vessel wall, causing "semi-lunar" activation.

Endovascular light has generally been delivered via laser devices. Laser light has many research conveniences, but involves capital and recurring maintenance costs that make it significantly less attractive outside research centers. Light-emitting diodes (LED) can deliver the required wavelengths for effective activation of PDT agents and make single-use, endovascular light activation catheters feasible. Rapid advances in LED technology have led to flexible, small diameter light arrays capable of meeting the variable requirements of endovascular intervention in both coronary and peripheral arterial beds.

As with other endovascular devices, developers of light source catheters used for PDT will need to solve problems related to ease of use, proximal and distal fall-off, overlap, and varying lumen diameters. Whether it is preferable to have a longer light emitter that covers a region of disease or a shorter light source that can be pulled back through diseased vessels is not yet clear. Arterial branches and bifurcations constitute obvious anatomical obstacles for stents. Light delivery catheters have the flexibility to negotiate branches and bifurcations; on the other hand, light dose may be unpredictable, with overlap as a potential concern.

Summary

Photodynamic therapy seems to offer broad applicability as either an adjunct to other endovascular procedures or as a means to treat de novo disease. At this juncture enough is known to imagine its potential without yet knowing its limitations. PDT could be an exciting tool for the emerging specialty of endovascular therapy, with potential applications in the heart, peripheral arteries, saphenous vein grafts, and arteriovenous grafts.

Endovascular biotechnology is transforming traditional relationships between medical specialties. It is also transforming traditional relationships between regulatory divisions, and between drug and device companies. Most importantly, it is transforming patient care. We hope PDT will be able to contribute importantly to these changes.

References

1. von Tappeiner H. On the action of fluorescent substances on infusoria according to the research of O. Raab. Münch Med Wochenschr 1900; 47:5–7.

2. Lipson RL, Baldes EJ, Olsen AM. The use of a derivative of hematoporphyrin in tumor detection. J Natl Cancer Inst 1961; 26:1–11.

3. Diamond I, Granelli S, McDonagh AF, et al. Photodynamic therapy of malignant tumors. Lancet 1972; ii:1175–1177.

4. Moan J, Berg K. The photodegradation of porphyrins in cells can be used to estimate the lifetime of singlet oxygen. Photochem Photobiol 1991; 53(4):549–553.

5. Moor AC. Signaling pathways in cell death and survival after photodynamic therapy. J Photochem Photobiol B 2000; 57(1): 1–13.

6. Kessel D, Luo Y. Photodynamic therapy: a mitochondrial inducer of apoptosis. Cell Death Differ 1999; 6(1):28–35.

7. Villanueva A, Dominguez V, Polo S, et al. Photokilling mechanisms induced by zinc(II)-phthalocyanine on cultured tumor cells. Oncol Res 1999; 11(10):447–453.

8. Plaetzer K, Kiesslich T, Krammer B, et al. Characterization of the cell death modes and the associated changes in cellular energy supply in response to AlPcS$_4$-PDT. Photochem Photobiol Sci 2002; 1(3):172–177.

9. Sakharov DV, Bunschoten A, van Weelden H, et al. Photodynamic treatment and H_2O_2-induced oxidative stress result in different patterns of cellular protein oxidation. Eur J Biochem 2003; 270:4859–4865.

10. LaMuraglia GM, Schiereck J, Heckenkamp J, et al. Photodynamic therapy induces apoptosis in intimal hyperplastic arteries. Am J Pathol 2000; 157:867–875.

11. Granville DJ, Cassidy BA, Ruehlmann DO, et al. Mitochondrial release of apoptosis-inducing factor and cytochrome c during smooth muscle cell apoptosis. Am J Pathol 2001; 159: 305–311.

12. Statius van Eps RG, Adili F, LaMuraglia GM. Photodynamic therapy inactivates cell-associated basic fibroblast growth factor: a silent way of vascular smooth muscle eradication. Cardiovasc Res 1997; 35:334–340.

13. Adili F, Statius van Eps RG, Flotte TJ, et al. Photodynamic therapy with local photosensitizer delivery inhibits experimental intimal hyperplasia. Lasers Surg Med 1998; 23:263–273.

14. Spears JR, Serur J, Shropshire D, Paulin S. Fluorescence of experimental atheromatous plaques with hematophorphyrin derivative. J Clin Invest 1983; 71:395–399.

15. Kessel D, Sykes E. Porphyrin accumulation by atheromatous plaques of the aorta. Photochem Photobiol 1984; 40(1): 59–61.

16. Yasunaka Y, Aizawa K, Asahara T, et al. In vivo accumulation of photosensitizers in atherosclerotic lesions and blood in atherosclerotic rabbits. Lasers Life Sci 1991; 4(1):53–65.

17   Hayashi J, Kuroiwa Y, Sato H, et al. Transadventitial localization of atheromatous plaques by fluorescence emission spectrum analysis of mono-L-aspartyl chlorin e6. Cardiovasc Res 1993; 27:1943–1947.

18   Hayashi J, Saito T, Sato H, et al. Direct visualization of atherosclerosis in small coronary arteries using the epifluorescence stereoscope. Cardiovasc Res 1995; 30:775–780.

19   Saito T, Hayashi J, Kawabe H, et al. Photodynamic treatment for atherosclerotic plaques of the rabbit abdominal aorta by the laparoscopic approach using a pheophorbide derivative. Med Electron Microsc 1996; 29:137–144.

20   Allison BA, Crespo MT, Jain AK, et al. Delivery of benzoporphyrin derivative, a photosensitizer, into atherosclerotic plaque of Watanabe heritable hyperlipidemic rabbits and balloon-injured New Zealand Rabbits. Photochem Photobiol 1997; 65(5):877–883.

21   Katoh T, Asahara T, Naitoh Y, et al. In vivo intravascular laser photodynamic lesions using a lateral direction fiber. Lasers Surg Med 1997; 20:373–381.

22   Amemiya T, Nakajima H, Katoh T, et al. Photodynamic therapy of atherosclerosis using YAG-OPO laser and porfimer sodium, and comparison with using argon-dye laser. Jpn Circ J 1999; 63(4):288–295.

23   Usui M, Asahara T, Naitoh Y, et al. Photodynamic therapy for the prevention of intimal hyperplasia in balloon-injured rabbit arteries. Jpn Circ J 1999; 63:387–393.

24   Uchimura N, Aizawa K, Nagae T, et al. In vivo accumulation of mono-L-aspartyl chlorin e6 in injured arteries after angioplasty. J Japan Soc Laser Surg Med 2000; 21(1):1–8.

25   Nagae T, Aizawa K, Uchimura N, et al. Endovascular photodynamic therapy using mono-L-aspartyl chlorin e6 to inhibit intimal hyperplasia in balloon-injured rabbit arteries. Lasers Surg Med 2001; 28:381–388.

26   Yamaguchi A, Woodburn KW, Hayase M, et al. Reduction of vein graft disease using photodynamic therapy with motexafin lutetium in a rodent isograft model. Circulation 2000; 102(suppl III):275–280.

27   Brown MS, Basu SK, Falck JR, et al. The scavenger cell pathway for lipoprotein degradation: specificity of the binding site that mediates the uptake of negatively charged LDL by macrophages. J Supramol Struct 1980; 13:67–81.

28   de VRies HE, Buchner B, Berkel TJC, Kuiper J. Specific interaction of oxidized low-density lipoprotein with macrophage-derived foam cells isolated from rabbit atherosclerotic lesions. Aterioscler Thromb Vasc Biol 1999; 19:638–645.

29   Aizawa K. Pathognostic image pattern of a spectrum of photosensitizers. Oyo Buturi 2001; 70(6):666–671.

30   Wada S, Sugiyama A, Yamamoto T, et al. Lipid accumulation in smooth muscle cells under LDL loading is independent of LDL receptor pathway and enhanced by hypoxic conditions. Arterioscler Thromb Vasc Biol 2002; 22:1712–1719.

31   Chen Z, Woodburn KW, Shi C, et al. Photodynamic therapy with motexafin lutetium induces redox-sensitive apoptosis of vascular cells. Arterioscler Thromb Vasc Biol 2001; 21:759–764.

32   Vogel S, Minshall RD, Pilipovic´M, et al. Albumin uptake and transcytosis in endothelial cells in vivo induced by albumin-binding protein. Am J Physiol Lung Cell Mol Physiol 2001; 281:1512–1522.

33   Prince MR, Deutsch T, Matthews-Roth MM, et al. Preferential light absorption in atheromas in vivo. J Clin Invest 1986; 78:295–302.

34   Usui M, Miyagi M, Fukasawa S, et al. A first trial in the clinical application of photodynamic therapy for the prevention of restenosis after coronary-stent placement. Lasers Surg Med 2004; 34(3):235–241.

35   Jenkins MP, Buonaccorsi GA, Mansfield R, et al. Reduction in the response to coronary and iliac artery injury with photodynamic therapy using 5-aminolaevulinic acid. Cardiovasc Res 2000; 45:478–485.

36   Mansfield RJR, Jenkins MP, Pai ML, et al. Long-term safety and efficacy of superficial femoral artery angioplasty with adjuvant photodynamic therapy to prevent restenosis. Br J Surg 2002; 89:1538–1539.

37   Lustig RA, Vogl TJ, Fromm D, et al. A multicenter phase I safety study of intratumoral photoactivation of talaporfin sodium in patients with refractory solid tumors. Cancer 2003; 98(8):1767–1771.

38   Pai M, Jamal W, Mosse A, et al. Inhibition of in-stent restenosis in rabbit iliac arteries with photodynamic therapy. Eur J Vasc Endovasc Surg 2005; 30(6):573–581.

39   Waksman R, Leitch I, Roessler J, et al. Intracoronary photodynamic therapy reduces neointimal growth without suppressing re-endothelialization in a porcine model. Heart 2006 (e-Pub).

40   Wakamatsu T, Saito T, Hayashi J, et al. Long-term inhibition of intimal hyperplasia using vascular photodynamic therapy in balloon-injured carotid arteries. Med Mol Morphol 2005; 38(4):225–232.

41   Cheung J, Todd M, Turnbull R, et al. Longer term assessment of photodynamic therapy for intimal hyperplasia: a pilot study. J Photochem Photobiol B 2004; 73(3):141–147.

42   Gabeler EE, van Hillegersberg R, Statius van Eps RG, et al. Endovascular photodynamic therapy with aminolaevulinic acid prevents balloon induced intimal hyperplasia and constrictive remodelling. Eur J Vasc Endovasc Surg 2002; 24(4):322–331.

43   Visona A, Angelini A, Gobbo S, et al. Local photodynamic therapy with Zn(II)-phthalocyanine in an experimental model of intimal hyperplasia. J Photochem Photobiol B 2000; 57(2–3):94–101.

44   Nyamekye I, Buonaccorsi G, McEwan J, et al. Inhibition of intimal hyperplasia in balloon injured arteries with adjunctive phthalocyanine sensitised photodynamic therapy. Eur J Vasc Endovasc Surg 1996;11(1):19–28.

45   LaMuraglia GM, ChandraSekar NR, Flotte TJ, et al. Photodynamic therapy inhibition of experimental intimal hyperplasia: acute and chronic effects. J Vasc Surg 1994; 19(2):321–329.

46   Adili F, Statius van Eps RG, Karp SJ, et al. Differential modulation of vascular endothelial and smooth muscle cell function by photodynamic therapy of extracellular matrix: novel insights into radical-mediated prevention of intimal hyperplasia. J Vasc Surg 1996; 23(4):698–705.

47   Adili F, Scholz T, Hille M, et al. Photodynamic therapy mediated induction of accelerated re-endothelialisation following injury to the arterial wall: implications for the prevention of postinterventional restenosis. Eur J Vasc Endovasc Surg 2002; 24(2):166–175.

48 Hayashi J, Saito T, Aizawa K. Change in chemical composition of lipids accumulated in atheromas of rabbits following photodynamic therapy. Lasers Surg Med 1997; 21(3): 287–293.

49 Kipshidze N, Petrosyan J. New trends in laser application: atherolysis. Int Angiol 1990; 9(2):111–116.

50 Overhaus M, Heckenkamp J, Kossodo S, et al. Photodynamic therapy generates a matrix barrier to invasive vascular cell migration. Circ Res 2000; 86(3):334–340.

51 Grant WE, Buonaccorsi G, Speight PM, et al. The effect of photodynamic therapy on the mechanical integrity of normal rabbit carotid arteries. Laryngoscope 1995; 105(8 Pt 1): 867–871.

52 Gabeler EE, Van Hillegersberg R, Sluiter W, et al. Arterial wall strength after endovascular photodynamic therapy. Lasers Surg Med 2003; 33(1):8–15.

53 Barger AC, Beeuwkes R, Lainey LL, Silverman KJ. Hypothesis: vasa vasorum and neovascularization of human coronary arteries. A possible role in the pathophysiology of atherosclerosis. N Engl J Med 1984; 310(3):175–177.

54 O'Brien K, McDonald TO, Chait A, et al. Neovascular expression of E-selectin, intercellular adhesion molecule-1, and vascular cell adhesion molecule-1 in human atherosclerosis and their relation to intimal leukocyte content. Circulation 1996; 93:672–682.

55 Fleiner M, Kummer M, Mirlacher M, et al. Arterial neovascularization and inflammation in vulnerable patients. Circulation 2004; 110:2843–2850.

56 Virmani R, Kolodgie FD, Burke AP, et al. Atherosclerotic plaque progression and vulnerability to rupture: angiogenesis as a source of intraplaque hemorrhage. Arterioscler Thromb Vasc Biol 2005; 25:2054–2061.

57 Moulton KS, Vakili K, Zurakowski D, et al. Inhibition of plaque neovascularization reduces macrophage accumulation and progression of advanced atherosclerosis. PNAS, 2003; 100:4736–4741.

58 Leon MB, Lu DY, Prevosti LG, et al. Human arterial surface fluorescence: atherosclerotic plaque identification and effects of laser atheroma ablation. J Am Coll Cardiol 1988; 12(1):94–102.

59 Keriakes DJ, Szyniszewski AM, Wahr D, et al. Phase 1 drug and light dose-escalation trial of motexafin lutetium and far-red light activation (phototherapy) in subjects with coronary artery disease undergoing percutaneous coronary intervention and stent deployment: procedural and long-term results. Circulation 2003; 108:1320–1315.

60 Rockson SG, Kramer P, Razavi M, et al. Photoangioplasty for human peripheral atherosclerosis: results of a phase 1 trial of photodynamic therapy with motexafin lutetium (Antrin). Circulation 2000; 102:2322–2324.

61 Jenkins MP, Buonaccorsi GA, Raphael M, et al. Clinical study of adjuvant photodynamic therapy to reduce restenosis following femoral angioplasty. Br J Surg 1999; 86:1258–1263.

62 Usui M, Fukasawa S, Takata R, et al. Photodynamic therapy with a locally delivered photosensitizer inhibits neointimal hyperplasia in animal and human subjects. Jpn J Interv Cardiol 2002; 17:375–381.

34

Angiogenesis and myogenesis

Shaker A. Mousa

Ischemia is known to promote angiogenesis, and the molecular mechanisms and growth factors involved have been thoroughly investigated. Angiogenesis and myogenesis occur concomitantly in regenerating muscles because of ischemia-induced cell death and inflammation. Therapeutic angiogenesis and vasculogenesis, which involve the administration of angiogenic growth factors, cytokines, or stem cells to stimulate collateral formation and improve myocardial perfusion, are being tested as alternative strategies for patients with medically intractable angina who are not candidates for mechanical revascularization therapies.

A variety of growth factors and chemokines convincingly increase the formation of small blood vessels in experimental models. Most clinical trials to date involve the transfer of vascular endothelial growth factor (VEGF) or fibroblast growth factor (FGF) using several delivery strategies.

The efficacy of gene transfer approaches to therapeutic angiogenesis is now being tested in clinical trials. Controlled phase II trials are providing positive but not definitive results. Gene therapy appears to be safe based on these data. Hard clinical endpoints, such as mortality, myocardial infarction, and the need for revascularization are lacking, as is long-term follow-up.

Myogenic cell transplantation into an infarcted region is intended to restore elasticity to the injured region and prevent cardiac thinning and dilatation. Several types of cultured cells have been transplanted into infarcted myocardium. However, mortality of cells after implantation in high fibrotic infarcted myocardium seems to be high because the oxygen and nutrient supply are limited within the scar. Furthermore, in current clinical trials the survival of the transplanted myogenic cells might be facilitated by the use of therapeutic angiogenesis. Hence, angiogenic therapy before myogenesis might be justified in future clinical trials.

Therapeutic angiogenesis is an emerging strategy for treating ischemic diseases by inducing new blood vessel growth in ischemic tissues. These therapies may be classified into four primary groups:

- Protein growth factors that stimulate newly sprouting vessels.
- Gene therapy to generate proteins that stimulate new vessel growth.
- Laser treatments that create channels in the myocardium, resulting in an angiogenic (wound) response.
- Small molecules that are driven from natural or synthetic sources that act directly or indirectly via endogenous pro-angiogenesis factors to promote angiogenesis.

There are now more than eight therapeutic angiogenesis agents in various stages of clinical trials. Clinical trials to date indicate that these agents are generally safe and well-tolerated. Despite the controversies surrounding gene therapy, delivery of naked DNA and adenoviral vectors encoding the angiogenic growth factor VEGF have been safely achieved in early phase I and II trials of patients with coronary and peripheral vascular disease. One striking finding from virtually all trials of angiogenic therapy is the placebo effect in reduction of angina, underscoring the need for controlled clinical trials and objective measurements. Presently, measurement of improvement following therapy involves nuclear perfusion scanning including single-photon emission computed tomography (SPECT), magnetic resonance imaging, exercise treadmill testing, and angiography. A number of phase II studies are underway to determine efficacy. A number of common cardiac drugs—such as lasix, bumetanide, captopril, isosorbide, and even aspirin—have been rediscovered to have antiangiogenic properties. The clinical significance of these drugs in modulating angiogenesis is not yet known.

Therapeutic angiogenesis is an experimental area of treatment for cardiac ischemia, which is a common symptom of coronary artery disease. Cardiac ischemia is usually a temporary situation in which the heart does not get enough oxygen. This lack of oxygen is often because of a blocked or obstructed coronary artery in the heart. *Angiogenesis* is the process by which new blood vessels are formed to supply the heart muscle with oxygen-rich blood. These new blood vessels are called *collaterals*.

The term "collaterals" should not be confused with the growth of the heart's coronary arteries or the aorta. Collaterals are smaller branches of blood vessels.

Angiogenesis is a natural process that occurs during healing. The goal with therapeutic angiogenesis is to stimulate the creation of blood cells through medical intervention. By doing this, researchers hope to increase the level of oxygen-rich blood reaching damaged areas of the heart.

Although more research is necessary, some researchers are hoping that therapeutic angiogenesis may one day offer the benefits of a bypass without open-heart surgery. The identification of angiogenic growth factors, such as VEGF and FGF, has fueled interest in using such factors to induce therapeutic angiogenesis. The results of numerous animal studies and clinical trials have offered promise for new treatment strategies for various ischemic diseases. Increased understanding of the cellular and molecular biology of vessel growth has, however, prompted investigators and clinicians alike to reconsider the complexity of therapeutic angiogenesis. The realization that formation of a stable vessel is a complex, multistep process may provide useful insights into the design of the next generation of angiogenesis therapy.

Angiogenesis is the growth of blood vessels from a pre-existing vessel bed. Clinical interest in the control of angiogenesis arises from two distinct quarters. In one case, the goal is to block the growth of new vessels as a means to suppress and/or regress tumor growth, or to suppress vessel proliferation in pathologies such as diabetes. In the second case, the objective is to induce or stimulate vessel growth in patients with conditions characterized by insufficient blood flow, such as ischemic heart disease, peripheral vascular diseases, and other diseases (Fig. 1). The latter applications are the focus of this chapter. Insufficient angiogenesis might occur because of the decrease of endogenous pro-angiogenesis factors (positive regulators) or increase in endogenous antiangiogenesis factors (negative regulators) or both (Table 1). We discuss some of the recent efforts to induce new

vessel growth and highlight challenges that have arisen regarding the means of delivery and efficacy of angiogenesis induction.

Therapeutic angiogenesis

There are several pro-angiogenic factors that promote angiogenesis (Table 2). Those include growth factors, hormone receptor agonists, pro-coagulants, extracellular matrix proteins, or glycosaminoglycans (GAGs).

Pro-angiogenesis factors

Both basic fibroblast growth factor (FGF-2) and VEGF-A have been used in attempts to stimulate angiogenesis.

Fibroblast growth factor

The FGF family consists of an ever-increasing number of peptide growth factors with diverse cellular targets and biological effects (1). Two family members, acidic FGF (FGF-1) and FGF-2, have a strong affinity for heparin and have been studied for their effects on vascular cells, including endothelial cells (ECs) and smooth muscle cells. Extensive evidence indicates that both FGF-1 and FGF-2 are potent angiogenic factors, providing support for their use as stimuli for therapeutic angiogenesis in vivo. It is also important to note that many cell types express one of the four FGF receptors and that FGF has been shown to have biological effects, which indicates that both FGF-1 and FGF-2 are potent angiogenic factors; this provides support for their use as stimuli for therapeutic angiogenesis in vivo. It is also important to note that many cell types express one of the four FGF receptors and that FGF has been shown to have biological effects in a number of cell systems, including induction of neurite outgrowth, suppression of skeletal muscle differentiation, and induction of bone formation and neuroprotection, to name just a few.

For patients with advanced symptomatic coronary artery disease that is not amenable to standard mechanical revascularization strategies, numerous innovative approaches are being developed. These approaches include promoting the growth of new blood vessels in the myocardium using several potential compounds, delivery vectors, and delivery mechanisms to the ischemic myocardium.

In numerous animal models, it has reportedly promoted angiogenesis, improved myocardial perfusion, and acutely improved endothelial vasodilatory function. In the present study, we report the impact of the administration of recombinant FGF-2 (rFGF-2) on stress and rest myocardial perfusion using gated SPECT myocardial perfusion imaging in a phase I trial in humans with advanced symptomatic coronary artery disease.

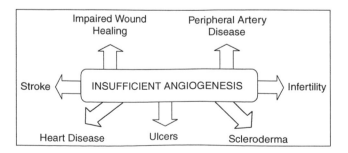

Figure 1
Diseases associated with insufficient angiogenesis.

Table 1   Endogenous pro- and antiangiogenic factors

Positive regulators	Negative regulators
VEGF-A (VPC)	Thrombospondin
VEGF-C	NK1, NK2, NK3 fragments of HGF
bFGF	TGF-beta-1
HGF	Heparin
Proteases and collagenases	Plasminogen (angiostatin)
Angiopoietin-1	High molecular weight kininogen (domain 5)
PDGF	Fibronectin (45-kD fragment)
EGF	EGF (fragment)
IGF-1	Alpha-2 antiplasmin (fragment)
IGF BP-3	Beta-thromboglobulin
Adenosine	TIMP 1,2
Extracellular matrix protein	Collagen fragments (endostatin)
Thyroid hormone	PF4
Procoagulants	

Abbreviations: bFGF, basic fibroblast growth factor; EGF, epidermal growth factor; HGF, hepatocyte growth factor; IGF, insulin-like growth factor; PDGF, platelet-derived growth factor; PF4, platelet factor-4; TGF, transforming growth factor; TIMP, tissue inhibitor of matrix metalloproteinase; VEGF, vascular endothelial growth factor.

Table 2   Pro-angiogenic factors

Angiopoietin-1
aFGF and bFGF
HGF/SF
Insulin
IL-8
Leptin
Placental growth factor
PDGF-BB
Thyroid hormone (T3, T4, and analogs)
Tissue factor/factor VIIa and other procoagulants
TGF-α and β
TNF-α
VEGF/VPF
Adenosine receptor agonists
Protease-activated receptor agonists
GAGs
Extracellular matrix proteins

Abbreviations: aFGF, acidic fibroblast growth factors; bFGF, basic fibroblast growth factors; GAGs, glycosaminoglycans; HGF, hepatocyte growth factor; IL-8, Interleukin-8; PDGF-BB, platelet-derived growth factor-BB; SF, scatter factor; TGF, transforming growth factor; TNF, tumor necrosis factor-alpha; VEGF, vascular endothelial growth factor; VPF, vascular permeability factor.

Hence, in patients with symptomatic advanced coronary artery disease, these preliminary data suggest that rFGF-2 attenuates the magnitude of stress-induced ischemia and improves resting myocardial blood flow among a subset of patients with resting hypoperfusion. The findings are consistent with a favorable but modest effect of therapeutic angiogenesis with this agent, resulting in improved myocardial blood supply and coronary flow reserve. Should these data be confirmed in upcoming and ongoing trials and if they are accompanied by improvements in clinical parameters, they may signal the beginning of an important new approach to patients with advanced symptomatic coronary artery disease: medical revascularization with agents promoting therapeutic angiogenesis.

Vascular endothelial growth factor-A

VEGF-A is the prototypic member of a family of secreted, homodimeric glycoproteins with EC-specific mitogenic activity and the ability to stimulate angiogenesis in vivo (2). VEGF-A also increases vascular permeability, with an effect 10,000 times more potent than that of the vasoactive substance histamine; VEGF-A was originally purified based on this property, and it was named vascular permeability factor (3). The VEGF-A family of polypeptides consists of a number of biochemically distinct isoforms (three isoforms in the mouse and up to five in humans) that are generated through alternative mRNA splicing of a single gene (4,5). The isoforms are named by the number of amino acids that comprise the proteins; the human isoforms include VEGF-121, VEGF-145, VEGF-165, VEGF-189, and VEGF-206.

Adenosine receptor agonists

Recent reports indicate that circulating endothelial progenitor cells (EPCs) may be recruited to sites of neovascularization where they differentiate into ECs. As we have previously demonstrated that adenosine A_{2A} agonists promote neovascularization in wounds (6,7), we sought to determine whether adenosine A_{2A} receptor agonist-augmented wound healing involves vessel sprouting (angiogenesis) or EPC recruitment (vasculogenesis) or both. Evidence is currently provided that an exogenous agent such as an adenosine A_{2A} receptor agonist increases neovascularization in the early stages of wound repair by increasing both EPC recruitment (vasculogenesis) and local vessel sprouting (angiogenesis) (6,7).

Thyroid hormone analogs

A recently identified thyroid hormone cell surface receptor on the extracellular domain of integrin alphaVbeta (3) leads to the activation of the mitogen-activated protein kinase (MAPK) signal transduction cascade in human cell lines. Examples of MAPK-dependent thyroid hormone actions are plasma membrane ion pump stimulation and specific nuclear events. These events include serine phosphorylation of the nuclear thyroid hormone receptor, leading to co-activator protein recruitment and complex tissue responses, such as thyroid hormone-induced angiogenesis. The existence of this cell surface receptor means that the activity of the administered hormone could be limited through structural modification of the molecule to reproduce only those hormone actions initiated at the cell surface (8,9).

In view of the evidence that thyroid hormone administration has angiogenic effects on the hypertrophic myocardium, the hypothesis that the capillary supply in the hypertrophic myocardium surviving infarction would be improved by administration of the thyroid hormone analog, di-iodothyroproprionic acid (DITPA) was tested. Subcutaneously administered DITPA to rats for 10 days following experimental infarction of the left ventricle (LV) resulted in increased capillary density in the remote region and the LV in the border region, indicating a more marked angiogenic response. In hearts with large infarcts, LV perfusion in the border region was higher in the DITPA group than in the nontreated rats. In the DITPA-treated group, cardiocyte size in the border region was positively correlated with that of the other regions, which contrasts with the negative correlations noted for the saline rats. These data suggest that DITPA therapy may improve maximal perfusion potential of the hypertrophied myocardium surviving a myocardial infarction, and it is selectively effective in the border region of hearts with large infarcts (10).

Glycosaminoglycans

Therapeutic angiogenesis with VEGF and FGF-2 provides an important clinical approach in ischemic myocardium, wound healing, and endometrial regeneration. In vitro and in vivo studies showed that a single growth factor may be insufficient for therapeutic angiogenesis. However, signals participate in the modulation of growth factor response, contribute to the architecture of the vasculature, and provide signals for the stabilization of mature capillary networks that are not well defined. The contributions of cell surface GAGs to some critical biological processes are now understood in significantly

molecular detail. However, the role of GAGs in angiogenesis is still not clear. In this study, we used an in vitro three-dimensional angiogenesis system in which human dermal microvascular ECs (HDMECs) are cultured on microcarrier beads and embedded in a three-dimensional gel to delineate the regulatory effect of synthetic oligosaccharides on angiogenesis. Using this assay, for the first time we demonstrated that a branched sulfated oligosaccharide (OS2) significantly enlarged the endothelial capillary network initiated by VEGF and FGF-2. Furthermore, the capillary network initiated by VEGF and FGF-2 lasted no more than seven days, but addition of OS2 significantly stabilized the capillary network of HDMEC for up to 20 days (11). OS2 alone had no effect on angiogenesis in vitro; it required angiogenic factors to initiate angiogenesis. In vivo, OS2 alone stimulated angiogenesis in the chick chorioallantoic membrane model. In conclusion, we suggest that chemically defined oligosaccharides played an important role in regulation of capillary structure, stability that might contribute to future angiogenesis therapy.

Preclinical studies

Current clinical trials of angiogenesis factors were preceded by a large number of studies using animal models of cardiac or peripheral ischemia. Early studies involved protein administration, whereas later efforts began to use gene therapy. In one early study using recombinant protein, a single intra-arterial injection of 500–1000 µg of VEGF-165 into rabbits with severe experimental hindlimb ischemia increased collateral vessels, as detected by angiography and histological analysis (12). Naked plasmid DNA injected directly into the skeletal muscle in a later study, using the same hindlimb ischemia model, also yielded increased collateral vessels, as determined by angiography. Although such reports of increased vessel growth and functional improvement in response to exogenously administered angiogenic factors are encouraging, it is essential to note that animal models such as the ischemic hindlimb model have definite limitations. Whereas the ischemia in the animal models is acute (produced by surgical procedure), the ischemia that characterizes the human disease often arises over an extended time and occurs in the context of complex atherosclerotic processes. The responses seen in the experimental models may thus be quite different in terms of the kinetics of vessel growth as well as the nature of the resultant vessels.

In a study assessing the effects of VEGF-A on myocardial ischemia in a porcine model of progressive coronary artery occlusion, VEGF-A was delivered by osmotic pump; magnetic resonance mapping revealed a reduction in the size of the ischemic zone and improved cardiac function (13). A single bolus injection was also found to produce significant improvements in myocardial blood flow and function (14). Myocardial ischemia in animals has also been treated with FGF. Delivery of FGF-2 via implantation of heparin-alginate beads led to an 80% reduction in infarct size and improved cardiac function in pigs with experimentally induced coronary artery constrictions, as compared with untreated controls (15). These studies were followed closely by the demonstration of gene therapy in a porcine model of stress-induced myocardial ischemia. Intracoronary injection of a recombinant adenovirus expressing another member of the FGF family, human FGF-5, led to improvements in stress-induced function and blood flow that were maintained for 12 weeks (16).

The identification of angiogenic growth factors, such as VEGF and FGF, has fueled interest in using such factors to induce therapeutic angiogenesis. The results of numerous animal studies and clinical trials have offered promise for new treatment strategies for various ischemic diseases. Increased understanding of the cellular and molecular biology of vessel growth has, however, prompted investigators and clinicians alike to reconsider the complexity of therapeutic angiogenesis. The realization that formation of a stable vessel is a complex, multistep process may provide useful insights into the design of the next generation of angiogenesis. Clinical interest in the control of angiogenesis arises from two distinct quarters. In one case, the goal is to block the growth of new vessels as a means to suppress and/or regress tumor growth, or to suppress vessel proliferation in pathologies such as diabetes. In the second case, the objective is to induce or stimulate vessel growth in patients with conditions characterized by insufficient blood flow, such as ischemic heart disease and peripheral vascular diseases. The latter applications are the focus of this review. We discuss some of the recent efforts to induce new vessel growth and highlight challenges that have arisen regarding the means of delivery and efficacy of angiogenesis induction.

Clinical trials

Results from basic research have proven that both VEGF-A and FGF-2 are potent angiogenic factors, and the use of these factors in animal models has indicated that they have therapeutic potential. The two factors have, therefore, been entered into clinical trials, testing their ability to provide angiogenesis therapy for various diseases in which new vessel growth is desirable. Both VEGF-A and FGF-2 have been tested in phase I clinical trials, with mixed results (17,18). Although phase I trials are not designed to test efficacy, many important insights regarding the potential obstacles in using angiogenic therapies have become evident.

Fibroblast growth factor

In one study, human recombinant FGF-2 was administered intraoperatively to areas of the coronary artery in 20 patients who were undergoing surgical revascularization (19). Angiographic analysis revealed evidence of collateralization. Local sustained release of high-dose (but not low-dose) FGF-2

to ischemic areas, in 24 patients during bypass surgery, led to a reduction in stress defect size (20). In a recent study involving 59 patients with coronary disease, the response to intravenous or intracoronary human recombinant FGF-2 was monitored by SPECT imaging (21). Perfusion was monitored at approximately one, two, and three months after growth factor administration. Analysis of global stress perfusion or inducible ischemia revealed a consistent and sustained reduction in the extent and severity of stress-inducible ischemia, as well as an improvement in resting perfusion in areas where there was a risk of ischemia.

Vascular endothelial growth factor

In an early phase I trial to test the safety and bioactivity of VEGF-A, naked VEGF-165 DNA was injected into the myocardium of five patients who had failed standard therapy. SPECT imaging demonstrated reduced ischemia (22). Adenoviral delivery of VEGF-121 to the myocardium of 21 patients by direct injection, either as an adjunct to coronary bypass grafting or as the sole therapy, led to improvement in the area injected, as measured by angiography; angina was also reduced (23). Administration of recombinant VEGF-121 improved function, as detected by SPECT (24). Furthermore, this study revealed a dose-dependent improvement in both stress perfusion and rest perfusion; there was an infrequent response in patients who received low-dose VEGF and an improvement in five of six patients who received high-dose VEGF. In a different approach, VEGF cDNA was delivered via liposomes by catheter to coronary arteries following angioplasty (25). While this phase I safety trial did not show an effect of VEGF-A on the degree of coronary ischemia, it did prove that the treatment was well tolerated. It is important to note that no phase II-controlled studies using defined and quantifiable endpoints have demonstrated efficacy of therapeutic angiogenesis. This highlights the main obstacles for assessing a therapeutic response to angiogenesis therapy, the reliability of the assessment methods, and the possible complications of the placebo effect. Thus, there is a critical need for more controlled trials and for the development of better defined and more quantifiable endpoints.

Mode of delivery

Delivery strategy is one of the most important variables when using angiogenic factors to treat pathological conditions. Expression of VEGF-A is tightly controlled during development, and slight changes in VEGF-A protein levels are associated with developmental abnormalities and embryonic lethality (26,27) Additionally, the unregulated expression of VEGF-A in the myocardium has been reported to produce deleterious cardiac effects in an animal model, causing cardiac failure and death (28). Clearly, if VEGF-A is to be used for therapeutic angiogenesis, tight control of its levels must be achieved.

Drug-eluting stents have been very effective. However, clinical concerns remain, despite the low thrombosis rates of 1% to 2%. Residual thrombosis can lead to a large myocardial infarction or frequently death. The thrombosis rates are quite similar with the Cypher, Taxus, and bare metal stents (BMSs). However, the question is whether the thrombosis can be reduced close to zero, without the patient taking antiplatelet drugs.

BMSs are usually well covered by an intimal hyperplasia. But, with drug-eluting stents, because of the potency of the drug being eluted, sometimes struts are found that are thinly or barely covered by intimal hyperplasia. Hence, the concern is actually a "vulnerable" stent strut. The polymer around the metal of the strut is usually quite thin and usually next to the blood stream, providing the potential for some of the metal strut to be exposed to the blood stream.

The stent struts are comprised of the metal and the polymer, and, over time, the drug disappears (e.g., with the Cypher stent) or some drug will remain (e.g., with the Taxus stent). Thus, there is the potential for some metal, polymer, and drug to remain exposed to the blood stream. Using high-resolution imaging techniques, intimal hyperplasia is seen when looking at BMS in vivo.

Factors that make a stent strut vulnerable, which may lead to thrombosis, jailing side branches, or breakage of the struts, include the following: polymer/drug coating dissolution, incomplete apposition, stent fracture, and overlap region.

Solutions to decrease thrombosis

Phosphorylcholine (PC) coating is a polymer that mimics the human chemistry of the cell membrane surface. The PC polymer is biocompatible, because it has hydrophobic areas that stick to each other and to the metal, and it is also cross-linked for strength. Its high water affinity allows for water to be attracted to its surface. PC-coated devices have a permanent water layer on the surface, again serving as a potentially biocompatible surface.

An uncoated device would have some thrombus and fibrin coating, but the PC-coated devices are clearly less attractive to blood cells and fibrin. These coatings do not seem to affect endothelialization, and within five days the device is covered with ECs. Potentially, these types of coatings may enhance the safety of the drug-eluting stent, because of the faster endothelialization and because they are more biocompatible.

In a baboon arteriovenous (AV)-fistula shunt model that tested PC-coated stents, platelet adhesion occurs much less frequently with the PC-coated stent, and there is no thrombus formation; conversely, thrombus quickly formed on the uncoated stent. Biocompatible coatings are likely to be part of the future, in terms of trying to help the stents essentially heal by themselves without any antiplatelet therapy.

Bioabsorbable materials

Bioabsorbable materials, such as polylactic acid as a bioabsorbable polymer and the drugs everolimus and biolimus, are being investigated. The safety of the materials have been shown in the FUTURE I FIH trial (everolimus) and the FUTURE II FIH trial (biolimus). A unique design with wells drilled into it, and using polylactide/glycolide and polyanhydrides to absorb drugs such as paclitaxel and use it as a material to deliver the drug is being developed.

Other potential materials that may be more bioinert and biocompatible are also being studied. Boston Scientific is working on iridium oxide coating. There are also other types of systems. For example, there are stents that use a special type of carbon coating, thus making the surface very inorganic. However, these may not have any elutive attributes.

The objective is to achieve a balance between using materials that can have drugs within them, elute the drugs, and have a surface material that can potentially coat the stent and make it more biocompatible. Another approach is making the stent itself disappear. These might be made of a magnesium-based alloy that essentially disappears over about six months.

Protein therapy

At present, the administration of protein seems to be preferable to gene therapy (17). This is mainly because dosage modulation in most clinical settings is far easier with purified protein than with gene therapy, which is hampered by the lack of an expression vector. Although protein therapy has many advantages, there are nevertheless technical problems associated with protein administration, including optimization of purification and formulation of delivery for single and/or multiple angiogenic factors.

Recent advances in drug-delivery methods using bioerodible polymer matrices will allow long-term sustained release of the growth factors (29). This will resolve one of the major problems associated with protein administration: namely, the limited tissue half-life of the purified angiogenic factors in patients. An important consideration, however, is that protein therapy is limited to secreted factors. Delivery of intracellular modulators for therapeutic angiogenesis, including transcription factors that control angiogenesis such as hypoxia-inducible factor-1 alpha (HIF-1α), is only possible through gene therapy.

Gene therapy

Viral vectors have been the most commonly used means of gene delivery for both VEGF-A and FGF-2. Gene therapy presents an attractive alternative to purified proteins because it offers the possibility of sustained production of one or more factors following a single administration. Furthermore, tissue-specific and highly localized production of the therapeutic factor is possible, through the use of tissue-specific promoters.

However, a variety of issues have implications for the use of viral vectors in gene therapy. Obvious potential concerns are the immune and inflammatory responses to viral vectors. Patients who received VEGF-121 via an adenoviral vector had increased levels of serum antiadenoviral neutralizing antibodies, but there was no report on an inflammatory response in these patients (27). The use of adenovirus-mediated gene therapy in treating brain tumors has been reported to lead to active brain inflammation as well as persistent (up to three months after treatment) transgene expression (30).

The lack of gene expression is another potential barrier. Some systems for inducible gene expressions have proved to be effective and safe in animal models (31), but they have not yet been tested in humans. Recent advances in stem cell research provide the possibility of combining gene therapy with ex vivo gene transfer into stem cells for angiogenesis therapy, as will be discussed later. If successful, this approach may overcome most of the obstacles presented by gene therapy.

Issues in therapeutic angiogenesis and potential solutions

Interpatient variability

It is not clear why some individuals develop a collateral circulation sufficient to compensate for their ischemic vascular disease whereas others do not. Certainly, features such as the extent of the disease and the time frame over which the ischemia develops are contributing factors. However, other previously unconsidered variables appear to play important roles.

Collateral vessel development, as measured by blood pressure, angiography, and vessel density, was significantly reduced in old (four to five years old) versus young (six to eight months old) animals (32), in a rabbit model of hind limb ischemia. EC dysfunction and reduced VEGF-A levels were the reasons suggested for the reduced collateral response. A subsequent study, demonstrating an age-dependent reduction in HIF-1α activity, provides one explanation for the lower VEGF-A expression in response to hypoxia in aged animals (33). A reduced response to hypoxia might translate into a weaker angiogenic response. This is supported by the fact that the extent of hypoxic induction of VEGF-A in monocytes correlates strongly with the presence of collateral vessels in patients (34).

It is possible that genetic variability may also play a significant role in an individual's ability to generate collateral vessels in response to ischemia, as well as the capacity to respond to an exogenous angiogenic agent. Not surprisingly, a recent report that assessed the angiogenic response in a murine corneal pocket model to a fixed dosage of FGF-2 in various strains of mice suggested that genetic backgrounds may influence angiogenic response (35). A nearly 10-fold range of response to the fixed dosage of FGF-2 was observed among different inbred strains of mice, suggesting that genetic variability may indeed play a significant role in determining the magnitude of angiogenic response to FGF-2.

Systemic effects

If VEGF-A delivery leads to significant circulating levels, as has been observed following myocardial transfection with VEGF-A's complementary DNA (cDNA) (36), then it may possibly affect angiogenesis elsewhere (37). Because plaque progression might be dependent on angiogenesis (38), investigators were prompted to examine the effect of VEGF-A administration on this process. Mice that were double-deficient in apolipoprotein-E and apolipoprotein-β100 were treated with a single intraperitoneal injection of VEGF-165 recombinant human protein (2 μg/kg). This led to significant increases in plaque area compared with untreated controls (39). In contrast, there has been no evidence of disease progression, to date, in 42 patients treated with intra-arterial gene transfer of naked VEGF-A cDNA. This has been delivered either to promote therapeutic angiogenesis (12 patients) or to accelerate re-endothelization (30 patients) (40). Although these observations suggest that human sensitivity to VEGF-A may be lower than in animal models, it will be necessary to study a larger cohort of patients, with appropriate controls, over a longer period to confirm this (41).

Vascular endothelial growth factor has also been shown to mediate the vessel growth that characterizes tumor expansion as well as the neovascularization that is associated with diabetic retinopathy. Although VEGF is produced locally in both of these circumstances, it is not known whether systemic administration of the factor could exacerbate these conditions by further stimulating vessel growth. Selection of the patient population that may benefit from angiogenic therapy may thus have to involve screening for coexisting conditions that could be activated or worsened by exposure to pro-angiogenic agents.

VEGF-A, FGF-1, and FGF-2 have all demonstrated systemic vascular effects. FGF-1 and FGF-2 have been shown to reduce blood pressure in a dose-dependent manner in rats (42). Similarly, VEGF-A has been reported to cause hypotension and death in pigs following an intracoronary bolus administration (43). Subsequent studies have revealed that VEGF-A administration causes greater vasodilatation of coronary vessels than serotonin or nitroglycerin, and it also causes tachyphylaxis via a nitric oxide-dependent mechanism (44). VEGF-A administration to the extremities of patients has also been associated with hypotension and edema (45). These side effects can be partly explained by the fact that VEGF-A is a potent vascular permeability factor.

VEGF-A isoforms in angiogenesis therapy

The five VEGF-A protein isoforms in humans (and at least three major isoforms in the mouse) have different biochemical and biological properties (46). It is therefore important to determine whether different VEGF-A isoforms give rise to different quality or quantity of vessels. Expression of the various isoforms during development is modulated both spatially and temporally (47), and observations from gene knockout studies have proven that these isoforms do not have equivalent biological functions during vessel development (47,48). Furthermore, there is considerable variability in the phenotype of vessels in tumors expressing different isoforms (49). For example, vessels within tumors expressing predominantly the VEGF-189 isoform, which has a strong heparin-binding affinity and thus is highly localized, are much less leaky than the vessels in tumors expressing the more diffusible VEGF-165 and VEGF-121 isoforms (50). It will be interesting and important to determine whether these observations from experimental systems can help predict the results of clinical trials, which primarily use the VEGF-165 isoform. Finally, as multiple VEGF-A isoforms are expressed during vascular development (47), it will also be important to determine whether the use of multiple isoforms in angiogenesis therapy will be necessary to replicate in vivo conditions.

Achieving vessel stability

The induction of new vessels to supply ischemic tissues is the primary goal of angiogenic therapy. Reaching this objective is, however, highly complex. Vessels formed in response to artificial angiogenic stimuli are prone to regression unless they are remodeled into mature, stable vessels (51). Thus, as the level of knowledge regarding the mechanisms of vessel growth and stabilization increases, there is increasing concern that the simple application of a bolus of angiogenic factor may be insufficient for stable vessel formation, or may even be dangerous.

Early studies involving the administration of VEGF-A showed angiographic evidence of new vessel formation, but these vessels did not persist, and they regressed within three months (45). It was recently reported that continuous delivery of VEGF-A into murine hearts by retroviral transfer led to the formation of aberrant vessels and hemangioma-like structures (28). One of the major problems encountered in the use of VEGF-A is that vessels formed are unstable and leaky (52). It has been speculated that VEGF-A alone may not be sufficient to form stable, mature vessels that are characterized by the recruitment of the perivascular mural cells, such as pericytes or smooth muscle cells (53). This process of vessel maturation is called arteriogenesis and is arguably the ideal way to form stable vessels for therapeutic purposes (54).

Administration of multiple factors

Various growth factors such as angiopoietin (ang)-1, platelet-derived growth factor, and transforming growth factor-β, as well as VEGF-A, are involved in arteriogenesis, and it may therefore be necessary to use combinations of these factors to obtain stable and mature vessels. Indeed, when VEGF-A and ang-1 are administered together in animal models, the resulting vessels are much more stable and less leaky than those that are induced by VEGF-A alone (55). Similarly, administration of submaximal doses of ang-1 and VEGF-A in a rabbit ischemic hindlimb model led to a stronger effect on resting and maximal blood flow and capillary formation than either of the agents alone (56).

Using a master switch gene

Another approach that addresses the involvement of multiple factors in therapeutic angiogenesis is the use of a so-called "master switch gene" of angiogenesis, such as HIF-1α. (57). This transcription factor can activate a collection of different genes that are involved in angiogenesis, including those encoding VEGF-A, VEGF receptor-1 (Flt-1), and ang-2 (58,59). It is hoped that using a "master switch gene" will result in more stable vessels, because the processes by which they are formed would resemble more closely those of normal vessel development.

Stem cells in therapeutic angiogenesis

Several recent discoveries have shifted the paradigm for myocardial regeneration and have fueled enthusiasm for a new frontier in the treatment of cardiovascular disease with stem cells. Fundamental to this emerging field is the cumulative evidence that adult bone marrow stem cells can differentiate into a wide variety of cell types, including cardiac myocytes and ECs. This phenomenon has been termed stem cell plasticity and is the basis for the explosive recent interest in stem cell-based therapies. Directed to cardiovascular disease, stem cell therapy holds the promise of replacing lost heart muscle and enhancing cardiovascular revascularization. Early evidence of the feasibility of stem cell therapy for cardiovascular disease came from a series of animal experiments demonstrating that adult stem cells could become cardiac muscle cells (myogenesis) and participate in the formation of new blood vessels (angiogenesis and vasculogenesis) in the heart after myocardial infarction. These findings have been rapidly translated to on-going human trials, but many questions remain.

The existence of circulating endothelial precursor (CEP) cells in adults has been reported (60–62). It has also been demonstrated that similar precursor cells may give rise to both ECs and perivascular mural cells (63). Furthermore, in an in vitro model of angiogenesis, normal vascular development has been shown to require the presence of the $CD45^+/c-Kit^+/CD34^+$ hematopoietic stem cells (64), which are similar and may be related to adult CEP cells.

It has been reported that CEP cells are able to participate in new vessel growth in a variety of animal models, including the rabbit ischemic hindlimb model (65). In patients with inoperable coronary disease, increased circulating VEGF-A resulting from transfection of myocardium with VEGF-165 cDNA led to significant mobilization of CEP cells (36). Another recent publication has shown that granulocyte-colony stimulating factor mobilized $CD34^+$ cells, including EC precursors with phenotypic and functional characteristics of embryonic angioblasts (66). When injected into rats with experimental myocardial infarction, these $CD34^+$ cells contributed to new vessel growth, which led to decreased cardiomyocyte apoptosis, reduced remodeling, and improved cardiac function.

Further studies of how CEP cells are released from bone marrow and to what extent they participate in postnatal angiogenesis will certainly provide valuable information regarding the therapeutic potential of CEP cells. The possibility of using CEP cells, both alone and in combination with different angiogenic growth factors, represents a promising means of obtaining stable vessels. Finally, because the use of CEP cells would allow easy ex vivo gene transfer, combining growth factor-induced therapeutic angiogenesis with gene therapy delivered via CEP should also be a promising approach.

Adult stem cells for cardiac repair

The real promise of a stem cell-based approach for cardiac regeneration and repair lies in the promotion of myogenesis and angiogenesis at the site of the cell graft to achieve both structural and functional benefits. Despite all of the progress and promise in this field, many unanswered questions

remain; the answers to these questions will provide the much-needed breakthrough to harness the real benefits of cell therapy for the heart in the clinical perspective. One of the major issues is the choice of donor cell type for transplantation. Multiple cell types with varying potentials have been assessed for their ability to repopulate the infarcted myocardium; however, only the adult stem cells, that is, skeletal myoblasts and bone marrow-derived stem cells, have been translated from the laboratory bench to clinical use (67–76). Which of these two cell types will provide the best option for clinical application in heart cell therapy remains arguable. With results pouring in from the long-term follow-ups of previously conducted phase I clinical studies, and with the onset of phase II clinical trials involving larger populations of patients, transplantation of stem cells as a sole therapy without an adjunct conventional revascularization procedure will provide a deeper insight into the effectiveness of this approach.

Myocardial circulatory insufficiency, cardiomyocyte necrosis, and apoptosis play important roles in many pathologic conditions of the heart. Therapeutic approaches aimed at promoting angiogenesis and growing new heart muscle fibers, currently undergoing intensive investigation and early clinical trials, therefore hold considerable promise for the future. Genes encoding angiogenic factors and angiogenic growth factor proteins, such as VEGF and FGF-2, are being delivered to the target tissue to induce growth of new blood vessels (77). For myogenesis, various progenitor and stem cells are being assessed as donor cells for implantation into the ventricular wall of injured hearts. Phase I and II clinical trials have already been undertaken for myocardial angiogenesis. Clinical studies into myogenesis have been recently initiated with implantation of autologous skeletal myoblasts into myocardial scar tissue (67). Although the results of phase I safety studies so far are promising, the establishment of efficacy requires rigorous phase II and III studies yet to come.

Myogenesis

Cellular myogenic and angiogenic therapy in cardiac or limb ischemia

For angiogenesis and vasculogenesis, the following cells can be proposed: ECs, bone marrow-derived stem cells, and circulating blood-derived progenitor cells. For myogenesis, skeletal myoblasts, smooth muscle cells, or fetal and neonatal cardiomyocytes can be used. The relative contribution of various sources of precursor cells in postnatal muscles and the factors that may enhance stem cell participation in the formation of new skeletal and cardiac muscle in vivo have been investigated by several groups. In postnatal muscle, skeletal muscle precursors (myoblasts) can be derived from satellite cells (reserve cells located on the surface of mature myofibers) or from cells lying beyond the myofiber (e.g., interstitial connective tissue or bone marrow).

Both of these categories of cells may have stem cell properties. In adult hearts (which previously were not considered capable of repair), the role of replicating endogenous cardiomyocytes and the recruitment of other stem cells into cardiomyocytes for new cardiac muscle formation has recently been reviewed. The main conclusions are that, although many endogenous cell types can be converted to contractile cells, the contribution of nonmyogenic cells to the formation of new postnatal muscle in vivo appears to be negligible. The recruitment of such cells to the myogenic lineage can be significantly enhanced by specific inducers and appropriate microenvironment. For myocardial repair, the participation of bone marrow-derived stem cells in the repair of damaged cardiac muscle motivates our group to start cell-based angiogenic and myogenic clinical trials.

Cell-based angiogenic therapy is an interesting and safe approach in comparison with the administration of growth factors in the form of proteins, which presents risks of systemic effects inducing problematic angiogenesis in the retina or the potentiation of growth and metastasis of occult tumors. Growth factor gene therapy also presents risks related with stability, unregulated expression, and adverse response to transfection vectors (78).

Clinical trial—rationale

To assess the feasibility of angiogenic cell therapy for patients with peripheral artery diseases, we organized a randomized controlled clinical trial using CD133$^+$ cells implanted in ischemic limbs. The goal of the study is to demonstrate that intramuscular implantation of autologous human CD133$^+$ cells into ischemic limbs effectively induces collateral vessel formation, improving function, and trophic ischemic lesions (79–81).

Endothelial progenitor cells can be sorted from the peripheral blood of patients with peripheral artery diseases and can be implanted into ischemic limbs in order to increase collateral vessel formation and to secrete various angiogenic factors or cytokines. Although this novel angiogenic cell therapy seems to be feasible, remote angiogenic actions should be considered as possible side effects, and the clinical efficacy should be tested by specific studies (79–81).

Inclusion criteria

Random adult patients with ischemia of the leg and without indication of surgical or percutaneous revascularization are selected to be injected with CD133$^+$ cells into the gastrocnemius of the ischemic limb. Side effects during cell mobilization from bone marrow are carefully evaluated (e.g., coagulation abnormalities).

Exclusion criteria

Patients presenting poorly controlled diabetes mellitus and proliferative retinopathy as well as patients presenting evidence of malignant disorder during the past five years.

Evaluation of efficacy and safety

The following studies are performed:

- Ankle-brachial index
- Transcutaneous oxygen pressure
- Rest pain
- Pain-free walking time
- Digital subtraction angiography
- Evaluation of cutaneous and muscular ischemic lesions.

Conclusion

As research into therapeutic angiogenesis progresses, new information regarding the control of vessel remodeling and stability will be incorporated into treatment strategies. Better designed studies and clinical trials that consider the issues discussed, coupled with well-defined and quantitative endpoints, will facilitate the development of novel and effective therapeutic approaches for ischemic diseases. Future preclinical and clinical studies will define the potential utility of pharmacotherapy versus gene therapy, cell therapy or perhaps the combinations in optimizing the treatment options for ischemic disorders.

References

1   Powers C, McLeskey SW, Wellstein A. Fibroblast growth factors, their receptors and signaling. Endocr Relat Cancer 2000; 7:165–197.

2   Leung DW, Cachianes G, Kuang W-J, et al. Vascular endothelial growth factor is a secreted angiogenic mitogen. Science 1989; 246:1306–1309.

3   Senger DR, Galli SJ, Dvorak AM, et al. Tumor cells secrete a vascular permeability factor that promotes accumulation of ascites fluid. Science 1983; 219:983–985.

4   Tischer E, Mitchell R, Hartman T, et al. The human gene for vascular endothelial growth factor. Multiple proteins are encoded through alternative axon splicing. J Biol Chem 1991; 266:11947–11954.

5   Shima DT, Kuroki M, Deutsch U, et al. The mouse gene for vascular endothelial growth factor. Genomic structure, definition of the transcriptional unit and characterization of transcriptional and post-transcriptional regulatory sequences. J Biol Chem 1996; 271:3877–3883.

6   Lutty GA, Mathews MK, Merges C, et al. Adenosine stimulates canine retinal microvascular endothelial cell migration and tube formation. Curr Eye Res 1998; 17:594–607.

7   Desai A, Victor-Vega C, Gadangi S, et al. Adenosine A2A receptor stimulation increases angiogenesis by down-regulating production of the antiangiogenic matrix protein thrombospondin 1. Mol Pharmacol 2005; 67:1406–1413.

8   Mousa SA, O'Connor L, Davis FB, et al. Proangiogenesis action of the thyroid hormone analog 3,5-diiodothyropropionic acid (DITPA) is initiated at the cell surface and is integrin mediated. Endocrinology 2006; 147:1602–1607.

9   Mousa SA, O'Connor LJ, Bergh JJ, et al. The proangiogenic action of thyroid hormone analogue GC-1 is initiated at an integrin. J Cardiovasc Pharmacol 2005; 46:356–360.

10 Tsurumi Y, Takeshita S, Chen D, et al. Direct intramuscular gene transfer of naked DNA encoding vascular endothelial growth factor augments collateral development and tissue perfusion. Circulation 1996; 94:3281–3290.

11 Mousa SA, Feng X, Xie J, et al. Synthetic oligosaccharide stimulates and stabilizes angiogenesis: structure–function relationships and potential mechanisms. J Cardiovasc Pharmacol 2006; 48:6–13.

12 Takeshita S, Zheng LP, Brogi E, et al. Therapeutic angiogenesis: a single intra-arterial bolus of vascular endothelial growth factor augments neovascularization in a rabbit ischemic hind limb model. J Clint Invest 1994; 93:662–670.

13 Pearlman JD, Hibberd MG, Chuang ML, et al. Magnetic resonance mapping demonstrates benefits of VEGF-induced myocardial angiogenesis. Nat Med 1995; 1:1085–1089.

14 Lopez JJ, Laham RJ, Stamler A, et al. VEGF administration in chronic myocardial ischemia in pigs. Cardiovasc Res 1998; 40: 272–281.

15 Harada K, Friedman M, Lopez JJ, et al. Vascular endothelial growth factor administration in chronic myocardial ischemia. Am J Physiol 1996; 270:H1791–H1802.

16 Giordano FJ, Ping P, McKirnan MD, et al. Intra-coronary gene transfer of fibroblast growth factor-5 increases blood flow and contractile function in an ischemic region of the heart. Nat Med 1996; 2:534–539.

17 Simons M, Bonow RO, Chronos NA, et al. Clinical trials in coronary angiogenesis: issues, problems, consensus: an expert panel summary. Circulation 2000; 102:E73–E86.

18 Thompson WD, Li WW, Maragoudakis M. The clinical manipulation of angiogenesis: pathology, side-effects, surprises, and opportunities with novel human therapies. J Pathol 2000; 190: 330–337.

19 Schumacher B, Pecher P, von Specht BU, et al. Induction of neoangiogenesis in ischemic myocardium by human growth factors: first clinical results of a new treatment of coronary heart disease. Circulation 1998; 97:645–650.

20 Laham RJ, Chronos NA, Pike M, et al. Intra-coronary basic fibroblast growth factor (FGF-2) in patients with severe ischemic heart disease: results of a phase I open-label dose escalation study. J Am Coll Cardiol 2000; 36:2132–2139.

21 Udelson JE, Dilsizian V, Laham RJ, et al. Therapeutic angiogenesis with recombinant fibroblast growth factor-2 improves stress and rest myocardial perfusion abnormalities in patients with severe symptomatic chronic coronary artery disease. Circulation 2000; 102:1605–1610.

22 Losordo DW, Vale PR, Symes JF, et al. Gene therapy for myocardial angiogenesis: initial clinical results with direct myocardial injection of phVEGF165 as sole therapy for myocardial ischemia. Circulation 1998; 98:2800–2804.

23 Rosengart TK, Lee LY, Patel SR, et al. Angiogenesis gene therapy: phase I assessment of direct intramyocardial administration of an adenovirus vector expressing VEGF121 cDNA to individuals with clinically significant severe coronary artery disease. Circulation 1999; 100:468–474.

24 Hendel RC, Henry TD, Rocha-Singh K, et al. Effect of intracoronary recombinant human vascular endothelial growth factor on myocardial perfusion: evidence for a dose-dependent effect. Circulation 2000; 101:118–121.

25 Laitinen M, Hartikainen J, Hiltunen MO, et al. Catheter-mediated vascular endothelial growth factor gene transfer to human coronary arteries after angioplasty. Hum Gene Ther 2000; 11:263–270.

26 Carmeliet P, Ferriera V, Breier G, et al. Abnormal blood vessel development and lethality in embryos lacking a single VEGF allele. Nature 1996; 380:435–439.

27 Miquerol L, Langille BL, Nagy A. Embryonic development is disrupted by modest increases in vascular endothelial growth factor gene expression. Development 2000; 127:3941–3946.

28 Lee RJ, Springer ML, Blanco-Bose WE, et al. VEGF gene delivery to myocardium: deleterious effects of unregulated expression. Circulation 2000; 102:898–901.

29 Langer R. Drug delivery and targeting. Nature 1998; 392 (suppl):5–10.

30 Dewey RA, Morrissey G, Cowsill CM, et al. Chronic brain inflammation and persistent herpes simplex virus 1 thymidine kinase expression in survivors of syngeneic glioma treated by adenovirus-mediated gene therapy: implications for clinical trials. Nat Med 1999; 5:1256–1263.

31 Bohl D, Naffakh N, Heard JM. Long-term control of erythropoietin secretion by doxycycline in mice transplanted with engineered primary myoblasts. Nat Med 1997; 3:299–305.

32 Rivard A, Fabre JE, Silver M, et al. Age-dependent impairment of angiogenesis. Circulation 1999; 99:111–120.

33 Rivard A, Berthou-Soulie L, Principe N, et al. Age-dependent defect in vascular endothelial growth factor expression is associated with reduced hypoxia-inducible factor 1 activity. J Biol Chem 2000; 275:29643–29647.

34 Schultz A, Lavie L, Hochberg I, et al. Inter-individual heterogeneity in the hypoxic regulation of VEGF: significance for the development of the coronary artery collateral circulation. Circulation 1999; 100:547–552.

35 Rohan RM, Fernandez A, Udagawa T, et al. Genetic heterogeneity of angiogenesis in mice. FASEB J 2000; 14:871–876.

36 Kalka C, Tehrani H, Laudenberg B, et al. VEGF gene transfer mobilizes endothelial progenitor cells in patients with inoperable coronary disease. Ann Thorac Surg 2000; 70: 829–834.

37 Ware JA. Too many vessels? Not enough? The wrong kind? The VEGF debate continues [letter; comment]. Nat Med 2001; 7:403–404.

38 Moulton KS, Heller E, Konerding MA, et al. Angiogenesis inhibitors endostatin or TNP-470 reduce intimal neovascularization and plaque growth in apolipoprotein E-deficient mice. Circulation 1999; 99:1726–1732.

39 Celletti FL, Waugh JM, Amabile PG, et al. Vascular endothelial growth factor enhances atherosclerotic plaque progression. Nat Med 2001; 7:425–429.

40 Isner JM. Still more debate over VEGF [letter to the editor]. Nat Med 2001; 7:639–640.

41 Dake MM. Reply to "Still more debate over VEGF" [letter to the editor]. Nat Med 2001; 7:640–641.

42 Cuevas P, Carceller F, Ortega S, et al. Hypotensive activity of fibroblast growth factor. Science 1991; 254:1208–1210.

43 Hariswala M, Horowitz JR, Esaof D, et al. VEGF improves myocardial blood flow but produces EDRF-mediated hypotension in porcine hearts. J Surg Res 1996; 63:77–82.

44 Lopez JJ, Laham RJ, Carrozza JP, et al. Hemodynamic effects of intracoronary VEGF delivery: evidence of tachyphylaxis and NO dependence of response. Am J Physiol 1997; 273:H1317–H1323.

45 Isner J, Peiczek A, Schainfeld R, et al. Clinical evidence of angiogenesis after arterial gene transfer of phVEGF165 in patients with ischaemic limb. Lancet 1996; 348:370–374.

46 Ferrara N, Davis-Smyth T. The biology of vascular endothelial growth factor. Endocrine Rev 1997; 18:4–25.

47 Ng Y-S, Rohan R, Sunday M, et al. Differential expression of VEGF isoforms in mouse during development and in the adult. Dev Dyn 2001; 220:112–121.

48 Carmeliet P, Ng Y-S, Nuyen D, et al. Impaired myocardial angiogenesis and ischemic cardiomyopathy in mice lacking the vascular endothelial growth factor isoforms VEGF164 and VEGF188. Nat Med 1999; 5:495–502.

49 Grunstein J, Masbad JJ, Hickey R, et al. Isoforms of vascular endothelial growth factor act in coordinate fashion to recruit and expand tumor vasculature. Mol Cell Biol 2000; 20:7282–7291.

50 Cheng S-Y, Nagane M, Su Huang H-J, et al. Intracerebral tumor-associated hemorrhage caused by overexpression of the vascular endothelial growth factor isoforms $VEGF_{121}$ and $VEGF_{165}$ but not $VEGF_{189}$. Proc Natl Acad Sci USA 1997; 94:12081–12087.

51 Darland DC, D'Amore PA. Blood vessel maturation: vascular development comes of age. J Clin Invest 1999; 103:157–158.

52 Dvorak HF, Nagy JA, Feng D, et al. Vascular permeability factor/vascular endothelial growth factor and the significance of microvascular permeability in angiogenesis. Curr Topics Microbiol Immunol 1999; 237:97–132.

53 D'Amore PA, Ng Y-S, Darland DK. Angiogenesis. Sci Med 1999; 6:44–53.

54 Buschmann I, Schaper W. The pathophysiology of the collateral circulation (arteriogenesis). J Pathol 2000;190:338–342.

55 Thurston G, Suri C, Smith K, et al. Leakage-resistant blood vessels in mice transgenically overexpressing angiopoietin-1. Science 1999; 286:2511–2514.

56 Chae JK, Kim I, Lim ST, et al. Coadministration of angiopoietin-1 and vascular endothelial growth factor enhances collateral vascularization. Arterioscler Thromb Vasc Biol 2000; 20:2573–2578.

57 Li J, Post M, Volk R, et al. PR39, a peptide regulator of angiogenesis. Nat Med 2000; 6:49–55.

58 Oh H, Takagi H, Suzuma K, et al. Hypoxia and vascular endothelial growth factor selectively upregulate angiopoietin-2 in bovine microvascular endothelial cells. J Biol Chem 1999; 274:15732–15739.

59 Semenza GL. HIF-1 and human disease: one highly involved factor. Genes Dev 2000; 14:1983–1991.

60 Asahara T, Murohara T, Sullivan A, et al. Isolation of putative progenitor endothelial cells for angiogenesis. Science 1997; 275:964–967.

61 Asahara T, Isner JM. Endothelial progenitor cells for vascular regeneration. J Hematother Stem Cell Res 2002; 11:171–178.

62 Shi Q, Rafii S, Wu MH, et al. Evidence for circulating bone marrow-derived endothelial cells. Blood 1998; 92:362–367.

63 Yamashita J, Itoh H, Hirashima M, et al. Flk1-positive cells derived from embryonic stem cells serve as vascular progenitors. Nature 2000; 408:92–96.

64 Takakura N, Watanabe T, Suenobu S, et al. A role for hematopoietic stem cells in promoting angiogenesis. Cell 2000; 102:199–209.

65 Asahara T, Masuda H, Takahashi T, et al. Bone marrow origin of endothelial progenitor cells responsible for postnatal vasculogenesis in physiological and pathological neovascularization. Circ Res 1999; 85:221–228.

66 Kocher AA, Schuster MD, Szabolcs MJ, et al. Neovascularization of ischemic myocardium by human bone-marrow-derived angioblasts prevents cardiomyocyte apoptosis, reduces remodeling and improves cardiac function. Nat Med 2001; 7:430–436.

67 Chachques JC, Cattadori B, Herreros J, et al. Treatment of heart failure with autologous skeletal myoblasts. Herz 2002; 27:570–578.

68 Chachques JC, Shafy A, Duarte F, et al. From dynamic to cellular cardiomyoplasty. J Cardiac Surg 2002; 17:194–200.

69 Chedrawy EG, Wang JS, Nguyen DM, et al. Incorporation and integration of implanted myogenic and stem cells into native myocardial fibers: anatomic basis for functional improvements. J Thorac Cardiovasc Surg 2002; 124:584–590.

70 Chiu RCJ. Therapeutic cardiac angiogenesis and myogenesis: the promises and challenges on a new frontier. J Thorac Cardiovasc Surg 2001; 122:851–852.

71 Cleland JG, Thygesen K, Uretsky BF, et al. ATLAS investigators: cardiovascular critical event pathways for the progression of heart failure: a report from the ATLAS study. Eur Heart J 2001; 22:1601–1612.

72 Fuchs S, Baffour R, Zhou YF, et al. Transendocardial delivery of autologous bone marrow enhances collateral perfusion and regional function in pigs with chronic experimental myocardial ischemia. J Am Coll Cardiol 2001; 37:1726–1732.

73 Hamano K, Li TS, Kobayashi T, et al. Therapeutic angiogenesis induced by local autologous bone marrow cell implantation. Ann Thorac Surg 2002; 73:1210–1215.

74 Hamano K, Li TS, Kobayashi T, et al. The induction of angiogenesis by the implantation of autologous bone marrow cells: a novel and simple therapeutic method. Surgery 2001; 130:44–54.

75 Hamano K, Nishida M, Hirata K, et al. Local implantation of autologous bone marrow cells for therapeutic angiogenesis in patients with ischemic heart disease: clinical trial and preliminary results. Jpn Circ J 2001; 65:845–847.

76   Jackson KA, Majka SM, Wang H, et al. Regeneration of ischemic cardiac muscle and vascular endothelium by adult stem cells. J Clin Invest 2001; 107:1395–1402.

77   Iwaguro H, Yamaguchi J, Kalka C, et al. Endothelial progenitor cell vascular endothelial growth factor gene transfer for vascular regeneration. Circulation 2002; 105:732–738.

78   Rajnoch C, Chachques JC, Berrebi A, et al. Cellular therapy reverses myocardial dysfunction. J Thorac Cardiovasc Surg 2001; 121:871–878.

79   Tateishi-Yuyama E, Matsubara H, Murohara T, et al. Therapeutic Angiogenesis using Cell Transplantation (TACT) Study Investigators: therapeutic angiogenesis for patients with limb ischaemia by autologous transplantation of bone-marrow cells: a pilot study and a randomized controlled trial. Lancet 2002; 360:427–435.

80   Taylor DA, Atkins BZ, Hungspreugs P, et al. Regenerating functional myocardium: improved performance after skeletal myoblast transplantation. Nat Med 1998; 4:929–933.

81   Vale PR, Losordo DW, Milliken CE, et al. Randomized, single blind, placebo-controlled pilot study of catheter-based myocardial gene transfer for therapeutic angiogenesis using left ventricular electromechanical mapping in patients with chronic myocardial ischemia. Circulation 2001; 103: 2138–2143.

35

Growth factor therapy

Munir Boodhwani, Joanna J. Wykrzykowska, and Roger J. Laham

Introduction

Despite improvements in the management of cardiovascular risk factors, as well as advances in percutaneous and surgical revascularization methods, coronary artery disease (CAD) affects over 13 million people in the United States and is responsible for one in every five deaths (1). In a large number of patients, CAD can be of such a diffuse and severe nature that repeated attempts at catheter-based interventions and surgical bypass may be unsuccessful in restoring normal myocardial blood flow. Up to 20% to 37% of the patients with ischemic heart disease cannot undergo either coronary artery bypass graft surgery (CABG) or percutaneous coronary intervention (PCI) or receive incomplete revascularization with these standard revascularization strategies (2–6). Furthermore, incomplete revascularization has been associated with increased mortality and poorer clinical outcome (7,8).

Therapeutic angiogenesis, using growth factors, aims to restore perfusion to chronically ischemic myocardium without intervening on the epicardial coronary arteries, particularly in patients in whom further mechanical revascularization in not possible (Fig. 1). Despite initial enthusiasm, therapeutic angiogenesis has not yet provided significant clinical benefit and is still reserved as an experimental treatment for patients who have failed conventional therapies.

The discordance between successful preclinical studies and disappointing clinical trials may be explained by a number of factors (9). First, angiogenesis is a complex process that involves interactions between a number of pro- and antiangiogenic mediators, the endothelium, and the extracellular matrix. It is therefore not surprising that single-agent growth factor therapy has not led to large functional improvements in patients. Second, patients with end-stage coronary disease are vastly different from the young and healthy animals in which preclinical testing is conducted. The presence of diabetes, hypercholesterolemia, and endothelial dysfunction can significantly limit the effect of growth factors on the angiogenic response (10,11). Third, the optimal delivery strategy, one that provides local delivery and prolonged exposure to an adequate dose of growth factor without causing unwanted effects, remains to be discovered. Finally, the lack of sensitive assays of myocardial angiogenesis limits our ability to detect small, subclinical changes that may be occurring in response to growth factor delivery. Despite these limitations, angiogenesis is a critical process that occurs in all humans and if appropriately modulated, can provide therapeutic benefit to the large population of patients suffering from end-stage CAD.

Growth factors for myocardial angiogenesis

Angiogenesis involves a complex molecular signaling cascade. A significant number of cytokines involved in this process have been identified including members of the fibroblast growth factor (FGF) family, vascular endothelial growth factor (VEGF) family, platelet-derived growth factor (PDGF) family, and angiopoietins (12). VEGFs and FGFs are the most widely studied and used for clinical studies, and will serve as the basis for this discussion.

Vascular endothelial growth factor

Vascular endothelial growth factors are a family of heparin-binding glycoproteins shown to act as mitogens for vascular endothelial cells as well as stimulants for the endothelial

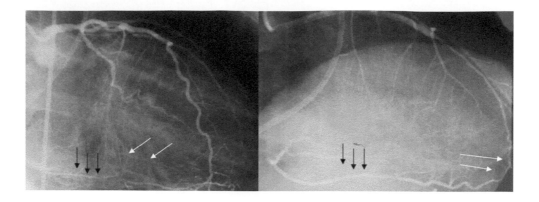

Figure 1
Coronary angiography in two patients who had an asymptomatic occlusion of the right coronary artery with extensive collaterals from the left coronary system. The right coronary artery (*black arrows*) fills by intramyocardial collaterals (*left, white arrows*) or large bore epicardial collaterals (*right, white arrows*) underscoring the native collateralization process.

progenitor cell mobilization from the bone marrow (13). The family of VEGF molecules includes VEGF (A–D) as well as placental growth factor (PIGF). These ligands interact with a number of different tyrosine kinase receptors (flt-1, flk-1, and flt-4) (12). VEGFs are expressed in cardiac myocytes and vascular smooth muscle and endothelial cells, with increased expression in the setting of vascular injury, acute and chronic ischemia, and hypoxia (14). Their actions are mediated through downstream activation of Akt and eventual release of nitric oxide (NO), and include vascular permeability,

increased endothelial cell growth and survival, and formation of tubular structures (12).

Preclinical data has provided evidence for VEGF as a pro-angiogenic agent in animal models of chronic myocardial ischemia (Fig. 2) with improvement in myocardial blood flow after VEGF treatment (15). Perivascular and intracoronary administration of VEGF has been demonstrated to improve myocardial flow and ventricular function in a porcine ameroid model of chronic ischemia (16) (Fig. 3). As the actions of VEGF are mediated, in large part, through NO release,

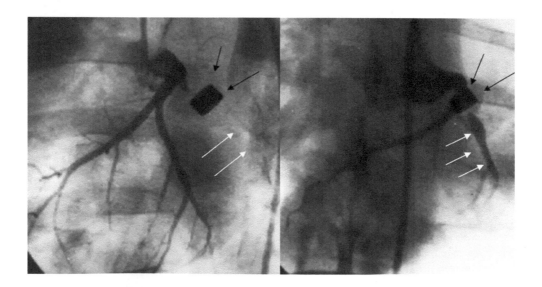

Figure 2
The most frequently used preclinical model for therapeutic angiogenesis is the porcine ameroid constrictor model. Shown here are angiograms from two animals with an ameroid constrictor (*black arrows*) placed on the left circumflex artery which results in total occlusion of the artery two to three weeks after placement. The angiogram on the left is from a control animal with no reconstitution of the left circumflex artery (*white arrows*). The angiogram on the right is from an animal that received perivascular vascular endothelial growth factor (VEGF) (via a pump) with prompt filling of the left circumflex artery (*white arrows*) by collaterals (both left→left and right→left). It is important to note that most of these experiments are performed on juvenile pigs.

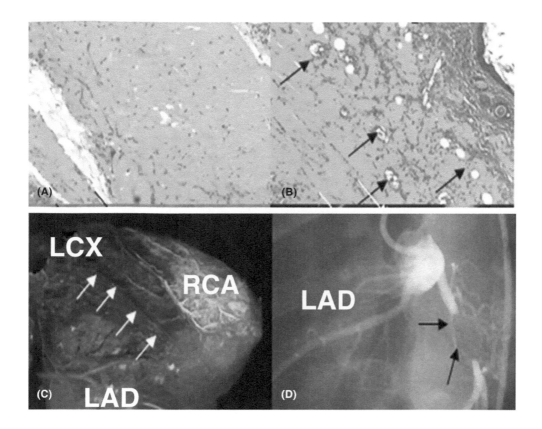

Figure 3

(*See color plate.*) Histological analysis in the ameroid constrictor model showing increased neovascularization after vascular endothelial growth factor (VEGF) administration (**B**) compared with control animal (**A**). Batson Casting (**C**) showing left circumflex artery in *blue*, left anterior descending in *red*, and right coronary artery in *white*. Left circumflex distribution is being supplied by collaterals from other territories. Corresponding angiography (**D**) of ameroid contrictor model of left circumflex artery occlusion and patent left anterior descending with bridging collaterals from the left anterior descending to the left circumflex artery territory. *Abbreviations*: LAD, left anterior descending coronery artery; LCX, Left circumflex artery; RCA, Right coronary artery.

disease states that lead to diminished bioavailable NO and endothelial dysfunction, for example, hypercholesterolemia are associated with impairment in growth factor-induced angiogenesis (11).

Hypotension, because of the release of NO and arteriolar vasodilation, is associated with intravenous and intracoronary VEGF administration and has proven to be dose-limiting in phase I trials (17). A theoretical risk associated with growth factor administration is the development of plaque angiogenesis that may precipitate the growth and destabilization of atherosclerotic plaques (17). Based on the well-documented role of angiogenesis in tumor biology, accelerated growth of primary tumors and stimulation of metastasis is another theoretical concern (18). Proliferative retinopathy in the diabetic population is another disease with potential for pathologic angiogenesis as a complication of growth factor therapy. These concerns provide support for local, rather than regional or systemic, delivery strategies. However, these matters so far have not become apparent clinically (19), though what has become apparent is the lack of efficacy of

VEGF in phase II clinical studies using intracoronary and intravenous administration.

Fibroblast growth factor

The FGF family consists of 23 proteins that are classified by their expression pattern, receptor-binding preference, and protein sequence (20,21). FGF is present in the normal myocardium (22). Its expression is stimulated by hypoxia (23) and hemodynamic stress (24). FGF-2 is a pluripotent molecule and modulates numerous cellular functions for multiple cell types. In the context of angiogenesis, it induces endothelial cell proliferation, survival, and differentiation, and is also involved in cell migration of endothelial cells, smooth muscle cells, macrophages, and fibroblasts (21). These effects are mediated through its interaction with the tyrosine kinase receptor FGFR1 which also leads to the downstream release of NO (25). Additionally, FGF-2 stimulates endothelial cells to produce a variety of proteases, including plasminogen activator and matrix metalloproteinases (26,27) that promote chemotaxis.

FGF was shown to induce angiogenesis in mature tissue by animal studies that demonstrated increased vascularity after intracoronary injections in acute coronary thrombosis models (28,29). In studies using the ameroid constrictor model of chronic myocardial ischemia, FGF-2 therapy using perivascular and intrapericardial delivery improved coronary blood flow and regional left ventricular function (30,31). Also, in studies using intracoronary infusions as the delivery method, improvements in myocardial perfusion and function were observed (32,33). Similar to VEGF, FGF-2 can cause acute vasodilation and hypotension. In addition to the potentially adverse effects of growth factors mentioned before, a significant long-term side effect of high-dose FGF administration is renal insufficiency as a result of membranous nephropathy accompanied by proteinuria (19).

Growth factor delivery

Two approaches have generally been used to achieve therapeutic angiogenesis: protein therapy and gene transfer which are briefly discussed next.

Protein therapy

The advantages of protein therapy include controlled delivery, established safety, predictable pharmacokinetics and tissue levels, and absence of long-term unexpected side effects (34–36). The main disadvantages of this strategy include short tissue half-life of most proteins and high cost of recombinant molecules, shortcomings potentially addressable with sustained delivery systems. An example of a sustained release system is the use of heparin alginate capsules for perivascular FGF-2 delivery in surgical angiogenesis trials (5). It is important to note that some angiogenic agents cannot be delivered as proteins and thus may necessitate gene transfer. Examples of such agents are hypoxia-inducible factor (HIF)-1α and PR39 (37,38), which are transcription factors involved in the angiogenic cascade. However, for FGFs and VEGFs, protein therapy may supersede gene transfer, especially given the limitations of current vectors.

Gene therapy

Gene transfer for angiogenesis relies on the ability of injected genetic material to provide sustained and effective expression of the desired protein in the targeted tissues. The target cells become "factories" for the desired angiogenic cytokines. The advantages of gene transfer include prolonged and sustained

expression of the protein in the target tissues, ability to express transcriptional factors, potential for regulated expression, and ability to express multiple genes simultaneously. The major shortcomings of gene transfer are the paucity of experience that has been achieved to date in clinical settings and the short- and long-term toxicities and side effects of various vectors that are incompletely understood. Furthermore, gene-based therapy can potentially cause detrimental sustained expression potentially leading to pathologic angiogenesis, inflammatory reaction to delivery vectors, and the potential for mutated pathogenic vectors (for viral therapy). Although the overall experience with protein-based (growth factor) therapy has been more extensive than gene transfer, several phase I and phase II studies involving gene therapy have recently been published (39–41).

Various vehicles and vectors exist for the transfer of target DNA to the cells and tissues of interest and are briefly discussed next.

Nonviral vectors

When naked DNA comes into contact with the cell membrane, only a small amount will enter the cell, leading to relatively low gene transfer efficiency (42). Therefore, a carrier or a virus vector is generally used to increase transfection efficiency and achieve adequate expression of the therapeutic agent. Plasmid or liposomal (43,44) complexes are the most commonly used carrier molecules. A small fraction of plasmid DNA enters the nucleus, where it persists in an episomal location (not integrated into the genome), resulting in limited duration of transgene expression in both proliferating and nonproliferating cells. The production and scale-up of plasmid and liposomal complexes is relatively easy, but low transfection efficiency and the short duration and low levels of transgene expression limit this approach. Phospholipid formulae such as 1,2-dioleoyl-sn-glycero-3-phosphoethanolamine-N-dodecanoyl/1,2-dioleoyl-sn- glycero-3-phosphocholine and cationic polymers such as poly-L-ornithine with galactose and the fusigenic peptide mHA2 (galactose-poly-L-ornithine-mHA2) can improve the transfection efficiency (44,45).

Viral vectors

Adenoviruses enter cells via specific receptors with subsequent lysosomal degradation releasing viral DNA into the cytoplasm, which makes its way to the nucleus, remaining in an extrachromosomal location. Replication-deficient adenoviruses are produced in vitro in specific packaging cells that complement gene products deleted from the viral genome to prevent in vivo replication (46–48). Adenoviruses have the advantage of easy production in high titers, relatively high transduction efficiency, and the ability to express in both proliferating and nonproliferating cells. However, both first- and second-generation adenoviral vectors are associated with a significant local inflammatory reaction that eventually extinguishes transgene expression. Circulating antiadenoviral antibody, common for some adenoviral subtypes, can greatly reduce the duration and magnitude of expression. Newer encapsidated (gutted) adenoviruses may produce less inflammatory reactions (49,50). These modifications also increase the capacity of these adenoviruses allowing them to carry full-length genes such as the dystrophin gene (49).

Recombinant *adeno-associated viruses* (AAV) are promising candidates as gene vectors, as they transduce nondividing cells and permit lasting transgene expression in a wide spectrum of tissues (51–58). However, AAV are difficult to produce, and they have a small expression cassette (54,56). Newer procedures for high throughput production, screening, and characterization of AAV vectors may circumvent the scalability problem (52) and the size limitation may be overcome by using a dual vector approach (54–56,58).

Retroviruses enter cells via specific receptors, following which viral RNA is reverse transcribed to DNA that is integrated into the cellular chromosomal architecture, leading to stable, prolonged, and high expression of the therapeutic transgene (59–61). Replication-deficient retroviruses are produced in vitro in specific packaging cell lines containing retroviral genes (G, P, E) that have been deleted from the retroviral genome. Retroviruses can only transduce dividing cells, thus limiting their target cell population (59–61). The second limitation of retroviruses is their low titer. In addition, the efficient insertion of genes by retroviruses is often complicated by transcriptional inactivation of the retroviral long terminal repeats (LTRs) and production of replication-competent retroviruses is feared. The development of lentivirus vectors has allowed efficient gene transfer to quiescent cells (49,62,63) and the development of pseudotyping has increased viral titers (64).

Cell-based therapy

Cell-based gene transfer is a promising new strategy that utilizes autologous cells or cell lines transfected with a transgene of interest to express that transgene in vivo. The advantage of such a system is to circumvent the inflammatory response by using autologous cells and achieve prolonged expression by stable transfection using various measures including electroporation, in vitro retroviral or lentiviral transfection (65–70). In addition, complex constructs can be built that would allow stable regulated expression and multiple transgene expression. There are numerous investigations in progress studying the use of cellular transplantation for myocardial regeneration or angiogenesis, using hematopoetic cells, skeletal myoblasts, and endothelial progenitor cells. The use of autologous cells carries the potential advantage of providing functional benefits that are independent of target

protein expression. This promising therapeutic strategy is discussed elsewhere in this text.

Delivery strategies

Delivery strategies can usually be classified as systemic (intravenous), local/regional infusion (intracoronary for myocardial angiogenesis and intra-arterial for limb angiogenesis), local periadventitial delivery (catheter-based or surgical implantation), and intramyocardial (catheter-based or surgical for myocardial therapy, intramuscular for peripheral vascular disease). Although a wealth of information exists regarding vector development and angiogenic potential of various cytokines, the delivery of these agents to the heart and peripheral vasculature has been arbitrarily chosen and tested for efficacy without optimizing the volume to be delivered, the rate of infusion or injection, the biocompatibility with materials used, and the optimal mode of delivery for each compound and vector. Different delivery methods have been utilized by different investigators for gene transfer to the heart and peripheral vasculature ranging from intracoronary (71), to epicardial (41) and endocardial (39) injections. Intravenous administration has not been advocated particularly with findings from several investigations that gene expression after intravenous administration of an adenoviral construct, the distribution was highest in the kidney followed by lung, liver, brain, and heart (72). Intracoronary administration of adenoviral vectors have been studied by several investigators (71,73–75); however, the majority of studies have been performed with intramuscular (limb) and intramyocardial delivery (heart) (76–78). These delivery strategies, nonetheless, have not been optimized for the vector and agent used, and basic parameters such as volume to be injected, needle depth, rate of injection, biocompatibility, and vehicle used are still under investigation.

Clinical studies of protein therapy

Phase I trials

The first phase I clinical trial of coronary angiogenesis demonstrated the safety of intramyocardial injection of 0.01 mg/kg of FGF-1 (79). A total of 40 patients undergoing CABG of the internal mammary artery (IMA) to left anterior descending coronary artery (LAD) were randomized to receive intramyocardial injections of either 0.01 mg FGF-1 or placebo. All the patients had further stenoses of the LAD distal to the anastomosis. Coronary angiography 12 weeks after treatment showed increased capillary refill in patients who received FGF-1 compared with control patients. Follow-up three years later confirmed the safety and efficacy of the FGF-1. Mortality was similar in the control and treatment groups. The capillary network seen at 12 weeks post-treatment persisted on angiography. Additionally, echocardiography suggested improved left ventricular ejection fraction (LVEF) (80).

A preliminary study of surgically delivered, intramyocardial FGF-2 that demonstrated the safety of this technique was followed by a phase II randomized, double-blind, placebo-controlled trial in which 24 patients undergoing CABG with ungraftable areas of myocardium were randomized to 10 μg FGF-2, 100 μg FGF-2, or placebo (5,35). Slow-release heparin-alginate microcapsules, which released FGF-2 over three to four weeks, were implanted into the ischemic and viable but ungraftable myocardial region. Follow-up averaged 16 months with clinical assessment and nuclear perfusion imaging. There were no reports of recurrent angina or repeat revascularizations for the 100-μg FGF-2 group versus three reports of recurrent angina and two repeat revascularizations in the control group. Significant reductions in nuclear defect size were observed in the 100-μg group (Fig. 4). After a mean follow-up of 32 months, significant benefits were reported in both myocardial perfusion and angina-free period in patients treated with growth factor at either dose compared with those receiving placebo. Nuclear perfusion scans revealed a persistent reversible or a new fixed defect in four of five patients who received placebo, versus only one of nine patients treated with FGF-2 ($P = 0.03$). In addition, among patients who received FGF-2, a trend toward improved LVEF was observed (81).

Phase I trials evaluating both intracoronary and intravenous administration of FGF-2 to examine the safety and efficacy of these less invasive methods of delivery have also been conducted (82). These were open label dose-escalating studies. Fifty-two patients with CAD and inducible ischemia who were deemed suboptimal candidates for either percutaneous transluminal coronary angioplasty (PTCA) or CABG received intracoronary FGF-2 at doses ranging from 0.33 μg/kg to 48 μg/kg. Hypotension was dose-limiting with 36 μg/kg being the maximally tolerated dose. At six months follow-up, patients reported improvement in quality of life assessments as well as reduced angina frequency and improved exertional capacity scores. Significant improvements were seen in exercise treadmill time, LVEF, target wall thickening, and myocardial perfusion as measured by magnetic resonance imaging (MRI). However, there was no correlation between the dose used and the efficacy parameters studied. The lack of a control group and the open label design of the study preclude conclusions as to the efficacy of the treatment. Another study evaluated intracoronary delivery of FGF-2 in a randomized, placebo-controlled, dose-escalated phase I trial (83). A total of 25 patients were randomized at a 2:1 ratio to a single intracoronary dose of FGF-2 or placebo. FGF-2 therapy was associated with hypotension in two patients and bradycardia in three patients. The FGF-2-treated group showed significantly increased epicardial coronary artery diameter compared with controls, but no improvement in treadmill exercise tolerance was observed.

Several phase I trials of the safety and tolerability of VEGF have also been conducted. Two trials investigated intravenous and intracoronary delivery of recombinant VEGF using dose escalation regimens (83–85) and a follow-up period up to 60 days. The results of these studies demonstrated that VEGF delivered by intracoronary and intravenous routes was well tolerated and suggested dose-dependent improvements in

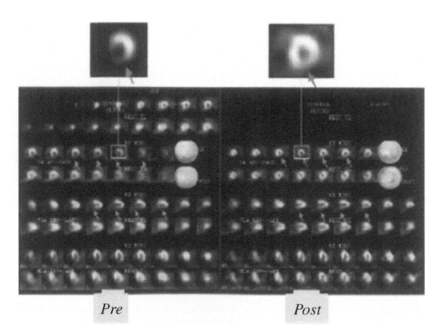

Pre   Post

Figure 4

Rest thalium (*bottom row*) and stress-SestaMibi (*upper row*) scans at baseline (*left*) and three months (*right*) after coronary artery bypass graft surgery (CABG) in a patient who received 100 μg of perivascular (intramyocardial) basic fibroblast growth factor (bFGF) showing improvement in inferolateral wall perfusion. *Source:* Adapted from Ref. 35.

myocardial blood flow by nuclear perfusion studies. As a whole, these results provide evidence for the safety of protein-based angiogenic therapy with VEGF and FGF and suggest the efficacy of this therapeutic modality.

Phase II trials

Despite the promising results seen in both preclinical and phase I trials, randomized, double-blind, controlled phase II trials have shown modest, if any, benefit. The VEGF in Ischemia for Vascular Angiogenesis (VIVA) trial was a multicenter, randomized, double-blind, placebo-controlled study of an intracoronary and intravenous regimen of recombinant VEGF (86,87). A total of 178 patients were randomized to low-dose, high-dose, or placebo groups. VEGF was delivered by an intracoronary infusion followed by intravenous infusions at three-day intervals. Treadmill exercise time was the primary endpoint. No significant improvements were reported in treadmill time or angina class in the treatment groups compared with controls at 60 days of follow-up. The VEGF infusions were well tolerated by patients in the treatment groups. Follow-up after one year revealed a trend in sustained improvement in angina class that was not statistically significant. No increased risk of cancer or myocardial infarction was apparent (86). Of note, all three groups in the VIVA trial had significant improvements in exercise treadmill time, angina class, and quality of life measures from baseline, which demonstrates the significance of the placebo effect in patients with end-stage CAD. Long-term follow-up of patients in clinical trials has shown persistence of the placebo effect for up to 30 months (88).

The FGF-2 Initiating Revascularization Support Trial (FIRST) was a multicenter, randomized, double-blind, placebo-controlled phase II study designed to examine the safety, pharmacokinetics, and efficacy of FGF-2 (89,90). A total of 337 patients who were poor candidates for percutaneous or surgical revascularization were randomized to treatment with 0, 0.3, 3, or 30 μg/kg doses of FGF-2 by intracoronary route. Exercise tolerance test time was the primary endpoint. The mean change in exercise tolerance test time was not significantly different after 90 or 180 days between treatment and control groups. However, a statistically significant benefit in treadmill time was shown in patients older than 63 years of age. Angina frequency was significantly reduced as determined by the Seattle Angina Questionnaire at 90 days, but the difference was no longer significant at 180 days because of continued improvement of the control group. No significant difference was observed in stress nuclear imaging.

Although the long-term follow-up of the randomized, double-blind controlled trial of surgical intramyocardial delivery of FGF-2 showed persistent improvement in time free of angina as well as nuclear perfusion at 32 months

in test patients versus control patients (81), the study population was small and a larger trial is needed to confirm these results.

These disappointing results can be attributed to a variety of factors. Recombinant proteins have a relatively short plasma half-life. Animal studies have demonstrated that <1% of ^{125}I-FGF-2 administered using the intracoronary route is deposited in the myocardium at one hour. Even less remains at 24 hours (36). Furthermore, the effect of growth factors is known to be diminished in the presence of endothelial dysfunction, a common finding in patients with coronary disease (10).

Clinical studies of gene therapy
Phase I trials

The first clinical trial included five patients with intractable angina and inoperable coronary disease that failed conventional medical management (91). Each patient received an intramyocardial injection of VEGF-165 plasmid through a small left anterior thoracotomy. There were no complications related to the administration of the plasmid. All five patients reported decreased nitroglycerin use between 10 and 60 days after treatment. Single photon emission computed tomography (SPECT)-sestamibi demonstrated improved blood flow and angiography showed increased collateral flow to previously ischemic areas. LVEF remained unchanged. This was followed by a larger nonrandomized uncontrolled, dose-escalating trial to assess the safety and bioactivity of intramyocardial delivery of the VEGF-165 plasmid (76). Twenty patients received the VEGF-165 plasmid and were followed for 180 days. There were no intraoperative complications but one patient suffered a cardiac arrest on the second postoperative day and died four months later secondary to aspiration pneumonia. Plasma VEGF levels were measured. The levels peaked at day 14 and returned to baseline by 90 days. Again, improvement was demonstrated on SPECT-sestamibi perfusion scans in 13 of the 17 patients studied at 60 days. Improvement in collateral filling was also demonstrated by angiography.

Rosengart et al. conducted a phase I clinical trial in 21 patients using direct intramyocardial injection of adenovirus encoding VEGF-121 (75,92). Fifteen patients received the therapy in conjunction with CABG and six received it as a sole therapy. Patients were followed for six months and there were no complications secondary to vector administration. Trends toward improvement in angina classification and treadmill exercise testing were seen at six months. Analysis of the Technetium (^{99m}Tc)-sestamibi images for wall motion at stress in the region of vector administration showed an improvement at 30 days in the majority of the patients. Coronary angiograms showed increased collaterals.

A phase I, open-label dose escalation study of VEGF-2 naked DNA delivered via direct myocardial injection through a thoracotomy was conducted by Fortuin et al. (41). Thirty patients with end-stage coronary disease were recruited and received 200, 800, or 2000 µg of naked plasmid DNA as sole therapy. There were no adverse effects and almost all patients in this open-label study experienced a reduction in angina frequency, Canadian Cardiovascular Society (CCS) angina class, and nitroglycerin use. However, there was no correlation between dose and clinical benefit and there was no angiographic evidence of angiogenesis.

Attempts to create a percutaneous method of gene delivery to the myocardium followed. The NOGA system is a catheter that electromechanically maps the myocardium to allow distinction between infracted and normal myocardium. The first study was a single blinded pilot study in which VEGF-2 plasmid DNA was delivered through intramyocardial injections in three patients and compared with three patients who received placebo injections (93). Reduction in angina frequency and nitroglycerin use was significantly lower in the patients who received the VEGF-2 plasmid versus the controls at one year follow-up. Significant decreases in the area of ischemia and improved perfusion scores were seen in test patients at 90 days after treatment.

Phase II Trials

The early success of the phase I trials led to follow-up with larger phase II double-blind placebo-controlled trials. Losordo et al. randomized 19 patients in a 2:1 ratio to either receive VEGF-2 plasmid injection or placebo via the NOGA system (94). Follow-up was performed at 12 weeks. CCS angina classification significantly improved in patients who were given the VEGF-2 plasmid injections versus no improvement in control subjects. Nitroglycerin use was decreased in both groups and was not statistically significant. The mean duration of exercise increased significantly at 12 weeks follow-up in phVEGF2-transfected patients but was unchanged in patients randomized to placebo. Electromechanical mapping demonstrated a reduction in the area of ischemic myocardium in the patients who received VEGF-2 plasmid injections. Patients in the control group demonstrated no change in the area of ischemia.

The Angiogenic Gene Therapy trial (AGENT) was a double-blinded, phase I/II trial using intracoronary infusion of increasing doses of adenovirus encoding for FGF-4 (95). Seventy-nine patients were randomized to receive either placebo or one of five doses of Ad5-FGF-4. At 12 weeks follow-up, exercise tolerance was not significantly increased in treatment groups over placebo. However, a subgroup analysis of patients with initial exercise tolerance tests (ETTs) of 10 minutes or less did show a

significant improvement in treated patients versus controls. There were no differences in stress-induced wall motion scores by echocardiography between baseline and 4 or 12 weeks. However, the AGENT III study was terminated early because of lack of effectiveness or likelihood of a positive outcome.

The Kuopio Angiogenesis Trial (KAT) was a randomized, double-blinded trial of intracoronary delivery of VEGF-165 gene transfer at the time of PTCA (40). A total of 109 patients were included in the study. Thirty-seven patients received VEGF adenovirus, 28 patients received VEGF plasmid liposome, and 38 control patients received Ringer's lactate solution. Although several patients had complications at the time of the procedure or soon after, none of these results were attributed to the gene therapy. Follow-up time was six months. Gene transfer to coronary arteries was feasible and well tolerated. The overall clinical restenosis rate was 6%. In quantitative coronary angiography analysis, the minimal lumen diameter and percent of diameter stenosis did not significantly differ between the study groups. However, myocardial perfusion showed a significant improvement in the VEGF-Adv-treated patients after the six-month follow-up. Some inflammatory responses were transiently present in the VEGF-Adv group, with transient fever and increases in serum C-reactive protein and lactate dehydrogenase levels. No increases were detected in the incidences of serious adverse events in any of the study groups.

The Euroinject One study (39) randomized 80 "no-option" (end-stage CAD) patients with stress-induced myocardial perfusion defects to intramyocardial plasmid gene transfer of VEGF-165 (0.5 mg) or placebo, delivered percutaneously via the NOGA catheter system. This double-blinded trial demonstrated an improvement in wall motion abnormalities but no improvement in myocardial perfusion, assessed by ^{99m}Tc sestamibi SPECT imaging. CCS angina class improved in both groups with no significant difference between the two groups.

Future prospects

Despite some disappointing initial results in clinical trials, therapeutic angiogenesis has the potential to provide new treatment strategies for patients with end-stage ischemic heart disease. Concerns regarding the safety of FGF and VEGF have not borne out in clinical trials. The trials described before have repeatedly demonstrated the safety of these agents as well as the safety of gene transfer. Angioma, neoplasms, plaque angiogenesis, and retinopathy have not been seen in the doses used in human trials.

There are a variety of reasons as to why some of these trials failed to show improvement with treatment. Patients selected for these trials are possibly the ones most likely to fail to respond to therapeutic angiogenic agents. They have had multiple percutaneous and surgical revascularization attempts and have comorbidities such as diabetes mellitus, hypercholesterolemia, and endothelial dysfunction which commonly accompany atherosclerotic disease. A diminished response to growth factor therapy has been demonstrated in the presence of endothelial dysfunction and may explain the disappointing results of clinical trials (10,11). Reversal of endothelial dysfunction by oral supplementation with L-arginine (a NO donor), in animal models, has been shown to improve the angiogenic response (96) and modulation of endothelial dysfunction may represent a novel strategy to enhance myocardial angiogenesis.

Endpoints of morbidity and mortality including myocardial infarction and death may provide objective measures of outcome. However, as these events occur at a low frequency, a prohibitively large study population may be required to show significant reductions in these outcomes. Changes in angina class, frequency, quality of life, and exercise tolerance are all somewhat subjective and therefore, susceptible to the powerful placebo effect observed in these patients. Adequate blinding, therefore, is critical to the ascertainment of a true therapeutic effect. The availability of a noninvasive, objective, and sensitive instrument to assess the efficacy of angiogenic therapy can help to address some of these issues. SPECT, positron emission tomography (PET), and MRI are potential candidates for such an instrument (Fig. 5).

The phase II trials reported to date have primarily focused on intravascular delivery, with a few exceptions. Phase I trials of intramyocardial protein as well as gene delivery have borne promising results. Adequately powered, randomized, double-blind, placebo-controlled trials of intramyocardial delivery techniques are needed. Although intravenous and intracoronary delivery techniques are less invasive than surgical techniques, they result in systemic release and side effects such as NO-mediated hypotension which limit the dose that is delivered. Intramyocardial delivery by a percutaneous, catheter-based or a minimally invasive surgical procedure is appealing for the ability to target desired areas of the heart with the adequate dose and duration of treatment while avoiding systemic effects. Furthermore, it has become clear that the timing and duration of growth factor therapy may be critical in inducing an angiogenic response (97). Thus, prolonged exposure to growth factors may be required, which would necessitate the use of sustained release systems or gene transfer for growth factor delivery.

Finally, multiagent therapy may be needed to modulate the complex process of angiogenesis in humans. A synergistic mechanism of action between growth factors in angiogenesis has been suggested (98). Gene transfer methods using transcription factors, such as HIF-1α, which regulates the expression of multiple angiogenic genes, may be an alternative strategy. As we further our knowledge of the basic mechanisms of angiogenesis and the techniques of angiogenic therapy, the strategies used in the design of technologies and clinical trials will be based on a more sound scientific foundation that may allow therapeutic angiogenesis to become a reality in the treatment of CAD.

References

1 Heart Disease and Stroke Statistics—2005 Update. American Heart Association, 2005.

2 Jones EL, Craver JM, Guyton RA, Bone DK, Hatcher CR, Jr, Riechwald N. Importance of complete revascularization in performance of the coronary bypass operation. Am J Cardiol 1983; 51(1):7–12.

3 McNeer JF, Conley MJ, Starmer CF, et al. Complete and incomplete revascularization at aortocoronary bypass surgery: experience with 392 consecutive patients. Am Heart J 1974; 88(2):176–182.

4 Folkman J. Angiogenic therapy of the human heart. Circulation 1998; 97(7):628–629.

5 Sellke FW, Laham RJ, Edelman ER, Pearlman JD, Simons M. Therapeutic angiogenesis with basic fibroblast growth factor: technique and early results. Ann Thorac Surg 1998; 65(6):1540–1544.

6 Moon MR, Sundt TM, 3rd, Pasque MK, et al. Influence of internal mammary artery grafting and completeness of revascularization on long-term outcome in octogenarians. Ann Thorac Surg 2001; 72(6):2003–2007.

7 Kleisli T, Cheng W, Jacobs MJ, et al. In the current era, complete revascularization improves survival after coronary artery bypass surgery. J Thorac Cardiovasc Surg 2005; 129(6):1283–1291.

8 Ellis SG, Chew D, Chan A, Whitlow PL, Schneider JP, Topol EJ. Death following creatine kinase-MB elevation after coronary intervention: identification of an early risk period: importance of creatine kinase-MB level, completeness of revascularization,

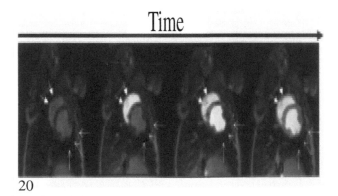

Time

20

Figure 5

Myocardial perfusion/contrast arrival as assessed using magnetic resonance imaging after bolus administration of gadodiamide. Time sequence display of selected short axis diastolic images shows contrast arrival to the right ventricle, the left ventricle, followed by left ventricular myocardium. The mean size of the delayed contrast arrival zone (underperfused area of myocardium) was reduced significantly after basic fibroblast growth factor (bFGF) administration (at 180 days). *Source:* Adapted from Ref. 82.

ventricular function, and probable benefit of statin therapy. Circulation 2002; 106(10):1205–1210.

9 Simons M, Bonow RO, Chronos NA, et al. Clinical trials in coronary angiogenesis: issues, problems, consensus: An expert panel summary. Circulation 2000; 102(11):E73–E86.

10 Ruel M, Wu GF, Khan TA, et al. Inhibition of the cardiac angiogenic response to surgical FGF-2 therapy in a Swine endothelial dysfunction model. Circulation 2003; 108(suppl 1):II335–II340.

11 Voisine P, Bianchi C, Ruel M, et al. Inhibition of the cardiac angiogenic response to exogenous vascular endothelial growth factor. Surgery 2004; 136(2):407–415.

12 Yancopoulos GD, Davis S, Gale NW, Rudge JS, Wiegand SJ, Holash J. Vascular-specific growth factors and blood vessel formation. Nature 2000; 407(6801):242–248.

13 Asahara T, Takahashi T, Masuda H, et al. VEGF contributes to postnatal neovascularization by mobilizing bone marrow-derived endothelial progenitor cells. Embo J 1999; 18(14):3964–3972.

14 Tofukuji M, Metais C, Li J, Franklin A, Simons M, Sellke FW. Myocardial VEGF expression after cardiopulmonary bypass and cardioplegia. Circulation 1998; 98(19 suppl):II242–II246; discussion II247–II248.

15 Harada K, Friedman M, Lopez JJ, et al. Vascular endothelial growth factor administration in chronic myocardial ischemia. Am J Physiol 1996; 270(5 Pt 2):H1791–1802.

16 Lopez JJ, Laham RJ, Stamler A, et al. VEGF administration in chronic myocardial ischemia in pigs. Cardiovasc Res 1998; 40(2):272–281.

17 Lopez JJ, Laham RJ, Carrozza JP, et al. Hemodynamic effects of intracoronary VEGF delivery: evidence of tachyphylaxis and NO dependence of response. Am J Physiol 1997; 273(3 Pt 2):H1317–H1323.

18 Folkman J. Angiogenesis in cancer, vascular, rheumatoid and other disease. Nat Med 1995; 1(1):27–31.

19 Post MJ, Laham R, Sellke FW, Simons M. Therapeutic angiogenesis in cardiology using protein formulations. Cardiovasc Res 2001; 49(3):522–531.

20 Faham S, Hileman RE, Fromm JR, Linhardt RJ, Rees DC. Heparin structure and interactions with basic fibroblast growth factor. Science 1996; 271(5252):1116–1120.

21 Detillieux KA, Sheikh F, Kardami E, Cattini PA. Biological activities of fibroblast growth factor-2 in the adult myocardium. Cardiovasc Res 2003; 57(1):8–19.

22 Casscells W, Speir E, Sasse J, et al. Isolation, characterization, and localization of heparin-binding growth factors in the heart. J Clin Invest 1990; 85(2):433–441.

23 Bernotat-Danielowski S, Sharma HS, Schott RJ, Schaper W. Generation and localisation of monoclonal antibodies against fibroblast growth factors in ischaemic collateralised porcine myocardium. Cardiovasc Res 1993; 27(7):1220–1228.

24 Schneider H, Huse K. Arterial gene therapy. Lancet 1996; 348(9038):1380–1381; author reply 1381–1382.

25 Slavin J. Fibroblast growth factors: at the heart of angiogenesis. Cell Biol Int 1995; 19(5):431–444.

26 Cuevas P, Carceller F, Ortega S, Zazo M, Nieto I, Gimenez-Gallego G. Hypotensive activity of fibroblast growth factor. Science 1991; 254(5035):1208–1210.

27 Sellke FW, Wang SY, Friedman M, et al. Basic FGF enhances endothelium-dependent relaxation of the collateral-perfused coronary microcirculation. Am J Physiol 1994; 267(4 Pt 2): H1303–H1311.

28 Battler A, Scheinowitz M, Bor A, et al. Intracoronary injection of basic fibroblast growth factor enhances angiogenesis in infarcted swine myocardium. J Am Coll Cardiol 1993; 22(7):2001–2006.

29 Yanagisawa-Miwa A, Uchida Y, Nakamura F, et al. Salvage of infarcted myocardium by angiogenic action of basic fibroblast growth factor. Science 1992; 257(5075):1401–1403.

30 Laham RJ, Rezaee M, Post M, et al. Intrapericardial delivery of fibroblast growth factor-2 induces neovascularization in a porcine model of chronic myocardial ischemia. J Pharmacol Exp Ther 2000; 292(2):795–802.

31 Harada K, Grossman W, Friedman M, et al. Basic fibroblast growth factor improves myocardial function in chronically ischemic porcine hearts. J Clin Invest 1994; 94(2):623–630.

32 Sato K, Laham RJ, Pearlman JD, et al. Efficacy of intracoronary versus intravenous FGF-2 in a pig model of chronic myocardial ischemia. Ann Thorac Surg 2000; 70(6):2113–2118.

33 Rajanayagam MA, Shou M, Thirumurti V, et al. Intracoronary basic fibroblast growth factor enhances myocardial collateral perfusion in dogs. J Am Coll Cardiol 2000; 35(2):519–526.

34 Simons M, Laham R. Therapeutic angiogenesis in myocardial ischemia. In: Ware J, Simons M, eds. Angiogenesis and Cardiovascular Disease. New York: Oxford University press, 1999:289–320.

35 Laham RJ, Sellke FW, Edelman ER, et al. Local perivascular delivery of basic fibroblast growth factor in patients undergoing coronary bypass surgery: results of a phase I randomized, double-blind, placebo-controlled trial. Circulation 1999; 100(18):1865–1871.

36 Laham RJ, Rezaee M, Post M, et al. Intracoronary and intravenous administration of basic fibroblast growth factor: myocardial and tissue distribution. Drug Metab Dispos 1999; 27(7):821–826.

37 Li J, Post M, Volk R, et al. PR39, a peptide regulator of angiogenesis. Nat Med 2000; 6(1):49–55.

38 Iyer NV, Kotch LE, Agani F, et al. Cellular and developmental control of O_2 homeostasis by hypoxia-inducible factor 1 alpha. Genes Dev 1998; 12(2):149–162.

39 Kastrup J, Jorgensen E, Ruck A, et al. Direct intramyocardial plasmid vascular endothelial growth factor-A165 gene therapy in patients with stable severe angina pectoris A randomized double-blind placebo-controlled study: the Euroinject One trial. J Am Coll Cardiol 2005; 45(7):982–988.

40 Hedman M, Hartikainen J, Syvanne M, et al. Safety and feasibility of catheter-based local intracoronary vascular endothelial growth factor gene transfer in the prevention of postangioplasty and in-stent restenosis and in the treatment of chronic myocardial ischemia: phase II results of the Kuopio Angiogenesis Trial (KAT). Circulation 2003; 107(21):2677–2683.

41 Fortuin FD, Vale P, Losordo DW, et al. One-year follow-up of direct myocardial gene transfer of vascular endothelial growth factor-2 using naked plasmid deoxyribonucleic acid by way of thoracotomy in no-option patients. Am J Cardiol 2003; 92(4):436–439.

42 MacColl GS, Novo FJ, Marshall NJ, Waters M, Goldspink G, Bouloux PM. Optimisation of growth hormone production by muscle cells using plasmid DNA. J Endocrinol 2000; 165(2):329–336.

43 Nishikawa M, Yamauchi M, Morimoto K, Ishida E, Takakura Y, Hashida M. Hepatocyte-targeted in vivo gene expression by

intravenous injection of plasmid DNA complexed with synthetic multi-functional gene delivery system. Gene Ther 2000; 7(7):548–555.

44   Shangguan T, Cabral-Lilly D, Purandare U, et al. A novel N-acyl phosphatidylethanolamine-containing delivery vehicle for spermine-condensed plasmid DNA. Gene Ther 2000; 7(9):769–783.

45   Atienza C, Jr., Elliott MJ, Dong YB, et al. Adenovirus-mediated E2F-1 gene transfer induces an apoptotic response in human gastric carcinoma cells that is enhanced by cyclin dependent kinase inhibitors. Int J Mol Med 2000; 6(1):55–63.

46   Bilbao R, Gerolami R, Bralet MP, et al. Transduction efficacy, antitumoral effect, and toxicity of adenovirus-mediated herpes simplex virus thymidine kinase/ ganciclovir therapy of hepatocellular carcinoma: the woodchuck animal model. Cancer Gene Ther 2000; 7(5):657–662.

47   Chen P, Kovesdi I, Bruder JT. Effective repeat administration with adenovirus vectors to the muscle. Gene Ther 2000; 7(7):587–595.

48   Lee EJ, Thimmapaya B, Jameson JL. Stereotactic injection of adenoviral vectors that target gene expression to specific pituitary cell types: implications for gene therapy. Neurosurgery 2000; 46(6):1461–1468; discussion 1468–1469.

49   Hartigan-O'Connor D, Amalfitano A, Chamberlain JS. Improved production of gutted adenovirus in cells expressing adenovirus preterminal protein and DNA polymerase. J Virol 1999; 73(9):7835–7841.

50   Dutheil N, Shi F, Dupressoir T, Linden RM. Adeno-associated virus site-specifically integrates into a muscle-specific DNA region. Proc Natl Acad Sci USA 2000; 97(9):4862–4866.

51   Drittanti L, Rivet C, Manceau P, Danos O, Vega M. High throughput production, screening and analysis of adeno-associated viral vectors. Gene Ther 2000; 7(11):924–929.

52   Hudde T, Rayner SA, De Alwis M, et al. Adeno-associated and herpes simplex viruses as vectors for gene transfer to the corneal endothelium. Cornea 2000; 19(3):369–373.

53   Sun L, Li J, Xiao X. Overcoming adeno-associated virus vector size limitation through viral DNA heterodimerization. Nat Med 2000; 6(5):599–602.

54   Duan D, Yue Y, Yan Z, Engelhardt JF. A new dual-vector approach to enhance recombinant adeno-associated virus-mediated gene expression through intermolecular cis activation. Nat Med 2000; 6(5):595–598.

55   Nakai H, Storm TA, Kay MA. Increasing the size of rAAV-mediated expression cassettes in vivo by intermolecular joining of two complementary vectors. Nat Biotechnol 2000; 18(5):527–532.

56   Rudich SM, Zhou S, Srivastava R, Escobedo JA, Perez RV, Manning WC. Dose response to a single intramuscular injection of recombinant adeno-associated virus-erythropoietin in monkeys. J Surg Res 2000; 90(2):102–108.

57   Hirata RK, Russell DW. Design and packaging of adeno-associated virus gene targeting vectors. J Virol 2000; 74(10):4612–4620.

58   Costello E, Munoz M, Buetti E, Meylan PR, Diggelmann H, Thali M. Gene transfer into stimulated and unstimulated T lymphocytes by HIV-1-derived lentiviral vectors. Gene Ther 2000; 7(7):596–604.

59   Palu G, Parolin C, Takeuchi Y, Pizzato M. Progress with retroviral gene vectors. Rev Med Virol 2000; 10(3):185–202.

60   Solaiman F, Zink MA, Xu G, et al. Modular retro-vectors for transgenic and therapeutic use. Mol Reprod Dev 2000; 56(2 suppl):309–315.

61   Marshall E. Improving gene therapy's tool kit. Science 2000; 288(5468):953.

62   Follenzi A, Ailles LE, Bakovic S, Geuna M, Naldini L. Gene transfer by lentiviral vectors is limited by nuclear translocation and rescued by HIV-1 pol sequences. Nat Genet 2000; 25(2):217–222.

63   Johnson LG, Olsen JC, Naldini L, Boucher RC. Pseudotyped human lentiviral vector-mediated gene transfer to airway epithelia in vivo. Gene Ther 2000; 7(7):568–574.

64   Cioffi L, Sturtz FG, Wittmer S, et al. A novel endothelial cell-based gene therapy platform for the in vivo delivery of apolipoprotein E. Gene Ther 1999; 6(6):1153–1159.

65   Powell C, Shansky J, Del Tatto M, et al. Tissue-engineered human bioartificial muscles expressing a foreign recombinant protein for gene therapy. Hum Gene Ther 1999; 10(4):565–577.

66   Su L, Lee R, Bonyhadi M, et al. Hematopoietic stem cell-based gene therapy for acquired immunodeficiency syndrome: efficient transduction and expression of RevM10 in myeloid cells in vivo and in vitro. Blood 1997; 89(7):2283–2290.

67   Zhang J, Russell SJ. Vectors for cancer gene therapy. Cancer Metastasis Rev 1996; 15(3):385–401.

68   Wei Y, Quertermous T, Wagner TE. Directed endothelial differentiation of cultured embryonic yolk sac cells in vivo provides a novel cell-based system for gene therapy. Stem Cells 1995; 13(5):541–547.

69   Tomita S, Li RK, Weisel RD, et al. Autologous transplantation of bone marrow cells improves damaged heart function. Circulation 1999; 100(19 suppl):II247–II256.

70   Kobayashi T, Hamano K, Li TS, et al. Enhancement of angiogenesis by the implantation of self bone marrow cells in a rat ischemic heart model. J Surg Res 2000; 89(2):189–195.

71   Giordano FJ, Ping P, McKirnan MD, et al. Intracoronary gene transfer of fibroblast growth factor-5 increases blood flow and contractile function in an ischemic region of the heart. Nat Med 1996; 2(5):534–539.

72   Iwatate M, Miura T, Ikeda Y, et al. Effects of in vivo gene transfer of fibroblast growth factor-2 on cardiac function and collateral vessel formation in the microembolized rabbit heart. Jpn Circ J 2001; 65(3):226–231.

73   Miao W, Luo Z, Kitsis RN, Walsh K. Intracoronary, adenovirus-mediated Akt gene transfer in heart limits infarct size following ischemia-reperfusion injury in vivo. J Mol Cell Cardiol 2000; 32(12):2397–2402.

74   Lai NC, Roth DM, Gao MH, et al. Intracoronary delivery of adenovirus encoding adenylyl cyclase VI increases left ventricular function and cAMP-generating capacity. Circulation 2000; 102(19):2396–2401.

75   Rosengart TK, Lee LY, Patel SR, et al. Angiogenesis gene therapy: phase I assessment of direct intramyocardial administration of an adenovirus vector expressing VEGF121 cDNA to individuals with clinically significant severe coronary artery disease. Circulation 1999; 100(5):468–474.

76   Symes JF, Losordo DW, Vale PR, et al. Gene therapy with vascular endothelial growth factor for inoperable coronary artery disease. Ann Thorac Surg 1999; 68(3):830–836; discussion 836–837.

77 French BA, Mazur W, Geske RS, Bolli R. Direct in vivo gene transfer into porcine myocardium using replication-deficient adenoviral vectors. Circulation 1994; 90(5):2414–2424.

78 Muhlhauser J, Jones M, Yamada I, et al. Safety and efficacy of in vivo gene transfer into the porcine heart with replication-deficient, recombinant adenovirus vectors. Gene Ther 1996; 3(2):145–153.

79 Schumacher B, Pecher P, von Specht BU, Stegmann T. Induction of neoangiogenesis in ischemic myocardium by human growth factors: first clinical results of a new treatment of coronary heart disease. Circulation 1998; 97(7):645–650.

80 Pecher P, Schumacher BA. Angiogenesis in ischemic human myocardium: clinical results after 3 years. Ann Thorac Surg 2000; 69(5):1414–1419.

81 Ruel M, Laham RJ, Parker JA, et al. Long-term effects of surgical angiogenic therapy with fibroblast growth factor 2 protein. J Thorac Cardiovasc Surg 2002; 124(1):28–34.

82 Laham RJ, Chronos NA, Pike M, et al. Intracoronary basic fibroblast growth factor (FGF-2) in patients with severe ischemic heart disease: results of a phase I open-label dose escalation study. J Am Coll Cardiol 2000; 36(7):2132–2139.

83 Henry TD, Rocha-Singh K, Isner JM, et al. Intracoronary administration of recombinant human vascular endothelial growth factor to patients with coronary artery disease. Am Heart J 2001; 142(5):872–880.

84 Hendel RC, Henry TD, Rocha-Singh K, et al. Effect of intracoronary recombinant human vascular endothelial growth factor on myocardial perfusion: evidence for a dose-dependent effect. Circulation 2000; 101(2):118–121.

85 Henry TD, Abraham JA. Review of preclinical and clinical results with vascular endothelial growth factors for therapeutic angiogenesis. Curr Interv Cardiol Rep 2000; 2(3):228–241.

86 Henry TD, Annex BH, McKendall GR, et al. The VIVA trial: vascular endothelial growth factor in ischemia for vascular angiogenesis. Circulation 2003; 107(10):1359–1365.

87 Ferguson JJ. Meeting highlights. Highlights of the 48th scientific sessions of the American College of Cardiology. Circulation 1999; 100(6):570–575.

88 Rana JS, Mannam A, Donnell-Fink L, Gervino EV, Sellke FW, Laham RJ. Longevity of the placebo effect in the therapeutic angiogenesis and laser myocardial revascularization trials in patients with coronary heart disease. Am J Cardiol 2005; 95(12):1456–1459.

89 Kleiman NS, Califf RM. Results from late-breaking clinical trials sessions at ACCIS 2000 and ACC 2000. American College of Cardiology. J Am Coll Cardiol 2000; 36(1):310–325.

90 Simons M, Annex BH, Laham RJ, et al. Pharmacological treatment of coronary artery disease with recombinant fibroblast growth factor-2: double-blind, randomized, controlled clinical trial. Circulation 2002; 105(7):788–793.

91 Losordo DW, Vale PR, Symes JF, et al. Gene therapy for myocardial angiogenesis: initial clinical results with direct myocardial injection of phVEGF165 as sole therapy for myocardial ischemia. Circulation 1998; 98(25):2800–2804.

92 Rosengart TK, Lee LY, Patel SR, et al. Six-month assessment of a phase I trial of angiogenic gene therapy for the treatment of coronary artery disease using direct intramyocardial administration of an adenovirus vector expressing the VEGF121 cDNA. Ann Surg 1999; 230(4):466–470; discussion 462–470.

93 Vale PR, Losordo DW, Milliken CE, et al. Randomized, single-blind, placebo-controlled pilot study of catheter-based myocardial gene transfer for therapeutic angiogenesis using left ventricular electromechanical mapping in patients with chronic myocardial ischemia. Circulation 2001; 103(17):2138–2143.

94 Losordo DW, Vale PR, Hendel RC, et al. Phase 1/2 placebo-controlled, double-blind, dose-escalating trial of myocardial vascular endothelial growth factor 2 gene transfer by catheter delivery in patients with chronic myocardial ischemia. Circulation 2002; 105(17):2012–2018.

95 Grines CL, Watkins MW, Helmer G, et al. Angiogenic Gene Therapy (AGENT) trial in patients with stable angina pectoris. Circulation 2002; 105(11):1291–1297.

96 Voisine P, Bianchi C, Khan TA, et al. Normalization of coronary microvascular reactivity and improvement in myocardial perfusion by surgical vascular endothelial growth factor therapy combined with oral supplementation of L-arginine in a porcine model of endothelial dysfunction. J Thorac Cardiovasc Surg 2005; 129(6):1414–1420.

97 Dor Y, Djonov V, Abramovitch R, et al. Conditional switching of VEGF provides new insights into adult neovascularization and pro-angiogenic therapy. Embo J 2002; 21(8):1939–1947.

98 Asahara T, Bauters C, Zheng LP, et al. Synergistic effect of vascular endothelial growth factor and basic fibroblast growth factor on angiogenesis in vivo. Circulation 1995; 92(9 suppl):II365–II371.

36

Cell transplantation for cardiovascular repair

Doris A. Taylor, Harald Ott, and Patrick Serruys

Introduction

Cardiovascular disease (CVD) has become a major health issue throughout the world, exceeding infection, as the leading cause of death worldwide (1,2). In the Western world, in particular, the United States, CVD exceeds the next five causes of death combined. Although there has been a reduction in mortality in several forms of CVD, including acute myocardial infarction (AMI), there has been little progress in treating heart failure (HF), a condition that affects 5 million people in the United States and 22 million worldwide (3). The increasing prevalence of HF directly relates to the improved survival of patients with acute coronary syndromes (nearly 40% of whom would manifest eventual HF by seven years) and by the significant reduction in sudden cardiac death owing to the use of internal cardio-defibrillators (ICDs) (1,4,5). However, the factor with the greatest impact on the incidence and prevalence of HF is its association with advanced aging. The number of people over 65 years of age in the United States would double in the next 25 years, and it is estimated that nearly 15% of this population will develop HF (1). These numbers clearly illustrate the need for the development of improved therapies throughout the continuum of this insidious disease process, that is, to intervene after acute injury, to prevent negative remodeling and to treat failing myocardium.

Translating cardiovascular repair is a process

Moving any novel therapeutic from bench to bedside requires multiple inter-related steps. The first step is the idea embodied in the basic science. Next, that idea must then be tested in clinically relevant preclinical models of disease. Only if those data are promising, should the idea progress to clinical studies, and if novel or unexpected issues arise, the idea may move in reverse from bedside to bench and when revised to move back again. Yet, even then, the continuum is not complete. A clinical "product" must be the ultimate goal or the treatment would never reach the bedside. At present, we are in iterations between bedside and bench. The first successful ideas have moved into clinical studies; early clinical safety and efficacy data are emerging and new insights are being garnered to force the next generation of preclinical innovations. The concept of a product is evolving, new business models are emerging, and multiple new therapeutic strategies are being evaluated. To dissect where we are in this continuum from bench to bedside, lets look back 5 to 10 years. Ten years ago, the concept of cardiac repair was virtually unheard of. No studies had been presented demonstrating the functional improvement of the myocardium, and only a few studies had been published suggesting that the injected cells could actually incorporate into damaged heart (6). It was not until 1998 that the first preclinical study was published demonstrating functional improvement of injured myocardium after transplantation of skeletal myoblasts (7). After that, the field virtually exploded. Within two years, a clinical trial had begun in Europe (8) in which skeletal myoblasts were delivered as an adjunct to coronary artery bypass grafting (CABG) in patients with HF, and now, six years later, multiple clinical trials using five to six different muscle-, bone marrow (BM)-, and blood-derived cell types have been reported (8–12).

In summary, this is a dynamic time in a new field: treatment strategies are being developed and modified almost daily; new cell types are being reported; novel delivery strategies are emerging; and slowly, we are dissecting the components of cellular cardiomyoplasty.

This explosion of trials for a novel therapy lies in the simplicity and straightforward nature. First, cell therapy offers an opportunity for the repair of the injury, rather than simply for the augmentation of the remaining uninjured heart often to its detriment. In other words, cell therapy provides hope of a solution to a previously unsolvable problem. Next, the treatment makes sense to patients. If cells normally die leading to HF after infarction, it could be attempted to either prevent them from dying as is a goal with current BM trials in early post-MI, or replace them, a current goal of virtually all trials? And because cell therapy to date primarily involves autologous cells, patients endorse it and often seek it out. From a clinical perspective, this innovative strategy provides a potential therapeutic option, where none existed previously. And as is often the case with novel strategies, it is exciting and prestigious to perform. These qualities together with the anticipated up to 5.3 billion dollar market potential have led scientists, companies, clinicians, and patients, into a plethora of first-in-man studies. As a result, within 10 years, we have moved from initiation of a new field to completed phase I clinical studies.

This rapid ascent also reflects the excitement and potential surrounding this promising therapy. The good news is that the field is moving rapidly. The bad news is that the field is sometimes moving without critical evaluation of the scientific underpinnings of the data. We have conflicting clinical outcomes—both negative and positive results with the same cells, in the same patients (13,14). We are realizing that outcome does not necessarily reflect the engraftment of cells. We have to invoke as yet unexplained "paracrine" effects of cells for repair.

Within the next few years, we should have the completion of both surgical and percutaneous phase I safety/feasibility studies with BM, blood, muscle, and possibly even fat-derived progenitor cells, and will likely see the initiation of at least one trial utilizing cardiac-derived cells. Furthermore, as more cells are described, more trials would emerge. It is very likely that when occurs cell types will segregate with the disease state; then as we gain more insights into when and how cells work, we will begin to choose the right cell for the right stage of the CVD continuum. In part, these would likely reflect the impact of phase II and even phase III data regarding the use of BM-derived stem cells in the acute and subacute setting of myocardial infarction and the use of myoblasts or mesenchymal cells in patients suffering from HF.

In addition to these definitive data, we should gain better insights into the myriad of components that are required for the successful completion of cardiac cell therapy: the choice of cell type, be it adult or embryonic, autologous or allogeneic, BM, blood, muscle, or fat derived; how to deliver the cells surgically (15), percutaneously, or simply intravenously; how to track cells (16), and how to monitor their effect(s) in patients. We will continue to see clinical data emerge regarding the use of stem cells in the continuum of diseases ranging from AMI through HF. We will begin to understand how the age of the patient (17), the time after injury, and perhaps even gender, impact the outcome. And as we do, we will likely have the opportunity to design cell therapy strategies that redefine the concept of "personalized" medicine.

Cell-based repair—what is the premise and what can be achieved?

The simplest tissue repair is endogenous. Exogenous cell therapy has allowed us to explore the idea of endogenous cardiac repair, a concept previously thought to be nonexistent. We realize now that virtually every organ in the body, including heart, is capable of ongoing maintenance throughout much of our lifetime and only with chronic disease, aging, or when overwhelmed by a catastrophic event does this repair process fail. Yet, this failure appears to occur more often in heart than in other organs. As we understand more about this endogenous cardiac process—what initiates it, what controls it, what allows it to work, and when it fails—we will begin to have other targets for repair. Manipulating those targets first preclinically and then clinically will become increasingly important as the field matures. Meanwhile, what can we learn from noncardiac repair that could apply to heart?

Successful endogenous cell-based repair of many noncardiac tissues can routinely occur after injury. For example, in bone, endogenous repair occurs *if* three simple premises are fulfilled: reduction, fixation, and perfusion (18). Although bone injuries are not usually ischemic in origin, the cascade of wound healing is similar to the process in myocardium: inflammation leads to the clearing of necrotic (bone) tissue and the formation of a fibrous scar. However, unlike in heart, the scar is then replaced by regenerating bone such that after a relatively short period, the bone is completely healed. Why does this succeed where endogenous cardiac repair fails? In bone repair, *mechanical stress has to be minimized*. When injured bone is insufficiently reduced or fixed, an unstable scar develops in a process similar to cardiac remodelling that ultimately results in heart failure. When perfusion is compromised, tissue necrosis leads to sequestration, chronic inflammation and pain—a process similar to chronic angina. Furthermore, in the absence of good perfusion, mature bone does not arise—similar to the need for angiogenesis to support new muscle formation in myocardium. Finally, *cells have to arrive at or home to the lesion*. Bone regeneration is ultimately performed by endogenous progenitor cells (osteoblasts and osteoclasts) that migrate into the lesion. In the injured myocardium, this appears to be the spot where the process breaks down. Rather than intensive colonization with the desired cardiac progenitor cells, the lesion is colonized primarily by fibroblasts, yielding collagen deposition and scar formation instead of nascent myocardium. This comparison with bone makes endogenous cell-based cardiovascular repair seem difficult if not impossible. We are facing patients with chronic disease often at a stage where endogenous repair has long failed and where failed repair has led to remodeling and worsening of the initial injury. At present, revitalizing endogenous repair remains an elusive but well-conceived goal. However, what is currently possible and what can be truly claimed as realistic is exogenous cell administration to promote cardiac and vascular repair.

In the past 15 years, an extensive amount of preclinical data has been on the *reparative* potential of cell transplantation in acute and chronic myocardial injury. Since the first preclinical report of *functional* repair after the injection of autologous skeletal myoblasts into the injured heart in 1998 (7), a variety of cell types or combinations (Table 1) have been proposed for transplantation during different stages of CVD (19). Preclinical data has been promising, and in at least one study, the amount of repair achieved with cell transplantation in HF is additive to current medical treatment (20). With the first cardiac clinical application in 2001 (8), the field rapidly moved from bench to bedside, and at present, we are gaining valuable information about the questions to ask and the early answers from both animal and human studies. To date, 19 clinical trials either in AMI (Table 2) or chronic HF have been published (21) (Table 3), including 13, where BM

cells were used (Table 4). The early results have led to optimism based on an improvement in left ventricular (LV) function and myocardial viability in addition to a clinical improvement that in some studies goes beyond the achievable effect of current treatment options. However, given the design of most of the early trials as safety and feasibility studies, we have to evaluate these promising results carefully even as we move into prospective randomized placebo-controlled trials.

Cell-based cardiac repair in 2006: the continued questions

The best cell type is unknown and likely varies with injury

The most prevalent question facing investigators is the choice of cell type. At present, no strong scientific rationale exists for this selection. Yet, developing such a rationale is critical if the therapy is to be optimized. Patients suffering from heart disease are a heterogeneous population, who present at

---

Table 1   Comparative preclinical studies

Study	Species	Model	Cell type	Outcome
Hutcheson et al. (82)	Rabbit	Cryoinjury	Skeletal myoblasts vs. fibroblasts	SKM superior to FB; SKMB improve systolic and diastolic function FB only improves diastolic
Thompson et al. (30)	Rabbit	Cryoinjury	Skeletal myoblasts vs. bone marrow mononuclear cells	No difference between SKMB and mononuclear bone marrow stem cells regarding LV function
Horackova et al. (28)	Guinea pig	LAD ligation	Skeletal myoblasts vs. cardiac fibroblasts vs. cardiomyocytes	Myotube formation in SKMB-treated animals; SKMB superior to CM and CFs regarding remodeling; functional improvement in SKMB-treated animals; no comparison regarding the LV function
Agbulut et al. (31)	Rat	LAD ligation	Human skeletal myoblasts vs. human AC133+	Myotubes in SKMB-treated group; no difference regarding the LV function
Ott et al. (29)	Rat	LAD ligation	Autologous skeletal myoblasts vs. BM-MNC	SKMB superior to isolated BM-MNC regarding LV function Combination of these cell types shows synergy

Experimental studies comparing different cell types in cellular cardiomyoplasty. Skeletal myoblasts have a higher myogenic potential, whereas bone marrow-derived stem cells seem to be more capable of inducing angiogenesis. Several cell types lead to functional improvement. One study suggests synergistic effects of different cell types in combined treatment.

Abbreviations: BM-MNC, bone marrow mononuclear cell; CF, cardiac fibroblast; CM, cardiomyocyte; FB, fibroblast; LAD, left anterior descending artery; LV, left ventricle; SKMB, skeletal myoblast.

Table 2 Cell therapy trials in patients with heart failure

Study	Cell type	Patients treated (n)	Delivery	LVEF (%)	Dose	Results
Menasche et al. (83)	SKMB	10	Transepicardial—without CABG of treated region	24 ± 4	$8.7 \pm 1.9 \times 10^8$	Global LVEF increased
Herreros et al. (84)	SKMB	11	Transepicardial—with CABG of treated region	36 ± 8	$1.9 \pm 1.2 \times 10^8$	Global LVEF, regional wall motion and viability increased
Siminiak et al. (85)	SKMB	10	Transepicardial—with CABG of treated region	25–40	$0.4–5.0 \times 10^7$	Global LVEF, regional wall motion increased
Chachques et al. (51)	SKMB	20	Transepicardial—without CABG of treated region	28 ± 3	$3.0 \pm 0.2 \times 10^8$	Global LVEF, regional wall motion and viability increased
Smits et al. (38)	SKMB	5	Transendocardial—guided by electromechanical mapping	36 ± 11	$2.0 \pm 1.1 \times 10^8$	Global LVEF, regional wall motion increased
Siminiak et al. (36)	SKMB	9	Transcoronary—venous	30–49	$17–106 \times 10^6$	Global LVEF improved in 6 of 9 cases
Stamm et al. (10,60)	CD133+	12	Transepicardial—without CABG of treated region	36 ± 11	$1–2.8 \times 10^6$	Global LVEF increased, LVEDV decreased
Schachinger et al. (9,61)	CPC BM-MNC	30 CPC 29 MNC	Intracoronary	40 ± 11	$1.7 \pm 0.8 \times 10^8$ $2.3 \pm 1.2 \times 10^7$	Global LVEF increased, LVEDV decreased in both cell-treated groups
Hamano et al. (86)	BM-MNC	5	Transepicardial—during CABG		$0.3–2.2 \times 10^9$	Perfusion increase in 3 of 5 patients
Tse et al. (41)	BM-MNC	8	Transendocardial—guided by electro mechanical mapping	58 ± 11	40-ml BM	Regional wall motion and perfusion increased; angina reduced
Fuchs et al. (42)	BM	10	Transendocardial—guided by electromechanical mapping	47 ± 10	$7.8 \pm 6.6 \times 10^7$	Increase in perfusion; angina reduced
Perin et al. (12,43)	BM-MNC	14	Transendocardial—guided by electromechanical mapping	30 ± 6	$3.0 \pm 0.4 \times 10^7$	Global LVEF, regional wall motion and perfusion increased; angina and NYHA class reduced

Comparison of clinical studies using myoblasts and bone marrow-derived cells for heart failure. Currently, myoblasts show greater potential to treat late-stage disease owing to their myogenic potential and contractility. In late-stage disease, bone marrow-derived stem cells have shown mainly angiogenic potential with less potential to differentiate into myogenic cells when in scar tissue.

Abbreviations: BM-MNC, bone marrow mononuclear cell; CABG, coronary artery bypass grafting; CPC, circulating progenitor cells; LV, left ventricle; LVED, left ventricular end-diastolic diameter; LVEDV, left ventricular end-diastolic volume; LVEF, left ventricular ejection fraction; NYHA, New York Heart Association; SKMB, skeletal myoblast.

Table 3 Cell therapy trials in patients with acute myocardial infarction

Study	Cell type	Patients treated (n)	Delivery	Time after AMI (days)	Dose	Results
Strauer et al. (11)	BM-MNC	10	Intracoronary	5–9	$2.8 \pm 2.2 \times 10^7$	Regional wall motion and perfusion increased; infarct size decreased; no change in LVEDV or global LVEF
TOPCARE-AMI (9,61,87)	CPC BM-MNC	30 CPC 29 MNC	Intracoronary	5 ± 2	$2.1 \pm 0.8 \times 10^8$ $1.6 \pm 1.2 \times 10^7$	Global LVEF, regional wall motion and coronary flow increased; LVEDV and infarct size decreased
Fernandez-Aviles et al. (88)	BM-MNC	20	Intracoronary	14 ± 6	$7.8 \pm 4.1 \times 10^7$	Global LVEF, regional wall motion increased; no change in LVEDV
Kuethe et al. (89)	BM-MNC	5	Intracoronary	6	$3.9 \pm 2.3 \times 10^7$	No change in global LVEF or regional wall motion
BOOST (62)	BM	30	Intracoronary	6 ± 1	$2.5 \pm 0.9 \times 10^8$	Global LVEF and regional wall motion increased; LVEDV and infarct size decreased
Chen et al. (90)	MSC	34	Intracoronary	18	$4.8–6.0 \times 10^{10}$	Global LVEF and regional wall motion increased; LVEDV and infarct size decreased
Vanderheyden et al. (91)	AC133+	12	Intracoronary	14 ± 6	$6.6 \pm 1.4 \times 10^6$	Global LVEF, regional wall motion and perfusion increased; accelerated atherosclerosis in one patient

Comparison of clinical studies using bone marrow and blood-derived cells after acute myocordian infarction to prevent the development of heart failure. Currently, bone marrow-derived stem cells show greater potential to treat early-stage disease, primarily owing to their angiogenic potential, leading to improved left ventricle protection and ultimately to better preserved function.

Abbreviations: AMI, acute myocardial infarction; BM-MNC, bone marrow mononuclear cell; BOOST, bone marrow transfer to enhance ST-elevation infarct regeneration; CPC, circulating progenitor cells; HF, heart failure; LV, left ventricle; LVED, left ventricular end-diastolic diameter; LVEDV, left ventricular end-diastolic volume; LVEF, left ventricular ejection fraction; MI, myocardial infarction; TOPCARE-AMI, transplantation of progenitor cells and regeneration enhancement in acute myocardial infarction.

Source: From Ref. 21.

different times after disease onset, and whose progenitor cell number and function may vary accordingly (22,23). Furthermore, cells differ in their phenotypic capacity and thus their therapeutic benefits are likely to differ. In conditions where chronic ischemia prevails, or where reperfusion is the primary objective, using cells with a high angiogenic potential but a low myogenic capacity may be of high priority. Under these conditions, multiple cell populations derived from BM or blood [mononuclear cells (MNC) (10), endothelial (9) or vascular progenitor cells (24), marrow angioblasts (25), or blood-derived multi-potent adult progenitor cells (26)] may suffice. In patients where the restoration of contractile function is the clinical goal (e.g., with end-stage ischemic HF) or at early times postinfarction, when blood flow has been restored but cardiocytes have died, delivering cells with contractile potential seems a more reasonable approach.

Under these conditions, naturally myogenic cells, such as skeletal myoblasts, cardiocytes, or any progenitor cell driven down a muscle lineage appear the logical first choice. However, the ultimate proof of any cell superiority will require side-by-side comparisons of cells in similar disease state studies, which to date are limited or nonexistent.

Although a few direct clinical comparisons have been made, several recent preclinical studies have been performed to compare the beneficial effects of different cell types for cellular cardiomyoplasty (Table 1). According to these, skeletal muscle-derived cell transplantation may be more effective than the transplantation of adult cardiomyocytes, dermal or cardiac fibroblasts, or BM-MNC in the subacute or chronic MI setting (27–29). This could reflect the greater survival of myoblasts than of cardiocytes; and/or an active impact of myoblasts on cardiac systolic function as compared with a

Table 4   A summary of clinical data with bone marrow mononuclear cells

Study	Cell type	Patients treated (n)	Delivery	Time after AMI (days)	Dose (×10⁶)	Baseline LVEF		Follow-up LVEF	
						Control	Cell treatment	Control	Cell treatment
Strauer et al. (11)	BM-MNC	10	Intracoronary	5–9	28	60	57	64	62
TOPCARE-AMI (9,61,87)	BM-MNC	29	Intracoronary	5	16	51	49	53.5	57
Fernandez-Aviles (88)	BM-MNC	20	Intracoronary	14	39	(–)	51	(–)	57
Kuethe (89)	BM-MNC	5	Intracoronary	6	39	42	45	44	44
BOOST (62)	BM	30	Intracoronary	6	250	51.3	50	52	56.7
Chen (90)	MSC	34	Intracoronary	18	4800	48	49	54	67
Vanderheyden (91)	AC133+	12	Intracoronary	14	6.6	44.3	45.0	48.6	52.1
Janssens (92)	BM-MNC	67	Intracoronary	1	172	46.9	48.5	49	51.8
ASTAMI (14,93)	BM-MNC	100	Intracoronary	5–8	(–)	46	46	48	47
REPAIR-AMI (93)	BM-MNC	104	Intracoronary	4	236	47	48	50	54
Perin (43)	BM-MNC	20	Endocardial		30	37	30	34	35
Wollert (62)	BM-MNC	60	Intracoronary	4.8	2460	51	50	52	57
Schachinger (61)	BM-MNC	204	Intracoronary	3–6	236	47	48	50	54
Mean					692	47.6	47.4	49.9	53.4
SEM					422	1.6	1.7	2.0	2.2

This table shows that although encouraging, mononuclear cell therapy, as it is currently practiced, does not lead to obvious large improvements in myocardial performance. However, cell number, time after injury, and delivery, all have the power to impact this outcome and as illustrated in this table, the variability in each parameter is significant. A consensus should be reached on time after injury, the dose and preparation of cells prior to injection, and the delivery method. Only by performing comparable studies will the field be able to critically evaluate both our successes and failures.

Abbreviations: AMI, acute myocardial infarction; BM-MNC, bone marrow mononuclear cell; LVEF, left ventricular ejection fraction; SEM, standard error of mean; TOPCARE-AMI, transplantation of progenitor cells and regeneration enhancement in acute myocardial infarction; MSC, mesenchymal stem cell.

passive effect of fibroblasts and other cells on compliance. Surprisingly, there was no functional difference between animals treated with skeletal muscle-derived cells and animals treated with BM stromal cells (30). However, this likely reflects the demonstrated differentiation of stromal cells into muscle-like cells within the infarct (22). More surprising is the similar outcome in animals treated with myoblasts or with AC133+ stem cells (31) where no muscle differentiation was demonstrated. This directly suggests that muscle formation is not the only factor contributing to the positive outcome, and illustrates our lack of understanding of the underlying mechanism(s) of cell-mediated repair. Of particular interest is the finding that a combined transplantation of BM-MNC with skeletal myoblasts increased the efficacy of each, suggesting a potential synergistic effect between the two cell types (29).

Developing the best cell(s) for cardiac repair is a dynamic process and one that clearly could vary with the injury. Looking back at bone fracture as an example of effective cell-based repair, the requirements for effective repair include *Perfusion* to allow cell survival, engraftment, and differentiation; *Fixation* to allow cells to stabilize the scar; and *Reduction* to minimize mechanical stress. In toto, the local milieu has to support the capacity of the implanted cell type. For example, in poorly perfused myocardium, myoblasts and undifferentiated BM cells survive where transplanted cardiomyocytes perish (32). Yet without optimal energy and in the absence of appropriate differentiation cues from surrounding myocardium, progenitor cells are not likely to differentiate down a contractile lineage. Thus, to optimize cardiomyocyte survival or to maximize cardiocyte cell differentiation, revascularization would likely be required. In fact, clinical evidence of this need could be inferred from the differing outcomes of clinical studies by Menasche et al. (33) versus those of Gavira et al. (34), where a minimal improvement in left ventricular ejection fraction (LVEF) was seen by Menasche after the administration of skeletal myoblasts as an adjunct to CABG in the *nonrevascularized* region of myocardium, whereas Gavira et al. showed significantly greater improvement when the same cells were delivered in the region revascularized by CABG. If these data are substantiated, revascularization either via angiogenic stem cell administration or traditional approaches could become an important aspect of cellular cardiomyoplasty for patients with ischemic heart disease. This type of multidisciplinary approach, based on a mechanistic understanding of cell behavior, will likely increase in importance.

Other mechanistic approaches to cell therapy can also be envisioned. For example, a characteristic of compensated cardiac hypertrophy is the reduction of mechanical stress—a clear call for cells that are able to stabilize scar. Mesenchymal BM cells, fibroblasts, and skeletal myoblasts (all mesoderm-derived progenitors) improve diastolic function and reduce wall stress (30). The BN-MNC, peripheral blood endothelial progenitor cells (EPCs), and umbilical cord blood (UCB) cells

have not demonstrated this potential to date. Thus, a mesenchymal-derived cell choice may be optimal in the setting of hypertrophy. However, early in the injury process, prior to significant remodeling, the choice of cell types may be broader. Many cell types appear capable of preventing LV dilatation to a certain extent; however, once severe dilatation has occurred, reduction or reverse remodeling (i.e., moving from a decompensated to a compensated state) may be difficult to achieve.

Optimal delivery varies with time after injury and cell type

Cell delivery is an important consideration of any study both from a safety and an efficacy perspective. Given a presumed need for cells to reach the site of injury to mediate repair, many early studies relied on precise surgical delivery of cells to allow direct visualization of the injured region (8). However, even early in the era of cell transplantation, attempts were made to deliver cells percutaneously—albeit with positive and negative results (35). More recently, percutaneous delivery has been applied more successfully either to deliver cells endoventricularly (12) or directly into the coronary arterial or venous circulation. Most recently, intravenous delivery has been utilized to deliver cells clinically (36). Although the ease of use is a major consideration, a larger issue is accurate, safe cell delivery to the necessary site(s) for repair. Unfortunately, science is not yet advanced to the point that we know the critical targets for repair. Yet, it stands to reason that local cardiac cell delivery is important; however, it is equally possible that nonlocal effects stimulate endogenous processes that culminate in repair. Conversely, it is possible that systemic delivery could generate a beneficial effect or it could simply increase the potential for adverse outcomes. And again, this may depend on cell type. Because it is the most well-studied cell and has been delivered via multiple routes, we will first discuss myoblast delivery followed by the BM data.

To date, the safety and feasibility of myoblast and BM cell therapy has been evaluated in a number of clinical studies with cells delivered either surgically as an adjunct to CABG or percutaneously as an adjunct to reperfusion or as a stand-alone treatment (Tables 2 and 3). Percutaneous delivery has been either endoventricular or intracoronary. Most recently, intravenous cell delivery has begun clinically. The first clinical trial using cell therapy to treat heart disease was initiated by Philippe Menasche et al. in 2000 (8). In this trial, an average of 870×10^6 autologous skeletal myoblasts were injected into nonrevascularizable, scarred LV as an adjunct to CABG. Over several years following transplantation, significant improvements in LV function were seen, including improved ejection fraction (EF) and regional wall thickening. The initial outcome was encouraging; however, no control group was included in the study and each patient received adjunctive revascularization at the time of cell transplantation. Four of 10 patients experienced ventricular tachycardia requiring Automatic Implantable Cardio-Defibrillator (AICD) implantation. Fortunately, none of the patients experienced fatal arrhythmia, and it is beginning to appear that appropriate prophylaxis can minimize electrical events (8). As a follow up, the Myoblast Autologous Graft in Ischemic Cardiomyopathy (MAGIC) trial has been initiated in 2003 as a phase 2 randomized clinical trial to examine CABG + myoblasts versus CABG alone in up to 300 patients in North America and Europe. As the field continued to progress after its inception and the number of CABG procedures decreased (in part owing to the use of drug-eluting stents), the MAGIC trial was halted in 2006. No safety reason was cited.

In a separate U.S. trial, where myoblasts were surgically injected concurrently with CABG ($n = 12$) or LVAD as a bridge to heart transplant ($n = 6$), patients showed improved myocardial perfusion and EF. Further, four of the five patients who underwent heart transplant showed areas of engrafted myoblasts within infarcted myocardium (37). In another late stage trial, skeletal myoblasts were injected as sole therapy (no CABG) in patients who were in symptomatic HF via a NOGA-guided catheter system (38). These patients showed improved wall motion and a trend toward increased EF over three to six months. Taken together, these data suggest that myoblasts can be delivered late in the disease process; can implant and survive within the infarcted myocardium; and improve both diastolic and systolic function.

One major drawback with surgical cell delivery is the invasiveness of the delivery process. The need for thoracotomy or sternotomy limits the potential patient population—in that patients with greatly reduced LV function will not easily tolerate this procedure.

Although surgical delivery allows a high cell volume to be administered and allows the surgeon to take steps to prevent regurgitation of the injected cell suspension, it is not appropriate for patients who do not require a sternotomy for either vascular bypass or assist device placement. Less invasive or nonsurgical approaches have thus been developed. These include thoracoscopic injection (39), ultrasound-guided coronary sinus injection (40), and endoventricular injection (12,41–43). Percutaneous catheter-based intracoronary delivery of BM cells has been safely reported in humans (11), and is supported by the evidence of cellular engraftment when employed in a rat model (44). However, with larger cells, such as mesenchymal cells, the risk of cellular embolization exists (45). Finally, the possibility of intravenous injection exists, for which success has been reported in rat models (46). However, in the chronic HF patient, the homing signal to the myocardial scar is very low and engraftment may therefore be too low to be of clinical benefit. In fact, early evidence suggests that after intravenous delivery, the majority of cells are extracted in the lung or spleen (47,48). The ideal delivery method, again, as the ideal cell type, may depend on

the clinical situation and the applied cell type. In the acute setting of a myocardial infarction when the homing signal to the scar is strong, the intravascular application of the stem cells should succeed. In the chronic setting of a remodeled, failing heart, targeted direct injection, either under direct or indirect vision or from the endoventricular approach, may be the optimal delivery route.

Expect the unexpected in new fields: unanticipated outcomes

Each cell type used to date has been associated with both positive and negative outcomes, and although several generic cell delivery issues have arisen, the majority of cell-safety issues appear to be cell-type specific. The generic issues primarily revolve around cell size and route of administration. For example, with large cells, such as BM stromal cells, skeletal myoblasts and fibroblasts, intravascular delivery poses specific problems not seen with smaller BM or peripheral blood hematopoietic fractions. After intravenous delivery of mesenchymal stem cells (MSCs), a large percentage of the cells are reported in the pulmonary bed followed by the liver, spleen, and kidney. Only a small proportion of the cells localize to the myocardium (49). Even more problematic, after intra-arterial delivery in normal canine heart, mesenchymal cells have been shown to result in micro-infarcts within the vascular bed downstream the injection site (45). Likewise, when myoblasts are injected into the coronary circulation, during the infusion period, transient ischemic episodes are evident via ST elevation, and only a small percentage of the cells are found in the myocardium several weeks later (35).

Specific safety issues have been reported for myoblasts (electrical instability), for mesenchymal stem cells (restenosis and microinfarction), and for granulocyte-colony stimulating factor (G-CSF)-mobilized BM progenitors [restenosis and major adverse cardiac events (MACE)].

A serious deleterious outcome associated to date primarily with myoblasts (and with thawed BM in chemotherapy patients) (50) is the incidence of cardiac electrical instability for a presumed transient period after cell delivery. These early reports of electrical instability in patients after the receipt of autologous skeletal myoblasts have led to doubts about the safety of these cells as a treatment in the injured heart. Patients who received myoblasts in the earliest clinical studies (33,38) were extremely ill patients with an expected high potential for negative electrical events. In fact, many of the patients who were included in the early trials met the Multicenter Automatic Defibrillator Implantation Trial MADIT-II criteria, which were presented after those trials began, and suggested that all patients who met those criteria be treated with AICDs. As a result, in more recent clinical studies, many investigators have only enrolled patients who receive AICDs

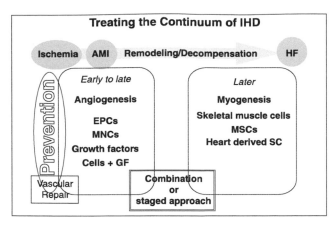

Figure 1

Treating the continuum of CVD from its acute onset to end-stage heart failure is likely to require different cell types at different stages of the disease. Early in the process, pro-angiogenic cells (e.g., bone marrow, peripheral blood or UCB-derived mononuclear cells or EPCs) or growth factors (that recruit these cells) may suffice. In later stages of CVD replacing underlying muscle is an additional consideration and pro-myogenic cells (e.g., skeletal muscle cells, mesenchymal cells and/or cardiac derived PCs) will likely be required. *Abbreviations*: CVD, cardiovascular disease; EPC, endothelial progenitor cell; MNC, mononuclear cell; MSC, mesenchymal stem cell; UCB, umbilical cord blood.

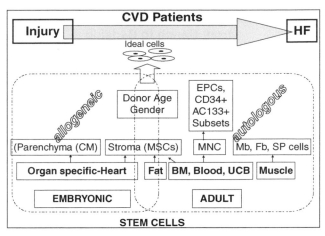

Figure 2

Choices involved in stem cell therapy. Choosing the right cell for the right patient at the right time in their disease process may be one of the most important decisions a clinician faces in this field. Embryonic cells although potentially very useful in the future, are not yet a clinical option in CVD. Thus adult derived cells are the only option at present. Adult cells can be either autologous or allogeneic. Autologous cells are generally thought to be safe, easy to isolate and administer, and decrease the need for immunosuppression, but are not an off-the-shelf choice. They require time needed for isolation and/or possible expansion of cells, and may be impacted by the age, disease state, and possibly even the gender of the patient. BMC, EPCs, and SKMB are the current autologous choices although others are in preclinical development. Allogeneic cells, although potentially immunogenic, offer an off the shelf potential. MSCs are the only allogeneic cell source currently in clinical evaluation. Fat, heart, and other tissues will likely pose future both autologous and allogeneic sources. *Abbreviations*: BM, bone marrow; CM, cardiomyocyte; CVD, cardiovascular disease; HF, heart failure; MNC, mononuclear cell; MSC, mesenchymal stem cell; UCB, umbilical cord blood.

or low-dose anti-arrhythmic agents prophylactically. This has reduced the reported incidence of adverse events significantly. In the MAGIC trial, as reported at the American Heart Association meeting in November 2004, the incidence of electrical instability in patients postmyoblast delivery was 10% lower than the initial 40% reported by the same group. Whether this is the result of a better selection of patients in the second study; the coadministration of anti-arrhythmic agents; or an improved safety profile of the cells, remains to be determined. Furthermore, Dib et al. have not reported an increased incidence of electrical instability after myoblast administration, nor have Chachques et al. in preclinical studies (51). Randomized controlled trials underway at present are the only way to address safety concerns and prove efficacy. Their results should be eagerly anticipated.

In contrast to that of myoblasts and mesenchymal cells, BM mononuclear or EPC delivery is primarily intracoronary (9). Presumably owing to the much smaller size of these angiogenic cells, their delivery has not been associated with significant adverse ischemic events. However, BM cell delivery has been associated with the theoretical potential for angiogenesis at unwanted sites, such as in occult tumors or retina. This unanticipated and potentially serious consequence illustrates our need to learn from our previous gene therapy colleagues and to expect the unexpected in this field.

Even when cells work: the mechanism is ill-defined

A myriad of preclinical and first-in-man clinical studies suggest that cell therapy has a positive effect on cardiac and vascular repair. In fact, in most studies, the tested cell types were found to be effective, even in the absence of the evidence of robust cell engraftment. This unexpected outcome defines how little we actually understand at present about the underlying mechanism(s) of cell-mediated repair. We attribute much repair to direct participation of the transplanted cells in angiogenesis or myogenesis, but in truth, despite promising clinical outcomes, relatively little clinical data exist to support this contention.

In fact, treating the continuum of CVD is likely to require different cell types at different stages of the disease. In situations where early ischemic injury occurs, treatment with pro-angiogenic cells (or growth factors to recruit proangiogenic cells) is likely to suffice. At present, the most commonly

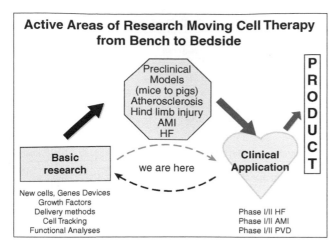

Figure 3

Moving cardiac repair from bench to bedside: what is next? Moving cell therapy from idea to product is an iterative process that requires the movement from bench to bedside and back again, requiring ongoing discussions between scientists and clinicians. The first clinical data have sent scientists and clinicians back to the bench to improve methods for isolation, storage, delivery, survival, tracking, and monitoring of cells and their clinical impact. A strong preclinical/clinical interaction is critical to minimize the time required and maximize the likelihood of success as novel techniques move forward.

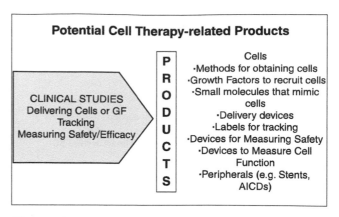

Figure 4

Cell therapy products are creating a new business model. Cell therapy is no longer simply a cell product. As the need for the tools to deliver, track, and monitor cells develops, new businesses are emerging around "systems for cardiac repair." No longer would the product be simply cells, instead it would likely become a method to isolate and deliver those cells, or a tool to track them, or a peripheral agent used to keep them alive or measure their effect. As a result, cell therapy is being practiced by groups ranging from individual hospitals to large multinational drug and device companies.

used pro-angiogenic cells are either those comprising the entire bone marrow mononuclear fraction (BMCs) or the endothelial progenitor cell (EPC) subset from BM or peripheral blood. In the future UCB is also likely to be a source of these cells. Both MNCs and EPCs are in clinical study in early disease stages (refractory angina to AMI). As CVD progresses, the need to replace underlying muscle arises. In this situation, pro-myogenic (muscle-forming) cells will likely be required. The first candidate in this class is commonly referred to as myoblasts but in actually is a mixture of skeletal muscle-derived progenitor cells, which have been in clinical study since 2000. More recently (in 2006), marrow-derived mesenchymal or stromal cells have begun to be used for myogenic repair. Furthermore, as the potential of cardiac-derived stem and progenitor cells continues to arise, these cells will likely form a ripe target for future investigation. Angiogenesis and myogenesis remain the two main targets of repair. However, preclinical and clinical data suggest that cell engraftment is not always directly related to outcome; thus, other underlying noncell-autonomous factors are being collectively called "paracrine" factors and being considered as future therapeutic targets. Although it is not yet clear what these factors are, small molecules that prevent apoptosis or promote cell survival (e.g., Akt-1, Bcl-1), growth factors that mobilize or recruit endogenous stem cells (e.g., G-CSF, SDF-1), and molecules that alter the inflammatory milieu will

all likely become increasingly important targets for therapeutic tools in the next few years. Meanwhile, the next-generation cell products are likely to include combinations of cells either given together or in staged approaches—as we realize that vascular supply without a functioning target, or muscle cells without blood supply are not likely to be capable of maximal functional contribution. Other newer cell products are expected to include combined cell and gene therapies to capitalize on the best of both. However, an ultimate next-generation target for cardiac repair will be the prevention or reversal of CVD by administering cells capable of vascular repair. Our group at the University of Minnesota (UMN) is currently evaluating this next generation scenario with promising results.

The advantage of this early promise is that the field is growing and more questions would be answered. An increasing understanding of cell differentiation and the process of endogenous cell-mediated repair will help us to better understand exogenous cell therapy. Direct cell-to-cell interaction (52), fusion of progenitor cells with cardiomyocytes (53), transdifferentiation of progenitor cells (54), and dedifferentiation of cardiomyocytes (55), are all discussed as potential mediators of the observed outcomes. Although clinical interest lies in developing effective and safe therapeutic tools, to develop, optimize, and tailor cell-based cardiovascular repair, we must better understand its mechanism(s) of action.

Cell therapy for prevention

Treating atherosclerosis to prevent ischemic heart disease

Ischemic heart disease (IHD) starts as a vascular disease. The ultimate goal of vascular repair is the prevention of end-organ damage by the restoration of vessel patency and/or regeneration of functional vasculature. Recent data suggest that atherosclerosis may be in part a result of a decreased endogenous repair potential and a decrease in progenitor cell numbers (24,56). Repeated intravenous injection of BM from young apoprotein E (ApoE)−/− mice prevented further progression of atherosclerotic lesions in old ApoE null mice. Injected cells differentiated into endothelial cells and engrafted in atherosclerotic lesions of recipient animals. Comparison of BM stem cell profiles showed a specific depletion of intermediate vascular progenitor cells (CD31+/CD45+), without parallel changes in more primitive stem cells (sca-1+,c-kit +, or CD34+) or mature vascular cells (VEGFR-2+), which most likely accounted for the age-related loss of BM-derived vascular repair capacity. Preliminary data suggesting that atherosclerotic changes are to some extent reversible, give hope that cell-mediated vascular repair may be an achievable goal in the prevention of IHD. A recent data analysis modeled the potential health effects of BM-derived EPC therapy using data from the 1950–1996 follow-up of the Framingham Heart Study. To model CVD mortality, progenitor cell therapy was applied at age 30, with the effect assumed to be a 10-year delay in atherosclerosis progression. This study suggests that progenitor cell therapy might increase life expectancy in the population as much as the complete elimination of cancer (in females, an additional 3.67 vs. 3.37 years; in males, an additional 5.94 vs. 2.86 years, respectively) (57).

When prevention fails: treating the vascular portion of ischemic heart disease

Although preventing IHD is the ultimate goal and thus the focus of early preclinical studies to treat vascular disease (24), treating the downstream consequences of IHD is more common at present. As stated earlier, one major premise of cell-based repair is the (re-)establishment of sufficient perfusion of the injury site. Vascular repair, or at a minimum, neovascularization of infarcted cardiac tissue must be achieved before contractility can be restored. Multiple nonmyogenic BM-derived cells have shown a high angiogenic potential. The BM-MNC (10), endothelial or vascular progenitor cells (24) from BM or blood (9), marrow angioblasts, (25) or blood-derived multi-potent adult progenitor cells

(26), may be applied to increase vascular density and tissue perfusion.

After promising results in experimental models of myocardial ischemia (58,59), multiple clinical trials were initiated. As in 2005, data from six clinical trials applying BM or peripheral blood-derived stem cells in patients with chronic HF and seven trials in patients with AMI were published (Tables 2 and 3). Stamm et al. injected 1.5×10^6 AC133 + BM stem cells into the infarct borderzone of patients, who underwent concurrent CABG. However, in contrast to myoblast studies, this study examined patients treated shortly after AMI. A total of 12 patients were treated, and they showed increased perfusion in treated areas and improved LV dimensions and EF compared with the controls (10,60). Further, unlike patients in myoblast trials, the improvements in this trial occurred without any incidence of electrical abnormalities. Whether this represents a difference in patient population, cell type, or even cell dose, remains unknown.

In a more preventive approach, a number of studies have been performed in an attempt to rescue myocardium and to prevent the development of HF (Table 3). These studies have primarily focused on percutaneous delivery of BM-derived stem cells after AMI. In the Transplantation of Progenitor Cells and Regeneration Enhancement in Acute Myocardial Infarction (TOPCARE-AMI) study, investigators injected $16 \pm 12 \times 10^6$ circulating progenitor cells (CPCs) or $213 \pm 75 \times 10^6$ bone marrow progenitor cells (BMCs) into the infarct artery of patients 4.9 ± 1.5 days after AMI. At four months post-therapy, LV end-diastolic volumes and EF improved in both cell groups compared with control patients who underwent standard treatment at the hospital during the same time but were not randomized into the TOPCARE study. No significant difference between CPC and BM groups was observed. By one year, EF was still significantly improved, infarct size was decreased, and there was no evidence of reactive hypertrophy. These results suggest favorable remodeling in response to cell therapy (61). Interestingly, similar results were seen between the cell-treated groups, despite the fact that a magnitude of more BMCs were injected than the CPCs. These data, when combined with the data by Stamm et al. earlier, suggest very favorable response to BM-derived stem cell therapy following AMI, with improved myocardial performance secondary to improved cardiac perfusion. These encouraging data also have provided the impetus for the initiation of randomized controlled trials using EPCs for the treatment of ST-segment elevation myocardial infarction (STEMI).

Although the data for the treatment of AMI are encouraging, what remains unclear is the response of late-stage cardiac injuries to BM stem cell therapy. To begin to address this, the TOPCARE-HF study, has been initiated. Given, the reduced number and migratory capacity of EPCs shown in preclinical studies (56) and the deficits in EPC number seen clinically in patients with severe coronary artery disease (CAD), it would be interesting to see if the cells from these patients are capable of improving the cardiac function.

In a randomized trial entitled BOne marrOw transfer to enhance ST-elevation infarct regeneration (BOOST trial) investigators compared 30 patients receiving optimal standard care following infarction to 30 patients receiving optimal standard care plus $24.6 \times 10^8 \pm 9.4 \times 10^8$ (mean $\pm$ SD) BMCs 4.8 ± 1.8 days after infarct. Six months after therapy, patients receiving BMCs showed significantly enhanced LVEF when compared with control patients. Further, systolic function was improved without any incidence of arrhythmic events or restenosis of stents (62). In Belgium, a recent clinical controlled trial compared the ability of autologous BM-derived cells (average of 172×10^6 MNCs) to a placebo for the ability to improve function after AMI. In this study, therapy with BM-derived cells was able to reduce infarct size, but no improvement in LV function was seen when compared with placebo treatment. In fact, over four months, the LVEF of the placebo group tended to improve more than the patients receiving BMCs, though results were not statistically significant (63).

When the vascular problem is not myocardium: treating peripheral vascular disease

Peripheral vascular disease (PVD) is becoming the second focus of cell-based repair. Similar to the therapy of CAD, peripheral vascular repair is currently limited to balloon angioplasty and ultimately surgical revascularization. Experimental data suggests that circulating stem cells may reflect the endogenous repair potential of vascular lesions in systemic atherosclerosis and aging (24). The number or function of EPCs may be related to progression or stabilization of athero- sclerotic lesions and is currently being evaluated as a biomarker for peripheral and coronary vascular disease (23,64). In PVD, the therapeutic focus clearly lies on restoration of perfusion to minimize tissue damage and achieve symptomatic relief, whereas the regeneration of functional muscle is secondary. Different cell types and delivery methods are currently evaluated (65). Preliminary studies applying direct intramuscular injection of BM-MNC and mesenchymal stem cells show promising results in increasing microvascular density and tissue perfusion and lead to an early move to clinical studies in 2002 (66). The Therapeutic Angiogenesis by Cell Transplantation (TACT) study investigators performed a randomized controlled trial in patients with peripheral artery disease, and reported a significant increase in transcutaneous oxygen pressure, rest pain, and pain-free walking time in 22 patients with leg ischemia after intramuscular injection of BM-derived MNCs (67). In a concomitant study, BM-MNC transplantation was found to improve endothelial dysfunction by increasing endothelium-dependent vasodilation in patients with limb ischemia (68).

Again, different cell types and delivery routes may apply in different stages of disease as the spectrum of patients suffering from PVD is at least as heterogeneous as in coronary vascular disease. With an increasing understanding of a potential role of stem cells in vasculogenesis and endogenous repair, we may be able to move toward manipulating cell mobilization or activation rather than simply exogenously delivering cells. Although cell mobilization studies (e.g., administration of G-CSF) are beyond the scope of this review, they should provide an exciting future direction for "cell-free" cell therapy.

Hurdles and opportunities

What have we learned from over 10 years of preclinical and six years of clinical research in this area? With the progress made to date, the field appears very promising and offers more opportunities than hurdles. Cardiovascular repair, more than ever, seems to be a reachable goal. Several obstacles remain before we can declare unfettered success. Moving cell therapy from bench to bedside is complex. As new cell types emerge and old ones find new applications, it is important to design a preclinical path that predicts clinical outcome. It will also be important as the field moves forward to compare cells in side-by-side studies. Beginning to dissect the physiology by which transplanted cells mediate repair is crucial. And finally, if we are to ultimately regenerate heart, we must continue to think outside the box and view cells as only one tool in our armamentarium moving into the 21st century. Cells plus genes, small molecules that replace the need for cells, and personalized genomics-based cell therapy are all medicines of the future that are as approachable today as cell therapy was in 1998. Considering new options, maximizing our understanding of cell effects and standardizing our approaches should provide us the tools to succeed where endogenous repair fails.

Hurdle #1—lack of data

A major hurdle is still a lack of definitive data describing how and when the cells are capable of repair. This may sound paradox, considering the number of preclinical studies and clinical studies that have been published in the field (i.e., 1235 Pubmed hits on keyword search for "heart" and "cell transplantation"). However, more than ten different cell types have been proposed and delivered using more than five different techniques in more than six models of acute or chronic injury in more than eight different species. This alone allows a minimal potential number of 2400 possible combinations to be tested. For us to determine the best cell would demand side-by-side comparisons in a given disease.

Only a few side-by-side comparisons of different cell populations have been performed (Table 1) (27–31). We lack direct comparisons of different cell types in clearly defined clinically relevant models of disease. Further, we lack data that evaluate time as an additional factor in treatment, time in disease progression and time in the dynamics of transplanted cells. Overall, there is a lack of standardization in the current preclinical approach to cell therapy; for example, cell types, doses, preclinical models and endpoints all differ. This may also explain the discrepancy between preclinical and clinical results. Attempts to standardize these parameters and to decide on a consensus will move us forward.

Several examples of current limitations in study design can be illustrated. To date, most cell studies have been accompanied by an additional revascularization procedure, either by coronary stenting or bypass grafting, making any functional improvement owing to cellular therapy nearly impossible to distinguish from the current standard of care. Although this may improve the outcome as discussed earlier, it makes interpretation extremely difficult in the absence of appropriate control studies. To date, only three studies have investigated the use of BM-MNCs (by endoventricular delivery), without an additional revascularization procedure, all in the setting of intractable ischemia (12,41,42). The need to establish appropriate controls in a novel area where the standard of care is ever changing, is an active area of debate in the field.

Another major experimental obstacle to the study of cell engraftment and fate is the poor engraftment (<10%) seen when the cells are administered by intracoronary, intravenous, and intracardiac routes. This is likely attributed to multiple factors, the most obvious being poor vascular supply to central infarct zones. In those experimental models with revascularized infarcts or ischemia/reperfusion injuries, the presence of inflammation, apoptotic signaling, and immunologic barriers likely contribute to graft loss. After intracoronary delivery, cellular engraftment should be limited to those cells capable of traversing the endothelial basement membrane, a characteristic not seen with skeletal myoblasts. Efforts to overcome graft loss are underway with less traumatic cell-application techniques, coadministration of angiogenic growth factors or hemangioblasts (69), and cellular transfection with prosurvival or heat shock genes, or antiapoptotic agents (e.g., AKT) (70).

Hurdle #2—lack of mechanistic understanding

Looking at the results of both preclinical and clinical studies, we recognize the potential of cardiac cell transplantation to alter outcomes. However, we have to admit that in most cases, we do not understand how different cell types improve LV function. Increases in microvascular density, diastolic and systolic function, and an attenuated remodeling, are all reported after the application of many different cell types, but the exact mechanisms are unclear. Only a few studies address the electrophysiologic fate of the injected cells (71,72). In these studies, skeletal myoblasts were found to be isolated from the surrounding myocardium, and they underwent severe

changes in their expression of voltage-gated channels. These results suggest that different mechanisms, other than active contractile function, may play a role in the effect of these cells. Most of the preclinical studies use global LV function and morphometry as major endpoints; however, to quantify the contractile improvement induced by cell transplantation, regional wall motion (7) needs to be addressed. The importance of paracrine effects (73,74) is more and more appreciated as a possible mainstay of cell-based repair. In summary, cell survival is limited, phenotype is often unknown, and direct effects of cells are debatable; yet myocardial function improves. Dissecting this paradox will be our greatest challenge going forward. Accepting that completely different cell types may improve LV function via multiple mechanisms, and understanding if and how differences impact outcome should enable us to find potential synergies between different cell types (71), and to move to better products for the future.

Hurdle #3—lack of "out of the box thinking"

The most common preclinical evaluation of cell therapy involves simple injection of a single cell into injured myocardium and follow up over days to weeks. Yet, most preclinical models do not account for the myriad of inputs (injury, atherosclerosis, hypertension, etc.) that impact clinical outcome or the multiple medical treatments in place. Only a single study has been reported evaluating cell therapy in relation to a current medical treatment (20), and this study showed significant interactions. Cell therapy might be effective, but the expectation that it will become the only solution for CVD is just not realistic. Looking at the development of other therapies we can expect that if effective, cell therapy will find its position among or in combination with other therapeutic modalities. As such, we should now begin to "think out of the box" to design studies evaluating cell therapy in a clinically relevant context or in conjunction with other state-of-the-art treatment modalities. These types of studies have begun, as indicated by the reports of combined cell and gene therapy studies designed to increase angiogenesis (74), upregulate genes to improve electrical integration (75), or to induce the production of protective factors (76).

Hurdle #4—the "gold rush"

The "gold rush" in clinical trials has to stop, and prospective randomized clinical trials with a central data registry must be conducted. Only if current standards for clinical trials are met, will cell therapy be taken seriously by a large, and of course, skeptical community. Creating a consensus for preclinical and clinical data standards and conducting the studies would enable us to gain comparable data and to progress more rapidly toward the development of clinically valuable tools. Recently, European investigators took this step (77). Although debate still continues as to whether large clinical trials should ensue, a consensus is emerging that controlled trials *will* occur and thus *should* occur in a standardized fashion led by investigators with experience in the field. The generation of a large registry comparable with those in surgical societies would allow us to evaluate the safety and efficacy of cell therapy, minimizing the biases that are inherent (and sometimes inevitable) in current study designs and allowing the application of statistical tools on this larger scale. The future is bright. Not only are there hurdles, but many opportunities as well.

Opportunity #1—from repair to prevention

Reducing the incidence of CVD. For the first time, we can begin to treat the underlying injury in damaged myocardium offering new potential for repair rather than palliative treatment of the remaining "healthy" myocardium. This offers tremendous opportunity to decrease the impact of HF worldwide. As we move forward, we also have the opportunity to treat vascular injury. Doing so could have profound effects on the incidence of and its downstream consequences globally. The final frontier for cell therapy is the prevention of cardiac disease (24,78). Our group has documented in animal studies that atherosclerosis can be slowed or decreased by the intravenous administration of BMCs (24). More recently, we have shown that gender is an important factor in this prevention and treatment. We found that, as in humans, there is a delayed onset of atherosclerotic disease in female ApoE null mice versus males and that a change in the stem cell population in the BM may account for this. We also found that female cells appear to be more potent in treating and preventing atherosclerosis than male cells. Expanding this understanding to the clinic could have profound implications for patients with CAD and PVD.

Opportunity #2—dissecting repair with state-of-the-art tools

Bringing molecular approaches to bear on cardiac cell therapy should allow us to better understand when and how cells contribute to the vague process we now call "repair" and thus allow us to design more specific approaches to intervene in the steps involved. The identification of signaling pathways involved in cardiomyocyte differentiation (79) and repair could allow us to predifferentiate cells to a designated atrial, ventricular, or pacemaker phenotype, or even to design small molecules to enhance specific endogenous progenitor cell proliferation and differentiation capacities within the damaged myocardium. Similarly, understanding the role of progenitor cells in vasculogenesis and nascent vessel formation could provide insights into the targets for the repair of ischemic or hibernating myocardium. Beginning to quantify global changes in gene expression that lead to the detrimental pathway(s) of remodeling and dilation (80) may also provide novel tools and potential molecular targets for therapeutic intervention. Finally, by approaching cardiac repair as a process parallel to cardiac development, and understanding myocardium at its richest capacity for repair (during early fetal development), we may ultimately be able to create systems in which cardiac repair is the norm rather than the exception.

Opportunity #3—multicenter trials

Progress in early clinical trials should prompt large-scale multicenter trials; however, these trials should rely heavily on the expertise of centers with successful phase I trials. As we learn that each step of the process is important—cell type, cell delivery, cell dose, cell functional capacity prior to injection, and perhaps even gender of the donor—it becomes imperative that we consider each of these parameters in designing new studies. To do so will be challenging—cell-based cardiac repair may not be a stand-alone treatment or may have synergistic effects with existing therapies. We have to be able to distinguish the effects of cell therapy from the current state-of-the-art treatment, a goal that is both ethically and scientifically demanding and may require large patient cohorts. Standardized patient populations, cell types, delivery methods, and endpoints developed and analyzed in core laboratories should allow the creation of central data registries to maximize the knowledge we gain and minimize patient risk and trial costs.

Opportunity #4—more cell types

The human heart is a complex organ comprised of myocardium, vasculature, and matrix electromechanically integrated to yield an efficient pump. When cell-based cardiac repair was initially proposed, skeletal myoblasts were the only myogenic progenitor cells that had been identified, isolated, and expanded in vitro. Since then, multiple populations of stem and progenitor cells have been described with different angio- and myogenic potential. The most popular at present are autologous, adult-derived progenitor cells derived from BM, blood, fat, muscle, or even adult myocardium. The ideal cell for myocardial repair should be able to withstand the harsh scar environment at the time of implantation but become a fully functioning cardiomyocyte or vascular cell over time. No progenitor cell currently used satisfies these criteria sufficiently. Therefore, it is important to keep evaluating novel cells with cardiomyocyte and vascular differentiation potential(s). The most promising new source of cells may be adult heart, from which multipotent cells have been derived. However, access and their scarcity may limit this option. Alternatively, UCB may provide a multipotent population of progenitors that could serve the same purpose. Finally, embryonic stem cells may become the source most likely to meet the demands of regenerating new heart. Yet, as we consider repair, it will be important to remember the need for electromechanical integration. Several proposed cell types have significantly different electrical properties than cardiomyocytes. These differences can lead to electrical abnormalities, including ventricular tachycardia. For cardiovascular cell therapy to reach its potential, it will be critical to electrically integrate transplanted cells into the surviving myocardium. This problem may be approached by genetically altering transplanted cells, by developing new adjunctive safety measures or preferably, by conditioning the transplanted cells to become true cardiomyocytes that can survive in an injury milieu. An ultimate goal may be to initiate a pathway of cardiocyte differentiation prior to implantation that would occur slowly enough to allow concomitant neovascularization to occur to provide nutrients for the emerging nascent myocardium.

Whatever cell type we choose, as repair drives our studies, it will likely open unexpected doors for discovery. We have already learned that cells themselves may not be required for cardiac repair. Investigators recently showed that postinfarction recovery in animals could be mimicked by media in which stem cells were grown (81). Thus, five years from now, we may be focused on small molecules, proteins, and peptides in addition to cells. Even so, cell therapy will likely survive. As much like gene therapy, the use of peptides or proteins would mean either choosing the "right" molecule or giving a cocktail of molecules, neither of which may be as effective as giving the ultimate protein cocktail, a living cell.

Cardiac regeneration: beyond the final frontier

Finally, in considering injured heart, the ultimate goal is to move beyond repair to regeneration. But, is it realistic to claim that a single cell type or even a combination of cell types will be capable of myocardial regeneration where endogenous repair has failed? The word "regeneration" expresses the true complexity of this goal; we would literally have to regenerate contractile cardiac muscle, mature, patent vascu-

lature, and integrated electrical conductance in a fibrous, dilated, and under-perfused scar. This is an enormous task which is currently not possible and will not likely occur in the near future. However, as we better understand the capacity of stem cells to generate each of these, we can begin to envision the future: a capacity to rebuild/replace dead, dying or missing cardiac tissues.

Conclusion

In summary, the future is bright, the potential is great, and the treatment options are increasing. However, even as the field progresses, we have a responsibility to promise patients (and the press) only what we can deliver, that is, to tell the truth about cardiac repair. At present, it is not a panacea. Functional improvements are modest and even then the best results are not yet validated in randomized controlled trials. Cell therapy is however a new alternative that warrants much further exploration.

This is an exciting time in the field of treating CVD. Cell transplantation opened a new frontier in cardiovascular medicine, providing physicians with techniques and treatment alternatives for a large patient population that extends beyond revascularization and metabolic control to reverse damage, which in many cases, has already been done. The concept of repairing or regenerating ischemic cardiac tissue is a fantastic possibility, and although many question its validity, it may eventually become a reality if we choose the right conditions and cell type. Although some researchers consider human trials premature at this point, cellular cardiomyoplasty with both BM and skeletal myoblasts has shown clinical benefit. Owing to the small study sizes and an inability at this point to standardize therapy, we are limited in our power to determine the best cell type, dose, and administration technique. However, the relevance of this therapy is evident to both clinicians and researchers alike. Both animal studies and clinical trials thus far have evoked both the scientific interest and promising results to warrant large-scale controlled clinical trials to determine the best and safest application of this technology, and to gain a better understanding of its mechanism(s).

To bring this field forward, we now have to come together and outline a plan for future studies. The diversity of cell types, application techniques, and disease stages can be a hurdle and an opportunity—only collaboration will allow us to move forward as a field instead of expanding information that cannot be combined or compared. We have the opportunity to create a new era in the treatment of CVD. Doing so would require continued bench to bedside and back to bench evaluations, as we learn from early clinical studies; find a consensus on preclinical models; and the design of clinical trials to maximize the potential of a 21st-century approach to repairing the injured heart.

Summary

Ten years ago, gene therapy was the promised panacea; approximately five years ago, clinical cell therapy broke into the headlines; and today, in 2006, cardiac repair is a possibility discussed with increasing frequency both scientifically and clinically. This enthusiasm reflects the idea that unlike gene therapy or its predecessors, cardiovascular cell therapy offers the first real potential to treat the underlying injuries associated with cardiac and vascular disease. By delivering appropriate reparative cells to an injury site, the potential exists to mitigate injury or even to begin to reverse damage. Based on their inordinate preclinical promise as myogenic or angiogenic precursors, skeletal muscle-, BM-, blood-, fat-, and even heart-derived progenitor cells have moved rapidly from bench toward early clinical studies. From their parallel paths, we are learning a number of useful lessons and have begun to visualize the hurdles to be overcome as we move these therapies forward.

It is now obvious that cell-based repair is feasible—both early and later in the CVD continuum. In fact, cell therapy may offer an unparalleled opportunity for cardiac and vascular functional improvement to millions living with CVD. Yet, many questions about the technology remain unanswered. Whether the best cell type, delivery method, or route of administration exists is unclear. The mechanisms associated with cardiovascular repair remain unknown, and, whether cell-based disease prevention is feasible is still unanswerable.

Now, five years into clinical investigation, but still early in the growth of the field, is the time to critically address the questions that have emerged even as we cautiously proceed clinically. Only by understanding our successes and failures will we be able to decrease unwanted clinical effects and fulfill the promise of the most exciting opportunity yet to treat CVD. This requires critical analysis of the early clinical data, call for increasing rigor in planning and completion of trials, modification of our assumptions as necessary, and until we understand cell therapy's potential, limit our promises to patients (and the press). Only by addressing unanswered questions, carefully limiting our promises, and rigorously performing iterative and innovative preclinical and clinical studies can we provide the surest opportunity for safely moving the field forward. In this chapter, we have defined gaps in our knowledge, described both hurdles and opportunities for success, posed questions that we believe can help shape the field, and finally have speculated on the new horizons in the field of cardiovascular repair.

Acknowledgments

This work was supported in part by NHLBI/National Institutes of Health awards to Dr. Taylor (R-01 HL-63346, HL-63703).

References

1 Miller LW, Missov ED. Epidemiology of heart failure. Cardiol Clin 2001; 19:547–555.

2 World Health Report. In: www.who.int/whr/en/, 2003.

3 Cohn JN, Francis GS. Cardiac failure: a revised paradigm. J Card Fail 1995; 1:261–266.

4 Moss AJ, Zareba W, Hall WJ, et al. Prophylactic implantation of a defibrillator in patients with myocardial infarction and reduced ejection fraction. N Engl J Med 2002; 346:877–883.

5 Moss AJ, Hall WJ, Cannom DS, et al. Improved survival with an implanted defibrillator in patients with coronary disease at high risk for ventricular arrhythmia. Multicenter Automatic Defibrillator Implantation Trial Investigators. N Engl J Med 1996; 335:1933–1940.

6 Chiu RC, Zibaitis A, Kao RL. Cellular cardiomyoplasty: myocardial regeneration with satellite cell implantation. Ann Thorac Surg 1995; 60:12–18.

7 Taylor DA, Atkins BZ, Hungspreugs P, et al. Regenerating functional myocardium: improved performance after skeletal myoblast transplantation. Nat Med 1998; 4:929–933.

8 Menasche P, Hagege AA, Scorsin M, et al. Myoblast transplantation for heart failure. Lancet 2001; 357:279–280.

9 Assmus B, Schachinger V, Teupe C, et al. Transplantation of Progenitor Cells and Regeneration Enhancement in Acute Myocardial Infarction (TOPCARE-AMI). Circulation 2002;106:3009–3017.

10 Stamm C, Westphal B, Kleine HD, et al. Autologous bone-marrow stem-cell transplantation for myocardial regeneration. Lancet 2003; 361:45–46.

11 Strauer BE, Brehm M, Zeus T, et al. Repair of infarcted myocardium by autologous intracoronary mononuclear bone marrow cell transplantation in humans. Circulation 2002; 106:1913–1918.

12 Perin EC, Dohmann HF, Borojevic R, et al. Transendocardial, autologous bone marrow cell transplantation for severe, chronic ischemic heart failure. Circulation 2003; 107:2294–2302.

13 Schachinger VES, Elsasser A, Haberbosch W, et al. Intracoronary infusion of bone marrow-derived progenitor cells in acute myocardial infarction: a randomized, double-blind, placebo-controlled muticenter trial (REPAIR-AMI). In: Scientific Sessions of the American Heart Association 2005. Internet communication, 2005.

14 Lunde KSS, Aakhus S, Arnesen H, Forfang K. Intracoronary injections of autologous mononuclear bone marrow cells in acute anterior wall myocardial infarction: the ASTAMI randomized controlled trial. In: Scientific Sessions of the American Heart Association 2005. Internet communication, 2006.

15 Ott HC, Brechtken J, Swingen C, et al. Robotic minimally invasive cell transplantation for heart failure. J Thorac Cardiothorac Surg 2006; 132:170–173.

16 van den Bos EJ, Wagner A, Mahrholdt H, et al. Improved efficacy of stem cell labeling for magnetic resonance imaging studies by the use of cationic liposomes. Cell Transpl 2003; 12:743–756.

17 Dimmeler S, Vasa-Nicotera M. Aging of progenitor cells: limitation for regenerative capacity? J Am Coll Cardiol 2003; 42:2081–2082.

18 Stuck WG, O'Donoghue DH, Rountree CR, et al. Progress in orthopedic surgery for 1946, fractures. Arch Surg 1949; 59(5):1139–1190.

19 Bonaros N, Yang S, Ott H, Kocher A. Cell therapy for ischemic heart disease. Panminerva Med 2004; 46:13–23.

20 Pouzet B, Ghostine S, Vilquin JT, et al. Is skeletal myoblast transplantation clinically relevant in the era of angiotensin-converting enzyme inhibitors? Circulation 2001; 104:1223–1228.

21 Wollert KC, Drexler H. Clinical applications of stem cells for the heart. Circ Res 2005; 96:151–163.

22 Hill JM, Zalos G, Halcox JP, et al. Circulating endothelial progenitor cells, vascular function, and cardiovascular risk. N Engl J Med 2003; 348:593–600.

23 Werner N, Kosiol S, Schiegl T, et al. Circulating endothelial progenitor cells and cardiovascular outcomes. N Engl J Med 2005; 353:999–1007.

24 Rauscher FM, Goldschmidt-Clermont PJ, Davis BH, et al. Aging, progenitor cell exhaustion, and atherosclerosis. Circulation 2003; 108:457–463.

25 Itescu S, Kocher AA, Schuster MD. Myocardial neovascularization by adult bone marrow-derived angioblasts: strategies for improvement of cardiomyocyte function. Heart Fail Rev 2003; 8:253–258.

26 Jiang Y, Jahagirdar BN, Reinhardt RL, et al. Pluripotency of mesenchymal stem cells derived from adult marrow. Nature 2002; 418:41–49.

27 Hutcheson KA, Atkins BZ, Hueman MT, Hopkins MB, Glower DD, Taylor DA. Comparison of benefits on myocardial performance of cellular cardiomyoplasty with skeletal myoblasts and fibroblasts. Cell Transpl 2000; 9:359–368.

28 Horackova M, Arora R, Chen R, et al. Cell transplantation for treatment of acute myocardial infarction: unique capacity for repair by skeletal muscle satellite cells. Am J Physiol Heart Circ Physiol 2004; 287:H1599–H1608.

29 Ott HC, Bonaros N, Marksteiner R, et al. Combined transplantation of skeletal myoblasts and bone marrow stem cells for myocardial repair in rats. Eur J Cardiothorac Surg 2004; 25:627–634.

30 Thompson RB, Emani SM, Davis BH, et al. Comparison of intracardiac cell transplantation: autologous skeletal myoblasts versus bone marrow cells. Circulation 2003; 108(suppl 1):II264–II271.

31 Agbulut O, Vandervelde S, Al Attar N, et al. Comparison of human skeletal myoblasts and bone marrow-derived CD133+ progenitors for the repair of infarcted myocardium. J Am Coll Cardiol 2004; 44:458–463.

32 Reinlib L, Field L. Cell transplantation as future therapy for cardiovascular disease? A Workshop of the National Heart, Lung, and Blood Institute. Circulation 2000; 101:e182–e187.

33 Menasche P, Hagege AA, Vilquin JT, et al. Autologous skeletal myoblast transplantation for severe postinfarction left ventricular dysfunction. J Am Coll Cardiol 2003; 41:1078–1083.

34 Gavira JJ, Herreros J, Perez A, et al. Autologous skeletal myoblast transplantation in patients with nonacute myocardial infarction: 1-year follow-up. J Thorac Cardiovasc Surg 2006; 131:799–804.

35 Taylor DA, Silvestry SC, Bishop SP, et al. Delivery of primary autologous skeletal myoblasts into rabbit heart by coronary infusion: a potential approach to myocardial repair. Proceedings of the Association of American Physicians, 1997; 109:245–253.

36 Siminiak T, Fiszer D, Jerzykowska O, et al. Percutaneous trans-coronary-venous transplantation of autologous skeletal myoblasts in the treatment of post-infarction myocardial contractility impairment: the POZNAN trial. Eur Heart J 2005; 26:1188–1195.

37 Dib N, McCarthy P, Campbell A, et al. Feasibility and safety of autologous myoblast transplantation in patients with ischemic cardiomyopathy. Cell Transplant 2005; 14:11–19.

38 Smits PC, van Geuns RJ, Poldermans D, et al. Catheter-based intramyocardial injection of autologous skeletal myoblasts as a primary treatment of ischemic heart failure: clinical experience with six-month follow-up. J Am Coll Cardiol 2003; 42:2063–2069.

39 Thompson RB, Parsa CJ, van den Bos EJ, et al. Video-assisted thoracoscopic transplantation of myoblasts into the heart. Ann Thorac Surg 2004; 78:303–307.

40 Thompson CA, Nasseri BA, Makower J, et al. Percutaneous transvenous cellular cardiomyoplasty. A novel nonsurgical approach for myocardial cell transplantation. J Am Coll Cardiol 2003; 41:1964–1971.

41 Tse HF, Kwong YL, Chan JK, Lo G, Ho CL, Lau CP. Angiogenesis in ischaemic myocardium by intramyocardial autologous bone marrow mononuclear cell implantation. Lancet 2003; 361:47–49.

42 Fuchs S, Satler LF, Kornowski R, et al. Catheter-based autologous bone marrow myocardial injection in no-option patients with advanced coronary artery disease: a feasibility study. J Am Coll Cardiol 2003; 41:1721–1724.

43 Perin EC, Dohmann HF, Borojevic R, et al. Improved exercise capacity and ischemia 6 and 12 months after transendocardial injection of autologous bone marrow mononuclear cells for ischemic cardiomyopathy. Circulation 2004; 110:II213–II218.

44 Saito T, Kuang JQ, Bittira B, Al-Khaldi A, Chiu RC. Xenotransplant cardiac chimera: immune tolerance of adult stem cells. Ann Thorac Surg 2002; 74:19–24; discussion 24.

45 Vulliet PR, Greeley M, Halloran SM, MacDonald KA, Kittleson MD. Intra-coronary arterial injection of mesenchymal stromal cells and microinfarction in dogs. Lancet 2004; 363:783–784.

46 Yeh ET, Zhang S, Wu HD, Korbling M, Willerson JT, Estrov Z. Transdifferentiation of human peripheral blood CD34+-enriched cell population into cardiomyocytes, endothelial cells, and smooth muscle cells in vivo. Circulation 2003; 108:2070–2073.

47 Aicher A, Brenner W, Zuhayra M, et al. Assessment of the tissue distribution of transplanted human endothelial progenitor cells by radioactive labeling. Circulation 2003; 107:2134–2139.

48 Barbash IM, Chouraqui P, Baron J, et al. Systemic delivery of bone marrow-derived mesenchymal stem cells to the infarcted myocardium: feasibility, cell migration, and body distribution. Circulation 2003; 108:863–868.

49 Chin BB, Nakamoto Y, Bulte JW, Pittenger MF, Wahl R, Kraitchman DL. III In oxine labelled mesenchymal stem cell SPECT after intravenous administration in myocardial infarction. Nucl Med Commun 2003; 24:1149–1154.

50 Alessandrino P, Bernasconi P, Caldera D, et al. Adverse events occurring during bone marrow or peripheral blood progenitor cell infusion: analysis of 126 cases. Bone Marrow Transpl 1999; 23:533–537.

51 Chachques JC, Herreros J, Trainini J, et al. Autologous human serum for cell culture avoids the implantation of cardioverter-defibrillators in cellular cardiomyoplasty. Int J Cardiol 2004; 95(suppl 1):S29–S33.

52 Koyanagi M, Brandes RP, Haendeler J, Zeiher AM, Dimmeler S. Cell-to-cell connection of endothelial progenitor cells with cardiac myocytes by nanotubes: a novel mechanism for cell fate changes? Circ Res 2005; 96:1039–1041.

53 Driesen RB, Dispersyn GD, Verheyen FK, et al. Partial cell fusion: a newly recognized type of communication between dedifferentiating cardiomyocytes and fibroblasts. Cardiovasc Res 2005; 68:37–46.

54 Yoon J, Shim WJ, Ro YM, Lim DS. Transdifferentiation of mesenchymal stem cells into cardiomyocytes by direct cell-to-cell contact with neonatal cardiomyocyte but not adult cardiomyocytes. Ann Hematol 2005; 84:715–721.

55 Matsuura K, Wada H, Nagai T, et al. Cardiomyocytes fuse with surrounding noncardiomyocytes and reenter the cell cycle. J Cell Biol 2004; 167:351–363.

56 Schmidt-Lucke C, Rossig L, Fichtlscherer S, et al. Reduced number of circulating endothelial progenitor cells predicts future cardiovascular events: proof of concept for the clinical importance of endogenous vascular repair. Circulation 2005; 111:2981–2987.

57 Kravchenko J, Goldschmidt-Clermont PJ, Powell T, et al. Endothelial progenitor cell therapy for atherosclerosis: the philosopher's stone for an aging population? Sci Aging Knowl Environ 2005; 2005:18.

58 Kocher AA, Schuster MJ, Szabolcs S, et al. Neovascularization of ischemic myocardium by human bone-marrow derived angioblasts prevents cardiomyocyte apoptosis, reduces remodeling and improves cardiac function. Nat Medicine 2001; 7:430–436.

59 Orlic D, Kajstura J, Chimenti S, et al. Bone marrow cells regenerate infarcted myocardium. Nature 2001; 410:701–705.

60 Stamm C, Kleine HD, Westphal B, et al. CABG and bone marrow stem cell transplantation after myocardial infarction. Thorac Cardiovasc Surg 2004; 52:152–158.

61 Schachinger V, Assmus B, Britten MB, et al. Transplantation of progenitor cells and regeneration enhancement in acute myocardial infarction: final one-year results of the TOPCARE-AMI Trial. J Am Coll Cardiol 2004; 44:1690–1699.

62 Wollert KC, Meyer GP, Lotz J, et al. Intracoronary autologous bone-marrow cell transfer after myocardial infarction: the BOOST randomised controlled clinical trial. Lancet 2004; 364:141–148.

63 Janssens S. Intracoronary autologous bone-marrow cell transfer after myocardial infarction: a double-blind, randomized, and placebo-controlled clinical trial. American College of Cardiology Scientific Sessions, 2005.

64 Fadini GP, Miorin M, Facco M, et al. Circulating endothelial progenitor cells are reduced in peripheral vascular complications of type 2 diabetes mellitus. J Am Coll Cardiol 2005; 45:1449–1457.

65 Opie SR, Dib N. Local endovascular delivery, gene therapy, and cell transplantation for peripheral arterial disease. J Endovasc Ther 2004; 11(suppl 2):II51–II62.

66 Iwase T, Nagaya N, Fujii T, et al. Comparison of angiogenic potency between mesenchymal stem cells and mononuclear cells in a rat model of hindlimb ischemia. Cardiovasc Res 2005; 66:543–551.

67 Tateishi-Yuyama E, Matsubara H, Murohara T, et al. Therapeutic angiogenesis for patients with limb ischaemia by autologous transplantation of bone-marrow cells: a pilot study and a randomised controlled trial. Lancet 2002; 360:427–435.

68 Higashi Y, Kimura M, Hara K, et al. Autologous bone-marrow mononuclear cell implantation improves endothelium-dependent vasodilation in patients with limb ischemia. Circulation 2004; 109:1215–1218.

69 Sakakibara Y, Nishimura K, Tambara K, et al. Prevascularization with gelatin microspheres containing basic fibroblast growth factor enhances the benefits of cardiomyocyte transplantation. J Thorac Cardiovasc Surg 2002; 124:50–56.

70 Mangi AA, Noiseux N, Kong D, et al. Mesenchymal stem cells modified with Akt prevent remodeling and restore performance of infarcted hearts. Nat Med 2003; 9:1195–1201.

71 Ott HC, Berjukow S, Marksteiner R, et al. On the fate of skeletal myoblasts in a cardiac environment: down-regulation of voltage-gated ion channels. J Physiol 2004; 558:793–805.

72 Leobon B, Garcin I, Menasche P, Vilquin JT, Audinat E, Charpak S. Myoblasts transplanted into rat infarcted myocardium are functionally isolated from their host. Proc Natl Acad Sci USA 2003; 100:7808–7811.

73 Vandervelde S, van Luyn MJ, Tio RA, Harmsen MC. Signaling factors in stem cell-mediated repair of infarcted myocardium. J Mol Cell Cardiol 2005; 39:363–376.

74 Suzuki K, Murtuza B, Smolenski RT, et al. Cell transplantation for the treatment of acute myocardial infarction using vascular endothelial growth factor-expressing skeletal myoblasts. Circulation 2001; 104:1207–1212.

75 Reinecke H, Minami E, Virag JI, Murry CE. Gene transfer of connexin43 into skeletal muscle. Hum Gene Ther 2004; 15:627–636.

76 Guttinger M, Padrun V, Pralong WF, Boison D. Seizure suppression and lack of adenosine A1 receptor desensitization after focal long-term delivery of adenosine by encapsulated myoblasts. Exp Neurol 2005; 193:53–64.

77 Bartunek J, Dimmeler S, Drexler H, et al. The consensus of the task force of the European Society of Cardiology concerning the clinical investigation of the use of autologous adult stem cells for repair of the heart. Eur Heart J 2006; 27:1338–1340.

78 Caplice NM, Bunch TJ, Stalboerger PG, et al. Smooth muscle cells in human coronary atherosclerosis can originate from cells administered at marrow transplantation. Proc Natl Acad Sci USA 2003; 100:4754–4759.

79 Koyanagi M, Haendeler J, Badorff C, et al. Non-canonical Wnt signaling enhances differentiation of human circulating progenitor cells to cardiomyogenic cells. J Biol Chem 2005; 280:16838–16842.

80 Kittleson MM, Minhas KM, Irizarry RA, et al. Gene expression analysis of ischemic and nonischemic cardiomyopathy: shared and distinct genes in the development of heart failure. Physiol Genomics 2005; 21:299–307.

81 Gnecchi M, He H, Liang OD, et al. Paracrine action accounts for marked protection of ischemic heart by Akt-modified mesenchymal stem cells. Nat Med 2005; 11:367–368.

82 Hutcheson KA, Atkins BZ, Hueman MT, Hopkins MB, Glower DD, Taylor DA. Comparing the benefits of cellular cardiomyoplasty with skeletal myoblasts or dermal fibroblasts on myocardial performance. Cell Transpl 2000; 9:359–368.

83 Menasche P. Myoblast-based cell transplantation. Heart Fail Rev 2003; 8:221–227.

84 Herreros J, Prosper F, Perez A, et al. Autologous intramyocardial injection of cultured skeletal muscle-derived stem cells in patients with non-acute myocardial infarction. Eur Heart J 2003; 24:2012–2020.

85 Siminiak T, Kalawski R, Fiszer D, et al. Autologous skeletal myoblast transplantation for the treatment of postinfarction myocardial injury: phase I clinical study with 12 months of follow-up. Am Heart J 2004; 148:531–537.

86 Hamano K, Nishida M, Hirata K, et al. Local implantation of autologous bone marrow cells for therapeutic angiogenesis in patients with ischemic heart disease: clinical trial and preliminary results. Jpn Circ J 2001; 65:845–847.

87 Britten MB, Abolmaali ND, Assmus B, et al. Infarct remodeling after intracoronary progenitor cell treatment in patients with acute myocardial infarction (TOPCARE-AMI): mechanistic insights from serial contrast-enhanced magnetic resonance imaging. Circulation 2003; 108:2212–2218.

88 Fernandez-Aviles F, San Roman JA, Garcia-Frade J, et al. Experimental and clinical regenerative capability of human bone marrow cells after myocardial infarction. Circ Res 2004; 95:742–748.

89 Kuethe F, Richartz BM, Sayer HG, et al. Lack of regeneration of myocardium by autologous intracoronary mononuclear bone marrow cell transplantation in humans with large anterior myocardial infarctions. Int J Cardiol 2004; 97:123–127.

90 Chen SL, Fang WW, Ye F, et al. Effect on left ventricular function of intracoronary transplantation of autologous bone marrow mesenchymal stem cell in patients with acute myocardial infarction. Am J Cardiol 2004; 94:92–95.

91 Vanderheyden MMS, Vandekerckhove B, De Bondt P, et al. Selected intracoronary CD133+ bone marrow cells promote cardiac regeneration after acute myocardial infarction. Circulation 2004; 110:324–325.

92 Janssens SDC, Bogaert J, Theunissen K, et al. Autologous bone marrow-derived stem-cell transfer in patients with ST-segment elevation myocardial infarction: double-blind, randomised controlled trial. Lancet 2006; 367:113–121.

93 Cleland JG, Freemantle N, Coletta AP, Clark AL. Clinical trials update from the American Heart Association: REPAIR-AMI, ASTAMI, JELIS, MEGA, REVIVE-II, SURVIVE, and PROACTIVE. Eur J Heart Fail 2006; 8:105–110.

37

Clinical trials in cellular therapy

Joanna J. Wykrzykowska, Munir Boodhwani, and Roger J. Laham

Introduction
Scope of the problem

Advances in pharmacotherapeutics, primary angioplasty, and stenting, which are reviewed in this textbook, have substantially decreased the mortality and morbidity of the acute coronary syndromes (ACS). However, of the 865,000 Americans who have an ACS, yearly, a substantial number will develop CHF resulting in 5 million heart failure patients (1). The mortality of ischemic cardiomyopathy and CHF remains high (50% at five years). Pharmacotherapy and surgical therapy, including biventricular pacers and left ventricle (LV) assist devices, along with transplantation itself, have not produced major survival benefit.

Regenerative potential of the heart

Recent challenge to the dogma that the heart is a terminally differentiated organ without the ability to regenerate, opened up an exciting new possibility of cellular transplant therapy to regenerate the infarcted myocardium, and thereby prevent the sequeli of ACS (2–4). During an ST elevation myocardial infarction, cytokines are elaborated that allow for the recruitment of both resident and circulating stem cells for cardiomyocyte regeneration (5,6). These endogenous mechanisms of repair are usually easily overwhelmed by the processes of apoptosis, fibrosis, and compensatory hypertrophy with consequent disadvantageous ventricular remodeling. In addition, the regenerative potential of the progenitors seems to be impaired by the aging of the host (7,8).

Definition of cellular therapy

Cellular cardiomyoplasty is a technique of delivering progenitor cells into the ischemic or infarcted (scarred) myocardium with the hope of restoring blood flow and contractility (9). Many cell types, including fetal cardiomyocytes, autologous skeletal myoblasts, adult cardiac myocytes, embryonic stem cells and both peripheral and autologous bone marrow (selected and unselected) stem cells (ABMSCs) were tested in various animal models. Preclinical trials of myogenesis are reviewed elsewhere in this text. However, clinical trials have been conducted, predominantly with autologous bone marrow–derived cells in acute setting of reperfusion therapy and skeletal myoblasts in the setting of chronic scar and myocardial dysfunction. Herein, we will review the clinical experience and outcomes of cardiomyoplasty trials.

Cell types
Bone marrow stem cells

Based on the expression of CD34 surface marker, bone marrow stem cells can be subdivided into hematopoetic progenitors that can give rise to endothelial cells and blood cells (10), and CD34-negative mesenchymal stem cells that can give rise to multiple lineages, including cardiomyocytes in vitro (11, 12). During acute myocardial infarction, these progenitor cells are mobilized in the periphery (13). In mouse models of myocardial infarction, both Lin-negative c-kit + cells and sca-1 + cells were capable of incorporating themselves as both endothelial cells and smooth muscle cells (support cells of neovessels), and cardiomyocytes (14). In our own work, we were able to show that matrigels within skeletal muscle injected with bone marrow cells are capable of forming new capillaries and vessels (Fig. 1). The identity of the pleuripotent stem cell and its lineage markers still remain elusive, however. In addition, their viability after intramyocardial injection into murine infarcted myocardium has been called into question with as few as 1% of the injected cells being viable four days postimplantation (15).

Skeletal myoblasts

Skeletal muscle cells are capable of regeneration and repair more readily than cardiac myocytes owing to the so-called satellite cells that can be readily mobilized at the time of injury (16). They are capable of easy expansion in culture; can be harvested easily from the autologous host; and are fairly resistant to hypoxia (17). The major drawback is that as the skeletal myocytes mature, they no longer form gap junctions and become electrically isolated, predisposing to re-entry arrhythmias (18). In addition, despite some encouraging data (19), the viability of dissociated myoblasts in suspension injected into myocardial scar deprived of appropriate trophic environment has been called into question (20). In our hands, skeletal myoblasts injected into canine myocardium could not be identified four weeks after implantation, and the needle tract caused fibrosis and scarring (Fig. 2).

Delivery methods and procedures

Bone marrow is aspirated usually under local anesthesia from the iliac crest. If bone marrow cells without enrichment for a particular population are used, very little processing is required. Some investigators enrich the monocyte population in endothelial progenitors by culturing for three days in endothelium-specific medium (21). Cells can not only be injected via surgical techniques intramyocardially, but also by several catheter-based approaches (intracoronary, intravenous, and intramyocardial from the LV cavity). Skeletal myoblasts are usually harvested from the thigh muscle under local anesthesia and undergo two to three weeks of expansion in culture before implantation. Injection approaches are limited to the intramyocardial route given the risk of embolization with intracoronary approach.

Clinical trials

Autologous bone marrow stem cell intracoronary injections in acute myocardial infarction

In the context of acute myocardial injury where the maximal restoration of blood flow to the ischemic/hibernating

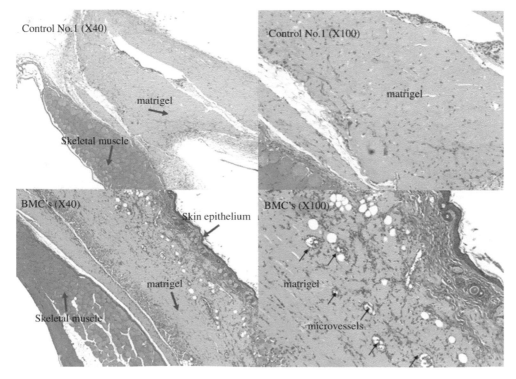

Figure 1

(*See color plate.*) Bone marrow cell-induced capillary and neovessel formation in the matrigel placed in the skeletal muscle of a dog. *Abbrevation*: BMC, bone marrow cell-induced.

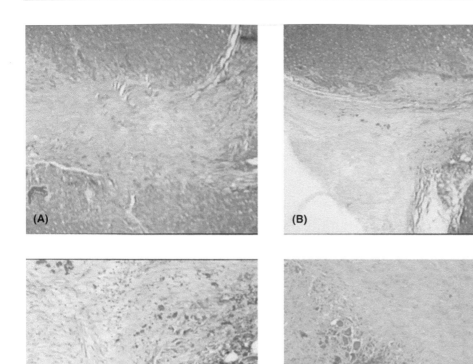

myocardium is the goal, bone marrow cells are optimal owing to their angiogenic potential and ability to either fuse with (22) or transdifferentiate (3) into cardiomyocytes. Improved collateral perfusion and regional myocardial function has been demonstrated in small animal (23,24) and large animal models of myocardial ischemia (25,26).

A total of 500 patients are studied so far who received either selected or unselected bone marrow stem cells. Until recently, most of these studies were small nonrandomized pilot studies. One of the earliest studies by Stauer et al. (27) enrolled 20 patients with transmural acute myocardial infarction with a mean duration of anginal pain of 12 hours. All patients underwent left coronary angiography and revascularization. Ten of the patients who consented to the study were assigned to the treatment with ABMSCs within five to nine days of their initial infarction. 1.5 to 4 million unselected ABMSCs were delivered via an over-the-wire intracoronary balloon catheter with six to seven repeated injections. The primary outcome was the left ventricular ejection fraction (LVEF) on left ventriculography and dobutamine echocardiography in addition to hemodynamic assessment at three months after treatment. Patients treated with ABMSCs had a significant decrease in the infarct size as assessed by the degree of wall motion abnormality on ventriculography at initial hospitalization and at three months (30 vs.

12%; $P = 0.005$). Infarct size remained the same in the nontreatment control group (20%). There was a statistically nonsignificant increase in the ejection fraction (EF) in both groups (57–62% in the treatment group and 60–64% in the control group; SD = 7–10%). The end-systolic but not end-diastolic volumes also decreased significantly in the treated patients. There was an increase in the ratio of the systolic pressure to end-diastolic volume on stress echocardiography. In addition, perfusion defect on thallium imaging decreased by 26% in the treatment group ($P = 0.016$). Thus, there was both an increase in perfusion, decrease in infarct size and hemodynamic improvement that could be attributed to the ABMSC transplant. Although the control group was not randomized, it was well matched to the treatment group. The effect of percutaneous transluminal coronary angioplasty (PTCA) on the outcomes was likely attenuated because of longer time to treatment from the time of symptom onset. The novel intracardiac injection technique was used to optimize the delivery and retention of cells in the myocardium. The timing of the injection within five to nine days of acute infarction, when there is still an expression of chemokines and cytokine, in addition to concomitant revascularization, likely were advantageous in promoting the angiogenesis effects of the ABMSCs. The study raised questions of standardization and optimization of the number of bone marrow cells transplanted, in addition to careful choice of timing of the intracoronary injection, given the kinetics of the inflammatory response in myocardial infarction (MI) (28).

The transplantation of progenitor cells and regeneration enhancement in acute myocardial infarction (TOPCARE-AMI) was initially a randomized study of 20 patients, which compared the bone marrow and peripheral blood-derived stem cell injection, and was later extended to include 60 patients (29,30). All the patients enrolled in the study had an acute ST elevation, MI treated with stenting and 2b3a inhibitors. A control nontreatment group consisted of 10 matched patients treated with similar revascularization technique within the institution. The 20 study patients were assigned randomly to receive either of the two cell types at 24 hours after the initial MI (time of cell harvest). Intracoronary cell injection was performed four days after the MI. Blood-derived cells were expanded in the media containing vascular endothelial growth factor (VEGF) and human plasma resulting in 90% endothelial cell population. Bone marrow cells were isolated by density gradient centrifugation and contained a heterogeneous progenitor cell population that was CD34 and CD45 positive. Primary outcomes were LVEF on ventriculography and stress ECHO cardiography, wall motion abnormalities, coronary blood flow reserve (CFR) on intracoronary Doppler, myocardial infarct size on fluorodeoxyglucose (FDG)-positron emission tomography (PET) scan at initial hospitalization and at four months post-MI. No elevation in serum inflammatory markers or troponin levels, attributable to stem cell intracoronary injections with balloon occlusion, was observed. There was no evidence of malignant arrhythmias and five of the 19 patients had an evidence of in-stent restenosis. Both the recipients of bone marrow and peripheral blood endothelial progenitors demonstrated 9% improvement (from 51% to 60%) in EF (P = 0.003), decrease in end-systolic but not end-diastolic volume and the degree of wall motion abnormalities in both the infarct per se and its border zone (P < 0.0001). The effect was more pronounced in the border zone. No such change was observed in the untreated controls. Ejection fractions increased by only 2.5% to 3% in the control group, which is in the range expected with revascularization alone (31). There was no further significant difference in the magnitude of the effect between the two cell types. Wall motion indexes improved at four months even in the patients who had in-stent restenosis. The CFR measurements demonstrated the normalization of perfusion in most patients, and some improvement in those patients with restenosis, suggesting angiogenic effects at the tissue perfusion level. FDG-PET viability study showed significant decrease in the infarct territory (increase in uptake from 54% to 63%; P < 0.0001) in the affected coronary territory. This study addressed some of the important safety issues of the cardiomyoplasty and the cell-delivery technique, such as arrhythmogenesis and the impact of vessel occlusion. When restenosis occurred, its rates were not markedly higher than in the baseline control group. The magnitude of improvement in

the EF was greater than that demonstrated by Stauer et al. (27). possibly because of earlier infusion time (four days after infarction). Neither of the studies addressed the contribution of ischemic conditioning from repeated balloon inflations as a potential contributor to the improvement in myocardial perfusion, as the control group did not undergo "sham" ballooning.

In the follow-up study, these patient were evaluated by cardiac magnetic resonance imaging (MRI) at four months to further delineate the mechanism of improvement in the LV function associated with cellular therapy (32). Late enhancement volume, that is, infarct volume, decreased by 20% over four months (P < 0.05). The regional EF within the infarcted areas and the global EF increased proportionally (r = 0.8; P < 0.001). There was further a correlation between the decrease in infarct volume (late enhancement) and improvement in wall thickening and wall motion score. Importantly, the initial size or transmural extent of infarction did not have an adverse impact on the improvement in function from cellular therapy. Full thickness infarcts improved their function as much as nontransmural infarct areas, which may suggest that this technology would be potentially beneficial in acute MI patients presenting with CHF and shock. These patients were excluded from all the current studies, and are a group that could possibly derive the greatest benefit. The cell number or type, that is, peripheral blood-derived endothelial progenitors versus bone-marrow derived unselected cells, on the other hand, did not impact the degree of improvement in function. The in vitro migratory response to angiogenic factors, such as VEGF and SDF-1 did appear to be a significant predictor. The use of functional cardiac MRI with its excellent ability to assess myocardial regional contractility (33) may be preferable in the future to other modalities in the assessment of the efficacy of cell therapy. The fact that the migratory capacity is important in mediating this effect would suggest that combining angiogenic factor gene or protein transfer with cellular therapy might enhance the beneficial effect of cardiomyoplasty. Although biologically sound, this proposition must be further evaluated in an in vivo setting. Lastly, it appears that contractility and not just perfusion improve within the infarct area itself and not in the peri-infarct zone alone is an important one. Caution must be exercised, however, in making a leap in logic and assuming that this is a direct result of the ability of progenitors to transdifferentiate into cardiomyocytes (3).

Long-term follow up over 12 months of additional 40 patients (total of 60) was recently completed for TOPCARE-AMI (30), and confirmed initial good safety profile and sustained improvement in EF and LV contractility by MRI. The total LV mass decreased the overall suggesting that deleterious compensatory hypertrophy and remodeling of adjacent myocardium did not occur. Restenosis rate remained at 21% and no lethal arrhythmia was reported.

More recently, Fernandez-Aviles et al. (34) enrolled 20 patients with extensive ST-elevation MI (>6 mm), treated with primary or rescue angioplasty and stenting for treatment with bone marrow stem cells at median time of 13 days after infarction. The patients were evaluated at 30 days and six months with stress echocardiography and functional MRI in addition to coronary angiography with LV gram and CFR. They were followed up to 21 months. Thirteen patients who refused treatment were used as matched controls. Patients were injected with >10 × the number of ABMSCs than in previous studies (70 million cells on average), but this did not result in markedly higher increases in EFs. CD34 + cells constituted only 1% of the injected population. The effects on the EF and contractility (wall thickening by MRI) were comparable with prior studies despite later time of injection (13 days when infarct scar is considered to have formed) (35). In vitro experiments accompanying this study showed that ABMSCs grown in the presence of murine cardiomyocytes displayed some of the cardiomyocyte surface markers. There was no clear and direct proof of whether these were contractile elements or whether these were a result of transdifferentiation or fusion with murine cardiomyocytes.

Bone marrow transfer to enhance ST-elevation infarct regeneration (BOOST) trial was the first prospective randomized trial of ABMSCs versus placebo in 60 patients with ST-elevation MI who were treated with percutaneous coronary intervention (PCI) (5). Patients had wall motion abnormality in two-thirds of the anterior, inferior, or lateral wall, but could not be in pulmonary edema/cardiogenic shock (baseline EF was 51–53% in both groups). 250 million ABMSCs were administered via intracoronary route five to six days post-MI to 30 patients. Primary end point was the EF change at six months post-treatment, as assessed by MRI. In keeping with the results of other studies, the EF increased by 6.7% in the treated group (50–56.7%), and remained unchanged in the control group (51.3–51%) treated with PCI alone ($P = 0.0026$). This was the first trial that controlled for the baseline benefit of PCI. The improvement in the global EF was observed in both older and younger patients, men and women, and regardless of whether right or left coronary territory was involved. Patients with greater symptom to PCI times seemed to benefit more. Similarly to TOPCARE-AMI, both patients with large and small baseline late-enhancement areas on MRI benefited. This benefit seemed to be greater in those patients with larger baseline defects. Unlike TOPCARE-AMI, the functional MRI demonstrated improvement in wall motion and wall thickening only in the peri-infarct border zone, but not in the infarct zone per se. Most recent communications report that the improvement in global EF is maintained at 18 months postinfarction. The trial confirmed good safety profile with comparable (30%) rates of in-stent restenosis between the two groups and no increase in the incidence of inducible ventricular tachycardia (VT) on electrophysiologic studies.

The only trial to date that was negative and failed to demonstrate any benefit of ABMSCs infusion was a small nonrandomized trial of five patients (36) with ST-elevation MI treated within six hours with primary or rescue PCI after failed thrombolysis. Thirty million cells were injected in a single injection. There was no improvement in the EF from baseline at three months on left ventriculography or stress echocardiography (42–44%; $P = NS$), wall motion or contractility index. The CFR improved from 1.7 to 2.5, but was not statistically significant (given $n = 5$). Ejection fractions increased to 46% (absolute increase of 4%) at 12-month follow up, but again this was not statistically significant. In general, the EFs in these five patients were 10% lower than in other studies indicating larger MI. This may possibly undermine the TOPCARE-AMI's claim that baseline infarct size was not a predictor of response to therapy. The time to PCI was shorter in this study possibly making the additional benefit of cell transplant difficult to demonstrate in only five patients.

Clearly, the preliminary phase I trials of ABMSCs in AMI show good safety profile and a promise in functional LV performance improvement, that is sustained long-term post-MI. Before any definitive claims can be made, large randomized trials of this therapy are needed. Two such multicenter trials, Reinfusion of Enriched Progenitor cells And Infarct Remodeling in Acute Myocardial Infarction (REPAIR-AMI) and Autologous Stem cell Transplantation in Acute Myocardial Infarction (ASTAMI) were recently presented at the American Heart Association meeting (November, 2005) (37). Reinfusion of enriched progenitor cells and infarct remodeling in acute myocardial infarction randomized 204 patients to 236 million bone marrow cell infusion versus supernatant injection four days after MI. Both the cellular therapy and the placebo group had a slight improvement in EF, but this improvement was somewhat greater in the treated group. The EF increased from 48% to 54% in the treated group and from 47% to 50% in the control group ($P = 0.02$). There was a slight difference in the number of patients requiring revascularization in the cell-therapy group. The clinical significance of these results is still uncertain and longer-term follow up would be needed to confirm the sustainability of these effects, especially in the face of contradictory results of the Norwegian ASTAMI trial. In contrast to REPAIR-AMI, this trial used sensitive imaging end points at six months after treatment with bone marrow stem cells. One hundred patients were randomized to stem cell injection versus placebo five to eight days after acute MI. By echocardiography, nuclear imaging, and the most sensitive cardiac MRI at six months postprocedure, there was no difference in the EF; in fact, the placebo group seemed to have greater improvement in function. The results of the trials reviewed here are summarized in Table 1.

Autologous bone marrow stem cells for chronic stable angina and ischemic cardiomyopathy without the option of revascularization

Initial experience with transmyocardial revascularization gave promising results in patients with refractory chronic angina

Table 1 Clinical trials of cellular therapy in acute myocardial infarction

Trial	NN	Cell dose	Delivery	Time post MI (days)	Outcome
Strauer	10 Tx + 10 Ctrl	28 million	IC	5–9	Decreased infarct size; improved perfusion; improved wall motion
TOPCARE-AMI	59 Tx + 11 Ctrl	200 million	IC	4	Increased EF, coronary flow, regional wall motion and decreased infarct size
Fernander-Aviles	20 Tx + 13 Ctrl	78 million	IC	14	Increased EF and wall motion
BOOST	30 Tx and 30 Ctrl	2.5 billion of nucleated bone marrow cells	IC	6	Increased EF and regional wall motion; no change in infarct size
Kuethe	5 Tx	40 million	IC	6	No effect
REPAIR-AMI	204	236 million	IC	4	Increased EF (5%) and less repeat revascularization
ASTAMI	100		IC	5–8	No effect

Abbreviations: ASTAMI, autologous stem cell transplantation in acute myocardial infarction; BOOST, bone marrow transfer to enhance ST-elevation infarct regeneration; Ctrl, control; EF, ejection fraction; IC, intracoronary; N, number; Tx, treated; REPAIR-AMI, reinfusion of enriched progenitor cells and infarct remodeling in acute myocardial infarction; TOPCARE-AMI, transplantation of progenitor cells and regeneration enhancement in acute myocardial infarction.

who were not candidates for traditional revascularization owing to the diffuse nature of their disease (38,39). The studies failed to account for a strong placebo effect observed in this group and the follow-up studies failed to show efficacy (40). The idea of using ABMSCs as potential sources of angiogenic factors has now been tested in several trials (41–44). Given that patients are not candidates for revascularization injection of the cells has to be accomplished via a transendocardial route with the guidance of electromechanical mapping (EMM) using a NOGA catheter or other intramyocardial injection catheters.

The first feasibility study to assess this new methodology enrolled eight patients with angina refractory to medical therapy (42). They were assessed with functional cardiac MRI at three months after the treatment. The EF was 57% at baseline and did not increase significantly. There was an improvement in the wall thickening (11%; $P = 0.004$) and wall motion (5.5%; $P = 0.008$) of the target wall, in addition to a decrease in hypoperfused myocardium (3.9%; $P = 0.004$). The EMM times approached 200 minutes. Fuchs et al. study (2003) (41) was a second feasibility pilot trial of 10 patients with chronic angina secondary to nonintervenable coronary disease but with EF above 30% (mean of 47%). Patients received 12 injections of ABMSCs via a transendocardial approach using EMM into the ischemic territory as determined by single photon emission computer tomography (SPECT). The outcomes assessed were EF change by

echocardiography at three months after the procedure, and a change in the size of reversible ischemia on SPECT, in addition to a change in the angina score. The EFs did not change. However, there was a decrease in the semi-quantitative stress scores on SPECT imaging within the injected segments ($P < 0.0001$). Angina score also improved in 8/10 patients. Importantly, there were no arrhythmic or procedural complications. The EMM time was 30 minutes.

The largest study to date of 21 patients was an open-label study with 14 patients who received treatment and seven who served as controls (44). Unlike in the pilot studies, the patients had to have an EF of less than 40% (both pilot studies enrolled patients with EFs > 40%). All patients had a demonstrable reversible defect by SPECT imaging. The group therefore represented a high mortality and morbidity patient population. The mean of 25 million cells were injected (split into 15 aliquots) into the area of viability and reversible defect as determined by unipolar voltage with NOGA catheter and by prior SPECT imaging, respectively. Notably control group patients did not undergo a sham procedure. The outcomes assessed were the change in cardiopulmonary exercise tolerance, echocardiographic EF and viability on SPECT at two months after treatment, in addition to angiographic LV function and EMM at four months. Again, the control group did not undergo the EMM assessment at four months. There was a significant decrease in the brain natriuretic peptide (BNP) levels and improvement in creatinine in the treated group at two months (BNP 282 vs. 565; $P = 0.06$; cr 1.1 vs. 1.62; $P = 0.03$). Patients in the treatment group had less anginal symptoms and increased exercise capacity [metabolic equivalent units (METs) went up from 5 to 6.7 in the treatment group and did not change in the control group; $P = 0.0085$]. There was a 6% increase in EF by echocardiography ($P = 0.027$). There was a reduction in the reversible defect by SPECT from 15% to 4.5% ($P = 0.022$) without a concomitant change in fixed defect percentage (ruling out the possibility that a decrease in the reversible defect was attributed to scar formation at the site of the injection). There was an increase in the ischemic area in the control group although the difference was not statistically significant. The improvement in the LV function was sustained at four months. The EMM also showed increased contractility in the injected regions (change in linear shortening 5.7 to 10.8; $P < 0.0005$). The authors hypothesized that the effect of ABMSCs injections was to the result of angiogenic properties of cells and hence better contractility of the hibernating myocardium. The use of EMM to guide the procedure was particularly useful to determine the viability of the tissue treated. The procedures were not associated with arrhythmia or myocardial injury or high incidence of perforation. The major limitation was the lack of sham procedure control, which raises the issue of placebo effect in interpreting the subjective NYHA class and exercise tolerance data. Improvement in SPECT imaging is reassuring, however.

More recently, the same authors extended their patient follow up to six and 12 months and attempted to stratify the magnitude of improvement by progenitor cell characteristics, that is, elucidate the potential mechanism of improvement (43). The BNP levels increased in both groups but not as markedly in the treatment group (BNP 507 vs. 740 at 12 months; $P = 0.08$). There was a persistent favorable difference in the NYHA class (2.7 vs. 1.4; $P = 0.01$) and exercise tolerance (METs 7.2 vs. 5.1; $P = 0.02$). There was no longer a difference in the EF between the two groups; however, the size of the reversible defect on repeat SPECT scans at 12 months was markedly smaller in the treated group (11% vs. 34%; $P = 0.01$). Monocyte and early hematopoietic cell phenotype correlated with better perfusion at six months by SPECT, particularly the monocyte lineage, suggesting their possible role in angiogenic factor secretion.

Similar to the experience in the acute MI setting, cellular therapy use in chronic angina patients needs validation in larger randomized trials that would allow for sham procedures to control for the placebo effect. In addition, although transendocardial administration with NOGA catheter appears to be an effective method of administration of cells, both preclinical and clinical studies are needed to establish the best approach that would allow for maximal cell survival and retention. As recently reviewed by Thompson (45), endoventricular catheters can be subject to motion owing to cardiac cycle, interference from the subvalvular apparatus or inadequate tract formation within the myocardium by the needle. One of the possible solutions to some of these limitations may be a use of the injections via the coronary sinus and the great cardiac vein using the guidance of intravascular ultrasound (IVUS) and an extendable nitinol needle (46). This approach may also shorten the procedure times (80–90 minutes as reported by Perin for EMM mapping). The results of the trials are summarized in Table 2.

Skeletal myoblast intramyocardial injection for ischemic myocardial dysfunction

In acute or chronic ischemia patients, angiogenic potential of transplanted cells is of the greatest importance. The patients with chronic nonviable scar and myocardial dysfunction are more likely to benefit from the cells that, either directly or indirectly (via paracrine effect) (47), improve the contractility of the treated myocardium (9). Autologous skeletal myoblasts have been successfully expanded in vitro and implanted in the myocardia of animals. Although they do not contract synchronously with the rest of the myocardium and do not integrate into it, they have been shown to improve contractility

Table 2 Clinical trials in cell therapy for chronic angina without revascularization options

Trial	N	Baseline EF	Cell dose	Delivery	Outcome
Tse	8 Tx	58%	40 ml	TEN-EMM	Decreased angina, increased perfusion, and regional wall motion
Fuchs	10 Tx	47%	78 million	TEN-EMM	Decreased angina and increased perfusion
Perin	14 Tx + 7 Ctrl	30%	30 million	TEN-EMM	Decreased angina and heart failure; increased perfusion, EF and regional wall motion

Abbreviations: Ctrl, control; *N*, number; TEN-EMM, transendocardial-electromechanical mapping; Tx, treated.

(48,49). The major drawback has been a need for manipulation in culture, need for epicardial implantation during an open surgical procedure, and most importantly, arrhythmogenic potential of these cell islands (50).

The first clinical study enrolled 10 patients with LVEF <35% and nonviable scar owing to past MI on FDG-PET and indication for coronary artery bypass grafting (CABG) (51). Myocytes were cultured from the patient's autologous vastus lateralis biopsy obtained two to three weeks before CABG. Eight hundred million myoblasts were injected via a 27-gauge needle epicardially during CABG into a scar supplied by a nongraftable diseased vessel. All patients were given prednisone postoperatively. Primary outcomes were patient safety and ability to obtain myocytes after culture. Left ventricular EF at one, three, and six months postprocedure was the secondary outcome. Sixty percent of the expanded cells were myogenic and 90% of them were viable. The patients had no major complications of the surgery but four of them developed inducible VT within 11–22 days and required automatic internal cardioverter-defibrillator (AICD). The LVEF increased from 23% to 32% (P = 0.002); however, this increase may have been to the result of revascularization alone. Both nonrevascularized segments that were transplanted with cells and those that were revascularized, improved their contractility, suggesting that myoblasts indeed improved contractility locally.

Another small pilot of 12 patients undergoing CABG with EFs between 25% and 45% and nonviable scar showed no need for AICD implantation and improvement in EF from mean of 35–53% at three months (P = 0.002) (52). It is unclear what contributed to this lower incidence of inducible VT, although the use of autologous patient plasma for muscle culture may have decreased the degree of inflammation around skeletal myoblasts, potentially caused by culture in fetal bovine serum. The suggestion that the risk of VT can be reduced by the use of autologous plasma is also shown in

another more recent study by Chachques et al. of 20 patients (53). A smaller number of myoblasts (200 million) were injected than in Menasche study, and appeared equally effective. In contrast to the Menasche study, the scar area was also revascularized making it more difficult to dissect the contribution of revascularization from myoblast transplant effect. The myoblast-treated areas had larger semi-quantitative improvement in wall motion than revascularized areas (wall motion score index 2.6 down to 1.6; P = 0.0001). The FDG-PET showed increase in the uptake in transplanted scar areas (from 0.126 to 0.231; P = 0.01). Similar change was observed in the revascularized areas (0.170–0.284; P = 0.014). Again, although this may imply the presence of viable myoblasts in the scar area, a definitive proof is lacking. It is possible that this improvement simply represents the effect of revascularization on hibernating myocardium that was previously undetected by FDG-PET and thought to be nonviable.

A small five-patient study (54) used a catheter-based transendocardial injection of skeletal myoblasts with EMM guidance and no concomitant revascularization. One of the patients developed long nonsustained ventricular tachycardia (NSVT), and an AICD was placed. There was a trend toward improvement in EF by echocardiography and LV angiography but not by MRI. Wall thickening in the injected areas showed significant improvement over untreated segments 0.9–1.8 mm; P = 0.008).

The longest follow up to date of patients status postskeletal myoblast implantation was 12 months (55). Ten patients undergoing CABG with low EFs were treated. Two patients developed NSVT in the postoperative period, necessitating amiodarone infusion, and all subsequent patients were placed on prophylactic amiodarone. Improvement in EF was similar to other studies and was sustained at 12 months.

In conclusion, skeletal myoblast implantations require better investigation into the efficacy of implantation and the viability of injected myocytes by possibly obtaining the biopsy data from

Table 3   Clinical trials of cell therapy in ischemic cardiomyopathy

Trial	N (Tx)	EF (%)	Dose	Delivery	Outcomes
Menasche	10	25	870 million	TEP-CABG	Increased EF and wall motion; Complications of VT (arrhythmia)
Herreros	11	36	190 million (in human serum)	TEP-CABG	Increased EF and wall motion and increased viability; no arrhythmias observed
Siminiak	10	25–40	50 million	TEP-CABG	Increased EF and wall motion
Chachques	20	28	300 million (in human serum)	TEP-CABG	Increased EF and wall motion and viability; no arrhythmias
Smits	5	36	200 million	TEN-EMM	Increased EF and wall motion

Abbreviations: Ctrl, control; EF, ejection fraction; N, number; TEP-CABG, transepicardial coronary artery bypass grafting; VT, ventricular tachycardia; TEN-EMM, transendocardial-electromechanical mapping; Tx, treated.

patients. It appears that the risk of arrhythmia is substantial and its etiology is still unclear. It may be prudent that the patients enrolled in further studies receive prophylactic AICDs which would offer not only treatment, but also potentially better recording and monitoring capabilities for different arrhythmias. The new EMM-guided catheters for epicardial implantation may offer less-invasive option for implantation than open-heart surgery. One such CellFix catheter allows for possible repeat administration of cells (56) and coadministration with angiogenic factors to improve survival. Larger safety and efficacy randomized trials are also needed to separate the effect of myoblast transplant from that of revascularization. Another option not yet investigated in human trials would be the use of adult cardiac myocytes for transplantation (57) or fetal cardiomyocytes, the supply of which is rather scarce (58). These cells may have a better chance of integrating with the rest of the myocardium and being less arrhythmogenic, potentially provide enhanced contractility. The results of cell therapy trials in ischemic myocardial dysfunction are summarized in Table 3.

Angiogenesis and cytokine clinical trials

The results of preclinical and clinical trials of angiogenic factor protein and gene therapy were recently reviewed by Losordo et al. (59,60), and are reviewed in detail elsewhere in this textbook. Here we will discuss the issues of synergistic coadministration of angiogenic factors and cytokine with cellular therapy. Fibroblast growth factor (FGF) Initiating RevaScularization Trial (FIRST) of intracoronary FGF-2 protein administration in 300 patients with coronary artery disease (CAD) did not show any advantage over placebo and demonstrated a substantial placebo effect (61). Similarly, a phase I trial of VEGF-2 gene therapy by direct myocardial injection showed no evidence of angiogenic effect by angiography (62). It is possible that the extracellular matrix or cellular vehicle is needed for sustained and effective administration of angiogenic factors. It is also possible that the angiogenic network elaborated after an MI is so elaborate that the administration of a single cytokine cannot replicate it. In addition, the endogenous endothelium may be too diseased to respond to angiogenic proteins, and new endothelial progenitor mobilization is needed for the process of angiogenesis and vasculogenesis to take place. Conversely, transplanted cells may also demonstrate better survival and retention when administered in their natural humoral and structural milieu rather than a suspension of cultured cells. Skeletal myoblast survival was demonstrated to be improved when fibrin biodegradable scaffold was used (63). Other tissue-engineering approaches to myocardial regeneration were recently reviewed by Nugent and Edelman (64). Our own laboratory is conducting preclinical trials of cardiomyoplasty for acute and chronic MI with myotissue transplantation. This technology

would provide the ultimate preservation of structure and angiogenic milieu of the transplanted cardiomyocytes (Fig. 3).

Another possibility for combining cytokine treatment and cell therapy was recently tested in the Myoblast Autologous Graft in Ischemic Cardiomyopathy (MAGIC) trial (65). In this prospective randomized trial of 27 patients undergoing stenting for acute MI effects of combining intracoronary infusion of unselected peripheral blood stem cells with the administration of intravenous granulocyte-colony stimulating factor (G-CSF). The hypothesis was that G-CSF would increase endothelial progenitor/stem cell mobilization from the bone marrow that usually occurs in the acute setting of MI (66), and that peripheral blood could be used instead of bone marrow for infusion. The trial was stopped prematurely, however, owing to increased incidence of in-stent restenosis in the patients treated with G-CSF. This safety concern outweighed the benefits on LVEF and exercise tolerance, in addition to recent evidence that G-CSF is capable of preventing the unfavorable ventricular remodeling (67).

Conclusions and future directions

Cellular therapy holds great promise, especially for patients with limited options, such as those with end-stage ischemic cardiomyopathy or refractory angina. It has the potential to reduce the incidence of LV dysfunction and heart failure. The results of small phase I trials conducted to date and summarized here are somewhat encouraging, but they clearly show the need for perfecting this technology before it can be widely applied. Similar to the early angiogenesis trials where small phase I studies showed some promise, but larger randomized phase II and III trials proved disappointing, we run a danger of disappointment with cellular therapy unless the mechanistic foundation is elucidated first, and the technology perfected based on this work (68). We need more research into the mechanisms of cellular therapy effects on ventricular performance, before embarking on larger randomized and appropriately controlled clinical trials. One of the fundamental issues that remains unresolved is the viability and survival of the injected cells that remain rather poor calling into question their direct contribution to the improvement in contractility, and suggesting that possibly the paracrine effect of apoptosis of these cells leads to the improvement in function. Many preclinical studies to date, including our own work, have shown this poor viability (Fig. 2). Cell delivery catheter technologies need to be developed further. Tissue-engineering technologies to construct matrix scaffolds, which would allow for better cell survival, need to be developed. The imaging techniques to allow for cell tracking and monitoring of their viability need to be developed further. Magnetic resonance imaging technology, allowing for gene and protein expression

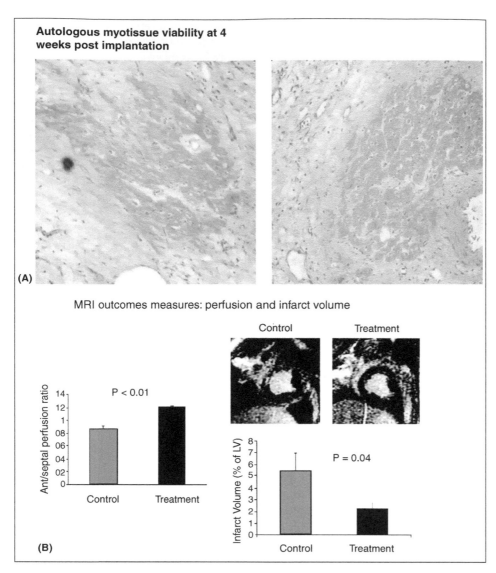

Autologous myotissue viability at 4 weeks post implantation

(A)

MRI outcomes measures: perfusion and infarct volume

Control   Treatment

P < 0.01

Ant/septal perfusion ratio

Control   Treatment

P = 0.04

Infarct Volume (% of LV)

Control   Treatment

(B)

Figure 3

(*See color plate.*) (**A**) Viability of myotissue (autologous myocardial septal biopsy tissue) implanted into anterior wall scar at four weeks postimplantation in a porcine model of myocardial infarction (MI). Twelve Yorkshire pigs underwent an anterior MI by balloon occlusion of the lactate dehydrogenase (LAD) and were randomized to the implantation of six to nine septal intact myocardial biopsy tissues into the anterior infarct area versus sham operation. Animals underwent cardiac magnetic resonance imaging (MRI) for anterior-wall perfusion and delayed enhancement imaging for infarct volume at four weeks postimplant and were subsequently sacrificed. Tissues were harvested for histology. (**B**) Bar graph showing the results of cardiac MRI showing increased perfusion in the anterior wall of treated animals as compared with the septal (nonimplanted) wall perfusion, and decreased infarction volume after myotissue implantation, as measured by delayed enhancement cardiac MRI in the same porcine model of MI.

imaging (69,70), would seem ideal for this purpose, in addition to being the most sensitive and specific technique of assessing the LV performance (wall motion, wall thickening, EF) and perfusion in addition to viability (late enhancement).

References

1   American Heart Association. Heart Disease and Stroke Statistics—Update 2004. 2004.

2   Beltrami AP, Barlucchi L, Torella D, et al. Adult cardiac stem cells are multipotent and support myocardial regeneration. Cell 2003; 114(6):763–776.

3   Orlic D, Kajstura J, Chimenti S, et al. Bone marrow cells regenerate infarcted myocardium. Nature 2001; 410(6829):701–705.

4   Nadal-Ginard B, Kajstura J, Anversa P, Leri A. A matter of life and death: cardiac myocyte apoptosis and regeneration. J Clin Invest 2003; 111(10):1457–1459.

5   Wollert KC, Meyer GP, Lotz J, et al. Intracoronary autologous bone-marrow cell transfer after myocardial infarction: the BOOST randomised controlled clinical trial. Lancet 2004; 364(9429):141–148.

6   Niam S, Cheung W, Sullivan PE, Kent S, Gu X. Balance and physical impairments after stroke. Arch Phys Med Rehabil 1999; 80(10):1227–1233.

7   Rauscher FM, Goldschmidt-Clermont PJ, Davis BH, et al. Aging, progenitor cell exhaustion, and atherosclerosis. Circulation 2003; 108(4):457–463.

8   Zhang H, Fazel S, Tian H, et al. Increasing donor age adversely impacts beneficial effects of bone marrow but not smooth muscle myocardial cell therapy. Am J Physiol Heart Circ Physiol 2005; 289(5):H2089–2096.

9 Taylor DA. Cell-based myocardial repair: how should we proceed? Int J Cardiol 2004; 95(suppl 1):S8–12.

10 Asahara T, Murohara T, Sullivan A, et al. Isolation of putative progenitor endothelial cells for angiogenesis. Science 1997; 275(5302):964–967.

11 Pittenger MF, Mackay AM, Beck SC, et al. Multilineage potential of adult human mesenchymal stem cells. Science 1999; 284(5411):143–147.

12 Makino S, Fukuda K, Miyoshi S, et al. Cardiomyocytes can be generated from marrow stromal cells in vitro. J Clin Invest 1999; 103(5):697–705.

13 Shintani S, Murohara T, Ikeda H, et al. Mobilization of endothelial progenitor cells in patients with acute myocardial infarction. Circulation 2001; 103(23):2776–2779.

14 Jackson KA, Majka SM, Wang H, et al. Regeneration of ischemic cardiac muscle and vascular endothelium by adult stem cells. J Clin Invest 2001; 107(11):1395–1402.

15 Toma C, Pittenger MF, Cahill KS, Byrne BJ, Kessler PD. Human mesenchymal stem cells differentiate to a cardiomyocyte phenotype in the adult murine heart. Circulation 2002; 105(1):93–98.

16 Mauro A. Satellite cell of skeletal muscle fibers. J Biophys Biochem Cytol 1961; 9:493–495.

17 Eckert P, Schnackerz K. Ischemic tolerance of human skeletal muscle. Ann Plast Surg 1991; 26(1):77–84.

18 Reinecke H, MacDonald GH, Hauschka SD, Murry CE. Electromechanical coupling between skeletal and cardiac muscle. Implications for infarct repair. J Cell Biol 2000; 149(3):731–740.

19 Ghostine S, Carrion C, Souza LC, et al. Long-term efficacy of myoblast transplantation on regional structure and function after myocardial infarction. Circulation 2002; 106(12 suppl 1): I131–136.

20 Fan Y, Maley M, Beilharz M, Grounds M. Rapid death of injected myoblasts in myoblast transfer therapy. Muscle Nerve 1996; 19(7):853–860.

21 Dimmeler S, Zeiher AM, Schneider MD. Unchain my heart: the scientific foundations of cardiac repair. J Clin Invest 2005; 115(3):572–583.

22 Murry CE, Soonpaa MH, Reinecke H, et al. Haematopoietic stem cells do not transdifferentiate into cardiac myocytes in myocardial infarcts. Nature 2004; 428(6983):664–668.

23 Fuchs S, Baffour R, Zhou YF, et al. Transendocardial delivery of autologous bone marrow enhances collateral perfusion and regional function in pigs with chronic experimental myocardial ischemia. J Am Coll Cardiol 2001; 37(6):1726–1732.

24 Kamihata H, Matsubara H, Nishiue T, et al. Implantation of bone marrow mononuclear cells into ischemic myocardium enhances collateral perfusion and regional function via side supply of angioblasts, angiogenic ligands, and cytokines. Circulation 2001; 104(9):1046–1052.

25 Kobayashi T, Hamano K, Li TS, et al. Enhancement of angiogenesis by the implantation of self bone marrow cells in a rat ischemic heart model. J Surg Res 2000; 89(2):189–195.

26 Ikenaga S, Hamano K, Nishida M, et al. Autologous bone marrow implantation induced angiogenesis and improved deteriorated exercise capacity in a rat ischemic hindlimb model. J Surg Res 2001; 96(2):277–283.

27 Strauer BE, Brehm M, Zeus T, et al. Repair of infarcted myocardium by autologous intracoronary mononuclear bone marrow cell transplantation in humans. Circulation 2002; 106(15):1913–1918.

28 Lee SH, Wolf PL, Escudero R, Deutsch R, Jamieson SW, Thistlethwaite PA. Early expression of angiogenesis factors in acute myocardial ischemia and infarction. N Engl J Med 2000; 342(9):626–633.

29 Assmus B, Schachinger V, Teupe C, et al. Transplantation of progenitor cells and regeneration enhancement in acute myocardial infarction (TOPCARE-AMI). Circulation 2002; 106(24):3009–3017.

30 Schachinger V, Assmus B, Britten MB, et al. Transplantation of progenitor cells and regeneration enhancement in acute myocardial infarction: final one-year results of the TOPCARE-AMI Trial. J Am Coll Cardiol 2004; 44(8):1690–1699.

31 Stone GW, Grines CL, Cox DA, et al. Comparison of angioplasty with stenting, with or without abciximab, in acute myocardial infarction. N Engl J Med 2002; 346(13):957–966.

32 Britten MB, Abolmaali ND, Assmus B, et al. Infarct remodeling after intracoronary progenitor cell treatment in patients with acute myocardial infarction (TOPCARE-AMI): mechanistic insights from serial contrast-enhanced magnetic resonance imaging. Circulation 2003; 108(18):2212–2218.

33 Kim RJ, Manning WJ. Viability assessment by delayed enhancement cardiovascular magnetic resonance: will low-dose dobutamine dull the shine? Circulation 2004; 109(21):2476–2479.

34 Fernandez-Aviles F, San Roman JA, Garcia-Frade J, et al. Experimental and clinical regenerative capability of human bone marrow cells after myocardial infarction. Circ Res 2004; 95(7):742–748.

35 Nian M, Lee P, Khaper N, Liu P. Inflammatory cytokines and postmyocardial infarction remodeling. Circ Res 2004; 94(12):1543–1553.

36 Kuethe F, Richartz BM, Sayer HG, et al. Lack of regeneration of myocardium by autologous intracoronary mononuclear bone marrow cell transplantation in humans with large anterior myocardial infarctions. Int J Cardiol 2004; 97(1):123–127.

37 Cleland JG, Freemantle N, Coletta AP, Clark AL. Clinical trials update from the American Heart Association: REPAIR-AMI, ASTAMI, JELIS, MEGA, REVIVE-II, SURVIVE, and PROACTIVE. Eur J Heart Fail 2006; 8(1):105–110.

38 Frazier OH, March RJ, Horvath KA. Transmyocardial revascularization with a carbon dioxide laser in patients with end-stage coronary artery disease. N Engl J Med 1999; 341(14):1021–1028.

39 Allen KB, Dowling RD, Fudge TL, et al. Comparison of transmyocardial revascularization with medical therapy in patients with refractory angina. N Engl J Med 1999; 341(14):1029–1036.

40 Saririan M, Eisenberg MJ. Myocardial laser revascularization for the treatment of end-stage coronary artery disease. J Am Coll Cardiol 2003; 41(2):173–183.

41 Fuchs S, Satler LF, Kornowski R, et al. Catheter-based autologous bone marrow myocardial injection in no-option patients with advanced coronary artery disease: a feasibility study. J Am Coll Cardiol 2003; 41(10):1721–1724.

42 Tse HF, Kwong YL, Chan JK, Lo G, Ho CL, Lau CP. Angiogenesis in ischaemic myocardium by intramyocardial autologous bone marrow mononuclear cell implantation. Lancet 2003; 361(9351):47–49.

43 Perin EC, Dohmann HF, Borojevic R, et al. Improved exercise capacity and ischemia 6 and 12 months after transendocardial

injection of autologous bone marrow mononuclear cells for ischemic cardiomyopathy. Circulation 2004; 110(11 suppl 1): II213–218.

44   Perin EC, Dohmann HF, Borojevic R, et al. Transendocardial, autologous bone marrow cell transplantation for severe, chronic ischemic heart failure. Circulation 2003; 107(18):2294–2302.

45   Thompson CA. Transvascular cellular cardiomyoplasty. Int J Cardiol 2004; 95(suppl 1):S47–49.

46   Thompson CA, Nasseri BA, Makower J, et al. Percutaneous transvenous cellular cardiomyoplasty. A novel nonsurgical approach for myocardial cell transplantation. J Am Coll Cardiol 2003; 41(11):1964–1971.

47   Leobon B, Garcin I, Menasche P, Vilquin JT, Audinat E, Charpak S. Myoblasts transplanted into rat infarcted myocardium are functionally isolated from their host. Proc Natl Acad Sci USA 2003; 100(13):7808–7811.

48   Taylor DA, Atkins BZ, Hungspreugs P, et al. Regenerating functional myocardium: improved performance after skeletal myoblast transplantation. Nat Med 1998; 4(8):929–933.

49   Jain M, DerSimonian H, Brenner DA, et al. Cell therapy attenuates deleterious ventricular remodeling and improves cardiac performance after myocardial infarction. Circulation 2001; 103(14):1920–1927.

50   Makkar RR, Lill M, Chen PS. Stem cell therapy for myocardial repair: is it arrhythmogenic? J Am Coll Cardiol 2003; 42(12):2070–2072.

51   Menasche P, Hagege AA, Vilquin JT, et al. Autologous skeletal myoblast transplantation for severe postinfarction left ventricular dysfunction. J Am Coll Cardiol 2003; 41(7):1078–1083.

52   Herreros J, Prosper F, Perez A, et al. Autologous intramyocardial injection of cultured skeletal muscle-derived stem cells in patients with non-acute myocardial infarction. Eur Heart J 2003; 24(22):2012–2020.

53   Chachques JC, Herreros J, Trainini J, et al. Autologous human serum for cell culture avoids the implantation of cardioverter-defibrillators in cellular cardiomyoplasty. Int J Cardiol 2004; 95(suppl 1):S29–33.

54   Smits PC, van Geuns RJ, Poldermans D, et al. Catheter-based intramyocardial injection of autologous skeletal myoblasts as a primary treatment of ischemic heart failure: clinical experience with six-month follow-up. J Am Coll Cardiol 2003; 42(12):2063–2069.

55   Siminiak T, Kalawski R, Fiszer D, et al. Autologous skeletal myoblast transplantation for the treatment of postinfarction myocardial injury: phase I clinical study with 12 months of follow-up. Am Heart J 2004; 148(3):531–537.

56   Chachques JC, Acar C, Herreros J, et al. Cellular cardiomyoplasty: clinical application. Ann Thorac Surg 2004; 77(3):1121–1130.

57   Koh GY, Soonpaa MH, Klug MG, Field LJ. Long-term survival of AT-1 cardiomyocyte grafts in syngeneic myocardium. Am J Physiol 1993; 264(5 Pt 2):H1727–733.

58   Soonpaa MH, Koh GY, Klug MG, Field LJ. Formation of nascent intercalated disks between grafted fetal cardiomyocytes and host myocardium. Science 1994; 264(5155):98–101.

59   Losordo DW, Dimmeler S. Therapeutic angiogenesis and vasculogenesis for ischemic disease: part II: cell-based therapies. Circulation 2004; 109(22):2692–2697.

60   Losordo DW, Dimmeler S. Therapeutic angiogenesis and vasculogenesis for ischemic disease. Part I: angiogenic cytokines. Circulation 2004; 109(21):2487–2491.

61   Simons M, Annex BH, Laham RJ, et al. Pharmacological treatment of coronary artery disease with recombinant fibroblast growth factor-2: double-blind, randomized, controlled clinical trial. Circulation 2002; 105(7):788–793.

62   Fortuin FD, Vale P, Losordo DW, et al. One-year follow-up of direct myocardial gene transfer of vascular endothelial growth factor-2 using naked plasmid deoxyribonucleic acid by way of thoracotomy in no-option patients. Am J Cardiol 2003; 92(4):436–439.

63   Christman KL, Vardanian AJ, Fang Q, Sievers RE, Fok HH, Lee RJ. Injectable fibrin scaffold improves cell transplant survival, reduces infarct expansion, and induces neovasculature formation in ischemic myocardium. J Am Coll Cardiol 2004; 44(3): 654–660.

64   Nugent HM, Edelman ER. Tissue engineering therapy for cardiovascular disease. Circ Res 2003; 92(10):1068–1078.

65   Kang HJ, Kim HS, Zhang SY, et al. Effects of intracoronary infusion of peripheral blood stem-cells mobilised with granulocyte-colony stimulating factor on left ventricular systolic function and restenosis after coronary stenting in myocardial infarction: the MAGIC cell randomised clinical trial. Lancet 2004; 363(9411):751–756.

66   Wojakowski W, Tendera M, Michalowska A, et al. Mobilization of CD34/CXCR4 + , CD34/CD117 + , c-met + stem cells, and mononuclear cells expressing early cardiac, muscle, and endothelial markers into peripheral blood in patients with acute myocardial infarction. Circulation 2004; 110(20):3213–3220.

67   Harada M, Qin Y, Takano H, et al. G-CSF prevents cardiac remodeling after myocardial infarction by activating the Jak-Stat pathway in cardiomyocytes. Nat Med 2005; 11(3):305–311.

68   Lee SU, Wykrzykowska JJ, Laham RJ. Angiogenesis: bench to bedside, have we learned anything? Toxicol Pathol 2006; 34(1):3–10.

69   Pearlman JD, Laham RJ, Post M, Leiner T, Simons M. Medical imaging techniques in the evaluation of strategies for therapeutic angiogenesis. Curr Pharm Des 2002; 8(16):1467–1496.

70   Jaffer FA, Weissleder R. Seeing within: molecular imaging of the cardiovascular system. Circ Res 2004; 94(4):433–445.

38

The heart failure patient

Basil S. Lewis and Mihai Gheorghiade

Introduction

Management of the heart failure (HF) patient presents a number of challenges to the interventional cardiologist. These include the pharmacologic management of heart failure and special considerations regarding the practical aspects of intervention, including the risk of intervention and the need for the preparation before intervention (HF management, hemodynamic support, renal function). Clinical decision-making regarding further treatment options may be different in the patient with HF.

Pharmacotherapy in the heart failure patient

Heart failure is a progressive syndrome, and optimal pharmacologic management is based on a detailed diagnosis, determination of the etiology, characterization of the clinical syndrome (systolic vs. diastolic) and careful monitoring of the response to pharmacologic therapy. There is a need to modify treatment in accordance with the patient's response to therapy.

Patients with left ventricular systolic dysfunction

Angiotensin-converting enzyme inhibitors

Pathophysiology Drugs acting on the renin–angiotensin–aldosterone system (RAAS) are the cornerstone of treatment in the management of the HF patient with systolic dysfunction. Angiotensin-converting enzyme (ACE) inhibitors interfere with the formation of angiotensin II, both at systemic and tissue level. In chronic HF, activation of the renin–angiotensin system has negative effects on the myocardium and on cardiovascular hemodynamics so that the preload and afterload are increased, and sodium and water are retained (1). The increased production of angiotensin II leads to ventricular hypertrophy, increased myocardial fibrosis, and apoptosis (2). Angiotensin-converting enzyme inhibitors stop the deleterious effects of angiotensin II, and lead to an improvement in the hemodynamic profile and a decrease in cardiac remodeling. They also increase the plasma concentrations of inflammatory cytokines (e.g., bradykinin), nitric oxide, and vasodilating prostaglandins (3).

Hemodynamic effects During treatment with ACE inhibitors, systemic vascular resistance is decreased along with the pulmonary capillary wedge pressure and right atrial pressure (4). End-diastolic and end-systolic dimensions are reduced. Long-term ACE inhibition decreases echocardiographic left ventricle (LV) dimensions and increases the shortening fraction (5).

Clinical effects Angiotensin-converting enzyme inhibitors improve symptoms, New York Heart Association (NYHA) functional class, and exercise capacity in patients with HF. The Captopril Multicenter Research Group (6) showed that captopril treatment improved the NYHA class in 61% of patients compared with only 24% of patients taking placebo over a 12-week period. Treadmill exercise time improved throughout the 12 weeks of the study in 24% of captopril-treated patients, but in none of the placebo-treated patients.

Therapy with ACE inhibitors is associated with a dramatic increase in survival in patients with NYHA class II–IV and in all patients with LV systolic dysfunction after an acute myocardial infarction, even those without the signs or symptoms of HF (Table 1) (7–9). After myocardial infarction, ACE inhibition attenuates ventricular dilation, reduces the incidence and hospitalization for HF, prevents recurrent ischemic events, and increase survival. The decreased recurrence of acute coronary events or stroke (10) with ACE-inhibitor therapy means that these drugs are an essential part of the therapeutic armamentarium in patients undergoing intervention in the circumstances of an acute coronary syndrome, and hence, perhaps in more than half the patients treated in a modern interventional center.

Practical use of ACE inhibitors   Based on the data from published trials, the 2005 American College of Cardiology/ American Heart Association (ACC/AHA) guidelines (11) recommend ACE inhibitors as first-line therapy for symptomatic HF with reduced systolic function and for asymptomatic LV dysfunction. In stage C HF, they should be used in conjunction with a diuretic to maintain the sodium balance and prevent the development of fluid overload. The ACC/AHA recommendations specify that ACE inhibitors should be initiated at very low dose and gradually uptitrated. Patients with HF should not generally be maintained on very low doses of an ACE inhibitor unless these are the only doses

Table 1   Angiotensin-converting enzyme inhibitor trials

Study	Selection criteria	Patients, n	Drug, dosage	Results
Chronic heart failure				
CONSENSUS (7)	NYHA IV cardiomegaly	253	*Enalapril,* 20-mg twice/day, vs. placebo	40% Reduction of overall mortality; significant improvement of NYHA class
SOLVD treatment (8)	NYHA I-IV LVEF < 35%	2569	*Enalapril,* 10-mg twice/day, vs. placebo	16% Reduction of overall mortality; fewer rehospitalizations for worsening HF
SOLVD prevention (9)	Asymptomatic LV dysfunction LVEF < 35%	4228	*Enalapril,* 10-mg twice/day, vs. placebo	No differences on mortality; significant reduction of worsening HF and hospitalizations
Postmyocardial infarction				
SAVE (86)	Acute MI within 3–16 days LVEF < 40% no overt HF	2231	*Captopril,* 50-mg/ three times a day, vs. placebo	19% Reduction of overall mortality; significant reduction of death, hospitalization, and recurrent myocardial infarction
AIRE (87)	Acute MI within 3–10 days Clinical evidence of HF	2006	*Ramipril,* 5-mg twice a day vs. placebo	27% Reduction of overall mortality; significant reduction of severe heart failure, myocardial infarction, and stroke
TRACE (88)	Acute MI within 3–7 days LVEF < 35%	2606	*Trandolapril,* 4-mg once per day, vs. placebo	22% Reduction of overall mortality; lower risk of cardiovascular death, severe HF, and sudden death
SMILE (89)	Acute MI within 24 hrs	1556	Zofenopril vs. placebo	26% Reduction of overall mortality

Abbreviations: AIRE, acute Infarction ramipril efficacy; CONSENSUS, cooperative north scandinavian enalapril survival study; HF, heart failure; LVEF, left ventricular ejection fraction; NYHA, New York Heart Association; SAVE, survival and ventricular enlargement; SMILE, survival of myocardial infarction long-term evaluation; SOLVD, studies of left ventricular dysfunction; TRACE, trandolapril cardiac evaluation study group.

that can be tolerated. Once the appropriate dose has been achieved, patients can be maintained on long-term therapy with an ACE inhibitor with little difficulty. Renal function and serum potassium should be assessed within one to two weeks of initiating therapy and every two to three months thereafter.

Adverse effects   The adverse effects of ACE-inhibitor use are related to angiotensin suppression (hypotension, increase in serum creatinine and potassium) and bradykinin potentiation (cough and angioedema). Initial hypotension would usually respond to a decrease in the dose of diuretic agent or the lowering of the ACE-inhibitor dose. If hypotension persists, the assessment of orthostatic changes in order to properly administer ACE inhibitors may be useful. Treatment should be reassessed if the levels of creatinine are >3.0 mg/dL or if serum potassium is >5.5 mEq/L. The development of a cough is a major reason for the discontinuation of the therapy, but ACE inhibitors should be stopped only if cough is persistent, and should be replaced with an angiotensin II receptor blocker. Pregnant patients should not be administered ACE inhibitors because of the danger of teratogenic effects. A history of angioedema or renal failure during previous exposure to this class of drugs, or severe hypotension with an immediate risk of cardiogenic shock, are contraindications to the prescription of this class of drug.

Beta blockers

Pathophysiology   Long-term and sustained activation of the sympathetic nervous system in the HF patient has detrimental effects on the cardiac function, and on the peripheral circulation, causing vasoconstriction (12) and possibly impairing sodium excretion by the kidney (13). Increased levels of plasma catecholamines cause myocyte hypertrophy and apoptosis (14–16). In the failing heart, there is a β-receptor downsensitizing and uncoupling with the intracellular signaling. Sympathetic activation has shown to be related to arrhythmogenesis and sudden death (17). β blockers act by inhibiting the adverse effects of sympathetic nervous system activation in patients with HF.

Hemodynamic effects   Shortly after the administration of this class of drugs, β-adrenergic blockade can decrease the ventricular contractility and impair sodium excretion, particularly in patients whose cardiac function is already compromised. These early adverse effects may be minimized by the use of β blockers with α-blocking properties; inversely, during long-term treatment, β blockers can improve cardiac performance (17,18). The administration of a β blocker for a longer period of time (three to six months) is associated with

an increase in the stroke volume and cardiac output and decreased pulmonary wedge pressure, right atrial pressure, heart rate, and systemic vascular resistance (19). Cardiac output, initially reduced by short-term treatment, was restored or increased during long-term treatment (20,21).

Left ventricular ejection fraction (LVEF) increases during long-term β-adrenergic blockade, and the magnitude of increase is larger than that with other treatments for HF. This improvement is particularly evident in HF patients who have viable but noncontractile myocardium and has generally been associated with a reduction in LV systolic and diastolic dimensions, suggesting a favorable effect on the process of ventricular remodeling.

Clinical effects   A large number of randomized, double-blind, placebo-controlled trials have shown that the long-term use of β blockers improves the clinical status in patients with HF (22–32) (Table 2) and the ACC/AHA guidelines (11) recommend that β blockers should be routinely prescribed to all patients with asymptomatic LV dysfunction or stable HF caused by LV systolic dysfunction (unless they have a contraindication or have been shown to be intolerant to treatment with these drugs). β blockers should also be used in patients with HF and preserved LV systolic function, particularly when those patients have hypertension, coronary artery disease (CAD) and/or atrial fibrillation.

β Blockers should be initiated at very low doses and increased at two-week intervals to achieve the target doses. Once the target dose is achieved, patients can generally be maintained on long-term treatment with little difficulty. Abrupt withdrawal of β blockers can lead to clinical deterioration and should be avoided, even in hospitalized patients who do not require inotropic support (11). Safe and feasible administration β blockers can be initiated in all classes of HF patients before hospital discharge, as proved in the Initiation Management Predischarge Process for Assessment of Carvedilol Therapy for Heart Failure (IMPACT-HF) trial (33).

Adverse effects   The adverse events associated with β blockers may be avoided by starting treatment at very low doses. However, treatment can be associated with complaints of fatigue and weakness, which usually resolve in a few weeks. Sometimes it is necessary to decrease the dose of the β blocker or diuretic. Symptomatic bradycardia is another serious adverse effect of β blockers, and requires a decrease in the dose or sometimes cardiac pacing to allow the use of this vital medication. Hypotension is another potential side effect; however, it is rarely seen as the therapy is started with a very low dose (3.25 mg twice a day for carvedilol, 1 mg for bisoprolol and 12.5 mg for extended release metoprolol). The administration of ACE inhibitor and diuretic at a different time of day than the β blocker can

Table 2 Major clinical trials with beta blockers

Study	Selection criteria	Patients, n	Drug, dosage	Results
Chronic heart failure				
MDC (22)	Idiopathic cardiomyopathy LVEF < 40%	383	*Metoprolol,* 100 to 150-mg twice or 3 times/day, vs. placebo	34% reduction of mortality and need of transplantation
U.S. Carvedilol Heart Failure Study (27)	NYHA II–IV LVEF < 35%	1094	*Carvedilol,* 25 to 50-mg twice/day, vs. placebo	Significant reduction of mortality and of hospitalization rates
CIBIS II (90)	NYHA III–IV LVEF < 35%	2647	*Bisoprolol,* 5 mg/day, vs. placebo	Significant reduction of mortality, sudden death, and hospitalization rates
MERIT-HF (24)	NYHA II–IV LVEF < 40%	3991	*Metoprolol succinate,* 200 mg/day, vs. placebo	Significant reduction of mortality, sudden death, and deaths for worsening HF
BEST (91)	NYHA III–IV LVEF < 35%	2708	*Bucindolol,* 50 to 100-mg twice/day, vs. placebo	No significant reduction of mortality; only in nonblack patients
COPERNICUS (30)	NYHA III–IV LVE < 35%	2289	*Carvedilol,* 25-mg twice/day, vs. placebo	Significant reduction of mortality; reduction of 24% of composite end points in mortality and rehospitalization
COMET (32)	NYHA class II–IV;LVEF < 35%; at least 1 admission for cardiovascular reason per year	3029	*Carvedilol,* 25-mg twice/day, vs. *Metoprolol* tartrate, 50-mg/day	Hazard ratio 0.83 in favor of carvedilol ($P = 0.0017$); absolute risk reduction 6%
Postmyocardial infarction				
CAPRICORN (31)	Acute myocardial infarction within 3 to 21 years; LVEF < 40%	1959	*Carvedilol,* 25-mg twice/day, vs. placebo	Significant reduction in mortality; absolute risk reduction 3%

Abbreviations: BEST, beta-blocker evaluation survival trial; CAPRICORN, carvedilol postinfarct survival control in left ventricular dysfunction; CIBIS II, Cardiac Insufficiency Bisoprolol Study II; COMET, Carvedilol or Metoprolol European Trial; COPERNICUS, carvedilol prospective randomized cumulative survival; HF, heart failure; LVEF, left ventricular ejection fraction; MDC, metoprolol in dilated cardiomyopathy; MERIT-HF, metoprolol controlled-release randomized intervention trial in congestive heart failure; NYHA, New York Heart Association.

minimize hypotension and dizziness. Patients who exhibit low systolic blood pressure should be evaluated for orthostatic changes. In the absence of orthostatic changes, these patients probably can safely tolerate the addition of β blockers to their ACE inhibitor and diuretic regimen. Administration of β blockers is contraindicated in patients with severe bronchospasm, symptomatic bradycardia, or advanced heart block in the absence of a pacemaker.

Aldosterone antagonists

Pathophysiology In HF patients, the levels of aldosterone are elevated, even in the presence of ACE inhibitors or angiotensin-receptor blockers (34,35). Aldosterone has detrimental effects in HF, such as causing potassium and magnesium loss, sodium retention, baroreceptor dysfunction, and myocardial fibrosis; it also decreases the neuronal uptake of norepinephrine, thereby enhancing the risk of cardiac arrhythmias (36).

Clinical effects   The effects of this drug class have been demonstrated in patients with HF and postmyocardial infarction with ventricular dysfunction (Table 3) (37,38). The Randomized Aldactone Evaluation Study (RALES) study was stopped after interim analysis revealed that the aldosterone antagonist was associated with a significant 30% relative reduction in both mortality and hospitalization for worsening HF. The side effects of spironolactone included gynecomastia or breast pain in 10% of men. Hyperkalemia had been thought to limit the combination of ACE inhibitors and potassium-sparing diuretics, but with careful monitoring, hyperkalemia was uncommon in both the placebo and spironolactone groups (37).

The result of the RALES study has been supported by the Eplerenone postacute myocardial infarction heart failure efficacy and survival study (EPHESUS) trial results (39), but the magnitude of improvement was smaller. In this trial, most patients were treated with β blockers. The mean eplerenone dose achieved (43-mg daily) produced a significant 15% reduction in the all-cause mortality and a significant 13% reduction in cardiovascular deaths or hospitalizations for cardiovascular causes. The benefit was more pronounced in the group of patients who received both ACE inhibitors/angiotensin II receptor blockers and β blockers, and did not exist in the patients who received neither class of drug. There was also a significant 21% reduction in the rate of sudden death from cardiac causes. The only significant complication in the eplerenone group was the rate of serious hyperkalemia (5.5% in the eplerenone vs. 3.9% placebo group).

Indications and clinical use of aldosterone antagonists.   Spironolactone should be added to treatment in patients with recent or current NYHA class IV symptoms, despite the use of ACE inhibitors, β blockers, digoxin, and diuretics as suggested in the ACC/AHA guidelines (11). Recent data suggest that aldosterone-blocking agents may also be used in patients with moderate HF. Contraindications to aldosterone antagonists include hyperkalemia (serum potassium levels >5 mEq/L) or renal insufficiency (creatinine >2.5 mg/dL).

Adverse effects   Renal function may deteriorate with the decreased circulating fluid volume, especially after the addition of another diuretic drug acting on the RAAS system, and careful monitoring of serum creatinine is essential. Serum potassium should be monitored within one week of initiation and at least every four weeks for the first three months and every three months thereafter. It should also be monitored at any dose change in spironolactone or if there is a change in concomitant medications that affects the potassium balance. The spironolactone dose (standard 25 mg per day) should be reduced if potassium levels are <5.4 mEq/L, and treatment should be discontinued if painful gynecomastia or serious renal dysfunction or hyperkalemia result.

Angiotensin II receptor blockers

Pathophysiology   Angiotensin-receptor blockers block the action of angiotensin II at the receptor level, and hence, block the effects of angiotensin II produced in addition by the chymase pathway. Current angiotensin II receptor blockers block the angiotensin II type I receptors (associated with hypertrophy and

Table 3   Trials with aldosterone-blocking drugs

Study	Selection criteria	Patients, n	Drug, dosage	Results
Chronic heart failure				
RALES (92)	NYHA III–IV LVEF < 35% Treatment with ACE inhibitors and loop diuretics	1663	*Spironolactone*, 25-mg daily, vs. placebo	Significant reduction of all causes of mortality; absolute risk reduction 11%; lower risk of hospitalization for worsening HF
Acute myocardial infarction				
EPHESUS (38)	AMI within 3–14 days LVEF < 40%; diabetes, signs of HF	6642	*Eplerenone*, 50-mg daily, vs. placebo	Significant reduction of all causes of mortality; absolute risk reduction 2.3%; reduction of rates of deaths and of hospitalization for cardiovascular causes

Abbreviations: ACE, angiotensin-converting enzyme; AMI, acute myocardial infarction; EPHESUS, eplerenone postacute myocardial infarction heart failure efficacy and survival study; HF, heart failure; LVEF, left ventricular ejection fraction; NYHA, New York Heart Association; RALES, randomized aldactone evaluation study.

remodeling) and enhance the activation of angiotensin II type 2 receptors, causing vasodilation (40). As some of the side effects of the ACE inhibitors, such as angioedema and dry nonproductive cough, may be bradykinin related, an angiotensin II receptor blocker could, theoretically, provide the same beneficial effects as an ACE inhibitor, with fewer side effects.

Effects on mortality and hospitalization   Table 4 summarizes the recent trials of angiotensin II receptor

blockers (41–48). In several clinical settings and placebo-controlled clinical trials of patients with chronic HF, angiotensin II receptor blockers produced hemodynamic, neurohormonal, and clinical effects similar to those obtained with ACE inhibitors. Among symptomatic HF patients with low LVEF enrolled in the Candesartan in Heart Failure: Assessment of Reduction in Mortality and Morbidity (CHARM-Added) trial, the addition of candesartan to a recommended dose of ACE inhibitor and other treatment individually reduced cardiovascular mortality and the risk of

Table 4   Trials with angiotensin-receptor blocking drugs

Study	Selection criteria	Patients, n	Drug, dosage	Results
Chronic heart failure				
ELITE (41)	Age > 65 years NYHA II–IV LVEF < 0.40	722	*Losartan*, 50 mg daily, vs. *Captopril*, 50 mg/3 times/day	Lower rates of deaths in Losartan group
ELITE II (42)	Age > 60 years NYHA II–IV LVEF < 0.40	3152	*Losartan*, 50 mg daily, vs. *Captopril*, 50 mg/3 times/day	No reduction of overall mortality; trend in reduction of sudden death and cardiac arrest in captopril group
Val-HeFT (43)	NYHA II–IV LVEF < 0.40 LV dilatation	5010	*Valsartan*, 160 mg twice/day, vs. placebo	No reduction in overall mortality; reduction of composite end point and number of hospitalization
CHARM-Added (47)	NYHA II–IV LVEF < 0.40 adjunctive to ACE inhibitors	2548	*Candesartan*, 32 mg/day vs. placebo	Absolute risk reduction 4%; trend toward lower in all cause mortality ($P = 0.086$)
CHARM-Alternative (46)	NYHA II–IV LVEF < 0.40 Intolerance to ACE inhibitors	2028	*Candesartan*, 32 mg/day vs. placebo	Absolute risk reduction 7%; trend toward lower in all cause mortality ($P = 0.11$)
Acute myocardial infarction				
OPTIMAAL (44)	Age > 50 years Acute MI with signs of HF LVEF < 0.35 or LV dilatation or anterior Q waves	5477	*Losartan*, 50 mg daily, vs. *Captopril*, 50 mg/3 times/day	No significant difference between the two groups; significant reduction of cardiovascular mortality in captopril group
VALIANT (48)	Acute MI within 24 hours 10 days; signs of HF; LVEF < 0.40; systolic BP >100 mmHg	14,703	Valsartan, 160 mg, daily vs. captopril, 50 mg, 3 times/day vs. captopril, 50 mg, 3 times/day plus valsartan, 160 mg, daily	No differences in all causes of mortality between valsartan and captopril; no differences in all causes of mortality between combined therapy vs. captopril.

Abbreviations: ACE, angiotensin-converting enzyme; CHARM, candesartan in heart failure; assessment of reduction in mortality and morbidity; ELITE, evaluation of losartan in the elderly; HF, heart failure; LVEF, left ventricular ejection fraction; MI, myocardial infarction; NYHA, New York Heart Association; OPTIMAAL, optimal trial in myocardial infarction with angiotensin II antagonist losartan; Val-HeFT, valsartan in heart failure trial; VALIANT, valsartan in acute myocardial infarction trial.

admission to hospital for HF, and reduced the risk of each of the secondary composite outcomes (47). The benefits of candesartan were similar in all predefined subgroups, with no evidence of heterogeneity of treatment effect, including patients receiving baseline β-blocker treatment.

Effects after myocardial infarction   In patients with evidence of LV dysfunction early after myocardial infarction, the Valsartan in Acute Myocardial Infarction Trial (VALIANT) (48) demonstrated that valsartan had a benefit that was not inferior to that of ACE inhibitors without an advantage in terms of tolerability. However, the addition of an angiotensin II receptor blocker to an ACE inhibitor did not improve the outcomes and resulted in more side effects.

Indications and use of angiotensin II receptor blockers   The ACC/AHA guidelines (11) recommend that angiotensin II receptor blockers should be used as an alternative first-line therapy if a patient is intolerant to ACE inhibitors with symptomatic LV dysfunction. The addition of an angiotensin II receptor blocker is advised in the case of persistent symptoms despite conventional therapy. In the recent ACC/AHA guidelines, the combination of an angiotensin II receptor blocker, an ACE inhibitor, and aldosterone is not recommended because of the adverse effects. When starting the therapy with angiotensin II receptor blockers, it is important to begin with the minimal dose and then double it. Blood pressure, potassium, and renal function should be assessed within two weeks after beginning therapy. For stable patients, it is reasonable to add β-blocking agents before full target doses of either ACE inhibitors or angiotensin II receptor blockers are reached.

Adverse effects   The adverse effects include hypotension, worsening renal function, and hyperkalemia. The ACE inhibitors should remain the first-choice treatment in patients after complicated acute myocardial infarction.

Diuretics

Pathophysiology   Non-potassium-sparing diuretics are the treatment of choice to reduce fluid retention and dyspnea. Acting at specific sites of nephrons, they inhibit sodium and water reabsorption. Loop diuretics act on the loop of Henle, producing a maximal diuretic effect equivalent to 20% to 25% of the filtered sodium load and promoting the free water clearance. Currently available loop diuretics include furosemide, bumetanide, torsemide, and ethacrynic acid. Because of their potency, they are generally effective in patients with advanced renal insufficiency (glomerular filtration rates <25 ml/min) (49).

Distal tubular diuretics, with the exception of metolazone, are generally six to eight times less potent than loop diuretics, and are usually reserved for hypertensive patients with mild fluid retention. They are less effective as the glomerular filtration rates decrease to levels <25–30 mL per minute. They are classified into potassium-wasting (thiazides, chlorthalidone, and metolazone) and potassium-sparing diuretics (triamterene, amiloride, and spironolactone, eplerenone). Potassium-wasting diuretics decrease sodium reabsorption in the cortical segment of the ascending limb of the loop of Henle and the distal convoluted tubule, and are associated with an increase in urinary potassium excretion. Potassium-sparing diuretics are not potent when used alone, but may be used to avoid the potassium-wasting effects of diuretics that act at more proximal nephron sites. Thiazides and distal tubule diuretics have longer half-lives that allow them to be given once daily or even every other day (e.g., metolazone). The plasma half-life of loop diuretics ranges from one to four hours. Once a dose of a loop diuretic has been administered, its effect dissipates before the next dose is given. During this time, the nephron avidly reabsorbs sodium, resulting in rebound sodium retention that nullifies the prior natriuresis (49). Combined diuretic therapy, using judicious doses of diuretics, acting (i) on the loop of Henle and also on the (ii) proximal and (iii) distal tubule, invariably produces adequate diuresis in patients resistant to individual drugs.

Clinical effects   Several trials have demonstrated the ability of diuretics to decrease the signs of fluid retention in patients with HF. In these short-term studies, diuretic use has led to a reduction in jugular venous pressures, pulmonary congestion, peripheral edema, and body weight, all observed within days (50–52). Diuretics have been shown to improve cardiac function, symptoms, and exercise tolerance in patients with HF. Diuretics activate the neurohormonal vasoconstrictor systems that have been implicated in the progression of the disease, increasing plasma renin activity and concentrations of angiotensin II, aldosterone, and norepinephrine (53). Long-term diuretic use also decreases the circulating concentrations of the vasodilating natriuretic peptides. This imbalance may partially explain the development of progressive diuretic resistance that may be a feature of advanced HF.

Indications   Appropriate administration of diuretics is crucial for the success of the other drugs being used. The ACC/AHA guidelines (11) recommend diuretics to be prescribed to all patients who have an evidence of fluid retention, and that they should be combined with an ACE inhibitor and a β blocker (and usually digoxin). Therapy is initiated with low doses, and the dose is increased until urine output increases and weight decreases, generally by 0.5–1.0 kg per day. The treatment goal is to eliminate the physical signs of fluid retention. Once fluid retention has resolved, treatment with the diuretic should be maintained to prevent the recurrence of volume overload. The dose should be adjusted periodically, allowing the patient to make changes in dose if weight increases or decreases beyond a specified range.

Adverse effects   Adverse effects include hypotension and/or diminished renal perfusion, leading to the development of prerenal azotemia or acute intrinsic renal failure that may resolve by decreasing the diuretic dose. Hypokalemia and hypomagnesemia may increase the risk of life-threatening ventricular arrhythmias in patients with HF, and may contribute to the incidence of sudden death, particularly during treatment with digoxin. Usually, the use in combination with ACE inhibitors, and if appropriate, spironolactone will minimize potassium loss. Magnesium and/or potassium supplements can be given as needed. If hypotension or azotemia is observed, the rapidity of diuresis could be reduced, but diuresis should be maintained until fluid retention is eliminated. Diuretics may also cause metabolic alkalosis, carbohydrate intolerance, hyperuricemia, hypersensitivity reactions, and acute pancreatitis. It is prudent to use the lowest dose of diuretic that helps control congestion and perhaps use torsemide, which has a more predictable bioavailability and may be safer than furosemide.

Digitalis

Pathophysiology   Digoxin exerts its effects by the inhibition of sodium-potassium adenosine triphosphatase (Na-K-ATPase). In the myocardium, this results in an increase in intracellular calcium and increased myocardial contraction (54). The inhibition of Na-K-ATPase in the vagal afferent fibers sensitizes the cardiac baroreceptors, reducing the sympathetic outflow from the central nervous system. By inhibiting Na-K-ATPase in the kidney, digoxin reduces the renal tubular reabsorption of sodium, resulting in the suppression of renin secretion from the kidneys (55,56). These observations have led to the hypothesis that digoxin acts in HF primarily by attenuating the activation of neurohormonal systems and not as a positive inotropic drug.

Clinical effects   In HF patients, digoxin has been proven to reduce symptoms, improve NYHA class, increase exercise time, modestly increase LVEF, enhance cardiac output, and decrease HF hospitalizations (56,57). The Randomized Assessment of Digoxin on Inhibitors of the Angiotensin-Converting Enzyme (RADIANCE) (58) and Prospective Randomized study Of Ventricular Failure and the Efficacy of Digoxin (PROVED) (59) trials demonstrated that these beneficial effects are lost when digoxin is withdrawn from the medical therapy. Digoxin withdrawal has been associated

with an increased hospitalization rate; decreased exercise time and LVEF; and increased heart rate, body weight, and cardiothoracic ratio on chest X ray.

Effects on mortality and hospitalization   The Digitalis Investigation Group (DIG) trial (60) tested the effects of digoxin on survival in patients with HF in normal sinus rhythm. The trial enrolled 7788 patients, of whom 87% had systolic dysfunction. They were randomized to a mean dose of 0.25 mg of digoxin or placebo, with a background therapy of ACE inhibitors and diuretic agents. Before enrollment, less than 50% of the patients were not receiving digoxin. For both groups, the all-cause mortality was 35%, and the cardiovascular mortality was 30%. There was a trend toward a decrease in mortality caused by HF in patients with a serum digoxin level of <1 ng/mL (60). In multivariable analysis, digoxin was associated with a significantly higher risk of death among women, but it had no significant effect among men. However, because serum digoxin concentrations were measured in less than 33% of patients at one month, the trial had insufficient statistical power to test whether the interaction between sex and digoxin therapy was independent of sex-based differences in serum digoxin concentration. Recent retrospective cohort analysis of the combined PROVED and RADIANCE databases indicates that patients with a low-serum digoxin concentration (0.5–0.9 ng/mL) were no more likely to have worsening symptoms of HF on maintenance of digoxin than those with moderate (0.9–1.2 ng/mL) or high (>1.2 ng/mL) serum digoxin concentrations (61). All serum digoxin concentration groups were significantly less likely to deteriorate during follow-up study compared with the patients withdrawn from digoxin.

Use of digoxin   Digoxin can be used to reduce symptoms in patients despite treatment with an ACE inhibitor and a β blocker. In patients not taking ACE inhibitors or β blockers, treatment with digoxin should not be stopped, but appropriate therapy with the neurohormonal antagonists should be instituted. In case of atrial fibrillation with a rapid ventricular rate, the β-blocker dose rather than the digoxin dose should be increased, because higher serum digoxin concentrations are associated with increased adverse effects. The digoxin dose should be low (0.125 mg per day), because this dose is shown to control the symptoms and is safe. The drug should be used cautiously in patients who are taking medications that can depress atrioventricular conduction and should not be used in patients with significant sinus or atrioventricular block, unless they have a pacemaker.

Adverse events   The major side effects include cardiac arrhythmias (e.g., ectopic and re-entrant cardiac rhythms and heart block); gastrointestinal symptoms (e.g., anorexia, nausea, and vomiting); and neurologic complaints (e.g., visual disturbances, disorientation, and confusion). Digitalis toxicity is commonly associated with serum digoxin levels >2 ng/mL, but they may occur with lower digoxin levels, especially if hypokalemia, hypomagnesemia, or hypothyroidism are present.

Hydralazine–isosorbide dinitrate

Pathophysiology Hydralazine and isosorbide dinitrate are effective vasodilators which may interfere with the biochemical and molecular mechanisms responsible for the progression of HF. Combined use may interfere with the development of nitrate tolerance (62).

Clinical benefits and effects on mortality and hospitalization Whether used alone or in combination, hydralazine and isosorbide dinitrate decrease the preload and afterload, decrease mitral regurgitation, improve cardiac output, increase exercise capacity, modestly increase LVEF, and prolong survival in patients with HF (63,64). V-Heart Failure Trial (HeFT) II (64) showed that enalapril had a major benefit on survival when compared with the combination of hydralazine–isosorbide dinitrate with enalapril in patients with predominantly NYHA class II–III. The African Americans in Heart Failure Trial (A-HeFT) (65) showed a beneficial effect of adding vasodilator therapy to African-American patients already treated with ACE inhibitors, β blockers, and spironolactone. There are no results with the same strategy in other patient groups.

Use of hydralazine–isosorbide dinitrate In the ACC/AHA guidelines (11), the combined use of hydralazine–isosorbide dinitrate may be considered as a therapeutic option in patients with reduced LV dysfunction already taking ACE inhibitors and β blockers and with persistent symptoms. Despite the lack of data about this vasodilator combination in patients who are intolerant of ACE inhibitors, the combined use of hydralazine and isosorbide dinitrate may be considered as an additive therapeutic option in such patients. However, compliance with this combination has generally been poor because of the large number of tablets required and the high incidence of adverse reactions.

Adverse events Adverse events are few and include headache and dizziness.

Calcium antagonists

Although calcium antagonists have anti-ischemic properties and cause systemic vasodilatation, they have not demonstrated sustained improvement in patients with HF, and

worsening symptoms and increased mortality have been reported, possibly because of their negative inotropic effect and reflex neurohormonal activation (66,67). Amlodipine and felodipine appear to have less negative inotropic effects and do not have the deleterious effects seen with first-generation drugs in this class. Amlodipine had no significant effect on the mortality in the subset of patients with coronary artery disease, as shown in the first Prospective Randomized Amlodipine Survival Evaluation (PRAISE I) (68). Based on the available data, calcium antagonists are not recommended for the treatment of HF (11). Diltiazem, verapamil, and nifedipine should be avoided in patients with HF with reduced systolic function. The vasculoselective agents, such as amlodipine, may be considered for the management of hypertension in patients with LV systolic dysfunction who are also receiving standard HF therapy.

Antiarrhythmic drugs

Pathophysiology Sudden cardiac death, frequently resulting from ventricular arrhythmias, accounts for 40–50% of mortality in these patients (69). After the increased mortality seen in the Cardiac Arrhythmia Suppression Trial (CAST) (70) and in CAST II (71), class I antiarrhythmics are currently contraindicated in the treatment of patients with HF (70). Amiodarone is an antiarrhythmic agent with low proarrhythmic potential and a favorable hemodynamic profile and in the Grupo de Estudio de la Sobrevida en la Insuficiencia Cardiaca en Argentina (GESICA) trial (72), amiodarone 300 mg per day, combined with standard therapy in patients with NYHA class II–IV, was associated with a 28% reduction in the risk of death and a 31% reduction in the combined risk of death or hospitalization for worsening HF in patients with advanced disease. There was a trend toward a reduction in the risk of death because of progressive HF and the risk of sudden death. The European Myocardial Infarct Amiodarone Trial (EMIAT) (73) assessed the effect of amiodarone versus placebo in patients after myocardial infarction with an LVEF <0.40%. Sudden death, however, was decreased by 35% with amiodarone, whereas the all-cause mortality was not reduced in these patients. A favorable interaction was apparent between the concomitant use of β blockers and cardiac mortality, independent of LV function. Because of the conflicting evidence and its known toxicity, the prophylactic use of amiodarone to prevent sudden cardiac death in patients with HF is not recommended in the current ACC/AHA guidelines (11). It should be used in combination with a β blocker and an implantable cardioverter defibrillator in patients with a history of sudden death, ventricular fibrillation, or sustained ventricular tachycardia. Patients on amiodarone therapy should be monitored for the occurrence of thyroid, ocular, pulmonary, or hepatic abnormalities. Thyroid and liver function tests, in addition to chest X-ray, should be assessed at baseline and every six months during therapy. Pulmonary function tests should be obtained at baseline and repeated only if the findings on follow-up chest X-ray are abnormal. Patients taking amiodarone, digoxin, and warfarin should be carefully monitored for drug interactions.

Atrial fibrillation is one of the most frequent arrythmias that HF patients experience. The Atrial Fibrillation Follow-up Investigation of Rhythm Management (AFFIRM) did not demonstrate any benefit from rhythm control in patients with HF or depressed LVEF (74). If indicated for the treatment of symptomatic atrial arrhythmias, amiodarone should be used because of its demonstrated safety in patients with HF. Device implantation rather than pharmacologic treatment is the mainstay of preventive therapy for sudden cardiac death among patients with HF (75).

Anticoagulation and antiplatelet drugs

Pathophysiology   In large studies, the risk of thromboembolism in clinically stable patients has been 1–3% per year, including those with very low LVEF and echocardiographic evidence of intracardiac thrombi (76,77). Because the benefit–risk ratio is low, anticoagulation is not justified in these patients. The Warfarin and Antiplatelet Therapy in Chronic Heart Failure (WATCH) study set out to evaluate the role of aspirin, clopidogrel, and warfarin to prevent major cardiovascular event and death in patients with HF, but low enrollment in the trial precluded definitive conclusions about efficacy. In the absence of definitive trials, it is not clear how anticoagulants should be prescribed in patients with HF. According to the ACC/AHA guidelines (11), anticoagulation with warfarin is justified in patients with HF and paroxysmal or chronic atrial fibrillation and/or a previous embolic event. It should not be prescribed in patients who are in normal sinus rhythm, even with a low LVEF. Antiplatelet treatment is generally recommended in patients with arterial disease, although the role of aspirin is still debated.

Treatment of comorbidity

A number of drugs should be avoided in HF, including antiarrhythmic agents, calcium channel blockers, antipsychotics, antihistamines, corticosteroids, and nonsteroidal anti-inflammatory drugs. Metformin and thiazolidinediones should be used with caution in HF with diabetes. Trials of statins have generally excluded patients with symptomatic HF, but two studies with morbidity and mortality outcomes in HF are now under way.

Anemia is a frequent finding in HF patients, and treatment improves outcome (78). There is a growing interest in the use of erythropoietic agents and iron supplementation to treat anemia in HF, and outcome trials are planned. Some patients with HF also have thiamine deficiency.

Patients with preserved systolic function

A few clinical trials are available to guide the management of patients with HF and relatively preserved LVEF (79–81). The CHARM-preserved trial evaluated the addition of candesartan to the treatment regimen for patients with symptomatic mild HF and relatively preserved LVEF, significantly reduced morbidity but did not reach the primary end point (45). In the absence of other controlled clinical trials, the management of these patients is based on the control of physiologic factors (blood pressure, heart rate, blood volume, and myocardial ischemia) that are known to exert important effects on ventricular relaxation (11). Many patients with HF and normal LVEF are treated with ACE inhibitors, β blockers, angiotensin II receptor blockers, digitalis, and diuretics because of the presence of comorbid conditions (i.e., atrial fibrillation, hypertension, diabetes mellitus, and coronary artery disease).

Special issues regarding heart failure patients in the interventional laboratory

Orthopnea

With proper pharmacotherapy and optimization of overall clinical status, most patients will be able to overcome the problem of orthopnea for the duration of interventional procedure. Diuretic therapy preintervention may be useful. In the very ill patient with hemodynamic compromise, and where intervention may lead to an improvement in cardiac function, supportive measure, such as intra-aortic balloon counterpulsation, pressure monitoring, or ventilation may be necessary during the acute phase of the illness.

Renal function

The contrast load may compound renal damage, common in HF patients, with consequent further fluid retention and worsening HF. A number of adjunctive treatments are currently recommended in the renal patient but none guarantee renal protection (82). The volume of contrast medium during intervention should be minimized and hypotension should be avoided.

Iso-osmolar or low-osmolar contrast medium is recommended, and it appears to be associated with a lower renal complication rate. Serum creatinine level should be measured 24 to 48 hours after the administration of the contrast medium. Nonsteroidal anti-inflammatory drugs and diuretics should be withheld for at least 24 hours before and after exposure to contrast medium, if possible, and adequate hydration guaranteed. Concomitant treatment with the antioxidant N-acetylcysteine (600-mg twice daily) may reduce the incidence of deterioration in renal function (83) but the results of clinical trials, although promising, have not all been consistent (84). Renal risk is compounded in the diabetic patient, where meticulous attention to detail regarding all these issues should be applied. Biguanides (such as metformin, which increases the acidotic load) should be avoided where possible prior to intervention (85).

Summary and conclusions

The HF patient presents a special challenge to the interventional cardiologist. The procedure may be challenging and complicated by technical difficulties regarding patient ability to undergo the procedure and complications, such as procedurally induced HF and renal failure. On the other hand the potential benefit of revascularization regarding survival in patients with HF owing to coronary disease is high and rewarding.

References

1. Bristow MR, Port JD, Kelly RA. Inhibitors of the renin-angiotensin-aldosterone system. In: Braunwald E, Libby P, Zipes DD, Zipes DP, eds. Heart Disease: A Textbook of Cardiovascular Medicine. Philadelphia: WB Saunders, 2001:582–583.
2. Bastien NR, Juneau AV, Ouellette J, Lambert C. Chronic AT I receptor blockade and angiotensin-converting enzyme (ACE) inhibition in (CHF 146) cardiomyopathic hamsters: effects on cardiac hypertrophy and survival. Cardiovasc Res 1999; 43:77–85.
3. Brown NJ, Ryder D, Gainer JV, Morrow JD, Nadeau J. Differential effects of angiotensin converting enzyme inhibitors on the vasodepressor and prostacyclin responses to bradykinin. J Pharmacol Exp Ther 1996; 279:703–712.
4. LeJemtel TH, Keung E, Frishman WH, Ribner HS, Sonnenblick EH. Hemodynamic effects of captopril in patients with severe chronic heart failure. Am J Cardiol 1982; 49:1484–1488.
5. Konstam MA, Kronenberg MW, Rousseau MF, et al. Effects of the angiotensin converting enzyme inhibitor enalapril on the long-term progression of left ventricular dilatation in patients with asymptomatic systolic dysfunction. SOLVD (Studies of Left Ventricular Dysfunction) Investigators. Circulation 1993; 88:2277–2283.
6. The-Captopril-Multicenter-Research-Group. A placebo-controlled trial of captopril in refractory chronic congestive heart failure. J Am Coll Cardiol 1983; 2:755–763.
7. The_CONSENSUS_Trial_Study_group. Effects of enalapril on mortality in severe congestive heart failure. Results of the Cooperative North Scandinavian Enalapril Survival Study (CONSENSUS). N Engl J Med 1987; 316:1429–1435.
8. The-SOLVD-Investigators. Effect of enalapril on survival in patients with reduced left ventricular ejection fractions and congestive heart failure. N Engl J Med 1991; 325:293–302.
9. The-SOLVD-Investigators. Effect of enalapril on mortality and the development of heart failure in asymptomatic patients with reduced left ventricular ejection fractions. N Engl J Med 1992; 327:685–691.
10. Heart_Outcomes_Prevention_Evaluation_Study_Investigators. Effects of ramipril on cardiovascular and microvascular outcomes in people with diabetes mellitus: results of the HOPE study and MICRO-HOPE substudy. Lancet 2000; 355:253–259.
11. Hunt SA, Abraham WT, Chin MH, et al. ACC/AHA 2005 Guideline update for the diagnosis and management of chronic heart failure in the adult: a report of the American College of Cardiology/American Heart Association Task Force on Practice Guidelines (Writing Committee to Update the 2001 Guidelines for the Evaluation and Management of Heart Failure): developed in collaboration with the American College of Chest Physicians and the International Society for Heart and Lung Transplantation: endorsed by the Heart Rhythm Society. Circulation 2005; 112:e154–235.
12. Smith KM, Macmillan JB, McGrath JC. Investigation of b1 adrenergic receptor subtypes mediating vasoconstriction in rabbit cutaneous resistance arteries. Br J Pharmacol 1997; 122:825–832.
13. Elhawary AM, Pang CC. b1-Adrenergic receptors mediate renal tubular sodium and water reabsorption in the rat. Br J Pharmacol 1994; 111:819–824.
14. Hasenfuss G, Holubarsch C, Blanchard EM, Mulieri LA, Alpert NR, Just H. Influence of isoproterenol on myocardial energetics: experimental and clinical investigations. Basic Res Cardiol 1989; 84:S147–S155.
15. Knowlton KU, Michel MC, Itani M, et al. The 1A -adrenergic receptor subtype mediates biochemical, molecular, and morphologic features of cultured myocardial cell hypertrophy. J Biol Chem 1993; 268:15374–15380.
16. Communal C, Singh K, Pimentel DR, Colucci WS. Norepinephrine stimulates apoptosis in adult rat ventricular myocytes by activation of the b-adrenergic pathway. Circulation 1998; 98:1329–1334.
17. Eichhorn EJ, Bristow MR. Medical therapy can improve the biologic properties of the chronically failing heart: a new era in the treatment of heart failure. Circulation 1996; 94:2285–2296.
18. Di Lenarda A, Sabbadini G, Salvatore L. Long-term effects of carvedilol in idiopathic dilated cardiomyopathy with persistent left ventricular dysfunction despite chronic metoprolol. The Heart-Muscle Disease Study Group. J Am Coll Cardiol 1999; 33:1926–1934.
19. Metra M, Giubbini R, Nodari S, Boldi E, Modena MG, Dei Cas L. Differential effects of beta-blockers in patients with heart failure: a prospective, randomized, double-blind comparison of the long-term effects of metoprolol versus carvedilol. Circulation 2000; 102:546–551.
20. Waagstein F, Caidahl K, Wallentin I, Bergh CH, Hjalmarson A. Long-term beta-blockade in dilated cardiomyopathy. Effects of short- and long-term metoprolol treatment followed by withdrawal and readministration of metoprolol. Circulation 1989; 80:551–563.

21 Olsen SL, Gilbert EM, Renlund DG, Taylor DO, Yanowitz FD, Bristow MR. Carvedilol improves left ventricular function and symptoms in chronic heart failure: a double-blind randomized study. J Am Coll Cardiol 1995; 25:1225–1231.

22 Waagstein F, Bristow MR, Swedberg K, et al. Beneficial effects of metoprolol in idiopathic dilated cardiomyopathy. Metoprolol in Dilated Cardiomyopathy (MDC) Trial Study Group. Lancet 1993; 342:1441–1446.

23 The-RESOLVD-Investigators. Effects of metoprolol CR in patients with ischemic and dilated cardiomyopathy. The randomized evaluation of strategies for left ventricular dysfunction pilot study. Circulation 2000; 101:378–384.

24 Hjalmarson A, Goldstein S, Fagerberg B, et al. Effects of controlled-release metoprolol on total mortality, hospitalizations, and well-being in patients with heart failure: the Metoprolol CR/XL Randomized Intervention Trial in congestive heart failure (MERIT-HF). MERIT-HF Study Group. JAMA 2000; 283:1295–302.

25 CIBIS-Investigators-and-Committees. A randomized trial of beta-blockade in heart failure. The Cardiac Insufficiency Bisoprolol Study (CIBIS). Circulation 1994; 90:1765–1773.

26 CIBIS-Investigators-and-Committees. The Cardiac Insufficiency Bisoprolol Study II (CIBIS-II): a randomised trial. Lancet 1999; 353:9–13.

27 Packer M, Bristow MR, Cohn JN, et al. The effect of carvedilol on morbidity and mortality in patients with chronic heart failure. U.S. Carvedilol Heart Failure Study Group. N Engl J Med 1996; 334:1349–1355.

28 Goldstein S, Fagerberg B, Hjalmarson A, et al. Metoprolol controlled release/extended release in patients with severe heart failure: analysis of the experience in the MERIT-HF study. J Am Coll Cardiol 2001; 38:932–938.

29 The-Beta-Blocker-Evaluation-of-Survival-Trial-Investigators. A Trial of the beta-blocker bucindolol in patients with advanced chronic heart failure. N Engl J Med 2001; 344:1659–1667.

30 Packer M, Coats AJ, Fowler MB, et al. Effect of carvedilol on survival in severe chronic heart failure. N Engl J Med 2001; 344:1651–1658.

31 Dargie HJ. Effect of carvedilol on outcome after myocardial infarction in patients with left-ventricular dysfunction: the CAPRICORN randomised trial. Lancet 2001; 357:1385–1390.

32 Poole-Wilson PA, Swedberg K, Cleland JG, et al. Comparison of carvedilol and metoprolol on clinical outcomes in patients with chronic heart failure in the Carvedilol Or Metoprolol European Trial (COMET): randomised controlled trial. Lancet 2003; 362:7–13.

33 Gattis WA, O'Connor CM, Gallup DS, Hasselblad V, Gheorghiade M. Predischarge initiation of carvedilol in patients hospitalized for decompensated heart failure: results of the Initiation Management Predischarge: Process for Assessment of Carvedilol Therapy in Heart Failure (IMPACT-HF) trial. J Am Coll Cardiol 2004; 43:1534–1541.

34 Struthers AD. Why does spironolactone improve mortality over and above an ACE inhibitor in chronic heart failure? Br J Clin Pharmacol 1999; 47:479–482.

35 Jorde UP, Vittorio T, Katz SD, Colombo PC, Latif F, Le Jemtel TH. Elevated plasma aldosterone levels despite complete inhibition of the vascular angiotensin-converting enzyme in chronic heart failure. Circulation 2002; 106:1055–1057.

36 Zannad F, Alla F, Dousset B, Perez A, Pitt B. Limitation of excessive extracellular matrix turnover may contribute to survival benefit of spironolactone therapy in patients with congestive heart failure: insights from the randomized aldactone evaluation study (RALES). Rales Investigators. Circulation 2000; 102:2700–2706.

37 Pitt B, Zannad F, Remme WJ, et al. The effect of spironolactone on morbidity and mortality in patients with severe heart failure. Randomized Aldactone Evaluation Study Investigators. N Engl J Med 1999; 341:709–717.

38 Pitt B, Remme W, Zannad F, et al. Eplerenone, a selective aldosterone blocker, in patients with left ventricular dysfunction after myocardial infarction. N Engl J Med 2003; 348:1309–1321.

39 Pitt B, Remme W, Zannad F, et al. The_Eplerenone Post–Acute Myocardial Infarction Heart Failure Efficacy and Survival Study Investigators. Eplerenone, a selective aldosterone blocker, in patients with left ventricular dysfunction after myocardial infarction. N Engl J Med 2003; 348:1309–1321.

40 Burnier M. Angiotensin II type 1 receptor blockers. Circulation 2001; 103:904–912.

41 Pitt B, Segal R, Martinez FA, et al. Randomised trial of losartan versus captopril in patients over 65 with heart failure (Evaluation of Losartan in the Elderly Study, ELITE). Lancet 1997; 349:747–752.

42 Pitt B, Poole-Wilson PA, Segal R, et al. Effect of losartan compared with captopril on mortality in patients with symptomatic heart failure: randomised trial—the Losartan Heart Failure Survival Study ELITE II. Lancet 2000; 355:1582–1587.

43 Cohn JN, Tognoni G. A randomized trial of the angiotensin-receptor blocker valsartan in chronic heart failure. N Engl J Med 2001; 345:1667–1675.

44 Dickstein K, Kjekshus J. Effects of losartan and captopril on mortality and morbidity in high-risk patients after acute myocardial infarction: the OPTIMAAL randomised trial. optimal trial in myocardial infarction with angiotensin II antagonist Losartan. Lancet 2002; 360:752–760.

45 Yusuf S, Pfeffer MA, Swedberg K, et al. Effects of candesartan in patients with chronic heart failure and preserved left-ventricular ejection fraction: the CHARM-Preserved trial. Lancet 2003; 362:777–781.

46 Granger CB, McMurray JJ, Yusuf S, et al. Effects of candesartan in patients with chronic heart failure and reduced left-ventricular systolic function intolerant to angiotensin-converting-enzyme inhibitors: the CHARM-Alternative trial. Lancet 2003; 362: 772–776.

47 McMurray JJ, Ostergren J, Swedberg K, et al. Effects of candesartan in patients with chronic heart failure and reduced left-ventricular systolic function taking angiotensin-converting-enzyme inhibitors: the CHARM-Added trial. Lancet 2003; 362:767–771.

48 Pfeffer MA, McMurray JJ, Velazquez EJ, et al. Valsartan, captopril, or both in myocardial infarction complicated by heart failure, left ventricular dysfunction, or both. N Engl J Med 2003; 349:1893–1906.

49 Brater DC. Pharmacology of diuretics. Am J Med Sci 2000; 319:38–50.

50 Patterson JH, Adams KF Jr, Applefeld MM, Corder CN, Masse BR. Oral torsemide in patients with chronic congestive heart failure: effects on body weight, edema, and electrolyte

excretion. Torsemide Investigators Group. Pharmacotherapy 1994; 14:514–521.

51 Cosin J, Diez J. Torasemide in chronic heart failure: results of the TORIC study. Eur J Heart Fail 2002; 4:507–513.

52 Murray MD, Deer MM, Ferguson JA, et al. Open-label randomized trial of torsemide compared with furosemide therapy for patients with heart failure. Am J Med 2001; 111:513–520.

53 Bayliss J, Norell M, Canepa-Anson R, Sutton G, Poole-Wilson P. Untreated heart failure: clinical and neuroendocrine effects of introducing diuretics. Br Heart J 1987; 57:17–22.

54 Gheorghiade M, Ferguson D. Digoxin: a neurohormonal modulator in heart failure? Circulation 1991; 84:2181–2186.

55 Kjeldsen K, Norgaard A, Gheorghiade M. Myocardial Na, K-ATPase: the molecular basis for the hemodynamic effect of digoxin therapy in congestive heart failure. Cardiovasc Res 2002; 55:710–713.

56 Eichhorn EJ, Gheorghiade M. Digoxin. Prog Cardiovasc Dis 2002; 44:251–266.

57 Tauke J, Goldstein S, Gheorghiade M. Digoxin for chronic heart failure: a review of the randomized controlled trials with special attention to the PROVED (Prospective Randomized Study of Ventricular Failure and the Efficacy of Digoxin) and RADIANCE (Randomized Assessment of Digoxin on Inhibitors of the angiotensin Converting Enzyme) trials. Prog Cardiovasc Dis 1994; 37:49–58.

58 Packer M, Gheorghiade M, Young JB, et al. Withdrawal of digoxin from patients with chronic heart failure treated with angiotensin-converting-enzyme inhibitors. RADIANCE Study. N Engl J Med 1993; 329:1–7.

59 Uretsky BF, Young JB, Shahidi FE, Yellen LG, Harrison MC, Jolly MK. Randomized study assessing the effect of digoxin withdrawal in patients with mild to moderate chronic congestive heart failure: results of the PROVED trial. PROVED Investigative Group. J Am Coll Cardiol 1993; 22:955–962.

60 The_Digitalis_Investigation_group. The effect of digoxin on mortality and morbidity in patients with heart failure. N Engl J Med 1997; 336:525–533.

61 Rathore SS, Curtis JP, Wang Y, Bristow MR, Krumholz HM. Association of serum digoxin concentration and outcomes in patients with heart failure. JAMA 2003; 289:871–878.

62 Bauer JA, Fung HL. Concurrent hydralazine administration prevents nitroglycerin-induced hemodynamic tolerance in experimental heart failure. Circulation 1991; 84:35–39.

63 Cohn JN, Archibald DG, Ziesche S, et al. Effect of vasodilator therapy on mortality in chronic congestive heart failure. Results of a Veterans Administration Cooperative Study (V-HeFT). N Engl J Med 1986; 314:1547–1552.

64 Cohn JN, Johnson G, Ziesche S, et al. A comparison of enalapril with hydralazine-isosorbide dinitrate in the treatment of chronic congestive heart failure. N Engl J Med 1991; 325:303–310.

65 Taylor AL, Ziesche S, Yancy C, et al. Combination of isosorbide dinitrate and hydralazine in blacks with heart failure. N Engl J Med 2004; 351:2049–2057.

66 Elkayam U, Amin J, Mehra A, Vasquez J, Weber L, Rahimtoola SH. A prospective, randomized, double-blind, crossover study to compare the efficacy and safety of chronic nifedipine therapy with that of isosorbide dinitrate and their combination in the treatment of chronic congestive heart failure. Circulation 1990; 82:1954–1961.

67 Goldstein RE, Boccuzzi SJ, Cruess D, Nattel S. Diltiazem increases late-onset congestive heart failure in postinfarction patients with early reduction in ejection fraction. The Adverse Experience Committee; and the Multicenter Diltiazem Postinfarction Research Group. Circulation 1991; 83:52–60.

68 Packer M, O'Connor CM, Ghali JK, et al. Effect of amlodipine on morbidity and mortality in severe chronic heart failure. Prospective Randomized Amlodipine Survival Evaluation Study Group. N Engl J Med 1996; 335:1107–1114.

69 Chakko CS, Gheorghiade M. Ventricular arrhythmias in severe heart failure: incidence, significance, and effectiveness of antiarrhythmic therapy. Am Heart J 1985; 109:497–504.

70 Echt DS, Liebson PR, Mitchell LB, et al. Mortality and morbidity in patients receiving encainide, flecainide, or placebo. The Cardiac Arrhythmia Suppression Trial. N Engl J Med 1991; 324:781–788.

71 The-Cardiac-Arrhythmia-Suppression-Trial-II-Investigators. Effect of the antiarrhythmic agent moricizine on survival after myocardial infarction. N Engl J Med 1992; 327:227–233.

72 Doval HC, Nul DR, Grancelli HO, Perrone SV, Bortman GR, Curiel R. Randomised trial of low-dose amiodarone in severe congestive heart failure. Grupo de Estudio de la Sobrevida en la Insuficiencia Cardiaca en Argentina (GESICA). Lancet 1994; 344:493–498.

73 Julian DG, Camm AJ, Frangin G, et al. Randomised trial of effect of amiodarone on mortality in patients with left-ventricular dysfunction after recent myocardial infarction: EMIAT. European Myocardial Infarct Amiodarone Trial Investigators. Lancet 1997; 349:667–674.

74 Wyse DG, Waldo AL, DiMarco JP, et al. A comparison of rate control and rhythm control in patients with atrial fibrillation. N Engl J Med 2002; 347:1825–1833.

75 Kadish A, Dyer A, Daubert JP, et al. Prophylactic defibrillator implantation in patients with nonischemic dilated cardiomyopathy. N Engl J Med 2004; 350:2151–2158.

76 Dunkman WB, Johnson GR, Carson PE, Bhat G, Farrell L, Cohn JN. Incidence of thromboembolic events in congestive heart failure. The V-HeFT VA Cooperative Studies Group. Circulation 1993; 87:VI94–101.

77 Cioffi G, Pozzoli M, Forni G, et al. Systemic thromboembolism in chronic heart failure. A prospective study in 406 patients. Eur Heart J 1996; 17:1381–1389.

78 Silverberg DS, Wexler D, Blum M, et al. Erythropoietin in heart failure. Semin Nephrol 2005; 25:397–403.

79 Zile MR, Brutsaert DL. New concepts in diastolic dysfunction and diastolic heart failure: Part I: diagnosis, prognosis, and measurements of diastolic function. Circulation 2002; 105:1387–1393.

80 Zile MR, Brutsaert DL. New concepts in diastolic dysfunction and diastolic heart failure: Part II: causal mechanisms and treatment. Circulation 2002; 105:1503–1508.

81 Aurigemma GP, Gaasch WH. Clinical practice. Diastolic heart failure. N Engl J Med 2004; 351:1097–1105.

82 Barrett BJ, Parfrey PS. Clinical practice. Preventing nephropathy induced by contrast medium. N Engl J Med 2006; 354:379–386.

83 Tepel M, van der Giet M, Schwarzfeld C, Laufer U, Liermann D, Zidek W. Prevention of radiographic-contrast-agent-induced reductions in renal function by acetylcysteine. N Engl J Med 2000; 343:180–184.

84   Nallamothu BK, Shojania KG, Saint S, et al. Is acetylcysteine effective in preventing contrast-related nephropathy? A meta-analysis. Am J Med 2004; 117:938–947.

85   Nawaz S, Cleveland T, Gaines PA, Chan P. Clinical risk associated with contrast angiography in metformin treated patients: a clinical review. Clin Radiol 1998; 53:342–344.

86   Pfeffer MA, Braunwald E, Moye LA, et al. Effect of captopril on mortality and morbidity in patients with left ventricular dysfunction after myocardial infarction. Results of the survival and ventricular enlargement trial. The SAVE Investigators. N Engl J Med 1992; 327:669–677.

87   The-Acute-Infarction-Ramipril-Efficacy-(AIRE)-Study-Investigators. Effect of ramipril on mortality and morbidity of survivors of acute myocardial infarction with clinical evidence of heart failure. The Acute Infarction Ramipril Efficacy (AIRE) Study Investigators. Lancet 1993; 342:821–828.

88   Kober L, Torp-Pedersen C, Carlsen JE, et al. A clinical trial of the angiotensin-converting-enzyme inhibitor trandolapril in patients with left ventricular dysfunction after myocardial infarction. Trandolapril Cardiac Evaluation (TRACE) Study Group. N Engl J Med 1995; 333:1670–1676.

89   Ambrosioni E, Borghi C, Magnani B. The effect of the angiotensin-converting-enzyme inhibitor zofenopril on mortality and morbidity after anterior myocardial infarction. The Survival of Myocardial Infarction Long-Term Evaluation (SMILE) Study Investigators. N Engl J Med 1995; 332:80–85.

90   CIBIS-II-Investigators-and-Committees. The Cardiac Insufficiency Bisoprolol Study II (CIBIS-II): a randomised trial. Lancet 1999; 353:9–13.

91   Beta-Blocker-Evaluation-of-Survival-Trial-Investigators. A trial of the beta-blocker bucindolol in patients with advanced chronic heart failure. N Engl J Med 2001; 344:1659–1667.

92   Pitt B, Zannad F, Remme W, et al. The effect of spironolactone on morbidity and mortality in patients with severe heart failure. Randomized Aldactone Evaluation Study Investigators. N Engl J Med 1999; 341:709–717.

39

The acute coronary syndrome patient

John F. Moran

In light of recent developments, a great deal of new material on the acute coronary syndrome (ACS) has been published in the last few years. The data focuses on the best treatment for the ACS patient in addition to diagnosis, prognosis, and risk stratification (1,2). The importance of this information is based on the prevalence of ACS and its complications (3). Nearly 1.7 million patients are hospitalized every year in the United States with ACS (4). Nearly 20 years ago, it was discussed that angiographic morphology of the stenosis was more important than the stenosis severity (5). From this angiographic viewpoint, clinical, biochemical, and histological information has developed for ACS patients.

The ACS patient can fit into one of the three clinical syndromes: unstable angina, non-ST segment elevation myocardial infarction (NSTEMI), and ST-segment elevation myocardial infarction (STEMI). These are differentiated by the threat or degree of myocardial necrosis. The chest pain accompanying the syndromes can be constricting, squeezing, burning, or a heavy feeling in the chest. It can occur across the chest and radiate to one or both arms and to the teeth, cheeks, and neck. It can go down the forearm to the fingers or in the interscapular area. The chest pain can be precipitated by exercise, excitement, stress, cold weather, or after meals. It is often relieved by rest or sublingual nitroglycerin. Any or all of these anatomic areas can be involved.

Atypical chest pain is more common in females. The females are more likely to have chest pain at rest, or sleep, or with periods of mental stress. They are more likely to have neck and shoulder pains. Fatigue, dyspnea, and nausea with vomiting are often present (6).

Braunwald's clinical classification of chest pain refines the discomforts of unstable angina (7). The severity of the chest pain is divided into three classes:

1. New onset angina pectoris or accelerated angina pectoris but no rest pain.
2. Angina pectoris at rest within the past month but not in the past 48 hours.
3. Angina at rest and within the past 48 hours.

The clinical circumstances can differ:

1. Developing in the presence of an extra cardiac condition that intensifies ischemia.
2. Angina can develop postmyocardial infarction before any treatment or after drug treatment.
3. Finally, unstable angina can develop with or without electrocardiographic changes.

This grouping of clinical syndromes are compatible with myocardial ischemia, and a prompt visit to the emergency department is indicated. Electrocardiograms in the emergency department would differentiate a NSTEMI from a STEMI, the latter suggesting a greater degree of myocardial ischemia.

The usual coronary risk factors are important as well. Hypertension, cigarette smoking, diabetes, hypercholesterolemia are the main coronary risk factors sought after in the history taken in the emergency department.

Antman developed a thrombosis in myocardial infarction (TIMI) risk score based on a database of 15,078 patients with STEMI or new onset of complete left bundle branch block (8). The score was validated in the TIMI 9 data set. Ten characteristics of these patients accounted for 97% of the predictive capacity of their multivariate model. These are included in the risk score (Table 1). Points were given for difference parameters as listed in Table 1. The risk score had a strong association with 30-day mortality. There was a greater >40-fold increase in mortality from TIMI risk score 0 to >8 at 30 days (Table 1) (8). The TIMI risk score is easy to apply and can be done at the bedside.

When clinical findings are added to biomarkers, these characteristics further define the high-risk patient who will especially benefit from an aggressive strategy. The patients presenting characteristics have an impact on early decision making, including transfer to a tertiary care center of the high-risk patient.

Table 1 TIMI risk score for ST-segment elevation myocardial infarction	
Age 65–74	2 points
>75	3 points
DM, HTN, angina	1 point
SBP <100	3 points
HR >100	2 points
Killip class II–IV	2 points
Weight <67 kg	1 point
Anterior STEMI at LBBB	1 point
Time to RX >4 hours	1 point
Risk score = Total	(0–14)

Abbreviations: DM, diabetes mellitus; HR, heart rate; HTN, hypertension; LBBB, left bundle branch block; SBP, systolic blood pressure; STEMI, ST-segment elevation myocardial infarction.

Biomarkers

Biomarkers help establish the presence of myocardial necrosis. There are nearly two dozen biomarkers currently under study. Most experience is with creatinine kinase, creatinine kinase MB, troponin I or T, and myoglobin. Others are under study (Fig. 1) (3). Two other biomarkers currently available are C-reactive protein (CRP) and brain natriuretic peptide (BNP).

Even minor elevations of troponin I or T have had prognostic importance. In the tactics TIMI 18 study, troponin levels between 0.1 ng/mL and more than 1.5 ng/mL were found in 60% of the 1821 patients (9). In this study, troponin T>0.1 ng/mL was found in 54% of the study patients. Patients with troponins greater than 0.1 were at a significantly increased risk of death or recurrent ischemia at 30 days (11.7% vs. 5.5%, *P* < 0.001) and at six months (20.1% vs. 14.2% *P* < 0.001). These values were independent of age, creatinine kinase (CK) MB, or electrocardiographic changes. In the Tactics TIMI 18 study, these patients with increased troponin levels benefited from an early invasive strategy with upstream tirofiban—a 39% relative risk reduction of the primary end point (9). Elevated troponins identified high-risk patients with more complicated coronary artery disease with thrombus (9). No benefits of an early aggressive strategy was seen in troponin negative patients. Higher troponin levels were associated with a greater thrombus burden.

Ohtani et al. used coronary angioscopy to evaluate 62 patients with ACS (10). These patients were divided into troponin-positive and troponin-negative patients. Higher troponin levels were associated with a greater thrombus burden. They found that the prevalence of thrombus, large thrombus, and yellow plaques were all higher in troponin T-positive patients than in negative patients.

Troponin levels are an important addition to stratify risk in the ACS patient with history and electrocardiographic changes. However, abnormal troponins are found in other conditions as well, notably pulmonary embolus and sepsis, when ACS patients are excluded. These authors suggest that elevated troponin levels are not specific for ACS (11). This requires clinical evaluation (Table 2).

Although troponin elevation suggests necrosis, biomarkers of myocardial ischemia are equally important. Ischemia-modified albumin was reported to be highly sensitive for a diagnosis of ischemia in patients with chest pain presenting to the emergency room (12). Further study needs to be done on this sensitive biomarker for myocardial ischemia.

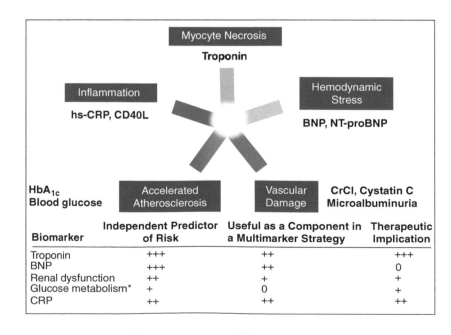

Biomarker	Independent Predictor of Risk	Useful as a Component in a Multimarker Strategy	Therapeutic Implication
Troponin	+++	++	+++
BNP	+++	++	0
Renal dysfunction	++	+	+
Glucose metabolism*	+	0	+
CRP	++	++	++

Figure 1
Predictors of risk, multimarker strategy, and therapeutic implications listed for their contribution to the atherosclerotic process. *Abbreviations*: BNP, brain natriuretic peptide; CRP, C-reactive protein; NT, N-terminal. *Source*: From Ref. 3.

Table 2 Nonthrombotic causes for elevated cardiac troponin level diagnosis

Demand ischemia
    Sepsis/systemic inflammatory response syndrome
    Hypotension
    Hypovolemia
    Supraventricular tachycardia/ atrial fibrillation
    Left ventricular hypertrophy
Myocardial ischemia
    Coronary vasospasm
    Intracranial hemorrhage or Stroke
    Ingestion of sympathomimetic agents
Direct myocardial damage
    Cardiac contusion
    Direct current cardioversion
    Cardiac infiltrative disorders
    Chemotherapy
    Myocarditis
    Pericarditis
    Cardiac transplantation
Myocardial strain
    Congestive heart failure
    Pulmonary embolism
    Pulmonary hypertension or emphysema
    Strenuous exercise
Chronic renal insufficiency

Transient myocardial ischemia was evaluated in 112 patients undergoing the Bruce protocol exercise stress testing. Technetium tetrofosmin scans were obtained and BNP levels were assessed before, during, and four hours after exercise (13). If patients had no inducible ischemia, BNP levels were low at baseline, 43 pg/mL, and unchanged during and after exercise. However, in patients with inducible ischemia, BNP levels rose from a median 62 to 92 pg/mL and nearly returned to baseline at four hours postexercise. Patients with severe ischemia had median BNP levels at baseline, 101 pg/mL and increased to 123 pg/mL. These were still elevated four hours postexercise to 115 pg/mL. Differences were based on the BNP levels. Patients with no ischemia (43 pg/mL), mild to moderate ischemia (60–92 pg/mL), and severe ischemia (101 pg/mL) were statistically different. These differences were increased with exercise stress (13).

In this study, N-terminal pro-BNP (NT-pro-BNP), circulating BNP, and N-terminal pro- atrial natriuretic peptide (NT-pro-ANP) were measured before and after exercise. The BNP levels are as given earlier. The BNP levels differed across the ischemic categories at all three time points. They shared an approximate 25% change from the baseline. Both NT-pro-BNP and NT-pro-ANP rose with ischemia but did not differ statistically in this study (13). The difference in BNP were more pronounced after exercise stress testing and were categorized as mild to moderate severity on the tetrosfosmin scan scores. Although coronary angiograms can demonstrate significant anatomic coronary artery disease, transient myocardial ischemia was associated with a brief release of BNP (13).

Ischemia results from an imbalance of oxygen supply and demand. In patients with ACS, multiple studies of atheroma have implicated inflammation as a critical part of the syndrome. Signs of inflammation in animal models and humans occur with lipid accumulation in the artery wall and plaque development. Plaque rupture and thrombosis have abruptly narrowed or occluded the coronary arteries precipitating ACS (14).

In many histologic studies, signs of inflammation occur with lipid deposition in the artery wall. An atherogenic diet can result in endothelial cells expressing surface adhesion molecules that would bind leukocytes. Superficial vascular cell adhesion molecule binds leukocytes found in atheroma, both human and animal. Augmented wall stress, that is, at arterial bifurcations, can promote smooth muscle cells to produce proteoglycans. Proteoglycans can retain and bind lipoprotein particles facilitating the oxidation of particles and thus promote inflammation at that site in the artery. Adherent leukocytes can penetrate the intima of the artery. Once inside the wall, monocytes scavenge lipids and become foam cells. T cells can elaborate tumor necrosis factor which would further stimulate macrophages, endothelial cells, and smooth muscle cells. The activated leukocytes produce more factors that promote smooth muscle cells and a dense extracellular matrix seen in the advanced atherosclerotic plaque. Macrophages also produce tissue factor, a major factor in thrombosis. Inflammation can lead to plaque disruption and thrombosis formation which can narrow or occlude the artery. Much evidence exists that shows inflammation is involved in plaque developments, progression, and thrombosis (14).

Many mediators of inflammation have been identified—cytokines: IL-6, tumor necrosis factor alpha; cell adhesion molecules: intracellular adhesion molecule-1 (ICAM-1), P-selectin; and acute phase reactants: CRP, fibrinogen, serum amyloid A, and soluble CD40 (Fig. 1) (3). Myeloperoxidase is an enzyme secreted from monocytes, neutrophils, and macrophages. A single measurement taken from patient with chest pain in the emergency department predicted the early risk of myocardial infarction and the risk of major cardiac of ends in the next 30 days to six months (15).

These authors felt that myloperoxidase was good for the prediction of ACS, because it is released by leukocytes, and is elevated and active in vulnerable plaques. It has also been mechanistically associated with factors that effect plaque development and stability. Myloperoxidase was independent of CRP in this study (15). Renal dysfunction and abnormal glucose metabolism were also the predictors of risk (2,3).

At this time, an important inflammatory biomarker is high sensitivity CRP. It can identify inflammation, and inflammation predicts the prognosis in patients with ACS (16). It is possible that CRP is a marker for atherosclerosis and not atherothrombosis. A study of 2554 patients with angina, but not myocardial infarction, found that CRP significantly correlated with the extent of coronary vascular disease. But it was a small association ($r = 0.02$–0.08). This suggested that the angiographic coronary artery disease and the level of CRP are independent. A high CRP and severe coronary artery disease had the highest risk in the five-year follow up. However, CRP retained a high predictive risk for myocardial infarction or death in the follow up regardless of the extent of coronary artery disease. There was a tenfold difference between the lowest level and the highest level of CRP (2.5% vs. 24%) (17). This suggests that CRP is a measure of the inflamed unstable plaque. The risk for myocardial infarction or death here was high if CRP was high and coronary artery disease less severe. In fact, this was a higher risk than the risk in those patients who had severe coronary artery disease and a low CRP level in this study (17).

The CRP and the inflammation it reflects play a key of role in plaque instability. Mauriello et al. studied 30 autopsy cases: 16 patients dying of acute myocardial infarction within 72 hours of symptom onset; five age-matched patients dying of cardiac causes but who had stable angina; and nine age-matched control cases dying of noncardiac causes who had no cardiac history (18). Autopsies were done within 12 to 24 hours of death. Morphometric analysis showed a greater plaque area in the acute myocardial infarction group compared with the other two groups of patients. A thrombus was found in all 16 patients with acute myocardial infarctions that involved the culprit artery and the infarcted myocardium. The cap of the plaque with the thrombus had ruptured in 14 cases and was attached to plaque erosion in two cases. The culprit plaque showed a necrotic lipid core, a thin fibrous cap, and a large inflammatory infiltrate of macrophage foam cells, CD68-positive and CD3-positive lymphocytes. In addition, the acute myocardial infarction group had 109 vulnerable plaques per patient compared with three or four vulnerable plaques in the other two groups of patients. There was no difference in inflammatory infiltrates between the ruptured and vulnerable plaques in the acute myocardial infarction group. Even stable plaques had more inflammation in the acute myocardial infarction group than the plaques in the other two groups of patients. The entire coronary tree of the acute myocardial infarction patient had three to four times the inflammatory infiltrates as the other two groups (18). This work suggests that a diffuse inflammatory process is at work in acute myocardial infarction. If the inflammatory process is diffuse, coronary blood flow could be reduced on a global basis.

Gibson et al. used the technique of corrected TIMI frame counts from the angiogram of patients with acute myocardial infarction enrolled in the four TIMI trials (TIMI 4, 10A, 10B, and 14) (19). The number of angiographic frames that the contrast needs to reach an anatomic landmark were counted. In all trials, the nonculprit artery frame count was 30.9 ± 15 at 90 minutes compared with a normal frame count of 21 ± 3.1. The nonculprit artery flow was 45% slower than normal. Abnormal nonculprit artery flow, 90 minutes after thrombolysis in three TIMI trials, was associated with more wall-motion abnormalities and a poorer outcome (19). The role of reinfarction is unclear but the presence of diffuse inflammation and multiple vulnerable plaques could be a significant finding.

In a comparison of thrombolysis and angioplasty, reinfarction after thrombolysis (6.3% compared with angioplasty 1.6%) worsens the patient's outcome (20). The improved outcome here was driven by a reduction in the rate of reinfarction. If coronary blood flow by cine frame count improved in the culprit artery, the flow also improved in the nonculprit arteries (19). This suggests that the active inflammatory infiltrate is a dynamic phenomenon.

In another study of 45 patients with ACS, the relationship between plaque rupture, CRP, and prognosis was investigated with intravascular ultrasound (21). These 45 patients had a first acute myocardial infarction with or without ST segment elevation. Intravascular ultrasound was performed in the patients before any percutaneous coronary intervention and within six hours of symptoms (21). The remaining coronary vasculature was examined within one month. Forty-five culprit arteries and 84 other coronary arteries were examined with intravascular ultrasound. They found that plaque ruptures in 47% of the arteries at the culprit site in the acute phase of the myocardial infarction. In addition, intravascular ultrasound revealed 17 occult plaque ruptures at remote sites in 24% of the patients (21). These findings suggest that some patients with acute myocardial infarctions have multiple plaque ruptures in other coronary arteries and the culprit artery.

The CRP levels were determined in these patients. It was higher in patients with plaque rupture (21 patients) compared with those without plaque rupture (24 patients)—3.1 ± 0.5 mg/L versus 1.9 ± 0.4 mg/L ($P = 0.04$). This suggests that an elevated CRP reflects an inflammatory process that can lead to plaque rupture. The CRP seems to have independent predictive capacity for identifying inflammation here. There is also a possibility that CRP may release factors that further weaken the plaque's fibrous cap and allow rupture or erosion (16).

Hong et al. studied the site of plaque ruptures in patients with three-vessel coronary artery disease utilizing intravascular ultrasound. They studied 206 patients scheduled for coronary intervention: 99 patients with STEMI, 37 with NSTEMI, 22 patients with Braunwald Class IIIB unstable angina, and 48 stable angina pectoris patients (22). Plaque ruptures in the left anterior descending coronary arteries occurred mostly in the segments 10 to 40 mm from the ostia (83%) as did the plaques in the right coronary artery, 10 to

40 mm from the ostia (48%). The left circumflex plaque ruptures were evenly distributed throughout the artery. Plaque ruptures follow the distribution of coronary artery disease as seen by the intravascular ultrasound. They also occurred at branch points or high stress areas (50%).

To study the interaction between atherothrombosis and inflammation, Monaco et al. selected 40 consecutive patients with Braunwald class IIIB unstable angina and 30 consecutive patients with severe peripheral arterial disease (23). They found more severe obstructive disease in the peripheral arterial disease patients than in the coronary arteries of the unstable angina patients. The levels of thrombin–antithrombin III complexes and d dimers were twice as high in peripheral arterial disease patients as in the unstable angina patients. However, the levels of CRP and IL-6 were significantly higher in patients with unstable angina than they were in peripheral arterial disease patients. Neutrophil activation and myeloperoxidase were also elevated in the unstable angina group. So more markers of thrombosis were found in the peripheral arterial disease patients with severe ischemic disease and more markers of inflammation in the unstable angina patients with lesser occlusive coronary artery disease (23). The data is graphed in Figure 2. Unstable angina had a marked up regulation of inflammatory markers. This suggests that the ACS may result from a transient upregulation of inflammation rather than the atherosclerotic burden. Still it is unclear at this time whether widespread coronary inflammation is a process that leads to plaque rupture or is the result of plaque rupture or both (24).

Plaque ruptures in the ACS setting are often involved with a diffuse process. Inflammation is involved in plaque growth and development in addition to complications of plaque rupture. These could be considered the result of injury. Well-known coronary risk factors can provide the impetus for plaque development. Cigarette smoking, hypertension, hyperlipidemia, hyperglycemia, or insulin resistance are noxious stimuli. The stimuli can facilitate monocyte attachment to endothelial cells. Eventually monocytes migrate to the subintimal space and become foam cells to initiate plaque development.

Multiple biomarkers are under study. Well-studied and commercially available biomarkers include CK-MB, troponin I or T, CRP, and BNP, and recently, myeloperoxidase. Each of these biomarkers is an independent predictor of death, myocardial infarction, or congestive heart failure. Utilizing the opus TIMI 16 patients, Sabatine et al. studied CRP, BNP, and troponin in 450 patients. These authors found a 30-day risk of death increased in proportion to the number of these biomarkers that were elevated at baseline (25). They validated the concept in the tactics TIMI 18 patients (26). These two trials of over 2000 patients with NSTEMI, troponin, CRP, and BNP provided independent prognostic information.

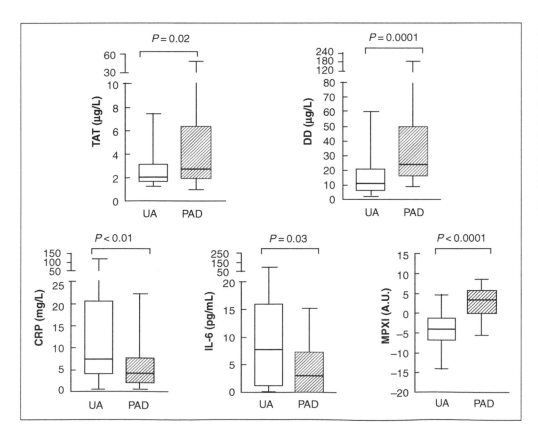

Figure 2

Graphs of the differences in the coagulation cascade and circulating biomarkers and unstable angina (*open bars*) and peripheral arterial disease (*shaded boxes*).
Abbreviations: CRP, C-reactive protein; DD, D-dimer; IL, interleukin; MPXI, myeloperoxidase index; TAT, thrombin–antithrombin. *Source*: From Ref. 23.

However, in addition, there was a doubling of mortality risk for each additional elevated biomarker (25).

Troponin assays are more sensitive than creatinine kinase for myocardial necrosis. Brain natriuretic peptide is released from the ventricles by increased wall stress. In ACS, BNP rises rapidly, and increased levels on days 2–7 identify patients with a poor survival (27). Mega et al. in the ENTIRE TIMI 23 study of 483 patients with STEMI evaluated CRP, BNP, and troponin I at baseline for their prognostic value (27). Troponin I or T are assays of myonecrosis, whereas CRP reflects the underlying inflammation, and BNP is elevated in left ventricular overload. In this study by Mega et al., BNP was a greater indication of mortality risk and risk assessment than either troponin or CRP. Troponin T, at the time of presentation, predicted two to three times the increase in mortality at 30 days, whereas elevated CRP was not predictive in the short term. Patients with high BNP had a greater mortality. The ENTIRE TIMI 23 trial showed full-dose Tenecteplase (TNK)-type tissue plasminogen activator, and enoxaparin had a 30-day mortality of 4.4%, whereas TNK and unfractionated heparin had a 30-day mortality of 15.9% (28). These also suggest that a high BNP identifies appropriate candidates for primary percutaneous coronary angioplasty (27).

These data support an earlier study on the important predictive value of BNP (29). The BNP levels predicted the risk of death and nonfatal cardiac events across the spectrum of ACS. The BNP levels were supportive of other high risk factors: age greater than 75 years; Killip class two, three, or four; ST-segment deviation greater than 1.0 mm; new complete left bundle branch block; troponin I, greater than 1.5 ng/mL (29).

There are differences in BNP levels according to age, body mass, gender, and renal function (30). In the Tactics TIMI 18 study, 34% of the patients were women. In that study, women had lower CK-MB, lower TnT and TnI levels, and higher hs-CRP and BNP levels (31).

There are also questions regarding the use of BNP and NT-pro-BNP. Richards et al. made a comparison study of BNP and NT-pro-BNP in 1049 patients with heart failure (32). They found a correlation coefficient that was very good ($r = 0.90$, $r^2 = 0.81$) between BNP and NT-pro-BNP. The values closely correlated and exhibited parallel changes across the range of left ventricular ejection fractions, age, and renal function. Neither marker was more influenced than the other by age, gender, or renal function. Nor was one more sensitive than the other. Brain natriuretic peptide may reflect more rapidly hemodynamic changes. But NT-pro-BNP may be more reliable if Natrecor is used as therapy (32). In the United States, 80% to 90% of the institutions use BNP, whereas in Europe, it is the reverse (31). The absolute values of BNP and NT-pro-BNP differ markedly and should not be used interchangeably. Hospitals ought to use one or the other.

These biomarkers represent a response to injury and may reflect the degree of ischemia. In a substudy of the platelet receptor inhibition for ischemic syndrome management (PRISM) trial, Heeschen et al. found that ACS patients with low

NT-pro-BNP at baseline showed no difference in the rate of death or MI between control and the Tirofiban-treated patients (33). However, a high borderline pro-BNP in ACS patients was associated with an increased event rate. These rates tended to be reduced by Tirofiban at 48 hours (0.5% vs. 2.5% $P < 0.02$) (33). These differences persisted up to 30 days of follow up. However, if Troponin T was negative and the NT-pro-BNP was elevated, these patients were at high risk but received no benefit from Tirofiban (33). If an elevated pro-BNP at baseline persisted at 72 hours, these patients had a mortality of 9.3% compared with a negative NT-pro-BNP patients of 0.6%. Serial measurements were valuable here.

Morrow et al. followed unstable angina patients with BNP levels up to four and twelve months. The BNP levels greater than 80 pg/mL were strongly associated with poor survival (34). A persistently elevated BNP of greater than 80 pg/mL was associated with the highest risk of death of new congestive heart failure. If the BNP was normal at baseline and greater than 80 pg/mL at four months, these patients had a fourfold increase in the risk of death or new congestive heart failure (34). This would suggest that BNP elevations reflect a greater ischemic burden or possibly left ventricular dysfunction. These data also suggest that important clinical prognostic information is available in serial BNP measurements. In the A to Z trial, simvastatin had no effect on the BNP levels. Patients in this trial were younger than 80 years and did not have significant renal disease. In their BNP model, CRP attenuated the relationship with death or new congestive heart failure (34). The A to Z trial compared high-dose simvastatin to a lower dose, whereas the pravastatin or atorvastatin evaluation and infection therapy (PROVE-IT) trial compared 80 mg of atorvastatin to 40 mg of pravastatin in patients with ACS (35).

In contrast to A to Z trial, the CRP levels fell from a median of 12.3 mg/L at baseline to 2.1 mg/L in the pravastatin group and 1.3 mg in the atorvastatin group in the PROVE-IT TIMI 22 trial (36). The primary end point of all caused death, myocardial infarction, and unstable angina requiring hospitalization was 26.3% in the pravastatin and 22.4% in the atorvastatin group. This represents a 16% reduction in the hazard ratio, favoring atorvastatin.

In the 80-mg simvastatin dose group in the A to Z trial, CRP levels fell from 20.1 to 1.7 at four months and 1.5 at eight months ($P < 0.001$) (36). Higher-dose simvastatin resulted in lower CRP levels. In PROVE-IT (35), A to Z (36), and MIRACL trials (37), higher doses of statin medications resulted in lower low-density cholesterol (LDL) and a better outlook. Higher doses of statin also caused greater falls in CRP levels. This suggests a role for inflammation in these ACS patients (37).

To further study the destabilized or possibly injured plaque, Toutouzas et al. measured plaque temperatures in 19 patients with ACS and 23 patients with stable angina (38). Temperature differences between the plaque and the proximal vessel wall were measured with a thermography catheter. Patients with ACS had greater temperature differences than patients with stable angina (ACS 0.11° vs. stable angina 0.05° *P* < 0.01). There were more plaques with elevated temperatures in the ACS group (84.2%) than in the stable angina group (30.4%). Moreover, patients treated with statins had lower temperature differences in nonculprit lesions than the untreated patients (38). The Dallas Heart Study compared coronary artery calcifications and CRP levels in 2726 patients with coronary risk factors (39). These investigators found a modest trend toward increasing CRP levels and coronary calcium scores. However, the relationship between the CRP levels and coronary artery calcium scores was not statistically significant after the analysis was adjusted for the traditional risk factors: body mass index, estrogen, and statin use. There was a strong relationship between female sex and body mass index (39). The CRP did not appear to be related to atherosclerotic burden but more so to stability and composition of the plaque (39).

The clinical setting of ACS places biomarkers in perspective. If not atherosclerotic burden, then the acute event and inflammation associated with it affect the biomarkers. The clinical presentation, the severity of inflammation with varying degrees of ischemia, and necrosis in addition to the amount of myocardium in jeopardy affect the degree of inflammation and subsequently the biomarkers. The coronary anatomy has been studied by intravascular ultrasound, angioscopy, coronary angiogram frame counts, plaque temperatures, and histology at autopsy. All point to a diffuse and hemodynamically unstable state. The value of biomarkers is their ability to suggest the need for aggressive therapy.

The ACS patient is identified by the history and physical examination and the electrocardiogram at baseline. Risk stratification begins here with evaluation, such as the TIMI risk score, as part of the history and physical. Further risk stratification is performed by an analysis of biomarkers. In this clinical setting, an elevated troponin suggests a degree of necrosis. If normal at baseline in the emergency room, serial troponins are now performed over the next several hours. An elevated BNP could be helpful in revealing congestion or perhaps a worsening prognosis. An elevated CRP in the ACS setting points to inflammation and leads to early administration of a high dose of statin medications. The data presented here suggest that the elevation of these biomarkers worsens prognosis. Of the nearly two dozen biomarkers under study, some will no doubt form a panel of biomarkers to help evaluate and stratify the risk of the ACS patients. Which biomarkers would be a part of that panel remains to be seen.

The importance of the biomarkers would lie in its direct aggressive therapy in a timely fashion. A recent meta-analysis of seven trials with 9212 patients showed that a routine invasive strategy was superior to a conservative strategy that brought patients to catheterization only if they had recurrent symptoms (40). The benefit of the routine invasive strategy occurred after hospital discharge. During the hospitalization, more death and myocardial infarction occurred in the routine invasive group. The use of biomarkers, glycoprotein IIb/IIIa inhibitors, and antithrombins in these ACS patients needs more research, especially in the early hospital management.

References

1 Schwartz GG, Olsson AG. The case for intensive statin therapy after acute coronary syndromes. Am J Cardiol, 2005; 96(suppl):F45–F53.
2 Schrier RW. Role of diminished renal function in cardiovascular mortality. J Am Coll Cardiol 2006; 47:1–8.
3 Giugliano RP, Braunwald E. The year in non-ST segment elevation acute coronary syndromes. J Am Coll Cardiol 2005; 46:906–919.
4 American Heart Association, Heart Disease and Stroke Statistics – 2005 update. Dallas, Texas. American Heart Association, 2005.
5 Fuster V. Acute coronary syndromes: the degree and morphology of coronary stenosis. J Am Coll Cardiol 2000; 35(suppl B):52B–54B.
6 Douglas PS, Ginsburg GS. The evaluation of chest pain in women. New Engl J Med 1996; 334:1311–1315.
7 Cannon CP, Braunwald E. Unstable Angina in Heart Disease, 6th ed. Chap. 36. In: Braunwald E, Zipes DP, Libby P, eds. Philadelphia: WB Saunders, 2001.
8 Morrow DA, Antman EM, Charlesworth A, et al. The TIMI risk score for ST elevation myocardial infarction: a convenient bedside clinical score for risk assessment at presentation. Circulation 2000; 102:2031–2037.
9 Morrow DA, Cannon CP, Rifai N, et al. Ability of minor elevations of troponin I and troponin T to predict benefit from an early invasive strategy in patients with unstable angina and non-ST elevation myocardial infarction. J Am Med Assoc 2001; 286:2405–2412.
10 Ohtani T, Yasunori U, Shimizu M, et al. Association between cardiac troponin T elevation and angioscopic morphology of culprit lesion patients with non-ST segment elevation acute coronary syndromes. Am Heart J 2005; 150:227–233.
11 Jeremias A, Gibson CM. Narrative review: alternative causes for elevated cardiac troponin levels when acute coronary syndromes are excluded. Ann Intern Med 2005; 142:786–791.
12 Sinha MK, Gaze DC, Collinson PO, et al. Role of "ischemia modified albumin" a new biochemical marker of myocardial ischemia in the early diagnosis of acute coronary syndromes. Emerg Med J 2004; 21:29–34.
13 Sabatine MS, Morrow DA, deLemos JA, et al. Acute changes in circulating natriuretic peptide levels in relation to myocardial ischemia. J Am Coll Cardiol 2004; 44:1988–1995.
14 Libby P, Ridker DM, Maseri A. Inflammation and atherosclerosis. Circulation 2002; 105:1135–1143.
15 Brennan ML, Penn MS, VanLempt F. Prognostic value of myloperoxidase in patients with chest pain. N Engl J Med 2003; 349:1595–1604.
16 Libby P. Act local, act global. Inflammation and the multiplicity of "vulnerable" coronary plaques. J Am Coll Cardiol 2005; 45:1600–1602.
17 Zebrack JS, Muhlstein JB, Horne BD, et al. C-reactive proteins and angiographic coronary artery disease: independent and additive predictors in subjects with angina. J Am Coll Cardiol 2002; 39:632–637.

18 Mauriello A, Sangiorgi G, Fratoni S, et al. Diffuse and active inflammation occurs in both vulnerable and stable plaques of the entire coronary tree. J Am Coll Cardiol 2005; 45:1585–1593.

19 Gibson CM, Ryan KA, Murphy SA, et al. Impaired coronary blood flow in nonculprit arteries in the setting of acute myocardial infarction. J Am Coll Cardiol 1999; 34:974–982.

20 Andersen HR, Nielsen TT, Rasmussen K, et al. Comparison of coronary angioplasty with fibromylitic therapy in acute myocardial infarction. N Engl J Med 2003; 349:733–742.

21 Tanaka A, Shimada K, Sano T, et al. Multiple plaque rupture and C-reactive protein in acute myocardial infarction. J Am Coll Cardiol 2005; 45:1594–1599.

22 Hong MK, Mintz GS, Whan Lee C, et al. The site of plaque rupture in native coronary arteries. J Am Coll Cardiol 2005; 46:261–265.

23 Monaco C, Rossi E, Milazzo D, et al. Persistent systemic inflammation in unstable angina is largely related to atherothrombotic burden. J Am Coll Cardiol 2005; 45:238–243.

24 Sabatine MS, Braunwald E. Another look at an age old question: which came first the elevated C-reactive protein or the atherothrombosis. J Am Coll Cardiol 2005; 45:244–245.

25 Sabatine MS, Morrow DA, de Lemos JA, et al. Multimarker approach to risk stratification in non-ST elevation acute coronary syndromes. Circulation 2002; 105:1760–1763.

26 Cannon CP, Weintraub WS, Demopoulos LA, et al. Comparison of an early invasive and conservative strategies in patients with unstable angina coronary syndromes treated with the glycoprotein IIb/IIIa inhibitor tirofiban. N Engl J Med 2001; 344:1879–1887.

27 Mega JL, Morrow DA, deLemos JA, et al. B-type natriuretic peptide at presentation and prognosis in patients with ST segment elevation myocardial infarction. J Am Coll Cardiol 2004; 44:335–339.

28 Antman EM, Louwerenburg HW, Baars HF, et al. Enoxoparin as adjunctive antithrombin therapy for ST elevation myocardial infarction. Circulation 2002; 105:1642–1649.

29 deLemos JA, Morrow DA, Bentley JA, et al. The prognostic value of B-type natriuretic peptides in patients with acute coronary syndrome. N Engl J Med 2001; 345:1014–1021.

30 Maisel A. The coming of age of natriuretic peptides. J Am Coll Cardiol 2006; 41:61–64.

31 Wiviott SD, Cannon CP, Morrow DA, et al. Differential expression of cardiac biomarkers by gender in patients with unstable angina/non-ST elevation myocardial infarction. Circulation 2004; 109:580–586.

32 Richards M, Nicholls MG, Espiner EA, et al. Comparison of B-type natriuretic peptides for assessment of cardiac function and prognosis in stable ischemic heart disease. J Am Coll Cardiol 2006; 47:52–60.

33 Heeschen C, Hamm CW, Mitrovic V, et al. N-terminal pro-B-type natriuretic peptide levels for dynamic risk stratification of patients with acute coronary syndromes. Circulation 2004; 110:3206–3212.

34 Morrow DA, deLemos JA, Blazing MA, et al. Prognostic value of serial B-type natriuretic peptide testing during follow-up of patients with unstable coronary artery disease. J Am Med Assoc 2005; 294:2866–2871.

35 Cannon CP, Braunwald E, McCabe CH, et al. Intensive versus moderate lipid lowering with statins after acute coronary syndromes. N Engl J Med 2004; 350:1495–1504.

36 de Lemos JA, Blazing MA, Wiviott SD, et al. Early intensive versus a delayed conservative simvastatin strategy in patients with acute coronary syndromes: phase Z of the A to Z trial. J Am Med Assoc 2004; 292:1307–1316.

37 Schwartz GG, Olsson AG, Ezekowitz MD, et al. Effects of Atorvastatin in early recurrent ischemic events in acute coronary syndromes: the MIRACL study: a randomized controlled trial. JAMA 2001; 285:1711–1718.

38 Toutouzas K, Drakopoulos M, Mitropoulos J, et al. Elevated plaque temperature in non-culprit de novo athermotous lesions of patients with acute coronary syndromes. J Am Coll Cardiol 2006; 47:301–306.

39 Khira A, deLemos JA, Peshock RM, et al. Relationship between C-reactive protein and subclinical atherosclerosis: the Dallas Heart Study. Circulation 2006; 113:38–43.

40 Mehta SR, Cannon CP, Fox KAA, et al. Routine versus selective invasive strategies in patients with acute coronary syndromes: a collaborative meta-analysis of randomized trials. J Am Med Assoc 2005; 293:2908–2917.

40

Cardiovascular interventional pharmacology in the diabetic patient

Mitchell D. Weinberg and George D. Dangas

Introduction

Diabetes is extremely prevalent within the United States, with more than 16 million confirmed cases and an additional 20 million cases of glucose intolerance. As the incidence of diabetes in this country is thought to be on the rise (1), coronary artery disease (CAD) in this group, which is the principal cause of death in this population, is expected to rise concomitantly (2). Clearly reflecting these trends, in over a 20-year period, the mortality rate in the United States from diabetes has risen more than 30% (3).

Pathogenesis of cardiac morbidity and mortality in diabetics

As a result of the hyperglycemia, hyperinsulinemia, dyslipidemia, and hypercoagulability associated with diabetes, diabetic patients are at particularly high risk for complications of atherosclerosis. Diabetes accelerates the natural course of the atherosclerotic process, precipitating more diffuse disease (4,5), increased rates of plaque ulceration and thrombosis (6), and a doubling of the five-year mortality rate when compared with nondiabetic CAD patients.

Moreover, currently, inflammation is being implicated as a driving force in the diabetic atherothromboembolic process. Increased concentrations of inflammatory markers such as C-reactive protein, tumor necrosis factor-alpha, platelet-derived soluble CD40 ligand, and upregulation of cellular adhesion molecules have been noted in blood samples of diabetic patients (7–10), and are a subject of great interest.

Percutaneous coronary intervention and related complications

Diabetic CAD, with its impressive prevalence and severity, is the frequent trigger of percutaneous coronary intervention (PCI) and, by extension, PCI-related complications. Approximately 25% of the revascularization procedures occurring in the United States are performed on diabetic patients (11). Diabetic patients are known to incur higher rates of restenosis, and, interestingly, higher rates of complete occlusive restenosis, than do nondiabetics (12). Occlusive restenosis has previously been documented to have markedly worse outcomes than nonocclusive restenosis (13). It has been theorized that occlusive restenosis plays a large role in both the increased number of target vessel revascularizations (TVRs) and the overall poorer long-term prognosis of the diabetic PCI group when compared with the nondiabetic PCI population (14).

Decreased reperfusion at the microvascular level might also contribute to the poorer prognosis of diabetic patients. Recent work in acute myocardial infarction (MI) has suggested that despite achieving comparable rates of thrombosis in myocardial infarction (TIMI)-3 flow, diabetics have poorer post-PCI myocardial reperfusion than nondiabetics, as evidenced by reduced ST-segment resolution and myocardial blush grade (15).

Angioplasty vs. surgery in diabetics

In nondiabetics with multivessel disease, trials comparing PCI and coronary artery bypass graft surgery (CABG) have shown identical rates of MI and mortality between the two, but have noted increased rates of repeat revascularization in the PCI group. As a result, choosing between PCI and CABG in nondiabetics only requires that one weigh the risk and burden of TVR, a risk that is believed to be diminishing in the postdrug-eluting stent era (16–18). Deciding between PCI and CABG in diabetics with multivessel disease, however, is more ambiguous.

The Bypass Angioplasty Revascularization Investigation (BARI) (19,20) revealed a significantly higher mortality in diabetics treated with PCI than with CABG. While these findings were supported in two other large registries (21,22), they were not duplicated in the BARI registry. Unlike BARI, the BARI registry was composed of those patients eligible but not randomized and found similar outcomes in diabetics treated with PCI or CABG (23). These findings, in conjunction with the advent of stenting since the start of the BARI trial, call into question the generalizability of the BARI results. In a subanalysis, the Arterial Revascularization Therapy Study (ARTS) trial specifically studied slotted metallic stents in diabetic patients and noted no difference in the combined endpoint of death, nonfatal MI, or stroke, but did note increased restenosis and TVR in the diabetes group (24,25). The recently presented ARTS 2 data, which compared sirolimus drug eluting stent (DES) with historical controls from the ARTS 1 trial, showed PCI with DESs to be as good as CABG. This finding is considered very significant and while the trial was nonrandomized, the results from the diabetic subgroup analysis are being eagerly awaited, as a greater portion of the PCI group was diabetic than ARTS 1 (26). Thus, the current data indicates that in the modern stent era the source of the majority of benefit conferred by CABG to the diabetic population is a decreased rate of restenosis-driven TVR. As such, similar to nondiabetics, before revascularizing a diabetic patient with multivessel disease, the clinician needs to weigh the burden of an open surgical procedure against an increased likelihood of TVR.

Pharmacology

Thus, as diabetic CAD continues to warrant a great number of PCIs and subsequent TVRs, interventional pharmacology in this population is of great interest. A number of agents which have been studied in detail in the nondiabetic population have been the subject of separate or substudy analysis in the diabetic population. Clearly, any pharmacological agent effective in improving PCI outcomes and reducing complications in the diabetic population is of vital importance.

Clopidogrel

In the PCI-CURE (Clopidogrel in Unstable Angina to Prevent Recurrent Events) trial, subgroup analysis of diabetic patients revealed only a nonsignificant trend toward benefit in the aspirin plus clopidogrel group compared with the aspirin plus placebo group. This benefit was noted to be less impressive in diabetics when compared with nondiabetics (27). The Credo (Clopidogrel for the Reduction of Events During Observation) trial studied individuals who were likely to receive PCI and randomized them to either a loading dose of clopidogrel followed by 12 months of clopidogrel or no loading dose and clopidogrel for only one month (28). There was only a trend toward benefit of prolonged clopidogrel therapy in the diabetic population (relative risk reduction, RRR = 11%), whereas the benefit observed in the nondiabetic population was significant (RRR = 33%). However, in a dedicated study among diabetics, clopidogrel was found to be more effective than aspirin in reducing recurrent ischemic events (29).

Platelet glycoprotein IIb/IIIa inhibitors

Platelet glycoprotein IIb/IIIa (GP IIb/IIIa) inhibitors impede the final common pathway of platelet activation—the bridging of GP IIb/IIIa with von Willebrand's factor and fibrinogen—and thus inhibit direct platelet to platelet binding, platelet activation, and, ultimately, platelet-based thrombus formation. Diabetics, noted to have approximately 3X the number of platelet surface GP IIb/IIIa receptors than nondiabetics, even in the setting of adequate glycemic control, should theoretically derive even greater benefit from GP IIb/IIIa (30). The main PCI-related benefit of IIb/IIIa inhibition was initially thought to reside in reduction of neointimal hyperplasia and, by extension, the diminution of TVR incidence. Using intravascular ultrasound to quantify in-stent intimal hyperplasia, both the Diabetes Abciximab steNT Evaluation (DANTE) study, which was limited to diabetics, and The Evaluation of ReoPro and Stenting to Eliminate Restenosis (ERASER) study, which examined both 12- and 24-hour abciximab infusions in the general population, did not reveal a reduction of in-stent intimal hyperplasia in any of the GP IIb/IIIa inhibitor treatment groups (31,32). Thus, alternative mechanisms likely explain GP IIb/IIIa inhibitor-mediated benefit.

The effects of GP IIb/IIIa inhibitors are not limited to direct antiplatelet activity. GP IIb/IIIa inhibitors are also thought to have anti-inflammatory effects. By suppressing CD40L, a member of the tumor necrosis-alpha family of proteins, GP IIb/IIIa inhibitors are thought to reduce platelet–leucocyte interactions. CD40L's binding to endothelial cells has been shown to upregulate cellular adhesion molecules (ICAM-1 and VCAM-1), matrix metalloproteinases, and tissue factor, all of which are thought to play a role in the inflammatory response resulting from endothelial injury.

The abciximab clinical trials, a group of prospective, randomized, double-blind trials, provided a large body of evidence supporting the use of platelet IIb/IIIa inhibitors during PCI in NSTE-ACS (non-ST-elevation acute coronary syndrome) (33–37). EPILOG (Evaluation in PTCA to Improve Long-term Outcome with abciximab GP IIb/IIIa blockade), EPIC (The Evaluation of c7E3 for Prevention of Ischemic Complications), EPISTENT (Evaluation of Platelet Inhibition in STENTing), ESPRIT (The Enhanced Suppression of the Platelet IIb/IIIa Receptor with Integrilin Therapy), and TARGET (do Tirofiban And ReoPro Give similar Efficacy Trial) all offered comparison of outcomes between nondiabetic and diabetic subjects. The first four of these trials noted similar benefit of GP IIb/IIIa inhibition in the diabetic and nondiabetic population at both 30 days (endpoint of death, MI, and urgent revascularization) and six months (death or MI). Perhaps most compellingly, the EPISTENT trial performed a prespecified analysis of clinical outcomes in diabetics who were assigned to strategies of stent implantation plus placebo, stent implantation plus abciximab, or angioplasty plus abciximab (38). There was a >50% reduction in death, nonfatal MI, or urgent revascularization rate at six-month follow-up in diabetic patients receiving a stent and abciximab compared with stent alone. Additionally, diabetics treated with stent plus abciximab were less likely to require repeat TVR (8.1%) than if they were treated with stent plus placebo (16.6%), or with angioplasty plus abciximab (18.4%, $P = 0.02$). This seemed to indicate that abciximab provided additive benefit to stent implantation with reduction of TVR in the diabetic population, a finding which was supported by the ADMIRAL (Abciximab before Direct angioplasty and stenting in Myocardial Infarction Regarding Acute and Long-term follow-up) trial (39), but not by the EPILOG diabetic substudy (40) or in the ESPRIT trial, which compared integrilin plus stent with placebo plus stent in diabetics (41). While it has been suggested that abciximab offers a unique reduction of TVR rates as a result of its effect on $\alpha v \beta 3$ or $\alpha M \beta 2$ receptors (which would explain for the nonresult in ESPRIT), no difference was noted between abciximab and integrillin in TARGET, making this less likely. TARGET did, however, note that abciximab was superior to tirofiban with respect to the primary 30-day endpoint in both diabetics and nondiabetics. This is currently used to justify the preferential use of abciximab in the PCI setting.

Of note, recent interest in the anti-inflammatory effects of GP IIb/IIIa inhibitors mentioned before has prompted speculation that certain GP IIb/IIIa inhibitors are more effective than others in reducing sCD40L (the soluble form of the protein). In vitro work has indicated that eptifibatide and tirofiban are possibly more effective in suppressing sCD40L than abciximab (42)—a finding which was supported in one recent small in vivo post-PCI study (43), but disputed by another (44). Looking at other inflammatory markers, a substudy of the EPIC trial noted the balloon angioplasty plus abciximab group to have decreased levels of CRP and IL-6 in the 24–48-hour period than did patients with balloon angioplasty alone (45).

Platelet glycoprotein IIb/IIIa inhibitors and clopidogrel

Given the study by Bhatt et al., which noted the superiority of plavix to aspirin in diabetics, and the aforementioned benefit of GP IIb/IIIa inhibitors, an analysis of clopidogrel in combination with abciximab, the current favorite of the GP IIb/IIIa inhibitors, in the diabetic population was warranted. The ISAR-SWEET trial (Intracoronary Stenting and Antithrombotic Regimen: Is Abciximab a Superior Way to Eliminate Elevated Thrombotic Risk in Diabetics) studied the use of abciximab in diabetic patients who were loaded with 600 mg of clopidogrel before receiving bare-metal stents (46). Abciximab plus clopidogrel was not shown to significantly impact mortality or rates of MI (Fig. 1), a result that was somewhat surprising given the impressive benefit conferred by GP IIb/IIIa inhibitors in EPISTENT. As ISAR-SWEET noted no reduction in mortality or recurrent MI but did reveal trends toward increased bleeding in those placed on concurrent clopidogrel and abciximab therapy, it supported limiting pre-PCI antiplatelet therapy to clopidogrel and aspirin.

Insulin/glucose insulin potassium infusion

Glucose insulin potassium (GIK) infusion has been suggested by some to offer additional myocardial salvage in the setting of an acute MI. Theoretically, GIK infusion provides glycolytic fuel to both the starving ischemic myocardium before intervention and the reperfused myocardium after PCI. It is also thought to decrease free fatty acid (FFA) levels and toxic FFA uptake by the ischemic myocardium.

Although the majority of randomized studies revealed only insignificant trends toward benefit in the general population, a meta-analysis of nine such studies performed from 1965 to 1987 (two were double-blinded and seven were open) revealed a significant mortality benefit with an odds ratio (OR) of 0.72 [95% confidence interval (CI) = 0.57–0.90] (47). In the four most recent trials in the general population to date (48–50), only one presented a significant mortality benefit in the GIK infusion group (51).

While the evidence for GIK infusion strategy in the general AMI population is sparse, the diabetes mellitus insulin-glucose infusion in acute myocardial infarction (DIGAMI) study group, which studied GIK infusion versus conventional therapy in diabetics, noted significant mortality reductions at three months and one year (52). However, whether this was a metabolic benefit of the acute GIK infusion or a result of strict glycemic control was impossible to interpret. The DIGAMI 2 investigators aimed to resolve this question by comparing three treatment strategies: (i) glucose–insulin infusion followed by insulin-based long-term glucose control; (ii) glucose–insulin

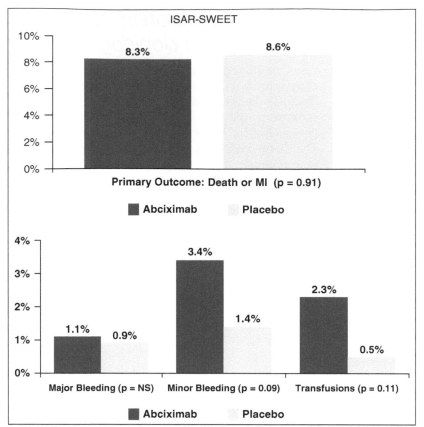

Figure 1

Intracoronary stenting and antithrombotic regimen: is abciximab a superior way to eliminate elevated thrombotic risk in diabetics. *Abbreviations*: MI, myocardial infarction; NS, nonsignificant. *Source*: Adapted from Ref. 46.

infusion followed by standard glucose control; and (*iii*) routine management based on local practice (53). And while this design should have been effective in isolating the source of DIGAMI 1's mortality benefit, DIGAMI 2 ran into considerable difficulty. First, problems with patient recruitment forced the early stoppage of the trial. Second, the established glucose targets in group 1 were never reached, and by the end of the trial glycemic control was similar in all three groups. The lack of benefit in patients with GIK infusion in DIGAMI 2 suggests that any benefit in the DIGAMI 1 treatment group was from superior glycemic control and not the initial GIK infusion. This concept has been supported by a recent study of insulin therapy/tight glycemic control in the critically ill, which evaluated glycemic control in surgical and trauma patients and noted a 34% mortality reduction in the more rigorously treated group (54).

Currently, the debate as to whether the beneficial effects of tight glycemic control with insulin regimens is because of decreased glucotoxicity or the beneficial metabolic effects of insulin is still ongoing. As such, while there is insufficient evidence to use intravenous insulin therapy in every case of acute MI, one should aggressively obtain adequate glycemic control in the diabetic acute MI patient. Of note, in DIGAMI 2, only a small percentage of patients underwent mechanical revascularization. Thus, from the interventionalist's perspective, this debate will remain unresolved until a randomized control trial is performed in the setting of consistent mechanical intervention.

Insulin sensitizers

While the thiazolidindiones enhance insulin-mediated glucose transport via binding to the peroxisome proliferator-activating receptor (PPAR-γ), the presence of this receptor in vascular smooth muscle cells, inflammatory cells, and endothelial cells likely facilitates the drug's ability to inhibit vascular smooth muscle cell proliferation, reduce inflammation, improve dyslipidemia, and, by extension, reduce in-stent restenosis.

A number of studies using intravascular ultrasound have demonstrated reductions of neointimal tissue proliferation after coronary stent implantation in patients taking glitazones (55,56). Two small randomized clinical trials of the glitazones administered after PCI, the first by Takagi et al. of troglitazone (which has since been pulled from the market) and the second by Choi et al. of rosiglitazone, demonstrated significant reduction in restenosis (57,58). Moreover, a recent small study showing decreased rates of stenosis in nondiabetics on pioglitazone therapy supports the notion that the glitazones confer benefit via mechanisms unrelated to glycemic control (59). Further large, prospective, randomized trials need to be conducted before glitazones are made the standard of care in the PCI setting.

Metformin, another agent with insulin-sensitizing effects, was found in retrospective analysis to have decreased rates of death and MI (OR = 0.29; $P = 0.007$ and OR = 0.31

$P = 0.002$) in diabetics undergoing coronary intervention. Interestingly, there was no difference in ischemia-driven TVR between the metformin and nonmetformin groups—suggesting that the mechanism of benefit from metformin was unrelated to intimal hyperplasia. The retrospective, nonrandomized nature of this study limits it utility, and further prospective studies are needed in this regard (60).

Heparin

The use of intravenous heparin during PCI is currently the standard of care. An indirect thrombin inhibitor, heparin requires antithrombin-III in order to initiate thrombin inhibition. While intravenous heparin is frequently used, its limitations, which include poor bioavailability, variable dose—response relationships, and erratic binding properties, have prompted the study of low-molecular weight heparins (LMWH) in the setting of PCI. These agents are promising in that they offer improved bioavailability, a steady dose—response relationship, and possibly less bleeding. While neither agent has been explicitly studied in diabetics, they are both regularly used in this population. Most recently, the superior yield of the new strategy of enoxaparin, revascularization, and glycoprotein IIb/IIIa inhibitors (SYNERGY) trial compared enoxaparin and unfractionated heparin in high-risk patients with ACS intended for an invasive strategy and did not reveal significant differences in the primary endpoints at 30 days, six months, or one year, but did note a modest excess of bleeding (61). Subgroup analysis of diabetic patients also noted no significant difference in rates of death or MI between the two modes of therapy at the predetermined follow-up periods. Until there is a dedicated trial of LMWH in diabetic patients with ACS going for invasive management, the interventionalist needs to weigh the convenience of administration offered by LMWH versus its accompanied modest increased risk of bleeding.

Of note, previous study has suggested that relative to nondiabetics, diabetics are less sensitive to intravenous heparin (62). Diabetics undergoing PCI and who have been administered heparin in the absence of abciximab have lower rates of ischemic events with activated clotting time (ACT) at increased levels (63). While in diabetics placed on heparin and abciximab elevated ACT ranges have been associated with trends toward decreased TVR rates (64), there is strong data from studies of diverse populations (~23% of patients with diabetes) that when the two are used in conjunction, lower ACT ranges (200–250 seconds) can be maintained to decrease the incidence of bleeding without incurring increased ischemic events (65,66). Further direct study of diabetics exposed to varying degrees of heparinization in the setting of GP IIb/IIIa inhibition needs to be performed to clarify this issue.

Statins and fenofibrates

High-dose statin therapy is of particular interest in the PCI population. While the mechanism of benefit is likely multifactorial, the well-documented anti-inflammatory role of statin therapy likely plays a large role (67). The use of high-dose statins has been correlated both with decreased serological measurements of inflammation (68), and more recently with reduced unstable plaque volume in intravascular ultrasound (IVUS) studies of ACS patients (69). Given these findings, high-dose statin therapy has been the subject of great interest. PROVE-IT TIMI-22 and treating to new targets (TNT) found a significant benefit in the primary outcome associated with high-dose statin therapy (70,71), the incremental decrease in end points through aggressive lipid lowering trial (IDEAL) and the A to Z trial failed to do so (72,73). While the value of high-dose statin therapy has not directly been addressed in the diabetic PCI population, the TIMI-PROVE IT study showed that diabetics treated with 80 mg of atorvastatin had an approximately 17% reduction in the combined endpoint of death, MI, stroke, angina requiring readmission, or revascularization at two years.

Most recently, in a substudy of the Lescol Intervention Prevention Study (LIPS) trial, diabetic patients treated with aggressive lipid-reducing therapy after PCI were noted to have a 51% reduced risk of future cardiovascular events at long-term follow-up (74). Of note, there was no difference in the rate of restenosis between the treatment and the control groups, and the benefit of fluvastatin in diabetics was based on reduction of long-term complications. Nevertheless, given the long-term findings in both of the studies, it is incumbent on the interventionalist to begin statin therapy in diabetic patients shortly after PCI.

Fenofibrates were found to slow the development of angiographic CAD in diabetics in the DAIS (Diabetes Atherosclerosis Intervention Study) study (75). While the diabetics undergoing PCI have yet to be evaluated, fenofibrates are being actively studied in the general diabetic population. The fenofibrate intervention and event lowering in diabetes (FIELD) randomized type 2 diabetics to placebo or fenofibrate. While there was no significant difference in the primary endpoint of coronary heart disease (CHD)-related-death or MI, the secondary endpoint of total cardiovascular events was significantly lower in the fenofibrate group (76). These results were possibly confounded by the asymmetric use of statins (17% and 7% in the placebo and fenofibrate groups, respectively) and will be remedied in the action to control cardiovascular risk in diabetes (ACCORD) trial, which will randomize diabetics already taking statins to either fenofibrate or placebo. Fenofibrates are currently an area of interest and will eventually need evaluation in the diabetic PCI setting.

Contrast-induced nephropathy

Contrast-induced nephropathy (CIN), defined as a serum creatinine increase of >25% relative to baseline, is associated with significant morbidity and mortality. The pathogenesis of CIN is thought to result from ischemia/nephrotoxicity mediated by either the generation of reactive oxygen-related species, renal vasoconstriction inducing medullary ischemia, or some combination of the two.

Preventing CIN is of particular importance in patients with diabetes and chronic kidney disease, as these are two of the most powerful independent risk factors for CIN (77). Diabetics are more susceptible to (CIN) than are the nondiabetics, and diabetics with pre-existing chronic kidney disease (CKD) are at even greater risk (78). In a recently proposed CIN risk-scoring system, patient characteristics such as diabetes, age >75, chronic congestive heart failure, admission with acute pulmonary edema, hypotension, anemia and chronic kidney disease; and various procedure-related characteristics including increasing volumes of contrast media, and intra-aortic balloon pump use were all found to reliably contribute to increased risk (79).

Methods of reducing CIN have focused on reducing the toxicity of the contrast media (CM) itself, and using various prophylactic pharmacologic regimens. Of the types of CM available, the low-osmolar iohexol induces less CIN than does the high-osmolar diatrizoate in both the CKD and diabetic population (80). By extension, many expected iodixanol, the iso-osmolar, dimeric, and nonionic CM to confer additional reno-protective benefit. Yet, no such benefit was noted in initial studies of low-risk patients and nondiabetics with renal failure (81–83). However, in the more recent nephrotoxicity in high-risk patients study of iso-osmolar nonionic contrast media (NEPHRIC) study, which examined diabetics with renal failure undergoing coronary or aortofemoral angiography, iso-osmolar iodixanol was found to be superior to the low-osmolar iohexol (84). Thus, iodixanol, at this point, is a reasonable choice in diabetics with prior renal insufficiency.

Of the prophylactic agents, hydration is unanimously endorsed. Its theorized mechanism of action is the enhancement of renal perfusion and, conversely, the minimization of ischemia. While it has become the standard of care based on a multitude of early trials (85,86), no large, prospective studies have been conducted. The optimal method of hydration has yet to be decided, with one study showing benefit of normal saline (0.9% NS) over half NS (0.45%) (87), and another study suggesting that 154 mEq/L of sodium bicarbonate is superior to NS alone. Of note, the total volume in the latter study was less than that was used in other trials, making it difficult to compare (88). Thus, currently, NS should be used unless the patient is highly intolerant to volume administration. In such a case, 154 mEq/L of sodium bicarbonate can be administered over a shorter time period.

N-acetylcysteine, probably the most studied agent used for CIN prophylaxis is thought to reduce oxidative damage. Tepel et al. found the prophylactic administration of 600 mg of N-acetylcysteine the day before and day of administration of iodinated contrast before computed tomographic (CT) scan in patients with CKD (Cr 2.4 ± 1.3) to decrease the incidence of CIN associated reduction in renal function (89). As N-acetylcysteine is virtually without toxicity, some have studied its administration in higher doses (1200 mg bid) and have demonstrated improved results (90). After Tepel et al., a multitude of studies have yielded varying results and prompted a set of meta-analyses which did the same (91–93). Thus, while formulating a definitive conclusion at the present time is difficult, 1200 mg of oral N-acetycysteine bid for two days in the peri-PCI period is without toxicity and, therefore, a reasonable choice.

A number of other agents have been studied but have not been found to yield significant benefit including dopamine, fenoldopam, diuretics dihydropyridine calcium channel blockers, and atrial natriuretic peptide.

Drug-eluting stents

Drug-eluting stents have been demonstrated to offer superior reduction of TVR rates when compared with nondrug-eluting stents in both the general (94,95) and the diabetic population (96). In the general population, sirolimus-eluting stents have been shown to be angiographically superior—with less late luminal loss than paclitaxel-eluting stents (97). However, whether sirolimus use correlates with clinically significant reductions in TVR is less clear, as it has been supported by some (97) but not others (98). In a dedicated study of diabetics, the Intracoronary Stenting and Angiographic Result: Do Diabetic Patients Derive Similar Benefit from Paclitaxel-Eluting and Sirolimus-Eluting Stents (ISAR-DIABETES), in which patients were randomized to either sirolimus or paclitaxel stents, showed a stronger association between decreased late luminal loss in the sirolimus group and improved TVR rates (99). While this suggests that stent choice might have true clinical significance in diabetic patients, the study was a noninferiority trial and not designed to make this distinction. Thus, a larger prospective trial powered to show superiority of sirolimus must be conducted before a real conclusion can be made. This particular field will become even more interesting (and complicated) with the emergence of new drug-eluting stents with sirolimus analogs. Dedicated studies in diabetic patents will be warranted.

Conclusion

At the present time, the management of diabetic patients requiring PCI is still being defined. Certainly, further studies in diabetics comparing drug-eluting stents with CABG in the setting of multivessel disease will help us delineate between the surgical and percutaneous forms of management. However, should percutaneous intervention continue to be used with such frequency, great efforts need to be made to define and enforce the use of adjuvant pharmacotherapy. GP IIb/IIIa inhibitors have been shown to be of significant benefit and should be considered strongly in diabetic patients. But the use of GP IIb/IIIa inhibitors in conjunction with clopidogrel has yet to show additional benefit. While there is now evidence supporting tighter glycemic management in the PCI setting, future prospective study comparing various hypoglycemic agents has to be performed before definitive guidelines can be offered. Glitazones also need to be studied both for their ability to reduce hyperglycemia and their possible role in the reduction of restenosis. Presently, LMWH, while more convenient, is not superior to intravenous heparin and is associated with an increased risk of bleeding. Improved lipid control is of considerable long-term benefit in the diabetic post-PCI setting, and should be initiated in the setting of the intervention. In the diabetic patient with CKD at high risk for CIN, hydration and high-dose N-acetylcysteine are recommended. Finally, while initial work in diabetics indicates the possible superiority of sirolimus to paclitaxel, this has yet to be adequately proven.

References

1 Mokdad AH, Ford ES, Bowman BA, et al. Prevalence of obesity, diabetes, and obesity-related health risk factors, 2001. JAMA 2003; 289:76–79.

2 Brun E, Nelson RG, Bennett PH, et al. Verona Diabetes Study. Diabetes duration and cause-specific mortality in the Verona Diabetes Study. Diabetes Care 2000; 23:1119–1123.

3 Mokdad AH, Ford ES, Bowman BA, et al. Diabetes trends in the U.S.: 1990–1998. Diabetes Care 2000; 23:1278–1283.

4 Waller BF, Palumbo PJ, Lie JT, Roberts WC. Status of the coronary arteries at necropsy in diabetes mellitus with onset after age 30 years. Analysis of 229 diabetic patients with and without clinical evidence of coronary heart disease and comparison to 183 control subjects. Am J Med 1980; 69:498–506.

5 Vigorita VJ, Moore GW, Hutchins GM. Absence of correlation between coronary arterial atherosclerosis and severity or duration of diabetes mellitus of adult onset. Am J Cardiol 1980; 46:535–542.

6 Silva JA, Escobar A, Collins TJ, Ramee SR, White CJ. Unstable angina. A comparison of angioscopic findings between diabetic and nondiabetic patients. Circulation 1995; 92:1731–1736.

7 Moreno PR, Murcia AM, Palacios IF, et al. Coronary composition and macrophage infiltration in atherectomy specimens from patients with diabetes mellitus. Circulation 2000; 102:2180–2184.

8 Marx N, Imhof A, Froehlich J, et al. Effect of rosiglitazone treatment on soluble CD40L in patients with type 2 diabetes and coronary artery disease. Circulation 2003; 107:1954–1957.

9 Bluher M, Unger R, Rassoul F, Richter V, Paschke R. Relation between glycaemic control, hyperinsulinaemia and plasma concentrations of soluble adhesion molecules in patients with impaired glucose tolerance or type II diabetes. Diabetologia 2002; 45:210–216.

10 Blankenberg S, Rupprecht HJ, Bickel C, et al. Circulating cell adhesion molecules and death in patients with coronary artery disease. Circulation 2001; 104:1336–1342.

11 Hammoud T, Tanguay JF, Bourassa MG. Management of coronary artery disease: therapeutic options in patients with diabetes. J Am Coll Cardiol 2000; 36:355–365.

12 Van Belle E, Abolmaali K, Bauters C, McFadden EP, Lablanche JM, Bertrand ME. Restenosis, late vessel occlusion and left ventricular function six months after balloon angioplasty in diabetic patients. J Am Coll Cardiol 1999; 34:476–485.

13 Mehran R, Dangas G, Abizaid AS, et al. Angiographic patterns of in-stent restenosis: classification and implications for long-term outcome. Circulation 1999; 100:1872–1878.

14 Stein B, Weintraub WS, Gebhart SP, et al. Influence of diabetes mellitus on early and late outcome after percutaneous transluminal coronary angioplasty. Circulation 1995; 91:979–989.

15 Prasad A, Stone GW, Stuckey TD, et al. Impact of diabetes mellitus on myocardial perfusion after primary angioplasty in patients with acute myocardial infarction. J Am Coll Cardiol 2005; 45:508–514.

16 Moses JW, Leon MB, Popma JJ, et al. SIRIUS Investigators. Sirolimus-eluting stents versus standard stents in patients with stenosis in a native coronary artery. N Engl J Med 2003; 349:1315–1323.

17 Stone GW, Ellis SG, Cox DA, et al. TAXUS-IV Investigators. A polymer-based, paclitaxel-eluting stent in patients with coronary artery disease. N Engl J Med 2004; 350:221–231.

18 Holmes DR Jr, Leon MB, Moses JW, et al. Analysis of 1-year clinical outcomes in the SIRIUS trial: a randomized trial of a sirolimus-eluting stent versus a standard stent in patients at high risk for coronary restenosis. Circulation 2004; 109:634–640.

19 The BARI Investigators. Seven-year outcome in the Bypass Angioplasty Revascularization Investigation (BARI) by treatment and diabetic status. J Am Coll Cardiol 2000; 35:1122–1129.

20 Influence of diabetes on 5-year mortality and morbidity in a randomized trial comparing CABG and PTCA in patients with multivessel disease: the Bypass Angioplasty Revascularization Investigation (BARI). Circulation 1997; 96:1761–1769.

21 Niles NW, McGrath PD, Malenka D, et al. Northern New England Cardiovascular Disease Study Group. Survival of patients with diabetes and multivessel coronary artery disease after surgical or percutaneous coronary revascularization: results of a large regional prospective study. Northern New England Cardiovascular Disease Study Group. J Am Coll Cardiol 2001; 37:1008–1015.

22 King SB 3rd, Kosinski AS, Guyton RA, Lembo NJ, Weintraub WS. Eight-year mortality in the Emory Angioplasty versus Surgery Trial (EAST). J Am Coll Cardiol 2000; 35:1116–1121.

23 The Bypass Angioplasty Revascularization Investigation (BARI) Investigators. Comparison of coronary bypass surgery with angioplasty in patients with multivessel disease. N Engl J Med 1996; 335:217–225.

24 Abizaid A, Costa MA, Centemero M, et al. Arterial Revascularization Therapy Study Group. Clinical and economic impact of diabetes mellitus on percutaneous and surgical treatment of multivessel coronary disease patients: insights from the Arterial Revascularization Therapy Study (ARTS) trial. Circulation 2001; 104(5):533–538.

25 Serruys PW, Unger F, Sousa JE, et al. Arterial Revascularization Therapies Study Group. Comparison of coronary artery bypass surgery and stenting for the treatment of multivessel disease. N Engl J Med 2001; 344:1117–1124.

26   Serruys PW, Ong AT, Colombo A, et al. Arterial Revascularization Therapies Part II: sirolimus-eluting stent for the treatment of patients with multivessel do novo coronary artery lesions. Late-breaking trial presented at the American College of Cardiology Scientific Session, 2005.

27   Mehta SR, Yusuf S, Peters RJ, et al. Clopidogrel in Unstable angina to prevent Recurrent Events trial (CURE) Investigators. Effects of pretreatment with clopidogrel and aspirin followed by long-term therapy in patients undergoing percutaneous coronary intervention: the PCI-CURE study. Lancet 2001; 358:527–533.

28   Steinhubl SR, Berger PB, Mann JT 3rd, et al. CREDO Investigators. Clopidogrel for the reduction of events during observation. Early and sustained dual oral antiplatelet therapy following percutaneous coronary intervention: a randomized controlled trial. JAMA 2002; 288:2411–2420.

29   Bhatt DL, Marso SP, Hirsch AT, Ringleb PA, Hacke W, Topol EJ. Amplified benefit of clopidogrel versus aspirin in patients with diabetes mellitus. Am J Cardiol 2002; 90:625–628.

30   Tschoepe D, Driesch E, Schwippert B, Nieuwenhuis HK, Gries FA. Exposure of adhesion molecules on activated platelets in patients with newly diagnosed IDDM is not normalized by near-normoglycemia. Diabetes 1995; 44:890–894.

31   Chaves AJ, Sousa AG, Mattos LA, et al. Volumetric analysis of in-stent intimal hyperplasia in diabetic patients treated with or without abciximab: results of the Diabetes Abciximab steNT Evaluation (DANTE) randomized trial. Circulation 2004; 109:861–866.

32   The ERASER Investigators. Acute platelet inhibition with abciximab does not reduce in-stent restenosis (ERASER study). Circulation 1999; 100:799–806.

33   The EPIC Investigators. Use of a monoclonal antibody directed against the platelet glycoprotein IIb/IIIa receptor in high-risk coronary angioplasty. N Engl J Med 1994; 330:956–961.

34   The EPILOG Investigators. Platelet glycoprotein IIb/IIIa receptor blockade and low-dose heparin during percutaneous coronary revascularization. N Engl J Med 1997; 336(24):1689–1696.

35   The CAPTURE Investigators. Randomised placebo-controlled trial of abciximab before and during coronary intervention in refractory unstable angina: the CAPTURE Study. Lancet 1997; 349:1429–1435.

36   Lincoff AM, Califf RM, Moliterno DJ, et al. Complementary clinical benefits of coronary-artery stenting and blockade of platelet glycoprotein IIb/IIIa receptors. Evaluation of Platelet IIb/IIIa Inhibition in Stenting Investigators. N Engl J Med 1999; 341:319–327.

37   Topol EJ, Moliterno DJ, Herrmann HC, et al; TARGET Investigators. Do Tirofiban and ReoPro Give similar efficacy trial. Comparison of two platelet glycoprotein IIb/IIIa inhibitors, tirofiban and abciximab, for the prevention of ischemic events with percutaneous coronary revascularization. N Engl J Med 2001; 344:1888–1894.

38   Marso SP, Lincoff AM, Ellis SG, et al. Optimizing the percutaneous interventional outcomes for patients with diabetes mellitus: results of the EPISTENT (Evaluation of Platelet IIb/IIIa Inhibitor for Stenting Trial) diabetic substudy. Circulation 1999; 100:2477–2484.

39   Montalescot G, Barragan P, Wittenberg O, et al. ADMIRAL Investigators. Abciximab before direct angioplasty and stenting in myocardial infarction regarding acute and long-term follow-up. Platelet glycoprotein IIb/IIIa inhibition with coronary stenting for acute myocardial infarction. N Engl J Med 2001; 344:1895–1903.

40   Kleiman NS, Lincoff AM, Kereiakes DJ, et al. Diabetes mellitus, glycoprotein IIb/IIIa blockade, and heparin: evidence for a complex interaction in a multicenter trial. EPILOG Investigators. Circulation 1998; 97(19):1912–1920.

41   O'Shea JC, Hafley GE, Greenberg S, et al. ESPRIT Investigators (Enhanced Suppression of the Platelet IIb/IIIa Receptor with Integrilin Therapy trial). Platelet glycoprotein IIb/IIIa integrin blockade with eptifibatide in coronary stent intervention: the ESPRIT trial: a randomized controlled trial. JAMA 2001; 285:2468–2473.

42   Nannizzi-Alaimo L, Alves VL, Phillips DR. Inhibitory effects of glycoprotein IIb/IIIa antagonists and aspirin on the release of soluble CD40 ligand during platelet stimulation. Circulation 2003; 107:1123–1128.

43   Welt FG, Rogers SD, Zhang X, et al. GP IIb/IIIa inhibition with eptifibatide lowers levels of soluble CD40L and RANTES after percutaneous coronary intervention. Catheter Cardiovasc Interv 2004; 61:185–189.

44   Furman MI, Krueger LA, Linden MD, et al. GPIIb-IIIa antagonists reduce thromboinflammatory processes in patients with acute coronary syndromes undergoing percutaneous coronary intervention. J Thromb Haemost 2005; 3:312–320.

45   Lincoff AM, Kereiakes DJ, Mascelli MA, et al. Abciximab suppresses the rise in levels of circulating inflammatory markers after percutaneous coronary revascularization. Circulation 2001; 104:163–167.

46   Mehilli J, Kastrati A, Schuhlen H, et al. Intracoronary Stenting and Antithrombotic Regimen: Is Abciximab a Superior Way to Eliminate Elevated Thrombotic Risk in Diabetics (ISAR-SWEET) Study Investigators. Randomized clinical trial of abciximab in diabetic patients undergoing elective percutaneous coronary interventions after treatment with a high loading dose of clopidogrel. Circulation 2004; 110:3627–3635.

47   Fath-Ordoubadi F, Beatt KJ. Glucose-insulin-potassium therapy for treatment of acute myocardial infarction: an overview of randomized placebo-controlled trials. Circulation 1997; 96:1152–1156.

48   Ceremuzynski L, Budaj A, Czepiel A, et al. Low-dose glucose-insulin-potassium is ineffective in acute myocardial infarction: results of a randomized multicenter Pol-GIK trial. Cardiovasc Drugs Ther 1999; 13:191–200.

49   van der Horst IC, Zijlstra F, van't Hof AW, et al. Zwolle Infarct Study Group. Glucose-insulin-potassium infusion inpatients treated with primary angioplasty for acute myocardial infarction: the glucose-insulin-potassium study: a randomized trial. J Am Coll Cardiol 2003; 42:784–791.

50   van der Horst IC, Timmer JR, Ottervanger JP, et al. GIPS Investigators. Glucose-insulin-potassium and reperfusion in acute myocardial infarction: rationale and design of the Glucose-Insulin-Potassium Study-2 (GIPS-2). Presented at the 2005 Annual Scientific Session of the American College of Cardiology, Orlando, FL, March 6–9, 2005.

51   Diaz R, Paolasso EA, Piegas LS, et al. Metabolic modulation of acute myocardial infarction. The ECLA (Estudios Cardiologicos Latinoamerica) Collaborative Group. Circulation 1998; 98:2227–2234.

52 Malmberg K, Ryden L, Efendic S, et al. Randomized trial of insulin-glucose infusion followed by subcutaneous insulin treatment in diabetic patients with acute myocardial infarction (DIGAMI study): effects on mortality at 1 year. J Am Coll Cardiol 1995; 26:57–65.

53 Malmberg K, Ryden L, Wedel H, et al. DIGAMI 2 Investigators. Intense metabolic control by means of insulin in patients with diabetes mellitus and acute myocardial infarction (DIGAMI 2): effects on mortality and morbidity. Eur Heart J 2005; 26:650–661.

54 van den Berghe G, Wouters P, et al. Intensive insulin therapy in the critically ill patients. N Engl J Med 2001; 345:1359–1367.

55 Takagi T, Yamamuro A, Tamita K, et al. Pioglitazone reduces neointimal tissue proliferation after coronary stent implantation in patients with type 2 diabetes mellitus: an intravascular ultrasound scanning study. Am Heart J 2003; 146:E5.

56 Takagi T, Akasaka T, Yamamuro A, et al. Troglitazone reduces neointimal tissue proliferation after coronary stent implantation in patients with non-insulin dependent diabetes mellitus: a serial intravascular ultrasound study. J Am Coll Cardiol 2000; 36:1529–1535.

57 Takagi T, Yamamuro A, Tamita K, et al. Impact of troglitazone on coronary stent implantation using small stents in patients with type 2 diabetes mellitus. Am J Cardiol 2002; 89:318–322.

58 Choi D, Kim SK, Choi SH, et al. Preventative effects of rosiglitazone on restenosis after coronary stent implantation in patients with type 2 diabetes. Diabetes Care 2004; 27:2654–2660.

59 Marx N, Wohrle J, Nusser T, et al. Pioglitazone reduces neointima volume after coronary stent implantation: a randomized, placebo-controlled, double-blind trial in nondiabetic patients. Circulation 2005; 112:2792–2798.

60 Kao J, Tobis J, McClelland RL, et al. Investigators in the Prevention of Restenosis with Tranilast and its Outcomes Trial. Relation of metformin treatment to clinical events in diabetic patients undergoing percutaneous intervention. Am J Cardiol 2004; 93:1347–1350, A5.

61 Mahaffey KW, Cohen M, Garg J, et al. SYNERGY Trial Investigators. High-risk patients with acute coronary syndromes treated with low-molecular-weight or unfractionated heparin: outcomes at 6 months and 1 year in the SYNERGY trial. JAMA 2005; 294:2594–2600.

62 Lee MS, Singh V, Nero T, et al. Diabetics achieve lower ACTs when given the same dose of heparin as non-diabetics during percutaneous coronary intervention (abstract). J Am Coll Cardiol 2003; 41:12A.

63 Chew DP, Bhatt DL, Lincoff AM, et al. Defining the optimal activated clotting time during percutaneous coronary intervention: aggregate results from 6 randomized, controlled trials. Circulation 2001; 103:961–966.

64 Kleiman NS, Lincoff AM, Kereiakes DJ, et al. Diabetes mellitus, glycoprotein IIb/IIIa blockade, and heparin: evidence for a complex interaction in a multicenter trial. EPILOG Investigators. Circulation 1998; 97:1912–1920.

65 Popma JJ, Prpic R, Lansky AJ, Piana R. Heparin dosing in patients undergoing coronary intervention. Am J Cardiol 1998; 82:9P–24P.

66 Tolleson TR, O'Shea JC, Bittl JA, et al. Relationship between heparin anticoagulation and clinical outcomes in coronary stent intervention: observations from the ESPRIT trial. J Am Coll Cardiol 2003; 41:386–393.

67 Libby P, Aikawa M. Stabilization of atherosclerotic plaques: new mechanisms and clinical targets. Nat Med 2002; 8:1257–1262.

68 Scott K, Gregory S, Anders O, et al. High dose atorvastatin enhances the decline in inflammatory markers in patients with acute coronary syndromes in the MIRACL study. Circulation 2003; 108:1560–1566.

69 Okazaki S, Yokoyama T, Miyauchi K, et al. Early statin treatment in patients with acute coronary syndrome: demonstration of the beneficial effect on atherosclerotic lesions by serial volumetric intravascular ultrasound analysis during half a year after coronary event: the ESTABLISH Study. Circulation 2004; 110:1061–1068.

70 LaRosa JC, Grundy SM, Waters DD, et al. Treating to New Targets (TNT) Investigators. Intensive lowering with atorvastatin in patients with stable coronary disease. N Engl J Med 2005; 352:1452–1435.

71 Cannon CP, Braunwald E, McCabe CH, et al. Pravastatin or Atorvastatin Evaluation and Infection Therapy—Thrombolysis in Myocardial Infarction 22 Investigators. Intensive versus moderate lipid lowering with statins after acute coronary syndromes. N Engl J Med 2004; 350:1495–1504.

72 Pedersen TR. The Incremental Decrease in End Points through Aggressive Lipid Lowering (IDEAL) trial. American Heart Association Scientific Sessions 2005; November 13–16, 2005; Dallas, Texas. Late Breaking Clinical Trials III.

73 de Lemos JA, Blazing MA, Wiviott SD, et al. A to Z Investigators. Early intensive vs a delayed conservative simvastatin strategy in patients with acute coronary syndromes: phase Z of the A to Z trial. JAMA 2004; 292(11):1307–1316.

74 Arampatzis CA, Goedhart D, Serruys PW, Saia F, Lemos PA, de Feyter P. LIPS Investigators. Fluvastatin reduces the impact of diabetes on long-term outcome after coronary intervention—a Lescol Intervention Prevention Study (LIPS) substudy. Am Heart J 2005; 149:329–335.

75 Diabetes Atherosclerosis Intervention Study Investigators. Effect of fenofibrate on progression of coronary-artery disease in type 2 diabetes: the Diabetes Atherosclerosis Intervention Study, a randomised study. Lancet 2001; 357(9260):905–910.

76 Keech A, Simes RJ, Barter P, et al. FIELD study investigators. Effects of long-term fenofibrate therapy on cardiovascular events in 9795 people with type 2 diabetes mellitus (the FIELD study): randomised controlled trial. Lancet 2005; 366(9500):1849–1861.

77 Rihal CS, Textor SC, Grill DE, et al. Incidence and prognostic importance of acute renal failure after percutaneous coronary intervention. Circulation 2002; 105:2259–2264.

78 Nikolsky E, Mehran R, Turcot D, et al. Impact of chronic kidney disease on prognosis of patients with diabetes mellitus treated with percutaneous coronary intervention. Am J Cardiol 2004; 94:300–305.

79 Mehran R, Aymong ED, Nikolsky E, et al. A simple risk score for prediction of contrast-induced nephropathy after percutaneous coronary intervention: development and initial validation. J Am Coll Cardiol 2004; 44:1393–1399.

80 Rudnick MR, Goldfarb S, Wexler L, et al. Nephrotoxicity of ionic and nonionic contrast media in 1196 patients: a randomized trial. The Iohexol Cooperative Study. Kidney Int 1995; 47:254–261.

81   Grynne BH, Nossen JO, Bolstad B, Borch KW. Main results of the first comparative clinical studies on Visipaque. Acta Radiol Suppl 1995; 399:265–270.

82   Carraro M, Malalan F, Antonione R, et al. Effects of a dimeric vs a monomeric nonionic contrast medium on renal function in patients with mild to moderate renal insufficiency: a double-blind, randomized clinical trial. Eur Radiol 1998; 8:144–147.

83   Jakobsen JA, Berg KJ, Kjaersgaard P, et al. Angiography with nonionic X-ray contrast media in severe chronic renal failure: renal function and contrast retention. Nephron 1996; 73:549–556.

84   Aspelin P, Aubry P, Fransson SG, Strasser R, Willenbrock R, Berg KJ. Nephrotoxicity in High-Risk Patients Study of Iso-Osmolar and Low-Osmolar Non-Ionic Contrast Media Study Investigators. Nephrotoxic effects in high-risk patients undergoing angiography. N Engl J Med 2003; 348:491–499.

85   Solomon R, Werner C, Mann D, D'Elia J, Silva P. Effects of saline, mannitol, and furosemide to prevent acute decreases in renal function induced by radiocontrast agents. N Engl J Med 1994; 331:1416–1420.

86   Eisenberg RL, Bank WO, Hedgock MW. Renal failure after major angiography can be avoided with hydration. AJR 1981; 136:859–861.

87   Mueller C, Buerkle G, Buettner HJ, et al. Prevention of contrast media-associated nephropathy: randomized comparison of 2 hydration regimens in 1620 patients undergoing coronary angioplasty. Arch Intern Med 2002; 162:329–336.

88   Merten GJ, Burgess WP, Gray LV, et al. Prevention of contrast-induced nephropathy with sodium bicarbonate: a randomized controlled trial. JAMA 2004; 291:2328–2334.

89   Tepel M, van der Giet M, Schwarzfeld C, Laufer U, Liermann D, Zidek W. Prevention of radiographic-contrast-agent-induced reductions in renal function by acetylcysteine. N Engl J Med 2000; 343:180–184.

90   Briguori C, Manganelli F, Scarpato P, et al. Acetylcysteine and contrast agent-associated nephrotoxicity. J Am Coll Cardiol 2002; 40:298–303.

91   Alonso A, Lau J, Jaber BL, Weintraub A, Sarnak MJ. Prevention of radiocontrast nephropathy with N-acetylcysteine in patients with chronic kidney disease: a meta-analysis of randomized, controlled trials. Am J Kidney Dis 2004; 43:1–9.

92   Kshirsagar AV, Poole C, Mottl A, et al. N-acetylcysteine for the prevention of radiocontrast induced nephropathy: a meta-analysis of prospective controlled trials. J Am Soc Nephrol 2004; 15:761–769.

93   Pannu N, Manns B, Lee H, Tonelli M. Systematic review of the impact of N-acetylcysteine on contrast nephropathy. Kidney Int 2004; 65:1366–1374.

94   Moses JW, Leon MB, Popma JJ, et al. Sirolimus-eluting stents versus standard stents in patients with stenosis in a native coronary artery. N Engl J Med 2003; 349:1315–1323.

95   Stone GW, Ellis SG, Cox DA, et al. One-year clinical results with the slow-release, polymer-based, paclitaxel-eluting TAXUS stent: the TAXUS-IV trial. Circulation 2004; 109:1942–1947.

96   Moussa I, Leon MB, Baim DS, et al. Impact of sirolimus-eluting stents on outcome in diabetic patients: a SIRIUS (SIRollmUS-coated Bx Velocity balloon-expandable stent in the treatment of patients with de novo coronary artery lesions) substudy. Circulation 2004; 109:2273–2278.

97   Windecker S, Remondino A, Eberli FR, et al. Sirolimus-eluting and paclitaxel-eluting stents for coronary revascularization. N Engl J Med 2005; 353:653–662.

98   Morice M-C, Serruys PW, Colombo A, et al. Eight-month outcome of the REALITY Study: a prospective, randomized, multi-center head-to-head comparison of the sirolimus-eluting stent (Cypher) and the paclitaxel-eluting stent (Taxus). Presented at the 2005 Annual Scientific Session of the American College of Cardiology, Orlando, FL, March 6–9, 2005.

99   Dibra A, Kastrati A, Mehilli J, et al. Paclitaxel-eluting or sirolimus-eluting stents to prevent restenosis in diabetic patients. N Engl J Med 2005; 353:663–670.

41

Atrial fibrillation during catheterization

Yves L. E. Van Belle, M. F. Scholten, and Luc J. Jordaens

Incidence and prevalence

It is evident that during all types of cardiac catheterization (Table 1) atrial fibrillation (AF) can occur and that several patients will present with preexisting AF. It is the most common type of arrhythmia in adults (1). The prevalence goes from less than 1% in persons younger than 60 years of age to more than 8% in those older than 80 years of age (2). The age-adjusted incidence for women is about half that of men.

The cardiac conditions most commonly associated with AF are rheumatic mitral valve disease, coronary artery disease, congestive heart failure, hypertension, hypertrophic cardiomyopathy, pericarditis, myocarditis, and congenital heart disease. It also occurs in cardiopulmonary disease such as pulmonary embolism and chronic obstructive pulmonary disease. Noncardiac causes include hyperthyroidism, hypoxic conditions, surgery, and alcohol intoxication. A predisposing condition exists in more than 90% of cases; the remaining cases have what is called lone AF. Comparing with age-matched controls, the relative risk for stroke is increased two- to sevenfold in patients with nonrheumatic AF, and the absolute risk for stroke is between 1% and 5% per year, depending on clinical characteristics. AF can be categorized as paroxysmal, persistent, or permanent.

Therapeutic options

Several treatment options are available when confronted with AF dependent on its clinical effect and duration. The hemodynamic effects and/or cardiac ischemia due to a rapid ventricular rate can seriously complicate a catheter procedure and can even be life threatening in some instances. Therefore, one goal can be to alleviate the clinical repercussions of the arrhythmia in order to finalize the procedure. The second goal is to restore sinus rhythm if possible. To achieve the first goal, a strategy called "rate control" might be sufficient if allowed by the hemodynamic

status. The second goal is more complex, but will be discussed as well. Whether sinus rhythm can be restored (rhythm control) is dependent on the risk for thromboembolic events.

Anticoagulation during catheter procedures in atrial fibrillation

During cardiac catheterization, intravenous anticoagulation is given to prevent venous thrombosis and left-sided emboli. In

Table 1   Interventions associated with atrial fibrillation
Coronary artery disease
Diagnostic coronary angiography
Percutaneous coronary intervention
Valvular pathology
Left–right catheterization
Balloon valvuloplasty
Cardiac arrhythmia
Diagnostic supraventricular or ventricular induction
Endocavitary ablation procedure (including pulmonary vein isolation)
Pericardial ablation procedure
Left auricular closure device
Congenital disease
Transcatheter closure of atrial or ventricular septal defect
Obliteration of anastomosis
Myocardial disease
Endocardial biopsy
Percutaneous transluminal septal alcoholization

some interventions, for example left-sided catheter ablations, a very high level of anticoagulation is required to prevent thrombus formation on the site of intervention (cf. Fig. 1). The risk of thrombosis and stroke is well known.

Patients with AF or atrial flutter (AFL) and impaired left atrial appendage (LAA) function are also potentially at high risk for thromboembolism and might therefore require anticoagulation (3). Approximately 90% of atrial thrombi in nonrheumatic AF are found in the LAA (4). Patients less than 60 years, without cardiovascular disease, however, have a low risk for stroke. Other factors, such as age and associated cardiovascular disease, therefore, play an important role. Platelet activation, on the other hand, probably does not play a significant role in thrombus formation in these patients (5). Five large, randomized trials of anticoagulation were pooled by The AF Investigators (6) and risk factors for stroke were defined. Age was shown to increase stroke risk by 1.4 per decade. Other risk factors include previous stroke or transient ischemic attack (TIA), hypertension, diabetes mellitus, congestive heart failure, ischemic or rheumatic heart disease, prior thromboembolism, and female gender. Patients with rheumatic heart disease, prosthetic heart valves, prior thromboembolism, and persistent atrial thrombus detected by transesophageal echocardiography (TEE) are considered to be at highest risk (7,8).

Echocardiography is useful in risk assessment for thromboembolism. TEE is superior in the detection of reduced flow velocities and spontaneous echo contrast in the left atrium and LAA (9). Patients with AF and complex atherosclerotic plaques in the aorta have a substantially higher risk for stroke (10,11).

Oral anticoagulation

Pooled data analysis for oral anticoagulation with coumadins (targeting an INR of 2.0 to 3.0) have shown a relative

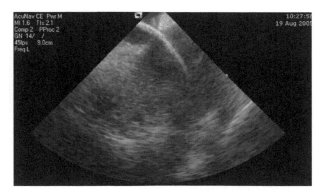

Figure 1
Intracardiac echocardiogram with transseptal sheath from right atrium (upper cavity) through the oval fossa in the left atrium. Attached to the sheath is a small clot, in spite of the administration of 5000 IU heparin before the puncture.

risk-reduction for stroke of between 62% and 70% (6,12). Several reports indicate that anticoagulation is actually underused in AF patients at high risk for thromboembolic complications (13,14). Possible explanations for this underuse are doubts about the effectiveness of anticoagulation, the fear of hemorrhagic complications such as intracerebral bleeding and the limitations of its use, such as frequent coagulation monitoring and interactions with other drugs. These fears also play a role in withholding oral anticoagulation at the time of catheterization. In patients with bioprosthetic valves and AF, similar levels of anticoagulation to those mentioned above seem adequate. In AF associated with mechanical valve prostheses, levels of anticoagulation recommended are less standardized, but what is clear is that the risks for thromboembolism depend on the type of valve inserted and its position (15,16). Accordingly, the target INR for these patients should be individualized and the presence or absence of AF has little influence on this targeting. Thromboembolic events after cardioversion in atrial tachyarrhythmias have been reported in 1% to 7% of patients not receiving prophylactic anticoagulation (17,18). Anticoagulation is recommended for three to four weeks before and after cardioversion for patients with AF of unknown duration and for AF of more than 48 hours duration (7). A reasonable alternative strategy is early cardioversion with a short period of anticoagulation therapy after exclusion of LA/LAA thrombi with TEE (7).

Anticoagulation in radiofrequency ablation of atrial fibrillation and atrial flutter

The treatment of AF entered a new era after the publication of the landmark observations of Haissaguerre et al (19). Both segmental ostial catheter ablation (20) and left atrial encircling ablation of the pulmonary veins (PVs) (21) have been reported to be successful in the treatment of AF. Radiofrequency (RF) ablation is a highly effective therapeutic approach in the treatment of typical isthmus- dependent AFL (22).

RF catheter ablation is complicated by thromboembolism in about 0.6% of patients (23). The risk of stroke from RF ablation may be higher in paroxysmal AF patients with prior TIA (24). As reflected by elevated plasma D-dimer levels, RF ablation has a thrombogenic effect that persists through the first 48 hours after the procedure (25). Activation of the coagulation cascade in RF ablation procedures is not related to the delivery of RF energy, but is related to the placement of intravascular catheters and to the duration of the ablation procedure (26,27). Furthermore, RF lesions themselves have been shown to be thrombogenic (28). The risk of a thromboembolic complication is higher for left-sided ablations

(1.8–2.0%) (23). By administering intravenous heparin immediately after introduction of the venous sheaths, hemostatic activation is significantly decreased (29). There is also a significant risk for thromboembolism in patients referred for ablation of typical AFL who have not been appropriately anticoagulated (30). Radiofrequency ablation of chronic AFL is associated with significant left atrial stunning (31).

The NASPE Policy Statement on catheter ablation (32) suggests anticoagulation for at least three weeks prior to ablation for AF and AFL for patients who are in these arrhythmias. Discontinuation of anticoagulants two to three days before the procedure is possible. For high-risk patients, heparin to cover this period should be considered (32). TEE shortly before pulmonary vein ablation to exclude left atrial thrombi is done routinely (33,34). Generally during left-sided ablation, heparin should be administered, aiming at an activated clotting time (ACT) of 250–300 seconds. Higher levels of anticoagulation (ACT >300 seconds) are used for pulmonary vein ablations (32). Experienced groups continue anticoagulation therapy at least three months after a successful ablation (33,35,36).

Rhythm control: cardioversion

Early cardioversion may be necessary in patients with hemodynamic compromise (acute pulmonary edema, worsening angina, or hypotension) in relation to uncontrolled AF (flow chart). Synchronized, direct current cardioversion is more effective and preferable to pharmacologic cardioversion under these circumstances. Intravenous anticoagulation should precede and follow the cardioversion (Fig. 2).

The necessity for urgent cardioversion is less well established in hemodynamically stable patients with AF. It may be wise to postpone cardioversion till the procedure is finished, and to limit the antiarrhythmic interventions to rate control. Despite this wisdom, the management of these patients has traditionally been dominated by a drive to restore and maintain sinus rhythm—the so-called rhythm-control strategy (37–39). From a short-term perspective, hemodynamic measurements may be more correct, and some procedures may require this. If cardioversion is performed in this, more or less elective, setting precaution to prevent emboli is warranted. TEE may be helpful to take a better and faster decision; there are procedures with a transesophageal probe in place, and the threshold to cardiovert can be low.

Electrical cardioversion of atrial fibrillation

This can be performed with the conventional external paddles or patches or with intracardiac or intraesophageal electrodes. Good sedation with diazepam, or short acting anesthesia with a product as etomidate can be sufficient. Propofol has cardiodepressive characteristics, making it less desirable under certain conditions.

Pharmacologic cardioversion of atrial fibrillation

Pharmacologic cardioversion appears to be most effective when initiated within seven days after the onset of AF. A large proportion of patients with recent-onset AF experience spontaneous cardioversion within 24 to 48 hours. This is less likely to occur when AF has persisted for more than seven days.

A systematic review of randomized controlled trials in patients with newly detected AF identified a number of antiarrhythmic drugs for which there was statistically significant evidence of benefit (1). In a limited number of comparative studies, flecainide was more effective than propafenone and procainamide, propafenone was superior to amiodarone, amiodarone was superior to quinidine, and quinidine was superior to sotalol.

Recommendations for pharmacologic therapy, according to the duration of AF, and the doses that should be used were published in 2001 by a task force of the ACC/AHA (7). In general, high doses of several drugs are more effective in producing cardioversion, but these doses are more prone to cause toxicity. As a result, direct current (DC) cardioversion has largely replaced aggressive pharmacologic therapy for primary cardioversion. However, antiarrhythmic drugs are commonly used to facilitate DC cardioversion (e.g., Ibutilide) and after the procedure to maintain sinus rhythm.

An overview of effective drugs is given below. During procedures, the time to conversion also plays an important role.

Flecainide

1. Class Ic agent that prolongs refractoriness and slows conduction in the atria, atrioventricular node (AV-node), His-Purkinje system, ventricles and accessory pathways. Predominantly blocks sodium channels in the activated state with rate-dependent block (40).
2. Bioavailability 90%–95%, T 1/2 13–19 hours, 2/3 hepatic metabolization, 1/3 renal excretion.
3. Therapeutic levels 0.2–1.0 µg/ml, through level <1.0. Prolongation of PR and QRS intervals when therapeutic levels are achieved.
4. Dosage: Oral, twice daily, initiation 100 mg twice daily up to 150 twice, rare 200 mg twice. Intravenous: 1 to 2 mg/kg over 10 minutes, then 0.15 to 0.25 mg/kg/hr.

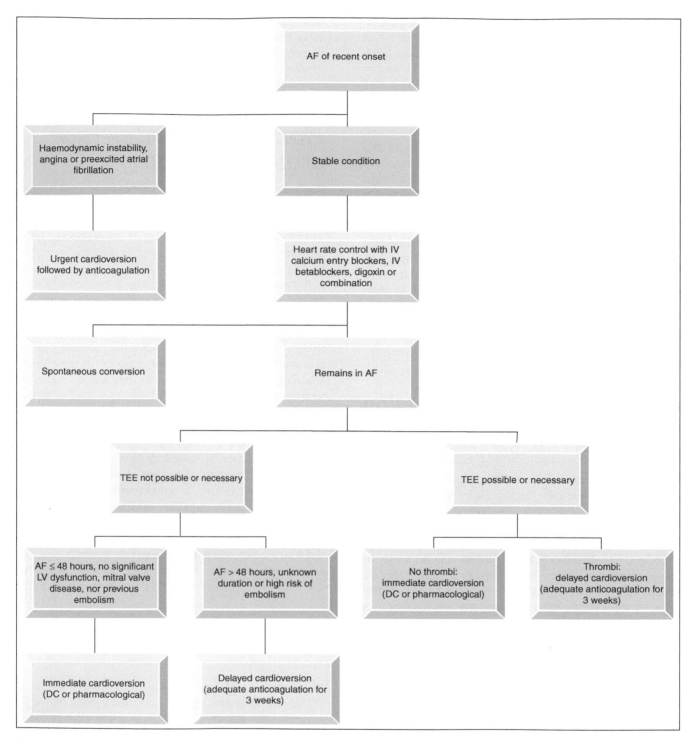

Figure 2
Flow chart for recent onset atrial fibrillation.

5. Intravenous flecainide (150 mg) converts recent onset AF in 55% to 65% of patients (41).
6. Cardiac proarrhythmic effects of flecainide include aggravation of ventricular arrhythmias and threat of sudden death as in the CAST study (42). The proarrhythmic effect is due to nonuniform slowing of conduction. Monitoring the QRS interval seems logical but no safety margins have been established. Furthermore, late proarrhythmic effects can

occur. In patients with pre-existing sinus node or AV conduction problems, there may be worsening of arrhythmia. In AF or AFL, the drug can cause the atrial rate to fall, with a subsequent rise of the ventricular rate: it should therefore always be prescribed with an AV-nodal depressing drug such as digitalis, betablockers, or verapamil to avoid fast AV conduction. Also, ventricular arrhythmias may be precipitated.

7. More effective than procainamide, sotalol, propafenone, and amiodarone (43–47).

Propafenone

1. Class Ic antiarrhythmic drug similar to flecainide, blocking sodium channels in both activated and inactivated states, additional weak betablocking effect.
2. T 1/2 2 to 12 hours, poor metabolizers 10 to 12 hours, steady state after 72 hours (T 1/2 of active metabolite).
3. Dosage: Oral 450 to 600 mg, iv: 1.5 to 2.0 mg/kg over 10 to 20 minutes.
4. Oral propafenone is an effective drug for conversion of AF to sinus rhythm (48,49). A review of the literature found that a single oral loading dose converted AF in 58% to 83% of patients, depending upon the duration of AF (50).
5. Increased mortality and cardiac arrest recurrence when structural heart disease (51).
6. Useful in reducing the ventricular response (52).

Ibutilide

1. Class III antiarrhythmic drug, which prolongs repolarization by inhibition of the delayed rectifier potassium current (I_{kr}) and by selective enhancement of the slow inward sodium current. Ibutilide has no known negative inotropic effects (53).
2. Only available as intravenous preparation
3. T 1/2 2 to 12 hours (54).
4. Dose- and concentration-related increase in the uncorrected and rate-corrected QT interval
5. Dosage: less than 60 kg—0.01 mg/kg infused over 10 minutes. If the arrhythmia does not terminate 10 minutes after the end of the infusion, a second bolus (same dose over 10 minutes) can be given. More than 60 kg—1 mg over 10 minutes. If arrhythmia does not terminate 10 minutes after the end of the infusion, a second bolus of 1 mg over 10 minutes can be given.
6. The acute AF conversion rate is higher with ibutilide than with placebo and can be expected to occur about 30 minutes after infusion (55,56). It is efficacious in the termination of AF and AFL with both single and repeated intravenous infusions (54). In patients with persistent AF or AFL, ibutilide has a conversion efficacy of 44% for a single dose and 49% for a second dose (56). Efficacy is higher in AFL than in AF and is related to an effect on the variability of the cycle length of the tachycardia (57) due to the phenomenon of reverse use dependence: prolongation of refractoriness becomes less pronounced at higher tachycardia rates.
7. Has the potential to provoke torsade de pointes. The rate of torsade de pointes ranged between 3.6% and 8.3% (55,56,58,59) and may be more common in women (59). Sustained episodes requiring cardioversion were seen in 1.7% to 2.4%. In addition to polymorphic VT, nonsustained monomorphic VT occurred in 3.2% to 3.6% (55,56). Therefore, continuous ECG monitoring for at least four hours after the infusion or until the QTc interval has returned to baseline.
8. In comparative studies, ibutilide has been more effective for AF reversion than procainamide (51% vs. 21% and 32% vs. 5%) (60,61) or intravenous sotalol (44% vs. 11%) (show Fig. 7) (53). It is as effective as amiodarone in cardioversion of AFL (1,62).
9. After cardiac surgery: dose-dependent effect in conversion of atrial arrhythmias with 57% conversion at a dose of 10 mg (63).
10. The drug is more effective when given as pretreatment prior to cardioversion (64).

Dofetilide

1. Useful, but not commercially available.

Amiodarone

1. Class III antiarrhythmic agent with additional classes I, II, III, and IV actions. Prolongs action potential duration and effective refractory period in all cardiac tissues.
2. Dosage: Oral: 1.2 to 1.8 g in divided doses until 10 g, then 200 to 400 mg/day or 30 mg/kg as a single daily dose. Intravenous: 5 to 7 mg/kg over 30 minutes, then 1.2 to 1.8 g in continuous infusion over 24 hour, then 200 to 400 mg daily (1).
3. Intravenous amiodarone has been reported to be effective, converting 60% to 70% of patients to sinus rhythm in some trials (65–67). The efficacy has been evaluated in studies with different durations of AF.
4. Oral amiodarone: A number of mostly small trials have evaluated the efficacy of oral amiodarone which, as with other drugs, appears to vary with the duration of AF (66,68). The SAFE-T trial of patients with persistent AF

who were on anticoagulation therapy showed that patients randomly assigned to amiodarone or sotalol had a higher frequency of cardioversion to sinus rhythm after one month compared to placebo. Patients who were still in AF underwent DC cardioversion of which efficacy was similar in all groups (69).

5. Cardiac side effects: Torsade de pointes (<0.5%), severe bradycardia (one-year risk of bradycardia 2.4% on amiodarone vs. 0.8% on placebo). Non-cardiac side effects: Pulmonary toxicity 1% per year with fatal cases: discontinue and treat symptomatically, hepatotoxicity 0.6%, periferal neuropathy 0.3%, hypothyroidism 6%, hyperthyroidism 0.9%. Routine toxicity screening is required. This includes periodic (usually every six months) measurement of thyroid (sensitive serum T4), hepatic (AST), and pulmonary function (chest X-ray), as well as clinical evaluation (70).

Procainamide

1. Intravenous procainamide converts 20% to 60% of cases to sinus rhythm, particularly if the AF is of recent onset. It can be used with caution (hypotension, QRS widening), when the more effective, previously described drugs are not available.

Quinidine

1. Should not be used in emergency settings (71).

Sotalol

1. Intravenous sotalol appears to be less effective than intravenous flecainide or ibutilide (47).
2. Oral sotalol less effective than quinidine for conversion of recent onset (<48 hours) AF and is comparable to amiodarone for conversion of AF of >48 hours in duration (69,72).

Digoxin

1. The rate of conversion with digoxin is no better than placebo. Digoxin may restore sinus rhythm when AF is due to heart failure (73,74). In this setting, reversion is the result of improved hemodynamics and a reduction in left atrial pressure.

Rate control: slowing conduction in the AV-node

Rate control can be effectively achieved using a betablocker, calciumantagonist, and/or digoxin either in monotherapy or combined as necessary. Caution must be taken that combining intravenous betablocker and calciumantagonist may cause severe depression of the left ventricular function and AV-node. In the setting of heart failure digoxin may be preferable since it has a positive inotropic effect, with diltiazem as a second choice agent.

Betablockers

Propranolol

1. Noncardioselective betablocker with a plasma half-life of one to six hours and a hepatic metabolisation.
2. Intravenous dose is 1 to 6 mg as needed.
3. Contraindications include hypotension, second and third degree heart block, cardiogenic shock and overt cardiac failure, peripheral ischemia, and bronchospasm.
4. Multiple drug interactions have been described with numerous compounds due to interference with hepatic clearance.

Metoprolol

1. β1-selective betablocker with a plasma half-life of three to seven hours and mainly hepatic elimination.
2. Bolus 2.5 to 5 mg over two minutes, repeated at five minutes interval up to 15 mg.
3. Contraindications: Hypotension, second and third degree heart block, cardiogenic shock and overt cardiac failure, and bronchospasm.
4. Drug interactions: Catecholamine-depleting drugs such as reserpine may have an additive effect in combination with betablockers. Drugs that inhibit CYP2D6 (quinidine, fluoxetine, paroxetine, and propafenone) increase metoprolol concentration.

Esmolol

1. Rapidly and very short acting betablocker (half life of nine minutes).

2. Bolus of 0.5 mg/kg over one minute followed by 50 μg/kg per minute. After four minutes another bolus can be given and infusion increased to 100 μg/kg per minute. Infusion rate can be increase to a maximum of 200 μg/kg per minute, guided by clinical response.
3. Contraindications include hypotension, peripheral ischemia, confusion, thrombophlebitis, skin necrosis from extravasation, bradycardia, second and third degree heart block, cardiogenic shock, overt heart failure, and bronchospasm.
4. Interactions with catecholamine depleting drugs and increases digoxin blood levels.

Calciumantagonists

Verapamil

1. Non-dihydropyridine calciumantagonist (Class IV AAD) that inhibits the calcium mediated depolarization of the AV-node, increasing the nodal effective refractory period and reducing ventricular rate in AF.
2. Can be given as a slow intravenous bolus of 5 to 10 mg over two to three minutes, repeated after 10 to 15 minutes. Acts within five minutes of intravenous administration. Plasma half-life is two to eight hours. Is metabolized in the liver by the P-450 system, with ultimately 75% renal and 25% gastrointestinal excretion.
3. Contraindications are hypotension, cardiogenic shock, marked bradycardia, second or third degree AV-block, Wolff-Parkinson-White (WPW) syndrome, wide complex tachycardia, VT and uncompensated heart failure.
4. Multiple drug interactions have been discribed (decreased serum concentrations of phenobarbital, phenytoin, sulfinpyrazone and rifampin, increased serum concentrations of quinidine, carbamazepine, cyclosporin). Important in this setting is that a marked interaction exists between digoxin and verapamil, increasing the serum concentrations of the former due to decreased renal excretion.

Diltiazem

1. Non-dihydropyridine calciumantagonist (Class IV AAD) with similar action as verapamil.
2. Initial intravenous dose is 0.25 mg/kg over two minutes followed by 0.35 mg/kg after 15 minutes as required. Continuous infusion rate after initial bolus of 5 to 10 mg/hr may be further increased to 15 mg/hr. Plasma

half-life is three to five hours, but may be longer in an elderly population.
3. Contraindications are similar to verapamil.
4. Drug interactions include rise in plasma concentration when concommittant administration with cimetidine and lowering of the concentration with barbiturates, phenytoin, rifampin. Digoxin levels may be variably affected, can rise.

Digoxin

1. Digoxin is a cardiac glycoside acting through inhibition of the sodium pump (Na/K-ATPase) causing a transient increase in intracellular sodium, which in turn promotes calcium influx by a sodium—calcium exchange mechanism resulting in an enhanced myocardial contractility. It also causes sinus slowing and atrioventricular nodal inhibition by parasympathetic activation, combined with a modest direct nodal inhibition. Digoxin inhibits sympathetic nerve discharge and inhibits renin release from the kidney with a natriuretic effect.
2. Intravenous loading with 500 μg produces a detectable effect in 5 to 30 minutes and becomes maximal in one to four hours. Additional doses of 250 μg can be given with six to eight hour intervals. Serum digoxin concentrations should be ranging from 0.8 to 2.0 ng/ml; however there can be a clinical benefit below this range. Sampling should be performed at least six to eight hours after the last dose.
3. Serum half-life is 36 hours, 70% by renal secretion, 30% hepatic/gastrointestinal.
4. Contraindications are hypertrophic obstructive cardiomyopathy (increase in inotropism can increase outflow tract obstruction), AF in WPW syndrome (can cause precipitation of the arrhythmia to ventricular fibrillation (VF) by preferential conduction over the accessory pathway), significant AV-block or sick sinus syndrome, hypokalemia (causes increased digoxin sensitivity and supraventricular/ventricular arrhythmia), thyreotoxicosis, postinfarction status (increased mortality). Caution should be exerted in renal failure, and coadministration of other drugs depressing sinus node or AV-nodal function.
5. Caution should be taken when administered in pulmonary disease because of the sensitivity to intoxication due to hypoxia, electrolyte disturbances and sympathetic discharge. Digoxin also experimentaly increases infarct size.
6. Drug interactions are multiple but of special interest is the interaction with other AADs such as quinidine and verapamil, both increasing the serum concentration.
7. Diuretics may induce hypokalemia, which sensitizes the heart to digoxin toxicity and stops the tubular excretion of the drug. Toxicity has gastrointestinal (nausea,

vomiting, anorexia, diarrhea), neurologic (malaise, fatigue, confusion, insomnia, facial pain, depression, vertigo, colored vision), and cardiac (palpitations, arrhythmias, syncope) effects, hypokalemia is also common in the typical patient. Digoxin arrhythmias range from AV-block and bradycardia, due to increased vagal tone, to accelerated atrial, junctional or ventricular arrhythmias, due to increased automaticity of junctional tissue in His-Purkinje tissue. Bidirectional tachycardia is rare but very suggestive. Blood level and electrolytes should be checked to confirm. Lidocaine can be given to reduce ventricular ectopy without increasing the AV-block, phenytoin reverses the latter (dose of 100 mg intravenously every five minutes to a total of 1000 mg or side effects). When faced with severe ventricular arrhythmias and thus life threatening intoxication, Digoxin-specific antibodies can be administered.

References

1 McNamara RL, et al. Management of atrial fibrillation: review of the evidence for the role of pharmacologic therapy, electrical cardioversion, and echocardiography. Ann Intern Med 2003; 139(12):1018–1033.

2 Majeed A, Moser K, Carroll K. Trends in the prevalence and management of atrial fibrillation in general practice in England and Wales, 1994–1998: analysis of data from the general practice research database. Heart 2001; 86(3):284–288.

3 Sakurai K, et al. Left atrial appendage function and abnormal hypercoagulability in patients with atrial flutter. Chest 2003; 124(5):1670–1674.

4 Odell JA, et al. Thoracoscopic obliteration of the left atrial appendage: potential for stroke reduction? Ann Thorac Surg 1996; 61(2):565–569.

5 Kamath S, et al. A study of platelet activation in atrial fibrillation and the effects of antithrombotic therapy. Eur Heart J 2002; 23(22):1788–1795.

6 Investigators AF. Risk factors for stroke and efficacy of antithrombotic therapy in atrial fibrillation. Analysis of pooled data from five randomized controlled trials. Arch Intern Med 1994; 154(13):1449–57.

7 Fuster V, et al. ACC/AHA/ESC Guidelines for the Management of Patients With Atrial Fibrillation: Executive Summary A Report of the American College of Cardiology/American Heart Association Task Force on Practice Guidelines and the European Society of Cardiology Committee for Practice Guidelines and Policy Conferences (Committee to Develop Guidelines for the Management of Patients With Atrial Fibrillation) Developed in Collaboration With the North American Society of Pacing and Electrophysiology. Circulation 2001; 104(17):2118–2150.

8 Group TEAFTS. Secondary prevention in non-rheumatic atrial fibrillation after transient ischaemic attack or minor stroke. Lancet 1993; 342(8882):1255–1262.

9 Pearson AC, et al. Superiority of transesophageal echocardiography in detecting cardiac source of embolism in patients with cerebral ischemia of uncertain etiology. J Am Coll Cardiol 1991; 17(1): 66–72.

10 Zabalgoitia M, et al. Transesophageal echocardiographic correlates of clinical risk of thromboembolism in nonvalvular atrial fibrillation. Stroke Prevention in Atrial Fibrillation III Investigators. J Am Coll Cardiol 1998; 31(7):1622–1626.

11 Tunick PA, et al. Effect of treatment on the incidence of stroke and other emboli in 519 patients with severe thoracic aortic plaque. Am J Cardiol 2002; 90(12):1320–1325.

12 Feinberg WM, et al. Prevalence, age distribution, and gender of patients with atrial fibrillation. Analysis and implications. Arch Intern Med 1995; 155(5):469–473.

13 Stafford RS, Singer DE. Recent national patterns of warfarin use in atrial fibrillation. Circulation 1998; 97(13):1231–1233.

14 Bungard TJ, et al. Why do patients with atrial fibrillation not receive warfarin? Arch Intern Med 2000; 160(1):41–46.

15 Stein PD. Antithrombotic therapy in valvular heart disease. Clin Geriatr Med 2001; 17(1):163–172, viii.

16 ACC/AHA guidelines for the management of patients with valvular heart disease. A report of the American College of Cardiology/American Heart Association. Task Force on Practice Guidelines (Committee on Management of Patients with Valvular Heart Disease). J Am Coll Cardiol 1998; 32(5):1486–1588.

17 Bjerkelund CJ, Orning OM. The efficacy of anticoagulant therapy in preventing embolism related to D.C. electrical conversion of atrial fibrillation. Am J Cardiol 1969; 23(2):208–216.

18 Arnold AZ, et al. Role of prophylactic anticoagulation for direct current cardioversion in patients with atrial fibrillation or atrial flutter. J Am Coll Cardiol 1992; 19(4):851–855.

19 Haissaguerre M, et al. Spontaneous initiation of atrial fibrillation by ectopic beats originating in the pulmonary veins. N Engl J Med 1998; 339(10):659–666.

20 Haissaguerre M, et al. Mapping-guided ablation of pulmonary veins to cure atrial fibrillation. Am J Cardiol 2000; 86(9 Suppl 1):K9–K19.

21 Pappone C, et al. Atrial electroanatomic remodeling after circumferential radiofrequency pulmonary vein ablation: efficacy of an anatomic approach in a large cohort of patients with atrial fibrillation. Circulation 2001; 104(21):2539–2544.

22 Passman R.S, et al. Radiofrequency ablation of atrial flutter: a randomized controlled study of two anatomic approaches. Pacing Clin Electrophysiol 2004; 27(1):83–88.

23 Zhou L, et al. Thromboembolic complications of cardiac radiofrequency catheter ablation: a review of the reported incidence, pathogenesis and current research directions. J Cardiovasc Electrophysiol 1999; 10(4):611–620.

24 Kok LC, et al. Cerebrovascular complication associated with pulmonary vein ablation. J Cardiovasc Electrophysiol 2002; 13(8):764–767.

25 Manolis AS, et al. Thrombogenicity of radiofrequency lesions: results with serial D-dimer determinations. J Am Coll Cardiol 1996; 28(5):1257–1261.

26 Dorbala S, et al. Does radiofrequency ablation induce a prethrombotic state? Analysis of coagulation system activation and comparison to electrophysiologic study. J Cardiovasc Electrophysiol 1998; 9(11):1152–1160.

27 Anfinsen OG, et al. The activation of platelet function, coagulation, and fibrinolysis during radiofrequency catheter ablation

in heparinized patients. J Cardiovasc Electrophysiol 1999; 10(4):503–512.

28 Khairy P, et al. Lower incidence of thrombus formation with cryoenergy versus radiofrequency catheter ablation. Circulation 2003; 107(15):2045–2050.

29 Anfinsen OG, et al. When should heparin preferably be administered during radiofrequency catheter ablation? Pacing Clin Electrophysiol 2001; 24(1):5–12.

30 Gronefeld GC, et al. Thromboembolic risk of patients referred for radiofrequency catheter ablation of typical atrial flutter without prior appropriate anticoagulation therapy. Pacing Clin Electrophysiol 2003; 26(1 Pt 2):323–327.

31 Sparks PB, et al. Left atrial "stunning" following radiofrequency catheter ablation of chronic atrial flutter. J Am Coll Cardiol 1998; 32(2):468–475.

32 Scheinman M, et al. NASPE policy statement on catheter ablation: personnel, policy, procedures, and therapeutic recommendations. Pacing Clin Electrophysiol 2003; 26(3):789–799.

33 Marrouche NF, et al. Phased-array intracardiac echocardiography monitoring during pulmonary vein isolation in patients with atrial fibrillation: impact on outcome and complications. Circulation 2003; 107(21):2710–2716.

34 Macle L, et al. Electrophysiologically guided pulmonary vein isolation during sustained atrial fibrillation. J Cardiovasc Electrophysiol 2003; 14(3):255–260.

35 Haissaguerre M, et al. Electrophysiological end point for catheter ablation of atrial fibrillation initiated from multiple pulmonary venous foci. Circulation 2000; 101(12):1409–1417.

36 Pappone C, et al. Circumferential radiofrequency ablation of pulmonary vein ostia: A new anatomic approach for curing atrial fibrillation. Circulation 2000; 102(21):2619–2628.

37 Hohnloser SH, Kuck KH, Lilienthal J. Rhythm or rate control in atrial fibrillation—Pharmacological Intervention in Atrial Fibrillation (PIAF): a randomised trial. Lancet 2000; 356(9244):1789–1794.

38 Wyse DG, et al. A comparison of rate control and rhythm control in patients with atrial fibrillation. N Engl J Med 2002; 347(23):1825–1833.

39 Van Gelder IC, et al. A comparison of rate control and rhythm control in patients with recurrent persistent atrial fibrillation. N Engl J Med 2002; 347(23):1834–1840.

40 Roden DM, Woosley RL. Drug therapy. Flecainide. N Engl J Med 1986; 315(1):36–41.

41 Reisinger J, et al. Flecainide versus ibutilide for immediate cardioversion of atrial fibrillation of recent onset. Eur Heart J 2004; 25(15):1318–1324.

42 Preliminary report: effect of encainide and flecainide on mortality in a randomized trial of arrhythmia suppression after myocardial infarction. The Cardiac Arrhythmia Suppression Trial (CAST) Investigators. N Engl J Med 1989; 321(6):406–412.

43 Donovan KD, et al. Intravenous flecainide versus amiodarone for recent-onset atrial fibrillation. Am J Cardiol 1995; 75(10):693–697.

44 Hohnloser SH, Zabel M. Short- and long-term efficacy and safety of flecainide acetate for supraventricular arrhythmias. Am J Cardiol 1992; 70(5):3A–9A; discussion 9A–10A.

45 Madrid AH, et al. Comparison of flecainide and procainamide in cardioversion of atrial fibrillation. Eur Heart J 1993; 14(8):1127–1131.

46 Martinez-Marcos FJ, et al. Comparison of intravenous flecainide, propafenone, and amiodarone for conversion of acute atrial fibrillation to sinus rhythm. Am J Cardiol 2000; 86(9):950–953.

47 Reisinger J, et al. Prospective comparison of flecainide versus sotalol for immediate cardioversion of atrial fibrillation. Am J Cardiol 1998; 81(12):1450–1454.

48 Boriani G, et al. Oral propafenone to convert recent-onset atrial fibrillation in patients with and without underlying heart disease. A randomized, controlled trial. Ann Intern Med 1997; 126(8):621–625.

49 Botto GL, et al. Conversion of recent onset atrial fibrillation with single loading oral dose of propafenone: is in-hospital admission absolutely necessary? Pacing Clin Electrophysiol 1996; 19(11 Pt 2):1939–1943.

50 Khan IA. Single oral loading dose of propafenone for pharmacological cardioversion of recent-onset atrial fibrillation. J Am Coll Cardiol 2001; 37(2):542–547.

51 Siebels J, et al. Preliminary results of the Cardiac Arrest Study Hamburg (CASH). CASH Investigators. Am J Cardiol 1993; 72(16):109F–113F.

52 Bianconi L, et al. Effects of oral propafenone administration before electrical cardioversion of chronic atrial fibrillation: a placebo-controlled study. J Am Coll Cardiol 1996; 28(3):700–706.

53 Vos MA, et al. Superiority of ibutilide (a new class III agent) over DL-sotalol in converting atrial flutter and atrial fibrillation. The Ibutilide/Sotalol Comparator Study Group. Heart 1998; 79(6):568–575.

54 Murray KT. Ibutilide. Circulation 1998; 97(5):493–497.

55 Abi-Mansour P, et al. Conversion efficacy and safety of repeated doses of ibutilide in patients with atrial flutter and atrial fibrillation. Study Investigators. Am Heart J 1998; 136(4 Pt 1):632–642.

56 Stambler BS, et al. Efficacy and safety of repeated intravenous doses of ibutilide for rapid conversion of atrial flutter or fibrillation. Ibutilide Repeat Dose Study Investigators. Circulation 1996; 94(7):1613–1621.

57 Guo GB, et al. Conversion of atrial flutter by ibutilide is associated with increased atrial cycle length variability. J Am Coll Cardiol 1996; 27(5):1083–1089.

58 Ellenbogen KA, et al. Efficacy of intravenous ibutilide for rapid termination of atrial fibrillation and atrial flutter: a dose-response study. J Am Coll Cardiol 1996; 28(1):130–136.

59 Gowda RM, et al. Female preponderance in ibutilide-induced torsade de pointes. Int J Cardiol 2004; 95(2–3):219–222.

60 Stambler BS, Wood MA, Ellenbogen KA. Antiarrhythmic actions of intravenous ibutilide compared with procainamide during human atrial flutter and fibrillation: electrophysiological determinants of enhanced conversion efficacy. Circulation 1997; 96(12):4298–4306.

61 Volgman AS, et al. Conversion efficacy and safety of intravenous ibutilide compared with intravenous procainamide in patients with atrial flutter or fibrillation. J Am Coll Cardiol 1998; 31(6):1414–1419.

62 Bernard EO, et al. Ibutilide versus amiodarone in atrial fibrillation: a double-blinded, randomized study. Crit Care Med 2003; 31(4):1031–1034.

63 VanderLugt JT, et al. Efficacy and safety of ibutilide fumarate for the conversion of atrial arrhythmias after cardiac surgery. Circulation 1999; 100(4):369–375.

64 Oral H, et al. Facilitating transthoracic cardioversion of atrial fibrillation with ibutilide pretreatment. N Engl J Med 1999; 340(24):1849–1854.

65 Cotter G, et al. Conversion of recent onset paroxysmal atrial fibrillation to normal sinus rhythm: the effect of no treatment and high-dose amiodarone. A randomized, placebo-controlled study. Eur Heart J 1999; 20(24):1833–1842.

66 Peuhkurinen K, et al. Effectiveness of amiodarone as a single oral dose for recent-onset atrial fibrillation. Am J Cardiol 2000; 85(4):462–465.

67 Vardas PE, et al. Amiodarone as a first-choice drug for restoring sinus rhythm in patients with atrial fibrillation: a randomized, controlled study. Chest 2000; 117(6): 1538–1545.

68 Tieleman RG, et al. Efficacy, safety, and determinants of conversion of atrial fibrillation and flutter with oral amiodarone. Am J Cardiol 1997; 79(1):53–57.

69 Singh BN, et al. Amiodarone versus sotalol for atrial fibrillation. N Engl J Med 2005; 352(18):1861–1872.

70 Connolly SJ. Evidence-based analysis of amiodarone efficacy and safety. Circulation 1999; 100(19):2025–2034.

71 Coplen SE, et al. Efficacy and safety of quinidine therapy for maintenance of sinus rhythm after cardioversion. A meta-analysis of randomized control trials. Circulation 1990; 82(4):1106–1116.

72 Ferreira E, Sunderji R, Gin K. Is oral sotalol effective in converting atrial fibrillation to sinus rhythm? Pharmacotherapy 1997; 17(6):1233–1237.

73 Falk RH, et al. Digoxin for converting recent-onset atrial fibrillation to sinus rhythm. A randomized, double-blinded trial. Ann Intern Med 1987; 106(4):503–506.

74 Jordaens L, et al. Conversion of atrial fibrillation to sinus rhythm and rate control by digoxin in comparison to placebo. Eur Heart J 1997; 18(4):643–648.

42

Contrast-induced nephropathy after percutaneous coronary interventions

Ioannis Iakovou

Contrast media (CM) are used to enhance visualization during diagnostic angiograms and to guide percutaneous coronary interventions (PCI). The increased use of PCI led to the increased number of patients receiving CM (1,2). However, use of CM is not without risks. Although some complications associated with CM are mild and transient, such as discomfort and itching, others are more serious such as anaphylaxis, hypotension, cardiovascular events, and renal dysfunction (1–3).

Contrast-induced nephropathy (CIN) is the most serious complication associated with the use of CM and can negatively affect long-term patient morbidity and mortality (4–10). CIN is usually defined as an *acute decline in renal function characterized by an absolute rise of 0.5 mg/dl (44 μmol/l) in serum creatinine (SCr) or a 25% increase from baseline, occurring after the systemic administration of CM in the absence of other risk factors such as atheroembolic disease, hypotension and low blood volume, surgery, or nephrotoxins* (1,2,6,7,10–13).

Typically, patients with CIN will experience changes in SCr 1–5 days following contrast exposure. The decline in renal function often occurs within 24–48 hours of CM, with peak elevations in SCr occurring after 3–5 days, and a return to baseline or near baseline in 7–10 days (1,2). While reduction in renal function is generally small and transient, some patients experience a more prolonged decrease and, in rare cases, require dialysis (5,14). The incidence of CIN varies among studies and is dependent on the definition, background risk, type, and dosage of CM, and imaging procedure. Whereas it is estimated to be 0.6–2.3% in the general population, it is higher in hospitalized patients (1–20%) and in patients with cardiovascular disease undergoing angiography procedures, ranging between 3.3% and 14.5% (1,2,5,14,15). These rates can be as high as 50% among patients with baseline renal dysfunction and diabetes (1,2,5,6,14–17). While most cases of CIN are characterized by seemingly small and transient changes in renal function, up to 30% of patients experiencing CIN might have some permanent decline in

renal function (4,5,7,9). More importantly, patients who develop CIN are at significantly higher risk of in-hospital and one-year mortality (2,7–9,13,18). The risk is even greater in patients with preexisting renal compromise (1,2,5,14,15).

The aim of the present article is to review the pathogenesis, the risk factors, and the outcomes of CIN and reviews current opinion on how best to prevent CIN.

Pathogenesis

The precise mechanisms behind the pathogenesis of CIN are as yet unclear. In vitro as well as animal studies suggest a combination of *toxic injury* to the renal tubules and *ischemic injury* (prerenal mechanism) partly mediated by reactive oxygen species (19,20). In addition, factors other than osmolality (such as viscosity, hydrophilicity) contribute substantially to the toxic effects of CM (20,21).

Increased perivascular hydrostatic pressure, high viscosity, or changes in vasoactive substances (i.e., endothelin, nitric oxide, and adenosine) might result in low blood flow in the medulla, which has a high demand for oxygen and thus produce ischemic injury (22–24). Similarly, factors impairing medullary vasodilation, such as nonsteroidal anti-inflammatory drugs, may worsen CIN (1,4,5,14,25,26). In addition, all water-soluble, nephrotropic, iodinated CM exert direct toxic effects on renal epithelial cells and might produce contrast-induced renal medullary ischemia (20,21). CM can also produce direct cytotoxic effects such as cytoplasmic vacuolization and lysosomal alteration in the proximal convoluted tubular cells and in the inner cortex of the kidneys (27). Animal studies have suggested that oxidant-mediated injury might arise due to an enhanced production of oxygen-free radicals concomitant with a reduction in the activity of the antioxidant enzymes, such as catalase and superoxide dismutase, in the renal cortex (28). Lipid peroxidation of biologic membranes might also be implicated and significant morphologic alterations in proximal tubules, along with elevated renal levels of malondialdehyde, a marker of lipid peroxidation, have been found in rats after exposure to iodinated CM (29).

Regarding ischemic injury, the deeper portion of the outer medulla of the kidney is particularly vulnerable, since this area is maintained at the verge of hypoxia, with pO_2 levels often as low as 20 mmHg (30). Possible mechanisms for medullary hypoxia and ischemia in response to CM exposure include: (1) CM might cause direct renal vasoconstriction and (2) CM might impair oxygen delivery indirectly by causing red blood cell aggregation (20,31,32).

Osmolality of contrast media and contrast-induced nephropathy

CM can be classified according to osmolality, which reflects the total particle concentration of the solution (the number of molecules dissolved in a specific volume) (1,2). CM with osmolality greater than that of blood may be more difficult for the kidney to excrete. Over the past 40 years, the osmolalities of available CM have been gradually decreased to physiologic levels. In the 1950s, only high-osmolar CM (e.g., diatrizoate)

with osmolality five to eight times that of plasma were available (1). In the 1980s, CM such as iohexol, iopamidol, and ioxaglate were introduced. While these are classified as the so-called low-osmolar CM, their osmolalities are two to three times greater than that of plasma (33). In the 1990s, isosmolar CM with the same physiologic osmolality as blood were developed (e.g., iodixanol) (33). Physiologic and chemical characteristics of water-soluble, iodinated CM are shown in Table 1.

Whether different types of CM have different mechanisms of nephrotoxicity or produce different degrees of renal effects have been the matter of intense scrutiny (5,25,33,34). Low-osmolar nonionic CM have long been known to have fewer direct cytotoxic effects compared to high-osmolar agents (35,36). However, controversial data have been reported by other investigators (35–38). Recently, Heinrich and Uder (39) have shown that nonionic dimeric CM have stronger direct cytotoxic effects on renal proximal tubular cells in vitro than nonionic monomeric CM. Experimental studies have suggested that iso-osmolar dimeric CM may worsen medullary hypoxemia more than low-osmolar CM, and even more than high-osmolar CM (40,41). A diminished transit time of the more highly viscous dimeric CM in the tubule might lead to a decrease of both glomerular filtration rate and renal blood flow by the compression of peritubular vessels (32). Moreover, the diminished tubular transit time of the nonionic dimers might result in an increased time for solute transport and increased oxygen utilization (42).

Table 1   Physiologic and chemical characteristics of water-soluble, iodinated contrast media

Ionicity	Osmotic class	Agent contrast	Iodine/particle (ratio)	Iodine concentration (mgI/kg)	Osmolality (mOsm/kg)	Viscosity (cPs at 37°C)
Ionic	High-osmolar monomers	Diatrizoate (renografin)	3/2 (1.5)	370; 300	1870; 1500	2.34; 5.2
	Low-osmolar dimers	Ioxaglate (hexabrix)	6/2 (3.0)	320	600	7.5
Nonionic	Low-osmolar monomers	Iohexol (omnipaque)	3/1 (3.0)	140–350	322–844	1.5–10.4
		Iomeprol (iomeron)		150–400	301–726	1.4–12.6
		Iopamidol (isovue)		250–370	524–796	3.0–9.4
		Iopentol (imagopaque)		150–350	310–810	1.7–12.0
		Iopromide (ultravist)		150–370	330–770	1.5–10.0
		Ioversol (optiray)		240–350	502–792	3.0–9.0
		Ioxilan (oxilan)		300–350	585–695	5.1–8.1
	Iso-osmolar dimers	Iodixanol (visipaque)	6/1	270–320	290	6.3–11.8
		Iotrolan (isovist)	(6.0)	240–300	270–290	3.9–8.5

Source: Modified from Ref. 20.

In summary, further studies are needed before iso-osmolar CM can be recommended in place of low-osmolar CM. Exceeding a volume of CM of 5 ml/kg of body weight divided by the SCr level in milligrams per deciliter strongly predicts nephropathy requiring dialysis (5,13).

Risk factors for contrast-induced nephropathy

Various conditions have been proposed as risk factors for CIN. However, it is uncertain to what extent these factors independently worsen renal function, as opposed to serving as markers for coexisting conditions. Chronic kidney disease (CKD) is a major determinant of CIN (5,7,19,43). McCullough et al. (44) reported that SCr levels rose by more than 25% in 14.5% of patients who underwent coronary angiography. On the contrary, in the absence of preexisting renal disease, the incidence is much lower. In a series of 1196 patients, Rudnick et al. (45) reported that only 8% of patients whose baseline SCr level was below 1.5 mg/dl (135 µmol/L) had an increase in the SCr level of more than 0.5 mg/dl, and none had an increase of more than 1 mg/dl (89 µmol/L). In another study by Freeman et al. (46), 0.8% of 1826 patients required dialysis after exposure to the CM; the baseline estimated creatinine clearance rate was below 47 mL/min/1.73 m^2 of body-surface area in all patients requiring dialysis. Serum creatinine levels rose by less than 1 mg/dl (89 µmol/L) in 29% of those requiring dialysis, indicating advanced preexisting kidney disease (46). Patients with preexisting renal dysfunction undergoing PCI are at increased risk for adverse outcomes compared with those with normal renal function (47). Similarly, an analysis of more than 130,000 elderly postmyocardial infarction patients found that one-year survival was progressively reduced as creatinine clearance declined (48). Acute renal failure occurring after cardiovascular procedures has been estimated to occur in 5–15% of patients. Nevertheless, patients who manifest mild CKD after exposure to CM who also have coronary artery disease may have a worse prognosis than patients without renal impairment. Their incidences of recurrent hospitalization, subsequent bypass surgery, and mortality are increased. Over a period of years, patients with mild CKD who had PCI were hospitalized more frequently than patients without (3.6% vs. 2.4%, p=0.003). After initial revascularization, more patients with chronic renal failure than without needed subsequent bypass surgery two years later (20% vs. 12%, respectively) (47). Best et al. (6) showed a renal function-dependent rise in the mortality rate in a study of more than 5000 patients. In patients with acute myocardial infarction undergoing PCI, moderate CKD compared with normal renal function at baseline was associated with a marked increase in mortality at 30 days (7.5% vs. 0.8%, p < 0.0001) and at one year (12.7% vs. 2.4%, p < 0.0001) (49). Among 7230 consecutive patients, CIN (≥25% or ≥0.5 mg/dl increase in preprocedure SCr 48 hours after the procedure) developed in 381 of 1980 patients

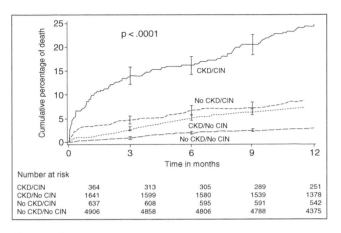

Figure 1

The prognostic significance of the proposed risk score for CIN extended to prediction of one-year mortality, as indicated by the results obtained from both the development and validation datasets. (*Solid bars*) development dataset; (*open bars*) validation dataset *Abbreviations*: CIN, contrast-induced nephropathy; CKD, chronic kidney disease. *Source*: From Refs. 7, 13.

(19.2%) with baseline CKD (estimated glomerular filtration rate <60 mL/min/1.73 m^2) and in 688 of 5250 patients (13.1%) without CKD. CIN was one of the most powerful predictors of one-year mortality in patients with preexisting CKD (odds ratio 2.37, 95% confidence interval 1.63 to 3.44) or preserved eGFR (odds ratio 1.78; 95% confidence interval 1.22 to 2.60) (Fig. 1) (7). Thus, regardless of the presence of CKD, baseline characteristics and periprocedural hemodynamic parameters predict CIN, and this complication is associated with worse in-hospital and one-year outcomes. Nevertheless, the additional burden of CIN in PCI patients with already compromised renal function markedly increases the risk of adverse outcomes.

Diabetes is a major risk factor for deterioration in renal function after angiography (2,7,13). Other factors variably associated with increased rates of CIN include *age over 75 years, anemia, female gender, periprocedural volume depletion, heart failure, cirrhosis, hypertension, proteinuria, concomitant use of nonsteroidal anti-inflammatory drugs, and intra-arterial injection* (2,4,5,7,10,13,14,19,43,44). In the setting of acute myocardial infarction or PCI, *hypotension* or use of an *intra-aortic balloon pump* has been associated with a higher rate of acute renal failure after exposure to a contrast medium (13,50). Finally, *high doses of CM* also increase the likelihood of renal dysfunction (51).

Clinical outcomes of contrast-induced nephropathy

If CIN occurs in PCI patients, its clinical course is usually benign, and spontaneous recovery of renal function ensues within one to two weeks (4–6,19,52). However, serious clinical consequences, including death, occur in certain patient subpopulations. Despite the widespread use of less toxic low osmolality CM for more than a decade, mortality rates associated with CIN have not decreased (4–6,19,52).

Patients with CIN developing post-PCI were observed to have a multitude of noncardiac in-hospital complications, including hematoma formation, pseudoaneurysms, stroke, coma, adult respiratory distress syndrome, pulmonary embolus, and gastrointestinal hemorrhage (5,53). Other frequent complications include serum electrolyte abnormalities and extrarenal comorbidities such as sepsis, respiratory failure, and bleeding. Episodes of bleeding as a result of acute renal deterioration affected about two-thirds (61%) of patients with CIN who later died during hospitalization (54). In another study, bleeding complications were shown to be significantly more frequent in PCI patients with CIN compared with those without CIN, with a respective 11.3% versus 4.8% of patients having gastrointestinal bleeding events (p = 0.02) and 42.8% versus 15.9% requiring blood transfusions (p = 0.001) (55). An analysis of almost 20,500 patients who underwent PCI showed that the 2% of patients who developed CIN had a 15-fold higher rate of major adverse cardiac events during hospitalization than patients without CIN. They also had a sixfold increase in myocardial infarction and a 11-fold increase in vessel reocclusion (p < 0.0001) (56). CIN requiring dialysis after PCI is rare; <1% of patients will require transient dialysis (acute hemodialysis, ultrafiltration, or peritoneal dialysis within five days of intervention) (44). These patients have a more complicated clinical outcome than patients who do not require dialysis, with a significantly higher rate of non-Q-wave myocardial infarction, creatinine kinase-myocardial band elevation, pulmonary edema, vascular complications such as gastrointestinal bleeding and they have significantly increased lengths of stay (1).

Probably as a result of the morbidities described, in-hospital mortality in PCI patients is significantly increased by CIN. Mortality was 5.5-fold higher in patients who developed CIN compared with control index patients in a study of more than 16,000 patients who underwent procedures using CM including CT of the head and body, and cardiac or peripheral angiography (54). These results have been verified by similar findings from other researchers (7,55). Patients who survive to discharge after an episode of CIN continue to be at high risk of adverse events during long-term follow-up, especially if dialysis is required. A study by Rihal et al. (53) showed that only 88% of patients who experienced CIN survived for one year, and only 55% survived for five years, compared with 96% and 85%, respectively, of patients without CIN (p < 0.0001). An even worse long-term outcome was found in patients requiring dialysis. The majority of patients (80%) in the study who developed CIN requiring permanent dialysis after coronary intervention did not survive for one year (44). This survival rate was confirmed in a later study that found a one-year mortality rate of 55% in patients undergoing PCI who required dialysis, compared with a 6% rate in the control group (p < 0.0001) (9). The patients receiving dialysis also had a higher rate of myocardial infarction (4.5% vs. 1.6%, p = 0.006).

Prevention of contrast-induced nephropathy

Evaluation of risk

The first steps in reducing the risk of kidney injury are to look for risk factors and review the indications for the administration of CM. Most risk factors for CIN can be detected by history taking and physical examination. Conditions such as dehydration can be at least partially corrected before exposure to the CM. The risk of a decline in kidney function after the administration of CM rises with the number of risk factors present (5,10,16,17,57). A useful tool in the form of validated risk-prediction model to be used in the routine clinical practice has been suggested by Mehran et al. and is summarized in Table 2 (13). The prognostic significance of the proposed risk score for CIN extended to prediction of one-year mortality, as indicated by the results obtained from both the development and validation datasets shown in Fig. 2. It is not necessary to measure the SCr levels of every patient before exposure to CM, but measurements should be made before intra-arterial use of the CM in patients with a history of kidney disease, proteinuria, kidney surgery, diabetes, hypertension, or gout (5,58). The creatinine clearance rate or the glomerular filtration rate should be estimated from the SCr level, according to either the Cockcroft–Gault or the Modification of Diet in Renal Disease formula to identify more accurately patients with values below 50 ml/min/1.73 m^2, who are at increased risk for nephropathy (50,59,60). Alternative imaging methods not requiring CM should be considered for use in patients with any risk factors. If CM has to be given, SCr levels should be measured 24 to 48 hours after administration of the CM. Because of the risk of lactic acidosis when CIN occurs in a patient with diabetes who is receiving metformin, it is prudent to withhold this agent until the glomerular filtration rate is greater than 40 mL/min/1.73 m^2 and for the 48 hours before exposure of the patient to the CM.

Volume expansion/administration of fluids

The administration of fluids is recommended to reduce the risk of CIN. However, data are lacking that specify the optimal fluid regimen. In a small trial reported by Trivedi et al. (61), SCr levels increased by more than 0.5 mg/dl in nine patients (34.6%) given water orally as compared with one (3.7%) given intravenous saline for 24 hours beginning

Table 2 Validation model to define contrast-induced nephropathy (CIN) risk score

Risk factor	Score
Hypotension	5
Intra-aortic balloon pump	5
Congestive heart failure	5
Age >75 years	4
Anemia	3
Diabetes	3
Volume of contrast medium	1 for each 100 mL
Serum creatinine >1.5 mg/dL	4
Or	
eGFR <60 mL/min/1.73 m^2	2 for 40 to <60 mL/min/1.73 m^2 4 for 20 to 39 mL/min/1.73 m^2 6 for <20 mL/min/1.73 m^2

Anemia: baseline hematocrit value <39% for men and >36% for women; congestive heart failure: class III/IV by New York Heart Association classification and/or history of pulmonary edema; Hypotension: systolic blood pressure <80 mmHg for at least 1 hr requiring inotropic support with medications or intra-aortic balloon pump (IABP) within 24 hours periprocedurally.
Abbreviation: eGFR, estimated glomerular filtration rate.
Source: From Ref. 13.

12 hours before administration of the CM, but the trial was stopped early after an unplanned interim examination of the data. Prolonged intravenous fluid therapy is difficult to administer for ambulatory procedures. Another small trial comparing the use of intravenous fluids for 12 hours (before and after administration of the contrast medium) with oral fluids plus a single intravenous bolus of fluid showed better results in the former group (62). However, the results of another trial were contradictory (63). In a study of 1620 patients comparing isotonic saline with 0.45% saline, each

given at 1 mL/kg of body weight per hour for 24 hours starting the morning of the procedure involving the CM, a rise in the SCr level of more than 0.5 mg/dL within 48 hours after administration of the CM was less likely in patients who were given isotonic saline (0.7% vs. 2.0%, p = 0.04) (64).

It has been hypothesized that alkalinization of tubular fluid might be beneficial by reducing the levels of pH-dependent free radicals. In a recently published study by Merten et al. (65), the creatinine level was less likely to rise more than 25% within two days after the administration of CM in patients who were given an infusion of isotonic sodium bicarbonate than in those given a saline infusion. However, there are methodologic concerns about these results. It is worth noting that the trial was terminated early because of a lower-than-expected rate of "events" in the bicarbonate group, but the timing of the interim analysis and the stopping rules were not prespecified, and the p value for the difference in event rates (p = 0.02) was higher than is standard for stopping a trial early.

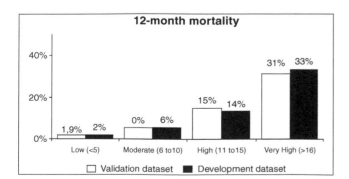

Figure 2
One-year survival after percutaneous coronary intervention in patients with or without chronic kidney disease and with or without contrast-induced nephropathy. *Source*: From Ref. 7.

Administration of agents

N-acetylcysteine

N-acetylcysteine has the potential to reduce the nephrotoxicity of CM through antioxidant and vasodilatory effects (66).

In a small trial by Tepel et al., SCr levels rose by more than 0.5 mg/dL in 2% of patients who received N-acetylcysteine as compared with 21% of patients in the control group (p < 0.01) (67,68). This event rate in the control group is unexpectedly high for patients who received low-dose intravenous low-osmolar CM. Subsequent trials have involved patients with reduced kidney function who underwent coronary angiography. Their results are inconclusive since the majority of these trials are burdened by methodologic problems; they are limited by low power and/or a lack of randomization (66,69–71). Recent meta-analyses suggest some benefit to N-acetylcysteine (66,69–73). However, this finding must be interpreted with caution, given the heterogeneous results of the individual trials, and the underrepresentation of small negative studies (74). In addition, the effect of N-acetylcysteine on outcomes other than minor changes in SCr levels is unknown. More data are needed before N-acetylcysteine can be strongly recommended for the prevention of CIN.

Hemodialysis or hemofiltration

Among patients with advanced kidney disease (mean creatinine clearance, 26 mL/min), an increase in SCr levels of at least 25% was significantly less common in patients randomly assigned to prophylactic hemofiltration before and after the administration of CM than in those assigned to receive fluid alone (5% vs. 50%, p < 0.001) (75). In-hospital death was also significantly less frequent in the hemofiltration group. However, the SCr level is directly altered by the intervention, and the relationship between the intervention and the reduced mortality rate is unclear. Thus, the role of hemodialysis in patients at high risk for CIN remains uncertain.

Other agents

Several other interventions have been proposed to reduce the risk of CIN, but data to support them are limited. Forced diuresis with furosemide, mannitol, dopamine, or a combination of these given at the time of exposure to the CM has been associated with similar or higher rates of CIN when compared to prophylactic fluids alone (4,5,76–79). Deleterious effects may be explained by negative fluid balance in some instances. In generally small randomized trials, the use of various vasodilators, including dopamine, fenoldopam, atrial natriuretic peptides, calcium blockers, prostaglandin E1, or a nonselective endothelin-receptor antagonist, has not been shown to reduce the risk of CIN in comparison with fluid therapy (5,80–83). On the contrary, a small randomized trial showed a lower frequency of creatinine increase in serum levels in patients given captopril for three days as compared with those given placebo (84). In another small trial, SCr levels were significantly less likely to increase within two to

five days of administration of the CM in patients who received ascorbic acid as an antioxidant than in those who received placebo (85). Theophylline and aminophylline have also been proposed as agents that may reduce the risk of CIN (4,5,86). A recent meta-analysis found that the mean rise in SCr levels was significantly lower [by 0.17 mg/dL (15 μmol/L)] at 48 hours after administration of the CM among patients receiving either of these medications than among those receiving placebo (86) However, the clinical importance of this finding is again questionable since there was heterogeneity among the studies included in this meta-analysis. Overall, no prophylactic administration of an agent has been shown conclusively to prevent clinically important CIN and confirmatory trials are required.

Clinical recommendations

1 Identify the patient at risk for CIN—For patients likely to have reduced kidney function a measurement of the SCr level and estimation of the glomerular filtration rate can be recommended. If the glomerular filtration rate is less than 50 mL/min/1.73 m^2, particularly in combination with other risk factors, consideration should be given to alternative imaging approaches.
2 Hydrate adequately—Additional fluids should be given; although the optimal regimen is uncertain, available data support a regimen of 0.9% saline at 1 mL/kg/hr intravenously from up to 12 hours before administration of contrast medium and for up to 12 hours after, with careful observation of fluid balance.
3 Discontinue nephrotoxic drugs—Nonsteroidal anti-inflammatory drugs and diuretics should be withheld for at least 24 hours before and after exposure to contrast medium, if possible. Metformin should be withheld for 48 hours before the administration of CM and until it is certain that CIN has not occurred.
4 Choose the CM with the lowest nephrotoxic effects—Low-osmolar CM have less effect on renal function than high-osmolar CM, and isosmolar CM have less effect on renal function than low-osmolar CM (LOCM) in high-risk patients with diabetes and renal insufficiency.
5 Check SCr levels 24 to 48 hours postprocedure.

Conclusions

CIN in at-risk patients is a clinical problem. The pathogenesis of CIN remains uncertain. The value of possible preventive strategies in reducing the risk of CIN and associated morbidity still is a matter of intense scrutiny and debate. Hydration has been shown consistently to prevent CIN, in contradiction to increased diuresis, hemodialysis, or pharmacologic prophylaxis.

References

1 McCullough P. Outcomes of contrast-induced nephropathy: experience in patients undergoing cardiovascular intervention. Catheter Cardiovasc Interv 2006; 67:335–343.

2 McCullough PA, Soman SS. Contrast-induced nephropathy. Crit Care Clin 2005; 21:261–280.

3 Thomsen HS, Morcos SK. Management of acute adverse reactions to contrast media. Eur Radiol 2004; 14:476–481.

4 Bagshaw SM, Culleton BF. Contrast-induced nephropathy: epidemiology and prevention. Minerva Cardioangiol 2006; 54:109–129.

5 Barrett BJ, Parfrey PS. Clinical practice. Preventing nephropathy induced by contrast medium. N Engl J Med 2006; 354:379–386.

6 Best PJ, Lennon R, Ting HH, et al. The impact of renal insufficiency on clinical outcomes in patients undergoing percutaneous coronary interventions. J Am Coll Cardiol 2002; 39:1113–1119.

7 Dangas G, Iakovou I, Nikolsky E, et al. Contrast-induced nephropathy after percutaneous coronary interventions in relation to chronic kidney disease and hemodynamic variables. Am J Cardiol 2005; 95:13–19.

8 Gruber SJ, Shapiro CJ. Nephropathy induced by contrast medium. N Engl J Med 2003; 348:2257–2259; author reply 2257–2259.

9 Gruberg L, Mehran R, Dangas G, et al. Acute renal failure requiring dialysis after percutaneous coronary interventions. Catheter Cardiovasc Interv 2001; 52:409–416.

10 Iakovou I, Dangas G, Mehran R, et al. Impact of gender on the incidence and outcome of contrast-induced nephropathy after percutaneous coronary intervention. J Invasive Cardiol 2003; 15:18–22.

11 Briguori C, Airoldi F, Morici N, et al. New pharmacological protocols to prevent or reduce contrast media nephropathy. Minerva Cardioangiol 2005; 53:49–58.

12 Kini AS, Mitre CA, Kamran M, et al. Changing trends in incidence and predictors of radiographic contrast nephropathy after percutaneous coronary intervention with use of fenoldopam. Am J Cardiol 2002; 89:999–1002.

13 Mehran R, Aymong ED, Nikolsky E, et al. A simple risk score for prediction of contrast-induced nephropathy after percutaneous coronary intervention: development and initial validation. J Am Coll Cardiol 2004; 44:1393–1399.

14 Aspelin P, Aubry P, Fransson SG, et al. Nephrotoxic effects in high-risk patients undergoing angiography. N Engl J Med 2003; 348:491–499.

15 Sanaei-Ardekani M, Movahed MR, Movafagh S, et al. Contrast-induced nephropathy: a review. Cardiovasc Revasc Med 2005; 6:82–88.

16 Bettmann MA. Contrast medium-induced nephropathy: critical review of the existing clinical evidence. Nephrol Dial Transplant 2005; 20(Suppl 1):i12–17.

17 Braun C, Birck R. Nephropathy induced by contrast medium. N Engl J Med 2003; 348:2257–2259; author reply 2257–2259.

18 Goldenberg I, Matetzky S. Nephropathy induced by contrast media: pathogenesis, risk factors and preventive strategies. CMAJ 2005; 172:1461–1471.

19 Barrett BJ. Contrast nephrotoxicity. J Am Soc Nephrol 1994; 5:125–137.

20 Schrader R. Contrast material-induced renal failure: an overview. J Interv Cardiol 2005; 18:417–423.

21 Rudnick MR, Kesselheim A, Goldfarb S. Contrast-induced nephropathy: how it develops, how to prevent it. Cleve Clin J Med 2006; 73:75–80, 83–87.

22 Heyman SN, Rosenberger C, Rosen S. Regional alterations in renal haemodynamics and oxygenation: a role in contrast medium-induced nephropathy. Nephrol Dial Transplant 2005; 20(Suppl 1):i6–11.

23 Korr KS, Reitman A. Renal implications of percutaneous coronary intervention. Semin Nephrol 2001; 21:36–46.

24 Liss P, Carlsson PO, Nygren A, et al. Et-A receptor antagonist BQ123 prevents radiocontrast media-induced renal medullary hypoxia. Acta Radiol 2003; 44:111–117.

25 Baker CS. Prevention of radiocontrast-induced nephropathy. Catheter Cardiovasc Interv 2003; 58:532–538.

26 Maeder M, Klein M, Fehr T, et al. Contrast nephropathy: review focusing on prevention. J Am Coll Cardiol 2004; 44:1763–771.

27 Rees JA, Old SL, Rowlands PC. An ultrastructural histochemistry and light microscopy study of the early development of renal proximal tubular vacuolation after a single administration of the contrast enhancement medium "Iotrolan". Toxicol Pathol 1997; 25:158–164.

28 Yoshioka T, Fogo A, Beckman JK. Reduced activity of antioxidant enzymes underlies contrast media-induced renal injury in volume depletion. Kidney Int 1992; 41:1008–1015.

29 Parvez Z, Rahman MA, Moncada R. Contrast media-induced lipid peroxidation in the rat kidney. Invest Radiol 1989; 24:697–702.

30 Brezis M, Rosen S. Hypoxia of the renal medulla—its implications for disease. N Engl J Med 1995; 332:647–655.

31 Heyman SN, Rosen S, Brezis M. Radiocontrast nephropathy: a paradigm for the synergism between toxic and hypoxic insults in the kidney. Exp Nephrol 1994; 2:153–157.

32 Liss P, Nygren A, Olsson U, et al. Effects of contrast media and mannitol on renal medullary blood flow and red cell aggregation in the rat kidney. Kidney Int 1996; 49:1268–1275.

33 Almen T. Visipaque—a step forward. A historical review. Acta Radiol Suppl 1995; 399:2–318.

34 Aspelin P, Aubry P, Fransson SG, et al. Cost-effectiveness of iodixanol in patients at high risk of contrast-induced nephropathy. Am Heart J 2005; 149:298–303.

35 Lautin EM, Freeman NJ, Schoenfeld AH, et al. Radiocontrast-associated renal dysfunction: a comparison of lower-osmolality and conventional high-osmolality contrast media. AJR Am J Roentgenol 1991; 157:59–65.

36 Lautin EM, Freeman NJ, Schoenfeld AH, et al. Radiocontrast-associated renal dysfunction: incidence and risk factors. AJR Am J Roentgenol 1991; 157:49–58.

37 Barrett BJ, Parfrey PS, Vavasour HM, et al. Contrast nephropathy in patients with impaired renal function: high versus low osmolar media. Kidney Int 1992; 41:1274–1279.

38 Carraro M, Malalan F, Antonione R, et al. Effects of a dimeric vs a monomeric nonionic contrast medium on renal function

in patients with mild to moderate renal insufficiency: a double-blind, randomized clinical trial. Eur Radiol 1998; 8:144–147.

39   Heinrich M, Uder M. Pathogenesis of contrast-induced nephropathy. AJR Am J Roentgenol 2005; 185:1079; author reply 1079.

40   Laissy JP, Menegazzo D, Dumont E, et al. Hemodynamic effect of iodinated high-viscosity contrast medium in the rat kidney: a diffusion-weighted MRI feasibility study. Invest Radiol 2000; 35:647–652.

41   Lancelot E, Idee JM, Couturier V, et al. Influence of the viscosity of iodixanol on medullary and cortical blood flow in the rat kidney: a potential cause of nephrotoxicity. J Appl Toxicol 1999; 19:341–346.

42   Ueda J, Nygren A, Hansell P, et al. Effect of intravenous contrast media on proximal and distal tubular hydrostatic pressure in the rat kidney. Acta Radiol 1993; 34:83–87.

43   Bridges CM, Swaroop VS, Cuddihy MT. Nephropathy induced by contrast medium. N Engl J Med 2003; 348:2257–2259; author reply 2257–2259.

44   McCullough PA, Wolyn R, Rocher LL, et al. Acute renal failure after coronary intervention: incidence, risk factors, and relationship to mortality. Am J Med 1997; 103:368–375.

45   Rudnick MR, Goldfarb S, Wexler L, et al. Nephrotoxicity of ionic and nonionic contrast media in 1196 patients: a randomized trial. The Iohexol Cooperative Study. Kidney Int 1995; 47:254–261.

46   Freeman RV, O'Donnell M, Share D, et al. Nephropathy requiring dialysis after percutaneous coronary intervention and the critical role of an adjusted contrast dose. Am J Cardiol 2002; 90:1068–1073.

47   Szczech LA, Best PJ, Crowley E, et al. Outcomes of patients with chronic renal insufficiency in the bypass angioplasty revascularization investigation. Circulation 2002; 105:2253–2258.

48   Shlipak MG, Heidenreich PA, Noguchi H, et al. Association of renal insufficiency with treatment and outcomes after myocardial infarction in elderly patients. Ann Intern Med 2002; 137:555–562.

49   Sadeghi HM, Stone GW, Grines CL, et al. Impact of renal insufficiency in patients undergoing primary angioplasty for acute myocardial infarction. Circulation 2003; 108:2769–2775.

50   Marenzi G, Lauri G, Assanelli E, et al. Contrast-induced nephropathy in patients undergoing primary angioplasty for acute myocardial infarction. J Am Coll Cardiol 2004; 44:1780–1785.

51   Cigarroa RG, Lange RA, Williams RH, et al. Dosing of contrast material to prevent contrast nephropathy in patients with renal disease. Am J Med 1989; 86:649–652.

52   Abizaid AS, Clark CE, Mintz GS, et al. Effects of dopamine and aminophylline on contrast-induced acute renal failure after coronary angioplasty in patients with preexisting renal insufficiency. Am J Cardiol 1999; 83:260–263, A5.

53   Rihal CS, Textor SC, Grill DE, et al. Incidence and prognostic importance of acute renal failure after percutaneous coronary intervention. Circulation 2002; 105:2259–2264.

54   Levy EM, Viscoli CM, Horwitz RI. The effect of acute renal failure on mortality. A cohort analysis. JAMA 1996; 275:1489–1494.

55   Gruberg L, Mintz GS, Mehran R, et al. The prognostic implications of further renal function deterioration within 48h of interventional coronary procedures in patients with

pre-existent chronic renal insufficiency. J Am Coll Cardiol 2000; 36:1542–1548.

56   Bartholomew BA, Harjai KJ, Dukkipati S, et al. Impact of nephropathy after percutaneous coronary intervention and a method for risk stratification. Am J Cardiol 2004; 93:1515–1519.

57   Boccalandro F, Anderson HV. Contrast-induced nephropathy: back to basics. J Invasive Cardiol 2003; 15:317–318.

58   Thomsen HS, Morcos SK. In which patients should serum creatinine be measured before iodinated contrast medium administration? Eur Radiol 2005; 15:749–754.

59   Cockcroft DW, Gault MH. Prediction of creatinine clearance from serum creatinine. Nephron 1976; 16:31–41.

60   Levey AS, Bosch JP, Lewis JB, et al. A more accurate method to estimate glomerular filtration rate from serum creatinine: a new prediction equation. Modification of Diet in Renal Disease Study Group. Ann Intern Med 1999; 130:461–470.

61   Trivedi HS, Moore H, Nasr S, et al. A randomized prospective trial to assess the role of saline hydration on the development of contrast nephrotoxicity. Nephron Clin Pract 2003; 93:C29–C34.

62   Bader BD, Berger ED, Heede MB, et al. What is the best hydration regimen to prevent contrast media-induced nephrotoxicity? Clin Nephrol 2004; 62:1–7.

63   Taylor AJ, Hotchkiss D, Morse RW, et al. PREPARED: Preparation for Angiography in Renal Dysfunction: a randomized trial of inpatient vs outpatient hydration protocols for cardiac catheterization in mild-to-moderate renal dysfunction. Chest 1998; 114:1570–1574.

64   Mueller C, Buerkle G, Buettner HJ, et al. Prevention of contrast media-associated nephropathy: randomized comparison of 2 hydration regimens in 1620 patients undergoing coronary angioplasty. Arch Intern Med 2002; 162:329–336.

65   Merten GJ, Burgess WP, Gray LV, et al. Prevention of contrast-induced nephropathy with sodium bicarbonate: a randomized controlled trial. JAMA 2004; 291:2328–2334.

66   Fishbane S, Durham JH, Marzo K, et al. N-acetylcysteine in the prevention of radiocontrast-induced nephropathy. J Am Soc Nephrol 2004; 15:251–260.

67   Tepel M, van der Giet M, Schwarzfeld C, et al. Prevention of radiographic-contrast-agent-induced reductions in renal function by acetylcysteine. N Engl J Med 2000; 343:180–184.

68   Tepel M, Zidek W. Acetylcysteine and contrast media nephropathy. Curr Opin Nephrol Hypertens 2002; 11:503–506.

69   Kshirsagar AV, Poole C, Mottl A, et al. N-acetylcysteine for the prevention of radiocontrast induced nephropathy: a meta-analysis of prospective controlled trials. J Am Soc Nephrol 2004; 15:761–769.

70   Nallamothu BK, Shojania KG, Saint S, et al. Is acetylcysteine effective in preventing contrast-related nephropathy? A meta-analysis. Am J Med 2004; 117:938–947.

71   Pannu N, Manns B, Lee H, et al. Systematic review of the impact of N-acetylcysteine on contrast nephropathy. Kidney Int 2004; 65:1366–1374.

72   Biondi-Zoccai GG, Lotrionte M, Abbate A, et al. Compliance with QUOROM and quality of reporting of overlapping meta-analyses on the role of acetylcysteine in the prevention of contrast associated nephropathy: case study. BMJ 2006; 332:202–209.

73 Boccalandro F, Amhad M, Smalling RW, et al. Oral acetylcysteine does not protect renal function from moderate to high doses of intravenous radiographic contrast. Catheter Cardiovasc Interv 2003; 58:336–341.

74 Bagshaw SM, McAlister FA, Manns BJ, et al. Acetylcysteine in the prevention of contrast-induced nephropathy: a case study of the pitfalls in the evolution of evidence. Arch Intern Med 2006; 166:161–166.

75 Marenzi G, Marana I, Lauri G, et al. The prevention of radiocontrast-agent-induced nephropathy by hemofiltration. N Engl J Med 2003; 349:1333–1340.

76 Baker CS, Wragg A, Kumar S, et al. A rapid protocol for the prevention of contrast-induced renal dysfunction: the RAPPID study. J Am Coll Cardiol 2003; 41:2114–2118.

77 Solomon R, Werner C, Mann D, et al. Effects of saline, mannitol, and furosemide to prevent acute decreases in renal function induced by radiocontrast agents. N Engl J Med 1994; 331:1416–1420.

78 Weisberg LS, Kurnik PB, Kurnik BR. Risk of radiocontrast nephropathy in patients with and without diabetes mellitus. Kidney Int 1994; 45:259–265.

79 Stevens MA, McCullough PA, Tobin KJ, et al. A prospective randomized trial of prevention measures in patients at high risk for contrast nephropathy: results of the P.R.I.N.C.E. Study.

Prevention of Radiocontrast Induced Nephropathy Clinical Evaluation. J Am Coll Cardiol 1999; 33:403–411.

80 Kurnik BR, Allgren RL, Genter FC, et al. Prospective study of atrial natriuretic peptide for the prevention of radiocontrast-induced nephropathy. Am J Kidney Dis 1998; 31:674–680.

81 Stone GW, McCullough PA, Tumlin JA, et al. Fenoldopam mesylate for the prevention of contrast-induced nephropathy: a randomized controlled trial. JAMA 2003; 290:2284–2291.

82 Wang A, Holcslaw T, Bashore TM, et al. Exacerbation of radiocontrast nephrotoxicity by endothelin receptor antagonism. Kidney Int 2000; 57:1675–1680.

83 Asif A, Preston RA, Roth D. Radiocontrast-induced nephropathy. Am J Ther 2003; 10:137–147.

84 Gupta RK, Kapoor A, Tewari S, et al. Captopril for prevention of contrast-induced nephropathy in diabetic patients: a randomised study. Indian Heart J 1999; 51:521–526.

85 Spargias K, Alexopoulos E, Kyrzopoulos S, et al. Ascorbic acid prevents contrast-mediated nephropathy in patients with renal dysfunction undergoing coronary angiography or intervention. Circulation 2004; 110:2837–2842.

86 Bagshaw SM, Ghali WA. Theophylline for prevention of contrast-induced nephropathy: a systematic review and meta-analysis. Arch Intern Med 2005; 165:1087–93.

43

Erectile dysfunction

Graham Jackson

Introduction

Erectile dysfunction (ED) is common and increases in incidence with age (Fig. 1). It is estimated that 140 million men worldwide currently experience ED to a variable degree and by 2025 the prevalence is predicted to rise to over 300 million men (1). The Massachusetts Male Aging Study (MMAS) identified a prevalence of ED in 52% of men aged 40 to 70 years. As ED increases with age men over 70 years of age have three times the incidence of men in their forties. ED is an important cause of relationships breaking down with the man losing self-esteem, feeling inadequate, and a failure. The frustration affects the partner, who must not be forgotten as part of the evaluation—it may be a man's problem but it is usually a couple's concern. While the commonest cause is organic, it is important not to compartmentalize ED—the organic cause may have psychologic consequences, especially depression, so that the management needs to embrace more than just trying to restore erectile function as a lot of psychosocial support is often needed.

When advising cardiac patients about sexual activity it is important to individualize the advice. We have a statistical framework to support our recommendations but each person being advised will have, as well as a general cardiac condition (e.g., be post myocardial infarction), varying degrees of effort restriction, determined by, for example, the size of the infarction. In addition, each person will have personal issues regarding safety of sex, treatment of ED, and their confidence in returning to normal activities including sex. As we advise on sex we need to remember that the problems may have preceded the cardiac event with important relationship issues as a consequence.

Cardiovascular response to sexual activity

Several studies have been performed using ambulatory ECG and blood pressure (BP) monitoring comparing the heart rate, ECG, and BP response to sexual activity with other normal daily activities (2). The energy requirement during sexual intercourse is not excessive for couples in a longstanding relationship. The average peak heart rate is 110–130 beats/min and the peak systolic BP 150–180 mmHg, resulting in a rate pressure product of 16,000–22,000. Expressed as a multiple of the metabolic equivalent (MET) of energy expenditure expanded in the resting state (MET = 1), sexual intercourse is associated with a work load of 2–3 METs before orgasm and 3–4 METs during orgasm. Younger couples, who are not usually the individuals we advise, may be more vigorous in their activity, expending 5–6 METs. The average duration of sexual intercourse is 5–15 minutes. Therefore, sexual intercourse is not an extreme or sustained cardiovascular stress for patients in a longstanding relationship who are comfortable with each other. Casual sexual intercourse, which must be separated from extramarital sexual intercourse with a longstanding "other partner", may involve a greater

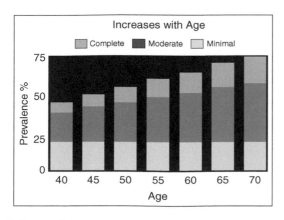

Figure 1
ED increases with age. *Source*: From Ref. 12.

Table 1 MET equivalents as a guide to relating daily activity to sexual activity

Daily activity	METs
Sexual intercourse with established partner	
Lower range (normal)	2–3
Lower range orgasm	3–4
Upper range (vigorous activity)	5–6
Lifting and carrying objects (9–20 kg)	4–5
Walking one mile (1.6 km) in 20 min on the level	3–4
Golf	4–5
Gardening (digging)	3–5
Do-it-yourself, wallpapering, etc.	4–5
Light housework, e.g., ironing, polishing	2–4
Heavy housework, e.g., making beds, scrubbing floors, cleaning windows	3–6

Abbreviation: MET, metabolic equivalent.

cardiac workload because of lack of familiarity and age mismatch (usually older men with a younger woman) leading to different levels of activity and expectations (3).

By using our knowledge of MET equivalents in the clinical setting we can advise on sexual safety by comparing sexual intercourse to other activities. Some of the daily activities and MET equivalents are shown in Table 1.

Exercise testing

Using METs, sexual intercourse is equivalent to 3–4 minutes of the standard Bruce treadmill protocol. Where doubts exist about the safety of sexual intercourse, an exercise test can help guide decision–making. If a person can manage at least four minutes on the treadmill without significant symptoms, ECG evidence of ischemia, a fall in systolic BP or dangerous arrhythmias, it will be safe to advise on sexual activity (3,4). Drory et al. (5,6) studied 88 men with CAD (off therapy) using ambulatory ECGs and bicycle exercise tests. On ambulatory ECGs one-third of the men had ischemia during sexual intercourse and all of them had ischemia on the bicycle exercise ECG. All patients without ischemia on the exercise test (n = 34) also had no ECG changes during sexual intercourse. All ischemic episodes during sexual intercourse were associated with an increasing heart rate identifying a potentially important therapeutic role for heart rate lowering drugs (β-adrenoreceptor antagonists, verapamil, diltiazem).

If a patient is unable to perform an exercise test because of mobility problems, a pharmacologic stress test should be utilized (e.g., Dobutamine stress echocardiography). A man who cannot achieve 3–4 METs should be further evaluated by angiography if appropriate (3).

Advice on METs in the clinical setting and relating this advice to sexual intercourse should also include advice on avoiding stress, a heavy meal or excess alcohol consumption prior to sexual intercourse.

I personally find the ability to walk a mile on the flat in 20 minutes without undue chest pain or breathlessness a useful clinical marker of physical ability equivalent to sex. Adding climbing up and down two flights of household stairs without symptoms is also helpful (one flight = about 13 steps). Many couples continue to be sexually active short of penetrative sexual intercourse, so if they are able to do so advice on treating ED is much easier. The importance of asking cannot be over emphasized (3).

Positions

As long as the couple are not stressed by the sexual position they use, there is no evidence of increased cardiac stress to a man or woman. Man on top, woman on top, side to side, oral sex, and masturbation are cardiologically equivalent. In homosexual relationships, other than casual, anal intercourse is not associated with increased cardiac stress provided proper lubrication is used and amyl nitrate ("poppers") are not used in the presence of a phosphodiesterase type-5 (PDE-5) inhibitor by the patient or partner.

Cardiac risk

There is only a small myocardial infarction risk associated with sex. The relative risk of a myocardial infarction (MI) during the two hours following sex is shown in Table 2 (7).

The baseline absolute risk of an MI during normal daily life is low—one chance in a million per hour for a healthy adult, and 10 chances in a million per hour for a patient with documented cardiac disease. Therefore, during the two hours post-sex, the risk increases to 2.5 in a million for a healthy adult and 25 in a million for a patient with documented cardiac disease, but, importantly, there is no risk

Table 2 Relative risk of MI during the two hours after sexual activity: physically fit equals sexually fit

Patient type	Relative risk (95% CI)
All patients	2.5 (1.7–3.7)
Men	2.7 (1.8–4.0)
Women	1.3 (0.3–5.2)
Previous MI	2.9 (1.3–6.5)
Sedentary life	3.0 (2.0–4.5)
Physically active	1.2 (0.4–3.7)

Abbreviations: CI, confidence interval; MI, myocardial infarction.

increase in those who are physically active (physically fit = sexually fit).

A similar study from Sweden reported identical findings (8). If we take a baseline annual rate of 1% for a 50-year old man, as a result of weekly sexual activity, the risk of an MI increases to 1.01% in those without a history of a previous MI and to 1.1% in those with a previous history.

Coital sudden death is very rare. In three large studies, sex activity-related death was 0.6% in Japan, 0.18% in Frankfurt, and 1.7% in Berlin. Extramarital (casual) sex was responsible for 75%, 75%, and 77%, respectively, and the victims were men in 82%, 94%, and 93% of cases, respectively (2). An older man with a younger woman was the commonest scenario.

Vasculogenic ED

Vascular diseases are the most common cause of ED with endothelial dysfunction now recognized as the common denominator (Fig. 2) (9). ED and coronary artery disease (CAD) share the same risk factors, which explains the endothelial link (Table 3) (10). However, before attributing ED to a purely vascular cause it is important to evaluate the patient thoroughly as other factors may be contributing to the problem or occasionally be the cause. As men age, there may be comorbid conditions which need to be addressed (endocrine, cellular, neural, or iatrogenic, e.g., drug therapy) and organic ED will have psychologic consequences needing counselling and support.

A large number of drugs, whether prescribed or recreational, can affect sexual function (3). These drugs include:

- Cardiovascular drugs: Thiazide diuretics, β-adrenoceptor antagonists, calcium channel antagonists, centrally acting agents (e.g., methyl-dopa, clonidine, reserpine, ganglion

Table 3	Shared risk factors for coronary artery disease and ED
Coronary artery disease	*ED*
Age	Age
Dyslipidemia	Dyslipidemia
Hypertension	Hypertension
Diabetes	Diabetes
Smoking	Smoking
Sedentary lifestyle	Sedentary lifestyle
Obesity	Obesity
Depression	Depression
Male sex	Coronary artery disease
	Peripheral vascular disease

Abbreviation: ED, erectile dysfunction.

blockers), digoxin, lipid-lowering agents, ACE inhibitors, recreational drugs, such as alcohol (ethanol), marijuana, amphetamines, cocaine, anabolic steroids, heroin (diamorphine);
- Psychotropic drugs: Major tranquillisers, anxiolytics and hypnotics, tricyclic antidepressants, selective serotonin reuptake inhibitors;
- Endocrine drugs: Antiandrogens, oestrogens, gonadotropin-releasing hormone analogues;
- Others: Cimetidine, ranitidine, metoclopramide, carbamazepine

The negative impact may be on erections, ejaculation, or sex drive. There is little evidence that changing cardiovascular drug therapy will restore erectile function, suggesting it is the underlying disease process that is more important. However, if there is a strong temporal relationship between the commencement of treatment and the onset of ED (2 − 4 weeks) it is logical to change therapy if it is safe to do so. Antihypertensive agents, especially thiazide diuretics, are the most frequently incriminated and a switch to angiotensin II receptor antiantagonists or α-adrenoceptor antagonists should be considered (11). Where drugs are prognostically important, such as ß-adrenoceptor antagonists post myocardial infarction, the decision to discontinue therapy should be approached with caution and only undertaken after considering overall risks (4).

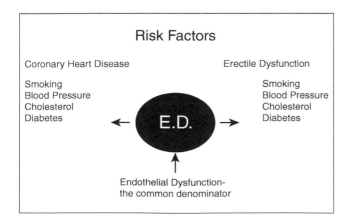

Figure 2

Risk factors for erectile dysfunction (ED) and coronary heart disease; Endothelial dysfunction (ED) = Erectile dysfunction (ED). *Source*: From Ref. 9.

ED and cardiovascular disease

MMAS (12) was a random sample, cross-sectional, observational study of 1709 healthy men aged 40–70 years to assess the impact of aging on a wide range of health-related issues. Fifty-two percent of respondents reported some degree of ED (17% mild, 25% moderate, 10% complete) with the prevalence increasing with age (Fig. 1). Cardiovascular disease was significantly associated with ED. The incidence was doubled in patients with hypertension, tripled in diabetic patients, and in those with established coronary disease it was quadrupled. Cigarette smoking increased the prevalence twofold for all of these conditions and a positive relationship was found for reduced high-density lipoprotein-cholesterol and ED.

The association between hyperlipidaemia and ED has been studied in apparently healthy men who complained of ED (13). Over 60% had hyperlipidaemia and 90% of these had evidence of penile arterial disease using Doppler ultrasound studies. Diabetes is commonly associated with ED with a prevalence of 50% (range 27–70% depending on age and disease severity). The onset of ED usually occurs within the first 10 years of the diagnosis of diabetes (14).

Men aged over 50 years with established CAD have an ED incidence of 40% and in those post myocardial infarction or post vascular surgery the incidence ranges from 39% to 64%, depending on diagnostic criteria (15).

ED as a marker of vascular disease

As ED and vascular disease share the same risk factors, the possibility arises that ED in otherwise asymptomatic men may be a marker of silent vascular disease, especially CAD (16). This has now been established to be the case and represents an important new means of identifying those at risk of vascular disease.

Pritzker (17) studies 50 asymptomatic men (other than ED) aged 40–60 years who had cardiovascular risk factors (multiple in 80%). An exercise ECG was abnormal in 28 men and subsequent coronary angiography in 20 men identified severe CAD in six, moderate two vessel disease in seven, and significant single vessel CAD in a further seven men. In a study of 132 men attending day case angiography, 65% had experienced ED before their CAD diagnosis had been made (18). ED also correlates with the severity of CAD with single vessel disease patients having less difficulty in obtaining an erection (19).

The smaller penile arteries (diameter 1−2 mm) suffer significant obstruction or endothelial disruption earlier from plaque burden than the larger coronary (3−4 mm), carotid (5−7 mm), or iliofemoral (6−8 mm) arteries; hence ED may be symptomatic before a coronary event (20). Addressing cardiovascular risk early after the presentation of ED and aggressive intervention to reduce risk may have long-term symptomatic and prognostic cardiac benefits (21). Most acute coronary syndromes follow from asymptomatic lipid-rich plaques rupturing and ED may therefore be a marker for reducing the risk of this happening (22).

In Montorsi et al's study of 300 men presenting with an acute coronary syndrome (mean age 62.5 years) the ED

prevalence was 49% (147/300) and in 99 (67%) the ED preceded the onset of cardiac symptoms by an average of three years (22). This time interval provides an important opportunity for risk reduction given the established benefits in both primary and secondary prevention of coronary disease and peripheral vascular disease.

Several studies have now reinforced the concept that endothelial dysfunction is the common denominator for ED and CAD (9). In one study 30 men with Doppler proven ED and no clinical evidence of cardiovascular disease (mean age, 46 years) were compared with 27 healthy age matched controls using flow-mediated brachial artery vasodilatation studies (23). The men with ED exhibited significantly lower brachial artery flow-mediated endothelium dependent vasodilatation (p < 0.05, Fig. 3) and endothelium-independent vasodilatation judged by a blunted response to 0.4 mg glyceryl trinitrate sublingually (p = 0.02). Looking at biochemical markers P-selection, ICAM-1, VCAM-1, and endothelin-1 concentrations were significantly greater in men with ED and no cardiovascular disease symptoms compared to men without ED (24). Asymmetric demethyl arginine (ADMA) is an endogenous competitive nitric oxide (NO) synthase inhibitor and is an independent risk marker for cardiovascular disease impairing the L-arginine-NO pathway. Recent studies have found elevated levels of ADMA in men with ED and CAD (25−27).

As the evidence accumulates that ED is a marker for asymptomatic CAD its importance as a barometer of the vasculature generally is being appreciated. Vlachopoulos et al. studied 50 asymptomatic men for CAD with ED and performed angiography in 47 (28). Nine (19%) had angiographic silent CAD. In a health screening program in Vienna 2869 men aged 20 to 80 years completed the International Index to Erectile Function (IIEF) questionnaire (29). Men with moderate to severe ED but not mild ED had a 10-year relative risk increase

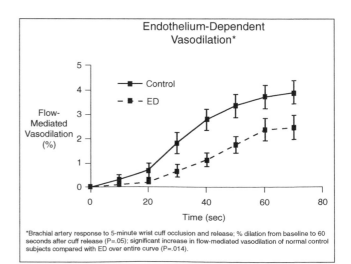

Figure 3

Men with ED and no cardiac symptoms demonstrate impaired endothelial function compared to controls. *Source*: From Ref. 13.

over 10 years of 65% for CAD and 43% for stroke. In the Prostate Cancer Prevention Trial 9457 men aged 55 or above were randomized to placebo and 8063 (85%) had no cardiovascular disease at entry (30). ED was present in 3816 (47%) at entry with a further 2420 developing ED after five years. Men with ED had a 25–45% increased risk of cardiovascular events during the nine-year study follow-up period.

The Second Princeton Consensus on Sexual Function concluded that the recognition of ED as a warning sign of silent vascular disease has led to the concept that a man with ED and no cardiac symptoms is a cardiac (or vascular) patient until proved otherwise. Therefore any asymptomatic man who presents with ED that does not have an obvious cause (e.g., trauma) should be screened for vascular disease and have blood glucose, lipids, and BP measured. Ideally, all patients at risk should undergo an elective exercise ECG to facilitate risk stratification (31,32).

Treating ED in patients with cardiovascular disease

Recognizing the need for advice on management of ED two consensus panels (UK and American) have produced similar guidelines dividing cardiovascular risk into three practical categories with management recommendations (3,4). The Princeton consensus guidelines have recently been updated (Table 4) (4). It is recommended that all men with ED should undergo a full medical assessment (Fig. 4). Baseline physical activity needs to be established and cardiovascular risk graded

low, intermediate, or high. Most patients with low or intermediate cardiac risk can have their ED managed in the outpatient or primary care setting.

There is no evidence that treating ED in patients with cardiovascular disease increases cardiac risk; however, this is with the proviso that the patient is properly assessed and the couple or individual (self-stimulation may be the only form of sexual activity) are appropriately counselled. Oral drug therapy is the most widely used because of its acceptability and effectiveness, but all therapies have a place in management. The philosophy is to always be positive during what, for many men and their partners, is an uncertain time.

Phosphodiesterase (PDE5) inhibitors

To say that sildenafil has transformed the management of ED would be a substantial understatement. Its mechanism of action by blocking the degradation of cGMP by PDE5 promotes blood flow into the penis and the restoration of erectile function (Fig. 5). Vardenafil and tadalafil have been added to this family of drugs (33,34). Because their mechanism of action is the same, there is no reason to assume that there will be any significant differences in ED effectiveness, but their half-life may be of cardiac clinical importance.

Hemodynamically, PDE5 inhibitors have mild nitrate-like actions (sildenafil was originally intended to be a drug for stable angina) (35). As PDE5 is present in smooth muscle cells throughout the vasculature and the NO/cGMP pathway is

Table 4 Risk from sexual activity in cardiovascular diseases: Second Princeton Consensus Conference

Low risk: typically implied by the ability to perform exercise of modest intensity without symptoms

Asymptomatic and <3 major risk factors (excluding gender)

  Major CVD risk factors include age, male gender, hypertension, diabetes mellitus, cigarette smoking, dyslipidemia, sedentary lifestyle, and family history of premature CAD

Controlled hypertension

  Betablockers and thiazide diuretics may predispose to ED

Mild, stable angina pectoris

  Noninvasive evaluation recommended

  Antianginal drug regimen may require modification

Postrevascularization and without significant residual ischemia

  ETT may be beneficial to assess risk

Post-MI (>6–8 wk), but asymptomatic and without ETT-induced ischemia, or postrevascularization

  If postrevascularization or no ETT-induced ischemia, intercourse may be resumed 3–4 weeks post MI

(Continued)

Table 4   Risk from sexual activity in cardiovascular diseases: Second Princeton Consensus Conference (*Continued*)

Mild valvular disease

    May include select patients with mild aortic stenosis

LVD (NYHA class I)

    Most patients are low risk

Intermediate or indeterminate risk: evaluate to reclassify as high or low risk

Asymptomatic and ≥3 CAD risk factors (excluding gender)

    Increased risk for acute MI and death

    ETT may be appropriate, particularly in sedentary patients

Moderate, stable angina pectoris

    ETT may clarify risk

MI >2 wk but <6 wk

    Increased risk of ischemia, reinfarction, and malignant arrhythmias

    ETT may clarify risk

LVD/CHF (NYHA class II)

    Moderate risk of increased symptoms

    Cardiovascular evaluation and rehabilitation may permit reclassification as low risk

Noncardiac atherosclerotic sequelae (peripheral arterial disease, history of stroke, or transient ischemic attacks)

    Increased risk of MI

    Cardiologic evaluation should be considered

High risk: defer resumption of sexual activity until cardiological assessment and treatment

Unstable or refractory angina

    Increased risk of MI

Uncontrolled hypertension

    Increased risk of acute cardiac and vascular events (i.e., stroke)

CHF (NYHA class III, IV)

    Increased risk of cardiac decompensation

Recent MI (<2 wk)

    Increased risk of reinfarction, cardiac rupture, or arrhythmias, but impact of complete revascularization on risk is unknown

High-risk arrhythmias

    Rarely, malignant arrhythmias during sexual activity may cause sudden death

    Risk is decreased by an implanted defibrillator or pacemaker

Obstructive hypertrophic cardiomyopathies

    Cardiovascular risks of sexual activity are poorly defined

    Cardiologic evaluation (i.e., exercise stress testing and echocardiography) may guide patient management

Moderate to severe valve disease

    Use vasoactive drugs with caution

Abbreviations: CAD, coronary artery disease; CHF, congestive heard failure; CV, cardiovascular; CVA, cerebrovascular accident; ED, erectile dysfunction; ETT, exercise tolerance test; LVD, left ventricular dysfunction; MI, myocardial infarction; NYHA, New York Heart Association.
Source: Adapted from Ref. 4.

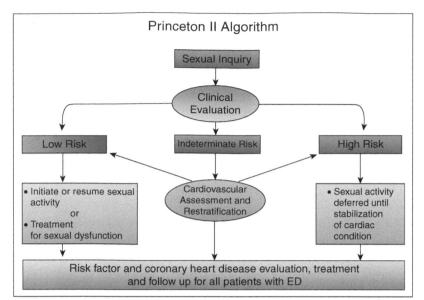

Figure 4
Princeton guidelines assessment algorithm.
Source: From Ref. 4.

involved in the regulation of BP, PDE5 inhibitors have a modest hypotensive action. In healthy men, a single dose of sildenafil 100 mg transiently lowered BP by an average of 10/7 mmHg with a return to baseline at six hours post dose. There was no effect on heart rate (35). As NO is an important neurotransmitter throughout the vasculature and is involved in the regulation of vascular smooth muscle relaxation, a synergistic and clinically important interaction with oral or sublingual nitrates can occur. A profound fall in BP can result. The mechanism involves the combination of nitrates increasing cGMP formation by activating guanylate cyclase and PDE5 inhibition decreasing cGMP breakdown by inhibiting PDE5. The concomitant administration of PDE5 inhibitors and nitrates is a contraindication to their use and this recommendation also extends to other NO donors such as nicorandil. Clinical guidelines regarding timing of sublingual

nitrate use post-PDE5 inhibitor are 12 hours for sildenafil and vardenafil (4). Tadalafil, with its long half-life, did not react with nitrates at 48 hours post use. Oral nitrates are not prognostically important drugs and they can therefore be discontinued and, if needed, alternative agents substituted (36). After oral nitrate cessation, and provided there has been no clinical deterioration, PDE5 inhibitors can be used safely. It is recommended that the cessation time interval prior to PDE5 inhibitor use is five half-lives which equals five days for the most popular once-daily oral nitrate agents.

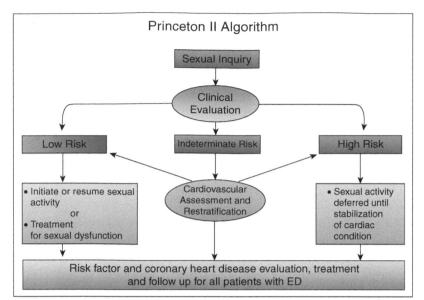

Figure 5
Mechanism of action of PDE5 inhibitors. *Abbreviations*: NO, nitric oxide; PDE5, phosphodieterase type 5.

Sildenafil

Sildenafil was the first oral treatment for ED and is the most extensively evaluated (35). Overall success rates in patients with cardiovascular disease of 80% or greater have been recorded with no evidence of tolerance. Patients with diabetes with or without additional risk factors, with their more complex, and extensive pathophysiology, have an average success rate of 60%. In randomized trials to date, open-label or outpatient monitoring studies the use of sildenafil is not associated with any excess risk of myocardial infarction, stroke, or mortality (38–40). In patients with stable angina pectoris there is no evidence of an ischemic effect due to coronary steal, and in one large, double-blind, placebo-controlled, exercise study sildenafil 100 mg increased exercise time and diminished ischemia (41). A study of the hemodynamic effects in men with severe CAD identified no adverse cardiovascular effects and a potentially beneficial effect on coronary blood flow reserve (42). Studies in patients with and without diabetes have demonstrated improved endothelial function acutely and after long-term oral dose administration, which may have implications beyond the treatment of ED (35). Sildenafil has also been shown to attenuate the activation of platelet IIb/IIIa receptor activity (43). Hypertensive patients on mono- or multiple therapy have experienced no increase in adverse events with the exception of doxazosin, a nonselective α-adrenoceptor antagonist. Occasional postural effects have occurred with sildenafil when taken within four hours of Doxazosin 4 mg; an advisory to avoid this time interval is now in place. Sildenafil has also been proven effective in heart failure patients who were deemed suitable for ED therapy (44). The incidence of ED in heart failure patients is 80%, making this finding of major clinical importance. On average, the sildenafil dose is 50 mg with 25 mg advised initially in those over 80 years of age because of delayed excretion. Sildenafil 100 mg is invariably needed in patients with diabetes. An empty stomach and avoiding alcohol or cigarette smoking facilitates the effect. Sildenafil 100 mg has no additional adverse cardiac effects above the 50 mg dose and should be routinely prescribed if the 50 mg dose after four attempts is not effective.

Sildenafil's short half-life makes it the drug of choice in patients with the more severe cardiovascular disease, allowing early use of support therapy if an adverse clinical event occurs.

Tadalafil

Tadalafil has also been extensively evaluated in patients with cardiovascular disease and has a similar safety and efficacy profile to sildenafil (45). Studies have shown no adverse effects on cardiac contraction, ventricular repolarization, or ischemic threshold. A similar hypotensive effect has been recorded with a dose of doxazosin 8 mg so caution is needed. As hypotension does not occur in the supine position and as tadalafil has a long half-life it is suggested that tadalafil is taken in the morning and doxazosin in the evening. There is no interaction of tadalafil with the selective α-adrenoceptor antagonist tamsulosin, which can, therefore, be prescribed as an alternative to doxazosin for symptomatic benign prostate hypertrophy (46).

Because of its long half-life, tadalafil may not be the first choice for the patients with more complex cardiovascular disease. However, as 80% of patients with cardiovascular disease stratify into low risk it is an alternative for the majority. Tadalafil 10 mg is equivalent to sildenafil 50 mg and 20 mg to 100 mg.

Of particular interest is the daily use of tadalafil 10 mg which, after one week because of its half-life, is equivalent to 16–18 mg at steady state. In on-demand failures a regular dosing regime has been successful in 60% without increased adverse effects (47). This increases the chance of success with important implications for the more difficult cases and its use post radical prostatectomy as a daily regime is encouraging. There is no evidence of increased cardiovascular risk with on-demand, three times weekly, or daily dosing (48).

Vardenafil

Since vardenafil has a very similar chemical structure to sildenafil, it is not surprising that it has a similar clinical profile. One study has reported no impairment of exercise ability in stable CAD patients receiving vardenafil 20 mg (49). Similar clinical efficiency for all three agents has been observed in patients with diabetes.

Other therapies

When oral agents are not effective, intracavernous injection therapy, transurethral alprostadil, or a vacuum pump are alternatives requiring specialized referral and advice (3,4). Warfarin is not a contraindication to vacuum pumps or injections but specialized training is needed. There is no evidence of increased cardiovascular risk from using any of these therapeutic options. If surgical intervention with general anesthetic is being anticipated, a full cardiologic risk evaluation is recommended.

Lifestyle factors

Lifestyle factors have been associated with ED in both cross-sectional and longitudinal studies. In particular, obesity and sedentary lifestyle are clear-cut risk factors for ED, both in men with comorbid illnesses such as hypertension and diabetes, and especially in men without overt cardiovascular disease (50). Other lifestyle factors, such as smoking and alcohol consumption, have been implicated in some, but not all, studies to date. Intervening on cardiovascular and lifestyle factors may have broader benefits beyond restoration of erectile function. This important concept needs careful consideration, as recent studies have implicated the role of the metabolic syndrome, obesity, insulin resistance, and lack of exercise as independent risk factors for both ED and cardiovascular disease (51,52).

The role of obesity in ED has been confirmed in large-scale, cross-sectional, and longitudinal studies (53,54). In a study in The Netherlands, 1700 Dutch men between the age of 50 and 75 were evaluated for the presence of ED and other health conditions (55). Body mass index (BMI) was found to be a significant predictor of ED, both as a single factor and in combination with other risk factors (e.g., lower urinary tract symptoms (LUTS), hypertension, diabetes).

Lack of physical activity is another lifestyle factor that has been strongly linked to the occurrence of ED in aging men. In the health professionals follow-up study (53), ED was associated with both increased BMI and decreased level of physical activity. Participants were categorized according to their level of exercise or physical activity. Higher levels of sedentary behavior (less physical activity) were found to be a strong, independent predictor of ED in this study. Frequent vigorous exercise was associated with an approximately 30% reduction in the risk for ED.

The effects of weight loss and exercise were examined further in a randomized intervention trial of lifestyle modification in men with obesity-related ED (56). This study compared two years of exercise and weight loss with an educational control in 110 obese men (mean BMI = 36.4 kg/m^2) with moderate to severe ED. Approximately one-third of men in the intervention group achieved normal levels of erectile function following treatment, compared with <5% of men in the control group. Changes in weight loss and exercise were shown to affect endothelial function, as measured by forearm brachial Doppler assessment, and were highly correlated with improvements in erection. Taken together, these studies strongly support the role of adverse lifestyle factors in the development and maintenance of ED. Obesity and lack of exercise, in particular, have been strongly implicated in a number of cross-sectional and longitudinal studies. At least one long-term prospective study has shown that lifestyle intervention can effectively restore erectile function in a substantial number of men with obesity-related ED, at least among those without significant medical comorbidities. For clinicians, the implications are clear that men with ED and other cardiovascular risk factors (e.g., obesity, sedentary lifestyle) should be counselled on lifestyle modification.

Androgens

The use of testosterone replacement therapy for the treatment of hypogonadism and ED may assist PDE5 inhibitors if they have failed to be effective (57). Testosterone levels within the normal range have neutral or potentially beneficial effects on the cardiovascular system (58). Androgen replacement therapy should be offered to men with CAD and hypogonadism if symptomatically appropriate. The absence of long-term studies needs to be addressed in terms of possible preventive properties on the vascular wall, reduction in low-density lipoprotein levels, and the reduction of insulin resistance in contrast to the increase in hematocrit and risk of exacerbating prostate cancer.

Nonarteritic anterior ischemic optic neuropathy (NAION)

The reports of the risk of "blindness" following PDE-5 inhibitor use has caused concern (59). Several case reports have linked PDE-5 inhibitors to NAION. No explanation as to the mechanism currently exists and it is most likely to be coincidental given the widespread use of PDE-5 inhibitors in men who are at risk being older and with vascular disease. The only identifiable risk factor is a small cup-disc ratio. It seems sensible to avoid PDE-5 inhibitors in those previous suffering NAION in one eye.

Summary

ED and vascular disease commonly coexist. They share the same risk factors and endothelial dysfunction is the common denominator. ED may develop in an otherwise asymptomatic male and be an important predictor of subsequent acute or chronic cardiac events. ED may therefore offer an opportunity for risk assessment and therapeutic intervention to reduce the chance of a subsequent cardiac presentation. Cardiac patients with ED need a careful assessment to judge the safety of sexual activity and suitability for ED treatment. Properly assessed and counselled patients can safely enjoy sexual activity. ED therapy with phosphodiesterase type five inhibitors is safe and effective providing the patient and partner are advised on their use and the importance of avoiding drug interactions, especially with nitrates.

Conclusion

ED is common in patients with cardiovascular disease and should be routinely enquired about. The cardiac risk of sexual activity in patients with cardiovascular disease is minimal in properly assessed patients. The restoration of a sexual relationship is a possibility for the majority of patients with cardiovascular disease and ED using oral PDE5 inhibitors, which have an excellent safety profile (avoiding nitrate use). ED is a marker for cardiovascular disease as well as its consequence; therefore, its identification (in the asymptomatic male) provides the opportunity to address other cardiovascular risk factors and detect silent but significant vascular pathology.

References

1 Ayta IA, McKinlay JB, Krane RJ. The likely worldwide increase in erectile dysfunction between 1995 and 2023 and some possible policy consequences. BJU Int 1999; 84:50–56.
2 Drory Y. Sexual activity and cardiovascular risk. Eur Heart J Suppl 2002; 4(Suppl. H):H13–H18.
3 Jackson G, Betteridge J, Dean J, et al. A systematic approach to erectile dysfunction in the cardiovascular patient: a consensus statement: update 2002. Int J Clin Pract 2002; 56:663–71.
4 Kostis JB, Jackson G, Rosen R, et al. Sexual Dysfunction and Cardiac Risk (the Second Princeton Consensus Conference). Am J Cardiol 2005; 96:313–321.

5 Drory Y, Fisman EZ, Shapira Y, et al. Ventricular arrhythmias during sexual activity in patients with coronary artery disease. Chest 1996; 109:922–924.

6 Drory Y, Shapira I, Fisman EZ, et al. Myocardial ischaemia during sexual activity in patients with coronary artery disease. Am J Cardiol 1995; 75:835–837.

7 Müller JE, Mittleman A, MacLure M, et al. Triggering myocardial infarction by sexual activity: low absolute risk and prevention by regular physical exercise. JAMA 1996; 275:1405–1409.

8 Müller J, Ahlbom A, Hulting J, et al. Sexual activity as a trigger of myocardial infarction: a case cross-over analysis in the Stockholm Heart Epidemiology Programme (SHEEP). Heart 2001; 86:387–390.

9 Solomon H, Man JW, Jackson G. Erectile dysfunction and the cardiovascular patient: endothelial dysfunction is the common denominator. Heart 2003; 89:251–254.

10 Billups KL. Endothelial dysfunction as a common link between erectile dysfunction and cardiovascular disease. Sex Health Rep 2004; 1:137–141.

11 Jackson G. Erectile dysfunction and hypertension.. Int J Clin Pract 2002; 56:491–492.

12 Feldman HA, Goldstein I, Hatzichristou DG, et al. Impotence and its medical and psychological correlates: results of the Massachusetts Male Aging Study. J Urol 1994; 151:54–61.

13 Kaiser DR, Billups K, Mason C, et al. Impaired brachial artery endothelium-dependent and -independent vasodilation in men with erectile dysfunction and no other clinical cardiovascular disease. J Am Coll Cardiol 2004; 43 (2):179–184.

14 Snow KJ. Erectile dysfunction in patients with diabetes mellitus: advances in treatment with phosphodiesterase Type 5 inhibitors. Br J Diab Vasc Dis 2002; 2:282–287.

15 Bortolotti A, Parazzini F, Colli E, et al. The epidemiology of erectile dysfunction and its risk factors. Int J Androl 1997; 20:323–334.

16 Kirby M, Jackson G, Betteridge J, et al. Is erectile dysfunction a marker for cardiovascular disease? Int J Clin Pract 2001; 55:614–618.

17 Pritzker M. The penile stress test: a window to the heart of the man [abstract]. Circulation 1999; 100:3751.

18 Solomon H, Man JW, Wierzbicki AS, et al. Relation of erectile dysfunction to angiographic coronary artery disease. Am J Cardiol 2003; 91:230–231.

19 Greenstein A, Chen J, Miller H, et al. Does severity of ischaemic coronary disease correlate with erectile function? Int J Impot Res 1997; 9:123–126.

20 Montorsi P, Montorsi F, Schulman CC. Is erectile dysfunction the 'Tip of the Iceberg' of a systemic vascular disorder? Eur Urol 2003; 44:352–354.

21 Kirby M, Jackson G, Simonsen U. Endothelial dysfunction links erectile dysfunction to heart disease? Int J Clin Pract 2005; 59:225–229.

22 Montrosi F, Briganti I, Salonia A, et al. Erectile dysfunction prevalence, time of onset and association with risk factors in 300 consecutive patients with acute chest pain and angiographically documented coronary artery disease. Eur Urol 2003; 44:360–365.

23 Virag R, Bouilly P, Frydman D. Is impotence an arterial disorder? A study of arterial risk factors in 440 impotent men. Lancet 1985; 1:181–184.

24 Bocchio M, Desideri G, Scarpelli P, et al. Endothelial cell activation in men with erectile dysfunction without cardiovascular risk factors and overt vascular damage. J Urol. 2004; 171:1601–1604.

25 Wierzbicki AS, Solomon H, Lumb PJ, et al. Asymmetric dimethyl arginine levels correlate with cardiovascular risk factors in patients with erectile dysfunction. Atherosclerosis 2006; 185:421–425.

26 Maas R, Wenske S, Zabel M, et al. Elevation of asymmetrical dimethylarginine (ADMA) and coronary artery disease in men with erectile dysfunction. Eur Urol 2005; 48:1004–1012.

27 Elesber AA, Solomon H, Lennon RJ, et al. Coronary endothelial dysfunction is associated with erectile dysfunction and elevated asymmetric dimethylarginine in patients with early atherosclerosis. Eur Heart J 2006; 27:824–831.

28 Vlachopoulos C, Rokkas K, Ioakeimidis N, et al. Prevalance of asymptomatic coronary artery disease in men with vasculogenic erectile dysfunction: a prospective angiographic study. Eur Urol 2005; 48:996–1003.

29 Ponholzer A, Temml C, Obermayr R, et al. Is erectile dysfunction an indicator for increased risk of coronary heart disease and stroke? Eur Urol 2005; 48:512–518.

30 Thompson IM, Tangen CM, Goodman PJ, et al. Erectile dysfunction and subsequent cardiovascular disease. JAMA 2005; 294:2996–3002.

31 Solomon H, Man J, Wierzbicki AS, et al. Erectile dysfunction: cardiovascular risk and the role of the cardiologist. Int J Clin Pract 2003; 57:96–99.

32 Jackson G, Rosen RC, Kloner RA, et al. The second Princeton consensus on sexual dysfunction and cardiac risk; new guidelines for sexual medicine. J Sex Med 2006; 3:28–36.

33 Brock GB, McMahon CG, Chen KK, et al. Efficiency and safety of tadalafil for the treatment of erectile dysfunction: results of integrated analysis. J Urol 2002; 168:1332–1336.

34 Porst H, Rosen R, Padma-Nathan H, et al. Efficacy and tolerability of vardenafil, a new selective phosphodiesterase type 5 inhibitor, in patients with erectile dysfunction: the first at home clinical trial. Int J Impot Res 2001; 13:192–199.

35 Gillies HC, Roblin D, Jackson G. Coronary and systemic haemodynamic effects of sildenafil citrate: from basic science to clinical studies in patients with cardiovascular disease. Int J Cardiol 2002; 86:131–141.

36 Kloner RA, Hutter AM, Emmick JT, et al. Time course of the interaction between tadalafil and nitrates. J Am Coll Cardiol 2004; 42:1855–1860.

37 Jackson G, Martin E, McGing E, et al. Successful withdrawal of oral long-acting nitrates to facilitate phosphodiesterase Type 5 Inhibitor use in stable coronary disease patients with erectile dysfunction. J Sex Med 2005; 2:513–516.

38 Padma-Nathan H (ed). Sildenafil citrate (Viagra) and erectile dysfunction: a comprehensive four year update on efficacy, safety, and management approaches. Urology 2002; 60(2B): 1–90.

39 Mittleman MA, MacClure M, Glasser DB. Evaluation of acute risk for myocardial infarction in men treated with sildenafil citrate. Am J Cardiol 2005; 96:443–446.

40 Jackson G, Gillies H, Osterloh I. Past, present and future: a 7-year update of Viagra (sildenafil citrate). Int J Clin Pract 2005; 59: 680–691.

41 Fox KM, Thadani U, Ma PTS, et al. Sildenafil citrate does not reduce exercise tolerance in men with erectile dysfunction and chronic stable angina. Eur Heart J 2003; 24:2206–2212.

42 Herrman HC, Chang G, Klugherz BD, et al. Haemodynamic effects of sildenafil in men with severe coronary artery disease. N Engl J Med 2000; 342:1662–1666.

43 Halcox JPJ, Nour KRA, Zalos G, et al. The effect of sildenafil on human vascular function, platelet activation and myocardial ischaemia. J Am Coll Cardiol 2002; 40:1232–1240.

44 Katz SD. Potential role of type 5 phosphodiesterase inhibition in the treatment of congestive heart failure. Congest Heart Fail 2003; 9:9–15.

45 Jackson G, Kloner RA, Costigan TM, et al. Update on clinical trials of tadalafil demonstrates no increased risk of cardiovascular adverse events. J Sex Med 2004; 1:161–167.

46 Kloner RA, Jackson G, Emmick JT, et al. Interaction between phosphodiesterase 5 inhibitor, tadalafil, and two alpha blockers, doxazosin and tamsulosin in healthy normotensive men. J Urol 2004; 172:1935–1940.

47 McMahon C. Comparison of efficacy, safety, and tolerability of on demand tadalafil and daily dosed tadalafil for the treatment of erectile dysfunction. J Sex Med 2006;2:415–424.

48 Kloner RA, Jackson G, Hutter AM, et al. Cardiovascular safety update of tadalafil: retrospective analysis of data from placebo-controlled and open-label clinical trials of tadalafil with as needed, three times-per-week or once-a-day dosing. Am J Cardiol 2006; 97:1778–1784.

49 Thadani U, Smith W, Nash S, et al. The effect of vardenafil, a potent and highly selective phosphodiesterase-5 inhibitor for the treatment of erectile dysfunction, on the cardiovascular response to exercise in patients with coronary artery disease. J Am Coll Cardiol 2002; 40:2006–2012.

50 Nicolosi A, Glasser DB, Moreira ED, et al. Prevalence of erectile dysfunction and associated factors among men without concomitant diseases: a population study. Int J Impot Res 2003; 15:253–257.

51 Esposito K, Giugliano D. Obesity, the metabolic syndrome and sexual dysfunction. Int J Impot Res 2005; 17:391–398.

52 Rosen RC, Fisher W, Eardley I, et al. The multinational men's attitudes of life events and sexuality (MALES) study; prevalence of erectile dysfunction and related health concerns in the general population. Curr Med Res Opin 2004; 20: 607–617.

53 Bacon CG, Mittleman MA, Kawachi I, et al. Sexual function in men older than 50 years of age; results from the health professionals follow-up study. Ann Intern Med 2003; 139: 161–168.

54 Blanker MH, Bosch JL, Groeneveld FP, et al. Erectile and ejaculatory dysfunction in a community-based sample of men 50–78 years old: prevalence, concerns and relation to sexual activity. Urology 2001; 57:763–768.

55 Blanker MH, Bohnen AM, Groeneveld FP, et al. Correlates for erectile and ejaculatory dysfunction in older Dutch men: a community-based study. J Am Geriatr Soc 2001; 49:436–442.

56 Esposito K, Giugliano F, Di Palo C, et al. Effect of lifestyle changes on erectile dysfunction in obese men: a randomized controlled trial. JAMA 2004; 291:1978–1984.

57 Shabsigh R, Kaufman JM, Steidle C, et al. Randomised study of testosterone gel as adjunctive therapy to sildenafil in hypogonadal men with erectile dysfunction who do not response to sildenafil alone. J Urol 2004; 172:658–663.

58 Muller M, Van Der Schouw YT, Thijssen JHH, et al. Endogenous sex hormones and cardiovascular disease in men. J Clin Endocrinol Metab 2003; 88:5076–5086.

59 Fraunfelder FW, Pomeranz HD, Egan RA. Non-arteritic anterior ischaemic optic neuropathy and sildenafil. Arch Ophthamol 2006; 124:733–734.

44

Peripheral arterial disease

Zoran Lasic and Michael R. Jaff

Introduction

The term "peripheral arterial disease" (PAD) covers a multitude of disorders involving arterial beds exclusive of the coronary arteries. There are numerous pathophysiologic processes that could contribute to the creation of stenoses or aneurysms of the noncoronary arterial circulation. Atherosclerosis represents the leading disease process affecting the aorta and its branch arteries. Patients undergoing percutaneous coronary intervention (PCI) who have PAD have been shown to have worse short- and long-term outcomes compared to patients without PAD (1–3). This chapter will cover pharmacotherapy and nonpharmacologic therapies for PAD involving lower extremities.

Cardiovascular risk reduction

The clinical manifestations of PAD are associated with reduction in functional capacity and quality of life, but because of the systemic nature of the atherosclerotic process there is a strong association with coronary and carotid artery disease. Consequently, patients with PAD have an increased risk of cardiovascular and cerebrovascular ischemic events [myocardial infarction (MI), ischemic stroke, and death] compared to the general population (4,5). In addition, these cardiovascular ischemic events are more frequent than ischemic limb events in any lower extremity PAD cohort, whether individuals present without symptoms or with atypical leg pain, classic claudication, or critical limb ischemia (6). Therefore, aggressive treatment of known risk factors for progression of atherosclerosis is warranted. In addition to tobacco cessation, encouragement of daily exercise and use of a low cholesterol, low salt diet, PAD patients should be offered therapies to reduce lipid levels, control blood pressure, control blood glucose in patients with diabetes mellitus, and offer other effective antiatherosclerotic strategies. A recent position paper

describing antiatherosclerosis strategies includes patients with PAD, viewed as a coronary artery equivalent (7).

Treatment of hyperlipidemia

A meta-analysis was performed on randomized trials assessing lipid-lowering therapy in 698 patients with PAD who were treated with a variety of therapies, including diet, cholestyramine, probucol, and nicotinic acid, for four months to three years (8). There was a significant difference in total mortality [0.7% in the treated patients, as compared with 2.9% in the patients given placebo (p = NS)], with an additional reduction in disease progression, as measured by angiography and the severity of claudication.

Two studies evaluated the effects of lipid-lowering therapy on clinical endpoints in the leg. The Program on the Surgical Control of the Hyperlipidemias was a randomized trial of partial ileal-bypass surgery for the treatment of hyperlipidemia in 838 patients (9). After five years, the relative risk (RR) of an abnormal ankle-brachial index value (ABI) was 0.6 (95% CI, 0.4 to 0.9, absolute risk reduction, 15% points, p < 0.01), and the RR of claudication or limb-threatening ischemia was 0.7 (95% CI, 0.2 to 0.9, absolute risk reduction, 7% points, p < 0.01), as compared with the control group.

In patients with PAD, therapy with a statin not only lowers serum cholesterol levels, but also improves endothelial function, as well as other markers of atherosclerotic risk, such as serum P-selectin concentrations (10,11).

In a subgroup of patients treated with simvastatin in the Scandinavian Simvastatin Survival Study, the RR of new claudication or worsening of preexisting claudication was 0.6 (95% CI, 0.4 to 0.9, absolute risk reduction, 1.3% points), as compared with patients randomly assigned to placebo (12).

Several studies have revealed that statins have a beneficial effect on exercise performance in patients with claudication (13). Statins also improve endothelial function and have other favorable metabolic effects, but the functional benefit of statins is not due to regression of atherosclerosis or gross change in limb hemodynamics.

The National Cholesterol Education Program classifies patients with PAD in the group of coronary heart disease (CHD) risk equivalents. Other coronary heart equivalents include abdominal aortic aneurysm, carotid artery disease (transient ischemic attacks or stroke of carotid origin or >50% obstruction of a carotid artery), diabetes mellitus, and patients with two or more risk factors for atherosclerosis which produces the 10-year risk for CHD >20% (14). Patients with PAD and low-density lipoprotein (LDL) cholesterol (LDL-C) of 100 mg/dL or greater should be treated with a statin, but when risk is very high, an LDL cholesterol goal of less than 70 mg/dl is an appropriate therapeutic option. Factors that place patients in the category of very high risk are the presence of established cardiovascular disease (CVD) plus (*i*) multiple major risk factors (especially diabetes), (*ii*) severe and poorly controlled risk factors (especially continued cigarette smoking), (*iii*) multiple risk factors of the metabolic syndrome [especially high triglycerides, that is greater than or equal to 200 mg/dL plus non-HDL cholesterol greater than or equal to 130 mg/dL with low-HDL cholesterol (less than or equal to 40 mg/dL)], and (*iv*) on the basis of the PROVE IT trial (15), patients with acute coronary syndromes (16,17).

Treatment of hypertension

Treatment of high blood pressure is indicated to reduce the risk of cardiovascular events (18). Betablockers, which have been shown to reduce the risk of MI and death in patients with coronary atherosclerosis (19), do not adversely affect walking capacity (20,21). These agents must be offered to patients with PAD who have already suffered a MI or have established coronary artery disease. Angiotensin-converting enzyme inhibitors reduce the risk of death and nonfatal cardiovascular events in patients with coronary artery disease and left ventricular dysfunction (22,23). The Heart Outcomes Prevention Evaluation trial found that in patients with symptomatic PAD, ramipril, a tissue-specific ACE-inhibitor reduced the risk of MI, stroke, or vascular death by approximately 25%, a level of efficacy comparable to that achieved in the entire study population (24). There is currently no evidence base for the efficacy of ACE inhibitors in patients with asymptomatic PAD, and thus, the use of ACE-inhibitor medications to lower cardiovascular ischemic event rates in this population must be extrapolated from the data on symptomatic patients. However, a recent small randomized prospective placebo-controlled trial of ramipril in patients with symptomatic PAD demonstrated a statistically significant improvement in pain-free walking distance when compared with placebo (25). ACC/AHA 2005 guidelines for the management of patients with PAD recommend that antihypertensive therapy should be administered to hypertensive patients with lower extremity PAD to achieve a goal of less than 140 mmHg systolic over 90 mmHg diastolic (nondiabetics) or less than 130 mmHg systolic over 80 mmHg diastolic (diabetics and individuals with chronic renal disease) to reduce the risk of MI, stroke, congestive heart failure, and cardiovascular death (26,27).

Treatment of diabetes mellitus

Intensive pharmacologic treatment of diabetes is known to decrease the risk for microvascular events such as nephropathy and retinopathy, but there is less evidence that it decreases macrovascular disease (28,29). DCCT/EDIC trial, however, demonstrated reduction in CVD (nonfatal MI, stroke, death from CVD, confirmed angina, or the need for coronary-artery revascularization) in patients with type 1 diabetes assigned to intensive diabetes treatment compared with conventional treatment by 42% (p = 0.02) (30). Patients with lower extremity PAD and both type 1 and type 2 diabetes should be treated to reduce their glycosylated hemoglobin (Hb A1C) to less than 7%, per the American Diabetes Association recommendation (31). Subanalysis of the UKPDS showed no evidence of a threshold effect of Hb A1C; a 1% reduction in Hb A1C was associated with a 35% reduction in microvascular endpoints, an 18% reduction in MI, and a 17% reduction in all-cause mortality. Frequent foot inspection by patients and physicians will enable early identification of foot lesions and ulcerations and facilitate prompt referral for treatment (32).

Homocysteine-lowering drugs

Patients with PAD have increased mortality risk from cardiovascular causes (4,5), which is significantly increased in the subgroup of patients with high serum homocysteine concentration (33,34). Association of a low ABI and high homocysteine level could be useful for identifying patients at excess risk for cardiovascular death (34). In spite of the efficacy in lowering homocysteine level with a folic acid supplement there is no evidence that reducing homocysteine concentration is beneficial in patients with CHD and PAD (26,35).

Antiplatelet and antithrombotic drugs

The Antithrombotic Trialists' Collaboration (ATC) investigated the effects of antiplatelet therapy in 287 studies involving

135,000 patients in comparison with antiplatelet therapy versus control and 77,000 in comparison with different antiplatelet regimens in patients at high risk of occlusive vascular events (36). "Serious vascular event" (nonfatal MI, nonfatal stroke, or vascular death) was less common in patients allocated to antiplatelet therapy by about one quarter; nonfatal MI was reduced by one-third, nonfatal stroke by one quarter, and vascular mortality by one-sixth (with no apparent adverse effect on other deaths). Aspirin was the most commonly studied antiplatelet drug, with doses of 75 to 150 mg daily at least as effective as higher daily doses. Clopidogrel-reduced serious vascular events by 10% (4%) compared with aspirin, which was similar to the 12% (7%) reduction observed with its analog ticlopidine.

Aspirin

Aspirin (acetylsalicylic acid—ASA) exerts its effect primarily by irreversibly inhibiting enzyme cyclo-oxygenase that blocks platelet synthesis of thromboxane A2—a promoter of platelet aggregation (37). The benefits of ASA in reducing cardiovascular death, MI, and stroke in patients with CHD (36) have led to the near universal use of this medication for patients undergoing PCI. Antithrombotic effects have been shown to be present at dosages between 50 and 100 mg/day, but the optimal dose for PCI has not been firmly established. Different aspirin doses compared in the ATC meta-analysis suggest that a daily dose of 75 to 150 mg is at least as effective as higher doses (>150 mg/day) and is less likely to cause gastrointestinal and bleeding complications (36).

When given in combination with warfarin or thienopyridine class of antiplatelet agents the ASA dose is usually lowered to 80 to 100 mg based on a post hoc analysis of data from the clopidogrel in unstable angina to prevent recurrent events (CURE), which showed similar efficacy but less major bleeding with the low dose (<100 mg) of ASA (38).

ASA nonresponsiveness or resistance is reported in 5% to 60% of patients (39,40). There is emerging clinical evidence that ASA resistance is associated with an increased risk of major adverse cardiovascular events. Five studies in patients with coronary peripheral, and/or cerebrovascular disease have reported a 1.8- to 10-fold increased risk of thrombotic events (41,42).

In the Physicians' Health Study aspirin treatment for primary prevention of PAD reduced the subsequent need for peripheral arterial surgery (43). Aspirin therapy significantly improved vascular-graft patency in 3226 patients with PAD who were treated surgically or with peripheral angioplasty during average follow-up to 19 months (43% reduction in the rate of vascular-graft occlusion: 25% in the control group as compared with 16% in the aspirin group) (44). Aspirin given as a monotherapy was as effective as the combination of aspirin and dipyridamole, sulfinpyrazone, or ticlopidine in preventing graft occlusion, without any difference between low-dose (75 to 325 mg/day) and high-dose aspirin (600 to 1500 mg/day).

The ACC/AHA guidelines state that ASA in daily doses of 75 to 325 mg is recommended as a safe and effective antiplatelet therapy to reduce the risk of MI, stroke, or vascular death in individuals with atherosclerotic lower extremity PAD (26).

Thienopyridines

Clopidogrel and ticlopidine are thienopyridine derivatives. They selectively and irreversibly inhibit the P2Y12 ADP receptor, which plays a critical role in platelet activation and aggregation (45). They work synergistically with ASA in providing greater inhibition of platelet aggregation than either agent alone (46). The inhibition of platelet aggregation by ticlopidine and clopidogrel is present after two to three days of therapy with ticlopidine 500 mg/day or clopidogrel 75 mg/day, and platelet function recovers in five to seven days after discontinuation owing to the synthesis of new platelets (47).

Clopidogrel

In the CAPRIE trial (Clopidogrel vs. Aspirin in Patients at Risk of Ischemic Events), clopidogrel reduced the risk of MI, stroke, or vascular death by 23.8% compared with aspirin in patients with PAD (48). Although this is an impressive reduction in major events, the benefits of clopidogrel over aspirin were identified as a subgroup analysis rather than a primary endpoint.

The Charisma trial evaluated antiplatelet treatment with aspirin alone compared with aspirin plus clopidogrel among high-risk patients with stable CVD (49). High-risk patients with established vascular disease included 37.4% with coronary disease, 27.7% with cerebrovascular disease, and 18.2% with symptomatic PAD. There was no difference in the primary endpoint of CV death, MI, or stroke between the clopidogrel plus aspirin group (6.8%) and the placebo plus aspirin group (7.3%, RR 0.93, p = 0.22). The secondary endpoint of death, MI, stroke or hospitalization for ischemic event was lower in the clopidogrel plus aspirin group (16.7% vs. 17.9%, RR 0.92, p = 0.04). The benefit of clopidogrel was evident in the symptomatic cohort (with documented CVD at enrollment) for the primary endpoint (6.9% for clopidogrel vs. 7.9% for placebo, RR 0.88, p = 0.046) but not in the asymptomatic cohort (6.6% for clopidogrel vs. 5.5% for placebo, RR 1.20, p = 0.20, interaction p = 0.045). Severe bleeding trended higher in the clopidogrel group (1.7% vs. 1.3%, RR 1.25, p = 0.09), while moderate bleeding was significantly higher in the clopidogrel group (2.1% vs. 1.3%, p < 0.001). There was no difference in intracranial hemorrhage (0.3% each). These findings suggest that dual antiplatelet therapy may not be beneficial in all patients at risk for CVD, but that in patients with established CVD, dual therapy may be effective in reducing subsequent events.

In the CURE study, 12,562 patients with acute coronary syndromes without ST-segment elevation have received ASA and clopidogrel 300 mg bolus, followed by 75 mg daily, versus ASA and placebo (50). The clopidogrel group had early reduction [within 24 hours of treatment—9.3% vs. 11.4%, RR reduction 20% (p < 0.001) in the primary endpoint death from cardiovascular cause, nonfatal MI, or stroke], which was sustained at one year, and was observed in all patients with acute coronary syndromes regardless of their level of risk. CURE patients who underwent PCI and were randomized to clopidogrel had a 31% RR reduction in death and MI compared with placebo-treated PCI patients (51).

The CREDO trial, which studied an elective population of patients who underwent PCI, showed benefits of clopidogrel (52). Patients were randomly assigned to receive a 300-mg clopidogrel loading dose (n = 1053) or placebo (n = 1063), 3 to 24 hours before PCI. Thereafter, all patients received clopidogrel, 75 mg/day, through day 28. The group loaded with clopidogrel was continued on active drug from day 28 through 12 months while the control group received placebo. Both groups received aspirin throughout the study. There was a significant 27% (p = 0.02) reduction in death, MI, or stroke in patients receiving clopidogrel, suggesting that clopidogrel therapy should be continued in addition to ASA for a minimum of nine months post PCI.

There was an increase in major bleeding with clopidogrel in both the CURE and CREDO trials. In CURE, those receiving clopidogrel had bleeding rates of 3.7% versus 2.7% (p = 0.001), most notably in those patients requiring CABG. In CREDO, there was only a trend toward more TIMI (thrombolysis in MI) major bleeding (8.8% vs. 6.7%, p = 0.07) and no excess bleedings among patients undergoing CABG.

Ticlopidine

Although the original stent thrombosis data were obtained with ticlopidine, its use has been virtually abandoned in the United States owing to its increased risk of neutropenia. A meta-analysis demonstrated that clopidogrel was associated with a significant reduction in the incidence of major adverse cardiac events (2.1% in the clopidogrel group and 4.04% in the ticlopidine group). After adjustment for heterogeneity in the trials, the odds ratio (OR) of having an ischemic event with clopidogrel, as compared with ticlopidine, was 0.72 (95% CI, 0.59–0.89, p = 0.002). Mortality was also lower in the clopidogrel group compared with the ticlopidine group −0.48% versus 1.09% (OR 0.55, 95% CI, 0.37–0.82, p = 0.003). The safety and tolerability of clopidogrel were superior to that of ticlopidine (53). This includes fewer rashes, gastrointestinal

side effects, as well as fewer hematologic complications (neutropenia). Ticlopidine use in the United States in patients undergoing PCI is mostly reserved for those patients with allergy or intolerance of clopidogrel.

Smoking cessation

Smoking cessation should be encouraged because it slows the progression of PAD to critical leg ischemia and reduces the risks of MI and death from vascular causes (54). Patients with CHD who stopped smoking had a 36% reduction in crude RR of mortality compared with those who continued smoking (RR 0.64, 95% CI, 0.58–0.71) (55). While smoking cessation does not improve maximal treadmill walking distance in patients with claudication based on a meta-analysis from published data (56), smoking cessation is critical in patients with thromboangiitis obliterans, because continued use is associated with a particularly adverse outcome (57). Physician advice coupled with frequent follow-up achieves one-year smoking cessation rates of approximately 5% compared with only 0.1% in those attempting to quit smoking without a physician's intervention (58). Pharmacologic interventions (nicotine replacement therapy and bupropion) should be encouraged because they achieve higher cessation rates at one year (16% and 30%, respectively) (59).

Treatment for claudication

Intermittent claudication decreases exercise capacity and overall functional capacity. Impaired walking ability is coupled with the inability to perform activities of daily living and results in a decrease in overall quality of life (60). Pharmacologic and nonpharmacologic measures aimed in improving mobility and consequently the quality of life is important treatment goals for patients with PAD.

Exercise

In patients with claudication, the most important nonpharmacologic treatment is a formal exercise-training program (61). An exercise program can significantly improve maximal walking time and overall walking ability (62). The optimal exercise program for improving distances walked without claudication pain involves intermittent walking to near-maximal pain over a period of at least six months based on meta-analysis from Gardner et al. (63). ACC/AHA guidelines recommend exercise training in duration for a minimum of 30 to 45 minutes, in sessions performed at least three times per week for a minimum of 12 weeks (ACC/AHA guidelines). Optimal results involve a motivated patient in a supervised setting, which represents a challenge for patients and health care providers because supervised exercise-training programs are not covered by medical insurance, which makes their extensive and long-term use difficult (64). The mechanism by which exercise improves leg symptoms is uncertain, but it does not appear to operate through improvement of the ABI or growth of collateral vessels (65).

Pharmacologic treatment for claudication

Cilostazol

The primary action of cilostazol is inhibition of phosphodiesterase type 3, which increases intracellular concentrations of cyclic AMP. Cilostazol inhibits platelet aggregation, the formation of arterial thrombi, and vascular smooth-muscle proliferation and causes vasodilatation (66–68). Since vasodilator and antiplatelet drugs do not improve claudication-limited exercise performance, the precise mechanism through which cilostazol exerts its effect in PAD is unknown. After 12 to 24 weeks of therapy patients treated with cilostazol improve maximal walking distance by 40% to 60% (69–73). In addition to improved walking capacity cilostazol improves health-related quality of life (74). Administered at the dose of 100 mg twice daily cilostazol is more effective than 50 mg twice daily (71,73). Although no trials have found a significant increase in major cardiovascular events in patients treated with cilostazol (an increased mortality was observed with other phosphodiesterase inhibitors such as milrinone), it remains contraindicated in individuals with coexistent heart failure because of its potential adverse effect in this population. The predominant side effect of cilostazol is headache, which affects 34% of patients taking 100 mg twice daily, as compared with 14% of patients taking placebo.

Pentoxifylline

Mechanism of action that provides symptom relief with pentoxifylline is poorly understood but is thought to involve red blood cell deformability as well as a reduction in fibrinogen concentration, platelet adhesiveness and whole blood viscosity (75). The recommended dose of pentoxifylline is 400 mg three times daily with meals. Pentoxifylline causes a marginal but statistically significant improvement in pain-free and maximal walking distance (a net benefit of 44 m in the maximal distance walked on a treadmill (95% CI, 0 14 to 0 74) based on meta-analyses of randomized, placebo-controlled, double-blind clinical trials (76). At the same time pentoxifylline does not increase the ABI at rest or after exercise (56). Pentoxifylline may be used to treat patients with intermittent claudication; however, it is likely to be of marginal clinical importance (56,77). *Medical* therapies whose effectiveness is not well established by evidence/opinion (Class IIb – ACC/AHA Guidelines).

L-arginine

Infusion of L-arginine produces systemic vasodilatation via stimulation of endogenous nitric oxide (NO) formation, which may improve vascular endothelial function and muscle blood flow in patients with PAD via the NO-cyclic GMP pathway in a dose-related manner (78). In patients with claudication, two weeks of treatment using a food bar enriched with L-arginine and a combination of other nutrients increased the pain-free walking distance 66% while the total walking distance increased 23% in the group taking two active bars per day. Improvements were not observed in the one active bar per day and placebo groups (79).

L-carnitine and propionyl-L-carnitine

Orally administered L-carnitine and propionyl-L-carnitine may have metabolic benefits by providing an additional source of carnitine to buffer the cellular acyl CoA pool. In this way, carnitine may enhance glucose oxidation under ischemic conditions and improve energy metabolism in the ischemic skeletal muscle. Propionyl-CoA generated from propionyl-L-carnitine may also improve oxidative metabolism through its anaphoretic actions in priming the Kreb's cycle, secondary to succinyl-CoA production.

After 180 days of treatment there was a significant improvement of $73 \pm 9\%$ (mean $\pm$ SE) in maximal walking distance in PAD patients treated with propionyl-L-carnitine compared to placebo (80). Propionyl-L-carnitine has been shown to improve treadmill performance and quality of life in patients with claudication. After six months of treatment, subjects randomly assigned to propionyl-L-carnitine increased their peak walking time by 162 ± 222 seconds (a 54% increase) as compared with an improvement of 75 ± 191 seconds (a 25% increase) for those on placebo ($p < 0.001$) (81).

Ginkgo biloba

Ginkgo biloba extract has been reported to improve symptoms of intermittent claudication. Meta-analysis of the efficacy of Ginkgo biloba extract for intermittent claudication based on the results of eight randomized, placebo-controlled, double-blind trials found a significant difference in the increase in pain-free walking distance in favor of Ginkgo biloba (weighted mean difference: 34 m, 95% CI, 26–43 m). Though the results showed statistical superiority of Ginkgo biloba extract compared to placebo in the symptomatic treatment of intermittent claudication, extent of the improvement was modest and of uncertain clinical relevance (82).

Prostaglandin

Vasodilators decrease arteriolar tone; however, numerous controlled trials have found no convincing evidence of clinical efficacy for any of these medications in patients with claudication (83). There are several potential pathophysiologic explanations for the lack of efficacy of these drugs in treating claudication. During exercise, resistance vessels dilate distal to a stenosis or occlusion in response to ischemia. Vasodilators have little effect on these already dilated vessels and may decrease resistance in unobstructed vascular beds, leading to a "steal" of blood flow away from underperfused muscles. Vasodilators can also lower systemic pressure, leading to a reduction in perfusion pressure. Thus, vasodilating medications do not favorably address the pathophysiology of claudication or result in a treatment benefit. The initial trial with oral prostaglandin beraprost showed an improvement of >50% in pain-free walking distance and maximum walking distances at six months compared to placebo (84).

A US study, however, showed that administration of beraprost did not improve the pain-free walking distance or the quality-of-life measures between the treatment groups (85).

Other therapies

A systematic review of the literature aimed to assess the effectiveness of any type of complementary therapy for intermittent claudication revealed that there is no evidence of effectiveness of acupuncture, biofeedback therapy, chelation therapy, $CO(2)$-applications and the dietary supplements of Allium sativum (garlic), omega-3 fatty acids and Vitamin E (86).

PAD is particularly common in patients with CAD undergoing PCI. PCI patients affected with PAD have an increased risk of major adverse cardiovascular events in addition to impaired ambulatory capacity and quality of life, compared with PCI patients without PAD. PAD is undertreated, especially in patients with asymptomatic PAD, with consideration to pharmacologic and nonpharmacologic therapies. Therefore it is important to recognize PAD in PCI patients so that they can be aggressively managed with regard to risk factor modification using pharmacologic approach in treating hypertension, hyperlipidemia, diabetes mellitus, and symptoms of PAD. Pharmacologic therapies should be coupled with a supervised exercise program and smoking cessation program.

References

1 Nikolsky E, Mehran R, Mintz GS, et al. Impact of symptomatic peripheral arterial disease on 1-year mortality in patients undergoing percutaneous coronary interventions. J Endovasc Ther 2004; 11(1):60–70.

2 Nallamothu BK, Chetcuti S, Mukherjee D, et al. Long-term prognostic implication of extracardiac vascular disease in patients undergoing percutaneous coronary intervention. Am J Cardiol 2003; 92(8):964–966.

3 Singh M, Lennon Ryan J, Darbar D. Effect of peripheral arterial disease in patients undergoing percutaneous coronary intervention with intracoronary stents. Mayo Clin Proc 2004; 79(9):1113–1118.

4 Criqui MH, Denenberg JO, Langer RD, et al. The epidemiology of peripheral arterial disease importance of identifying the population at risk. Vasc Med 1997; 2:221–226.

5 Ness J, Aronow WS. Prevalence of coexistence of coronary artery disease, ischemic stroke, and peripheral arterial disease in older persons, mean age 80 years, in an academic hospital-based geriatrics practice. J Am Geriatr Soc 1999; 47: 1255–1256.

6 Weitz JI, Byrne J, Clagett GP, et al. Diagnosis and treatment of chronic arterial insufficiency of the lower extremities a critical review. Circulation 1996; 94:3026–3049.

7 Smith SC Jr, Allen J, Blair SN, et al. AHA/ACC guidelines for secondary prevention for patients with coronary and other atherosclerotic vascular disease: 2006 update: endorsed by the National Heart, Lung, and Blood Institute. Circulation 2006; 113(19):2363–2372.

8 Leng GC, Price JF, Jepson RG. Lipid-lowering for lower limb atherosclerosis (Cochrane review). In: The Cochrane Library. Oxford, England: Update Software, 2001.

9 Buchwald H, Bourdages HR, Campos CT, et al. Impact of cholesterol reduction on peripheral arterial disease in the Program on the Surgical Control of the Hyperlipidemias (POSCH). Surgery 1996; 120:672–679.

10 Khan F, Litchfield SJ, Belch JJ. Cutaneous microvascular responses are improved after cholesterol-lowering in patients with peripheral arterial disease and hypercholesterolaemia. Adv Exp Med Biol 1997; 428:49–54.

11 Kirk G, McLaren M, Muir AH, et al. Decrease in P-selectin levels in patients with hypercholesterolaemia and peripheral arterial occlusive disease after lipid-lowering treatment. Vasc Med 1999; 4:23–26.

12 Pedersen TR, Kjekshus J, Pyorala K, et al. Effect of simvastatin on ischemic signs and symptoms in the Scandinavian Simvastatin Survival Study (4S). Am J Cardiol 1998; 81: 333–335.

13 Mohler ER III, Hiatt WR, Creager MA. Cholesterol reduction with atorvastatin improves walking distance in patients with peripheral arterial disease. Circulation 2003; 108(12): 1481–1486.

14 National Cholesterol Education Program (NCEP) Expert Panel on Detection, Evaluation, and Treatment of High Blood Cholesterol in Adults (Adult Treatment Panel III). Third Report of the National Cholesterol Education Program (NCEP) Expert Panel on Detection, Evaluation, and Treatment of High Blood Cholesterol in Adults (Adult Treatment Panel III) final report. Circulation 2002; 106:3143–3421.

15 Cannon CP, Braunwald E, McCabe CH, et al. Pravastatin or Atorvastatin Evaluation and Infection Therapy-Thrombolysis in Myocardial Infarction 22 Investigators. Intensive versus moderate lipid lowering with statins after acute coronary syndromes. N Engl J Med 2004; 350:1495–1504.

16 MRC/BHF Heart Protection Study of cholesterol lowering with simvastatin in 20,536 high-risk individuals, a randomised placebo-controlled trial. Lancet 2002; 360:7–22.

17 Grundy SM, Cleeman JI, Merz CN, et al. Implications of recent clinical trials for the National Cholesterol Education Program Adult Treatment Panel III guidelines Arterioscler Thromb Vasc Biol 2004; 24:e149–e161.

18 Psaty BM, Smith NL, Siscovick DS, et al. Health outcomes associated with antihypertensive therapies used as first-line agents, a systematic review and meta-analysis. JAMA 1997; 277:739–745.

19 Hennekens CH, Albert CM, Godfried SL, et al. Adjunctive drug therapy of acute myocardial infarction evidence from clinical trials. N Engl J Med 1996; 335:1660–1667.

20 Radack K, Deck C. Beta-adrenergic blocker therapy does not worsen intermittent claudication in subjects with peripheral arterial disease, a meta-analysis of randomized controlled trials. Arch Intern Med 1991; 151:1769–1776.

21 Heintzen MP, Strauer BE. Peripheral vascular effects of beta-blockers. Eur Heart J 1994; 15(suppl C):2–7.

22 Pfeffer MA, Braunwald E, Moye LA, et al. Effect of captopril on mortality and morbidity in patients with left ventricular dysfunction after myocardial infarction, results of the Survival And Ventricular Enlargement trial. N Engl J Med 1992; 327:669–677.

23 Gustafsson F, Torp-Pedersen C, Kober L, et al. TRACE Study Group Trandolapril Cardiac Event. Effect of angiotensin converting enzyme inhibition after acute myocardial infarction in patients with arterial hypertension. J Hypertens 1997; 15:793–798.

24 Yusuf S, Sleight P, Pogue J, et al. Heart Outcomes Prevention Evaluation Study Investigators Effects of an angiotensin-converting-enzyme inhibitor, ramipril, on cardiovascular events in high-risk patients N Engl J Med 2000; 342:145–153.

25 Ahimastos AA, Lawler A, Reid CM, et al. Brief communication: ramipril markedly improves walking ability in patients with peripheral arterial disease. Ann Int Med 2006; 144:660–664.

26 Hirsch AT, Haskal ZJ, Hertzer NR, et al. ACC/AHA 2005 guidelines for the management of patients with peripheral arterial disease (lower extremity, renal, mesenteric, and abdominal aortic): executive summary a collaborative report from the American Association for Vascular Surgery/Society for Vascular Surgery, Society for Cardiovascular Angiography and Interventions, Society for Vascular Medicine and Biology, Society of Interventional Radiology, and the ACC/AHA Task Force on Practice Guidelines (Writing Committee to Develop Guidelines for the Management of Patients With Peripheral Arterial Disease) endorsed by the American Association of Cardiovascular and Pulmonary Rehabilitation; National Heart, Lung, and Blood Institute; Society for Vascular Nursing; TransAtlantic Inter-Society Consensus; and Vascular Disease Foundation. J Am Coll Cardiol 2006; 47(6):1239–1312.

27 Chobanian AV, Bakris GL, Black HR, et al. Seventh report of the Joint National Committee on Prevention, Detection, Evaluation, and Treatment of High Blood Pressure. Hypertension 2003;42(6):1206–1252. Epub 2003 Dec 1.

28 Effect of intensive diabetes management on macrovascular events and risk factors in the Diabetes Control and Complications Trial. Am J Cardiol 1995; 75:894–903.

29 UK Prospective Diabetes Study (UKPDS) Group. Intensive blood-glucose control with sulphonylureas or insulin compared with conventional treatment and risk of complications in patients with type 2 diabetes (UKPDS 33). Lancet 1998; 352: 837–853.

30 Nathan DM, Cleary PA, Backlund JY, et al. Diabetes Control and Complications Trial/Epidemiology of Diabetes Interventions and Complications (DCCT/EDIC) Study Research Group. Intensive diabetes treatment and cardiovascular disease in patients with type 1 diabetes. N Engl J Med 2005; 353(25):2643–2653.

31 Standards of medical care for patients with diabetes mellitus Diabetes Care 2003; 26(suppl 1):S33–S50.

32 Donohoe ME, Fletton JA, Hook A, et al. Improving foot care for people with diabetes mellitus, a randomized controlled trial of an integrated care approach. Diab Med 2000; 17:581–587.

33 Graham IM, Daly LE, Refsum HM, et al. Plasma homocysteine as a risk factor for vascular disease: the European Concerted Action Project. JAMA 1997; 277:1775–1781.

34 Lange S, Trampisch HJ, Haberl R, et al. Excess 1-year cardiovascular risk in elderly primary care patients with a low ankle-brachial index (ABI) and high homocysteine level. Atherosclerosis 2005; 178(2):351–357.

35 Bonaa KH, Njolstad I, Ueland PM, et al. NORVIT Trial Investigators. Homocysteine lowering and cardiovascular events after acute myocardial infarction. N Engl J Med 2006; 354(15):1578–1588.

36 Collaborative meta-analysis of randomised trials of antiplatelet therapy for prevention of death, myocardial infarction, and stroke in high risk patients. BMJ 2002; 324:71–86.

37 Awtry EH, Loscaizo J. Aspirin. Circulation 2000; 101: 1206–1218.

38 Peters R, Mehta SR, Fox KA, et al. Effects of aspirin dose when used alone or in combination with clopidogrel in patients with acute coronary syndromes: observations from the Clopidogrel in Unstable angina to prevent Recurrent Events (CURE) study. Circulation 2003; 108: 1682–1687.

39 Howard PA. Aspirin resistance. Ann Pharmacother 2002; 36:1620–1624.

40 Bhatt DL. Aspirin resistance: more than just a laboratory curiosity. J Am Coll Cardiol 2004; 43:1127–1129.

41 Eikelboom JW, Hirsh J, Weitz JI, et al. Aspirin-resistant thromboxane biosynthesis and the risk of myocardial infarction, stroke, or cardiovascular death in patients at high risk for cardiovascular events. Circulation 2002; 105:1650–1655.

42 Grundmann K, Jaschonek K, Kleine B, et al. Aspirin non-responder status in patients with recurrent cerebral ischemic attacks. J Neurol 2003; 250:63–66.

43 Goldhaber SZ, Manson JE, Stampfer MJ, et al. Low-dose aspirin and subsequent peripheral arterial surgery in the Physicians' Health Study. Lancet 1992; 340:143–145.

44 Collaborative overview of randomised trials of antiplatelet therapy. II. Maintenance of vascular graft or arterial patency by antiplatelet therapy. BMJ 1994; 308:159–168.

45 Andre P, Delaney SM, LaRocca T, et al. P2Y12 regulates platelet adhesion/activation, thrombus growth, and thrombus stability in injured arteries. J Clin Invest 2003; 112:398–406.

46 Herbert JM, Dol F, Bernat A, et al. The antiaggregating and antithrombotic activity of clopidogrel is potentiated by aspirin in several experimental models in the rabbit. Thromb Haemost 1998; 80:512–518.

47 Weber AA, Braun M, Hohlfeld T, et al. Recovery of platelet function after discontinuation of clopidogrel treatment in healthy volunteers. Br J Clin Pharmacol 2001; 52: 333–336.

48 CAPRIE Steering Committee. A randomised, blinded, trial of clopidogrel versus aspirin in patients at risk of ischaemic events (CAPRIE). Lancet 1996; 348:1329–1339.

49 Bhatt DL, Fox KA, Hacke W, et al. Clopidogrel and aspirin versus aspirin alone for the prevention of atherothrombotic events. N Engl J Med 2006; 354(16):1706–1717.

50 Yusuf S, Zhao F, Mehta SR, et al. Effects of clopidogrel in addition to aspirin in patients with acute coronary syndromes without ST-segment elevation. N Engl J Med 2001; 345(7):494–502.

51 Mehta SR, Salim Y, Peters RJG, et al. Effects of pretreatment with clopidogrel and aspirin followed by long-term therapy in patients undergoing percutaneous coronary intervention: the PCI-CURE study. Lancet 2001; 358:527–533.

52 Steinhubl SR, Berger PB, Mann JT III, et al. Clopidogrel for the Reduction of Events During Observation. Early and sustained dual oral antiplatelet therapy following percutaneous coronary intervention: a randomized controlled trial. JAMA 2002; 288:2411–2420.

53 Bhatt DL, Bertrand ME, Berger PB, et al. Meta-analysis of randomized and registry comparisons of ticlopidine with clopidogrel after stenting. J Am Coll Cardiol 2002; 39(1):9–14.

54 Quick CRG, Cotton LT. The measured effect of stopping smoking on intermittent claudication. Br J Surg 1982; 69(Suppl):S24–S26.

55 Critchley JA, Capewell S. Mortality risk reduction associated with smoking cessation in patients with coronary heart disease: a systematic review. JAMA 2003; 290(1):86–97.

56 Girolami B, Bernardi E, Prins MH, et al. Treatment of intermittent claudication with physical training, smoking cessation, pentoxifylline, or nafronyl: a meta-analysis. Arch Intern Med 1999; 159:337–345.

57 Olin JW. Thromboangiitis obliterans (Buerger's disease) N Engl J Med 2000; 343:864–869.

58 Law M, Tang JL. An analysis of the effectiveness of interventions intended to help people stop smoking. Arch Intern Med 1995; 155:1933–1941.

59 Jorenby DE, Leischow SJ, Nides MA, et al. A controlled trial of sustained-release bupropion, a nicotine patch, or both for smoking cessation N Engl J Med 1999; 340:685–691.

60 Khaira HS, Hanger R, Shearman CP. Quality of life in patients with intermittent claudication. Eur J Vasc Endovasc Surg 1996; 11:65–69.

61 Nehler MR, Hiatt WR. Exercise therapy for claudication. Ann Vasc Surg 1999; 13:109–114.

62 Leng GC, Fowler B, Ernst E. Exercise for intermittent claudication. Cochrane Database Syst Rev 2000;2:CD000990.

63 Gardner AW, Phoelman ET. Exercise rehabilitation programs for the treatment of claudication pain: a meta-analysis. JAMA 1995; 274:975–980.

64 Regensteiner JG, Meyer TJ, Krupski WC, et al. Hospital vs home-based exercise rehabilitation for patients with peripheral arterial occlusive disease. Angiology 1997; 48:291–300.

65 Stewart KJ, Hiatt WR. Exercise training for claudication. N Engl J Med 2002; 347:1941–1951.

66 Kohda N, Tani T, Nakayama S, et al. Effect of cilostazol, a phosphodiesterase III inhibitor, on experimental thrombosis in the porcine carotid artery. Thromb Res 1999; 96:261–268.

67 Igawa T, Tani T, Chijiwa T, et al. Potentiation of anti-platelet aggregating activity of cilostazol with vascular endothelial cells. Thromb Res 1990; 57:617–623.

68 Tsuchikane E, Fukuhara A, Kobayashi T, et al. Impact of cilostazol on restenosis after percutaneous coronary balloon angioplasty. Circulation 1999; 100:21–26.

69 Dawson DL, Cutler BS, Meissner MH, et al. Cilostazol has beneficial effects in treatment of intermittent claudication results from a multicenter, randomized, prospective, double-blind trial. Circulation 1998; 98:678–686.

70 Money SR, Herd JA, Isaacsohn JL, et al. Effect of cilostazol on walking distances in patients with intermittent claudication caused by peripheral vascular disease. J Vasc Surg 1998; 27:267–274.

71 Beebe HG, Dawson DL, Cutler BS, et al. A new pharmacological treatment for intermittent claudication results of a randomized, multicenter trial. Arch Intern Med 1999; 159:2041–2050.

72 Dawson DL, Cutler BS, Hiatt WR, et al. A comparison of cilostazol and pentoxifylline for treating intermittent claudication. Am J Med 2000; 109:523–530.

73 Strandness Jr DE, Dalman RL, Panian S, et al. Effect of cilostazol in patients with intermittent claudication randomized, double-blind, placebo-controlled study. Vasc Endovasc Surg 2002; 36:83–91.

74 Regensteiner JG, Ware Jr JE, McCarthy WJ, et al. Effect of cilostazol on treadmill walking, community-based walking ability, and health-related quality of life in patients with intermittent claudication due to peripheral arterial disease meta-analysis of six randomized controlled trials. J Am Geriatr Soc 2002; 50:1939–1946.

75 Jacoby D, Mohler ER III. Drug treatment of intermittent claudication. Drugs 2004; 64(15):1657–1670.

76 ACSM's Guidelines for Exercise Testing and Prescription. In: Franklin BA, ed. Baltimore, MD, Lippincott: Williams & Wilkins, 2000.Girolami B, Bernardi E, Prins MH, et al. Treatment of intermittent claudication with physical training, smoking cessation, pentoxifylline, or nafronyla meta-analysis. Arch Intern Med 1999; 159:337–345.

77 Hood SC, Moher D, Barber GG. Management of intermittent claudication with pentoxifylline meta-analysis of randomized controlled trials. CMAJ 1996; 155:1053–1059.

78 Schellong SM, Boger RH, Burchert W, et al. Dose-related effect of intravenous L-arginine on muscular blood flow of the calf in patients with peripheral vascular disease: a H2 150 positron emission tomography study. Clin Sci (Lond) 1997; 93(2):159–165.

79 Maxwell AJ, Anderson BE, Cooke JP. Nutritional therapy for peripheral arterial disease: a double-blind, placebo-controlled, randomized trial of Heart Bar. Vasc Med 2000; 5(1):11–19.

80 Brevetti G, Perna S, Sabba C, et al. Propionyl-L-carnitine in intermittent claudication: double-blind, placebo-controlled, dose titration, multicenter study. J Am Coll Cardiol 1995; 26(6):1411–1416.

81 Hiatt WR, Regensteiner JG, Creager MA, et al. Propionyl-Lcarnitine improves exercise performance and functional status in patients with claudication. Am J Med 2001;110(8): 616–622.

82 Pittler MH, Ernst E. Ginkgo biloba extract for the treatment of intermittent claudication: a meta-analysis of randomized trials. Am J Med 2000;108(4):276–281.

83 Coffman JD. Vasodilator drugs in peripheral vascular disease. N Engl J Med 1979; 300:713–717.

84 Lievre M, Morand S, Besse B, et al. Oral beraprost sodium, a prostaglandin I(2) analogue, for intermittent claudication: a

double-blind, randomized, multicenter controlled trial. Circulation 2000; 102:426–431.

85 Mobler ER III, Hiatt WR, Olin JW, et al. Treatment of inter-mittent claudication with beraprost sodium, an orally active prostaglandin 12 analogue: a double-blinded, randomized, controlled trial. J Am Coll Cardiol 2003; 41(10): 1679–1686.

86 Pittler MH, Ernst E. Complementary therapies for peripheral arterial disease: systematic review. Atherosclerosis 2005; 181(1):1–7. Epub 2005 Mar 31.

45

Pharmacotherapy peri-percutaneous coronary intervention

Waqas Ullah, Rakesh Sharma, and Carlo Di Mario

Introduction

Since Andreas Grüntzig described the first percutaneous coronary intervention (PCI) in 1978 (1), the field has progressed immeasurably in both equipment and pharmacotherapy. The overall trend with regard to the latter has been for improved strategies aimed at inhibition of platelet aggregation and the clotting cascade. This has led to better outcomes by reduction of the ischemic complications associated with the procedure.

The current evidence regarding the available agents in a PCI setting is summarized in Table 2. A practical flowchart based on our recommendations is provided in Table 3.

Antiplatelet agents

Aspirin

Aspirin inhibits platelet aggregation by reducing production of thromboxane A2 through inhibition of the enzyme cyclo-oxygenase-1. Initial studies of aspirin often combined its administration with dipyridamole. Aspirin either with or without dipyridamole was found to reduce the incidence of coronary thrombosis during percutaneous transluminal coronary angioplasty (2), and the combination was found to reduce the incidence of Q-wave infarction compared to placebo (3). The combination of dipyridamole and aspirin has lost favor as the addition of dipyridamole has been found to confer no additional benefit (4). With respect to actual dose of aspirin used peri-PCI, there have not been any randomized trials looking into this issue. Subgroup analysis based on aspirin dosing (range 75 to 325 mg) of patients with non-ST elevation myocardial infarction (NSTEMI) acute coronary

syndrome (ACS) in the Clopidogrel in Unstable Angina to Prevent Recurrent Ischemic Events (CURE) trial has demonstrated that higher doses of aspirin do not confer additional benefit but are conversely associated with an increased risk of bleeding complications (5).

Thienopyridines

Thienopyridines reduce platelet aggregation by inhibiting the activity of the adenosine diphosphate receptor.

The addition of ticlopidine to aspirin has been shown to have a synergistic effect on the inhibition of platelet aggregation after stent insertion (6), and this combination has also been found to be superior in terms of prevention of in-stent thrombosis to both aspirin alone and aspirin combined with warfarin (7). However, due to the rare but serious side effect of agranulocytosis associated with ticlopidine (8), and its slow onset of action, ticlopidine is no longer used in most countries. The combination of clopidogrel and aspirin has been proved to be as effective as aspirin and ticlopidine in the prevention of intrastent thrombosis (9).

The PCI-clopidogrel as adjunctive reperfusion therapy trial was a randomized control trial of the use of clopidogrel in patients treated with fibrinolysis for an ST-segment elevation myocardial infarction (STEMI) who went on to have a PCI (10). In this trial, patients given clopidogrel prior to PCI had better indices of infarct-related artery patency. These patients also had lower rates of preprocedural recurrent myocardial infarction (MI) and a significantly decreased incidence of the combined endpoint of recurrent MI, cardiovascular death or cerebrovascular accident at 30 days. PCI-CURE studied NSTEMI patients who were randomized to receive either placebo or a 300 mg loading dose of clopidogrel, followed by regular doses, with PCI carried out a median of 6 days later (11). Those in the treatment group had lower rates of preprocedure MI and refractory ischemia. These patients also had a significant reduction in the combined endpoint of cardiovascular death, MI, and urgent target vessel revascularization at 30 days, and this was extended to the longer period of follow-up (the median length of the latter being eight months). Clopidogrel has also been studied among elective patients. The Clopidogrel for the Reduction of Events During Observation (CREDO) trial found no significant benefit at 28 days from preloading patients with clopidogrel a range of 3 to 24 hours prior to PCI (12). In this study, clopidogrel was continued for a year, leading to a significant decrease in the combined endpoint of stroke, MI, and death at this time point. There was also a suggestion that there may be additional benefit from clopidogrel given greater than six hours prior to PCI, with a nonsignificant improvement in the combined endpoint (p = 0.51).

The three trials above all used a 300-mg loading dose followed by 75-mg maintenance dose, yet CREDO (12) failed to demonstrate the same shorter term benefits. While this may be because of the higher risk patients studied in the other trials (10,11), the results relating the outcome to the timing of clopidogrel administration may be the key. In the Atorvastatin for Reduction of MYocardial Damage during Angioplasty-2 (ARMYDA-2) trial, comparison was made of a 300 mg to a 600 mg loading dose of clopidogrel given four to eight hours prior to PCI (13). This trial showed a significantly lower incidence of peri-procedural MI in the latter group. These results demonstrate the faster onset of action of the higher loading dose of clopidogrel. Kandzari et al. examined the pharmacokinetics after administration of a 600 mg dose given at different time points (from two to three hours or earlier) pre-PCI in elective patients (14). They found that there was no difference, at 30 days, in the combined endpoint of death, MI or urgent revascularization between patients given clopidogrel two to three hours pre-PCI and those who started it sooner. These trials therefore suggest an advantage from the higher loading dose of clopidogrel when PCI is to be performed within eight hours.

It is with respect to clopidogrel that there is a significant point of variance in the pharmacotherapeutic management between bare-metal stents and the newer, drug-eluting stents. In the case of the former, no benefit has been found to a course of clopidogrel longer than one month in elective cases, on direct comparison of a one month and six-month course (15). With drug-eluting stents, there is a concern that delayed endothelialization will lead to an increased risk of stent thrombosis. For this reason, trials have empirically used longer clopidogrel regimens, three months for sirolimus-eluting stents (16) and six months for paclitaxel-eluting stents (17). While no trials are available where comparison has been made between different lengths of treatment, the importance of uninterrupted antiplatelet therapy is propounded by the association between discontinuation of

clopidogrel and stent thrombosis (18,19). A longer course of clopidogrel treatment is recommended in the ACS setting on the basis of the PCI-CURE trial; in this study, patients with NSTEMI-ACS were given clopidogrel for up to 12 months (11).

Our own practice in terms of the length of treatment with clopidogrel is to prescribe a one month course of clopidogrel for bare metal stents and a one year course for drug-eluting stents. In the case of all ACS, a one year course is given. These practices are concordant with the current European guidelines, where a month is also recommended for bare metal stents, 6–12 months for drug-eluting stents and 9–12 months of clopidogrel for ACS cases (20).

Cilostazol

Cilostazol is a phosphodiesterase inhibitor that reduces platelet aggregation, vascular smooth muscle proliferation and also has vasodilatory effects. Earlier studies comparing cilostazol and aspirin to ticlodipine and aspirin identified no significant increase in the subacute stent thrombosis rate (21–23). Indeed, the latter has been supported by comparison of this combination to clopidogrel and aspirin (24). Two recent trials, however, have demonstrated that a much higher proportion of patients develop subacute stent thrombosis when taking cilostazol as compared with ticlodipine (25,26). The data from these trials are summarized in Table 1.

Glycoprotein IIb/IIIa inhibitors

Glycoprotein IIb/IIIa receptors are present on the surface of activated platelets. Fibrinogen and von Willebrand Factor are able to cross link platelets through these receptors, leading to their aggregation (Fig. 1). Glycoprotein IIb/IIIa (Gp IIb/IIIa) inhibitors are the most potent and fastest acting anti-platelet agents available. After the unfavorable results of trials with oral agents, only three commercially available drugs (all given parenterally) are presently available in this class: abciximab (ReoPro), eptifibatide (Integrilin), and Tirofiban (Aggrastat).

Abciximab use peri-PCI has been well studied in the setting of STEMI. A meta-analysis of 8 trials using abciximab in the context of primary-PCI has demonstrated a significant reduction in mortality in the context of primary PCI at both 30 days and longer term (6 or 12 month) follow-up (27). In this analysis there was also a reduced reinfarction rate at 30 days with abciximab and no increased risk of bleeding complications. Data also suggests that an early infusion (in the ambulance or immediately after admission) can be beneficial when compared to administration at the time of the procedure. The Chimeric 7E3 Antiplatelet Therapy in Unstable Angina REfractory to Standard Treatment (CAPTURE) trial was the first to demonstrate the benefit of abciximab among patients with unstable angina, with a lower rate of the

Table 1 A comparison of the rates of subacute stent thrombosis in trials comparing cilostazol with ticlodipine or clopidogrel

| | Patients with subacute stent thrombosis (%) | | |
	Clopidogrel	Ticlodipine	Cilostazol
Park 1999 (21)	N/A	0/243	2/247
Tanabe 2000 (22)	N/A	0/50	0/54
Kamishirado 2002 (23)	N/A	2/65	0/65
Sekiguichi 2004 (25)	N/A	1/138	8/144
Takeyasu 2005 (26)	N/A	1/321	8/321
Total (Ticlodipine trials)	N/A	4/817 (0.49%)	18/831 (2.17%)
Lee 2005 (24)	2/345		3/344
Total (Thienopyridine trials)	6/1162 (0.52%)		21/1175 (1.79%)

The first total is a comparison of ticlodipine and aspirin to cilostazol and aspirin; the second total compares the results for thienopyridines and aspirin to cilostazol and aspirin.

combined endpoint of death, MI and urgent intervention (driven by a lower rate of non-Q wave MI), but a higher bleeding rate (28). In the evaluation of platelet IIb/IIIa inhibitor for stenting (EPISTENT) trial, abciximab was shown to be of benefit in a wider range of patients following stent implantation (elective and urgent cases), with the incidence of bleeding reduced by the use of weight-adjusted, low-dose heparin administration. This trial showed that abciximab reduced the incidence of the combined endpoint of mortality, MI and urgent revascularization (major adverse cardiovascular events, MACE). EPISTENT (29) had the merit of replicating in the era of universal stent usage the

results obtained in the earlier CAPTURE and EPIC (30) trials (which were conducted in the balloon angioplasty era). Unfortunately, no attempt was made to explore whether the 12 hour infusion shown to be more beneficial than the bolus alone in the EPIC study was still necessary when the risk of postprocedural abrupt occlusion was nearly abolished through the use of stents.

Mortality benefit for Gp IIb/IIIa inhibitors during PCI has been demonstrated on meta-analysis for abciximab (31) and this class of agents as a whole (32). These agents have also been shown, on meta-analysis, to reduce rates of MI and urgent revascularization post-PCI (33).

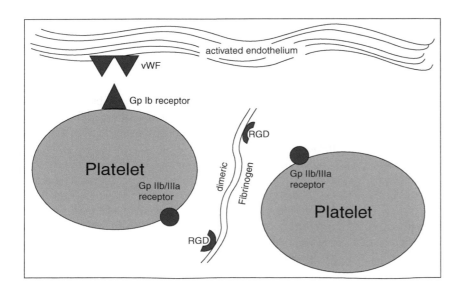

Figure 1
Fibrinogen and von Willebrand Factor are able to cross link platelets through binding to glycoprotein IIb/IIIa receptors present on the surface of activated platelets, leading to their aggregation. *Abbreviations*: Gp, glycoprotein; RGD, Arg-Gly-Asp.

Some of the results with abciximab were duplicated using the small molecules eptifibatide and tirofiban. These are intrinsically cheaper than abciximab which is produced using recombinant DNA technology for its production.

The enhanced suppression of platelet receptor IIb/IIIa using integrilin therapy (ESPIRIT) trial of nonurgent PCI demonstrated a significant reduction in the incidence of post-PCI MI at 30 days but not death or urgent target vessel revascularization using eptifibatide in terms of MACE (34). However, this trial randomized patients to receive placebo in the control arm.

To date, of the Gp IIb/IIIa inhibitors, only abciximab and tirofiban have been compared directly. The Do Tirofiban and ReoPro Give Similar Efficacy (TARGET) trial, a randomized double-blind trial of urgent and elective PCI (excluding patients in cardiogenic shock or with STEMI), demonstrated that abciximab significantly reduced the incidence of MACE at 30 days compared to tirofiban (35). In further analysis it was noted that the only point of significant difference was in the incidence of nonfatal MI, and that the benefit of abciximab in terms of MACE at 30 days was only present in ACS patients. No mortality benefit has been found at one year among those patients treated with abciximab instead of tirofiban (36). The tirofiban dosing regimen used in the TARGET trial (10 μg/kg bolus followed by 0.15 μg/kg/min infusion) has been found to be suboptimal for platelet inhibition in one small study (37). This issue has been addressed further in a recent observational trial which demonstrated no difference compared to abciximab in MACE incidence at six months when a higher tirofiban dosing regimen was used (25 μg/kg bolus followed by 0.15 μg/kg/min infusion) (38).

The main concern with the use of Gp IIb/IIIa inhibitors is the risk of hemorrhage and thrombocytopenia. On meta-analysis, major hemorrhage was significantly more likely with abciximab than with either tirofiban (standard regimen) or eptifibatide (33). The TARGET trial demonstrated abciximab to predispose to thrombocytopenia when compared to tirofiban (35). Regardless, thrombocytopenia (platelet count <20,000/μl) is rare (<3%) and can often be treated conservatively, without the need for platelet transfusions.

Clopidogrel use peri-PCI has gained popularity and its interaction with Gp IIb/IIIa inhibitors has been investigated for all three agents. The intracoronary stenting and antithrombotic regimen–rapid early action for coronary treatment (ISAR-REACT) trial studied low/intermediate risk patients given clopidogrel 600 mg at least two hours before the PCI along with aspirin, and randomized them to receive abciximab or placebo (39). This trial showed that patients receiving abciximab had a significantly higher incidence of profound thrombocytopenia (less than 20,000 platelets per mm³) and required more blood transfusions than the placebo group. In terms of 30 day MACE incidence, there was no difference between the two groups. This lack of benefit was further confirmed by Claeys et al., who demonstrated that these results were achieved despite abciximab's addition resulted in greater inhibition of platelet aggregation (40). A re-evaluation of the ISAR-REACT patients at one year continued to show a lack of advantage conferred by abciximab (41). It should be noted however that these trials did not include high-risk patients and so it may not be appropriate to extrapolate these results to this group which has been investigated separately in the ISAR-REACT 2 trial.

The combination of tirofiban with clopidogrel and aspirin on the other hand, in the small (109 elective patient) troponin in planned PTCA/stent implantation with or without administration of the glycoprotein IIb/IIIa receptor antagonist tirofiban study, has been shown to significantly reduce MACE incidence at nine months compared to clopidogrel and aspirin alone (42). This was associated with significantly lower levels of Troponin release at 12 and 24 hours in the tirofiban group although differences that were not maintained at 48 hours. In comparison to the two abciximab/clopidogrel combination studies this study did use a slightly lower dose of clopidogrel [375 mg loading as opposed to the 600 mg ISAR-REACT (39) loading or 300 mg plus 150 mg loading (40)] but the influence of this on the results is unclear.

In view of the widespread use of clopidogrel peri-PCI, it is important to elucidate the interaction between this and Gp IIb/IIIa inhibitors. A lack of synergistic benefit would not be unexpected as clopidogrel ultimately exert its effects on platelet aggregation through the Gp IIb/IIIa receptor (43). Still, Gp IIb/IIIa antagonists do have a more potent and consistent inhibitory action platelet aggregation than clopidogrel.

Anticoagulants

Heparin

The two forms of heparin available are unfractionated heparin (UFH) and low molecular weight heparin (LMWH). Both exert their anticoagulant effect on the clotting cascade by enhancing the activity of antithrombin. In the case of LMWH this is by enhancing the binding of antithrombin to factor Xa and so inhibiting the function of the latter; UFH not only shares this effect but also enhances the inhibition of thrombin through antithrombin (44).

UFH is the most commonly employed anticoagulant peri-PCI. UFH suffers from several shortcomings as reviewed by Kokolis et al. (45) and Rebeiz et al. (8). These drawbacks include the variability of its anticoagulant effect necessitating monitoring of clotting indices, its ability to activate platelets causing a paradoxical pro-coagulant effect, and the possibility of inducing heparin-induced thrombocytopenia (HIT).

The main cause of debate at present with regard to UFH centers on the amount used peri-PCI. The level of anticoagulation produced by UFH is measured by the activated partial thromboplastin time and activated clotting time (ACT), the latter being available in the cardiac catheter laboratory as a near-patient test.

A meta-analysis of earlier trials found the risk of complications associated with PCI to be closely related to the ACT, with a target ACT of 350–375 suggested (45). Higher ACTs were associated with increased bleeding risks. ACTs above and below this range were both associated with an increased incidence of death, MI and urgent revascularization at 7 days. The reason for the association between ischemic complications and elevated ACTs is believed to be a consequence of heparin's platelet activating properties at higher doses. The trials summated in this meta-analysis were from an era prior to the widespread adoption of stents, thienopyridines, and Gp IIa/IIIb inhibitors. A more recent meta-analysis of four trials involving 9974 patients demonstrated different relationships, most likely due to the change in practices in the interim (46). In this meta-analysis, a lack of correlation was found between the ACT and ischemic complications at 48 hours. A correlation was found with the total heparin dose, with doses above 5000 units associated with increased ischemic complications. With the heparin dose adjusted for weight, every 10 U/kg increase in dose, up to 90 U/kg, was associated with a significant increase in the risk of ischemic complications. There was no significant association between ACT and rates of major bleeding. For a combination of major and minor bleeding, increasing ACTs up to 365 were associated with an increasing rate of major/minor bleeding but above this the rate actually decreased. When looking from a dosing point of view, there was a relationship between increasing heparin dose and rates of major/minor bleeding. With regard to weight-indexed dosing, there was a significant increase in the bleeding risk with every 10 U/kg increase in dose. Based on these findings, in the context of oral and intravenous antiplatelet therapies and stenting, the suggestion is that lower heparin doses may not compromise efficacy and may in fact be safer. Moreover, the ACT itself may not be as useful a marker of optimal UFH use peri-PCI compared to the actual UFH dose given.

LMWHs mainly inhibit factor Xa through antithrombin, although they have varying degrees of associated indirect thrombin inhibiting activity. In the latter respect they share the disadvantage of UFH of being unable to inhibit clot-associated thrombin. The advantages of LMWH over UFH include a more predictable anticoagulant effect requiring less monitoring, and reduced incidence of HIT.

Of the LMWH, the most extensively studied with regard to PCI is enoxaparin. The National Investigators Collaborating on Enoxaparin (NICE) trials examined the use of intravenous enoxaparin peri-PCI in elective and urgent patients (47). These trials were observational studies without a control group: patients from other trials served as historical controls for comparison. NICE-1 examined 828 patients treated with 1 mg/kg of intravenous enoxaparin at the time of PCI (47). Similar efficacy and safety was found to equivalent patients treated with UFH in the previous EPISTENT trial. NICE-4 investigated patients treated with 0.75 mg/kg of intravenous enoxaparin and concomitant abciximab (47). The results also compared favorably with respect to death, infarction and urgent revascularization at 30 days as well as bleeding complications on comparison to patients treated with abciximab and UFH from the EPISTENT and evaluation of PTCA to improve long-term outcome by c7E3 GP IIb/IIIa receptor blockade trials (48).

Among elective patients, trials have also examined the combination of enoxaparin with eptifibatide (49,50) or tirofiban (50) and similarly found no significant differences between UFH and 0.75 mg/kg intravenous enoxaparin.

The above trials have investigated intravenous enoxaparin. The pharmacokinetics of enoxaparin in PCI (PEPCI) study found that anti-Xa levels, a measure of LMWH activity, were within target range two to eight hours after a dose of subcutaneous enoxaparin (51). Anti-Xa levels could be kept in the target range for a further two hours by an additional intravenous bolus of 0.3 mg/kg. The SYNERGY (52) trial of ACS patients compared UFH to an enoxaparin regimen as suggested by the PEPCI (51) trial. Among these patients, those who had received their last dose of subcutaneous enoxaparin over eight hours prior to PCI were given an additional intravenous bolus. In the SYNERGY trial, no difference in the incidence of ischemic events during PCI was noted between UFH and subcutaneous LMWH, and there was an increased incidence of major bleeding in the LMWH group (52). The observation that an increased bleeding risk compared to UFH was noted in this trial rather than those investigating intravenous enoxaparin may be indicative of a less predictable bioavailability of this route of administration, or perhaps a need for dose reduction.

On the whole, while not demonstrating superiority of LMWH with regard to bleeding complications, death, infarction, and urgent revascularization over UFH, the above results do support its noninferiority. In view of LMWH's simplicity of use in ACS, which makes most centers prefer it to UFH, it is important to recognize it as an acceptable alternative to UFH when the patient must be treated soon after their last subcutaneous dose.

Fondaparinux

Fondaparinux is a pure inhibitor of factor Xa, which exerts its effect through antithrombin. This compares with UFH and LMWH both of which have additional activity against thrombin to a greater and lesser degree, respectively. To date one trial has been published investigating fondaparinux use peri-PCI. Compared to UFH, no significant increase in bleeding complications or a composite of all cause mortality, MI, urgent revascularization, and need for bailout Gp IIb/IIIa antagonist was demonstrated (53). Whether this agent will have any advantage over LMWH or UFH is to be established.

Direct thrombin inhibitors

Direct thrombin inhibitors (DTIs) inhibit thrombin directly rather than through the indirect, antithrombin-mediated pathway utilized by UFH and LMWH. Unlike heparin, they can inhibit clot-bound thrombin and do not induce HIT. While heparin-based anticoagulation can be reversed using protamine, there is no such agent for DTIs: this is especially a concern for lepirudin which, unlike bivalirudin, binds to thrombin irreversibly and so has a longer half life. With bivalirudin, the effect almost disappears after two hours which helps planning the timely removal of arterial sheaths. Bivalirudin has been the subject of a large trial, randomized evaluation in PCI linking angiomax to reduced clinical events-2 (REPLACE-2), involving 6010 patients (54). Randomization was either to UFH and Gp IIb/IIIa (abciximab or eptifibatide) or to bivalirudin with the option of Gp IIb/IIIa use if there were procedural or angiographic complications. Patients with unstable ischemic syndromes or acute-MI were excluded. There was no difference in the combined endpoint of death, MI, and urgent repeat revascularization at 30 days. While the latter suggested equivalence in efficacy with UFH, a reduced incidence of major and minor bleeding with bivalirudin suggested that it held safety advantages over UFH. At six months, the rates of death, MI, and revascularization were no difference between the two groups and this lack of difference in mortality was also present at one year (55).

A meta-analysis of DTIs compared to UFH in ACS has shown that there is a significant decrease in the combined endpoint of death and MI at 30 days, with the significance driven by the improvement in MI incidence in the former group (56). There was no significant decrease in mortality itself. The benefit of DTIs compared to heparin was only found in those patients undergoing early (within 72 hours) PCI as opposed to those managed conservatively or treated with PCI after this. There was also significantly less major bleeding in patients receiving DTIs rather than UFH. These results suggest that DTI may have increased safety and efficacy for those undergoing early PCI for ACS. The results from REPLACE-2 (54) would seem to extend this benefit to a wider group of patients and additionally suggests that a more parsimonious use of Gp IIb/IIIa agents may be possible. The acute catheterization and urgent intervention triage strategy trial has explored the use of bivalirudin in highly unstable syndromes, also in combination with LMWH, with results just presented. The harmonizing outcomes with revascularization

and stents trial will answer the same question in STEMI patients undergoing primary PCI.

Lipid-lowering medication

In a small (81 patients) retrospective analysis, patients on lipid-lowering medication (statins, fibrates, or niacin derivatives) at the time of PCI had a significantly lower incidence of adverse events during the procedure, such as emboli and dissections, as compared to those not taking such agents (57). A high-total cholesterol, low-density lipoprotein, or ratio of low to high-density lipoprotein were also associated with increased adverse events.

A prospective trial of ACS patients undergoing PCI (119 patients) showed that those on statins at the time of PCI had significantly reduced incidence of peri-procedural myocardial necrosis as determined by CK or CK-MB level (58). At six months, these patients also had a lower incidence of the combined endpoint of death, MI, target vessel revascularization, and hospital admission for unstable angina. The patients who were on statins were significantly less likely to have hyperlipidemia at the time of PCI. The incidence of the combined endpoint was not increased by patients being hyperlipidemic at six months, or reduced by patients being on statin therapy at six months. Instead the relationship was with being on a statin prior to PCI, suggesting the importance of pretreatment.

he ARMYDA study of 153 low-risk elective PCI demonstrated that pretreatment of patients with a week of atorvastatin prior to PCI resulted in significantly less release of markers of myocardial damage such as Troponin, myoglobin, and CK-MB compared to placebo (59). This was associated with a decrease in the rate of peri-procedural MI. It is postulated that this effect of atorvastatin may relate to its anti-inflammatory properties.

Conclusions

A summary of the discussions above regarding the various trials can be found in Table 2. Table 3 details our recommendations with regard to pharmacotherapy peri-PCI, which includes an attempt to offer advice in the cases where trial evidence is lacking.

There is a wealth of data currently available regarding different agents to use peri-PCI and yet, as with any field, there remain unanswered questions particularly concerning long term treatment after drug eluting stents. It is the task of the physician to tailor these therapies to the specific clinical situations with which they are presented. In this article, as well as reviewing the currently available evidence, we have also provided our own recommendations for the use of the

Table 2 A comparison of the different drugs used peri-percutaneous coronary intervention

Drug	Patient type	Dosing	Main findings and conclusions
Aspirin	All PCI	75–325 mg	Reduced incidence of coronary thrombosis (2) and Q-wave infarct (3)
Dipyridamole	No longer recommended	No longer recommended	No additional benefit when given with aspirin (4)
Ticlopidine	Only if intolerant to clopidogrel	At least 250 mg bd	Synergistic with aspirin in reducing platelet aggregation (6) and reducing instent restenosis (7) Concern over associated incidence of agranulocytosis (8,9), frequent gastric intolerance and skin rashes Sequential FBC required at follow-up
Clopidogrel	STEMI (10), NSTEMI (11), Elective PCI (12)	300 mg loading dose (10–12) unless PCI to be performed within eight hours in which case 600 mg recommended	As effective as ticlopidine in preventing stent thrombosis (9) Reduced incidence of adverse hematologic reactions compared to ticlodipine (9)
Cilostazol	Elective (21–25) and emergency (22–26) PCI	100 mg twice daily	Possibility of increased subacute stent thrombosis rate (21–26)
Gp IIb/IIIa inhibitors	See below	See below	Mortality benefit in the context of PCI (32) Decreased MI and urgent revascularization rates post-PCI (33)
Abciximab	STEMI (27), unstable angina (28),elective PCI (29)	0.25 mg/kg followed by 0.125 μg/kg/min infusion Benefit in low/intermediate risk patients following clopidogrel pretreatment debated (39,40)	Significant benefit (27–29) especially with respect to mortality (27) and reinfarction (27,28) Increased risk of major bleeding and thrombocytopenia compared to other Gp IIb/IIIa inhibitors (33)
Epitifibatide	ACS (not including STEMI) (60), nonurgent PCI (34)	Two 180 μg/kg boluses 10 min apart and 2 μg/kg/min infusion (34)	Studies comparing efficacy to other members of this class awaited
Tirofiban	ACS (not including STEMI) (61)	25 μg/kg bolus and 0.15 μg/kg/min infusion—may be more effective than standard regimen of 10 μg/kg bolus and 0.15 μg/kg/min infusion (37,38)	Beneficial in one trial evaluating use in patients with non-STEMI ACS, but no benefit in another investigating patients with ACS including STEMI Abciximab associated with more favorable outcome at 30 days (35) [no mortality benefit at one year (36)]. This superiority may be abrogated by the higher tirofiban dosing regimen (38)
UFH	All PCI	Dose of UFH more predictive of complications than ACT value (46)	Variable anticoagulant effect (needing monitoring), platelet activation causing paradoxical pro-coagulant effect, HIT, unable to bind clot-bound thrombin (8,44)
LMWH	Elective and urgent PCI (47,49,50)	1 mg/kg intravenous enoxaparin (0.75 mg/kg if used with Gp IIb/IIIa) (47,49,50)	Similar efficacy to UFH with no increase in adverse events (47,49,50) Unable to bind clot-bound thrombin (8,44)
Fondaparinux	Urgent and elective PCI (53)	Optimal dosing still being determined	Similar efficacy and safety to UFH (53)
DTI	Elective PCI (54), ACS (56) past HIT	Dependent on agent used	Able to bind clot-bound thrombin, do not induce HIT (8,44) May have benefit compared to UFH among ACS patients (56)
Lipid lowering medication	Elective PCI (59)	Dependent on agent used	Pretreatment with atorvastatin associated with decreased peri-PCI myocardial infarction (59)

Abbreviations: ACS, acute coronary syndrome; DTI, direct thrombin inhibitor; Gp IIb/IIIa, glycoprotein IIb/IIIa; HIT, heparin induced thrmobocytopenia; LMWH, low molecular weight heparin; NSTEMI, non-ST elevation myocardial infarction; PCI, percutaneous coronary intervention; STEMI, ST elevation myocardial infarction; UFH, unfractionated heparin.

Table 3   Practical tips for drug administration peri-percutaneous coronary intervention

Drug	Dose	Recommendation
Pre-PCI		
Aspirin	75–100 mg	Start at least 48 hours before procedure Consider 250 mg i.v. if PCI to be performed sooner than this
Clopidogrel	75 mg	300 mg loading dose if not already on treatment, with 600 mg loading if PCI expected to occur within eight hours
Glycoprotein IIb/IIIa inhibitors		In the case of unstable angina or NSTEMI, the preferred agents are epitifabatide/tirofiban. Abciximab is the preferred agent in the cases of STEMI
Sedation		Avoidance of doses inducing respiratory sedation and hypotension is recommended. Agents such as midazolam with a rapid onset and offset of action are preferred
Proton pump inhibitors		Low threshold in the cases of previous gastric problems (e.g., ulcers, diaphragmatic hernias) and in the cases of microcytic anemia of unknown cause
During PCI		
Heparin	50–75 mg/kg Avoid additional boluses > 30 mg/kg	Preferred agent in the cases of chronic total occlusion. Recommend checking ACT after five minutes and then every hour. Target ACT of 200–250 s. Keep as close as possible to 200 s if used in conjunction with Gp IIb/IIIa inhibitors. Higher target (250–300 s) recommended if filters are used. Avoid routine infusion after PCI (associated with increased bleeding events with little benefit)
Enoxaparin	0.5 mg/kg i.v.	No additional boluses if within four to six hours of subcutaneous injection
Bivalirudin	0.75 mg/kg bolus plus 1.75 mg/kg per hour for the duration of PCI	Excellent alternative to heparin in elective cases. Trial results pending for unstable syndromes. Adjust dose according to renal function. Not enough data in acute MI and after enoxaparin. Stop after removal of intracoronary wires. Remove sheath after two hours unless closure devices are used
Glycoprotein IIb/IIIa inhibitors	Abciximab 0.25 mg/kg or high dose bolus epitifibatide or tirofiban	If infusion already started, continue same Gp IIb/IIIa inhibitor started pre-PCI. Low threshold for administering in the cases of thrombus containing lesions in the context of unstable angina; no reflow/slow reflow after PCI; treatment of diffuse disease, and in diabetes mellitus. Caution (not needed or risky) for treatment of SVGs, CTO or lesions at risk of perforation. In the case of abciximab, consider withholding infusion if normal flow is obtained with a good result after stenting and the patient is fully loaded with clopidogrel
Nitrates	Preferred agents: isosorbide dinitrate 1–3 mg and nitroglycerine 100–300 μg	Use intracoronarily to appropriately size the balloons and stent, and to prevent coronary spasm during wire/balloon manipulation. Not effective/contraindicated in the treatment of secondary spasm. Avoid pressure drop in no reflow/slow flow
Sodium nitroprusside	40–100 μg in three minutes	Preferred agent in the cases of no reflow/slow reflow. Always selective infusion (or better subselective infusion via intracoronary catheter). Strict BP monitoring required during administration. Needs to be available for the cases of degenerate SVG or lesions containing thrombus

(Continued)

Table 3 Practical tips for drug administration peri-percutaneous coronary intervention (*Continued*)

Drug	Dose	Recommendation
Adenosine	20–100 µg	Have the same indications as sodium nitroprusside Can cause sinus arrest/AV block when high doses are used, especially in the RCA (an effect which is reversible within seconds)
Verapamil	1–2 mg	Same indications as sodium nitroprusside and adenosine but associated with more prolonged hypotension/bradycardia
Post-PCI		
Aspirin	75–100 mg od	Lifelong Higher doses are advantageous only to prolong the effect in the cases of withheld doses, but are associated with increased bleeding complications with no reduction in the incidence of thrombotic events
Clopidogrel	75 mg od	Continue for 28–30 days after bare metal stent insertion but 9 to 12 months in the cases of ACS In the cases of proven resistance (<50% in vitro platelet inhibition) consider doses of 150 mg od. Also consider higher dose in the cases of previous stent thrombosis For drug-eluting stents, continue for six months (but consider stopping after two to three months for sirolimus eluting stents for simple lesion treatment). For indications outside major drug eluting/sirolimus eluting stent trials (Sirius/Taxus IV, long lesions, bifurcations, ostial, SVGs, CTO etc.) the most frequent empirical approach is to prolong treatment for 9–12 months Where thrombosis would be catastrophic, such as in left main or single remaining vessel intervention, a more prolonged treatment perhaps even lifelong—can be considered until the risk of late stent thrombosis is better defined
Lipid lowering agents, beta blockers, angiotensin converting enzyme inhibitors, angiotensin receptor blockers, other antihypertensives, antihyperglycemic medications		Titrate according to most recent guidelines
Warfarin		If systemic anticoagulation is strongly indicated based on high thrombo-embolic risk (cases of mechanical valve prosthesis, left ventricular thrombus, active deep vein thrombosis, high-risk atrial fibrillation), stop warfarin three to four days pre-PCI and anticoagulate with unfractionated heparin or enoxaparin. Warfarin can be restarted the evening after the procedure with a loading dose Consider the possibility of stopping clopidogrel (or aspirin) after one month in the case of nondrug eluting stents, or two to three months in drug eluting stents. If the indication for warfarin is less robust, such as AF at low embolic risk, consider stopping warfarin permanently or until double antiplatelet treatment is no longer required

Abbreviations: ACS, acute coronary syndrome; ACT, activated clotting time; BP, blood pressure; CTO, chronic total occlusion; i.v., intravenous; MI, myocardial infarction; NSTEMI, non-ST-segment elevation myocardial infarction; PCI, percutaneous coronary intervention; RCA, right coronary artery; STEMI, ST-segment elevation myocardial infarction; SVGS, saphenous vein grafts.

various agents available: in doing so it is hoped this will facilitate the decision making process.

References

1 Grüntzig A. Transluminal dilatation of coronary-artery stenosis. Lancet 1978; 1(8058):263.

2 Barnathan ES, Schwartz JS, Taylor L, et al. Aspirin and dipyridamole in the prevention of acute coronary thrombosis complicating coronary angioplasty. Circulation 1987; 76(1): 125–134.

3 Schwartz L, Bourassa MG, Lesperance J, et al. Aspirin and dipyridamole in the prevention of restenosis after percutaneous transluminal coronary angioplasty. N Engl J Med 1988; 318(26): 1714–1719.

4 Lembo NJ, Black AJ, Roubin GS, et al. Effect of pretreatment with aspirin versus aspirin plus dipyridamole on frequency and type of acute complications of percutaneous transluminal coronary angioplasty. Am J Cardiol 1990; 65(7):422–426.

5 Peters RJ, Mehta SR, Fox KA, et al. Clopidogrel in unstable angina to prevent recurrent events (CURE) trial investigators. Effects of aspirin dose when used alone or in combination with clopidogrel in patients with acute coronary syndromes: observations from the clopidogrel in unstable angina to prevent recurrent events (CURE) study. Circulation 2003; 108(14):1682–1687.

6 Rupprecht HJ, Darius H, Borkowski U, et al. Comparison of antiplatelet effects of aspirin, ticlopidine, or their combination after stent implantation. Circulation 1998; 97(11):1046–1052.

7 Leon MB, Baim DS, Popma JJ, et al. A clinical trial comparing three antithrombotic-drug regimens after coronary-artery stenting. Stent anticoagulation restenosis study investigators. N Engl J Med 1998; 339(23):1665–1671.

8 Rebeiz AG, Adams J, Harrington RA. Interventional cardiovascular pharmacotherapy: current issues. Am J Cardiovasc Drugs 2005; 5(2):93–102.

9 Müller C, Buttner HJ, Petersen J, Roskamm H. A randomized comparison of clopidogrel and aspirin versus ticlopidine and aspirin after the placement of coronary-artery stents. Circulation 2000; 101(6):590–603.

10 Sabatine MS, Cannon CP, Gibson CM. Clopidogrel as adjunctive reperfusion therapy (CLARITY)-thrombolysis in myocardial infarction (TIMI) 28 investigators. Effect of clopidogrel pretreatment before percutaneous coronary intervention in patients with ST-elevation myocardial infarction treated with fibrinolytics: the PCI-CLARITY study. JAMA 2005; 294(10):1224–1232.

11 Mehta SR, Yusuf S, Peters RJ, et al. Clopidogrel in unstable angina to prevent recurrent events trial (CURE) investigators. Effects of pretreatment with clopidogrel and aspirin followed by long-term therapy in patients undergoing percutaneous coronary intervention: the PCI-CURE study. Lancet 2001; 358(9281):527–533.

12 Steinhubl SR, Berger PB, Mann JT 3rd, et al. CREDO investigators. Clopidogrel for the reduction of events during observation. Early and sustained dual oral antiplatelet therapy following percutaneous coronary intervention: a randomized controlled trial. JAMA 2002; 288(19):2411–2420.

13 Patti G, Colonna G, Pasceri V, Pepe LL, Montinaro A, Di Sciascio G. Randomized trial of high loading dose of clopidogrel for reduction of periprocedural myocardial infarction in patients undergoing coronary intervention: results from the ARMYDA-2 (Antiplatelet therapy for Reduction of MYocardial Damage during Angioplasty) study. Circulation 2005; 111(16):2099–2106.

14 Kandzari DE, Berger PB, Kastrati A. ISAR–REACT study investigators. Influence of treatment duration with a 600-mg dose of clopidogrel before percutaneous coronary revascularization. J Am Coll Cardiol 2004; 44(11):2133–2136.

15 Pekdemir H, Cin VG, Camsari A, et al. A comparison of 1-month and 6-month clopidogrel therapy on clinical and angiographic outcome after stent implantation. Heart Vessels 2003; 18(3):123–129.

16 Moses JW, Leon MB, Popma JJ, et al. SIRIUS investigators. Sirolimus-eluting stents versus standard stents in patients with stenosis in a native coronary artery. N Engl J Med 2003; 349(14):1315–1323.

17 Stone GW, Ellis SG, Cox DA, et al. A polymer-based, paclitaxelleluting stent in patients with coronary artery disease. N Engl J Med 2004; 350:221–231.

18 Iakovou I, Schmidt T, Bonizzoni E, et al. Incidence, predictors, and outcome of thrombosis after successful implantation of drug-eluting stents. JAMA 2005; 293(17):2126–2130.

19 Kuchulakanti PK, Chu WW, Torguson R, et al. Correlates and long-term outcomes of angiographically proven stent thrombosis with sirolimus- and paclitaxel-eluting stents. Circulation 2006; 113(8):1108–1113.

20 Silber S, Albertsson P, Aviles FF, et al. Task force for percutaneous coronary interventions of the European Society of Cardiology. Guidelines for percutaneous coronary interventions. The task force for percutaneous coronary interventions of the European Society of Cardiology. Eur Heart J 2005; 26(8):804–847.

21 Park SW, Lee CW, Kim HS, et al. Comparison of cilostazol versus ticlopidine therapy after stent implantation. Am J Cardiol 1999; 84(5):511–514.

22 Tanabe Y, Ito E, Nakagawa I, Suzuki K. Effect of cilostazol on restenosis after coronary angioplasty and stenting in comparison to conventional coronary artery stenting with ticlopidine. Int J Cardiol 2001; 78(3):285–291.

23 Kamishirado H, Inoue T, Mizoguchi K, et al. Randomized comparison of cilostazol versus ticlopidine hydrochloride for antiplatelet therapy after coronary stent implantation for prevention of late restenosis. Am Heart J 2002; 144(2):303–308.

24 Lee SW, Park SW, Hong MK, et al. Comparison of cilostazol and clopidogrel after successful coronary stenting. Am J Cardiol 2005; 95(7):859–862.

25 Sekiguchi M, Hoshizaki H, Adachi H, Ohshima S, Taniguchi K, Kurabayashi M. Effects of antiplatelet agents on subacute thrombosis and restenosis after successful coronary stenting: A randomized comparison of ticlopidine and cilostazol. Circ J 2004; 68(7):610–614.

26 Takeyasu N, Watanabe S, Noguchi Y, Ishikawa K, Fumikura Y, Yamaguchi I. Randomized comparison of cilostazol vs ticlopidine for antiplatelet therapy after coronary stenting. Circ J 2005; 69(7):780–785.

27 De Luca G, Suryapranata H, Stone GW, et al. Abciximab as adjunctive therapy to reperfusion in acute ST-segment elevation

myocardial infarction: a meta-analysis of randomized trials. JAMA 2005; 293(14):1759–1765.

28 The CAPTURE Investigators. Randomised placebo-controlled trial of abciximab before and during coronary intervention in refractory unstable angina: the CAPTURE study. Lancet 1997; 349(9063):1429–1435.

29 The EPISTENT Investigators. Randomised placebo-controlled and balloon-angioplasty-controlled trial to assess safety of coronary stenting with use of platelet glycoprotein-IIb/IIIa blockade. Lancet 1998; 352(9122):87–92.

30 Lefkovits J, Ivanhoe RJ, Califf RM, et al. Effects of platelet glycoprotein IIb/IIIa receptor blockade by a chimeric monoclonal antibody (abciximab) on acute and six-month outcomes after percutaneous transluminal coronary angioplasty for acute myocardial infarction. EPIC investigators. Am J Cardiol 1996; 77(12):1045–1051.

31 Topol EJ, Lincoff AM, Kereiakes DJ, et al. Multi-year follow-up of abciximab therapy in three randomized, placebo-controlled trials of percutaneous coronary revascularization. Am J Med 2002; 113(1):1–6.

32 Karvouni E, Katritsis DG, Ioannidis JP. Intravenous glycoprotein IIb/IIIa receptor antagonists reduce mortality after percutaneous coronary interventions. J Am Coll Cardiol 2003; 41(1):26–32.

33 Brown DL, Fann CS, Chang CJ. Meta-analysis of effectiveness and safety of abciximab versus eptifibatide or tirofiban in percutaneous coronary intervention. Am J Cardiol 2001; 87(5): 537–541.

34 Novel dosing regimen of eptifibatide in planned coronary stent implantation (ESPIRIT): a randomised placebo-control trial. The Lancet 2000; 356, 9247.

35 Topol EJ, Moliterno DJ, Herrmann HC, et al. TARGET investigators. Comparison of two platelet glycoprotein IIb/IIIa inhibitors, tirofiban and abciximab, for the prevention of ischemic events with percutaneous coronary revascularization. N Engl J Med 2001; 344(25):1888–1894.

36 Mukherjee D, Topol EJ, Bertrand ME, et al. Mortality at 1 year for the direct comparison of tirofiban and abciximab during percutaneous coronary revascularization: do tirofiban and ReoPro give similar efficacy outcomes at trial 1-year follow-up. Eur Heart J 2005; 26(23):2524–2528.

37 Kimmelstiel C, Badar J, Covic L, et al. Pharmacodynamics and pharmacokinetics of the platelet GPIIb/IIIa inhibitor tirofiban in patients undergoing percutaneous coronary intervention: implications for adjustment of tirofiban and clopidogrel dosage. Thromb Res 2005; 116(1):55–66.

38 Gunasekara AP, Walters DL, Aroney CN. Comparison of abciximab with "high-dose" tirofiban in patients undergoing percutaneous coronary intervention. Int J Cardiol 2005 [Epub ahead of print].

39 Kastrati A, Mehilli J, Schuhlen H, et al. Intracoronary stenting and antithrombotic regimen-rapid early action for coronary treatment study investigators. A clinical trial of abciximab in elective percutaneous coronary intervention after pretreatment with clopidogrel. N Engl J Med 2004; 350(3):232–238.

40 Claeys MJ, Van der Planken MG, Bosmans JM, et al. Does pretreatment with aspirin and loading dose clopidogrel obviate the need for glycoprotein IIb/IIIa antagonists during elective coronary stenting? A focus on peri-procedural myonecrosis. Eur Heart J 2005; 26(6):567–575.

41 Schomig A, Schmitt C, Dibra A, et al. Intracoronary stenting and antithrombotic regimen-rapid early action for coronary treatment study investigators. One year outcomes with abciximab vs. placebo during percutaneous coronary intervention after pretreatment with clopidogrel. Eur Heart J 2005; 26(14):1379–1384.

42 Bonz AW, Lengenfelder B, Strotmann J, et al. Effect of additional temporary glycoprotein IIb/IIIa receptor inhibition on troponin release in elective percutaneous coronary interventions after pretreatment with aspirin and clopidogrel (TOPSTAR trial). J Am Coll Cardiol 2002; 40(4):662–668.

43 Geiger J, Brich J, Honig-Liedl P, et al. Specific impairment of human platelet P2YAC ADP receptor—Mediated signaling by the antiplatelet drug clopidogrel. Arterioscler Thromb Vasc Biol 1999; 19(8):2007–2011.

44 Kokolis S, Cavusoglu E, Clark LT, Marmur JD. Anticoagulation strategies for patients undergoing percutaneous coronary intervention: Unfractionated heparin, low-molecular-weight heparins, and direct thrombin inhibitors. Prog Cardiovasc Dis 2004; 46(6):506–523.

45 Chew DP, Bhatt DL, Lincoff AM, et al. Defining the optimal activated clotting time during percutaneous coronary intervention: Aggregate results from 6 randomized, controlled trials. Circulation 2001; 103(7):961–966.

46 Brener SJ, Moliterno DJ, Lincoff AM, Steinhubl SR, Wolski KE, Topol EJ. Relationship between activated clotting time and ischemic or hemorrhagic complications: analysis of 4 recent randomized clinical trials of percutaneous coronary intervention. Circulation 2004; 110(8):994–998.

47 Kereiakes DJ, Grines C, Fry E, et al. NICE 1 and NICE 4 investigators. National investigators collaborating on enoxaparin. Enoxaparin and abciximab adjunctive pharmacotherapy during percutaneous coronary intervention. J Invasive Cardiol 2001; 13(4):272–278.

48 The EPILOG Investigators. Platelet glycoprotein IIb/IIIa receptor blockade and low-dose heparin during percutaneous coronary revascularization. N Engl J Med 1997; 336:1689–1696.

49 Bhatt DL, Lee BI, Casterella PJ, et al. Safety of concomitant therapy with eptifibatide and enoxaparin in patients undergoing percutaneous coronary intervention: results of the coronary revascularization using integrilin and single bolus enoxaparin study. J Am Coll Cardiol 2003; 41(1):20–25.

50 Madan M, Radhakrishnan S, Reis M, et al. Comparison of enoxaparin versus heparin during elective percutaneous coronary intervention performed with either eptifibatide or tirofiban (the ACTION Trial). Am J Cardiol 2005; 95(11): 1295–1301.

51 Martin JL, Fry ET, Sanderink GJ, et al. Reliable anticoagulation with enoxaparin in patients undergoing percutaneous coronary intervention: the pharmacokinetics of enoxaparin in PCI (PEPCI) study. Catheter Cardiovasc Interv 2004; 61(2):163–170.

52 Ferguson JJ, Califf RM, Antman EM, et al. SYNERGY trial investigators. Enoxaparin vs unfractionated heparin in high-risk patients with non-ST-segment elevation acute coronary syndromes managed with an intended early invasive strategy: primary results of the SYNERGY randomized trial. JAMA 2004; 292(1):45–54.

53 Mehta SR, Steg PG, Granger CB, et al. ASPIRE investigators. Randomized, blinded trial comparing fondaparinux with

unfractionated heparin in patients undergoing contemporary percutaneous coronary intervention: Arixtra Study in percutaneous coronary intervention: a randomized evaluation (ASPIRE) pilot trial. Circulation 2005; 111(11):1390–1397.

54   Lincoff AM, Bittl JA, Harrington RA, et al. REPLACE-2 investigators. Bivalirudin and provisional glycoprotein IIb/IIIa blockade compared with heparin and planned glycoprotein IIb/IIIa blockade during percutaneous coronary intervention: REPLACE-2 randomized trial. JAMA 2003; 289(7):853–863.

55   Lincoff AM, Kleiman NS, Kereiakes DJ, et al. REPLACE-2 investigators. Long-term efficacy of bivalirudin and provisional glycoprotein IIb/IIIa blockade vs heparin and planned glycoprotein IIb/IIIa blockade during percutaneous coronary revascularization: REPLACE-2 randomized trial. JAMA 2004; 292(6):696–703.

56   Sinnaeve PR, Simes J, Yusuf S, et al. Direct thrombin inhibitors in acute coronary syndromes: effect in patients undergoing early percutaneous coronary intervention. Eur Heart J 2005; 26(22):2396–2403.

57   Ferguson MA, Romick BG, Carter LI, De Geare VS. Relation of the use of lipid-lowering medications prior to percutaneous coronary intervention to the incidence of intraprocedural adverse angiographic events. Am J Cardiol 2005; 95(8): 978–980.

58   Chang SM, Yazbek N, Lakkis NM. Use of statins prior to percutaneous coronary intervention reduces myonecrosis and improves clinical outcome. Catheter Cardiovasc Interv 2004; 62(2):193–197.

59   Pasceri V, Patti G, Nusca A, Pristipino C, Richichi G, Di Sciascio G; ARMYDA investigators. Randomized trial of atorvastatin for reduction of myocardial damage during coronary intervention: results from the ARMYDA (Atorvastatin for Reduction of MYocardial Damage during Angioplasty) study. Circulation 2004; 110(6):674–678.

60   The PURSUIT Trial Investigators. Inhibition of platelet glycoprotein IIb/IIIa with eptifibatide in patients with acute coronary syndromes. N Engl J Med 1998, 339:436–443.

61   The PRISM-PLUS Study Investigators. Inhibition of the platelet glycoprotein IIb/IIIa receptor with tirofiban in unstable angina and non-Q-wave myocardial infarction. N Engl J Med 1998; 338(21):1488–1497.

46

Pharmacologic management of patients with CTO interventions

David R. Holmes, Jr

Patients with chronic total occlusion (CTO) represent a significant problem for interventional cardiology. Interest in this group dates back to the earliest days of the field (1–4). The presence of a chronic total occlusion identified patients in whom the chances of a successful procedure were decreased compared with those patients who treated for a subtotal stenosis. In addition, failure was not necessarily benign because of the potential for coronary perforation which can lead to tamponade or compromise of collaterals to the distal vessel which could lead to infarction. Because of these issues, the presence of a chronic total occlusion was the most common reason for deferral of percutaneous coronary intervention (PCI) in early studies instead patients with chronic total occlusions were preferentially treated with coronary artery bypass graft surgery (CABG). In a more recent single-center registry series of 8004 consecutive patients undergoing diagnostic catheterization from 1990 to 2000, a chronic total occlusion was found in 52% of patients with significant coronary artery disease. Patients with a chronic total occlusion had more frequent hypertension and peripheral vascular disease. The ejection fraction was significantly less 53 ± 16% versus 60 ± 14% (p < 0.001), and multivessel disease was significantly more common 66% versus 42% (p < 0.001). Twelve percent of patients had more than one chronic total occlusion. Typically, the occlusion involved the RCA (64%) followed by the circumflex (35%) and then the LAD (28%). In this more recent series, using multivariate analysis, the presence of a chronic total occlusion remained the strongest predictor against selection of PCI (OR 0.26, 95% CI 0.22–0.31, p < 0.0001) (5).

Because of the frequency with which chronic total occlusion occurs, there has been intense interest in developing and studying new approaches. These efforts have been spurred on by the finding in multiple series that successful PCI of a chronic occlusion is associated with a survival benefit as well as improvement in LV function. In an early study, Suero et al. (6) evaluated in-hospital and longer-term outcome in 2007 consecutive patients undergoing PCI for a CTO from 1980 to 1999 (Fig. 1A and 1B). These were matched with patients treated for a subtotal stenosis using a propensity analysis. For both cohorts, the 10-year survival was similar —71.2% for CTO patients and 71.4% for non-CTO patients. In patients with a CTO, the outcome of the procedure was a very important determinant of survival; in those patients with successful CTO treatment, 10-year survival was 73.5% compared with patients with a failed procedure in whom the 10-year survival was only 65.1% (p = 0.001).

More recent series have also documented a survival advantage (7–9). Hoye et al. in 874 consecutive patients with a CTO found a five-year survival in 93.5% of patients with successful revascularization versus 88.0% in these patients with failed revascularization (p = 0.02). In a Canadian registry of 1458 patients at seven year, successful recanalization of a chronic total occlusion was associated with improved survival as well as lower rates of PCI and/or CABG (9). In addition to survival advantage, both regional and global left ventricular function is improved in patients with successful treatment of a chronic total occlusion (10). This improvement may depend on whether the patient had a prior infarction in the distribution of the occlusion (11). If prior infarction resulted in frank myocardial necrosis, then recanalization may not improve the function; however, many patients with chronic occlusion have preservation of regional wall function.

Despite the potential for improved outcome in patients treated percutaneously for chronic total occlusion, in many laboratories, these procedures are undertaken sparingly. Abbott et al. (12) analyzed 2000 patients undergoing PCI in four sequential waves of patients from 1997 to 2004. In this group, 5173 lesions were attempted. In the first cohort treated from 1997 to 1998, 9.6% of treated lesions were chronic total occlusions; in the last cohort from 2004, the percentage of lesions treated that were chronic total occlusions had decreased to 5.7% (p < 0.0001) (Fig. 2). Procedural success declined from 79.7% to 71.4% during those same time periods. Procedural success rates such as this may be an over estimate because series of chronic total occlusion cases contain only patients in whom the

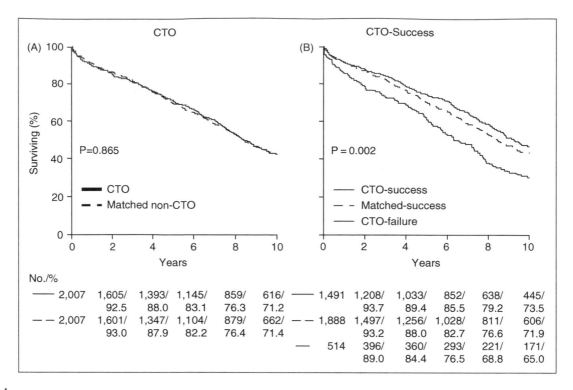

Figure 1

Long-term outcome of patients undergoing attempted PCI of a chronic total occlusion. (A) Outcome of chronic total occlusion versus non-chronic total occlusion patients. (B) Outcome of successful versus unsuccessful treatment of a chronic total occlusion. Successful treatment is associated with a survival advantage. *Abbreviation*: CTO, chronic total occlusion.

interventional cardiologist thought that successful recanalization was possible. There are multiple reasons for the decrease in frequency of performing procedures for CTO at the centers, but among the most prominent are the low success rates, procedural complexity, and time and resource utilization. In addition, recently because of the duration of procedures, excess radiation exposure has been documented (13,14).

The most common reason for failure of a chronic total occlusion is inability to cross with a guidewire. The pathologic basis for this has been studied (15–17). Srivatsa et al. (15) evaluated the histologic correlates of angiographic total coronary artery occlusion in an autopsy series of 61 patients with

96 angiographic chronic total occlusions. They analyzed the occlusion segments for histologic composition and for the presence of neovascular channels. They identified that fibro-calcific intimal plaque increased with increasing age of the occlusion and that neovascular channels were related to the extent of inflammation. Micro channels particularly advential channels may make entry into the true lumen difficult (Fig. 3). Entry into and dilatation of these advential collaterals could result in vessel perforation. Another finding in chronic total occlusion is a fibrotic hard cap which is sometimes calcified. These hard caps may be difficult or even impossible to cross. A final large component is collagen-rich extracellular matrix (17). The entire longitudinal picture is often underlying plaque

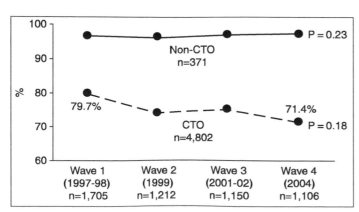

Figure 2

Dynamic wave registry of four separate time intervals. Attempts at CTO recanalization have been decreased. *Abbreviation*: CTO, chronic total occlusion.

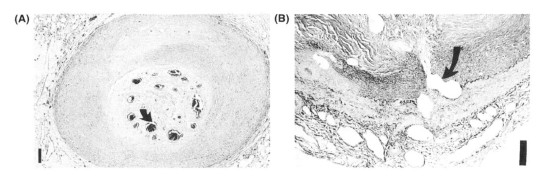

Figure 3

Histologic specimens of chronic coronary arterial occlusions with (A) large central neovascular channels (*arrow*) or (B) extensive media/adventitial collaterals.

and then multiple layers of matrix and thrombus which build up to form the occlusion (16).

The specific anatomy of the occlusion has a major impact on outcome of attempted percutaneous revascularization. Correlates of decreased success rates include older age of the occlusion, the presence of an abrupt cut off, the presence of a large patent side branch at the site of occlusion, and the presence of bridging collaterals. There are some patients in whom there are central intraplaque vessels (15,18,19). These may be associated with improved success rates.

These problems have led to the development and testing of new approaches, both mechanical and pharmacologic

Table 1 New mechanical approaches for CTO revascularization

New approaches

    Double wire
    Anchoring balloon
    Retrograde via collaterals
    Re-entry techniques

Dedicated guidewires

    Hydrophilic guidewires
    Tapered tip guidewires
    Stiff guidewires with variable stiffness (3–12 gms)

New devices

    Frontrunner blunt microdissection catheter
    Radiofrequency ablation with optical
    Coherence reflectometry guidance
    Laser guidewire
    High frequency ultrasound

New visualization adjuncts

    Preprocedural multislice CT
    Forward looking ultrasound

Abbreviations: CT, computed tomography; CTO, chronic total occlusion.

(Table 1). The mechanical approaches are very variable and range from new stiffer and/or coated guidewires, lasers, forward-looking ultrasound and ablative catheters. In addition, new guide catheter techniques and totally new approaches such as retrograde approaches through collaterals have been tested in specialized expert centers. These new catheter techniques have been reviewed elsewhere and are not the scope of this chapter on pharmacology (20). One item for emphasis is the use of drug-eluting stents. As the field has evolved, bare metal stents for chronic total occlusion were found to be substantially superior to conventional PTCA in reducing restenosis and reducing subsequent recurrent occlusion. More recently, there has been great interest in drug-eluting stents (21–27). This has culminated in a randomized trial which has been reported to show improvement in outcome compared with bare metal stents (26).

Pharmacologic approaches are also evolving. Some of these approaches are aimed at making the procedure safer and avoiding complications; others are aimed at improving initial success rates or preventing reocclusion or restenosis.

Pharmacologic approaches to optimize initial safety

The most important safety concerns are the potential for perforation which could result in tamponade or compromise of collaterals which can result in infarction. In current PCI practice with its reliance on drug eluting stent (DES), dual antiplatelet therapy with aspirin (ASA) and a thienopyridine (usually clopidogrel) is standard. These should be used in all patients. Pre-procedure administration of the thienopyridine should be given, if possible.

IIb/IIIa platelet glycoprotein inhibitors are widely used in some institutions, particularly in the setting of complex interventions. However, in the setting of chronic total occlusion, these agents should not be used until the occlusion has successfully been crossed. This minimizes the potential for bleeding should perforation occur. In addition if guidewire perforation does occur, even if the procedure is eventually successful and the guidewire can be seen entering the distal vessel, IIb/IIIa agents should be avoided. If crossing a complete occlusion is achieved without complications, a IIb/IIIa agent can then be administered particularly if the vessel is small or has other complex features.

Heparin is the standard treatment for conventional PCI. Recently, bivalirudin has been promoted extensively as an alternative. The latter has several advantages; it can be given as a single bolus, ACTs are not measured, and the half life is very short. In the setting of chronic total occlusion, bivalirudin has some significant disadvantages, namely although the half life is short, it cannot be reversed; in addition, chronic total occlusion cases are often long and would require additional dosing of bivalirudin which can increase costs substantially. Accordingly, unfractionated heparin should remain as the standard.

Pharmacologic agents to optimize initial success

Recognition that the usual reason for failure with chronic total occlusions is inability to cross with a guidewire; there has been interest in softening the occlusion. This is based on a robust experience in the treatment of peripheral arterial occlusions with thrombolytic therapy (29–33). In that setting, intravenous thrombolytic therapy was used initially to soften the occluded segment and make subsequent PTA easier and more successful. The field soon migrated to using intra arterial infusions of urokinase to decrease hemorrhagic complications and improve success rates. This has widely been used for iliac, femoral, and poplitial occlusions. The specific dose and duration of therapy have varied, but even for long chronic total occlusions, it has been found to be effective although bleeding remains a problem particularly during longer duration of occlusion; the bleeding may be in part related to the need for heparin.

Application of this concept has been expanded to the treatment of coronary arterial chronic total occlusion, the aim being the same as in the periphery to soften the occlusion and facilitate guidewire passage (34–37). Zidar et al. (36) reported on a randomized trial of prolonged intracoronary urohinase for chronic total occlusion of native coronary arteries. This study included 101 patients with an occlusion >3 mo. Patients were pre-treated with ASA and then given 10,000 U of IV heparin. Urohinase was infused after initial attempts at crossing the occlusion with a guidewire. The urohinase was administered for approximately eight hour with a split dosing through the guide catheter and the infusion catheter which were positioned proximal to the site of occlusion. One of three doses was used for a total of 800,000 U, 16 million U or 3.2 million U over the eight hour. Following infusion, the patient was returned to the catheterization laboratory for an additional attempt at guidewire passage. After urohinase infusion, angioplasty was successful in 53%. Patients receiving higher doses of urohinase had more bleeding although the numbers were too small to reach statistical significance. Follow up angiographic rates were low but the target vessel was patent in 91%; however, restenosis rates were high.

Subsequent to this study, Abbas et al. (37) reported on 85 patients who had a history of failed attempt at recanalization of a chronic coronary occlusion in whom at the time of repeat intervention, pre-procedural intracoronary fibrin-specific lytic therapy was used. In this group, either weight-adjusted alteplase (tPA, Genentech, San Francisco, CA; 0.025–0.05 mg/kg/hr; 2 mg/hr for weight ≤60 kg, 3 mg/hr for weight 61 to ≤80 kg, 4 mg/hr for weight 81 to ≤105 kg, and 5 mg/hr for weight ≥105 kg) or standard dose tenecteplase (TNK) (Genentech; 0.5 mg/hr) was administered for eight hour with an infusion catheter positioned at the face of the chronic total occlusion (Fig. 4). All of the occlusions were greater than three month in duration and 62% involved the right coronary artery. Despite the fact that all of the patients had had a previous failed attempt at recanalization, the procedure after lytic therapy was successful in 54%. Among the failed cases, inability to cross the occlusion with a guidewire was the most common reason for failure (97%). Procedural complications were relatively infrequent and included 5% with dissections that did not result in perforation or tamponade, groin hematoma in 8%, and positive biomarkers with elevation of total CK with an increase in MB fraction seen in 5%. This approach appears promising in these patients with previously failed attempts and will be tested in a larger trial.

Recently, there has been in the use of other pharmacologic agents to modify the chronic total occlusion and render it more suitable for treatment (38–40). An animal model has been developed for testing these new approaches. In this rabbit model, thrombin is injected into an isolated portion of the femoral artery. After recovery, during the next two to four month, the thrombus is replaced by collagen which results in a chronic total occlusion.

Using this rabbit model, a purified human grade collagenase was tested (39). Similar to the human situation, an over-the-wire balloon angioplasty catheter was advanced and positioned immediately proximal to the part of occlusion. The collagenase was administered through the central lumen for 24 hour. Following this, guidewire recanalization was attempted using conventional coronary guidewires. In the series of 10 CTO treated in this way, passage of the guidewire was successful in all 10. A wire-induced dissection was identified in two animals; despite that the wire eventually crossed into the distal vessel.

For this study, multiple doses of collagenase were used. The author studied the effect of the collagenase on subcutaneous

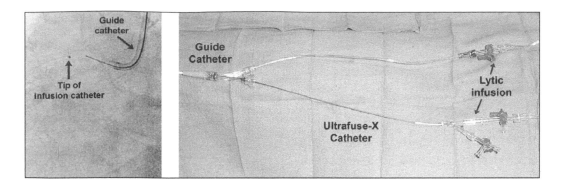

Figure 4

Approach used for subselective infusion prior to attempted PCI of a RCA. (*Left*) The RCA has been intubated with a guiding catheter, and a small infusion catheter advanced to the beginning of the occlusion. (*Right*) Both guide catheter and infusion catheter are used to deliver material. Both must be secured to avoid displacement. Ostial occlusion lesions are not suitable for this approach.

bruising. With higher doses, there was more extensive bruising but no significant differences in hemoglobin at 24 hours. Vessel wall structure remained intact.

This approach has considerable potential in the human arena although multiple details need to be worked out including the optimal duration of local arterial therapy. This detail has major implications for patient care. Infusions for up to six hour may be reasonably well tolerated; beyond this window, they become increasingly complicated. Prolonged heparin if required to maintain guide and sub-selective catheter patency may be associated with increased bleeding.

Conclusions

Chronic total occlusions remain one of the last great problems (or opportunities) for interventional cardiology. Despite their frequency, current success rates are still quite low even in selected patients; the dominant reason for failure is inability to cross with a guidewire. New mechanical approaches continue to be evaluated. In addition to these, new pharmacologic strategies are being developed to facilitate initial safe passage of the guidewire. These have the potential to improve success rates. Resolution of this problem will open up the doors for many patients with chronic coronary artery disease to undergo a percutaneous revascularization procedure rather than CABG.

References

1   Holmes DR Jr, Vlietstra RE, Reeder GS, et al. Angioplasty in total coronary artery occlusion. JACC 1984; 3:845–849.

2   Bell MR, Berger PB, Bresnahan JF, et al. Initial and long term outcome of 354 patients after coronary balloon angioplasty of total coronary artery occlusion. Circulation 1992; 85: 1003–1011.

3   Safian RD, McCabe CH, Sipperly ME, et al. Initial success and long-term follow-up of percutaneous transluminal coronary angioplasty in chronic total occlusions versus conventional stenoses. Am J Cardiol 1988; 61:23G–28G.

4   Ivanhoe RJ, Weintraub WS, Douglas JS Jr., et al. Percutaneous transluminal coronary angioplasty of chronic total occlusions. Primary success, restenosis and long-term clinical follow-up. Circulation 1992; 85:106–115.

5   Christofferson RD, Lehmann KG, Martin GV, et al. Effect of chronic total coronary occlusion on treatment strategy. Am J Cardiol 2005; 95:1088–1091.

6   Suero JA, Marso SP, Jones PG, et al. Procedural outcomes and long term survival among patients undergoing percutaneous coronary intervention of a chronic total occlusion in native coronary arteries: a 20 year experience. JACC 2001; 38:409–414.

7   Noguchi T, Miyazaki S, Morii I, et al. Percutaneous transluminal coronary angioplasty of chronic total occlusions. Determinants of primary success and long-term clinical outcome. Catheter Cardiovasc Inter 2000; 49:258–264.

8   Hoye A, van Domburg RT, Sonnenschein K, Serruys, PW. Percutaneous coronary intervention for chronic total occlusions: the Thoraxcenter experience 1992–2002. Eur Heart J 2005; 26:2630–2636.

9   Ramanathan K, Gao M, Nogareda GJ, et al. Successful percutaneous recanalization of a non acute occluded coronary artery predicts clinical survival and outcome. Circulation 2001; 104:415A.

10   Ermis C, Boz A, Tholakanahalli V, et al. Assessment of percutaneous coronary intervention on regional and global left ventricular function in patients with chronic total occlusions. Can J Cardiol 2005; 21:275–280.

11   Chung CM, Nakamura S, Tanaka K, et al. Effect of recanalization of chronic total occlusions on global and regional left ventricular function in patients with or without previous myocardial infarctions. Catheter Cardiovasc Interv 2003; 60:368–374.

12   Abbott JD, Kip KE, Vlachos HA, et al. Recent trends in the percutaneous treatment of chronic total artery occlusions. Am J Cardiol 2006; 97:1691–1696.

13   Suzuki S, Furui S, Kohtake H, et al. Radiation exposure to patient's skin during percutaneous coronary intervention for various lesions including chronic total occlusion. Circulation 2006; 70:44–48.

14   Kuon E, Empen K, Rohde D, Dahm JB. Radiation exposure to patients undergoing percutaneous coronary

interventions: are current reference values too high. Herz 2004; 29: 208–217.

15 Srivatsa SS, Edwards WD, Boos CM, et al. Histologic correlates of angiographic chronic total coronary occlusion. JACC 1995:29:955–963.

16 Meier B. Chronic total occlusions. In Topol EJ editor Textbook of Interventional Cardiology 4th Edition Philadelphia PA Saunders 2003; 303–316.

17 Katsuda S, Okada Y, Minamoto T, et al. Collagens in human atherosclerosis: immunohistochemical analysis using collagen type specific antibodies. Arterioscler Thromb 1992; 12:494–502.

18 Katsuragawa M, Fujiwara H, Miyamae M, et al. Histologic studies in percutaneous transluminal coronary angioplasty for chronic total occlusion: comparison of tapering and abrupt types of occlusion and short and long occluded segments. JACC 1993; 21:604–611.

19 Strauss BH, Segev A, Wright GA, et al. Microvessels in chronic total occlusions: pathways for successful guidewire crossing? J Interv Cardiol 2005; 18:425–436.

20 Fung A, Hamburger JN. The chronic total occlusion In Ellis S and Holmes 3rd Edition Strategic Approaches in Coronary Interventions. 2005:366–373.

21 Ge L, Iakovou I, Cosgrove J, et al. Immediate and mid-term outcomes of Sirolimus eluting stent implantation for chronic total occlusions. Eur Heart J 2005; 26:1056–1062.

22 Rohel BM, Suttorp MJ, Laarman GL. Primary stenting of occluded native coronary arteries: final results of the primary stenting of occluded native coronary arteries (PRISON) study. Am Heart J 2004; 147:H1–H5.

23 Hoye A, Tanabe K, Lemos A, et al. Significant reduction in restenosis after the use of Sirolimus eluting stents in the treatment of chronic total occlusions. JACC 2004; 43:1954–1958.

24 Olivari Z, Rubertelli P, Piscione F, et al. TOAST-GISE Investigators. Immediate results and one-year clinical outcome after percutaneous coronary interventions in chronic total occlusions: data from a multicenter, prospective, observational study (TOAST-GISE). J Am Coll Cardiol 2003; 41: 1672–1678.

25 Migliorini A, Moschi G, Vergara R, et al. Drug-eluting stent supported percutaneous coronary intervention for chronic total coronary occlusion. Catheter Cardiovasc Interv 2006; 67:344–348.

26 Rahel BM, Laarmen GJ, Suttorp MJ, et al. Primary stenting of occluded native coronary arteries II—rationale and design of the PRISON II study: a randomized comparison of bare metal stent implantation with Sirolimus-eluting stent implantation for the treatment of chronic total coronary occlusions. Am Heart J 2005; 149:e1–e3.

27 Olivari Z, Rubartelli P, Piscione, F, et al. Immediate results and one-year clinical outcome after percutaneous coronary interventions in chronic total occlusions: data from a multicenter, prospective, observational study (TOAST-GISE). J Am Coll Cardiol 2003; 41:1672–1678.

28 Braim MR, Gert JL, Maarten JS, et al. Primary stenting of occluded native coronary arteries II—rationale and design of the PRISON II Study: a randomized comparison of bare metal stent implantation with sirolimus-eluting stent implantation for the treatment of chronic total coronary occlusions. Circulation 2006; 114:921–928.

29 Poliwoda H, Alexander K, Buhl V, et al. Treatment of chronic arterial occlusions with streptokinase. N Engl J Med 1969; 280:689–692.

30 Martin M, Schoop W, Weitler E. Streptokinase in chronic arterial occlusive disease. JAMA 1970; 211:1169–1173.

31 Verstraete M, Vermlen J, Donati MB. The effect of streptokinase infusion on chronic arterial occlusions and stenoses. Ann Intern Med 1971; 74:377–382.

32 Lupattelli L, Barzi F, Corneli P, et al. Selective thrombolysis with low-dose urokinase in chronic arteriosclerotic obstructions. Cardiovasc Intervent Radiol 1988; 11:123–126.

33 Motarjeme A, Gordon G, Bodenhagen K. Thrombolysis and angioplasty of chronic iliac artery occlusions. J Vasc Intervent Radiol 1995; 6:665–725.

34 Ajluni SC, Jones D, Zidar FJ, et al. Prolonged urokinase infusion for chronic total native coronary occlusions: clinical, angiographic, and treatment observations. Cathter Cardiovasc Diagn 1995; 34:106–110.

35 Razavi MK, Wong H, Kee ST, et al. Initial clinical results of tenecteplase (TNK) in catheter-directed thrombolytic therapy. J Endovasc Ther 2002; 9:593–598.

36 Zidar FJ, Kaplan BM, O'Neill WW, et al. Prospective randomized trial of prolonged intracoronary urokinase infusion for chronic total occlusions in native arteries. J Am Coll Cardiol 1996; 27:1406–1412.

37 Abbas AE, Brewington SD, Dixon SR, et al. Intracoronary fibrin-specific thrombolytic infusion facilitates percutaneous recanalization of chronic total occlusion. JACC 2005; 46:793–798.

38 Segev A, Strauss BH. Novel approaches for the treatment of chronic total occlusions. J Interv Cardiol 2004; 17:411–416.

39 Segev A, Nili N, Qiang B, et al. Human-grade purified collagenase for the treatment of experimental arterial chronic total occlusion. Cardiovasc Revasc Med 2005; 6:65–69.

40 Strauss BH, Goldman L, Qiang B, et al. Collagenase plaque digestion for facilitating guidewire crossing in chronic total occlusions. Circulation 2003; 108:1259–1262.

47

Newer pharmacologic approaches targeting receptors and genes

Omer M. Iqbal, Debra Hoppensteadt, and Jawed Fareed

Introduction

The emergence of pharmacogenomic-guided drug development has led to novel approaches in the effective management of patients and ensured individualized therapy tailored to the needs of one and all, at the right dosage and right time. The entire human genome is now completely mapped. Gene expression profiling and identification of the single nucleotide polymorphism (SNP) will enable effective diagnosis of various diseases, and has a role in preclinical phases of drug development, in developing markers for adverse drug interactions and desired pharmacologic effects. Newer drugs can be withdrawn from the drug development pipeline should they exhibit hepatic metabolism requiring CYP450 enzymes known to manifest SNPs resulting in adverse drug reactions. Vogel for the first time introduced the term, pharmacogenetics, in 1959 (1), which refers to the analysis of monogenetic variants that define an individual's response to a drug, and aims to deliver the right drug at right dosage to a right patient by using DNA information. The variable drug response in different patients may be the result of genetic differences in drug metabolism, drug distribution, and drug target proteins (2). Pharmacogenetics refers to the entire library of genes that determine drug efficacy and safety. There are approximately three billion base pairs in the human genome that code for at least 30,000 genes. Although the majority of basepairs are identical from individual to individual, only 0.1% of the basepairs contribute to individual differences. Three consecutive basepairs form a codon that specifies the amino acids that constitute the protein. Genes represent a series of codons that specifies a particular protein. At each gene locus, an individual carries two alleles, one

from each parent. If there are two identical alleles, it is referred to as a homozygous genotype, and if the alleles are different, it is heterozygous. Genetic variations usually occur as SNPs and occur on an average of at least once every 1000 basepairs, accounting to approximately three million basepairs distributed throughout the entire genome. Genetic variations that occur at a frequency of at least 1% in the human population are referred to as polymorphisms. Genetic polymorphisms are inherited and monogenic; they involve one locus and have interethnic differences in frequency. Rare mutations occur at a frequency of less than 1% in the human population. Other examples of genetic variations include insertion–deletion polymorphisms, tandem-repeats, defective splicing, aberrant splice site, and premature stop codon polymorphisms. Pharmacogenomics, through the discovery of new genetic targets, is expected to improve the quality of life and control the healthcare costs by treating specific genetic subgroups and by avoiding adverse drug reactions and by decreasing the number of treatment failures. The evolution and the concepts of pharmacoeconomic-based pharmacogenomics and pharmacogenetics should be widely known and practiced. Pharmacogenomics and cheminformatics should become a part of the current study designs of prospective clinical trials. Pharmacogenomic and pharmacogenetic data should be included in the investigational new drug (IND) applications, thereby enabling the food and drug administration (FDA) to evaluate its true impact on pharmacoeconomics resulting in drastic reduction in the healthcare expenditure worldwide. Pharmacogenomics provides a significant paradigm shift in the management of patients and provides a means to increase the quality of medical care.

Single nucleotide polymorphism

Pharmaceutical industries are very much interested in pharmacogenomics as a means to reduce the costs and the time involved in conducting the clinical trials and to improve the efficacy of drugs tailored to the individual patient need. Although the genetic association studies are used to establish links between polymorphic variation in the coagulation Factor V gene and deep vein thrombosis (DVT), this approach of "susceptibility genes" that has a crucial role in the likelihood of developing a disease has enabled identification of other genes (3). Variations in a drug metabolizing enzyme gene, thiopurine methyltransferase (TPMT), have been linked to adverse drug reactions (4). Similarly, variants in a drug-target, 5-lipoxygenase, (ALOX5) have been linked to variations in drug response (5). Through linkage disequilibrium (LD) or nonrandom association between SNPs in proximity to each other, tens of thousands of anonymous SNPs are identified and mapped. These anonymous genes may fall either within susceptibility genes or in noncoding DNA between genes. Through LD, the associations found that with these anonymous SNP markers can identify a region of the genome that may harbor a particular susceptibility gene. Through positional cloning, the gene and the SNP can be revealed conferring the underlying associated condition or disease (6). Numerous companies have now developed DNA microarrays (biochips) of different genes of interest that could be used in high-throughput sequencing in a population to detect common or uncommon genetic variants. These DNA-based diagnostic microarrays, which are targeted for patient care, must be accurate, high-throughput, reproducible, flexible, and inexpensive. Efforts should be made to improve the sensitivity as well as to reduce the costs of identifying polymorphisms by direct sequencing. It is important to understand the genetic variability in genes in relation to the safety and efficacy of any drug. The functional consequences of nonsynonymous SNPs can be predicted by a structure-based assessment of amino acid variation (7).

Pharmacogenomics in coagulation disorders

According to the SNP Map Working Group (Nature 2001), there are 1.42 million SNPs; one SNP per 1900 bases; 60,000 SNPs within exons; two exonic SNPs per gene (1/1080 bases); 93% of genetic loci contain two SNPs. Because each person is different at one in 1000–2000 bases, SNPs are responsible for human individuality. A list of genes involved in coagulation disorders is given in Table 1.

The various polymorphisms in different coagulation proteins are discussed subsequently.

Table 1 List of genes involved in coagulation disorders

Clone ID	Name	Gene title
22040	MMP9	Matrix metalloproteinase 9 (gelatinase B, 92-Kd gelatinase, 92-Kd type IV collagenase)
26418	EDG1	Endothelial differentiation, sphingolipid G-protein-coupled receptor
32609	LAMA4	Laminin, alpha 4
34778	VEGF	Vascular endothelial growth factor
40463	PDGFRB	Platelet-derived growth factor (PDGF) receptor, betapolypeptide
41898	PTGDS	Prostaglandin D2 synthase (21 Kd, brain)
44477	VCAM1	Vascular cell adhesion molecule 1
45138	VEGFC	VEGF factor C
49164	VCAM1	Vascular cell adhesion molecule 1
49509	EPOR	Erythropoietin receptor
49665	EDNRB	Endothelin receptor type B
49920	PTDSS1	Phosphatidylserine synthase 1
51447	FCGR3B	Fc fragment of IgG, low affinity IIIb, receptor for Z(CD16)
66982	PLGL	Plasminogen-like
67654	PDGFB	PDGF-betapolypeptide [Simian sarcoma viral (v-sis) oncogene homolog]
71101	PROCR	Protein C receptor, endothelial (EPCR)
71626	ZNF268	Zinc finger protein 268

(Continued)

Table 1   List of genes involved in coagulation disorders (*Continued*)

Clone ID	Name	Gene title
768246	G6PD	Glucose-6-phosphate dehydrogenase
85678	F2	Coagulation factor II
85979	PLG	Plasminogen
120189	PSG4	Pregnancy-specific beta-1-glycoprotein 4
121218	PF4	Platelet factor 4
127928	HBP1	HMG-box containing protein 1
130541	PECAM1	Platelet/endothelial-cell adhesion molecule (CD31 antigen)
131839	FOLR1	Folate receptor 1 (adult)
135221	S100P	S100 calcium-binding protein P
136821	TGFB1	Transforming growth factor, beta 1
137836	PDCD10	Programmed cell death 10
138991	COL6A3	Collagen, type VI, alpha 3
139009	FN1	Fibronectin 1
142556	PSG2	Pregnancy-specific beta-1-glycoprotein 2
143287	PSG11	Pregnancy-specific beta-1-glycoprotein 11
143443	TBXAS1	Thromboxane A synthase 1
149910	SELL	Selectin E (endothelial adhesion molecule 1)
151662	P11	Protease, serine, 22
155287	HSPA1A	Heatshock 70Kd protein 1A
160723	LAMC1	Laminin, gamma 19 formerly LAMB2
179276	FASN	Fatty acid synthase
180864	ICAM5	Intercellular adhesion molecule 5, telencephalin
184038	SPTBN2	Spectrin, beta, nonerythrocytic 2
191664	THBS2	Thrombospondin 2
194804	PTTPN	Phosphatidylinositol transfer protein
196612	MMP12	Matrix metalloproteinase 1 (interstitial collagenase)
199945	TGM2	Transglutaminase 2 (C polypeptide, protein-glutamine-gamma-glutamyltransferase)
205185	THBD	Thrombomodulin
210687	AGTR1	Angiotensin receptor 1
212429	TF	Transferrin
212649	HRG	Histidine-rich glycoprotein
234736	GATA6	GATA-binding protein 6
240249	APLP2	Amyloid beta (A4) precursor-like protein 2
241788	FGB	Fibrinogen, B betapolypeptide
243816	CD36	CD36 antigen (collagen type 1 receptor, thrombospondin receptor)
245242	CPB2	Carboxypeptidase B2 (Plasma, carboxypeptidase U)
260325	ALB	Albumin
261519	TNFRSF5	TNF-receptor (superfamily, member 5)
292306	LIPC	lipase, hepatic

(*Continued*)

Table 1   List of genes involved in coagulation disorders (*Continued*)

Clone ID	Name	Gene title
296198	CHS1	Chediak-Higashi syndrome 1
310519	F10	Coagulation factor X
340644	ITGB8	Integrin, beta 8
343072	ITGB1	Integrin, beta 1 (finronectin receptor, beta polypeptide, antigen CD29 includes MDF2, MSK12)
345430	PIK3CA	Phosphoinositide 3 kinase, catalytic, alpha polypeptide
589115	MMP1	Matrix metalloproteinase 1 (interstitial collagenase)
666218	TGFB2	Transforming growth factor, beta 2
712641	PRG4	Proteoglycan 4 (megakaryocyte-stimulating factor, articular superficial zone protein)
714106	PLAU	Plasminogen activator, urokinase
726086	TFPI2	Tissue factor pathway inhibitor (TFPI) 2
727551	IRF2	Interferon regulatory factor 2
753211	PTGER3	Prostaglandin E receptor 3 (subtype EP30)
753418	VASP	Vasodilator-stimulated phosphoprotein
753430	ATRX	Alpha Thalassemia/mental retardation syndrome X-linked RAD54 (S. cerevisiae) homolog
754080	ICAM3	Intercellular adhesion molecule 3
755054	IL18R1	Interleukin 18 receptor 1
758266	THBS4	Thrombospondin 4
770462	CPZ	Carboxypeptidase Z
770670	TNFAIP3	Tumor necrosis factor (TNF), alpha-induced protein 3
770859	ITGB5	Integrin, beta 5
776636	BHMT	Betaine-homocysteine methyltransferase
782789	AVPR1A	Arginine vasopressin receptor 1A
785975	F13A1	Coagulation factor XIII, A1 polypeptide
788285	EDNR A	Endothelial receptor type A
809938	TACSTD2	Matrix metalloproteinase 7 (matrilysin, uterine)
810010	PDGFRL	PDGF-receptor-like
810017	PLAUR	Plasminogen activator, urokinase receptor
810117	ANXA11	Annexin A11
810124	PAFAH1B3	Platelet-activating factor acetylhydrolase, isoform 1b, gamma subunit (29 Kd)
810242	C3AR1	Complement component 3a receptor 1
810512	THBS1	Thrombospondin 1
810891	LAMA5	Laminin, alpha 5
811096	ITGB4	Integrin, beta 4
811792	GSS	Glutathione synthetase
812276	SNCA	Synuclein, alpha (non-A4 component of amyloid precursor)
813757	FOLR2	Folate receptor 2 (fetal)
813841	PLAT	Plasminogen activator, tissue serine (or cysteine) proteinase inhibitor, Clade E (nexin, plasminogen activator inhibitor type 1), member 1
814378	SPINT2	Serine protease inhibitor, kunitz type 2

(*Continued*)

Table 1 List of genes involved in coagulation disorders (*Continued*)

Clone ID	Name	Gene title
814615	MTHFD	Methylene tetrahydrofolate dehydrogenase (NAD-dependent), methylenetetrahydrofolate cyclohydrolase
825295	LDLR	low-density lipoprotein-receptor (familial hypercholesterolemia)
840486	vWF	von Willebrand factor
842846	TIMP2	Tissue inhibitor of metalloproteinase-2
1813254	F2R	Coagulation factor II (thrombin) receptor

Fibrinogen

Various polymorphisms have been identified in all the three genes located on the long arm of chromosome 4 (q23–32). However, the two dimorphisms in the β-chain gene, namely the HaeIII polymorphisms (a G→A substitution at position −455 in the 5′ promoter region and the BcII polymorphism in the 3′ untranslated region, are of major importance and are in LD with each other. The −455G/A substitution in different investigations was found to be a determinant of plasma fibrinogen levels (8,9) and linked the fibrinogen gene variation to the risk of arterial disease. Because of conflicting reports from different studies, this association between fibrinogen gene variation and arterial disease is controversial. The α-chain Thr-312 Ala polymorphism has been reported to increase the stability of the clot (10). Specific factor XIIIa inhibitors may play an important role in decreasing clot stability.

Prothrombin

The coagulation Factor II (prothrombin) G20210A mutation occurring in 2% of the population is located in the 3′ UTR of the coagulation Factor II propeptide near a putative polyadenylation site (11). It is associated with increased levels of prothrombin resulting in DVT, recurrent miscarriages, and portal vein thrombosis in cirrhotic patients (13–16). Anticoagulant drugs, such as Factor Xa inhibitors or tissue factor pathway inhibitor (TFPI), should be developed to prevent thrombosis in these conditions. The interactive role of hormone replacement therapy and prothrombotic mutations has been reported to cause the risk of nonfatal myocardial infarction in postmenopausal women (17).

Factor V Leiden R506Q

This mutation (G1691A), occurring in 8% of the population and referring to specific G→A substitution at nucleotide 1691 in the gene for Factor V, is cleaved less efficiently (10%) by activated protein C. This results in DVT, recurrent miscarriages, portal vein thrombosis in cirrhotic patients, early kidney transplant loss, and other forms of venous thromboembolism (12,14,15,17). A dramatic increase in the incidence of thrombosis is seen in women who are taking oral contraceptives. Both prothrombin G20210 and Factor V Leiden in the presence of major risk factors may contribute to atherothrombosis. Antithrombin drugs may play a crucial role in the management of these thrombotic disorders. The Factor V Leiden allele is common in Europe, with a population frequency of 4.4%. The mutation is very rare outside Europe with a frequency of 0.6% in Asia Minor (18).

Factor VII

Polymorphisms in the Factor VII gene, especially the Arg-353Gln mutation in exon 8 located in the catalytic domain of Factor VII, influence plasma Factor VII levels. The Gln-353 allele caused a strong protective effect against the occurrence of myocardial infarction (19). Further research in this area is warranted to understand the role of Factor VII in determining arterial thrombotic risk. Since the Factor VIIa/tissue factor (TF) is the initial coagulation pathway, much attention has been given in blocking this pathway by developing Factor VIIa inhibitors and TFPI (20). NAPc2 and NAP-5 are two of the anticoagulant proteins isolated from the hookworm nematode, Ancylostoma caninum. NAPc2 is currently undergoing Phase II clinical trials for prevention of venous thromboembolism in patients with elective knee arthroplasty. NAPc2 binds to a noncatalytic site on Factor X or Xa and inhibits Factor VII. NAP-5 inhibits Factor Xa and the Factor VII/TF complex after prior binding to Factor Xa.

Factor VIII

Increased Factor VIII activity levels are associated with increased risk of arterial thrombosis. However, no specific polymorphisms in the Factor VIII gene have been determined.

Von Willebrand factor

Although increased plasma von Willebrand factor (vWF) levels have been attributed to increased risk of arterial thrombotic events, no gene polymorphisms in vWF have been identified.

Factor XIII

Factor XIII SNP G→T in exon 2 causes a Val/Leu change at position 34. The Val34Leu polymorphism increases the rate of thrombin activation of Factor XIII and causes increased and faster clot stabilization (21,22). The Leu34 allele has been shown to play a protective role against arterial and venous thrombosis (23,24).

Specific Factor XIIIa inhibitors, such as tridegin and others mentioned earlier, may provide an interesting and novel approach to preventing fibrin stabilization. It is important to identify this polymorphism since the Leu34 variant associated with increased Factor XIIIa activity reduces the activity of thrombolytic therapy (21,22).

Polymorphisms in the natural anticoagulant system

Genetic defects in the antithrombin, protein C and protein S in arterial diseases are not completely understood and may not contribute to the risk of arterial thrombosis.

Thrombomodulin

Thrombomodulin mutations are more important in arterial diseases than in venous diseases. The thrombomodulin polymorphism, G→A substitution at nucleotide position 127 in the gene, has been studied regarding its relation with the arterial disease. The 25 Thr allele has been reported to be more prevalent in male patients with myocardial infarction than the control population (25). Polymorphism in the thrombomodulin gene promoter (−33 G/A) influences the plasma soluble thrombomodulin levels and causes increased risk of coronary heart disease (26). Carriership of the −33A allele was also reported to cause increased occurrence of carotid atherosclerosis in patients less than 60 years (27).

Tissue factor pathway inhibitor

Sequence variation of the TFPI gene has been reported. The four different polymorphisms reported are: pro-151Leu, Val-264Met, T384C exon 4, and C-33T intron 7 (28,29).

The Val264Met mutation causes decreased TFPI levels (29). It is reported that the Pro-151Leu replacement is a risk factor for venous thrombosis (30). A polymorphism in the 5′ UTR of the TFPI gene (−287 T/C did not alter the TFPI levels and did not influence the risk of coronary atherothrombosis (31). It has been recently reported that the −33T→C polymorphism in the intron 7 of the TFPI gene influences the risk of venous thromboembolism, independently of the Factor V Leiden and prothrombin mutations, and its effect is mediated by increased total TFPI levels (32).

Endothelial protein C receptor

A 23 bp insertion in exon 3 of the endothelial protein C receptor (EPCR) gene has been reported to predispose patients to the risk of coronary atherothrombosis (33). Further studies are needed to relate the polymorphisms in the EPCR gene to thrombotic diseases.

Platelet surface gene polymorphisms

Various polymorphisms of the platelet surface proteins, such as glycoprotein (GP) Ia-IIa, GPIb-V-IX, and GPIIb/IIIa have been reported. Afshar-Kharghan et al. (34) have recently reported a gene polymorphism in the Kozac sequence of the GpIbα receptor. Definition of the role of these polymorphisms in arterial diseases is warranted.

Platelet receptor GPIbα and immobilized vWF interactions cause rolling of platelets on the damaged endothelium facilitating platelet activation. These interactions in occluded atherosclerotic arteries or ruptured atherosclerotic plaques cause arterial thrombosis (35). Mutations of GPIbα and vWF cause four different types of bleeding disorders enhancing or reducing complex formation. The receptor complex consists of GPIbα, GPIbβ, IX, and V. Through GPIbα, the complex is anchored to the cytoskeleton. The vWF protein forms large multimers, which are found in plasma and subendothelial cell matrix and are released from the storage granules upon activation of platelets and endothelial cells. GPIbα and vWF have two contact sites and may serve as primary useful targets for the development of drugs for the treatment or prophylaxis of arterial thrombosis (36,37).

Methylene tetrahydrofolate reductase gene

A common polymorphism C677T, seen in the methylenetetrahydrofolate reductase (MTHFR) gene causing hyperhomocysteinemia is considered to be a potential risk factor for both venous and arterial thrombotic diseases.

Cardiovascular genomics

Cardiovascular healthcare can be personalized. The complete mapping of the human genome has brought out novel technologies that allow genome-wide interrogation of SNPs. Several other technologies such as transcriptomics (gene expression profiles), proteomics (proteomes), metabolomics (metabolomes) would go hands in gloves with genomics (human genome sequence), in making the personalized healthcare possible. The first autosomal dominant gene for coronary artery disease and myocardial infarction, reported recently, was a deletion mutation in a member of the myocyte enhancer Factor 2 transcription factor family (MEF2A), discovered in a single large family of which 13 members had coronary artery disease, and nine had myocardial infarction (38). Large case control association studies of candidate genes for myocardial infarction or premature coronary artery disease have been carried out. The various candidate genes include the gap junction protein, alpha 4, 37 kDa gene (GJA4) or connexin 37, p22 (phox) (39); plasminogen activator inhibitor-1, stromelysin-1 (39); lymphotoxin-alpha (40); alpha-adducing (ADD1), cholesteryl ester transfer protein (CETP), paraoxonase-1,2, apolipoprotein C-III (41); 5-lipoxygenase activating protein (FLAP), apolipoprotein E (42); low-density lipoprotein-related protein-1, matrix metalloproteinase 3 gene (MMP3), angiotensin-1 converting enzyme, methylene tetrahydrofolate reductase, Factor VII, P-selectin (SELP, fibrinogen-beta, thrombopoietin, GP-Ib alpha, interleukin-1 receptor antagonist, thrombospondin 2 and 4, and plasminogen activator inhibitor 2 (43).

Expression profiling of RNA

Gene variants may be associated with the disease; however, it does not specify that a disease phenotype will be present. While the information in the DNA may not be altered, RNA, an intermediate gene product from DNA transcription, might change in response to environmental, intracellular, and extracellular stimuli. Using microarrays the entire transcriptome comprising 25,000 transcripts can be interrogated. The RNA profile can help to subclassify disease, for example heart failure (44,45), and predict response to different therapies or to identify genes associated with a clinical outcome.

Genomics and sudden cardiac death

Although cardiac arrhythmias involve the electrical conduction system of the heart including the sinus node, atrioventricular

node and bundle of His and the Purkinje system and eventually the electrical current has to pass in the cardiomyocytes. In order to facilitate such a transmission to the cardiomyocytes, it involves the functional roles of ionic currents, ion channels, structural proteins, and gap junctions. Genetic defects are known to involve the subunits of the ion channels. So far 429 genes encoding ion channel proteins in humans have been identified (46). Of the 429 genes, 170 encode potassium channels, 38 calcium channels, 29 sodium channels, 58 chloride channels, and 15 encode glutemate receptors (47). Ion channels have quite a complex functional network and are known to not only regulate membrane potentials but also regulate cell volume and hormone secretion (48,49). Sudden cardiac death in younger patients (<35 years) is mainly due to genetic causes. Atrial fibrillation has been mapped to nine chromosomal loci involving four genes. The adenosine monophosphate-activated protein kinase gene is responsible for the Wolff-Parkinson-White syndrome. The long QT syndrome and the Brugada syndrome are due to the involvement of other genes defects primarily in sodium and potassium channels in the heart (50).

Eradication of cardiovascular disease and future prospects

Eradication of cardiovascular disease is the long-term goal of cardiovascular genomics. As the aging population continues to grow, the actual number of persons who die from cardiovascular disease remained nearly constant at about three quarters of a million per year during the period 1970–1998 (51,52). However, the cardiovascular death in women has declined less than men. Furthermore, the growing incidence of obesity worldwide would lead to diabetes and metabolic syndrome and should sound a major alarm for heightened risk of cardiovascular morbidity and mortality.

Cardiovascular genomics and biomedical engineering

Keeping pace with the pharmacogenomics and metabolomics, the advances in molecular imaging have contributed significantly to the understanding of cardiovascular system. The display and quantification of the molecular and cellular targets have become possible with the development of chemical and biologic probes to monitor the activity of molecular pathways, and development of molecular imaging techniques. For example, the optical coherence tomography (OCT) helps in measuring the macrophage content of arterial plaques enabling prognosis and guiding therapy (53), radiolabeled antibodies against epitopes on low-density lipoproteins such as I-125 MDA2 used in animals to assess disease severity (54), magnetic resonance imaging, fluorescence imaging, bioluminescence imaging, positron emission/single photon emission computed tomography (PET/SPECT) and ultrasound techniques to image enzymes (e.g., cathepsins B,D,K,S, and MMPs), receptors (e.g., GPCRs, integrins), and endothelial cells (e.g., E-selectin, VCAM) apoptosis (phosphatidylserine), angiogenesis (VCAM), and thrombosis (fibrin, thrombin) (55). Furthermore, visualization of clot formation and angiogenesis may be possible through application of magnetic resonance nanoparticles targeting directly to fibrin and integrins (56). Other applications of molecular imaging are in the fields of cancer and inflammatory diseases as well as atherosclerosis, heart failure, and thrombosis for early detection of disease, monitoring of disease progression, and to monitor response to therapy (55).

Polymorphisms in candidate genes related to hemostasis, thrombosis, lipid metabolism, inflammation, and cell matrix adhesion have been known to be useful in risk assessment of cardiovascular diseases. However, recent report on multilocus candidate gene polymorphisms and risk of myocardial infarction, a population-based, prospective genetic analysis concluded that after correction for multiple comparisons, the addition of genetic information observed had a little impact on myocardial infarction risk prediction models (57). Realizing the fact that the analyses in this study were not designed to directly address the potential for gene−environmental interactions, further studies need to be done to better understand the haplotypic effect, gene–gene interactions, and gene–environment interactions in the pathophysiology of athero-thrombosis. This would be a potential focus of intense research in the postgenomic era. Analyzing Zee et al.'s study, Reitsma commented that the study although based on the very large Physicians Health Study lacks power and includes data on about 500 cases and 2000 controls, which is too little to detect small but clinically relevant genetic risk factors or a combination of risk factors (58).

Reitsma further commented that study performed by Zee et al. did not include a variant gene encoding leukotriene A4 hydrolase, which has recently been reported to confer the risk of myocardial infarction particularly in Africans and Americans (59). Furthermore, Lysenko et al reported that future Type 2 diabetes, a major risk factor for cardiovascular disease, could be detected by a combination of peroxisome proliferator-activated receptor gamma (PPARG) and CALPAIN (CAPN) genotypes in susceptible individuals with high plasma glucose and body mass index (60). Interestingly, even though the PPARG polymorphism came up positive in Zee et al's study, this result was rejected after correction for multiple testing (58).

Pharmacogenetic-based dosing of oral anticoagulants

Improved prediction of maintenance warfarin dose is linked to SNPs in the vitamin K epoxide reductase complex subunit

I gene (VKORC1) (61–63). The different high- and low-dose haplotypes can be identified by screening for haplotype tag SNPs (61). Warfarin dose can also be predicted by CYP2C9 genotype (64,65). While VKORKC1 haplotype accounts for 21–25% of the variation and by the addition of CYP2C9*2 and 3 genotype improved the prediction model to 31% (64), considering the narrow therapeutic range and life-threatening thrombotic and bleeding complications, prior screening of VKORKC1 and CYP2C9 enables dose selection and monitoring strategies. Considering some studies that have reported population differences in VKORKC1 and CYP2C9 haplotypes, Marsh et al identified the frequency of genotype combinations across world populations of four haplotype tag SNPs for VKORKC1 (861, 5808, 6853, and 9041) and CYP2C9 (*2 and *3) (61,64,66,67) using prosequencing (61,64). Using Rieder et al.'s criteria to determine high- and low-dose VKORKC1 haplotype groups (61) and incorporating Gage et al.'s dose-limiting CYP2C9 genetic variation (64), Marsh et al concluded that Asians and Caucasian populations had the highest incidence (86% and 55%, respectively) of "low-dose" individuals from either VKORKC1 or CYP2C9 variants (from at least one VKORKC1 or haplotype A or CYP2C9 variant allele) (67). Eighteen percent of the Caucasian population had a combination of at least one VKORKC1 haplotype A and at least one CYP2C9 variant (67). Hence, caution is required to identify the predictive SNPs and haplotypes in all populations before proposing pharmacogenetic-based warfarin dosing regimens (67).

Dual functionality of factor V

Factor V through its APC resistant properties is well known to have a strong prothrombotic effect (68). Factor V also has anticoagulant properties, as it participates in the degradation of Factor VIIIa by APC and Protein S (69,70). Cleavage of FV by APC at position 506 is essential for FV to function as a cofactor. Thus, FV Leiden, lacking the APC cleavage site at position 506, is not capable of inactivating FVIII and hence procoagulant through yet another mechanism. The APC cofactor function of FV and the FXa cofactor role of FVa are the two opposing functions, which render FV-derived proteins manifest dual functions, viz., more procoagulant and less anticoagulant functions. This dual functionality of FV is important since there is a relatively high frequency of FV Leiden mutations in Caucasian population. Interestingly, heterozygous carriers of FV Leiden were reported to be protected against death from sepsis (71) although the survival benefits in both humans and mice are not as strong as initially reported (72,73). Besides FV Leiden variation at Arg 506, variations at Arg306, the other major cleavage sites in FV include FV Hong Kong (R306G, Arg306Gly, A1090G) and FV Cambridge (R306T, Arg306Thr, G1091C) (74,75) and were shown to have mild form of APC resistance in vitro (76,77). Factor V

Liverpool is a variant displaying APC resistance (78). The dual function of FV, the thrombotic function (79,80), and the anticoagulant side (81) need further research, especially because of the polymorphic nature of protein V-derived proteins.

COL4A1 Mutations and predisposition to hemorrhagic stroke

It has recently been reported that mutation in the mouse Col4a1 gene, encoding procollagen type IV α1, a basement membrane protein, predisposes both newborn and adult mice to intracerebral hemorrhage. A COL4A1 mutation was identified in a human family with small-vessel disease (82). It was concluded that persons with COL4A1 mutations might be predisposed to intracerebral hemorrhage especially after environmental stress (82).

Conclusions

Pharmacogenomic-based personalized practice of medicine is expected to reduce the number of adverse drug effects, and drug failure rates thereby dramatically reducing the total healthcare costs. Ethical concerns with gene therapy requiring transgenic manipulations of germline cells may be minimized by focusing on somatic gene transfer instead of the germline. Advances in pharmacogenomics, metabolomics, transcriptomics, and molecular imaging techniques will revolutionize the practice of medicine in the future, provided these advancements are embraced and adapted by the physicians. Those days are not too far off, when a physician will first see the genetic profile of the patient before examining the patient and then providing personalized medical care (83).

References

1 Vogel F. Moderne probleme der Humangenetik. Ergebn Inn Med Klinderheilk 1959; 12:52–125.

2 Evans WE, Relling MV. Pharmacogenomics: translating functional genomics into rational therapeutics. Science 1999; 286:481–491.

3 MacCarthy JJ, Hilfiker R. The use of single nucleotide polymorphisms maps in pharmacogenomics. Nat Biotechnol 2000; 18:505–508.

4 Krynetski EY, Evans WE. Pharmacogenetics as a molecular basis of individualized drug therapy: the thiopurine S-methyltransferase paradigm. Pharm Res 1999; 16:342–349.

5 Drazen JM, Yandava CN, Dube L, et al. Pharmacogenetic association between ALOX5 promoter genotype and the response to asthma treatment. Nat Genet 1999; 22:168–170.

6 Collins FS. Positional cloningL let's not call it reverse anymore. Nat Genet 1992; 1:3–6.

7 Daniel Chasman R, Adams M. Predicting the functional consequences of non-synonymous single nucleotide polymorphisms: structure-based assessment of amino acid variation. J Mol Biol 1996; 307:683–706.

8 Humphries SE, Ye S, Talmud P, et al. European Atherosclerosis Research Study: genotype at the fibrinogen locus (G-455–Aβ gene) is associated with differences in plasma fibrinogen levels in young men and women from different regions in Europe. Evidence for gender-genotype-environment interaction. Arterioscler Thromb Vasc Biol 1995; 15:96–104.

9 Nishiuma S, Katio K, Yakushijin K, et al. Genetic variation in the promoter of the β-fibrinogen gene is associated with ischemic stroke in a Japanese population. Blood Coagul Fibrinolysis 1998; 9:373–379.

10 Muszbeck L, Adany R, Mikkola H. Novel aspects of blood coagulation Factor XIII. Structure, distribution, activation and function. Crit Rev Clin Lab Sci 1996; 33:357–421.

11 Poort SW, Rosendaal FR, Reitsma PH, et al. A common genetic variation in the 3'-untranslated region of the prothrombin gene is associated with elevated plasma prothrombin levels and an increase in venous thrombosis. Blood 1996; 88:3698–3703.

12 Manucci PM. The molecular basis of inherited thrombophilia. Vox Sang Suppl 2000; 2:39–45.

13 Soria JM, Almasy L, Souto JC, et al. Linkage analysis demonstrates that the prothrombin G20210A mutation jointly influences the plasma prothrombin levels and risk of thrombosis. Blood 2000; 95(9):2780–2785.

14 Folka ZJ, Lambropoulos AF, Saravelos H, et al. Factor V Leiden and prothrombin G20210 mutations but no methylenetetrahydrofolate reductase C677T are associated with recurrent miscarriages. Hum Reprod 2000; 15(2):458–462.

15 Amitrano L, Brancacio V, Guardascione MA, et al. Inherited coagulation disorder in cirrhotic patients with portal vein thrombosis. Hepatology 2000; 31(2):345–348.

16 Psaty BM, Smith NL, Lemairre RN, et al. Hormone replacement therapy, prothrombotic mutations and the risk of incident non-fatal myocardial infarction in postmenopausal women. JAMA 2001; 285:906–913.

17 Ekberg H, Swensson PJ, Simanaitis M, et al. Factor V R506Q mutation (activated protein C resistance) is additional risk factor for early renal graft loss associated with acute vascular rejection. Transplantation 2000; 69(8):1577–1581.

18 Rees DC, Cox M, Clegg JB. World distribution of Factor V Leiden. Lancet 1995; 346:1133–1134.

19 Iacovelli L, Di Castelnuovo A, de Knijff P, et al. Alu-repeat polymorphism in the tissue-type plasminogen activator (tPA) gene, tPA levels and risk of familial myocardial infarction (MI). Fibrinolysis 1996; 10:13–16.

20 Furie B, Burie BC. Molecular and cellular biology of blood coagulation. N Engl J Med 1992; 326:800–806.

21 Wartiovaara U, Mikkola H, Szoke G, et al. Effect of Val34Leu polymorphism on the activation of the coagulation factor XIIIA. Thromb Haemost 2000; 84:595–600.

22 Ariens RAS, Philippou H, Nagaswami C, et al. The Factor XIII V34L polymorphism accelerates thrombin activation of Factor XIII and affects crosslinked fibrin structure. Blood 2000; 96:988–995.

23 Kohler HP, Stickland MH, Ossei-Gernig N, et al. Association of a common polymorphism in the Factor XIII gene with myocardial infarction. Thromb Haemost 1998; 79:8–13.

24 Wartiovaara U, Perola M, Mikkola H, et al. Association of Factor XIII Va34Leu with decrease risk of myocardial infarction in Finnish males. Atherosclerosis 1999; 142:295–300.

25 Goggen CJM, Kunz G, Rosebdaal FR, et al. A mutation in the thrombomodulin gene 127G to A coding for Ala25Thr and the risk of myocardial infarction in men. Thromb Haemost 1998; 80:743–748.

26 Li YH, Chen JH, Wu HL, et al. G-33A mutation in the promoter region of thrombomodulin gene and its association with coronary artery disease and plasma soluble thrombomodulin levels. Am J Cardiol 2000; 85:8–12.

27 Li YH, Chen CH, Yeh PS, et al. Functional mutation in the promoter region of thrombomodulin gene in relation to carotid atherosclerosis. Atherosclerosis 2001; 154:713–719.

28 Kleesiek K, Schmidt M, Gotting C, et al. A first mutation in the human tissue factor pathway inhibitor gene encoding [P151L] TFPI. Blood 1998; 92:3976–3977.

29 Moatti D, Seknadji P, Galand C, et al. Polymorphisms of the tissue factor pathway inhibitor (TFPI) gene in patients with acute coronary syndromes and in healthy subjects: impact of the V264M substitution on plasma levels of TFPI. Arterioscler Thromb Vasc Biol 1999; 19:862–869.

30 Kleesiek K, Schmidt M, Gotting C, et al. The 536C→T transition in the human tissue factor pathway inhibitor (TFPI) gene is statistically associated with a higher risk for venous thrombosi. Thromb Haemost 1999; 82:1–5.

31 Moatti D, Haidar B, Fumeron F, et al. A new T-287C polymorphism in the 5′ regulatory region of the tissue factor pathway inhibitor gene. Association study of the T-287C and 3-399T polymorphisms with coronary artery disease and plasma TFPI levels. Thromb Haemost 2000; 84:244–249.

32 Ameziane N, Seguin C, Borgel D, et al. The −33T→C polymorphism in intron 7 of the TFPI gene influences the risk of venous thromboembolism. Independently of Factor V Leiden and Prothrombin mutations. Thromb Haemost 2002; 88:195–199.

33 Merati GB, Biguzzi F, Oganesyan N, et al. A 23 bp insertion in the endothelial protein C receptor (EPCR) gene in patients with myocardial infarction and deep vein thrombosis. Thromb Haemost 1999; 82:507.

34 Afshar-Kharghan V, Khoshnevis-Als M, Lopez J. A Kozac sequence polymorphism is a major determinant of the surface levels of a platelet adhesion receptor. Blood 1999; 94(1):186–191.

35 Higashi MK, Veenstra DL, Kondo LM, et al. Association between CYP2C9 genetic variants and anticoagulation-related outcomes during warfarin therapy. JAMA 2002; 287(13):1690–1698.

36 Goto S. Role of von Willebrand factor for the onset of arterial thrombosis. Clin Lab 2001; 47:327–334.

37 Huisinga EG, Tsuji S, Romjin RAP, et al. Structures of glycoprotein Ibα and its complex with von Willebrand Factor A1 domain. Science 2002; 297:1176–1179.

38 Wang L, Fan C, Topol E, et al. Mutation of MEF2A in an inherited disorder with features of coronary artery disease. Science 2003; 302:1578–1581.

39 Yamada Y, Izawa H, Ichihara S, et al. Prediction of the risk of myocardial infarction from polymorphisms in candidate genes. N Engl J Med 2002; 347:1916–1923.

40 Ozaki K, Ohnishi Y, Iida A, et al. Functional SNPs in the lymphotoxin alpha gene that are associated with susceptibility to myocardial infarction. Nat Genet 2002; 32:650–654.

41 Tobin MD, Braund PS, Burton PR, et al. Genotypes and haplotypes predisposing to myocardial infarction: a multilocus case-control study. Eur Heart J 2004; 25:459–467.

42 Helgadottir A, Manolescu A, Thorleifsson G, et al. The gene encoding 5-lipoxygenase activating protein confers risk of myocardial infarction and stroke. Nat Genet 2004; 36:233–239.

43 McCarthy JJ, Parker A, Salem R, et al. Large scale association analysis for identification of genes underlying premature coronary heart disease: cumulative perspective from analysis of 111 candidate genes. J Med Genet 2004; 41:334–341.

44 Liew CC, Dzau VJ. Molecular genetics and genomics of heart failure. Nat Rev Genet 2004; 5:811–825.

45 Kittleson MM, Minhas KM, Irizarry RA, et al. Gene expression analysis of ischemic and nonischemic cardiomyopathy. Shared and distinct genes in the development of heart failure. Physiol Genomics 2005; 21:299–307.

46 Xu J, Chen Y, Li M. High-throughput technologies for studying potassium channels—progresses and challenges. Circ Res 2004; 3:32–38.

47 Yellen G. The voltage-gated potassium channels and their relatives. Nature 2002; 419:35–42.

48 Jan LY, Jan YN. Cloned potassium channels from eukaryotes and prokaryotes. Annu Rev Neurosci 1997; 20:91–123.

49 Jan LY, Jan YN. Structural elements involved in specific K+ channel functions. Annu rev Physiol 1992; 54:537–555.

50 Roberts R. Genomics and cardiac arrhythmias. J Am Coll Cardiol 2006; 47:9–21.

51 Centers for disease control, National Center for Health Statatistics. Available at: http://www.cdc.gov/needphp/burdenbook2002/. Accessed July 18:2005.

52 American Heart Association. 2001 Heart and Stroke Statistical Update. Dallas, TX: American Heart Association, 2000.

53 MacNeill BD, Jang IK, Bouma BE, et al. Focal and multi-focal plaque macrophage distributions in patients with acute and stable presentations of coronary artery disease. J Am Coll Cardiol 2004; 44:972–979.

54 Tsimikas S, Paluski W, Halpern SE, et al. Radiolabeled MDA2, an oxidation-specific, monoclonal antibody, identifies native atherosclerotic lesions in vivo. J Nucl Cardiol 1999; 6:41–53.

55 Jaffer FA, Weissleder R. Seeing within: molecular imaging of the cardiovascular system. Circ Res 2004; 94:433–445.

56 Lanza GM, Winter PM, Caruthers SD, et al. Resonance molecular imaging with nanoparticles. J Nucl Cardiol 2004; 11:733–743.

57 Zee RYL, Cook NR, Cheng S, et al. Multi-locus candidate gene polymorphisms and risk of myocardial: a population-based, prospective genetic analysis. J Thromb Haemost 2006; 4:341–348.

58 Reitsma PH. When is cardiovascular genomics delivering on its promise? J Thromb Haemost 2006; 4:339–340.

59 Helgadottir A, Manolescu A, Helgason A, et al. A variant of the gene encoding leukotriene A4 hydrolase confers ethnicity-specific risk of myocardial infarction. Nat Genet 2006; 38:68–74.

60 Lysenko V, Almgren P, Anevski D, et al. Genetic prediction of future type 2 diabetes. PLOS Med 2005; 2:e345.

61 Rieder MJ, Reiner AP, Gage BF. Effect of VKORKC1 haplotypes on transcriptional regulation and warfarin dose. NEJM 2005; 352:2285–2293.

62 D'Andrea G, D'Ambrosio RL, Di Perna P, et al. A polymorphism in the VKORKC1 gene is associated with an interindividual variability in the dose-anticoagulant effect of warfarin. Blood 2005; 105:645–649.

63 Scone EA, Khan TI, Wynne HA, et al. The impact of CYP2C9 and VKORKC1 genetic polymorphism and patient characteristics upon warfarin dose requirements: proposal for a new dosing regimen. Blood 2005; 106:2329–2333.

64 Gage BF, Eby C, Milligan PE, et al. Use of pharmacogenetics and clinical factors to predict the maintenance dose of warfarin. Thromb Haemost 2004; 91:87–94.

65 Shikata E, Ieiri I, Ishiguru S, et al. Association of pharmacokinetics (CYP2C9) and pharmacodynamics (factors II, VII, IX, and X; protein S and C; and gamma-glutamyl carboxylase) gene variants with warfarin sensitivity. Blood 2004; 103:2630–2635.

66 Veenstra DL, You JH, Rieder MJ, et al. Association of vit K epoxide reductase complex I (VKORKC1) variants with warfarin dose in a Hong Kong Chinese patient population. Pharmacogenet Genomics 2005; 15:687–691.

67 Marsh S, King CR, Porche-Sorbet RM, et al. Population variation in VKORKC1 haplotype structure. J Thromb Haemost 2006; 4:473–474.

68 Dahlback B, Carlsson M, Svensson PJ. Familial thrombophilia due to a previously unrecognized mechanism characterized by poor anticoagulant response to activated protein C: prediction of a cofactor to activated protein C. Proc Natl Acad Sci USA 1993; 90:1004–1008.

69 Nicolaes GAF, Dahlback B. Factor V and thrombotic disease. Description of a Janus-faced protein. Arterioscler Thromb Vasc Biol 2002; 22:530–538.

70 Castoldi E, Rosing J. Factor V Leiden: a disorder of factor V anticoagulant function. Curr Opin Hematol 2004; 11:176–181.

71 Kerlin BA, Yan SB, Isermann BH, et al. Survival advantage associated with heterozygous Factor V Leiden mutation in patients with severe sepsis and in mouse endotoxemia. Blood 2003; 102:3085–3092.

72 Yan SB, Nelson DR. Effect of factor V Leiden polymorphism in severe sepsis and on treatment with recombinant human activated protein C. Crit Care Med 2004; 32:S239–S246.

73 Weiler H, Kerlin B, Lytle MC. Factor V Leiden polymorphism modifies sepsis outcome: evidence from animal studies. Crit Care Med 2004; 32:S233–S238.

74 Chan WP, Lee CK, Kwong YL, et al. A novel mutation of Arg306 of factor V gene in Hong Kong Chinese. Blood 1998; 91:1135–1139.

75 Williamson D, Brown K, Luddington R, et al. Factor V Cambridge: a new mutation (Arg306→Thr) associated with resistance to activated protein C. Blood 1998; 91:1140–1144.

76 Norstrom E, Thorelli E, Dahlback B. Functional characterization of recombinant FV Hong Kong and FV Cambridge. Blood 2002; 100:524–530.

77 van der Neut Kolfschotten M, Dirven RJ, Vos HL, et al. The activated protein C (APC)-resistant phenotype or APC cleavage site mutants of recombinant factor V in a reconstituted plasma model. Blood Coagul Fibrinolysis 2002; 13:207–215.

78 Mumford AD, McVey JH, Morse CV, et al. Factor V 1359T: a novel mutation associated with thrombosis and resistance to activated protein C. Br J Haematol 2003; 123:496–501.

79 Kamphuisen PW, Rosendal FR, Eikenboom JC, et al. Factor V antigen levels and venous thrombosis risk profile, interaction with factor V Leiden, and relation with factor VIII antigen levels. Arterioscler Thromb Vasc Biol 2000; 20:1382–1386.

80 Asselta R, Tenchini ML, Duga S. Inherited defects of coagulation factor V: the hemorrhagic side. J Thromb Haemost 2006; 4:26–34.

81 Vos HL. Inherited defects of coagulation Factor V: the thrombotic side J Thromb Haemost 2006; 4:35–40.

82 Gould DB, Phalan C, van Mil SE, et al. Role of COL4A1 in small-vessel disease and hemorrhagic stroke. N Engl J Med 2006; 354:1489–1496.

83 Iqbal O. Pharmacogenomics in anticoagulant drug development. Pharmacogenomics 2002; 3(6):823–828.

48

Carotid artery stenting

Amir Halkin, Sriram S. Iyer, Gary S. Roubin, and Jiri Vitek

Introduction

Carotid artery stenting (CS), a less invasive intervention than carotid endarterectomy (CEA), has emerged as a safe and effective method for revascularization of extra-cranial carotid artery stenosis. Recent observational (1–4) and randomized (5,6) trials in well-defined patient subsets have shown that the risk of major procedure-related complications, i.e., stroke and death, is comparable when these interventions are performed in skilled hands. In patients at high risk for CEA, carotid stenting has been established as the revascularization strategy of choice (4). Multicenter, randomized trials [carotid revascularization endarterectomy vs. stent trial (CREST); asymptomatic carotid stenosis stenting versus endarterectomy trial (ACT 1)] are in progress to assess the applicability of carotid stenting in a broader clinical spectrum, i.e., asymptomatic patients with severe carotid artery stenosis and patients at low surgical risk with CEA.

With the ongoing refinement of endovascular devices and techniques for carotid revascularization, catheter-based therapy has become technically feasible in most patients. Notwithstanding, appropriate case selection is required to ensure procedural safety. Here within we review new concepts pertaining to patient selection and technical procedural considerations that we consider crucial for enhancing clinical outcomes following carotid stenting.

The evolution of endovascular carotid revascularization: historical perspectives

Carotid revascularization, initially by CEA, was introduced in early 1950s as a method to prevent stroke due to atherosclerosis of the carotid bifurcation and internal carotid artery (ICA). At least four prospective randomized trials have demonstrated that CEA compared with medical therapy reduces the risk of stroke in patients with carotid artery stenosis (7–10), with the magnitude of clinical benefit dependent on symptom status, lesion severity, and the risk of surgery-related complications. While perioperative death and stroke rates were low in the highly selected patients enrolled in these trials, the risk for other complications causing significant morbidity was not negligible. For example, in the North American Symptomatic Carotid Endarterectomy trial (NASCET) cranial nerve damage and serious medical complications occurred in 5.6% and 8.1% of patients, respectively (11,12).

Effective application of carotid angioplasty began in the mid 1970s (13,14) and rapidly developed during the following two decades (15–19). The first rigorous, prospective study of carotid stenting entailing independent neurologic evaluation at baseline and at 30 days post procedure was instigated in 1994 (20). This study, as well as the experience of others (21,22), demonstrated that in the hands of experienced operators carotid stenting resulted in acceptable outcomes. While stenting compared with balloon angioplasty significantly enhanced the safety and late outcomes (primarily the risk of restenosis) of endovascular carotid revascularization, atherembolism from the intervention site remained the Achilles heel of catheter-based interventions. The development of embolic protection methods has in large provided an answer to this problem. From Vitek's early description of innominate artery angioplasty with occlusive balloon protection of the common carotid artery (CCA) (23), through pioneering work by Theron (24) and Henry (25), distal (26) and proximal (27) antiembolic protection technology has developed with impressive rapidity. The availability of multiple embolic protection systems has been shown in many single and multicenter registries to confer a remarkably low risk of embolic complications following carotid stenting (28–32). Thus, the technical feasibility of carotid stenting, its simplicity compared with CEA and the low morbidity afforded by distal protection devices and refinements in the process of case selection have accelerated the acceptance and utilization of this procedure.

Clinical outcomes and the impact of embolic protection devices

Procedural neurologic complications are due primarily to embolization of atheromatous material from the aortic arch or the carotid intervention site (31,33,34). Embolic protection devices (EPDs) that eliminate liberated atheromatous debris from the circulation have had a significant impact on the safety of carotid stenting, and a number of such protection devices have recently been introduced and are under clinical evaluation (26). In the European Arbeitsgemeinschaft Leitende Kardiologische Krankenhausärzte (ALKK; n = 1483) registry (35), use of an EPD (n = 668) compared with no such use (n = 815) was associated with significantly lower in-hospital rates of stroke (1.7% vs. 4.1%, p = 0.007) and stroke or death (2.1% vs. 4.9%, p = 0.004). Our own group's experience in more than 1300 carotid stent procedures has recently been presented (36). In a prospective registry, carotid stenting procedures with (n = 538) versus without (n = 775) embolic protection were associated with lower 30-day rates of any stroke (1.9% vs. 5.8%, respectively, p = 0.0003) and stroke or death (2.4% vs. 6.5%, respectively, p = 0.001). Utilization of embolic protection was the strongest multivariate predictor of freedom from periprocedural stroke. The impact of EPD use on stroke risk was most pronounced in patients >80 years (n = 220), in whom 30-day rates of any stroke or major stroke were significantly lowered by EPD use (6.6% vs. 15.4%, p = 0.02; 0.8% vs. 2.3%, p < 0.001, respectively). A meta-analysis of earlier studies has reported similar findings (37). Most recently, the stent-supported percutaneous angioplasty of the carotid artery versus endarterectomy (SPACE) randomized controlled trial, comparing carotid stenting with CEA in symptomatic patients (n = 1200) has been published (5). With EPDs used in only 27% of patients randomized to endovascular therapy, the rates of the 30-day composite endpoint (all-cause mortality or any ipsilateral stroke) was 6.84% in carotid stenting patients (vs. 6.34% in CEA patients, p = NS, OR = 1.09, 95% CI, 0.69–1.72).

Randomized trial data suggest that unprotected carotid angioplasty can be performed with results comparable to those of CEA (5,6), and some authors have suggested that filter-type EPDs use might be associated with an increased propensity to embolism (38). Nevertheless, we believe that utilization of embolic protection should be considered the standard of care in carotid stenting. When use of an EPD is precluded by anatomical factors, alternative treatment strategies (CEA, medical therapy) must be strongly considered.

Late neurologic events (occurring more than 30 days following angioplasty) and restenosis complicating carotid stenting are rare. In the stenting and angioplasty with protection in patients at high risk for endarterectomy (SAPPHIRE) trial, the one-year rate of major ipsilateral stroke following carotid stenting was 0.0% (vs. 3.5% with CEA, p = 0.02) (4). In the prospective carotid stenting registry reported by Roubin

et al. follow-up, available in 99.6% of 528 patients, ranged from six months to five years (mean 17 months) (1). Freedom from any ipsilateral stroke after the first postprocedural month was ≈99% and the rate of restenosis requiring reintervention was only 3%. Gray et al. performed clinical follow-up and serial imaging studies in 136 patients after carotid stenting, demonstrating angiographic restenosis in four patients (3.1%) at six-month follow-up, an additional two cases between six and twelve months, with no further restenosis or any major ipsilateral strokes at two-year follow-up (39). Bosiers et al. recently reported the long-term outcomes of 2167 patients undergoing successful carotid angioplasty (stenting rate in ≈95%). At five-year follow-up, approximately 85% of patients were alive and free from ipsilateral stroke, with restenosis rates <4% (40). Other centers have also witnessed low rates of late adverse events, with long-term freedom of death, ipsilateral major stroke, or restenosis in excess of 95% (41). The available data thus demonstrate that in a broad spectrum of patients, the excellent early results of carotid stenting are durable in the long term.

Indications

Candidates for carotid revascularization include patients with symptomatic carotid lesions and asymptomatic patients, usually diagnosed as the result of a screening procedure. In general, the indications for carotid revascularization are dependent on the symptomatic status of the patient and on lesion severity, and are similar for the endovascular and surgical strategies (Table 1) (42–45).

Carotid stenting is particularly useful in the presence of specific clinical and/or anatomical features indicative of a high risk for perioperative complications after CEA. The randomized SAPPHIRE trial compared CEA with carotid stenting with use of an EPD in 334 patients considered at high risk for open surgical intervention due to coexistent vascular disease or medical comorbidities (4). Enrollment required lesion severity ≥50% in symptomatic patients, or ≥80% in asymptomatic patients (the latter accounting for ≈71% of the trial population). Though by intention to treat the differences in one-year rates of the individual major adverse events rates favoring carotid stenting over CEA did not attain statistical significance [death (7.4% vs. 13.5%, p = 0.08), any stroke (6.2% vs. 7.9%, p = 0.60), major ipsilateral stroke (0.6% vs. 3.3%, p = 0.09), myocardial infarction (3.0% vs. 7.5%, p = 0.07)], the composite endpoint occurred significantly less frequently with carotid stenting than with CEA (12.2% vs. 20.1%, respectively, 0.053). At one year, the requirement for repeated carotid revascularization procedures was lower in patients treated with stenting versus CEA (0.6% vs. 4.3%, p = 0.04). Notably, carotid stenting was entirely devoid of cranial nerve injury, which occurred in 5.3% of CEA patients. Recent prospective registries of carotid stenting in patients at high risk for CEA are consistent with the SAPPHIRE trial, reporting

Table 1 Indications for carotid artery revascularization

Indication level	Symptomatic stenosis	Asymptomatic stenosis
Proven	70–99% stenosis	>60% stenosis
	Periprocedural complication risk <6%	Periprocedural complication risk <3%
		Life expectancy >5 yrs
Acceptable	50–69% stenosis	>60% stenosis
	Periprocedural complication risk <3%	Periprocedural complication risk <3%
		Simultaneous CABG
Unacceptable	<29% stenosis	<60% stenosis
	Or	Or
	Periprocedural complication risk >6%	Periprocedural complication risk >5%
		No indication for CABG

Abbreviation: CABG, coronary artery bypass graft surgery.
Source: From Refs. 42–45.

30-day major adverse event rates <8% (2,3). Thus, patients who have serious comorbid medical and/or anatomical conditions that increase the risk from an open surgical approach or general anesthesia should be primary candidates for carotid stenting. These conditions include advanced age, significant cardiac and pulmonary disease, prior neck irradiation or radical surgery, restenosis following endarterectomy, contralateral carotid occlusion, high lesions behind the mandible and low lesions that would require thoracic exposure. Randomized trials comparing carotid stenting and CEA in patients at low surgical risk are in progress.

Carotid stenting has a number of notable relative contraindications. In patients who are intolerant of or noncompliant with antiplatelet agents, CEA should be strongly considered. Similarly, in patients planned for a major surgical procedure within three to four weeks that will require the cessation of antiplatelet therapy, CEA may be a better option than carotid stenting. A large thrombus burden as well as specific angiogrpahic findings discussed in detail below should be excluded prior to carotid stenting. Intracranial arterial stenoses, arteriovenous malformations, or stable aneurysms are not necessarily contraindications for CS. However, in the latter case, stringent control of blood pressure and careful modulation of anticoagulation is mandatory. While contrast nephropathy is an important consideration in all patients exposed to radiographic dye, this seldom represents a contraindication to carotid stenting since experienced operators should rarely require ≥75 cc of contrast material to complete the procedure.

Patient selection

The risk of stroke due to carotid artery stenosis treated conservatively is primarily dependent on two features: (i) Angiographic lesion severity; (ii) patient symptom status

(7,9,45,46). In this regard, it is important to note that the methods for the measurement of the degree of carotid stenosis have varied among trials, so that application of the ECST methodology results in greater degrees of stenosis for a given lesion than the NASCET methodology (44,47). It is also noteworthy that the risk of periprocedural complications following CEA appears to be largely independent of the degree of the stenosis (10), and the available data suggest that the same holds true for carotid stenting (unless the lesion contains a large thrombus load) (1,40,48).

Symptomatic patients

Given the demonstrated benefit of revascularization over medical therapy in the management of severely stenotic lesions [70–99% diameter stenosis by the NASCET criteria (44,47,49)] associated with recent ipsilateral symptoms (<6 mo), CEA in these patients has been considered indicated when the periprocedural risk of death or stroke is <6% (43). The same is applicable to carotid stenting. Available data demonstrate that the rates of periprocedural death or disabling stroke following carotid stenting are generally below 6%, even without the universal use of EPDs (1,5,50) and in patients high risk for CEA (2–4).

The risk of recurrent ipsilateral neurologic events with medical management is much lower for moderate (50–69% by the NASCET criteria) compared with severe carotid lesions (10). Since the potential benefit of any revascularization procedure is dependent on lesion severity (45) in patients with moderate or borderline stenoses the risk-benefit ratio of carotid stenting should carefully be weighed.

Asymptomatic patients

Stroke prevention in asymptomatic patients requires special consideration. The risk of stroke in the territory of an asymptomatic carotid stenosis is closely related to angiographic lesion severity (46). In the European Carotid Surgery Trial (ECST), the three-year rates of ipsilateral stroke with asymptomatic lesions less or greater than 70% stenosis were approximately 2% and 5.7%, respectively (46). In the medical treatment arms of ACAS and ACST, five-year rates of death or ipsilateral stroke were similar at ≈12% (7). Thus, for clinical benefit to be derived by an asymptomatic patient with a severely stenotic carotid lesion, periprocedural rates of death or stroke following carotid revascularization must not exceed 3% (9). Given the high prevalence of asymptomatic carotid disease (51,52), the

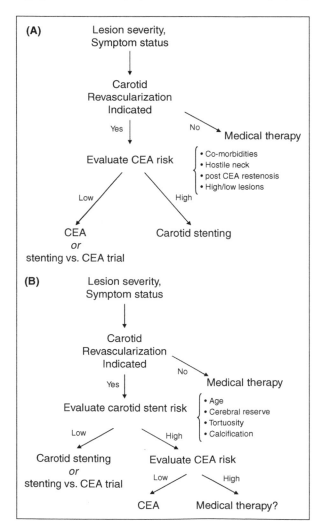

Figure 1

Decision-making in the management of carotid artery stenosis based upon symptom status, lesion severity, and estimated procedural risks. The conventional paradigm for treatment assignment is depicted in the top panel. The proposed new paradigm in the bottom panel. *Abbreviation*: CEA, carotid endarterectomy.

optimal application of carotid stenting in this patient subset must be rigorously defined (see "3% Rule" below).

Due to the very low event rates in patients with asymptomatic lesions of moderate severity (<60% diameter stenosis), it is unknown whether currently available interventional techniques can improve long-term outcomes over those achievable with optimal medical management. Also unresolved are the indications for carotid stenting in asymptomatic individuals with contralateral carotid occlusion (53) and those undergoing major cardiac or vascular surgery (54).

The 3% rule

As explained above, arotid artery revascularization can be justified in the asymptomatic patient only if the procedure can be accomplished with a complication rate ≤3% (9), a principle underlying the "3% Rule" coined by one of the authors (SI). With the widespread availability of CEA and carotid stenting, candidates for carotid revascularization have generally been selected for either procedure based on the presumed surgical risk (the "conventional paradigm", depicted in Fig. 1, top panel). Low-risk surgical patients would usually be referred for CEA or be enrolled in a randomized clinical trial of surgery versus stenting. Patients considered at high risk for open surgery were often referred for carotid stenting, arbitrarily considered a low-risk intervention since little attention had been given to definition of the risks associated with the latter procedure. However, it is of crucial importance to recognize the risks of carotid stenting and to realize that in certain patients (easily identified by readily available clinical and angiographic features), particularly those with asymptomatic lesions, the risks of procedure-related major adverse events might exceed the long-term risk of ipsilateral stroke with medical therapy. We believe that for the full clinical potential of carotid stenting to be realized, a paradigm shift needs to be implemented in the process of procedural-risk stratification and selection of patients for revascularization. This applies both to clinical practice and to the design and inclusion criteria of randomized trials. Clinical decision-making based upon these principles is outlined in the lower panel of Figure 1.

Implementing the 3% rule

In determining the risk of death or stroke associated with carotid stenting it is of critical importance to recognize four factors that have been associated with increased procedural complications following carotid stenting (Table 2). The most important of these factors is advanced age. In the lead-in phase of the multicenter CREST trial, the risk of 30-day stroke or death among 749 patients was directly related to age (<60 years, 1.7%; 60–69 years, 1.3%; 7079, 5.3%; >80 years, 12.1%, p = 0.006). Though the risk attributable to advanced age in this analysis appeared to be independent

Table 2 Clinical and angiographic features associated with increased risk for peri-procedural complications following CS

T	Risk factor	Features
Clinical	Advanced age	≥80 yrs
	Decreased cerebral reserve	Dementia
		Prior (remote) stroke
		Multiple lacunar infarcts
		Intracranial microangipathy
Angiographic	Excessive tortuosity	≥2 90°-bends within 5 cm of the lesion
	Heavy calcification	Concentric circumferential calcification, width ≥3 mm

Abbreviation: CS, carotid stenting.
Source: From Refs. 42–45.

of other clinical (e.g., gender, symptom status), angiographic (e.g., lesion severity), or procedural (e.g., use of distal protection devices) factors (55), it is likely that increasing prevalence of the other factors listed in Table 2 with advanced age accounts, at least partly, for this association. Decreased cerebral reserve is another important factor when considering the risk of carotid stenting. Carotid revascularization (carotid stenting or CEA) is usually associated with some degree of cerebral embolization that is generally well tolerated in patients with good cerebral reserve. However, patients with prior strokes, lacunar infarcts, microangiopathy, or dementia of varying stages are much more likely to experience neurologic deficits after carotid stenting. This risk is markedly amplified in the presence of an isolated hemisphere with lack of good collateral support.

While some lesion characteristics (e.g., degree of stenosis, length) indicate potential technical difficulties, the two most important anatomic findings portending an increased procedural risk are vascular tortuosity and heavy concentric calcification. Excessive tortuosity is defined as two or more bend points exceeding 90°, within a 5 cm segment spanning the lesion, including the takeoff of the ICA from the CCA (Fig. 2). Excessive tortuosity increases the difficulty of access to the lesion, may not permit device delivery, and can prevent distal positioning of an EPD with a "landing zone" sufficient for stent placement. These factors expose the patient to the risks of atheroembolism from the arch, air embolism, excessive contrast administration, bifurcation plaque disruption, and ICA dissection. Importantly, tortuosity should be assessed after the sheath (or guide catheter) has been placed in the CCA, since forces by the catheter directed toward the unyielding base of the cranium tend to exaggerate ICA tortuosity. Finally, heavy calcification is an important predictor of complications. This is defined as concentric calcification, ≥3 mm in width and deemed by at least two orthogonal views to be circumferentially situated around lesion (Fig. 3).

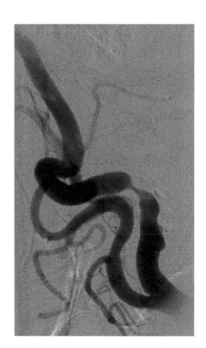

Figure 2
Vascular tortuosity predicting adverse events following carotid stenting. (See text for definition.)

Heavy calcification, especially in combination with arterial tortuosity, causes difficulties in tracking devices, lesion dilation, stent positioning, and achieving adequate stent expansion. In our experience, the presence of two or more of the risk factors listed in Table 2 is an important adverse prognosticator in patients undergoing carotid stenting. Although special techniques generally result in a satisfactory angiographic outcome, the risk of neurologic adverse events exceeds the "3% Rule" and is thus prohibitive.

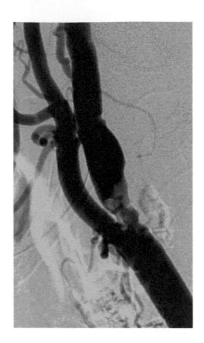

Figure 3
Heavy lesion calcification predicting adverse events following carotid stenting. (See text for definition.)

Procedural considerations

The protocol for carotid stenting has been described in detail previously (56). The following technical and procedural factors have proved important in ensuring a facile and complication-free carotid stenting procedure.

Periprocedural monitoring and management

With respect to preprocedural therapy, adequately dosed dual antiplatelet therapy is key. Patients must receive either a combination of clopidogrel 75 mg and aspirin 325 mg for five days prior to carotid stenting, or alternatively, loading doses of clopidogrel (600 mg) and aspirin (650 mg) at least four hours prior to the procedure. On the day of the procedure oral antihypertensive therapy is withheld and adequate volume status is ensured. Mild sedation may be offered to anxious patients but for the vast majority reassurance and adequate local anesthesia are all that is necessary. Avoiding sedatives enhances neurologic monitoring and limits hypotension. Continuous monitoring of pulse oximetry, intra-arterial pressure, and heart rhythm are essential as is meticulous control of hemodynamics. Intravenous atropine (0.6–1.0 mg) should be administered following placement of the sheath in the CCA to suppress bradycardic responses to balloon inflation and stent implantation. Hypotension is invariably noted after balloon dilatation of the stent, particularly in elderly patients with heavily calcified stenoses, and is generally benign. However, aggressive volume expansion, intravenous phenylephrine, and occasionally dopamine infusions are sometimes necessary. Blood pressure elevation after the relief of the stenosis can also occur and should be treated using intravenous nitroglycerine, nitroprusside, or labetalol. If distal protection is with an occlusion-aspiration system, blood pressure should be lowered *before* deflating the occlusive balloon to prevent the potential consequences of hyperperfusion (57). Anticoagulation therapy with carotid stenting is vital, but it is equally important to note that modest anticoagulation levels should be targeted. Either heparin (70 IU/kg initial bolus, targeting an activated clotting time of 200–250 sec) or bivalirudin (0.75 mg/kg bolus, followed by a maintenance infusion of 1.75 mg/kg/hr) are administered immediately with sheath insertion. Prolonged infusion of anticoagulant drugs is unnecessary and these are stopped immediately following stent deployment. Glycoprotein IIb/IIIa antagonists are not routinely used (58).

The use of 6Fr femoral sheaths and arteriotomy closure devices allows for early ambulation. This counteracts the bradycardia and hypotension commonly associated with carotid stenting. Postprocedural intensive care monitoring is unnecessary although patients should be followed in a monitored environment by staff familiar with the postprocedural course and groin access site management. Remaining sheaths should be removed as early as possible, once the activated clotting time has fallen below 150 sec. Hypotension should be treated aggressively and causes unrelated to baroreceptor responses (e.g., retroperitoneal hemorrhage) should be considered and managed promptly.

Procedural stages

The extent of diagnostic angiography is determined by the anatomic information obtained by preprocedural noninvasive studies, but should at the very least include an accurate evaluation of lesion severity; the carotid bifurcation, ipsilateral intracranial anatomy, and the anatomy of the CCA. If a balloon-occlusive EPD is to be used, it is mandatory to ensure adequate collateral flow from the contralateral carotid or posterior circulations. For diagnostic angiography, a double-curved 5Fr catheter (VTK, Cook Inc.) and a 0.038-inch angled-tip hydrophilic-coated wire are used (59). In >98% of patients this system enables safe selective catheterization of the CCA, ICA and ECA, both subclavian arteries and at least one vertebral artery. The same catheterization technique is used to introduce a 6F 90 cm sheath (Shuttle, Cook Inc.) into the CCA, generally delivered over a soft-tipped, stiff 0.035-inch guidewire (e.g., Supracore, Guidant Inc.) positioned in the ECA. The tip of the sheath is positioned in the distal CCA. "Guiding-shots" of the lesion immediately following sheath placement are performed, since ICA tortuosity might be more pronounced by the sheath (Fig. 3, top panel). Next, the lesion is crossed with a 0.014-inch guidewire, usually that of the EPD. The EPD is deployed in a distal segment of the cervical ICA. Next, the lesion is dilated with an undersized coronary balloon ("predilatation"). The stent is the deployed and subsequently "postdilated" with a conservatively sized, low profile balloon. Finally, the EPD is removed and final angiography is performed. Using contemporary rapid exchange ("monorail") systems the entire process should take as little as 10 to 15 minutes.

Special considerations

Catheter placement

Modifications of the catheter placement technique may be required when the lesion is located in the distal segments of the CCA or if the ECA cannot be catheterized. In these cases, the tip of the 5Fr catheter and guidewire (Amplatz Super Stiff J-wire, MediTech) assembly over which the 6Fr sheath is placed in the CCA is kept below the lesion or bifurcation. In cases of significant aortic arch elongation or CCA tortuosity, inability to access the ECA might result in insufficient support for sheath placement. Placing guidewires and catheters at or across the lesion to provide adequate support markedly increases the risk of embolic complications.

Crossing the lesion

Wiring the lesion and device delivery can be technically challenging. It is critical to minimize the number and volume of contrast injections into the brain, since this alone predisposes to neurologic events. At times, due to extreme angulation at its takeoff, the ICA might not be amenable to wiring. In more complex and calcified lesions, a 7Fr sheath will provide superior support. At all times the position of the sheath should be monitored to prevent its prolapse back into the arch. Appropriately shaped 5Fr catheters (125 cm right Judkin's or internal mammary catheters) can be advanced through the guiding sheath so that the tip points into the ostium of the ICA, facilitating wire entry. The EPD has to be placed at least ≥ 2 cm cephalad to the stenosis to accommodate the tip of the stent delivery system and satisfactory coverage of the lesion. With heavy calcification, it can be technically difficult or even impossible to advance the EPD beyond the lesion. In these situations, placement of a second ("buddy") wire and gentle dilatation of the lesion with an undersized balloon can facilitate delivery of the system. Anticipating this situation

and having the necessary equipment available minimizes cerebral ischemia. Frequently used for this purpose are 0.014-inch coronary guidewires (e.g., Balance, Guidant Inc.) through an over-the-wire low profile angioplasty balloon (e.g., Maverick, 2.0 × 40 mm, Boston Scientific). Following inflation, the balloon catheter is used to exchange the wire for a more supportive type (e.g., Stabilizer-Plus, Cordis Inc.). This guidewire will usually straighten the ICA permitting delivery of the EPD beyond the lesion, though it might result in significant spasm reducing flow. The tip of any wire used is placed close to the skull base so the operator must ensure its control in order to avoid distal vessel trauma. Depending on the severity of ICA tortuosity, "buddy wires" can be removed after the protection device has been placed. Alternatively, the "buddy wire" can be withdrawn after the stent has been positioned, following stent deployment and postdilated ("jailed buddy wire"), or even after retrieval of the protection device. This can be important since resistance to stent delivery might cause the sheath to prolapse into the arch, a problem that can be eliminated by the "buddy wire."

Predilatation

Lesion dilation prior to stenting is strongly recommended. Experimental work has shown that less debris is liberated from the lesion site when pre dilation is performed (29), and clinical experience suggests that this strategy is associated with a reduction in lower rates of neurologic complications (40). Atherembolism is increased when predilation is performed with large (0.035-inch compatible) balloons, so low-profile coronary balloons should be selected. When full deflation is ensured, these balloons "re-wrap" well without residual winging so that the risk of vessel wall trauma during balloon withdrawal is reduced. If the lesion is preocclusive, it is preferable to gradually step up the balloon size to minimize plaque disruption and distal embolization. In these situations, predilatation is first performed using a 2.0 mm balloon followed by a second inflation of a 3.5–4.0 mm balloon. In rare cases, mainly in heavily calcified lesions, a 5 mm balloon might be required to enable stent delivery. Long balloons (30–40 mm in length) are preferred to avoid "watermelon seed effect."

Stent selection and deployment

Self-expanding stents are routinely used because balloon-expandable stents are prone to deformation by external compression. The nominal diameter of the self-expanding stent chosen should be at least 1–2 mm larger than the largest diameter of the treated segment, usually the CCA, and 10 mm stents are used in almost all cases (oversizing the stent relative to the diameter of the ICA produces no adverse effects and provides effective trapping of plaque, thereby reducing the risk for embolization). Stent length should be adequate to cover the entire lesion, typically located at the origin or proximal segment of the ICA, such that it usually extend from the distal CCA to a healthy segment of the ICA, covering the origin of the ECA. For the large majority of cases, a stent 30 mm in length by 10 mm in diameter will provide complete lesion coverage and facilitates facile, accurate placement using "road mapping," or bone landmarks.

Though randomized trial data are not available, some have suggested that in symptomatic patients stents of the closed cell design might afford superior clinical outcome (60). Clearly, such observational data must be considered hypothesis generating and further research is necessary before device design can be selected based upon clinical and/or angiographic features.

The use of contrast injections for stent positioning should be avoided, since embolic events from air trapping may occur. Positioning the distal end of the stent in kinks and tortuosities of the ICA should be avoided. These tortuosities can be rarely eliminated, and tend to be displaced distally and exaggerated by the stiff stent. Covering the origin of the ECA with the stent is not associated with adverse clinical consequences. Follow-up arteriograms have shown that the ECA remains patent with only few exceptions.

Postdilatation

This is a critical step and requires careful attention since it is at this stage that embolic events are most likely to develop. The risk of embolization is minimized by conservative sizing of the balloon (5 mm) and by performing a single inflation. The balloon should be deflated slowly. Mild residual stenoses (≤20%) or persistence of an ulcer at the lesion site should be accepted, since aggressive stent dilatation can produce cerbral embolization.

EPD removal

Removal of balloon-occlusive EPDs is preceded by aspiration of 50–60 ml of blood using a dedicated catheter. Filter-based EPDs are removed using a dedicated retrieval catheter. Difficulties in advancing the retrieval catheter through the stent are at time eliminated by having the patient rotate his/her neck. Rarely, the filter can become obstructed by large amounts of embolic material and blood flow in the ICA is interrupted. Facile technique and optimal antiplatelet therapy prevent this complication in most cases.

Final angiographic assessment

Careful attention must be paid to the segment of the ICA that contained the EPD. Rarely, the embolic protection device causes a dissection in the distal ICA. The risk of this complication is probably greater with balloon-occlusive devices then with filter-based devices. It is not unusual to encounter spasm and kinks in ICA segments distal to the site of intervention, particularly in tortuous vessels. These are generally alleviated by guidewire removal and withdrawal of the guiding sheath to the proximal. A small dose of intra-arterial nitroglycerine (100–200 μg) is occasionally needed. Stent-related distal edge dissections are rare.

Postdischarge therapy and surveillance

In our practice, most patients are discharged on clopidogrel (75 mg daily) for one month. Patients treated for lesions related to prior neck irradiation are prescribed clopidogrel for one year. In the absence of contraindications, aspirin (100–325 mg daily) is prescribed indefinitely. Patients should have a baseline postprocedural ultrasound duplex study within one month following carotid stenting. This serves as a reference for later follow-up evaluations for potential restenosis. Not infrequently, flow velocities within the stent are elevated immediately after the procedure, despite documented good angiographic results. Evidence to date suggests that this finding neither predicts excessive progression of neointimal proliferation nor restenosis (61). Magnetic resonance angiography is not useful for follow-up purposes because of signal dropout due to the metallic stent. Computed tomographic angiography has shown some promise (62) and may prove to be the modality of choice for follow-up post carotid stenting. Significant angiographic restenosis (>80%) is an uncommon finding, occurring in 3–6% of patients (1,40,63). Restenosis is more common in patients initially treated for radiation-induced or post-CEA lesions, and can usually be managed by balloon dilatation or repeated stenting (Fig. 4).

Procedural complications

Potential complications of carotid stenting are listed in Table 3.

Bradyarrhythmias (including asystole) and/or *hypotension* are frequent in CS, usually occur during balloon inflations and generally respond promptly to balloon deflation. Prevention is by adequate hydration, conservative balloon sizing, premedication with atropine and early ambulation. Although some advocate the routine prophylactic use of temporary transvenous pacemakers in CS (64,65), we consider the risks of this procedure to outweigh any potential benefit. In one series (n = 114), a transvenous pacemaker was required in 9.6% (66), though in our experience this is needed far less frequently. Permanent pacemaker requirement is exceptionally rare. Occasionally, patients require short-term treatment

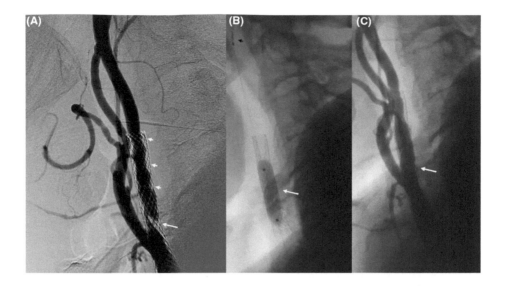

Figure 4

Cartoid in-stent restenosis. This patient underwent stenting of the right internal carotid artery (ICA) in 2000 and was followed by serial doppler studies. A scan performed in 2002 did not indicate significant obstruction within the stent. A repeat doppler study in 2005 indicated a severe stenosis of the proximal ICA, a finding confirmed by angiography (**A**), revealing a severe discrete lesion within the stent in the proximal ICA (*arrow*), with mild irregularities of its distal portion (*arrowheads*). Using a filter-based EPD (Accunet, Guidant) (**B**, *arrowhead*), the lesion was dilated with a 3.5 × 20 mm (Maverick2, Boston Scientific), followed by deployment of a 7–10 × 30 mm self-expanding nitinol stent (Acculink, Guidant Corp.) and post-stent dilatation with a 5.0 × 20 mm balloon (Gazelle, Boston Scientific) (**B**, *arrow*). The procedure resulted in the elimination of the severe proximal lesion (**C**, *arrow*). The mild distal irregularities within the stent were intentionally left untreated.

with ephedrine for symptomatic bradycardia. Hypotension may last from hours to days dependent on baroreceptors sensitivity, the stent used, and whether bilateral carotid stenting was performed. The degree of hypotension tends to be more pronounced following treatment of heavily calcified lesion. Although some reports differ (67), we find that with the aforementioned preventive measures postprocedural hypotension usually requires no specific intervention. Bed rest, sedation, or narcotics exacerbate hypotension and interfere with rapid ambulation and recovery. Importantly, alternative causes of hypotension including bleeding complications should be sought.

Table 3 Potential peri-procedural complications in CS

	Minor	*Major*
Vascular access	Groin hematoma	Retroperitoneal hemorrhage
	Femoral artey pseudoaneurysm	
Hemodynamic/arrhythmic	Hypotension	
	Transient bradycardia	
Cerebrovascular	Carotid spasm	Carotid dissection
	Compromise of ECA ostium	Carotid perforation
	Hyperfusion syndrome	Hyperperfusion syndrome
	Contrast encephalopathy	Acute stent thrombosis
	Transient symptomatic cerebral ischemia	Major ischemic stroke
	Global	Cerebral hemorrhage
	Focal	

Abbreviations: CS, carotid artery stenting; ECA, external carotid artery.

Hyperperfusion syndrome, characterized by headache, a confusional state, and at times focal neurological deficits, occurs in some patients, particularly those with a history of hypertension or those treated for high-grade stenoses (>90%) with concomitant severe contralateral carotid disease (68). This condition may not be associated with angiographic abnormalities, although CT or MR imaging will often show mild hemispheric swelling with effacement of sulci or suggest "luxury perfusion." With meticulous blood pressure control, symptoms usually resolve within 24 hours. However, some patients develop life-threatening cerebral hemorrhage. Management involves blood pressure control (preferably avoiding direct vasodilators) and reversal of anticoagulation. *Contrast encephalopathy* is a rare syndrome in which the ipsilateral hemisphere is overexposed to contrast material resulting in profound neurological deficits. CT characteristically shows marked contrast staining in the basal ganglia and the cortex. Angiography is normal. With good hydration and control of blood pressure, patients usually recover within 24–48 hours. *Transient cerebral ischemia* is a syndrome caused by cerebral deprivation of blood flow during occlusion of the carotid artery with the balloon or EPD in patients with an isolated hemisphere or in those with occlusion of the contralateral ICA (the contralateral hemisphere supplied through the anterior communicating artery). Sudden loss of consciousness, pseudo-seizures and paresis are common and completely reverse on prompt balloon deflation and restoration of blood flow. In these anatomical situations balloon-occlusive EPDs are contraindicated.

Though rare, major complications can occur even when carotid stenting is meticulously performed with an EPD. Carotid dissection or perforation is usually technique-related complications. *Carotid dissection* is most serious when it involves the ICA distal to the stent. This generally occurs when the distal edge of the stent is deployed near a severe kink but can also develop when the a balloon is infalted beyond the distal edge of the stent, when stiff peripheral balloons or stent delivery systems are advanced through bends points, or by the EPD at the site of its deploymeny. Distal dissections are best treated with appropriately sized flexible stents. A less common dissection site is in the CCA and is caused by the tip of the guiding sheath. This complication can be treated, if necessary, with another stent. *Carotid perforation* is an extremely rare event caused by balloon oversizing, usually in a misguided attempt to optimize the final angiographic appearance. Perforation can be sealed with heparin reversal, inflation of a soft balloon or a covered stent. *Stent thrombosis* is a potentially catastrophic event that is uncommon (<0.005%) with appropriate doses of antiplatelet agents and adherence to stenting techniques (elimination of significant inflow or outflow obstruction, ensuring that the proximal and distal edges of the stent are anchored in normal arterial segments, proper sizing of self-expanding stents and ensuring apposition to the vessel wall).

Major ischemic stroke due to distal embolization is the commonest serious complication of carotid stenting. Neurologic monitoring throughout the procedure is imperative (69). Changes in neurological status should initiate immediate measures to optimize blood pressure, volume status, and oxygenation as well as an evaluation of the cervical and intracranial vasculature to identify alternative causes of neurologic status changes (e.g., lesion recoil, guidewire-induced spasm, dissection). The stenting procedure should be quickly and efficiently completed. If a change in neurological status does not resolve and there are no signs of embolism on intracranial angiography, a CT scan should be performed immediately to rule out intracerebral hemorrhage. If intracranial embolus is detected, appropriate steps are taken to recanalize the occluded vessel as soon as possible. *Cerebral hemorrhage* is a devastating complication of CS. Cerebral hemorrhage has been associated with at least one, but usually a combination, of the following factors: treatment of a preocclusive lesion with severe contralateral disease (in the setting of the hyperperfusion syndrome); excessive anticoagulation; poorly controlled hypertension; stentingng after a recent (<2 wk) ischemic stroke; and presence of a vulnerable aneurysm. If a cerebral hemorrhage is suspected, the procedure should be terminated. Sudden loss of consciousness preceded by a headache in the absence of intracranial vessel occlusion and presence of moderate mass effect should alert the operator to this devastating event. Anticoagulation should be reversed if possible and an emergency CT scan should be performed. Blood pressure control and supportive measures are generally the only therapeutic options.

Conclusion

Carotid stenting with the use of an EPD has evolved as a safe and effective method for revascularization of the extracranial carotid bifurcation. In patients at high risk for complications due to CEA, carotid stenting has proven the intervention-of-choice. Randomized trials comparing the endovascular and open surgical methods in standard-risk CEA patients and asymptomatic individuals are continuing active enrollment. Until the results of these trials are available, careful patient selection, based on readily available clinical and angiographic features, must be exercised for this procedure to fulfill the potential it holds for stroke prevention. Individuals not considered ideal candidates for carotid stenting, especially asymptomatic patients and those with a low-CEA operative risk, should be offered well-validated surgical or medical alternatives.

References

1   Roubin GS, New G, Iyer SS, et al. Immediate and late clinical outcomes of carotid artery stenting in patients with

symptomatic and asymptomatic carotid artery stenosis: a 5-year prospective analysis. Circulation 2001; 103:532–537.

2   Gray WA. The ARCHeR trials: final one year results: Presented at the Annual American College of Cardiology Scientific Sessions, New Orleans, March 2004.

3   Withlow P. Registry Study to evaluate the Neuroshield Bare-Wire Cerebral Protection System and X-Act Stent in patients at high risk for Carotid Endarterectomy (SECuRITY). Presented at the Annual Transcatheter Therapeutics Scientific Sessions, Washington, DC, September 2003.

4   Yadav JS, Wholey MH, Kuntz RE, et al. Protected carotid-artery stenting versus endarterectomy in high-risk patients. N Engl J Med 2004; 351:1493–1501.

5   Ringleb PA, Allenberg J, Bruckmann H, et al. 30 day results from the SPACE trial of stent-protected angioplasty versus carotid endarterectomy in symptomatic patients: a randomised non-inferiority trial. Lancet 2006; 368: 1239–1247.

6   Endovascular versus surgical treatment in patients with carotid stenosis in the Carotid and Vertebral Artery Transluminal Angioplasty Study (CAVATAS): a randomised trial. Lancet 2001; 357:1729–1737.

7   Halliday A, Mansfield A, Marro J, et al. Prevention of disabling and fatal strokes by successful carotid endarterectomy in patients without recent neurological symptoms: randomised controlled trial. Lancet 2004; 363:1491–1502.

8   Beneficial effect of carotid endarterectomy in symptomatic patients with high-grade carotid stenosis. North American Symptomatic Carotid Endarterectomy Trial Collaborators. N Engl J Med 1991; 325:445–453.

9   Endarterectomy for asymptomatic carotid artery stenosis. Executive Committee for the Asymptomatic Carotid Atherosclerosis Study. JAMA 1995; 273:1421–1428.

10 Randomised trial of endarterectomy for recently symptomatic carotid stenosis: final results of the MRC European Carotid Surgery Trial (ECST). Lancet 1998; 351:1379–1387.

11 Paciaroni M, Eliasziw M, Kappelle LJ, Finan JW, Ferguson GG, Barnett HJ. Medical complications associated with carotid endarterectomy. North American Symptomatic Carotid Endarterectomy Trial (NASCET). Stroke 1999; 30:1759–1763.

12 Ferguson GG, Eliasziw M, Barr HW, et al. The North American Symptomatic Carotid Endarterectomy Trial: surgical results in 1415 patients. Stroke 1999; 30:1751–1758.

13 Mathias K. [A new catheter system for percutaneous transluminal angioplasty (PTA) of carotid artery stenoses]. Fortschr Med 1977; 95:1007–1011.

14 Mathias K, Mittermayer C, Ensinger H, Neff W. [Percutaneous catheter dilatation of carotid stenoses—animal experiments (author's transl)]. Rofo 1980; 133:258–261.

15 Belan A, Vesela M, Vanek I, Weiss K, Peregrin JH. Percutaneous transluminal angioplasty of fibromuscular dysplasia of the internal carotid artery. Cardiovasc Intervent Radiol 1982; 5:79–81.

16 Bockenheimer SA, Mathias K. Percutaneous transluminal angioplasty in arteriosclerotic internal carotid artery stenosis. AJNR Am J Neuroradiol 1983; 4:791–792.

17 Hasso AN, Bird CR, Zinke DE, Thompson JR. Fibromuscular dysplasia of the internal carotid artery: percutaneous transluminal angioplasty. AJR Am J Roentgenol 1981; 136:955–960.

18 Wiggli U, Gratzl O. Transluminal angioplasty of stenotic carotid arteries: case reports and protocol. AJNR Am J Neuroradiol 1983; 4:793–775.

19 Tsai FY, Matovich V, Hieshima G, et al. Percutaneous transluminal angioplasty of the carotid artery. AJNR Am J Neuroradiol 1986; 7:349–358.

20 Roubin GS, Yadav S, Iyer SS, Vitek J. Carotid stent-supported angioplasty: a neurovascular intervention to prevent stroke. Am J Cardiol 1996; 78:8–12.

21 Diethrich EB, Ndiaye M, Reid DB. Stenting in the carotid artery: initial experience in 110 patients. J Endovasc Surg 1996; 3:42–62.

22 Wholey MH, Al-Mubarek N. Updated review of the global carotid artery stent registry. Catheter Cardiovasc Interv 2003; 60:259–266.

23 Vitek JJ, Raymon BC, Oh SJ. Innominate artery angioplasty. AJNR Am J Neuroradiol 1984; 5:113–114.

24 Theron J, Courtheoux P, Alachkar F, Bouvard G, Maiza D. New triple coaxial catheter system for carotid angioplasty with cerebral protection. AJNR Am J Neuroradiol 1990; 11:869–874; discussion 875–877.

25 Henry M, Amor M, Henry I, et al. Carotid stenting with cerebral protection: first clinical experience using the PercuSurge GuardWire system. J Endovasc Surg 1999; 6:321–331.

26 Ohki T, Veith FJ. Critical analysis of distal protection devices. Semin Vasc Surg 2003; 16:317–325.

27 Parodi JC, La Mura R, Ferreira LM, et al. Initial evaluation of carotid angioplasty and stenting with three different cerebral protection devices. J Vasc Surg 2000; 32:1127–1136.

28 Reimers B, Corvaja N, Moshiri S, et al. Cerebral protection with filter devices during carotid artery stenting. Circulation 2001; 104:12–15.

29 Ohki T, Marin ML, Lyon RT, et al. Ex vivo human carotid artery bifurcation stenting: correlation of lesion characteristics with embolic potential. J Vasc Surg 1998; 27:463–471.

30 Jaeger H, Mathias K, Drescher R, et al. Clinical results of cerebral protection with a filter device during stent implantation of the carotid artery. Cardiovasc Intervent Radiol 2001; 24:249–256.

31 Al-Mubarak N, Roubin GS, Vitek JJ, Iyer SS, New G, Leon MB. Effect of the distal-balloon protection system on microembolization during carotid stenting. Circulation 2001; 104:1999–2002.

32 Guimaraens L, Sola MT, Matali A, et al. Carotid angioplasty with cerebral protection and stenting: report of 164 patients (194 carotid percutaneous transluminal angioplasties). Cerebrovasc Dis 2002; 13:114–119.

33 Cremonesi A, Manetti R, Setacci F, Setacci C, Castriota F. Protected carotid stenting: clinical advantages and complications of embolic protection devices in 442 consecutive patients. Stroke 2003; 34:1936–1941.

34 Mas JL, Chatellier G, Beyssen B. Carotid angioplasty and stenting with and without cerebral protection: clinical alert from the Endarterectomy Versus Angioplasty in Patients With Symptomatic Severe Carotid Stenosis (EVA-3S) trial. Stroke 2004; 35:e18–20.

35 Zahn R, Mark B, Niedermaier N, et al. Embolic protection devices for carotid artery stenting: better results than stenting without protection? Eur Heart J 2004; 25:1550–1558.

36 Weisz G. Distal protection devices improve the safety of carotid artery stenting. Analysis of Over 1350 Procedures. Circulation 2003; 108 (suppl IV):IV-605. [Abstract].

37 Kastrup A, Groschel K, Krapf H, Brehm BR, Dichgans J, Schulz JB. Early outcome of carotid angioplasty and stenting with and without cerebral protection devices: a systematic review of the literature. Stroke 2003; 34:813–819.

38 Vos JA, van den Berg JC, Ernst SM, et al. Carotid angioplasty and stent placement: comparison of transcranial Doppler US data and clinical outcome with and without filtering cerebral protection devices in 509 patients. Radiology 2005; 234:493–499.

39 Gray WA, White HJ, Jr, Barrett DM, Chandran G, Turner R, Reisman M. Carotid stenting and endarterectomy: a clinical and cost comparison of revascularization strategies. Stroke 2002; 33:1063–1070.

40 Bosiers M, Peeters P, Deloose K, et al. Does carotid artery stenting work on the long run: 5-year results in high-volume centers (ELOCAS Registry). J Cardiovasc Surg (Torino) 2005; 46:241–247.

41 Wholey MH, Tan WA, Eles G, Jarmolowski C, Cho S. A comparison of balloon-mounted and self-expanding stents in the carotid arteries: immediate and long-term results of more than 500 patients. J Endovasc Ther 2003; 10:171–181.

42 Goldstein LB, Adams R, Becker K, et al. Primary prevention of ischemic stroke: a statement for healthcare professionals from the Stroke Council of the American Heart Association. Circulation 2001; 103:163–182.

43 Biller J, Feinberg WM, Castaldo JE, et al. Guidelines for carotid endarterectomy: a statement for healthcare professionals from a special writing group of the Stroke Council, American Heart Association. Stroke 1998; 29:554–562.

44 Albers GW, Hart RG, Lutsep HL, Newell DW, Sacco RL. AHA Scientific Statement. Supplement to the guidelines for the management of transient ischemic attacks: a statement from the Ad Hoc Committee on Guidelines for the Management of Transient Ischemic Attacks, Stroke Council, American Heart Association. Stroke 1999; 30:2502–2511.

45 Barnett HJ, Taylor DW, Eliasziw M, et al. Benefit of carotid endarterectomy in patients with symptomatic moderate or severe stenosis. North American Symptomatic Carotid Endarterectomy Trial Collaborators. N Engl J Med 1998; 339:1415–1425.

46 Risk of stroke in the distribution of an asymptomatic carotid artery. The European Carotid Surgery Trialists Collaborative Group. Lancet 1995; 345:209–212.

47 Rothwell PM, Gutnikov SA, Warlow CP. Reanalysis of the final results of the European Carotid Surgery Trial. Stroke 2003; 34:514–523.

48 Mathur A, Roubin GS, Iyer SS, et al. Predictors of stroke complicating carotid artery stenting. Circulation 1998; 97:1239–1245.

49 Eliasziw M, Smith RF, Singh N, Holdsworth DW, Fox AJ, Barnett HJ. Further comments on the measurement of carotid stenosis from angiograms. North American Symptomatic Carotid Endarterectomy Trial (NASCET) Group. Stroke 1994; 25:2445–2449.

50 Wholey MH, Wholey M, Mathias K, et al. Global experience in cervical carotid artery stent placement. Catheter Cardiovasc Interv 2000; 50:160–167.

51 Pujia A, Rubba P, Spencer MP. Prevalence of extracranial carotid artery disease detectable by echo-Doppler in an elderly population. Stroke 1992; 23:818–822.

52 Ellis MR, Franks PJ, Cuming R, Powell JT, Greenhalgh RM. Prevalence, progression and natural history of asymptomatic carotid stenosis: is there a place for carotid endarterectomy? Eur J Vasc Surg 1992; 6:172–177.

53 Baker WH, Howard VJ, Howard G, Toole JF. Effect of contralateral occlusion on long-term efficacy of endarterectomy in the asymptomatic carotid atherosclerosis study (ACAS). ACAS Investigators. Stroke 2000; 31:2330–2334.

54 Paciaroni M, Caso V, Acciarresi M, Baumgartner RW, Agnelli G. Management of asymptomatic carotid stenosis in patients undergoing general and vascular surgical procedures. J Neurol Neurosurg Psychiatry 2005; 76:1332–1336.

55 Hobson RW II, Howard VJ, Roubin GS, et al. Carotid artery stenting is associated with increased complications in octogenarians: 30-day stroke and death rates in the CREST lead-in phase. J Vasc Surg 2004; 40:1106–1111.

56 Vitek JJ, Roubin GS, Al-Mubarek N, New G, Iyer SS. Carotid artery stenting: technical considerations. AJNR Am J Neuroradiol 2000; 21:1736–1743.

57 Coutts SB, Hill MD, Hu WY. Hyperperfusion syndrome: toward a stricter definition. Neurosurgery 2003; 53:1053–1058; discussion 1058–1060.

58 Chan AW, Yadav JS, Bhatt DL, et al. Comparison of the safety and efficacy of emboli prevention devices versus platelet glycoprotein IIb/IIIa inhibition during carotid stenting. Am J Cardiol 2005; 95:791–795.

59 Vitek JJ. Femoro-cerebral angiography: analysis of 2,000 consecutive examinations, special emphasis on carotid arteries catheterization in older patients. Am J Roentgenol Radium Ther Nucl Med 1973; 118:633–647.

60 Hart JP, Peeters P, Verbist J, Deloose K, Bosiers M. Do device characteristics impact outcome in carotid artery stenting? J Vasc Surg 2006; 44:725–730; discussion 730–731.

61 Roffi M, Chan A, Yadav J. Can ultrasound accurately predict restenosis after carotid artery stenting? (Abstract). Circulation 2001; 104:II-583.

62 Leclerc X, Gauvrit JY, Pruvo JP. Usefulness of CT angiography with volume rendering after carotid angioplasty and stenting. AJR Am J Roentgenol 2000; 174:820–822.

63 Bergeron P, Roux M, Khanoyan P, Douillez V, Bras J, Gay J. Long-term results of carotid stenting are competitive with surgery. J Vasc Surg 2005; 41:213–221.

64 Harrop JS, Sharan AD, Benitez RP, Armonda R, Thomas J, Rosenwasser RH. Prevention of carotid angioplasty-induced bradycardia and hypotension with temporary venous pacemakers. Neurosurgery 2001; 49:814–820; discussion 820–822.

65 Bush RL, Lin PH, Bianco CC, Hurt JE, Lawhorn TI, Lumsden AB. Reevaluation of temporary transvenous cardiac pacemaker usage during carotid angioplasty and stenting: a safe and valuable adjunct. Vasc Endovascular Surg 2004; 38:229–235.

66 Wholey MH, Jarmolowski CR, Eles G, Levy D, Buecthel J. Endovascular stents for carotid artery occlusive disease. J Endovasc Surg 1997; 4:326–338.

67 Qureshi AI, Luft AR, Sharma M, et al. Frequency and determinants of postprocedural hemodynamic instability after carotid angioplasty and stenting. Stroke 1999; 30:2086–2093.

68 Abou-Chebl A, Yadav JS, Reginelli JP, Bajzer C, Bhatt D, Krieger DW. Intracranial hemorrhage and hyperperfusion syndrome following carotid artery stenting: risk factors, prevention, and treatment. J Am Coll Cardiol 2004; 43: 1596–1601.

69 Gomez CR, Roubin GS, Dean LS, et al. Neurological monitoring during carotid artery stenting: the Duck Squeezing Test. J Endovasc Surg 1999; 6:332–336.

49

Anticoagulants in peripheral vascular interventions

Rajesh M. Dave, Azim Shaikh, and Mubin Syed

Introduction

There are no anticoagulants with defined indications for use during percutaneous peripheral intervention (PPI). The endovascular treatment of peripheral arterial disease expands from simple procedures such as renal artery stenting to more complex interventions such as those required to treat acute critical limb ischemia (CLI), deep vein thrombosis (DVT), and acute stroke. The disease states range from focal severe atherosclerotic stenosis to thrombus-laden lesions within diffusely diseased large to small lumen arteries. Depending on the complexity of the PPI, total procedure time also varies from relatively short to very long. All these factors must be considered when deciding the optimal choice of anticoagulant for a peripheral vascular intervention.

Procedural anticoagulants currently in use are unfractionated heparin (UFH) and bivalirudin. While UFH is the most widely used anticoagulant during PPI, there is no consistent dosing regimen and dose response variability demands diligence in monitoring the therapeutic response and duration. Bivaluridin is intended for use with aspirin and has been studied only in patients receiving concomitant aspirin therapy.

PPI is becoming a more frequent first line approach for the treatment of renal, iliac, femoral, femoropopliteal, and tibial vascular diseases. Since the introduction of angioplasty, great progress has been made in technology for use in these procedures. These include laser atherectomy, nitinol stents, thrombectomy devices, and radiation therapy. Despite technological advances, progress in anticoagulant therapy was halted until the availability of direct thrombin inhibitors (DTI).

Indirect thrombin inhibitors

Unfractionated heparin

UFH is the oldest and most widely utilized agent in PPI. It was discovered by McLean in 1916 (1). It is a mixture of sulfated monopolysacharrides with molecular weight ranging from 3000 to 30,000 daltons, with a mean molecular weight of 15,000 daltons (2). Standard UFH is derived from porcine or bovine intestinal mucosa or bovine lung.

Heparin acts indirectly at multiple points within the coagulation cascade. Its major anticoagulant effect is via interaction with its requisite co-factor, antithrombin III (AT). The heparin–AT complex inactivates factors IXa, Xa, and XIIa, and binds thrombin at its active site to prevent the conversion of fibrinogen to fibrin (3). Heparin also prevents fibrin stabilization through the inhibition of fibrin stabilization factor. Heparin has no fibrinolytic activity and therefore is ineffective as a thrombolytic (4,5).

Heparin is administered intravenously at the start of a PPI procedure either as a standard bolus injection or, as more appropriately, a weight-adjusted dose regimen. No consistent dosing regimen has been tested in a well-controlled study. The anticoagulant effect of heparin during PPI should be monitored by the activated clotting time (ACT).

Clinical indications

UFH anticoagulation is routinely used during vascular and cardiac surgery, for the prophylaxis and treatment of DVT, for the prevention of pulmonary embolism in surgical patients, and in patients with atrial fibrillation and recent embolization (6).

Adverse reactions

Heparin is associated with an increased risk of bleeding either due to over anticoagulation or the occurrence of heparin inducted thrombocytopenia. The risk of major bleeding associated with heparin is reported to be 0% to 7% (7,8). The long-term administration of UFH may also be associated with osteopenia. Other reported adverse effects include skin lesions, priaprism, and elevated liver enzymes.

The most devastating complication is heparin induced thrombocytopenia (HIT) (1). In contrast with other immune mediated thrombocytopenia, HIT is associated with thrombosis.

Therapeutic limitations

The anticoagulant activity of UFH varies among patients and therefore has a narrow therapeutic index, unpredictable pharmacokinetics, and requires frequent monitoring of the ACT. The optimal ACT for minimizing both ischemic and hemorrhagic complications during PPI in patients not treated with a glycoprotein IIb/IIIa inhibitor or thrombolytic is approximately 300 seconds.

Advantages of UFH

The primary advantage of UFH as an anticoagulant is the relatively low unit cost and familiarity with its use and monitoring by staff members during the intervention. Another important consideration in the selection of UFH is the availability of a reversal agent, protamine, in an unfortunate event of major bleeding due to a procedural vascular perforation.

Protamine

As an endovascular specialist, it is important to be familiar with the use of protamine in an emergent situation. Protamine is a low molecular weight protein that has an anticoagulant effect when administered alone. However when given in the presence of heparin, a stable salt forms to effect a loss of anticoagulant activity of both drugs. Heparin is highly acidic and forms a strong bond with the highly basic protamine molecules, forming an inactive complex. Protamine has a rapid onset of action; within five minutes of administration, it begins to neutralize heparin. It should he administered slowly over 10 minutes, with a goal of one milligram of protamine to neutralize every 90 units of heparin. Further dosing should be guided by coagulation studies.

Too rapid of an administration of protamine can have serious side effects, including hypotension and anaphylaxis. Pulmonary hypertension, shortness of breath, flushing, and urticaria have all been associated with rapid administration. Patients with allergies to fish products may be allergic to protamine.

Direct thrombin inhibitors

The direct thrombin inhibitor (DTI) is a new class of antithrombotic with the potential for improving outcomes in endovascular interventions. Thrombin is a central enzyme in hemostasis. Its multiple roles include the conversion of fibrinogen to fibrin, further amplification of the coagulation cascade, and activation of platelets. The treatment of many thrombotic disorders in cardiovascular medicine is directed toward thrombin inhibition. Heparin has historically been used as a primary treatment of such disorders, although there are several limitations that control its clinical utility including extensive protein binding and an inability to inactivate platelet bound Factor Xa and fibrin bound thrombin.

The thrombin molecule contains the following three binding sites:

1. A catalytic site responsible for the cleavage of substances (active site);
2. A substrate recognition site that also functions as the binding site for the AT-heparin complex—AT complex (exosite 1); and
3. A heparin binding domain (exosite 2) (10,11).

Heparin bound to exosite 2 bridges more fibrin onto thrombin and renders the heparin–fibrin–thrombin complex inaccessible to inhibition by AT. Such fibrin bound thrombin serves as a reservoir of thrombogenic activity capable of converting Factors V and VIII to their activated form, converting fibrinogen to fibrin, activating Factor XIII, and attenuating fibrinolysis (12). Bound thrombin also continues to activate platelets through thromboxane A_2 independent mechanisms not inhibited by aspirin (13).

Platelet bound Factor Xa is similarly resistant to inactivation by heparin–AT complex, serving as a source of further thrombin generation. Therefore, drugs such as heparin cannot fully attenuate the thrombotic process, a potentially important concern at the site of arterial injury or foreign body placement in the form of a self-expanding or balloon expandable stent.

A DTI offers several advantages over conventional heparin. They act independent of AT and are capable of inactivating free and clot-bound thrombin equally well. As a group, these agents inhibit thrombus growth and thrombin-mediated platelet activation. Several direct thrombin inhibitors have now been studied in clinical trials.

Bivalirudin

The active substance in bivalirudin (Hirulog), a direct thrombin inhibitor, is a 20-amino acids ynthetic peptide based on the hirudin template. In the Hirulog angioplasty study, 4098 patients with unstable or post infarction angina were randomized to bivalirudin or heparin before PTCA (14). The conclusion of this study was that there was no difference in the 30-day primary endpoint with either treatment. Patients randomized to Hirulog, however, did have a statistically significant reduced incidence of bleeding-related complications.

Hence, bivalirudin concurrently reduced both ischemia-driven and bleeding complications.

In the REPLACE-2 trial, 6010 PTCA patients were randomized to bivalirudin with provisional GP IIb/IIIa inhibitor use versus the current standard of heparin and planned GP IIb/IIIa inhibitor use (15). Patients in both groups were also pretreated with aspirin. Stents were used in approximately 85% of patients, and approximately 86% of patients were pretreated with thienopyridines (ticlopidine or clopidogrel). A 30-day composite endpoint of death, myocardial infarction (MI), urgent revascularization, or major in-hospital bleeding occurred in 9.2% of patients in the bivalirudin arm versus 10% of the patients in the heparin plus GP IIb/IIIa arm. Major bleeding rates were 2.4% in the bivalirudin arm versus 4.1% in the heparin and GP IIb/IIIa arm (p < 0.001). The investigators concluded that bivalirudin was effective in reducing the incidence of acute ischemic events with the added advantage of less bleeding.

Bivalirudin use in peripheral interventions

The Angiomax Peripheral Procedure Registry of Vascular Events (APPROVE), a prospective, open-label single arm study, evaluated bivalirudin in 505 patients undergoing renal, iliac, or femoral artery intervention (16). Bivalirudin was administered as a 0.75 mg/kg bolus followed by a 1.75 mg/kg/hr infusion for the duration of the produce.

The primary endpoint was procedural success defined as ≤20% residual stenosis. Secondary endpoints included death, MI, unplanned revascularization, or surgical intervention for ischemia, amputation through 30 days and major bleeding. Aspirin was administered in 96.8% of the patients and clopidogrel to 95% of the patients.

In-hospital procedural success was achieved in 95% of patients. At 30 days, the incidence of the composite of death/MI/unplanned revascularization/amputation was 1.2%. In-hospital major bleeding occurred in 2.2% of the patients. In this study however, patients with a serum creatinine >4 mg/dl were excluded. No dose adjustment was made for renal insufficiency. There was no correlation between clinical outcome and the degree of renal impairment.

In addition to the APPROVE trial, three single center studies have reported successful use of bivalirudin with similar outcomes during PPI (17,18,19). The results of these studies are summarized in Table 1.

In summary, bivalirudin use during PPI is safe and may prove to have an advantage over heparin. However, we caution the use of bivalirudin during PPI procedures attempting to cross and treat chronic total occlusions where the risk of perforation is substantial with an indication for immediate reversal of anticoagulation. There is no known antidote to bivalirudin.

Thrombolytic agents and antiplatelet therapy, including GPIIb/IIIa inhibitors, are an important modality in the treatment of peripheral arterial disease. The following section presents the latest published data supporting the use of these relatively new drugs during PPI.

Thrombolytics

Thrombolytic agents belong to the family of drugs called plasminogen activators. The mechanism of action of these agents results in the breakdown of plasminogen to form fibrinolytic plasmin. The formed plasmin enzymatically dissolves thrombus and degrades particular coagulation and complement plasma proteins. Direct acting agents are currently under investigation and include alfimeprase and plasmin. These drugs directly degrade fibrin within a blood clot due to their strong proteolytic activity, in contrast to the currently available plasminogen activators, which are dependent on the conversion of clot bound plasminogen to form plasmin.

The management of acute arterial and vascular graft occlusions by the intra-arterial local administration of fibrinolytic agents has emerged as an alternative and a frequent adjunct to surgical or endovascular therapy in a select group of patients. It is important to understand that there is no regulatory approval or labeling indication for the use of these drugs in the treatment of peripheral vascular disease.

Absolute contraindications for thrombolytic agents include recent stroke or recent transient ischemic attack (TIA) (although low dosage regimens might be considered in desperate cases), active or recent bleeding, and significant coagulopathy. Relative contraindications include recent neurosurgery (<3) or cranial trauma, resuscitation or trauma in the last 10 days, uncontrolled high blood pressure (>180 SBP, >110 DBP), recent puncture of noncompressible vessel, and intracranial tumor or recent eye surgery.

Urokinase

Urokinase (UK) was the first of the thrombolytic agents to appear in widespread use in the 1990s (20). UK is a naturally occurring thrombolytic produced by renal parenchyma and is therefore found in human urine. It has a plasma half-life of 15 minutes and when administered intravenously, it is rapidly removed from circulation by hepatic clearance.

UK is nonantigenic and its mechanism of action is much more direct compared with that of streptokinase. UK cleaves plasminogen, by first-order reaction kinetics, to form plasmin. It is pH and temperature stable. The lack of circulating neutralizing antibodies and its direct mechanism of action allow for a predictable dose response relationship.

Table 1   In-hospital clinical outcomes with bivalirudin in recent PPI studies

	Eres A n = 150 n *(%)*		*Allie DE* n = 255 n *(%)*		*Shammas NW* n = 131 n *(%)*	
Death	3	(2.0)	0	(0.0)	0	(0.0)
MI	0	(0.0)	0	(0.0)	0	(0.0)
Revascularization	1	(0.8)	0	(0.0)	0	(0.0)
Amputation	0	(0.0)	0	(0.0)	0	(0.0)
Major bleeding[a]	7	(4.7)	4	(1.6)	2	(4.2)
Minor bleeding[a]	3	(2.0)	8	(3.1)	0	(0.0)

[a]The definition of bleeding varied between trials.
Abbreviation: PPI, peripheral intervention.

Controversy exists regarding the actual thrombolytic effect of UK when administered in vivo. Experimental studies suggest exogenous fibrinolysis as the main pathway of thrombolysis (21). However, laboratory findings in treated patients have indicated less fibrinolytic response suggesting activity within thrombus also. In clinical practice, UK has produced similar results to streptokinase with less bleeding complications.

UK was voluntarily withdrawn by Abbott Laboratories in 1999 when the FDA alerted the company about potential viral contamination in its manufacturing process. In October 2002, the FDA approved the reintroduction of UK (Abbokinase®) to the market after Abbott made significant changes to its quality control and manufacturing practices.

Urokinase is intended for intravenous use only and indicated for the treatment of pulmonary embolism, coronary artery thrombosis, and intravenous catheter clearance. Typical dosages in peripheral arterial disease consist of an infusion at a rate ranging from 60,000 IU/hr to 240,000 IU/hr infused directly into the thrombus.

Rochester trial

Ouriel et al. conducted this important equally randomized trial in which 114 patients presenting with acute lower limb ischemia (≤7 days) received either catheter-directed UK or underwent surgical revascularization (22). The primary endpoints were limb salvage and survival at 12 months. The amputation-free survival rates at one year were statistically significant at 75% and 52%, respectively. Other results of Rochester Trial are summarized in Table 2.

Although there was no statistical difference in limb salvage, 12-month mortality was higher in surgical group. The authors attributed the higher mortality to cardiopulmonary complications. This is an important fact considering that many CLI

patients do have associated morbidities such as coronary heart disease, diabetes, cerebrovascular disease, and renal insufficiency.

Thrombolysis or peripheral arterial surgery (TOPAS) trial

The findings of Rochester Trial led to a two-phase randomized prospective multicenter trial known as the TOPAS Trial. Phase 1 was designed as a dose ranging study where 213 patients with lower extremity arterial occlusion of less than 14 days duration were randomized to receive one of three doses of recombinant UK (2000 IU/min, 4000 IU/min, or 6000 IU/min) for four hours followed by 2000 IU/min for 44 hours versus surgical revascularization (23). The 4000 IU/min regimen was found to be the most effective when safety and efficacy was considered. Amputation free survival was similar in both groups but patients who underwent thrombolytic infusion required much less surgical intervention. However, bleeding complications were higher in UK group compared to surgery.

In the larger second phase of the TOPAS Trial, 544 patient patients with acute limb ischemia of less than 14 days duration were randomized to receive either catheter-directed recombinant UK or operative revascularization (24). The summary of results is described in Table 3. Amputation-free survival rates in UK group were 72% at 6 months and 65% at one year compared to 75% and 70%, respectively, in the surgical group. By one year the surgical group had undergone 30% more surgical procedures compared to the UK group. However, bleeding complications were again more frequent in UK group compared to surgery (12.5% vs. 5.5%, p = 0.005). It is important to note that the bleeding rate was considerably less in patients who did not require concomitant heparin therapy.

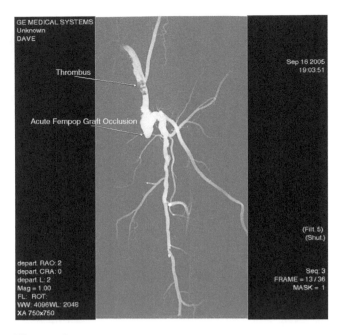

Figure 1
Patient presents with acute lower extremity ischemia,
thrombotic lesion in common femoral artery with
femoropopliteal bypass occlusion.

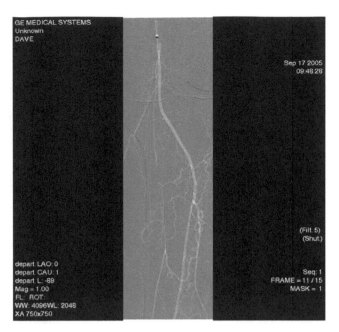

Figure 3
Crossing of femoropopliteal occlusion and selective angiography
of the graft demonstrates large thrombus burden.

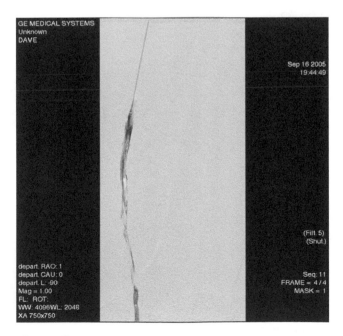

Figure 2
Distal reconstitution of popliteal artery via collaterals.

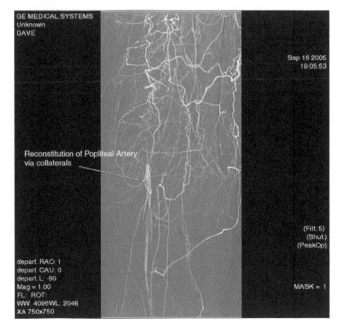

Figure 4
Placement of infusion catheter across the entire length of the
occlusion. A critical step in the procedure.

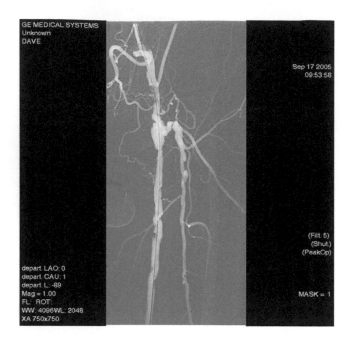

Figure 5
Post 12 hours lysis with 0.5 mg/hr tPA through infusion catheter and IV heparin.

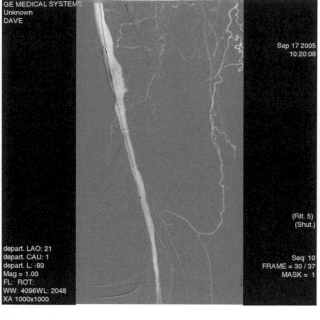

Figure 7
Post balloon angioplasty and nitinol stent placement at distal end of graft.

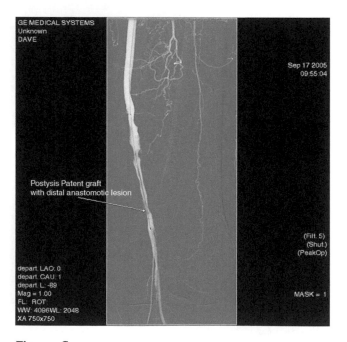

Figure 6
After thrombolysis distal anastomotic disease is uncovered.

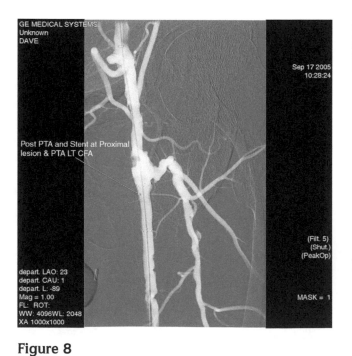

Figure 8
Post balloon angioplasty and nitinol stent placement at proximal graft occlusion site.

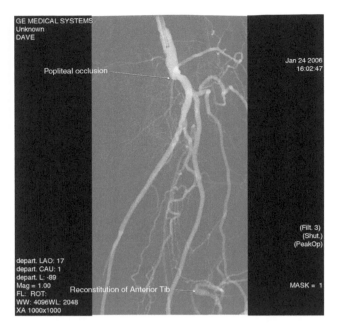

Figure 9
Patient with severe claudication and complex popliteal artery occlusion.

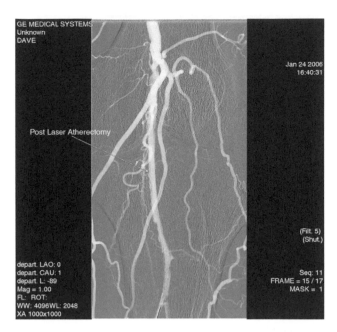

Figure 11
Post laser atherectomy and percutaneous transluminal angioplasty of popliteal artery as well as tibioperoneal trunk. IV heparin used as an anticoagulant with pretreatment with aspirin and clopidogrel.

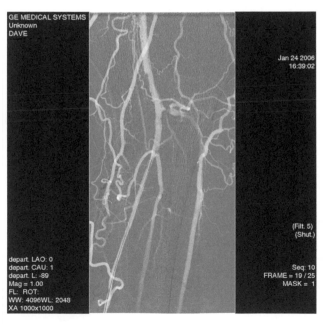

Figure 10
Post laser atherectomy and percutaneous transluminal angioplasty of popliteal artery as well as tibioperoneal trunk. IV heparin used as an anticoagulant with pretreatment with aspirin and clopidogrel.

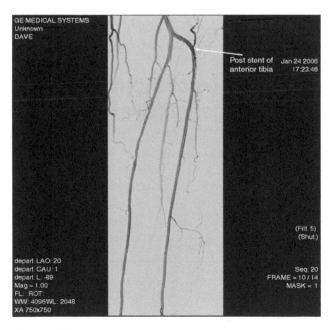

Figure 12
Reconstruction of anterior tibial artery with balloon angioplasty and nitinol stent in the proximal segment of anterior tibial artery.

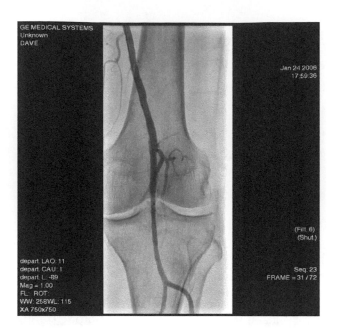

Figure 13
Final result at popliteal occlusion postnitinol stent placement.
at follow up complete resolution of symptoms.

During the time that UK was unavailable, increased experience and familiarity were gained with other agents, such as recombinant tissue plasminogen activator (rt-PA) and reteplase.

Alteplase (recombinant tissue plasminogen activator)

Tissue plasminogen activator (t-PA) is an endogenous serine protease synthesized and secreted by the vascular endothelium. It is present in all human tissues. With the exception of liver and spleen, tissue concentration correlates directly with vascularity.

t-PA is a direct plasminogen activator. Its main advantage is its high affinity for clot-bound fibrin. t-PA specifically binds to fibrin within a formed thrombus and enzymatically converts surface-bound plasminogen to plasmin. Two forms of t-PA are recognized, single- and double-chain, and both are commercially available. Both contain enzymatic activity. The endogenous single-chain molecule is converted by plasmin to a double-chain plasmin molecule.

Alteplase was the first commercially available recombinant tissue-type plasminogen activator (rt-PA) (25). It has a plasma half-life of less than five minutes and is metabolized by the liver. This agent was initially hailed as fibrin-specific unlike its precursors (urokinase and streptokinase). It was thought that this would result in a better safety profile, but this has not been born out in either the coronary or the peripheral experience, where actually there may be a higher bleeding risk as infusion time increases. Alteplase is currently indicated for use in the treatment of myocardial infarction, acute ischemic stroke, and pulmonary embolism.

STILE trial

The STILE (Surgery versus Thrombolysis for the Ischemic Lower Extremity) Trial compared catheter-directed lysis to surgery as well as differences in outcome between rt-PA and UK (26). This study enrolled patients with acute limb ischemia as well as chronic limb ischemia. Dosages of rt-PA were initial infusion of 0.1 mg/kg/hr followed by 0.05 mg/kh/hr for 12 hours. UK was given as 250,000 IU bolus followed by 4000 IU/min for four hours and then reduced to 2000 IU/min for 36 hours. Outcomes of this trial are summarized in Tables 4 and 5.

Endpoints measured included death, ongoing or recurrent ischemia, major amputation, and major morbidity. The trial was halted early after first interim analysis. This was driven by the failure of catheter-directed lysis in patients with chronic native artery occlusions.

Table 2 Major observations from the rochester trial

	Thrombolytic therapy (n = 57)	Surgical therapy (n = 57)	p value
Limb salvage at 12 months	82%	82%	1.00
Survival at 12 months	84%	58%	0.01
Hospitalization (median)	11 days	11 days	1.00
Major bleeding	11%	6%	0.06
Intracranial bleed	2%	0	NS
Hospital cost	$15,672	$12,253	0.02

Abbreviation: NS, not significant.

Table 3 TOPAS trial—summary of results

	Urokinase p_x (n = 272)	Surgery (n = 272)
Early		
Recanalization	80%	—
Complete lysis	68%	—
Hospitalization (median)	10 days	10 days
Major hemorrhage	13%	6%[b]
Intracranial bleed	1.6%	0%
1 year		
Major amputation	15%	13%
Death	20%	17%
Amputation-free survival	65%	70%
Open surgical procedures	351	590
Percutaneous procedures	135	70

[a]Percentages rounded except for intracranial bleed.
[b]$p = 0.005$.
Abbreviation: TOPAS, thrombolysis or peripheral arterial surgery.

In patients with acute limb ischemia, there was a significant reduction in major amputation and significantly improved amputation-free survival in the lysis group. Surgical treatment fared better in chronic limb ischemic group. Detailed analysis did not demonstrate differences in efficacy and safety between UK and rt-PA. However, lysis infusion time was shorter in rt-PA group compared to UK.

Once again, bleeding complications were higher with lysis compared to surgery. These complications occur early in the course of thrombolytic infusion. The duration of therapy was not longer in patients who experienced bleeding. One important observation was lower fibrinogen levels (188 mg/dL vs. 310 mg/dL, $p = 0.01$) and the partial thromboplastin time (PTT) was longer (114 seconds vs. 58 seconds; $p = 0.26$) in patients with bleeding complication, suggesting more a severe coagulopathy. Our current clinical practice guidelines include monitoring fibrinogen levels; if it falls below 150 mg/dl we decrease the dose of lytic infusion by 50% and if below 100 mg/dl, we discontinue the lytic infusion.

Reteplase

Reteplase is a second-generation recombinant tissue plasminogen activator, which lacks portions of the original alteplase. The chemical structure results in a smaller molecule having less fibrin specificity and a longer half-life than alteplase. Studies from Ouriel et al. and Castaneda et al. demonstrated

a good efficacy and safety profile comparable to alteplase in the peripheral circulation (27,28).

Reteplase is indicated for acute myocardial infarction. Due to its longer half-life of 13–16 minutes it can be administered as double bolus injections. This treatment option is of no value in peripheral arterial thrombus, where continuous infusion is the norm. Typical dosage is 0.25 to 0.5 units/hr. Castaneda et al. evaluated 101 arterial occlusions in 87 patients using three different dosing regimens of reteplase: 0.5 u/hr, 0.25 u/hr, and 0.125 u/hr. Concomitant heparin was administered in all patients. Thrombolytic success was achieved in 86.7%, 83.8%, and 85.3%, respectively. The 0.5 u/hr group received more reteplase and had higher bleeding complications while the 0.125 u/hr group required longer infusion times to achieve a successful outcome.

Kiproff et al. demonstrated efficacy of pulsed spray reteplase in 18 acute ischemic limb patients using 0.5 u/hr dosing (29). Clinical success was achieved in 89% of patients with the average time of lysis reported as 26.9 hr.

Tenecteplase

Tenecteplase-tPA (TKNase™) is a bioengineered mutant of rt-PA. The mutations were directed at three sites on the molecule to affect pharmacological improvements relative to native rt-PA. These alterations created a molecule with a longer half-life, increased fibrin specificity, and increased resistance to plasminogen activator inhibitor-1 (PAI-1) (30). TKNase can be administered by single bolus injection with less systemic plasminogen/plasmin interaction and more rapid reperfusion. These features may be beneficial in reducing bleeding complications. Tenecteplase is currently indicated for use in mortality reduction associated with acute myocardial infarction.

Early experience with this lytic in the treatment of peripheral arterial disease has been promising with equivalent safety and efficacy to alteplase (31,32). Burkart et al. published their initial experience in 13 patients with arterial occlusion and five with venous thrombosis. TNK-tPA was administered at a rate of 0.25 mg/hr with restoration of flow in all patients. The clinical success with respect to limb salvage or symptom relief was achieved in 11 of 13 (85%) patients and four out of the five patients with venous thrombosis. There were no intracranial bleeding complications.

Glycoprotein IIb/IIIa inhibitors

The use of GPIIb/IIIa inhibitors has been extensively studied in numerous large randomized controlled trials involving percutaneous coronary intervention (PCI). The advantages of their use in the coronary circulation that can theoretically

Table 4 STILE trial—outcome at one month duration of ischemia (53-3) (intention-to-treat analysis)

Event	Surgery (n = 135)		Thrombolysis (n = 240)		P Value
	No.	%	No.	%	
Duration of Ischemia: 0–14 days (count)	39		73		
Composite clinical outcome	21	53.8	43	61.4	0.459
Death	2	5.1	3	4.3	0.810
Major amputation	7	17.9	4	5.7	0.061
Ongoing/recurrent ischemia	15	38.5	34	48.6	0.328
Major morbidity	10	25.6	15	21.4	0.598
Life-threatening hemorrhage	0	0	4	5.7	0.157
Perioperative complications	8	20.5	7	10	0.098
Renal failure	0	0	0	0	—
Anesthesia complications	0	0	0	0	—
Vascular complications	1	2.6	5	7.1	0.293
Post intervention wound complications	1	2.6	5	7.1	0.293
Duration of Ischemia >14 days (count)	96		170		
Composite clinical outcome	28	29.2	107	62.9	<0.001
Death	4	4.2	5	2.9	0.617
Major amputation	2	2.1	9	5.3	0.218
Ongoing/recurrent ischemia	20	20.8	99	58.2	<0.001
Major morbidity	13	13.5	34	20	0.169
Life-threatening hemorrhage	1	1.0	9	5.3	0.080
Perioperative complications	5	5.2	7	4.1	0.712
Renal failure	1	1	3	1.8	0.618
Anesthesia complications	1	1	0	0	—
Vascular complications	4	4.2	18	10.6	0.063
Postintervention wound complications	3	3.1	8	4.7	0.526

crossover into the peripheral circulation include decreased distal microembolization, decreased vascular thrombus formation, decreased abrupt closure at the site of intervention, increased efficacy of thrombolytic therapy, and decreased long-term target vessel revascularization in diabetic subjects.

Glycoprotein IIb/IIIa receptor inhibitors include abciximab, eptifibatide, and tirofiban. These drugs disrupt the platelet aggregation cascade by inhibiting the binding of fibrinogen to the platelet membrane. The use of these drugs is established in the coronary vasculature through large randomized controlled trials. However, in peripheral disease no large studies have been conducted to prove their efficacy. It has been suggested that in peripheral vascular interventions their use may be justified when heparin is likely to be inadequate in preventing acute intraprocedural thrombosis. Such examples would include infrapopliteal angioplasty or long segment superficial femoral artery stenosis or occlusion. The current practice of administering dual-platelet function inhibitors (i.e., aspirin and clopidogrel) prior to any PPI may obviate any clinical benefit to the administration of a GPIIb/IIIa inhibitor.

Abciximab

Abciximab was the first commercially available GPIIb/IIIa receptor inhibitor. Abciximab is a monoclonal Fab immunoglobulin fragment that binds to the glycoprotein receptor on the platelet membrane. The half-life of abciximab

Table 5 STILE trial—death and amputation outcome at six months by duration of ischemia (53-4)

| | 0–14 Days | | | | | >14 Days | | | | |
| | Surgery | | Lysis | | | Surgery | | Lysis | | |
	No.	%	No.	%	p value	No.	%	No.	%	p value
Intent-to-treat (count)	40		72			101		174		
Death/amputation	15	7.5	11	15.3	0.01	10	9.9	31	17.8	0.08
Death	4	10	4	5.6	0.45	8	7.9	12	6.9	0.81
Major amputation	12	30	8	11.1	0.02	3	3	21	12.1	0.01
Per-protocol (count)	36		50			89		143		
Death/amputation	13	36.1	7	14	0.02	9	10.1	30	21	0.03
Death	4	11.1	3	6	0.45	7	7.9	12	8.4	0.99
Major amputation	10	27.8	5	10	0.04	3	3.4	20	14	0.01

is less than 10 minutes with a second phase half-life of 30 minutes. The antiplatelet effect lasts for up to 48 hours and low levels of GPIIb/IIIa inhibition may last for up to 15 days.

Abciximab is indicated for PCI and ACS (acute coronary syndrome) if PCI is planned within 24 hours. It is infused intravenously as a weight-based bolus of 0.25 mg/kg (about 17 mg). This is followed by a continuous IV infusion at 0.125 mcg/kg/min (max = 10 mcg/min) for 12 hours. The adverse reaction of mild thrombocytopenia occurs in 4.2% of patients versus 2.0% of patients receiving placebo. Severe thrombocytopenia (<50,000 per microliter) occurs in 1.0% of patients versus 0.4% of patients receiving placebo (33).

Abciximab binds to other integrins (a class of cell surface receptors involved in platelet aggregation) such as avB3 (vitronectin receptor) and the leukocyte integrin MAC-I (34). This could theoretically reduce the inflammatory response from vessel wall injury and the resulting intimal hyperplasia. This has not been proven in any large scale clinical trial.

One randomized control trial involving the use of abciximab during PPI demonstrated no long-term benefit in stent patency for complex superficial femoral lesions (35). However, a larger prospective, double-blind, placebo-controlled designed study that involved 98 patients showed that adjunctive administration of abciximab had a favorable effect on patency and clinical outcome in patients undergoing complex femoropopliteal catheter interventions not hampered by serious bleeding (36).

Eptifibatide

Eptifibatide is a lower molecular weight molecule than abciximab. It is derived from a peptide constituent of venom from the southeastern pigmy rattlesnake. This agent binds competitively to the GPIIb/IIIa receptor. It therefore has a much shorter receptor blockade and plasma half-life of 2.5 hr. This drug is eliminated by the kidney and the dosage must be adjusted in renal insufficiency.

Eptifibatide is indicated for PCI. Dosing is 180 mg/kg bolus followed by a 2.0 mg/kg/min infusion with a second 180 mg/kg bolus 10 minutes after the first bolus for 18–24 hr.

Eptifibatide has been shown to be safe and feasible for peripheral interventions (37). The INFLAME trial showed that markers of inflammation are reduced by using eptifibatide when performing peripheral interventions (38). There has been no data yet to suggest improved clinical outcomes or patency.

Tirofiban

Tirofiban is another low molecular weight nonpeptide drug, which was designed using X ray crystallography. It is a competitive inhibitor of the GPIIb/IIIa receptor. The drug plasma half-life is one to six hours. Tirofiban is excreted by the kidney. Tirofiban is indicated for use in ACS.

Dosing is 0.10 mg/kg followed by 0.15 mg/kg for 18–24 hr. Renal insufficiency patients with a creatinine clearance <30 mL/min should receive half the dose. Adverse reactions could include thrombocytopenia (<100,000) in 0.5% of patients (39).

In the peripheral circulation there has been no large study demonstrating the benefit of tirofiban as stand alone therapy. A trend toward improved outcomes was demonstrated in a study using combined therapy with bivalirudin and tirofiban for CLI (40).

Combination therapy

Combination therapy with a thrombolytic agent and GPIIb/IIIa inhibitor has been studied in acute MI. Various randomized trials (TAMI-8, IMPACT, INTRO AMI, TIMI-14, SPEED, GUSTO V) in the coronary literature have shown that combination therapy reduced thrombolysis time and permitted a reduction of thrombolytic doses by 25% to 50% of the normal dose. This is explained by the fact that thrombus is composed of both fibrin and platelets. Thrombolytics only address the fibrin component of acute thrombus. Furthermore, thrombolytics may actually activate platelets directly resulting in additional thrombus formation. Therefore, the addition of GPIIb/IIIa inhibition facilitates the efficiency of the thrombolytic agent. It is also known that GPIIb/IIIa inhibition alone can actually dissolve platelet rich clot (41,42,43).

There are several small studies examining this concept of thrombolytic infusion with GPIIb/IIIa inhibition to reduce lytic infusion time and improve efficacy as summarized below. This concept is not universally proven in these studies. A larger randomized trail is needed to examine this concept before a clinical practice recommendation can be made.

Tepes et al. reported the first clinical experience with abciximab and urokinase combination therapy in the peripheral circulation (44). Schweizer et al. used abciximab and rt-PA versus rt-PA with ASA in an 84 patient trial and found a significantly shorter duration of thrombolytic infusion was required to achieve lytic success in the combination group as well as improved clinical endpoints of less re-hospitalization, re-intervention, and amputation compared to ASA and heparin (45).

Duda et al. prospectively studied 70 patients in the PROMPT trial of UK and abciximab versus UK alone. The trial showed the combination therapy resulted in a decreased infusion time, improved amputation free survival, and improved open surgery free survival at 90 days (46). Interestingly, a post hoc economic analysis of the PROMPT trial found an economic benefit to combination therapy at 90 days based on endpoints of amputation free survival, survival without open surgery, lack of major amputation and lack of major complications. The extra cost of abciximab was more than offset by the decreased costs through improved patient outcomes (47).

Yoon et al. retrospectively compared the clinical outcomes of 17 patients who received eptifibatide and rt-PA to an age-matched group of patients who received only rt-PA. The study demonstrated a significantly decreased thrombolytic dose in the combination group (9.0 +/- 4.4 mg vs. 38.9 +/- 30.7 mg) (48). Syed et al. reported that intra-arterial eptifibatide infusion with reteplase can be successful in restoring blood flow in the presence of chronic arterial thrombus (49).

With combination therapy using reteplase and abciximab, a prospective double center study of 50 patients was reported by Drescher et al (50). Recently, however, the 74 patient RELAX trial comparing reteplase and abciximab combination therapy to reteplase monotherapy found no significant difference in safety and efficacy in all major clinical end points (death, amputation, PTA/stent, surgical revascularization). The trial did demonstrate a decreased rate of distal embolic event in the combination group (51).

Very limited clinical data is available for tenecteplase and eptifibatide combination therapy. A small 16 patient study did show feasibility of combining these agents with positive efficacy and safety (52). However, there was a negative safety correlation with the use of abciximab with tenecteplase in a recent 37 patient study (53).

A 60 patient study comparing treatment with abciximab and rt-PA to treatment with tirofiban with rt-PA found no difference in bleeding complications, re-hospitalization, re-intervention, or amputation rate. The duration of lysis was only slightly shorter in the abciximab group but this was not clinically relevant (149.7 + 18 vs. 139.3 +31.3 min) (54). The 50 patient APART trial recently compared reteplase plus abciximab or urokinase plus abciximab and found overall no significant differences except a decreased thrombolysis time in the urokinase and abciximab group (120 min vs. 200 min, p = 0.001) (55).

References

1   McLean J. The thromboplastic action of cephalin. Am J Physiol 1916; 41:250–257.

2   Johnson EA, Mulloy B. The molecular weight range of mucosal heparin preparations. Carbohydr Res 1976; 51:119–127.

3   Rosenberg RD, Lam L. Correlation between structure and function of heparin. Proc Natl Acad Sci USA 1979; 76:1218–1222.

4   Hirsh J, Warkentin TE, Shaughnessy SG, et al. Heparin and low-molecular-weight heparin: mechanisms of action, pharmacokinetics, dosing, monitoring, efficacy, and safety. Chest 2001; 119(1 suppl):64S–94S.

5   Weitz JI, Crowther M: Direct thrombin inhibitors. Thromb Res 2002; 106:V275–V284.

6   Hirsh j, Anand SS, Halperin JL, Fuster V. Guide to Anticoagulant therapy: heparin. Circulation 2001; 103:2994–3018.

7   Levine MN, Raskob G, Landefeld S, Kearon C. Hemorrhagic complications of anticoagulant treatment. Chest 2001; 119(1 suppl):108S–121S.

8   Wester JP, de Valk HW, Nieuwenhuis HK, et al. Risk factors for bleeding during treatment of acute venous thromboembolism. Thromb Haemost 1996; 76:682–688.

9   Gupta AK, Kovacs MJ, Sauder DN. Heparin-induced thrombocytopenia. Ann Pharmacotherapy 1998; 32:55–59.

10 Weitz JI, Crowther M: Direct thrombin inhibitors. Thromb Res 2002; 106:V275–284.

11 Wiggins BS, Spinler S, Wittkowsky AK, Stringer KA. Bivalirudin. a direct thrombin inhibitor for percutaneous transluminal coronary angioplasty. Pharmacotherapy 2002; 22:1007–1018.

12   Bates SM, Weitz JI. Direct thrombin inhibitors for treatment of arterial thrombosis: Potential differences between bivalirudin and hirudin. Am J Cardiol 1998; 82:12–18.

13   Direct thrombin inhibitors in acute coronary syndromes: Principal results of a meta-analysis based on individual patients' data. Lancet 2002; 359:294–302.

14   Bittl JA, Strony J, Brinker JA, et al. Treatment with bivalirudin (Hirulog) as compared with heparin during coronary angioplasty for unstable or postinfarction angina. Hirulog Angioplasty Study Investigators. N Engl J Med 1995; 333:764–769.

15   Lincoff AM, Bittl JA, Harrington RA, et al. and for the REPLACE-2 Investigators. bivalirudin and provisional glycoprotein IIb/IIIa blockade compared with heparin and planned glycoprotein IIb/IIIa blockade during percutaneous coronary intervention: REPLACE-2 randomized trial. JAMA 2003; 289:853–863.

16   Alle D, Hall P, Shammas N, et al. The Angiomax peripheral procedure registry of vascular events trial (APPROVE): In hospital and 30-day results. J Invas Cardiol 2004; 16:651–656.

17   Eres A. Use of bivalirudin as the foundation anticoagulant during percutaneous peripheral interventions. J Invas Cardiol 2006; 18:125–128.

18   Allie D, Lirtzman M, Watt DH, et al. Bivalirudin as a foundation anticoagulant in peripheral vascular disease: a safe and feasible alternative for renal and iliac interventions. J Invasive Cardiol 2003; 15:334–342.

19   Shammas N, Lemke J, Dippel E et al. Bivalirudin in peripheral vascular interventions: A single center experience. J Invas Cardiol 2003; 15:401–404.

20   Comerota AJ, Rao AK, Throm RC, et al. A prospective, randomized, blinded, and placebo-controlled trial of intraoperative intraarterial urokinase infusion during lower extremity revascularization: Regional and systemic effects. Ann Surg 1993; 218:534.

21   Varadi A, Patthy L. Location of plasminogen-binding sites in human fibrin(ogen). Biochemistry 1983; 22:2240–2246.

22   Ouriel K, Shortell C, DeWeese J, et al. A comparison of thrombolytic therapy with operative revascularization in the initial treatment of acute peripheral arterial ischemia. J Vasc Surg 1994; 19:1021.

23   Ouriel K, Veith FJ, Sasahara AA, et al. Thrombolysis or peripheral artery surgery: phase I results. J Vasc Surg 1996; 23:64–75.

24   Ouriel K, Veith FJ, Sasahara AA. A comparison of recombinant urokinase with vascular surgery as initial treatment for acute arterial occlusion of the legs. N Engl J Med 1998; 338:1105–1111.

25   Goldhaber SZ, Kessler CM, Heit J, et al. Randomized controlled trial of recombinant tissue plasminogen activator versus urokinase in the treatment of acute pulmonary embolism. Lancet 1988; 2:293–298.

26   The Stile Investigators. Results of a prospective randomized trial evaluating surgery versus thrombolysis for ischemia of the lower extremity. Ann Surg 1994; 220:251–268.

27   Ouriel K, Katzen B, Mewissen M, et al. Reteplase in the treatment of peripheral arterial and venous occlusions: a pilot study. J Vasc Interv Radiol 2000; 11(7):849–854.

28   Castaneda F, Swischuk JL, Li R, Young K, Smouse B, Brady T. Declining-dose study of reteplase treatment for lower extremity arterial occlusions. J Vasc Interv Radiol 2002; 13(11):1093–1098.

29   Kiproff PM, Yammine K, Potts JM, et al. Reteplase infusion in the treatment of acute lower extremity occlusions. J Thromb Thrombolysis 13:75–79, 2002.

30   McCluskey ER, Refino CJ, Zioncheck TF, et al. Tenecteplase: Biochemistry, pharmacology, and clinical experience. In Sasahara AA, Loscalzo J (eds): New Therapeutic Agents in Thrombosis and Thrombolysis, 2nd ed. New York: Marcel Dekker, 2003:501–511.

31   Razavi MK, Wong H, Kee ST, Sze DY, Semba CP, Dake MD. Initial clinical results of tenecteplase (TNK) in catheter-directed thrombolytic therapy. J Endovasc Ther 2002; 9(5):593–598.

32   Burkart DJ, Borsa JJ, Anthony JP, Thurlo SR. Thrombolysis of occluded peripheral arteries and veins with tenecteplase: a pilot study. J Vasc Interv Radiol 2002; 13(11):1099–1102.

33   Dasgupta H, Blankenship JC, Wood GC, Frey CM, Demko SL, Menapace FJ. Thrombocytopenia complicating treatment with intravenous glycoprotein IIb/IIIa receptor inhibitors: a pooled analysis. Am Heart J 2000; 140(2):206–211.

34   Scarborough RM, Kleiman NS, Phillips DR. Platelet glycoprotein IIb/IIIa antagonists. What are the relevant issues concerning their pharmacology and clinical use? Circulation 1999; 100(4):437–444.

35   Ansel GM, Silver MJ, Botti CF Jr, et al. Functional and clinical outcomes of nitinol stenting with and without abciximab for complex superficial femoral artery disease: a randomized trial. Catheter Cardiovasc Interv 2006; 67(2):288–297.

36   Dorffler-Melly J, Mahler F, Do DD, Triller J, Baumgartner I. Adjunctive abciximab improves patency and functional outcome in endovascular treatment of femoropopliteal occlusions: initial experience. Radiology 2005; 237(3):1103–1119.

37   Rocha-Singh KJ, Rutherford J. Glycoprotein IIb-IIIa receptor inhibition with eptifibatide in percutaneous intervention for symptomatic peripheral vascular disease: the circulate pilot trial. Catheter Cardiovasc Interv 2005; 66(4):470–473.

38   Shammas NW, Dippel EJ, Lemke JH, et al. Eptifibatide in peripheral vascular interventions: results of the Integrilin Reduces Inflammation in Peripheral Vascular Interventions (INFLAME) trial. J Invasive Cardiol 2006 18(1):6–12.

39   Merlini PA, Rossi M, Menozzi A, et al. Thrombocytopenia caused by abciximab or tirofiban and its association with clinical outcome in patients undergoing coronary stenting. Circulation 2004; 109(18):2203–2206. Epub 2004 Apr 26.

40   Allie DE, Hebert CJ, Lirtzman MD, et al. A safety and feasibility report of combined direct thrombin and GP IIb/IIIa inhibition with bivalirudin and tirofiban in peripheral vascular disease intervention: treating critical limb ischemia like acute coronary syndrome. J Invasive Cardiol 2005; 17(8):427–432.

41   Gold HK, Garabedian HD, Dinsmore RE, et al. Restoration of coronary flow in myocardial infarction by intravenous chimeric 7E3 antibody without exogenous plasminogen activators. Observations in animals and humans. Circulation 1997; 95(7):1755–1759.

42   Rerkpattanapipat P, Kotler MN, Yazdanfar S. Images in cardiovascular medicine. Rapid dissolution of massive intracoronary thrombosis with platelet glycoprotein IIb/IIIa receptor inhibitor. Circulation 1999; 99(22):2965. No abstract available.

43   Berkompas DC. Abciximab combined with angioplasty in a patient with renal artery stent subacute thrombosis. Cathet Cardiovasc Diagn 1998; 45(3):272–274.

44 Tepe G, Duda SH, Erley CM, Schott U, Huppert PE, Claussen CD. [The adjuvant use of the monoclonal antibody c7E3 Fab in peripheral arterial thrombolysis] Rofo 1997; 166(3):254–257. German.

45 Schweizer J, Kirch W, Koch R, Muller A, Hellner G, Forkmann L. Short- and long-term results of abciximab versus aspirin in conjunction with thrombolysis for patients with peripheral occlusive arterial disease and arterial thrombosis. Angiology 2000; 51(11):913–923.

46 Duda SH, Tepe G, Luz O, et al. Peripheral artery occlusion: treatment with abciximab plus urokinase versus with urokinase alone—a randomized pilot trial (the PROMPT Study). Platelet receptor antibodies in order to manage peripheral artery thrombosis. radiology 2001; 221(3):689–696.

47 Duda SH, Tepe G, Luz O, et al. Peripheral artery occlusion: treatment with abciximab plus urokinase versus with urokinase alone–a randomized pilot trial (the PROMPT Study). platelet receptor antibodies in order to manage peripheral artery thrombosis. Radiology 2001; 221(3):689–696.

48 Yoon HC, Miller FJ Jr. Using a peptide inhibitor of the glycoprotein IIb/IIIa platelet receptor: initial experience in patients with acute peripheral arterial occlusions. AJR Am J Roentgenol 2002; 178(3):617–622.

49 Syed, MI, Shaikh, A. Combination thrombolysis/GPIIbIIIa inhibition in chronic peripheral thrombosis- A case report. New Deve- lopments in Vascular Disease. Vol 1, (4) Spring 2003: 12–17.

50 Drescher P, McGuckin J, Rilling WS, Crain MR. Catheter-directed thrombolytic therapy in peripheral artery occlusions: combining reteplase and abciximab. AJR Am J Roentgenol 2003; 180(5):1385–1391.

51 Ouriel K, Castaneda F, McNamara T, et al. Reteplase monotherapy and reteplase/abciximab combination therapy in peripheral arterial occlusive disease: results from the RELAX trial. J Vasc Interv Radiol 2004; 15(3):229–238.

52 Burkart DJ, Borsa JJ, Anthony JP, Thurlo SR. Thrombolysis of acute peripheral arterial and venous occlusions with tenecteplase and eptifibatide: a pilot study.

50

Repair of AAAs

Alexandra A. MacLean and Barry T. Katzen

Introduction

Fifteen years ago, the only option for patients with large abdominal aortic aneurysms (AAA) that required either elective or emergent repair was an open surgical approach using a transperitoneal or retroperitoneal incision. Now with the advent of endovascular approaches to aortic diseases, many patients, especially those in the high-risk groups, have a minimally invasive option to permit repair of aortic aneurysms, dissections, pseudoaneurysms, and ruptures.

The endovascular procedure is most frequently used to treat infrarenal AAAs that are a leading cause of death in the older population. As our population ages, we will encounter AAAs more frequently than ever before. An aneurysm is defined by a size greater than 5 cm or 2.5 times the normal diameter of the native artery. Most aneurysms begin below the renal arteries and end close to the iliac bifurcation. More complicated AAAs exist involving the suprarenal aorta and visceral vessels and extending into the iliac arteries. The prevalence of AAAs is 3% to 10% for patients older than 50 years (1). They occur more frequently in men and reach a peak incidence close to the age of 80 years. AAA rupture is associated with an 80% to 90% mortality rate and therefore the focus of AAA treatment is on intervening before the aneurysm ruptures; elective repair has mortality rate of less than 5%.

The first endovascular repair of an AAA in a human was performed by Parodi in 1991. He made an endograft by combining a prosthetic vascular graft with expandable Palmaz stents (2). Since this milestone, the field has undergone immense growth and has benefited from many technologic advances that have permitted a wider application of this treatment modality. The patient population that has benefited most has been the population at high risk for open surgical repair. These patients have severe comorbidities including and not limited to old age, renal, heart, and pulmonary diseases.

Endovascular aneurysm repair (EVAR) of AAAs, results in a quick recovery, can be done under local anesthesia and has fewer systemic complications than open surgical repair. The goal of this chapter is to describe patient and aneurysm selection factors, the procedure and endografts, review clinical trials, outcomes and complications and address some of the controversial and challenging areas of EVAR with a view to the future.

Patient selection factors

Abdominal aortic aneurysms can present as an incidental asymptomatic finding on imaging or with symptoms, most prominently, back and abdominal pain. The asymptomatic aneurysms can be detected during routine physical examination but are more likely found during workup for other complaints or as part of a screening program for patients who are at high risk for developing AAAs (positive family or personal history of aneurysms). Intervention is indicated for symptomatic aneurysms regardless of size, and asymptomatic aneurysms with a size greater than 5 cm in diameter or with an increase in size greater than 10% per year as these groups have the greatest chance of rupture. Controversy exists as to when to intervene in females with aneurysms less than 5 cm diameter. Given smaller native aorta in this group, the aneurysmal dilatation can be greater than 2.5 times the diameter of the native aorta and less than 5 cm in diameter. Given the smaller native aorta in this group, the aneurysmat dilatation can be greater than 2.5 times the diameter of the native aorta and less than 5 cm in diameter. This smaller size of aneurysm may put the patient at equivalent risk of rupture.

There are patient selection factors for EVAR of AAAs that set this procedure apart from open repair. The durability of the open repair is well known and has been demonstrated in multiple clinical studies. EVAR on the other hand requires routine and frequent follow-up with ultrasound examination and or CT scans to evaluate the repair for the development of complications that require secondary interventions. The patient must be able to commit to this follow-up routine in order to be eligible for the procedure. In general, patients who are young with few comorbidites are still advised to undergo open surgical repair because of the demonstrated longevity of the repair and ease of follow-up. EVAR has become the procedure of choice for patients at high risk for open repair given an older age and other morbidities (3).

Aneurysm assessment

The aneurysm and aorta are assessed with a 3D reconstruction CT scan or aortography with a calibrated catheter (Table 1, Fig. 1). The fitness of the femoral arteries is evaluated as the access route. They should be greater than 7 mm in diameter and free from extensive atherosclerotic or stenotic disease.

The anatomy of the proximal neck is important; the length of aneurysm free aorta from the most caudal renal artery to the beginning of aneurysmal dilatation must be at least 15 mm to permit adequate seal of the device to a segment of normal aorta. In addition, the angulation of the neck is ideally less than 60°. The placement of an endovascular device is not possible when the neck is too large. The size limitation comes from the need to have device sizes that can be packaged into sheaths deliverable through the femoral artery. The shape of the neck is described as tapered, reverse tapered, or straight, with the latter being ideal.

The distal landing zone is evaluated for the location of the hypogastric artery and presence of iliac aneurysms. Once again, an area adequate for seal of the device to the iliac artery is located, usually 20 mm in length. If a common iliac aneurysm precludes landing the device proximal to the takeoff of the hypogastric artery, then the patient's circulation is evaluated for preoperative embolization of the hypogastric artery. This will permit the device to land distal to the hypogastric artery and backflow from this artery is eliminated by the embolization.

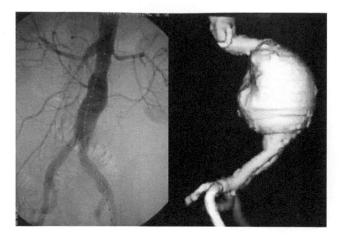

Figure 1
(*Left*) Angiogram of infrarenal abdominal aortic aneurysms (AAA) with marker catheter in place; (*Right*) 3D CT reconstruction of an infrarenal AAA.

The visceral vessels are evaluated for patency because the required coverage of the inferior mesenteric artery mandates that blood supply to the viscera be adequate from other sources (celiac and superior mesenteric arteries). With experience, some of these contraindications can be overcome with suprarenal attachment devices, additional cuffs, and limbs, but for the nascent EVAR physician the contraindications should be acknowledged and adherence to the fundamental principles of endovascular device implantation will permit good outcomes.

EVAR technology

Endograft design is derived directly from the traditional grafts used in open aortic surgery. The endograft body comes in one piece (unibody) or as a bifurcated graft (Fig. 2). The unibody endograft is designed to land into one of the iliac arteries, thereby necessitating contralateral iliac occlusion and a femoro-femoral bypass graft. Most of the procedures carried out today use a bifurcated graft that comes with extensions into the limbs and additional cuffs. This design provides greater flexibility for matching the device to the particular aneurysm features. The early endografts were unsupported throughout the body with stents at the proximal and distal ends. Today, the endografts have a metal skeleton throughout the graft providing a supported structure. The metal skeleton is covered with a fabric [polyester or polytetrafluoroethylene (PTFE)]. To prevent slippage of the endograft, it is secured either by radial force or additional hooks and barbs. The majority of the endografts are designed to fixate and seal to a 15 mm segment of normal infrarenal native aorta. The device is deployed with either a self-expanding or balloon-expanding mechanism.

Table 1   Assessment and contraindications
CT scan assessment for EVAR eligibility
Proximal neck: diameter, length, angle.
Presence or absence of thrombus
Distal landing zone: diameter and length
Iliac arteries: presence of aneurysms and occlusive disease
Access arteries (common, external and femoral arteries):
Diameter, presence of occlusive disease
Contraindications for EVAR
Short proximal neck
Thrombus presence in proximal landing zone
Conical proximal neck
Greater than 120° angulation of the proximal neck
Critical inferior mesenteric artery
Significant iliac occlusive disease
Tortuosity of iliac vessels
Abbreviation: EVAR, endovascular aneurysm repair.

The many permutations of these features have led to the generation of multiple devices employing a variety of concepts and approaches (Table 2). Two devices are no longer available (Ancure and Vanguard/Stentor) but are mentioned because some patients had these implanted and these may be encountered in the clinical setting. Four devices are currently FDA approved for commercial use in the United States (AneuRx, Excluder, Zenith, and PowerLink); the other devices are in clinical trials or in use in Europe.

With multiple devices available and increased clinical and technical experiences, it is apparent that each device has its own advantages and disadvantages. The best results can come from optimizing the type of endograft to specific anatomy of a given patient. This is less important in patients with 'ideal' anatomic features, but when features such as neck angulation, calcification, access tortuosity are encountered, one device may to superior to another for dealing with the challenging anatomy. On some occasions suprarenal attachment may be necessary and desirable, in others infrarenal fixation may be sufficient.

The procedure: start to finish

Once the patient is selected and the appropriate device is in hand to deal with the particular aneurysm morphology, the patient is brought into the interventional or operating room suite for the procedure. The procedure is now performed by interventional radiologists, cardiologists, and vascular surgeons with the patient under general, regional, or local anesthesia (4). The femoral arteries are accessed by either open surgical incisions or percutaneously. An aortogram is performed to

---

Table 2	Endo devices

Available or in trials/development
    AneuRx (Medtronic, Santa Rosa, CA, U.S.A.)
    Excluder (W.L. Gore, Flagstaff, AZ, U.S.A.)
    Zenith (Cook Inc., Bloomington, IN, U.S.A.)
    PowerLink (Endologix, Irvine, CA, U.S.A.)
    Talent (Medtronic, Santa Rosa, CA, U.S.A.)
    Fortron (Cordis Corp., Johnson and Johnson,
    Miami, FL, U.S.A.)
    Lifepath (Edwards Lifesciences, Irvine, CA, U.S.A.)
    Quantum (Cordis Corp., Johnson and Johnson, Miami, FL)
    Enovus (Trivascular, Santa Rosa, CA, U.S.A.)
No longer available
    Ancure (Guidant Corp., Indianapolis, IN, U.S.A.)
    Vanguard/Stentor (Boston Scientific Corp., Natick,
    MA, U.S.A.)

---

locate the renal and hypogastric arteries. The main body is then inserted through either femoral arteriotomy but the largest and most disease free femoral artery is preferred. The patient is anticoagulated as at this point in the procedure blood flow to the legs is interrupted by the size of the sheath; heparin or a direct thrombin inhibitor (e.g., bivalirudin) may be used (5). The location of the renal arteries with respect to the top of the endograft is reassessed. The endograft is then deployed. Next the limbs are inserted through each groin into the respective leg of the endograft. Once again the location of the hypogastric arteries is verified before the limbs are landed just proximal to their orifices or distally if the hypogastric was embolized preoperatively. A completion angiogram is performed and examined for the development of complications, especially Type I endoleaks. If further intervention is required, it is done at this point. Finally, the groins are closed either with sutures or with the aid of one of many percutaneous closure devices. The distal pulses are examined and documented for further vascular monitoring.

Endograft challenges
Ruptured aneurysm

A ruptured AAA is a devastating event with an overall mortality rate of greater than 90% and 40% to 70% of those patients who make it to the hospital alive die (1). An endovascular approach to ruptured aneurysms has been developed and involves the rapid deployment of a proximal occlusion balloon through the brachial artery to sit in the descending thoracic aorta. Some of the key maneuvers include permissive hypotension, placement of the brachial wire under local anesthesia, performance of a diagnostic angiogram, and of course, readiness for conversion to an open procedure if necessary (6,7). The patients who undergo endovascular repair have to be stable enough to have a CT scan performed preoperatively. In one study, the thirty day mortality rate was 10.8% for this approach and the late conversion rate was 9% and was attributed to mainly infection issues and device migration (8). Survival was 89.1% at one year and 69.9% at four years. This was compared with a thirty-day mortality rate of 35% for patients undergoing open repair of ruptures.

Difficult neck

The difficult neck comes in a variety of types: angulated, conical, stenotic (Fig. 3). The angulated neck makes wire passage challenging, but this can be overcome with the use of flexible sheaths and if necessary brachial artery insertion of the initial wire for retrieval from the femoral artery. In addition, the angulation often straightens during endograft placement and

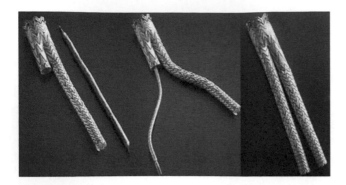

Figure 2
Abdominal aortic aneurysms bifurcated supported stent graft
(Excluder, Gore).

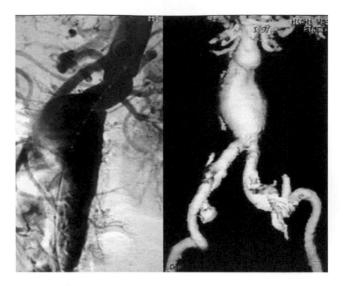

Figure 3
(*Left*) Angulated proximal aortic neck; (*Right*) tortuous iliac
arteries.

therefore the ability to judge the exact postprocedure
location of the graft is difficult, especially with respect to the
renal arteries.

The conical neck can be viewed as a cone with an increasing diameter from the renals to the aneurysm sac. This neck
is a challenge for endograft sizing and achievement of graft
seal to nonaneurysmal aorta. The first issue is often dealt with
by decreasing the amount of the usual graft oversizing from
the normal 20% to 10% to 15%; this reduces stretching the
narrower portion of the conical neck. Endografts that require
balloon expansion, as opposed to radial force, may facilitate
graft seal when dealing with the conical neck.

The third type of challenging neck is the stenotic neck.
Once again, the issue centers on the importance of sizing the
graft correctly. If the graft is oversized for the stenotic portion,
graft infolding may occur. On the other hand, if the graft is
undersized, then the neck may seal but the remainder of the
repair does not fit properly, leading to endoleak and possible
graft migration.

Difficult iliac arteries

Access to the aorta is usually obtained through the femoral
arteries, either by percutaneous methods or by surgical
exposure. The presence of tortuous or atherosclerotic
iliac arteries makes the insertion of wires and sheaths through
the arteriotomy difficult and potentially risky (Fig. 3). CT
scan imaging techniques often do not adequately show iliac
artery anatomy. Even arteriography cannot reliably measure
areas of stenosis. 3D CT scan reconstructions with the
ability to insert a virtual sheath help tackle the challenge of
preoperative imaging and measuring of iliac arteries.
Sometimes it is necessary to access the brachial artery to
pass the initial wire into the femoral artery (9) or access
the iliac artery or aorta through a retroperitoneal incision
with the addition of a conduit to facilitate endograft
insertion (10).

Small iliac arteries are encountered in 8% of the population and most are found in women (11). Some arteries can be
dilated but not without risk of dissection and rupture.
Therefore, a patient with an external iliac artery smaller than
7 mm should undergo either open repair or have the endograft inserted through the larger common iliac artery or aorta.
Stenotic iliac arteries can also be dilated but with the same
risks of dissection and rupture. Aneurysmal iliac disease is a
challenging anatomical feature especially for adequate endograft distal landing and sealing and may require coverage of
the hypogastric artery.

EVAR complications

One of the distinguishing differences between EVAR and
open repair is the higher rate of graft related complications
with EVAR (12). Some occur during or soon after the procedure whereas others are only noticed during the graft
surveillance period (Table 3). Reporting standards have been
established to permit comparison of complications (13). The
analysis of the Lifeline Registry (2664 EVAR cases and 334
open surgical cases) showed that the thirty-day operative
mortality rates for the two groups were similar at 1.7% for
EVAR and 1.4% for open surgical. The freedom from rupture
was also similar for the two groups at one year: 99.8% and
100% and there was no difference in AAA-related death rates
(14). Greenhalgh in the report from the EVAR 1 trial noted
that complication rate was 41% for EVAR patients and 9% for
open surgical patients within four years of the procedure (15).
The aneurysm-related death rate was 4% for EVAR patients
and 7% for open surgical patients. The all-cause mortality
rates were similar for the two groups (28%).

Table 3 Complications

Early
  Type I proximal and distal endoleaks
  Type IV endoleak
  Device related complications
  Inability to deploy stent
  Arterial complications
  Systemic complications
  Cardiac
  Cerebral
  Pulmonary
  Renal
  Access site and lower limb complications
  Bleeding, hematoma, false aneurysm
  Arterial thrombosis
  Death
  Conversion
  Rupture
Late
  Endoleaks: I (a, b), II, III
  Aneurysm growth greater than or equal to 8 mm
  Late AAA-related death
  Death
  Conversion
  Rupture
Classification of endoleaks
  Attachment site leaks
    Proximal end of endograft
    Distal end of endograft
    Iliac occluder (plug)
  Branch leaks (without attachment site connection
    Simple or to-and-fro (from only one patent branch)
    Complex or flow-through (with two or
    more patent branches)
  Graft defect
    Junctional leak or modular disconnect
    Fabric disruption (midgraft hole)
      Minor (<2 mm; e.g., suture holes)
      Major (≥2 mm)
  Graft wall (fabric) porosity (<30 days after graft
  placement)

Access complications

Access problems occur with either the percutaneous approach or open surgical approach to the vessels for endograft insertion. The femoral artery may be injured and require immediate repair with a patch or replacement of a segment. In addition, distal thrombosis may occur from the blockage of the flow into the lower extremities by the sheath and inadequate anticoagulation. This highlights the importance of noting the preoperative pulse examination, so that the postoperative findings can be correctly interpreted. As with any groin procedure, lymph leaks, wound infections and hematomas can occur and vary from the benign that resolves to the serious that requires further intervention (re-exploration, evacuation, muscle flaps, etc.).

Device problems

Device design evolves to remedy problems associated with structural integrity. There have been reports of fabric erosion (16), hook fractures (17), and component separation (18).

Surgical conversion

Primary surgical conversion occurs within the first postoperative 30 days and secondary surgical conversion occurs any time after that. In an examination of the EUROSTAR (European Collaborators on Stent/graft Techniques for aortic Aneurysm Repair) registry, 2.6% of the 1871 patients required conversion and in 38 patients this occurred in the first postoperative month (primary conversion) (19). Eleven patients underwent open surgical repair during a mean follow-up period of eight months (secondary conversion) and rupture was the most frequent reason for this. Kong et al. examined secondary conversion for the 594 patients in the Excluder clinical trials and noted that 2.7% of the patients underwent late open conversion; no conversions occurred in the first year after the procedure. Freedom from conversion was 96.7% at forty-eight months postoperative. The major indication noted was the development of endotension in the absence of a demonstrable endoleak.

Endoleaks

Endoleaks are a major concern for those engaged in EVAR (Table 3, Fig. 4). This phenomenon describes the continuation of blood flow into the extragraft portion of the aneurysm (20). Endoleaks are related to the graft itself or other factors such as the presence of large patent lumbar arteries (21). The presence of an endoleak increases the chance of rupture. Diagnostic imaging plays an important role in the detection of endoleaks: intraprocedural angiograms, surveillance CT scans, or duplex ultrasounds.

The management of endoleaks varies according to the type: type I and III endoleaks should be addressed expediently, and type IV endoleaks usually resolve. The treatment algorithm for

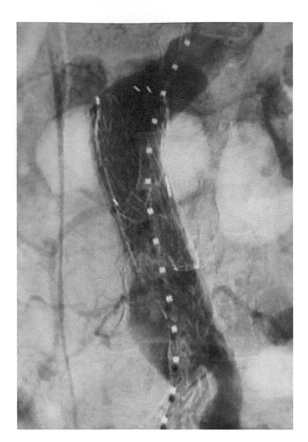

Figure 4
Type IA endoleak noted on completion angiogram.

type II endoleaks is not straightforward as these endoleaks may resolve on their own over time. If a type I endoleak is noted on the completion angiogram, a stent-graft cuff or extension is immediately placed to facilitate better seal. A similar treatment plan is undertaken if the type I endoleak is noted in the post-operative period. Type II endoleaks can be followed and intervention planned if the endoleak does not resolve; some physicians suggest a follow-up CT scan at six months and if the endoleak is present, then the patent artery is either embolized or surgically ligated. Other physicians will only treat type II endoleaks if it is accompanied with sac enlargement. Gelfand et al. examined the clinical significance of type II endoleaks by analyzing data from 10 EVAR trials (22). The authors found that approximately half of the endoleaks disappeared within 12 months. This paper delineated situations when type II endoleak intervention is warranted: AAA sac enlargement after six months, increased sac pressure (>20% of systolic BP), presence of leak greater than 12 months after procedure.

Endograft limb occlusion

This is an infrequently encountered problem, occurring in less than 5% of patients, but its morbidity is serious leading to

extremity loss (23). Small limb diameter and graft extension to the external iliac artery, as opposed to the common iliac, is a risk factor for the development of limb occlusion. Fifty percent of the thromboses occurred within 30 days of the procedure and almost 70% required intervention: surgical (femorofemoral, axillary-femoral, axillary-bifemoral bypasses) and/or endoluminal techniques (rheolytic and pharmacologic thrombolysis).

Graft kinks

Stent-graft kinks are more often seen when unsupported endografts are used (24). This complication occurred in 3.7% of the patients in the EUROSTAR registry and was associated with type I and III endoleaks, graft stenosis, graft limb thrombosis, graft migration, and conversion to open repair (25). In addition, women with angulated AAA necks were atmost risk for stent-graft kink. This problem is usually managed with stenting of the kink.

Sac enlargement

The AneuRx clinical trial was analyzed by Zarins to describe the phenomenon of aneurysm sac enlargement (26). Twelve percent of the patients experienced aneurysm sac enlargement and these patients were older and usually had an endoleak. When patients with endoleaks were analyzed, 17% had sac enlargement whereas only 2% of patients without endoleaks had the same finding. Elevated pressure within the aneurysm sac, also known as endotension, has been reported as one mechanism that is responsible for sac enlargement (27). This finding is documented when the intra-aneurysm pressure is measured during follow-up angiography. Endotension can exist without an endoleak.

Device migration

The AneuRx trial has also been analyzed to determine the frequency of stent migration and identify risk factors (21,28). Ninety-four of 1119 patients had evidence of stent migration that occurred a mean of 30 months after EVAR. Low initial deployment, below the renals, and short proximal fixation length are the identifiable risk factors. In this study, 68% of the patients required no treatment whereas 23 patients had extender modules placed and seven patients underwent surgical conversion. Surgical conversion was examined in a single center study of 640 patients by Verzini (29). This group found that early conversion (within 30 days) was performed in nine patients and late conversion was carried out in 29. At six years after EVAR the risk of undergoing a conversion was 9%. A study by Tonnessen et al. examined device migration at mid- and long-term timepoints with the AneuRx and Zentih endografts (30). The AneuRx device had a significantly higher incidence of migration than the Zenith device. At three and four years out from the procedure, the migration rate was 22% and 28%, respectively, for AneuRx and only 2.4% for Zenith. In addition, a greater proportion of the migrated AneuRx endografts had dilated necks compared with the nonmigrated AneuRx endografts. One of the conclusions was that devices with active fixation design (e.g., Zenith) may be protective against migration. Also, a significant proportion of patients with endograft migration required intervention and so this one again highlights the importance of long-term surveillance.

Extremity and visceral ischemia

Ischemia to the viscera and extremities can also occur and the signs can be subtle (decreased pulses, mild abdominal pain, buttock claudication) or alarmingly obvious (lower extremity mottling, severe abdominal pain, elevated creatinine phosphokinase levels, or gastrointestinal bleeding) (31). Lower extremity ischemia can result from problems at the femoral access site (dissection, atheroembolization) or from issues with the endograft (limb occlusion, kinking). The former often requires surgical intervention whereas the latter can be managed by interventional techniques like placing additional stents. The endograft covers the inferior mesenteric artery and if the remainder of the visceral and hypogastric circulation is poor or compromised can lead to colonic ischemia. In addition, spinal cord ischemia can manifest in paresis or paralyis due to the coverage of intercostals arteries; this complication is rare but serious.

Surveillance

The recommended surveillance routine is for a CT scan at 1, 6, and 12 months and annually thereafter. If an endoleak is detected, the frequency of the scans increases to every six months until resolution of the endoleak is detected. Investigators have compared duplex ultrasound with CT scan for surveillance and found that CT scan is superior for endoleak detection (32). Since endoleaks are an important complication with therapeutic implications, CT scans should be used rather than duplex examination for repair surveillance.

MRI has been investigated as a useful way to follow these patients. It has advantages over CT scan surveillance because it does not put renal function at risk in this older population. It should especially be entertained in patients with preexisting renal insufficiency (33). Endograft surveillance methods now

include the use of an implanted sensor to measure sac pressure to assess for the development of endotension (34,35). The advances in EVAR technology have been accompanied by a greater understanding of the basic science of aneurysmal disease and cross-fertilization has occurred. For example, Curci has been studying the relationship between the secretion of matrix metalloproteinases (MMPs) and AAAs (36). He has measured increased levels in the aneurysmal rather than the normal arterial wall. This finding led physicians to develop a new method for endograft surveillance: the lack of a decrease in MMP-3 and MMP-9 levels should alert the physician to possibility of a failing endograft repair (37). Advances in the basic science of aneurysm disease are helping us better manage this disease.

EVAR outcomes and trial results

Examination of outcomes of endovascular AAA repair comes from mainly two sources: databases and clinical trials.

Eurostar registry

The EUROSTAR Registry was started in 1996 and has continued to provide a substantial amount of data especially for outcome analyses. Data come from 135 vascular centers in Europe (38–40).

Outcomes in patients greater than or equal to eighty years old have been analyzed and compared to those less than 80 years (41). The octogenarians more frequently had heart, kidney, and lung disease preoperatively and a greater proportion was deemed not fit for surgery compared with the younger group of patients. The thirty-day and in-house mortality rate for octogenarians was significantly higher than the younger group: 5% versus 2%. In addition, this group of patients had higher device-related and systemic complication rates. Finally, aneurysm related and all cause mortality rates were significantly higher for this older group of patients.

Dream trial

The Dream trial examined outcomes two years following open or endovascular repair of AAAs (42). The cumulative survival rates for the two groups were similar: 89.6% (open), 89.7% (endovascular). There was no significant difference in aneurysm related mortality. The study concluded that the early advantage of EVAR is no longer present after one year following intervention.

EVAR 1 and 2 trials

Results of the EVAR trial 1 were recently published and describe the outcomes of 543 patients who were anatomically suitable for EVAR and fit for open repair but ultimately underwent EVAR and 539 patients who had open repair (15). The authors found that EVAR is more expensive, had a higher number of complications and reinterventions but it resulted in a 3% better aneurysm survival rate. The EVAR trial 2 then examined those patients who were unfit for open repair and underwent either EVAR or no intervention (43). The 30-day operative mortality rate in the EVAR group was 9% and in the no intervention group the rupture rate was nine per 100 person years. There was no significant difference in either aneurysm-related mortality or all-cause mortality.

EVAR future directions and controversies

The future of EVAR is not fully determined; many questions remain unanswered. Some help will come from the results of ongoing clinical trials. The impact of endotension and the viability of pressure monitoring will become clearer once more intragraft sensor data becomes available. In addition, the utility of fenestrated transrenal endografts is an area of great interest. We will soon see if this is a solution to short proximal aortic necks and suprarenal aneurysms (44). With this new technology and low mortality rate physicians are investigating whether we should be treating smaller aneurysms and clinical trials are being conducted to address this issue (45,46). As the design of EVAR devices evolves and our facility using them improves, the one thing that will not change is the importance of appropriate patient selection.

References

1   Rutherfor RB, ed. Vascular Surgery, 6th ed. Amsterdam, Netherlands: Elsevier, 2005.
2   Parodi JC, Palmaz JC, Barone HD. Transfemoral intraluminal graft implantation for abdominal aortic aneurysms. Ann Vasc Surg 1991; 5(6):491–499.
3   Hua HT, Cambria RP, Chuang SK, et al. Early outcomes of endovascular versus open abdominal aortic aneurysm repair in the National Surgical Quality Improvement Program-Private Sector (NSQIP-PS). J Vasc Surg 2005; 41(3):382–389.
4   Parra JR, Crabtree T, McLafferty RB, et al. Anesthesia technique and outcomes of endovascular aneurysm repair. Ann Vasc Surg 2005; 19(1):123–129.
5   Katzen BT, Ardid MI, MacLean AA, et al. Bivalirudin as an anticoagulation agent: safety and efficacy in peripheral interventions. J Vasc Interv Radiol 2005; 16(9):1183–1187; quiz 7.
6   Lee WA, Hirneise CM, Tayyarah M, et al. Impact of endovascular repair on early outcomes of ruptured abdominal aortic aneurysms. J Vasc Surg 2004; 40(2):211–215.
7   Ohki T, Veith FJ. Endovascular therapy for ruptured abdominal aortic aneurysms. Adv Surg 2001; 35:131–151.
8   Hechelhammer L, Lachat ML, Wildermuth S, et al. Midterm outcome of endovascular repair of ruptured abdominal aortic aneurysms. J Vasc Surg 2005; 41(5):752–757.
9   Criado FJ, Wilson EP, Abul-Khoudoud O, et al. Brachial artery catheterization to facilitate endovascular grafting of abdominal aortic aneurysm: safety and rationale. J Vasc Surg 2000; 32(6):1137–1141.
10 Carpenter JP. Delivery of endovascular grafts by direct sheath placement into the aorta or iliac arteries. Ann Vasc Surg 2002; 16(6):787–790.
11 Wolf YG, Arko FR, Hill BB, et al. Gender differences in endovascular abdominal aortic aneurysm repair with the AneuRx stent graft. J Vasc Surg 2002; 35(5):882–886.
12 Elkouri S, Gloviczki P, McKusick MA, et al. Perioperative complications and early outcome after endovascular and open surgical repair of abdominal aortic aneurysms. J Vasc Surg 2004; 39(3):497–505.
13 Chaikof EL, Blankensteijn JD, Harris PL, et al. Reporting standards for endovascular aortic aneurysm repair. J Vasc Surg 2002; 35(5):1048–1060.
14 Lifeline registry of endovascular aneurysm repair: long-term primary outcome measures. J Vasc Surg 2005; 42(1):1–10.
15 Greenhalgh RM, Brown LC, Kwong GP, et al. Endovascular aneurysm repair versus open repair in patients with abdominal aortic aneurysm (EVAR trial 1): randomised controlled trial. Lancet 2005; 365(9478):2179–2186.
16 Teutelink A, van der Laan MJ, Milner R, et al. Fabric tears as a new cause of type III endoleak with Ancure endograft. J Vasc Surg 2003; 38(4):843–846.
17 Najibi S, Steinberg J, Katzen BT, et al. Detection of isolated hook fractures 36 months after implantation of the Ancure endograft: a cautionary note. J Vasc Surg 2001; 34(2): 353–356.
18 Maleux G, Rousseau H, Otal P, et al. Modular component separation and reperfusion of abdominal aortic aneurysm sac after endovascular repair of the abdominal aortic aneurysm: a case report. J Vasc Surg 1998; 28(2):349–352.
19 Cuypers PW, Laheij RJ, Buth J. Which factors increase the risk of conversion to open surgery following endovascular abdominal aortic aneurysm repair? The EUROSTAR collaborators. Eur J Vasc Endovasc Surg 2000; 20(2):183–189.
20 White GH, Yu W, May J. Endoleak—a proposed new terminology to describe incomplete aneurysm exclusion by an endoluminal graft. J Endovasc Surg 1996; 3(1):124–125.
21 Veith FJ, Baum RA, Ohki T, et al. Nature and significance of endoleaks and endotension: summary of opinions expressed at an international conference. J Vasc Surg 2002; 35(5):1029–1035.
22 Gelfand DV, White GH, Wilson SE. Clinical significance of type II endoleak after endovascular repair of abdominal aortic aneurysm. Ann Vasc Surg 2006; 20(1):69–74.
23 Carroccio A, Faries PL, Morrissey NJ, et al. Predicting iliac limb occlusions after bifurcated aortic stent grafting: anatomic and device-related causes. J Vasc Surg 2002; 36(4):679–684.
24 Carpenter JP, Neschis DG, Fairman RM, et al. Failure of endovascular abdominal aortic aneurysm graft limbs. J Vasc Surg 2001; 33(2):296–302; discussion 3.

25 Fransen GA, Desgranges P, Laheij RJ, et al. Frequency, predictive factors, and consequences of stent-graft kink following endovascular AAA repair. J Endovasc Ther 2003; 10(5): 913–918.

26 Zarins CK, Bloch DA, Crabtree T, et al. Aneurysm enlargement following endovascular aneurysm repair: AneuRx clinical trial. J Vasc Surg 2004; 39(1):109–117.

27 Lin PH, Bush RL, Katzman JB, et al. Delayed aortic aneurysm enlargement due to endotension after endovascular abdominal aortic aneurysm repair. J Vasc Surg 2003; 38(4):840–842.

28 Zarins CK, Bloch DA, Crabtree T, et al. Stent graft migration after endovascular aneurysm repair: importance of proximal fixation. J Vasc Surg 2003; 38(6):1264–1272; discussion 72.

29 Verzini F, Cao P, De Rango P, et al. Conversion to open repair after endografting for abdominal aortic aneurysm: causes, incidence and results. Eur J Vasc Endovasc Surg 2006; 31(2):136–142.

30 Tonnessen BH, Sternbergh WC, 3rd, Money SR. Mid- and long-term device migration after endovascular abdominal aortic aneurysm repair: a comparison of AneuRx and Zenith endografts. J Vasc Surg 2005; 42(3):392–400; discussion-1.

31 Maldonado TS, Rockman CB, Riles E, et al. Ischemic complications after endovascular abdominal aortic aneurysm repair. J Vasc Surg 2004; 40(4):703–709; discussion 9–10.

32 Raman KG, Missig-Carroll N, Richardson T, et al. Color-flow duplex ultrasound scan versus computed tomographic scan in the surveillance of endovascular aneurysm repair. J Vasc Surg 2003; 38(4):645–651.

33 Engellau L, Albrechtsson U, Hojgard S, et al. Costs in follow-up of endovascularly repaired abdominal aortic aneurysms. Magnetic resonance imaging with MR angiography versus EUROSTAR protocols. Int Angiol 2003; 22(1):36–42.

34 Baum RA, Carpenter JP, Cope C, et al. Aneurysm sac pressure measurements after endovascular repair of abdominal aortic aneurysms. J Vasc Surg 2001; 33(1):32–41.

35 Ellozy SH, Carroccio A, Lookstein RA, et al. First experience in human beings with a permanently implantable intrasac pressure transducer for monitoring endovascular repair of abdominal aortic aneurysms. J Vasc Surg 2004; 40(3): 405–412.

36 Curci JA, Thompson RW. Adaptive cellular immunity in aortic aneurysms: cause, consequence, or context? J Clin Invest 2004; 114(2):168–171.

37 Sangiorgi G, D'Averio R, Mauriello A, et al. Plasma levels of metalloproteinases-3 and -9 as markers of successful abdominal aortic aneurysm exclusion after endovascular graft treatment. Circulation 2001; 104(12 suppl 1):I288–I295.

38 Berg P, Kaufmann D, van Marrewijk CJ, et al. Spinal cord ischaemia after stent-graft treatment for infra-renal abdominal aortic aneurysms. Analysis of the Eurostar database. Eur J Vasc Endovasc Surg 2001; 22(4):342–347.

39 Fransen GA, Vallabhaneni SR Sr, van Marrewijk CJ, et al. Rupture of infra-renal aortic aneurysm after endovascular repair: a series from EUROSTAR registry. Eur J Vasc Endovasc Surg 2003; 26(5):487–493.

40 Peppelenbosch N, Buth J, Harris PL, et al. Diameter of abdominal aortic aneurysm and outcome of endovascular aneurysm repair: does size matter? A report from EUROSTAR. J Vasc Surg 2004; 39(2):288–297.

41 Lange C, Leurs LJ, Buth J, et al. Endovascular repair of abdominal aortic aneurysm in octogenarians: an analysis based on EUROSTAR data. J Vasc Surg 2005; 42(4):624–630; discussion 30.

42 Blankensteijn JD, de Jong SE, Prinssen M, et al. Two-year outcomes after conventional or endovascular repair of abdominal aortic aneurysms. N Engl J Med 2005; 352(23):2398–2405.

43 Endovascular aneurysm repair and outcome in patients unfit for open repair of abdominal aortic aneurysm (EVAR trial 2): randomised controlled trial. Lancet 2005; 365(9478): 2187–2192.

44 Verhoeven EL, Prins TR, Tielliu IF, et al. Treatment of short-necked infrarenal aortic aneurysms with fenestrated stent-grafts: short-term results. Eur J Vasc Endovasc Surg 2004; 27(5): 477–483.

45 Cao P. Comparison of surveillance vs Aortic Endografting for Small Aneurysm Repair (CAESAR) trial: study design and progress. Eur J Vasc Endovasc Surg 2005; 30(3):245–251.

46 Zarins CK, Crabtree T, Arko FR, et al. Endovascular repair or surveillance of patients with small AAA. Eur J Vasc Endovasc Surg 2005; 29(5):496–503; discussion 4.

51

Interventions for structural heart disease

Ralph Hein, Neil Wilson, and Horst Sievert

Transcatheter ablation of septal hypertrophy

Approximately 25% of all patients with hypertrophic cardiomyopathy (HCM) have latent left ventricular outflow obstruction with an intraventricular gradient (1). Pathophysiologic features are asymmetric hypertrophy of the septum and a systolic anterior movement of the anterior leaflet. Medical treatment includes betablockers, and calcium antagonists of the verapamil type. Approximately 5–10% of the patients with outflow obstruction are refractory to such negative inotropic therapy (2). Positive inotropic drugs such as digitalis or sympathomimetics are strictly contraindicated. In the presence of atrial fibrillation, anticoagulation therapy should be started. Since endocarditis is more common in patients with HCM because of turbulence in the left ventricle, prophylactic antibiotics should be administered for periods of potential bacteraemia.

Subvalvular myectomy has a reported success of more than 90% with a mortality rate of less than 2%, but this therapy is not applicable to every patient. Transcatheter ablation of septal hypertrophy has been performed since 1994 as a reasonable option for obstructive HCM patients. An increasing number of reports claim efficacy comparable to that of the surgical approach (3).

Patients with a high risk of surgical morbidity and mortality and those who suffer from pharmacologic side effects under conservative treatment should be considered for transcatheter alcohol ablation. NYHA classification, left ventricular gradient, and a septal thickness exceeding 16 mm are indications for intervention. NYHA or CCS class II patients with a minimum resting gradient of 50 mmHg are candidates for this procedure as well as class III and IV patients with a resting gradient of more than 30 mmHg or a provoked gradient greater than 60 mmHg (4,5).

The initial stage of the procedure entails measurement of the peak to peak intraventricular gradient at rest. Induced extrasystolic beats can unmask a potentially higher gradient.

Stepwise application (until a heart rate of about 110 bpm is achieved) of isoproterenol 200 mcg in 50 cc of saline can be used to increase the pressure gradient in sedated patients. Following administration of heparin, the target vessel for alcohol dilution is probed by catheter. The target vessel is almost always the first septal branch of the left anterior descending artery. Balloon inflation isolates the vessel, occluding blood flow. Retrograde leakage of alcohol back into the left anterior descending has to be avoided. An echo contrast study is performed to confirm effective occlusion and thus obviate this complication. Intravenous analgesia should be administered before alcohol injection to diminish chest pain.

Slow application of 0.2–1.5 mL of alcohol through the inflated balloon catheter induces necrosis of the myocardium, which is seen as an obvious contrast enhancement on echocardiography. If the gradient post instillation of alcohol remains above 30 mmHg, the balloon may be positioned more proximally in the vessel or a second septal perforating artery may be treated in the same way.

In some cases, tissue edema of the affected myocardium may temporarily increase the outflow gradient during the early days of follow-up. During subsequent months remodeling of the outflow tract is usually observed, resulting in a progressive reduction in gradient. Several studies have documented the efficacy of alcohol septal ablation (6–8), demonstrating improvement in functional class and exercise capacity.

Possible complications include massive myocardial infarction due to retrograde flow around the occlusion balloon, complete heart block, ventricular fibrillation, stroke, dissection of the left anterior descending artery, and right coronary artery thrombosis. Though high grade atrioventricular blockage occurs relatively frequently, procedural mortality rate is low (0–4%) and severe complications are rare and often avoidable (7–10).

Creatinine kinase levels should be assessed frequently during the stay in the coronary care unit and may rise up to 1500 U/l. After the procedure there may be some risk of thrombus formation in the area of ablation. Some operators prescribe aspirin (100 mg/day, p.o.) for four weeks postinterventionally.

LAA occlusion

The left atrial appendage (LAA) is a muscular cavity discharging into the left atrium. It is the prevalent location for intracardiac thrombus (11). If atrial fibrillation cannot be eliminated with medical therapy or an ablation procedure then life-long anticoagulation is necessary. Usually patients with chronic atrial fibrillation are anticoagulated with coumadin type drugs. Many patients however have contraindications to anticoagulation like intracerebral aneurysms, hemorrhagic diathesis, gastrointestinal lesions, and liver dysfunction. For such patients interventional closure of the LAA may be a therapeutic alternative, and has been performed now for almost five years. There are currently three devices under investigation:

1. PLAATO device (ev3, Inc., Plymouth, MN)
2. Amplatzer occluder (AGA Medical Corporation, Golden Valley, MN)
3. Watchman device (Atritech, Inc., Minneapolis, MN)

1. The PLAATO device (Fig. 1) was the first device to be implanted in a human LAA in August 2001. Its nitinol framework features a tissue-anchoring system on the struts to maintain the correct position once deployed. The orifice of the LAA is sealed by a nonthrombogenic polytetrafluoroethylene membrane excluding the appendage from the blood circulation and allowing tissue adhesion.

The morphology and diameter of the appendage are very variable; hence, detailed preinterventional imaging with transesophageal echocardiography (TEE) and angiography is important. Thrombus in the appendage is obviously a strict contraindication to the procedure and should be excluded by transesophageal echo before attempting closure. The orifice diameter of the appendage should range between 13 and 27 mm to achieve a stable device position.

To access the LAA transseptal puncture is necessary. Angiography is performed for further morphologic measurements. The PLAATO system is engaged via a delivery catheter and unfolded in the appendage. Compression of 10% is mandatory and at least two rows of anchors should be engaged into the surrounding tissue.

In July 2005, the PLAATO Feasibility Study reported good implantation results with this device with an acceptable complication rate (12).

For premedication aspirin 300 mg twice a day 48 hours prior to the procedure and a loading dose of clopidogrel 300 mg (or ticlopidine 250 mg) is recommended. Endocarditis prophylaxis with a first generation cephalosporin (e.g., cefuroxime, 1, 5 g, i.v.) should be administered before and after intervention. After transseptal puncture, 10,000 units of heparin are administered. An activated clotting time of 200–300 seconds is desirable.

Postprocedure, clopidogrel (75 mg/day, p.o.) and endocarditis prophylaxis for the first six months is suggested. Aspirin (300–325 mg/day, p.o.) should be prescribed indefinitely.

2. A variety of Amplatzer devices are applicable for LAA occlusion including the atrial and ventricular septal defect devices, the patent foramen ovale devices, the patent ductus arteriosus devices, and other arteriovenous fistulae devices. A special fabric-free LAA plug is currently under investigation (Fig. 2).

The characteristic feature of all Amplatzer devices is the nitinol wire mesh. There are two possible methods of implantation. Either the device is placed entirely into the appendage or the distal disc is expanded in the neck and the proximal disc in the left atrium. The risk of residual shunting around the device is increased when it is totally inserted into the LAA with no part protruding into the atrium. The Amplatzer occluder series holds the widest spectrum of device sizes (4 to 40 mm). The device is attached to a delivery cable and can simply be opened or recollapsed into the delivery catheter. Release is by unscrewing the device after first testing stability with simple traction.

Intravenous antibiotics are given before and after the procedure. Five thousand to ten thousand units of heparin should be administered after transseptal puncture. Aspirin (100–300 mg/day, p.o.) and clopidogrel (75 mg/day, p.o.) is prescribed for the following six months as well as endocarditis prophylaxis. A TEE is performed at six months. If the LAA is completely occluded, no further anticoagulation is required.

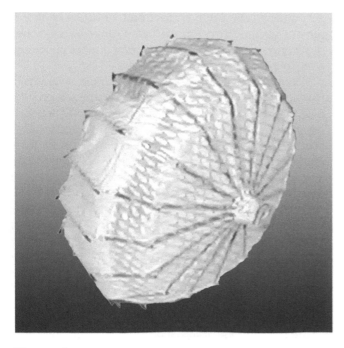

Figure 1
PLAATO left atrial appendage device.

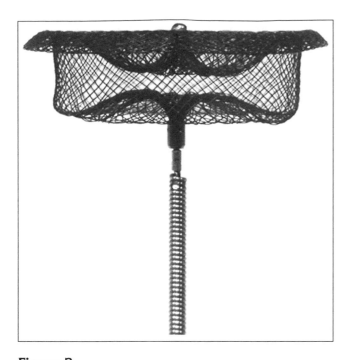

Figure 2
Amplatzer left atrial appendage plug.

Aspirin therapy should be continued to prevent thrombus formation outside the LAA.

3. The Watchman implant (Fig. 3) is the latest device to be used for occlusion of the LAA.

The nitinol frame structure incorporates a permeable 160 micron PET filter on the proximal face of the device to encourage endothelialization. Fixation barbs on the surface anchor the device to the LAA wall. The filter is released distal to the LAA ostium. Clinical experience is limited with this device (13).

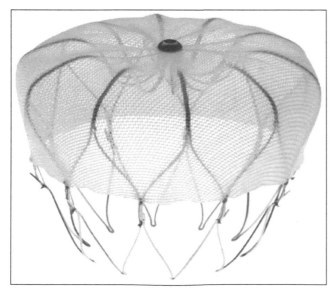

Figure 3
Watchman left atrial appendage device.

Intravenous antibiotics are given before and after the procedure. Endocarditis prophylaxis is recommended for six months. Coumadin type drugs should be administered at least for 45 days after the Watchman implantation procedure with an INR between two and three in combination with 100 mg aspirin. When complete endothelialization is likely with no or only little flow through the device, coumadin can be discontinued and clopidogrel 75 mg/day is given until six months follow-up examination. In the absence of thrombus or flow in the appendage at TEE at six months, clopidogrel is stopped and aspirin therapy 100 mg/day is continued indefinitely. If thrombus formation is seen, obviously coumadin therapy is restarted.

Valvuloplasty

Percutaneous valvuloplasty was introduced during the early 1980s as a method for treatment of stenotic valves (14). Since then, with the improvement in wire and balloon technology and expertise, it is the method of choice for almost all patients with severe pulmonary stenosis and for younger patients with congenital noncalcified aortic valve stenosis. Mitral balloon valvuloplasty is widely applicable and efficacious in postrheumatic mitral stenosis. Tricuspid valvuloplasty is rarely performed as severe rheumatic stenosis of this valve is rarely seen.

Pulmonary stenosis

Congenital abnormalities of pulmonary valve morphology including fused valve commissures, unicuspid and bicuspid valves, leaflet thickening, or valve dysplasia may occur in isolation or combination to cause narrowing of the valve. Without treatment, chronic right ventricular hypertension leads to severe hypertrophy and ultimately right ventricular failure, tricuspid regurgitation, and atrial and ventricular tachyarrhythmias.

The first report of percutaneous balloon dilation of a pulmonary valve was published in 1982 (14). Today the transcatheter approach has largely replaced surgical valvulotomy for pure stenosis. Surgery is only necessary when balloon dilatation was not successful or other heart abnormalities demand an open heart procedure.

Exercise intolerance and dyspnea are the predominant symptom. Doppler systolic gradient on echocardiography of 50 mmHg or more is generally accepted as a clear indication for intervention, accepting that invasive gradients measured in a sedated or anesthetized patient are likely to be less than the Doppler gradient for reasons of timing and a reduced cardiac output. After puncture of the femoral vein, a multipurpose catheter is used to document right ventricular and pulmonary artery pressures, with a pullback across the pulmonary valve to measure the peak-to-peak systolic gradient. A right ventricular angiogram is performed in an right anterior oblique (RAO) and/or lateral projection to localize the valve and to measure the size of the valve annulus. A multipurpose catheter is then advanced to one of the branch pulmonary arteries and an exchange length guidewire positioned in a distal branch. An appropriate sized balloon catheter is advanced into the right ventricle and positioned across the pulmonary valve. The balloon diameter should measure about 1.2–1.5 times the size of the valve annulus. Balloon inflation is performed until the waist is abolished, signaling effective disruption of the stenotic valve leaflets. After dilation, the pressure gradient across the valve is measured; a reduction to less than half the predilation gradient is accepted as an effective result. However, some patients, especially those with the more severe obstruction, display a "reactive" infundibular dynamic obstruction after valvuloplasty. In this case, the initial fall in gradient may seem disappointing, but providing the operator is confident that an appropriate sized balloon was used, the gradient will fall further in the weeks following valvuloplasty as the right ventricular hypertrophy regresses.

Complications reported with this type of intervention are rare. Rupture of the annulus is reported. The tricuspid valve may also be damaged if a large diameter balloon catheter has been passed inadvertently through the tricuspid valve chordae. After inflation, the balloon is relatively bulky and as it is removed the tricuspid valve apparatus may be disrupted causing regurgitation. A procedure-associated death rate of 0.24% and a major complication rate of 0.35% were found in a large study comprising 822 balloon pulmonary valvuloplasty procedures (15).

Aortic stenosis

The commonest cause of stenosis in patients below 60 years of age is a congenitally bicuspid aortic valve with fused commissures and/or dysplastic leaflets. Over time calcification and fibrosis may cause the valve to become rigid and obstructive. Coexisting regurgitation of these valves is common.

The number of patients with a rheumatic type of stenosis has decreased in recent years. Rheumatic valve disease causes fusion and thickening of the commissures, which in turn accelerates calcification and fibrosis.

A third type of stenosis of a degenerative nature occurs in patients above 70 years of age in whom the commissures stay separated but the valve excursion is impeded at the base of the leaflets. Clinical symptoms may include syncope, dyspnea, or angina. Advanced stages of this disease can cause heart failure and sudden death.

Surgery has been the preferred option for patients with severe stenosis. The options are either a commissurotomy or, in patients with significant regurgitation or severe calcification,

valve replacement or a pulmonary autograft procedure, the Ross operation.

After successful experience with pulmonary balloon valvuloplasty, aortic balloon valvuloplasty has gained acceptance (16–18). The aim of aortic valvuloplasty is to reduce the transvalvular gradient to a subintervention level. An efficacious result is generally accepted as a pressure gradient less than 50 mmHg and an increase in valve area of 100%. The acute results of dilation are comparable to pulmonary procedures though the complication rate is considerably higher. Aortic regurgitation, embolic events, arrhythmias, and progressive heart failure have all been reported during intervention or follow-up. Recurrent stenosis is the highest among patients with severe calcification (19), which has been addressed by the development of transcutaneous valve replacement (for further information see the section "valve replacement").

Mitral stenosis

Mitral stenosis is seen typically as a consequence of chronic rheumatic fever. Isolated congenital mitral stenosis is very rare and not suitable for balloon valvuloplasty. Clinical symptoms depend on the degree of obstruction. Dyspnea, atrial fibrillation, embolic events, pulmonary edema, and right heart decompensation may occur and are all indications for treatment. Surgery and catheter intervention provide similar results. Balloon valvuloplasty produces best results in patients with little or no calcification of the mitral leaflets (20–23).

Since the first steps in transluminal balloon dilation of mitral valves in 1982 (24) numerous techniques have been described. One method is to access the left atrium with a transseptal puncture from the venous side (antegrade). Another way is to advance the catheter via the aorta into the left ventricle and perform the valvulotomy from the arterial side (retrograde). The use of two dilation balloons introduced via the transseptal approach is a common technique described by Bonhoeffer using a monorail-type system over a single guidewire (25).

Minor degrees of mitral regurgitation are relatively common after valvuloplasty of the mitral valve. More severe regurgitation requiring early surgical repair or replacement may also occur. Restenosis is seen after both surgical and interventional valvuloplasty on the mitral valve in longer-term follow-up (26,27). The valve area usually increases approximately from 1 to 1.8–2.2 cm^2 (28).

Tricuspid stenosis

Isolated tricuspid stenosis is very rare and almost always associated with chronic rheumatic fever. Techniques to dilate this valve are based on those for mitral dilation.

During all valvuloplasty interventions antibiotics (e.g., cefuroxime, 1, 5 g, i.v.) are administered. Patients allergic to penicillin should receive vancomycin 1 g intravenously. Most physicians perform transcatheter valvuloplasty in the fasting state under mild sedation. Substances that are frequently used are meperidine, promethazine, and chlorpromazine, given intramuscularly or intermittent doses of midazolam (0.05 to 0.1 mg/kg, i.v.) and/or fentanyl (0.5 to 1.0 μg/kg, i.v.). Some operators also apply ketamine or general anesthesia for all interventional cases.

Following transseptal left heart catheterization, systemic anticoagulation is achieved by the intravenous administration of 100 U/kg of heparin.

Mitral valve repair

Transcutaneous mitral valve repair has been developed for patients with significant valve regurgitation. A frequent etiology of regurgitation is myocardial infarction causing ventricular dilation, rupture of chordae, or dysfunctional papillary muscles. Additionally mitral valve prolapse, dilated cardiomyopathy, or rheumatic/bacterial endocarditis can result in a regurgitant mitral valve. Chronic regurgitation is tolerated by many patients for quite a long time but eventually symptoms of dyspnea, palpitations, edema, and severe arrhythmias emerge.

Indications for surgical intervention include regurgitation with NYHA III–IV symptoms or NHYA >II with atrial fibrillation refractory to conservative treatment. Several surgical techniques are effective. The "Alfieri stitch" or "edge to edge" technique is of interest because one of the percutaneous mitral valve repair techniques is based on an equivalent principle (29,30). Currently two methods for transcatheter mitral valve repair are investigated in clinical trials:

1. Edge-to-edge repair
2. Transcatheter annuloplasty

1. In 1991, the surgical variant of the edge-to-edge repair technique was first tried in patients that were not suitable for complex mitral valve repair (29). This procedure is still performed with the intention of sewing together part of the free edges of the anterior and posterior valve leaflets in such a way as to construct a double orifice valve to decrease regurgitation.

The edge-to-edge transcatheter mitral valve repair system consists of a steerable guide catheter and a steerable clip or suture delivery system. From a venous approach, a transseptal puncture is employed to access the left atrium. The delivery system is maneuvered through the mitral valve into the left ventricle and aligned perpendicular to the line of valve coaptation. The EVEREST 1 trial featured first data on transcatheter mitral repair with this technique using a clip (31). In 89% the implantation procedure was successful reducing

mitral regurgitation in 67% of the patients to levels under II°. However, 25% of these patients required surgery within two months after the intervention.

2. The concept of percutaneous transvenous mitral annuloplasty is to place a relatively stiff rod or stent into the coronary sinus (CS) to achieve a configuration change of the dilated mitral annulus. This procedure is feasible due to the fact that the posterior mitral annulus is separated from the CS and great cardiac vein (GCV) only by a thin band of atrial muscle and connective tissue. Preinterventional assessment of the anatomical relationships between the CS and mitral annulus by magnetic resonance imaging, CT scan, or 3D echocardiography is helpful for this procedure. The rod is positioned under fluoroscopic guidance through the CS and GCV to an appropriate position. By straightening the venous vessels, the posterior leaflet converges to the anterior leaflet thereby reducing regurgitation. A new CS probe, which applies heat energy to the mitral annulus, is being developed to denaturize collagen fibers in the adjacent mitral annulus producing a shrinkage effect that decreases the valve dilation, potentially reducing regurgitation. Perforation and tamponade, coronary occlusion, sinus thrombosis, or device migration are all potential complications of this procedure. Short- and mid-term follow-up results are expected (32,33).

With annuloplasty procedures heparin and endocarditis prophylaxis should be administered before the procedures. When the edge-to-edge technique is performed, heparin should not be administered until the transseptal puncture has been performed. Regular follow-up examination, anticoagulation, and endocarditis prophylaxis are recommended after mitral repair procedures.

Valve replacement

Currently transcatheter replacement of heart valves is limited to the aortic and pulmonary valves.

Hywel Davies reported of temporarily treatment of aortic regurgitation with a parachute valve mounted onto a catheter tip in 1965 (34). Twenty-seven years later Andersen and his colleagues described the first experience with a bioprosthetic valve attached to a wire-based stent and mounted on a balloon valvuloplasty catheter (35). In 2002, Alain Cribier performed the first transcatheter valve implantation in an elderly patient with inoperable aortic stenosis using a prototype of a stent-mounted, pericardial, tricuspid aortic valve (36).

Approaching the aortic valve with a catheter can be achieved via the venous (antegrade, transseptal) or the arterial routes (retrograde) (37,38). The delivery assembly is positioned within the diseased native valve. Before expansion of the valve mounted balloon rapid pacing (>200 beats/min) is performed to lower stroke volume during the implantation sequence. The balloon is inflated fixing the stented valve to the implantation site. Immediately after balloon deflation pacing is discontinued and the balloon removed leaving the valve in position. Reported complications in this group of patients with very high comorbidity are renal failure, pericardial tamponade, stroke, injury to the mitral valve and atrial septum, paravalvular regurgitation, valve migration and cardiogenic shock.

Residual regurgitation after reparative surgery of congenital heart disease is the most frequent indication for pulmonary valve replacement. Bonhoeffer reported early results in 2000 (39,40). Since then, over 100 patients have undergone this procedure. Extensive diagnostic imaging is performed before pulmonary valve implantation to delineate anatomy, and quantify the regurgitation and right ventricular function. The pulmonary valve is a bovine jugular vein valve mounted within a platinum iridium stent. It is advanced on a double-balloon delivery system via the femoral vein into the right atrium, through the tricuspid valve and into the right ventricular outflow tract.

Once the correct position of the valve-stent assembly is identified angiographically, the inner and outer balloons are inflated sequentially, and subsequently deflated and removed. Occasionally, it is necessary to perform further deployment of the valve using a high pressure, noncompliant balloon system.

The procedures may be performed under local anesthesia and mild sedation or general anesthesia with heparin anticoagulation. Aspirin (160 mg, p.o.) and a loading dose of clopidogrel (300 mg, p.o.) are administered 24 hours before intervention for the aortic valve. Antibiotics (e.g., first generation cephalosporin, i.v.) are given before the procedure and continued for 48 hours. After the procedure aspirin is continued for three to six months.

Post-surgical and post-myocardial infarction ventricular septal defect

The vast majority of ventricular septal defects (VSD) are congenital. Acquired VSDs are almost always a consequence of septal rupture following myocardial infarction, traumatic VSDs as a consequence of sharp or blunt chest trauma are exceptionally rare. Typically the post myocardial infarction ventricular septal defect (PMIVSD) occurs within the first week after the event (41). In the current era of thrombolysis about 0.2% of patients develop a VSD as a result of septal necrosis. Medical management of these patients is limited and carries a 30-day mortality of 94% compared with 47% who were treated surgically (42).

A residual VSD following surgical closure occurs in 10% to 40% of patients depending on its location (43). Selected patients are suitable for a transcatheter approach. Interventional closure of selected muscular VSD has been possible for some years using the Rashkind (44) and subsequent generation devices (Clamshell, CardioSEAL). Currently the Amplatzer muscular,

membranous, and the new perimembranous device (Fig. 4) are by far the most widely applied. The CardioSEAL-STARflex occluder or Nit-Occlud Coils may also be used for this purpose.

Before intervention clinical condition often warrants intra-aortic balloon pump and revascularization or stenting of the infarct-related artery. For VSD closure either the transvenous or the transarterial approach can be used to access the defect. Commonly an arteriovenous circuit is established. This increases wire stability and thus facilitates positioning of the delivery sheath. The appropriate device size is selected and positioned within the defect. Care is taken that the device does not impinge on important related structures such as the aortic, mitral, and tricuspid valves. The morphology of the post infarction VSDs is complex thus residual shunting is often seen and mortality remains high. While the procedure may be life saving in some circumstances, procedural failure and residual flow are commoner than with congenital defects (for further information on congenital VSD closure see chap. 62).

Post infarction patients need to be treated with long-term antiplatelet therapy. Aspirin (100 mg/day, p.o.) reduces the mortality rate within one year post infarction by 15% and the risk for reinfarction by 30%. Additionally, clopidogrel (75 mg/day, p.o.) may be administered. Supplementary clopidogrel therapy for at least nine months also improves prognosis (45). The risk of thrombus formation in the affected myocardium is high. Anticoagulation for three months with a target INR of 2.0–3.0 is recommended by some operators.

Patent foramen ovale

Persistence of patent foramen ovale (PFO) into adulthood carries a risk of paradoxical embolization. This risk is accentuated

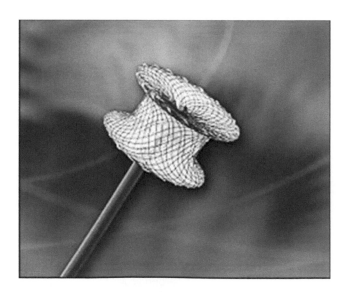

Figure 4
Amplatzer post myocardial infarction ventricular septar defects (VSD) occluder.

if the PFO is associated with an atrial septal aneurysm (46). Therapeutic options to prevent embolism are a lifelong application of anticoagulant drugs, surgical closure, or catheter intervention. Despite efficacious new generation antiplatelet and anticoagulation drugs there is nevertheless a risk of recurrent embolic events. Additionally, 2–5% of the patients on anticoagulant drugs will encounter significant bleeding complications per year (47).

Surgery for PFO closure lowers the rate of cerebrovascular events per year and carries a mortality of less than 1%, but is associated with significant morbidity. Transcatheter closure of PFO is a standard technique for many interventional cardiologists. Low morbidity, efficacy approaching 100% at follow-up, and the avoidance of scar, make transcatheter closure the procedure of choice. All double disc devices (see later) are introduced via the femoral vein and advanced within a delivery catheter through the PFO into the left atrium. Here the distal disc of the occluder is released and carefully withdrawn to the left side of the atrial septum. The proximal disc is deployed on the right side of the septum. Effective positioning is confirmed on fluoroscopy and transesophageal or intracardiac echo and the device subsequently released from its delivery system.

Following devices are either standard PFO devices or constitute emerging methods for PFO closure:

1. Amplatzer PFO occluder (AGA Medical Corporation, Golden Valley, MN)
2. Helex occluder (W.L. Gore & Associates, Flagstaff, AZ)
3. Premere occluder (St Jude Medical, Maple Grove, MN)
4. CardioSEAL-STARflex occluder (NMT Medical, Inc., Boston, MA)
5. BioSTAR (NMT Medical, Inc., Boston, MA)
6. PFX Closure System (Cierra, Inc., Redwood City, CA)

1. The Amplatzer occluder (Fig. 5) is probably the most widely used device in this indication. This double disc device

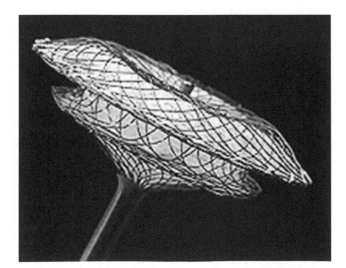

Figure 5
Amplatzer PFO occluder.

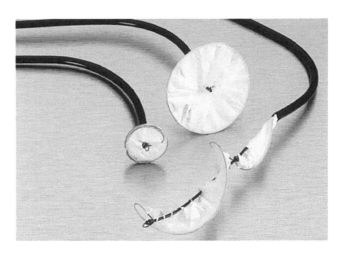

Figure 6
Helex PFO occluder.

consists of self-expandable nitinol wire mesh. Both discs contain patches of polyester fabric for enhanced defect occlusion. Compared to other Amplatzer devices, the PFO occluder features a thinner connection waist and is available in sizes of 18, 25, and 35 mm. Most frequently the 18 and 25 mm devices are implanted, but the 35 mm occasionally is useful in patients with a large ASA.

Before insertion the device needs to be evacuated from air by expanding and refolding the wire mesh in saline. Once accomplished, the device is loaded into the delivery catheter and percutaneously introduced. Self-expansion of the left and right atrial discs is achieved by pushing the delivery cable and retrieving the catheter stepwise. After checking for proper device position and configuration, the device is released.

2. The Helex device differs from the common double umbrella concept (Fig. 6). Expanded polytetrafluoroethylene (ePTFE) patch material is bonded to a single strand of nitinol wire. When fully constituted the device conforms in a circular fashion with two discs held together by an integrated eyelet mechanism. This mechanism also provides visibility under fluoroscopy and ensures flat alignment of the discs to the left and right aspects of the atrial septum. Due to its round edges, ePTFE material and the fine nitinol wire, this device has a low rate of complications. The device remains elongated in a linear form when loaded in the catheter and forms $1\frac{1}{4}$ turns on each side of the septum after deployment. A security suture is attached to the proximal eyelet allowing device retrieval even after release.

3. The Premere PFO occluder (Fig. 7) is another self-expanding double disc device specifically designed for PFO closure. The right-sided anchor is constructed of nitinol between two layers of knitted polyester fabric connected by a flexible polyester braided tether to the left atrial anchor. The left atrial anchor consists of four radiating arms without polyester layers to improve tissue absorption and to minimize thrombus formation. Since the distance between the anchors

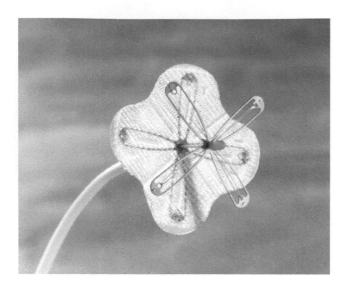

Figure 7
Premere PFO occluder.

adapts to the tunnel length, this device is suitable for long-tunnel type PFOs. Until the abovementioned tether is cut, the anchors are fully retrievable. This device was first used in November 2003.

4. The CardioSEAL occluder features eight wire spring arms that form two rectangular discs. Each disc is covered with a knitted polyester patch. The CardioSEAL-STARflex septal repair system (Fig. 8) is an advanced version, which has nitinol coil microsprings connecting the opposing arms of the left and right atrial discs. These springs enable self-centering of the device to obtain improved adjustment to the septal anatomy.

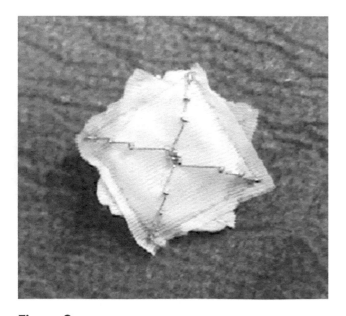

Figure 8
CardioSEAL-STARflex device.

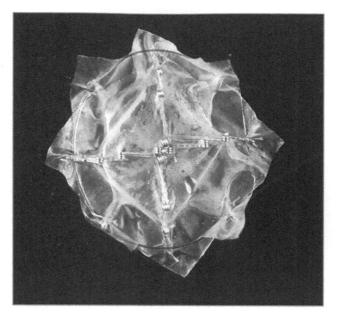

Figure 9
BioSTAR persistence of patient foramenovale (PFO) occluder.

5. The BioSTAR occluder (Fig. 9) evolved from the CardioSEAL-STARflex design. It is a prototype of a bioactive device that uses tissue-engineered collagen matrix derived from the submucosal layer of the porcine small intestine (Organogenesis Inc., Canton, MA) as its "fabric". The device is 90% absorbable and has a very low profile encouraging tissue overgrowth and decreased thrombogenicity. The BioSTAR occluder features drug eluting capabilities for heparin or growth factors. This device is currently in clinical trials.

6. The PFX Closure system (Fig. 10) does not involve the implantation of a device. The method of action involves the sealing of the flap valve of the foramen ovale to the atrial septum. The distal end of the catheter consists of an electrode composed of a metallic wire framework and covered by an elastomeric vacuum housing. A retractable outer sleeve confines the electrode from the surrounding blood. The system is introduced transvenously and positioned in the right atrium. The electrode is guided toward the overlapping septum primum and secundum. Both parts of the atrial septum are engaged by inducing a vacuum within the elastomeric housing. After confirming the position of the electrode by TEE or ICE, a monopolar radiofrequency energy impulse is triggered, welding the tissues of septum primum and septum secundum together. This procedure was first performed in 2005 and is currently under procedural and technical evaluation (48).

It has become recognized that PFO device closure not only significantly decreases the incidence of paradoxical embolism (47), but can also reduce the incidence of migraine in susceptible patients. Fifty-five percent of patients with aura and 62% of those without aura experienced a reduction of

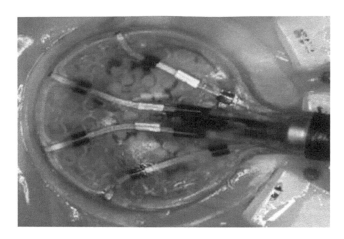

Figure 10
PFX electrode.

headache frequency after PFO closure (49). The MIST study (http://www.migraine-mist.org) found out that PFO closure might achieve a mean reduction in headache burden of 50 hours per month. In this study, 42% of the patients with migraine experienced a 50% reduction in headache.

Reported major procedural and post procedural complications include frame fracture, device embolization, or the need for surgical retrieval. Depending on the operator experience, the method and the morphology of the PFO, the procedure time constitutes approximately 20–40 minutes. The hospital stay is rarely more than a single overnight stay; many patients undergo PFO closure as a day case procedure.

Before intervention heparin is administered (100 U/kg) in addition to endocarditis prophylaxis (e.g., cefuroxime, 1,5 g, i.v.). Endocarditis prophylaxis is repeated after the procedure. Aspirin (100 mg, p.d.) and clopidogrel (75 mg/day, p.o.) are prescribed for six months after implantation. The incidence of thrombus formation varies between devices (50). If thrombus is seen during follow-up, coumadin therapy should be commenced.

References

1   Maron MS, Olivotto I, Betocchi S, et al. Effect of left ventricular outflow tract obstruction on clinical outcome in hypertrophic cardiomyopathy. N Engl J Med 2003; 348: 295–303.

2   Maron BJ, Bonow RO, Cannon RO III, et al. Hypertrophic cardiomyopathy. Interrelations of clinical manifestations, pathophysiology, and therapy (2). N Engl J Med 1987; 316 (14):844–852. Review.

3   Gietzen FH, Leuner CJ, Obergassel L, et al. Role of transcoronary ablation of septal hypertrophy in patients with hypertrophic cardiomyopathy, New York Heart Association functional class III or IV, and outflow obstruction only under provocable conditions. Circulation 2002; 106:454–459.

4   Maron BJ, McKenna WJ, Danielson GK, et al. Task Force on Clinical Expert Consensus Documents. American College of Cardiology; Committee for Practice Guidelines. European Society of Cardiology. American College of Cardiology/European Society of Cardiology clinical expert consensus document on hypertrophic cardiomyopathy. A report of the American College of Cardiology Foundation Task Force on Clinical Expert Consensus Documents and the European Society of Cardiology Committee for Practice Guidelines. J Am Coll Cardiol 2003; 42:1687–1713.

5   Seggewiss H. Medical therapy versus interventional therapy in hypertropic obstructive cardiomyopathy. Curr Control Trials Cardiovasc Med 2000; 1:115–119.

6   Kim JJ, Lee CW, Park SW, et al. Improvement in exercise capacity and exercise blood pressure response after transcoronary alcohol ablation therapy of septal hypertrophy in hypertrophic cardiomyopathy. Am J Cardiol 1999; 83(8): 1220–1223.

7   Knight C, Kurbaan AS, Seggewiss H, et al. Nonsurgical septal reduction for hypertrophic obstructive cardiomyopathy: outcome in the first series of patients. Circulation 1997; 95(8):2075–2081.

8   Gietzen FH, Leuner CJ, Raute-Kreinsen U, et al. Acute and long-term results after transcoronary ablation of septal hypertrophy (TASH). Catheter interventional treatment for hypertrophic obstructive cardiomyopathy. Eur Heart J 1999; 20(18):1342–1354.

9   Lakkis NM, Nagueh SF, Dunn JK, et al. Nonsurgical septal reduction therapy for hypertrophic obstructive cardiomyopathy: one-year follow-up. J Am Coll Cardiol 2000; 36:852–855.

10 Kuhn H, Seggewiss H, Gietzen FH, et al. Catheter-based therapy for hypertrophic obstructive cardiomyopathy. First in-hospital outcome analysis of the German TASH Registry. Z Kardiol 2004; 93:23–31.

11 Blackshear JL, Odell JA. Appendage obliteration to reduce stroke in cardiac surgical patients with atrial fibrillation. Ann Thorac Surg 1996; 61:755–759.

12 Ostermayer SH, Reisman M, Kramer PH, et al. Percutaneous left atrial appendage transcatheter occlusion (PLAATO system) to prevent stroke in high-risk patients with non-rheumatic atrial fibrillation: Results from the international multi-center feasibility trials. J Am Coll Cardiol 2005; 46(1):9–14.

13 Sick P, Ulrich M, Muth G, et al. Universität Leipzig, Herzzentrum GmbH, Leipzig; Herzzentrum Siegburg; Krankenhaus der Barmherzigen Brüderk, Trier. Erste klinische Erfahrungen mit dem WATCHMAN® Verschlußsystem für das linke Vorhofohr zur Verhinderung thromboembolischer Komplikationen bei Patienten mit nicht valvulärem Vorhofflimmern. Z Kardiol 2005; 94(Suppl 1). Abstract V241.

14 Kan JS, White RI Jr, Mitchell SE, et al. Percutaneous balloon valvuloplasty: a new method for treating congenital pulmonary-valve stenosis. N Engl J Med 1982; 307(9):540–542.

15 Stanger P, Cassidy SC, Girod DA, et al. Balloon pulmonary valvuloplasty: results of the valvuloplasty and angioplasty of congenital anomalies registry. Am J Cardiol 1990; 65(11): 775–783.

16 Lababidi Z, Wu JR, Walls JT. Percutaneous balloon aortic valvuloplasty: results in 23 patients. Am J Cardiol 1984; 53(1):194–197.

17 Cribier A, Savin T, Saoudi N, et al. Percutaneous transluminal valvuloplasty of acquired aortic stenosis in elderly patients: an alternative to valve replacement? Lancet 1986; 1(8472): 63–67.

18 Sievert H, Kaltenbach M, Bussmann WD, et al. Percutaneous valvuloplasty of the aortic valve in adults. Dtsch Med Wochenschr 1986; 111(13):504–506. German.

19 Otto CM, Mickel MC, Kennedy JW, et al. Three-year outcome after balloon aortic valvuloplasty. Insights into prognosis of valvular aortic stenosis. Circulation 1994; 89(2):642–650.

20 Lock JE, Khalilullah M, Shrivastava S, et al. Percutaneous catheter commissurotomy in rheumatic mitral stenosis. N Engl J Med 1985; 313(24):1515–1518.

21 Al Zaibag M, Ribeiro PA, Al Kasab S, et al. Percutaneous double-balloon mitral valvotomy for rheumatic mitral-valve stenosis. Lancet 1986; 1(8484):757–761.

22 Reyes VP, Raju BS, Wynne J, et al. Percutaneous balloon valvuloplasty compared with open surgical commissurotomy for mitral stenosis. N Engl J Med 1994; 331(15):961–967.

23 Sievert H, Kober G, Bussmann WD, et al. Catheter valvuloplasty in mitral valve stenosis. Dtsch Med Wochenschr 1989; 114(7):248–252. German.

24 Inoue K, Owaki T, Nakamura T, et al. Clinical application of transvenous mitral commissurotomy by a new balloon catheter. J Thorac Cardiovasc Surg 1984; 87(3):394–402.

25 Bonhoeffer P, Esteves C, Casal U, et al. Percutaneous mitral valve dilatation with the Multi-Track System. Catheter Cardiovasc Interv 1999; 48(2):178–183.

26 Block PC, Palacios IF, Block EH, et al. Late (two year) follow-up after percutaneous mitral balloon valvotomy. Am J Cardiol 1992; 69:537–541.

27 Hung JS, Chern MS, Wu JJ, et al. Short and long-term results of catheter balloon percutaneous transvenous mitral commissurotomy. Am J Cardiol 1991; 67:854–862.

28 Ribeiro PA, al Zaibag M, Abdullah M. Pulmonary artery pressure and pulmonary vascular resistance before and after mitral balloon valvotomy in 100 patients with severe mitral valve stenosis. Am Heart J 1993; 125(4):1110–1114.

29 Maisano F, Torracca L, Oppizzi M, et al. The edge-to-edge technique: a simplified method to correct mitral insufficiency. Eur J Cardiothorac Surg 1998; 13:240–245.

30 Alfieri O, Maisano F, De Bonis M, et al. The double-orifice technique in mitral valve repair: a simple solution for complex problems. J Thorac Cardiovasc Surg 2001; 122:674–681.

31 Feldman T, Wasserman HS, Herrmann HC, et al. Percutaneous mitral valve repair using the edge-to-edge technique: six-month results of the EVEREST Phase I Clinical Trial. J Am Coll Cardiol 2005; 46:2134–2140.

32 Liddicoat JR, Mac Neill BD, Gillinov AM, et al. Percutaneous mitral valve repair: a feasibility study in an ovine model of acute ischemic mitral regurgitation. Catheter Cardiovasc Interv 2003; 60:410–416.

33 Maniu CV, Patel JB, Reuter DG, et al. Acute and chronic reduction of functional mitral regurgitation in experimental heart failure by percutaneous mitral annuloplasty. J Am Coll Cardiol 2004; 44:1652–1661.

34 Davies H. Catheter mounted valve for temporary relief of aortic insufficiency. Lancet 1965; 1:250.

35 Andersen HR, Knudsen LL, Hasenkam JM. Transluminal implantation of artificial heart valves. Description of a new expandable aortic valve and initial results with implantation by catheter technique in closed chest pigs. Eur Heart J 1992; 13(5):704–708.

36 Cribier A, Eltchaninoff H, Bash A, et al. Percutaneous transcatheter implantation of an aortic valve prosthesis for calcific aortic stenosis: first human case description. Circulation 2002; 106(24):3006–3008.

37 Cribier A, Eltchaninoff H, Tron C, et al. Early experience with percutaneous transcatheter implantation of heart valve prosthesis for the treatment of end-stage inoperable patients with calcific aortic stenosis. J Am Coll Cardiol 2004; 43(4):698–703.

38 Webb JG, Chandavimol M, Thompson CR, et al. Percutaneous aortic valve implantation retrograde from the femoral artery. Circulation 2006; 113(6):842–850.

39 Bonhoeffer P, Boudjemline Y, Saliba Z et al. Transcatheter implantation of a bovine valve in pulmonary position. A lamb study. Circulation 2000; 102:813–816.

40 Bonhoeffer P, Boudjemline Y, Saliba Z et al. Percutaneous replacement of pulmonary valve in a right-ventricle to pulmonary-artery prosthetic conduit with valve dysfunction. Lancet 2000; 356:1403–1405.

41 Topaz O, Taylor AL. Interventricular septal rupture complicating acute myocardial infarction: from pathophysiologic features to the role of invasive and noninvasive diagnostic modalities in current management. Am J Med 1992; 93(6):683–688. Review.

42 Crenshaw BS, Granger CB, Birnbaum Y, et al. Risk factors, angiographic patterns, and outcomes in patients with ventricular septal defect complicating acute myocardial infarction. GUSTO-I (Global Utilization of Streptokinase and TPA for Occluded Coronary Arteries) Trial Investigators. Circulation 2000; 101(1):27–32.

43 Killen DA, Piehler JM, Borkon AM, et al. Early repair of postinfarction ventricular septal rupture. Ann Thorac Surg 1997; 63(1):138–142.

44 Lock JE, Block PC, McKay RG, et al. Transcatheter closure of ventricular septal defects. Circulation 1988; 78:361–368.

45 Fox KA, Mehta SR, Peters R, et al. Clopidogrel in Unstable angina to prevent Recurrent ischemic Events Trial. Benefits and risks of the combination of clopidogrel and aspirin in patients undergoing surgical revascularization for non-ST-elevation acute coronary syndrome: the Clopidogrel in Unstable angina to prevent Recurrent ischemic Events (CURE) Trial. Circulation 2004; 110(10):1202–1208.

46 Mas JL, Arquizan C, Lamy C. Patent Foramen Ovale and Atrial Septal Aneurysm Study Group: recurrent cerebrovascular events associated with patent foramen ovale, atrial septal aneurysm or both. N Eng J Med 2001; 345:1740–1746.

47 Khairy P, O'Donnell CP, Landzberg MJ. Transcatheter closure versus medical therapy of patent foramen ovale and presumed paradoxical thromboemboli: a systematic review. Ann Intern Med 2003; 139(9):753–760.

48 Skowasch M, Hein R, Buescheck F, et al. Non-Implant Closure of Patent Foramen Ovale: First-in-Man Results. Am J Cardiol 2005; 96(suppl 7A):101H.

49 Schwerzmann M, Wiher S, Nedeltchev K, et al. Percutaneous closure of patent foramen ovale reduces the frequency of migraine attacks. Neurology 2004; 62(8):1399–1401.

50 Krumsdorf U, Ostermayer S, Billinger K, et al. Incidence and clinical course of thrombus formation on atrial septal defect and patient foramen ovale closure devices in 1,000 consecutive patients. J Am Coll Cardiol 2004; 43(2):302–309. Review.

52

Pharmacologic use of ethanol for myocardial septal ablation

George D. Dangas, Edwin Lee, and Jeffrey W. Moses

Hypertrophic cardiomyopathy, a primary myocardial disorder of sacromeric proteins with an autosomal dominant pattern of inheritance is characterized by asymmetric hypertrophy of the septum with or without dynamic obstruction of the outflow tract (1,2). The prevalence in the general population is estimated as 1:500 and it is the most common monogenic cardiac disorder. Annual mortality in an unselected population is reported to be about 1% to 2%, and sudden death is the most common cause. Sudden death is assumed to be due to idiopathic ventricular arrhythmias, but hemodynamic factors and myocardial ischemia may be involved as well.

Hemodynamics

The most characteristic hemodynamic feature of hypertrophic cardiomyopathy is the dynamic intraventricular pressure gradient (3). Obstruction to left ventricular ejection occurs in the left ventricular outflow tract due to the contraction of the basal aspect of an asymmetrically hypertrophied interventricular septum resulting in a subaortic pressure gradient. As the ventricle contracts the subaortic flow velocity increases. The acceleration of blood flow through the narrowed outflow tract causes a pressure drop that draws the anterior leaflet of the mitral valve towards the ventricular septum due to a Venturi effect, exacerbating the outflow obstruction and contributing to mitral incompetence. Outflow obstruction is a dynamic phenomenon. Patients with hypertrophic cardiomyopathy may not have a systolic pressure gradient at rest but can have one provoked with the Valsava maneuver or an extrasystole. There is a variability and heterogeneity of hemodynamics among affected patients and even within the same patient over time.

The dynamic outflow obstruction leads to the characteristic spike-and-dome arterial pressure waveform seen most evidently in the proximal aorta (Fig. 1). The early spike is due to a rapid ventricular ejection from the hypercontractile myocardium, and the pressure dip and subsequent doming of the pulse reflect the dynamic outflow obstruction. This is seen following conditions that increase the dynamic gradient, such as an extrasystole, the Valsalva maneuver, or administration of beta-adrenergic agonists or vasodilators. The narrowing in pulse pressure of the spike-and-dome arterial waveform following an extra-systole is known as the Brockenbrough-Braunwald sign. Associated diastolic dysfunction is common with increased diastolic filling pressure evident in the contour of the left ventricular diastolic pressure tracing.

Treatment options

The treatment strategy in patients with severe symptoms unresponsive to maximum medical management and a significant outflow tract obstruction is the reduction of the myocardial septum either by surgery or alcohol ablation (4–6).

Surgery

Surgical myectomy involves incision into and resection of small portions of the hypertrophied septum resulting in a significant reduction or abolition of intramyocardial gradients and reduction in mitral incompetence. Patients report a significant reduction in disabling symptoms and improvement in exercise capacity, and the benefit is usually sustained. The complications are few and the postoperative mortality is

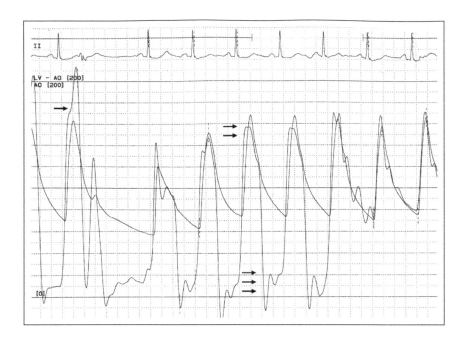

Figure 1
Demonstration of the typical hemodynamic evaluation of hypertrophic cardiomyopathy. Equipment used: single end-hole pigtail catheter, a femoral arterial sheath at least one size larger than the catheter, and two pressure transducers (one at the femoral sheath side port and the other at the pigtail catheter). The catheter is initially seated beyond the stenosis and a pressure gradient is documented, as well as the spike-and-dome configuration during systolic ventricular pressure rise can be observed while the arterial systolic pressure upstroke is steep (*single black arrow*). While the catheter is pulled back, the gradient essentially disappears while the catheter is still inside the left ventricular cavity as documented by the diastolic part of the pressure curve. Finally, the catheter is pulled outside the ventricle and the two transducers document essentially identical pressures (small differences are due to the aortic to femoral pressure wave potentiation). This pullback maneuver is pathognomonic for subaortic obstruction and needs to be performed very slowly and taking special care to avoid provoking a series of ventricular extra-systoles that will obviate the above-described evaluation.

1–3% when myectomy are performed by experienced surgeons in a comprehensive care setting. Long-term survival in patients with obstructive hypertrophic cardiomyopathy and severe symptoms postsurgical myectomy was equivalent to that of the general population (7). Surgical myectomy patients had reduced all cause mortality and sudden cardiac death compared to nonoperated obstructive hypertrophic cardiomyopathy patients (7), suggesting that myectomy may reduce mortality risk in severely symptomatic patients with obstructive hypertrophic cardiomyopathy.

Septal Ablation

Septal alcohol ablation, first reported in 1995 (4), has evolved to become a relatively common procedure with >4000 patients having been treated. This procedure consists of injecting absolute alcohol into a septal perforator to create necrosis and permanent myocardial infarction (MI) in the proximal septum. Subsequent intramyocardial scarring (8) leads to progressive left ventricular wall thinning, restricted septal excursion, enlargement of the outflow tract and consequent reduction in obstruction and mitral regurgitation, thus mimicking the remodeling that results from surgical myectomy.

Selection of patients

Selection of patients for septal ablation includes those with severe symptoms (i.e., New York Heart Association functional class III or IV) *despite appropriately adjusted medical therapy*, with a documented resting left ventricular outflow tract gradient >30 mmHg or a provocable gradient ≥60 mmHg and septal thickness of at least 18 mm. Patients at high risk of surgical morbidity or mortality, including patients of advanced age or with insufficient motivation for surgery, and those with other important comorbidities or other conditions that will likely limit long-term survival are candidates for septal ablation (Table 1).

Patients who have not obtained a satisfactory result after surgical myectomy may also be candidates for septal ablation. Selected patients with advanced function class II with obstructive symptoms that interfere with their occupation may also be candidates for intervention.

Patients with the non-obstructive form of hypetrophic cardiomyopathy should not undergo septal ablation. Patients with congential anomalies of the mitral valve apparatus, associated heart lesions (e.g., advanced multivessel coronary artery disease) requiring surgical correction, unfavorable distribution of septal hypertrophy with mild proximal thickening, basal septal wall thickness <18 mm, or anatomically unsuitable septal perforators should not be candidates for septal ablation.

Table 1   Patient selection criteria for septal alcohol ablation

Severe symptoms (NYHA or CCS class III or IV) despite appropriate drug therapy
NYHA or CCS class II with a resting gradient of >50 or >30 mmHg and ≥100 mmHg with physiological exercise
Symptoms resulting from left ventricular obstruction after discontinuing medication because of intolerable side effects
Resting left ventricular outflow gradient of >30 mmHg or a provocable gradient ≥60 mmHg
Previous unsatisfactory surgical myectomy or pacemaker therapy
Septal thickness >18.5 mm

Abbreviations: CCS, Canadian Cardiovascular Score; NYHA, New York Heart Association.

Ablation techniques

Detailed baseline coronary angiography, left ventriculography, hemodynamic measurements, and measurement of resting/provocable gradients should precede any attempt at septal ablation. Angiography allows for identification of suitable target septal perforators, preferably a large first septal perforator. Ventriculography is useful for demonstrating the degree of mitral regurgitation and location of the dynamic outflow obstruction. Initial hemodynamic assessment assures that the level of obstruction is subaortic. Contrast echocardiography is essential as it enhances the effectiveness and safety of septal ablation (9).

Left ventricular pressure measurements are monitored continuously by use of a 5F end-hole pig-tail catheter in the left ventricular apex and a 6F femoral sheath in order to be able to assess the gradient. If the outflow gradient is absent or small under the basal conditions, the magnitude of provocable obstruction is most appropriately assessed with maneuvers (Valsalva, ventricular pacing, extrasystoles, physiological exercise, amyl nitrate). The inability to elicit any provocable gradient is a contraindication to the procedure.

Dobutamine, an inotropic and catecholamine-inducing drug and a powerful stimulant of subaortic gradients in normal hearts and cardiac conditions other than hypertrophic cardiomyopathy, is not recommended to provoke outflow gradients for assessing the appropriateness of septal ablation (1).

If the gradient is indeed confirmed, a 6 or 7Fr sheath is placed in the left coronary artery from the contralateral femoral artery, in order to reliably assess the ascending aortic pressure even in the presence of intracoronary wires and a balloon inside it (Fig. 2).

A guidewire and subsequently a balloon catheter (2.0–2.5 mm in diameter) are advanced into the septal perforator. Identification of the target territory is performed by contrast echocardiography to determine the most appropriate septal perforator for ethanol infusion by showing echo contrast localization in the area of maximal septal bulge when the target septal is injected with contrast (preferably at the point of mitral leaflet near-contact with the septum). The guidewire is then removed and dilute Optison (1:10) is injected through the inflated balloon lumen to echocardiographically visualize the septal territory perfused by the target septal perforator. The appropriate area of outflow obstruction should be opacified with little spillover to other areas.

Once Optison injection confirms appropriate placement, a small amount of angiographic contrast is infused through the inflated balloon to confirm stasis in the septal perforator and also to document the absence of reflux into the left anterior descending artery during balloon inflation. One to two milliliters of ethanol (100% dehydrated ethanol) is then injected slowly into the target septal artery through the balloon lumen in 0.5–1.0 milliliter amounts at a rate of approximately 1 ml/min, under continuous fluoroscopy in order to surveil for possible balloon displacement (Fig. 2). Throughout the course of balloon inflation, the patency of the downstream left anterior descending artery should be monitored with occasional contrast injection through the guiding catheter. Following the outflow tract gradient response, the coronary balloon remains inflated for 5–10 minutes after the final administration of ethanol to insure that no alcohol refluxes into the left anterior descending artery. After the procedure, repeated hemodynamic and angiographic studies should be performed. "No-flow" at the site of the injected target septal perforator indicates successful alcohol ablation. Hemodynamic measurements are repeated 10 minutes after balloon deflation.

Because of the possibility of developing bradycardia from high-degree atrioventricular block as a consequence of the procedure, a temporary pacemaker should be placed. If the gradient is not adequately reduced, consideration then can be given to repeating the injection or injecting alcohol in an adjacent septal perforating branch, bearing in mind that each additional amount of alcohol increases the risk of atrioventricular block.

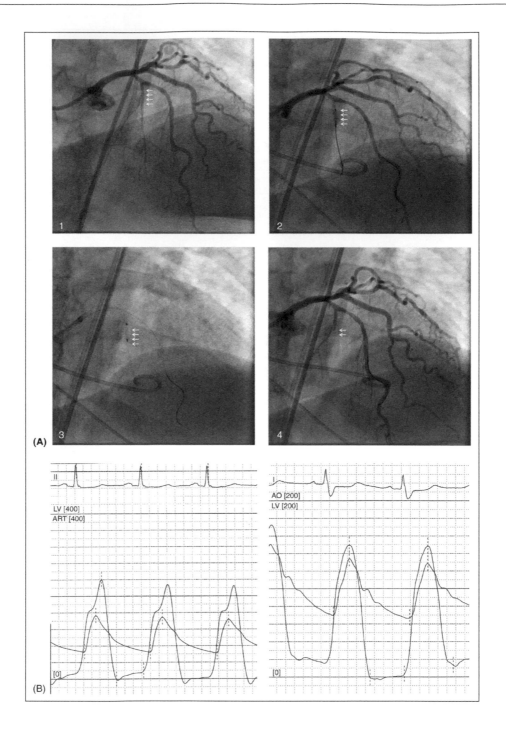

Figure 2

(A) Four stop-frames of an alcohol septal ablation have been captured. Note the presence of a pigtail catheter in the left ventricle and a temporary pacemaker in the right ventricle. Spot-1 depicts the dominant proximal septal perforator. Spot-2 shows the selective catheterization of this septal branch with a 0.014 inch wire and an "over-the-wire balloon," while another wire has been placed in the left anterior descending artery. Spot-3 depicts the way slow, selective injections are delivered selectively in the septal branch through the balloon, after the septal perforator wire has been removed. A test injection with contrast is first performed to ensure absence of back-flow in the left anterior descending artery; contrast echocardiography is then performed after selective contrast injection in order to verify the myocardial distribution of this septal branch in relation to the hypertrophied septal area; another radiographic contrast injection is then performed to verify continued absence of back-flow (spill) in the left anterior descending artery; finally, ethanol injections are performed in 0.5 to 1 ml increments with verification of absence of back-flow before any repeat injection. (B) Hemodynamic documentation of the pre- and post-procedure pressure tracings in this case. On the left side, the pressure scale is up to 400 mmHg and a gradient >60 mmHg is documented; the spike-and-dome configuration of the left ventricular pressure tracing is observed, as well as a steep upstroke of the arterial pressure. On the right side, a small residual gradient is observed (<20 mmHg); note that the pressure scale is now up to 200 mmHg.

Postprocedure care

Following septal ablation, patients should be monitored in a coronary care unit for 24 to 48 hours and the temporary pacing wire should be removed at the end of this period in the absence of atrioventricular block. Patients may then be transferred to a telemetry unit for monitoring of arrhythmias. Total hospitalization is usually for three to five days to monitor for occurrence of complete heart block that would require a permanent pacemaker. A sizeable infarction is induced with alcohol ablation and causes creatinine phosphokinase to peak at 1000 to 1500 one day after the ablation. Patients should be maintained on aspirin indefinitely.

Various drugs

In preparation for chest discomfort during alcohol injection, prophylactic analgesic medication (eg. fentanyl 25 mm IV) is administered. Antithrombotic prophylaxis with intravenous, weight-adjusted heparin is given to maintain an activated clotting time of 200 to 250 seconds.

Acute results

Procedural success is defined by an acute reduction in resting and/or provoked left ventricular outflow gradient by 50% or to <20 mmHg, which can be achieved in the short term in approximately 90% of treated patients (Tables 2 and 3) (10,11). The immediate post-ablation gradient reduction is probably due to alcohol-mediated septal necrosis and stunning. Progressive decrease in the gradient across the outflow on long-term follow-up is secondary to septal thinning and ventricular remodeling.

Long-term results

Successful septal ablation leads to significant improvement in objective tests of exercise performance in terms of treadmill exercise time and peak oxygen consumption in follow-up studies over 3 to 18 months (Table 2) (11–15). Significant and sustained improvement in echocardiographic measures of diastolic function are seen up to two years which may account for the improved functional status after septal ablation (16).

The three-month (11) and one-year (10) results of both surgical myomectomy and alcohol septal ablation were comparable, however, surgical myomectomy was superior to ablation in terms of improved exercise test parameters (Table 1) (14). Studies indicate maintenance of clinical and hemodynamic benefits from two-year follow-up studies (17,18) and more recently up to five-year follow-up (Table 2) (19).

Patients with increased outflow gradients prior to discharge after initial success of septal ablation that improves at three-month follow-up and that remains less than 50% at one-year follow up have been reported (20). At present, it is not known whether the timing of maximal outflow gradient reduction after surgical myectomy or septal ablation is important in reducing morbidity and mortality. The small mean differences in reduction of the LV outflow gradient between surgery and septal ablation may be important, as the severity of left ventricular outflow tract gradient is an independent risk factor for functional deterioration (21).

Predictors of an unsatisfactory outcome after septal ablation (persistent symptoms with a less than 50% reduction in the left ventricular outflow tract gradient) includes baseline higher outflow tract gradients, fewer septal arteries injected with alcohol, lower peak creatine kinase, smaller septal area opacified by contrast echocardiography, and higher residual gradient in the catheterization laboratory after septal ablation. Of note, age, New York Heart Association, or Canadian Cardiovascular Score functional class, exercise capacity, septal thickness, left ventricular filling pressures, mitral regurgitation severity, and ventricular function were not determinants of unsuccessful outcome (22).

Implications on arrhythmogenicity

Conduction system defects, a common complication of septal ablation can be associated with a incidence of complete heart block ranging from 10% to 33% (23) compared to a <1% incidence of complete heart block after surgical myectomy (6,24) (Table 4). Because specific, but different, portions of the ventricular septum are affected by each procedure, patients with baseline right bundle branch block are more likely to need long-term pacing after surgical myectomy, whereas those with baseline left bundle branch block are more likely to need pacing after septal ablation (25). Patients who develop acute complete heart block or new intraventricular conduction defects during septal ablation are at high risk of developing subacute complete heart block and should therefore have temporary pacing support for at least 48 hours after septal ablation (26).

Other risk factors for complete heart block were left bundle branch block, first degree atrioventricular block, female gender, volume of alcohol, and number of septal perforators treated (27–29).

Concerns of increased ventricular arrhythmias created by scarring remaining from spetal ablation have been raised. However, there is no evidence for increased arrhythmogenicity as assessed by serial electrophysiological studies

Table 2 Summary of studies comparing surgical myectomy and septal ablation

Study	No. of patients	F/U months	Mean NYHA or % in NYHA Class III/IV		LVOT gradient, mmHg		Peak O$_2$ consumption, ml/kg/min		Exercise workload, watts	
			Pre	Post	Pre	Post	Pre	Post	Pre	Post
Van der Lee, 2005 (33)		12								
Myectomy	29		2.8 ± 0.4	1.3 ± 0.4[a]	100 ± 20	17 ± 14[a]				
Ablation	43		2.4 ± 0.5	1.5 ± 0.7[a]	101 ± 34	23 ± 19[a]				
Nagueh, 2001 (10)		12								
Myectomy	41		78%	2%[a]	78 ± 20	4 ± 7[a]	20.8 ± 4.9	26.2 ± 6.5[a]		
Ablation	41		90%	0%[a]	76 ± 23	8 ± 15[a]	18.9 ± 5.7	22.2 ± 5.3[a]		
Qin, 2001 (11)		3								
Myectomy	26		3.3 ± 0.5	1.5 ± 0.7[a]	62 ± 43	11 ± 6[a]				
Ablation	25		3.5 ± 0.5	1.9 ± 0.7[a]	64 ± 39	24 ± 19[a]				
Firoozi, 2002 (14)		12								
Myectomy	24		2.4 ± 0.6	1.5 ± 0.7[a]	83 ± 23	17 ± 12[a]	16.4 ± 5.8	23.1 ± 7.1[a,b]	130 ± 57	161 ± 60[a,b]
Ablation	20		2.3 ± 0.5	1.7 ± 0.8[a]	91 ± 18	21 ± 12[a]	16.2 ± 5.2	19.3 ± 6.1[a]	121 ± 53	137 ± 51

Note: Pre indicates preintervention; post indicates postintervention.
[a]p < 0.05 versus baseline values.
[b]p < 0.05 versus septal ablation.
Abbreviation: NYHA, New York Heart Association.

Table 3 Summary of septal ablation follow-up studies

Study	No. of patients	F/U, months or Mean ± SD	Mean NYHA class or percent of patients in NYHA Class III/IV		LVOT gradient, mmHg		Exercise duration/sec		Exercise/ Watts		VO₂	
			Pre	Post	Pre	Post	Pre	Post	Pre	Post	Pre	Post
Knight, 1997 (34)	18	3			67 (48–87)	22 (12–32)ᵃ	418 (273–563)	452 (283–621)			24.2 (18.4–30.0)	26.8 (19.1–34.5)
Lakkis, 1998 (35)	33	1.4	3.0 ± 0.5	0.9 ± 0.6ᵃ	49 ± 33	9 ± 19*	286 ± 193	421 ± 181ᵃ				
Gietzen, 1999 (18)	50	10.6 ± 5.6	3.0 ± 0.3	1.7 ± 0.6ᵃ	45 ± 38	5 ± 7ᵃ			69 ± 29	88 ± 34ᵃ	13 ± 4	16 ± 6ᵃ
Ruzyllo, 2000 (36)	25	10.4 ± 1.8	2.8 ± 0.5	1.2 ± 0.5ᵃ	84.5 ± 31.4	32.4 ± 25.8	571.9 ± 192.2	703.5 ± 175.4ᵃ			14.6 ± 5.2	20.5 ± 8.6ᵃ
Lakkis, 2000 (23)	50	12			74 ± 23	6 ± 18ᵃ	271 ± 160	407 ± 211ᵃ				
Faber, 2000 (13)	25	30 ± 4	2.8 ± 0.6	1.2 ± 1.0ᵃ	60 ± 38	3 ± 6ᵃ			67 ± 74	105 ± 40*		
Boekstegers, 2001 (12)	50	18	2.8 ± 0.6	1.7 ± 0.7ᵃ	80 ± 33	17 ± 15ᵃ						
Gietzen, 2002 (15)	45	10 ± 8	3.1 ± 0.3	1.7 ± 0.6ᵃ	ᵇ111 ± 44ᵇ	†24 ± 24ᵃ			66 ± 29	85 ± 27ᵃ	13.3 ± 4.6	16.0 ± 5.3
	84	10 ± 8	3.1 ± 0.2	1.5 ± 0.6ᵃ	81 ± 33	16 ± 20ᵃ			73 ± 31	94 ± 37ᵃ	14.8 ± 4.5	16.6 ± 6.0ᵃ
Shamin, 2002 (37)	64	36.0 ± 15.6			64 ± 36	16 ± 15ᵃ	366 ± 168	600 ± 192ᵃ			18.4 ± 5.8	30.0 ± 4.4ᵃ
Faber, 2004 (9)	312	3	2.9 ± 0.5	1.5 ± 0.6ᵃ					94 ± 51	115 ± 43ᵃ	18 ± 4	21 ± 6ᵃ
Faber, 2005 (38)	242	4.9 ± 2.3	2.8 ± 0.7	1.7 ± 0.7ᵃ	57 ± 31	20 ± 21ᵃ						
Fernandes, 2005 (19)	130	43.2 ± 16.8	3.0 ± 0.4	1.2 ± 0.6ᵃ	74 ± 30	4 ± 13ᵃ	322 ± 207	443 ± 200ᵃ				
Yoerger, 2006 (20)	47	12	2.9 ± 0.7	1.7 ± 0.9ᵃ	98 ± 48	22 ± 29ᵃ						

Note: Pre indicates preintervention; post indicates postintervention.
ᵃp <0.05 versus baseline values.
ᵇProvocable left ventricular outflow tract gradient.

Table 4   Reported complication after surgical myectomy or septal ablation

Study	Procedure	No. of patients	F/U, months or mean ± SD	Death, n (%)	Late cardiac mortality, n (%)	Acute MI n (%)	Ventricular fibrillation, n (%)	Permanent pacing, n (%)	Reintervention, n (%)
Van der Lee, 2005 (33)	Myectomy	29	12	0 (0)		0 (0)	0 (0)	0 (0)	1 (3)
	Ablation	43		2 (5)		1 (2)	6 (14)	4 (9)	4 (9)
Nagueh, 2001 (10)	Myectomy	41	12	0 (0)				1 (2)	
	Ablation	41		1 (2)				9 (22)	
Qin, 2001 (11)	Myectomy	26	3	0 (0)				2 (8)	0 (0)
	Ablation	25		0 (0)				6 (24)	6 (24)
Firoozi, 2002 (14)	Myectomy	24	12	1 (4)				1 (4)	
	Ablation	20		1 (4)				3 (15)	
Talreja, 2004 (25)	Myectomy	117		0 (0)				4 (3)	
	Ablation	58		0 (0)				66 (12)	
Knight, 1997 (34)	Ablation	18	3	0 (0)		1 (6)	2 (11)		
Lakkis, 1998 (35)	Ablation	33	1.4	0 (0)				11 (33)	
Gietzen, 1999 (18)	Ablation	50	10.6 ± 5.6	2 (4)				19 (38)	
Ruzyllo, 2000 (36)	Ablation	25	10.4 ± 1.8	0 (0)		3 (12)	0 (0)	4 (16)	
Lakkis, 2000 (23)	Ablation	50	12	2 (4)	1 (2)			11 (22)	7 (14)
Faber, 2000 (13)	Ablation	25	30 ± 4	1 (4)			1 (4)	5 (20)	3 (12)
Boekstegers, 2001 (12)	Ablation	50	18	0 (0)				5 (10)	
Gietzen, 2002 (15)	Ablation	45	10 ± 8	0 (0)	0 (0)			12 (27)	
		84	10 ± 8	0 (0)	0 (0)			21 (25)	
Shamin, 2002 (37)	Ablation	64	36.0 ± 15.6					17 (27)	
Faber, 2004 (9)	Ablation	312	3	4 (1)					
Faber, 2005 (38)	Ablation	242	4.9 ± 2.3	3 (1)					
Fernandes, 2005 (19)	Ablation	130	43.2 ± 16.8	2 (2)	3 (2)				17 (13)

Abbreviations: ICD, internal cardiac defibrillator; MI myocardial infarction; SCD, sudden cardiac death.

before and after septal ablation (18). There was also no increase in the incidence of ventricular arrhythmias or sudden cardiac death in all of the follow-up studies of septal ablation (Table 4).

Dose of alcohol

The amount of alcohol injected depends on the contrast echocardiographic estimated size of the target area, extent of septal thickness, as well the hemodynamic effect required (30). Lower doses of ethanol (1 to 2 ml) injected into the target septal branch reduces the size of myocardial necrosis and has comparable hemodynamic reduction and clinical outcome as usual doses (2 to 4 milliliters) (31,32). Injection of smaller doses of ethanol (one to 2 mL) over longer time periods (5 to 10 min) can decrease the higher incidence of CHB after septal ablation (27).

Complications

Septal ablation related mortality at experienced centers is currently 1% to 2%, similar to that of surgical myectomy (Table 4). Conduction system abnormalities are relatively common complications of septal ablation. Permanent right bundle branch block occurs in about 50% of patients and transitory complete heart block in 60% and permanent pacemakers required for high grade atrioventricular block in about 5% to 20%. Concerns of late occurrence of complete heart block following septal ablation mandates in-patient monitoring for 4 to 5 days.

Chest pain during septal ablation commonly occurs and is effectively managed by analgesic therapy. Intensive care unit monitoring is employed routinely postprocedure in anticipation of ventricular arrhythmias during the initial period of myocardial injury. Prophylactic antiarrhythmic therapy has not been used in our center.

A profound complication of septal ablation is anterior MI due to ethanol reflux from the septal perforator down the left anterior descending artery. This can be avoided by careful position of the balloon and angiographic monitoring. Other rare complications include coronary dissection, perforation, thrombosis, and spasm.

Conclusions

Ethanol has been used successfully for selective ablation of the hypertrophied septum in hyperthrophic cardiomyopathy patients with refractory symptoms on maximal medical therapy. This technique is less invasive than surgical myomectomy, and patient suitability depends on the angiographic delineation of the septal perforators and the distribution of their myocardial perfusion territory as assessed by contrast echocardiography. Both the interventional and the surgical techniques have not been tested against medical therapy or in a prospective, controlled long-term follow-up study. Although the interventional procedure appears simple, it should be conducted with meticulous technique and great attention to all the details because it could have rare, albeit very serious complications.

References

1   Maron BJ, McKenna WJ, Danielson GK, et al. American College of Cardiology/European Society of Cardiology clinical expert consensus document on hypertrophic cardiomyopathy. A report of the American College of Cardiology Foundation Task Force on Clinical Expert Consensus Documents and the European Society of Cardiology Committee for Practice Guidelines. J Am Coll Cardiol 2003; 42:1687–1713.

2   Maron MS, Olivotto I, Betocchi S, Casey SA, Lesser JR, Losi MA, Cecchi F, Maron BJ. Effect of left ventricular outflow tract obstruction on clinical outcome in hypertrophic cardiomyopathy. N Engl J Med 2003; 348:295–303.

3   Fang J, Eisenhauer A. Profiles in cardiomyopathy and congestive heart failure. Textbook: Grossman's Cardiac Catheterization, Angiography, and Intervention. Seventh Edition. Lippincott Williams & Wilkins, 2005.

4   Sigwart U. Non-surgical myocardial reduction for hypertrophic obstructive cardiomyopathy. Lancet 1995; 346:211–214.

5   Maron BJ, Dearani JA, Ommen SR, et al. The case for surgery in obstructive hypertrophic cardiomyopathy. J Am Coll Cardiol 2004; 44:2044–2053.

6   Nishimura RA, Holmes DR, Jr. Clinical practice. Hypertrophic obstructive cardiomyopathy. N Engl J Med 2004; 350: 1320–1327.

7   Ommen SR, Maron BJ, Olivotto I, et al. Long-term effects of surgical septal myectomy on survival in patients with obstructive hypertrophic cardiomyopathy. J Am Coll Cardiol 2005; 46:470–476.

8   Raute-Kreinsen U. Morphology of necrosis and repair after transcoronary ethanol ablation of septal hypertrophy. Pathol Res Pract 2003; 199:121–127.

9   Faber L, Seggewiss H, Welge D, et al. Echo-guided percutaneous septal ablation for symptomatic hypertrophic obstructive cardiomyopathy: 7 years of experience. Eur J Echocardiogr 2004; 5:347–355.

10 Nagueh SF, Ommen SR, Lakkis NM, et al. Comparison of ethanol septal reduction therapy with surgical myectomy for the treatment of hypertrophic obstructive cardiomyopathy. J Am Coll Cardiol 2001; 38:1701–1706.

11 Qin JX, Shiota T, Lever HM, et al. Outcome of patients with hypertrophic obstructive cardiomyopathy after percutaneous transluminal septal myocardial ablation and septal myectomy surgery. J Am Coll Cardiol 2001; 38:1994–2000.

12 Boekstegers P, Steinbigler P, Molnar A, et al. Pressure-guided nonsurgical myocardial reduction induced by small septal infarctions in hypertrophic obstructive cardiomyopathy. J Am Coll Cardiol 2001; 38:846–853.

13 Faber L, Meissner A, Ziemssen P, Seggewiss H. Percutaneous transluminal septal myocardial ablation for hypertrophic obstructive cardiomyopathy: long term follow up of the first series of 25 patients. Heart 2000; 83:326–331.

14 Firoozi S, Elliott PM, Sharma S, et al. Septal myotomy-myectomy and transcoronary septal alcohol ablation in hypertrophic obstructive cardiomyopathy. A comparison of clinical, haemodynamic and exercise outcomes. Eur Heart J 2002; 23:1617–1624.

15 Gietzen FH, Leuner CJ, Obergassel L, et al.. Role of transcoronary ablation of septal hypertrophy in patients with hypertrophic cardiomyopathy, New York Heart Association functional class III or IV, and outflow obstruction only under provocable conditions. Circulation 2002; 106:454–459.

16 Jassal DS, Neilan TG, Fifer MA, et al. Sustained improvement in left ventricular diastolic function after alcohol septal ablation for hypertrophic obstructive cardiomyopathy. Eur Heart J 2006.

17 Mazur W, Nagueh SF, Lakkis NM, et al. Regression of left ventricular hypertrophy after nonsurgical septal reduction therapy for hypertrophic obstructive cardiomyopathy. Circulation 2001; 103:1492–1496.

18 Gietzen FH, Leuner CJ, Raute-Kreinsen U, et al. Acute and long-term results after transcoronary ablation of septal hypertrophy (TASH). Catheter interventional treatment for hypertrophic obstructive cardiomyopathy. Eur Heart J 1999; 20:1342–1354.

19 Fernandes VL, Nagueh SF, Wang W, et al. A prospective follow-up of alcohol septal ablation for symptomatic hypertrophic obstructive cardiomyopathy—the Baylor experience (1996–2002). Clin Cardiol 2005; 28:124–130.

20 Yoerger DM, Picard MH, Palacios IF, et al. Time course of pressure gradient response after first alcohol septal ablation for obstructive hypertrophic cardiomyopathy. Am J Cardiol 2006; 97:1511–1514.

21 Kofflard MJ, Ten Cate FJ, van der Lee C, et al. Hypertrophic cardiomyopathy in a large community-based population: clinical outcome and identification of risk factors for sudden cardiac death and clinical deterioration. J Am Coll Cardiol 2003; 41:987–993.

22 Chang SM, Lakkis NM, Franklin J, et al. Predictors of outcome after alcohol septal ablation therapy in patients with hypertrophic obstructive cardiomyopathy. Circulation 2004; 109:824–827.

23 Lakkis NM, Nagueh SF, Dunn JK, et al, Spencer WH III3rd. Nonsurgical septal reduction therapy for hypertrophic obstructive cardiomyopathy: one-year follow-up. J Am Coll Cardiol 2000; 36:852–855.

24 McCully RB, Nishimura RA, Tajik AJ, et al. Extent of clinical improvement after surgical treatment of hypertrophic obstructive cardiomyopathy. Circulation 1996; 94:467–471.

25 Talreja DR, Nishimura RA, Edwards WD, et al. Alcohol septal ablation versus surgical septal myectomy: comparison of effects on atrioventricular conduction tissue. J Am Coll Cardiol 2004; 44:2329–2332.

26 Chen AA, Palacios IF, Mela T, et al. Acute predictors of subacute complete heart block after alcohol septal ablation for obstructive hypertrophic cardiomyopathy. Am J Cardiol 2006; 97:264–269.

27 Chang SM, Nagueh SF, Spencer WH III, et al. Complete heart block: determinants and clinical impact in patients with hypertrophic obstructive cardiomyopathy undergoing nonsurgical septal reduction therapy. J Am Coll Cardiol 2003; 42:296–300.

28 Faber L, Seggewiss H, Welge D, et al. [Predicting the risk of atrioventricular conduction lesions after percutaneous septal ablation for obstructive hypertrophic cardiomyopathy]. Z Kardiol 2003; 92:39–47.

29 Kern MJ, Holmes DG, Simpson C, Bitar SR, Rajjoub H. Delayed occurrence of complete heart block without warning after alcohol septal ablation for hypertrophic obstructive cardiomyopathy. Catheter Cardiovasc Interv 2002; 56:503–507.

30 Seggewiss H. Medical therapy versus interventional therapy in hypertropic obstructive cardiomyopathy. Curr Control Trials Cardiovasc med 2000; 1:115–119.

31 Veselka J, Prochazkova S, Duchonova R et al. Alcohol septal ablation for hypertrophic obstructive cardiomyopathy: Lower alcohol dose reduces size of infarction and has comparable hemodynamic and clinical outcome. Catheter Cardiovasc Interv 2004; 63:231–235.

32 Veselka J, Duchonova R, Prochazkova S, et al. Effects of varying ethanol dosing in percutaneous septal ablation for obstructive hypertrophic cardiomyopathy on early hemodynamic changes. Am J Cardiol 2005; 95:675–678.

33 van der Lee C, ten Cate FJ, Geleijnse ML, et al. Percutaneous versus surgical treatment for patients with hypertrophic obstructive cardiomyopathy and enlarged anterior mitral valve leaflets. Circulation 2005; 112:482–488.

34 Knight C, Kurbaan AS, Seggewiss H, et al. Nonsurgical septal reduction for hypertrophic obstructive cardiomyopathy: outcome in the first series of patients. Circulation 1997; 95:2075–2081.

35 Lakkis NM, Nagueh SF, Kleiman NS, et al. Echocardiography-guided ethanol septal reduction for hypertrophic obstructive cardiomyopathy. Circulation 1998; 98:1750–1755.

36 Ruzyllo W, Chojnowska L, Demkow M, et al. Left ventricular outflow tract gradient decrease with non-surgical myocardial reduction improves exercise capacity in patients with hypertrophic obstructive cardiomyopathy. Eur Heart J 2000; 21:770–777.

37 Shamim W, Yousufuddin M, Wang D, et al. Nonsurgical reduction of the interventricular septum in patients with hypertrophic cardiomyopathy. N Engl J Med 2002; 347:1326–1333.

38 Faber L, Seggewiss H, Gietzen FH, et al. Catheter-based septal ablation for symptomatic hypertrophic obstructive cardiomyopathy: follow-up results of the TASH-registry of the German Cardiac Society. Z Kardiol 2005; 94:516–523.

Epilogue: Anticoagulant management of patients undergoing interventional procedures

Jawed Fareed

Over the past decade, interest in anticoagulant, antiplatelet, and thrombolytic drugs has grown dramatically, as evident by a continual increase in the number of drugs introduced for both preclinical and clinical development. Several comprehensive reviews have provided a timely coverage of new therapeutic agents in thrombosis and thrombolysis, focusing on such topics as new heparins, synthetic heparinomimetic agents, antithrombin agents, anti-Xa agents, biotechnology-derived antithrombotic proteins, antiplatelet drugs, and novel thrombolytic agents. The developments are so fast that periodic updates on the newly available information on these agents are needed. The outstanding scientific research and development activities in the academic centers and pharmaceutical industry have resulted in a steady flow of new products from various groups. Third-party validation of the products developed and extensive clinical trials has been carried out globally to validate the claims on the safety and efficacy of the newer drugs. The results of these studies also constitute a significant portion of the progress reported at scientific forums. Through their fast track and revised policies, the regulatory bodies such as the European Medicine Evaluation Agency, U.S. Food and Drug Administration (US FDA), and other regional agencies have continually contributed to the timely evaluation and approval of new drugs by providing input at various stages of drug development. Such close interactions have facilitated the clarification of various issues related to drug development and, in fact, have accelerated the approval process of many new drugs such as low molecular weight heparins (LMWs), synthetic heparin pentasaccharide (Arixtra), and newer antithrombin agents. Many new antiplatelet drugs and thrombolytic agents have also gained approval for multiple indications. The concept of polytherapy, including a combination of different drugs, has been introduced.

The introduction of stents in interventional cardiology has added a new dimension in the management of acute coronary syndrome and related disorders. Moreover, stents are now commonly used in the management of vascular and ischemic disorders in expanded indications. Initial attempts to coat stents with anticoagulant drugs have met with limited success; however, such approaches are still carried out. Drug-coated stents have also been introduced and until recently were widely used. Antiproliferative agents such as Taxol and Sirolimus have also been employed; however, their use has resulted with unexpected thrombotic complications. A recent US FDA panel has reviewed this matter and recommended that drug-coated stent implanted patients should be simultaneously treated with antithrombotic agents.

Over the past few years, interest in anticoagulant drugs has grown significantly, as evidenced by a constant increase in the number of drugs introduced for both preclinical and clinical development. The excellent scientific research and development activities in the laboratories of the pharmaceutical industry have resulted in a steady flow of new products from various groups. Several new antithrombotics and anticoagulants have been introduced during the past five years for clinical evaluation. Third-party validation of developed products and well-designed clinical trials has been carried out in various academic medical centers. The results of these studies also constitute a significant portion of the progress reported at scientific meetings, and many important results have become available since the inception of this publication. Through its fast-track drug approval and revised policies, the FDA has provided expeditious mechanisms to the pharmaceutical industry, along with open-platform meetings, to discuss regulatory issues in the optimal development of new anticoagulant, antithrombotic, and thrombolytic drugs. The FDA and its representatives have continually contributed to the timely availability of new drugs by providing input at various stages of drug development. This input also has helped to clarify various issues related to new drug development and, in fact, has accelerated the approval process for many newer drugs, such as the LMWHs, ReoPro, and recombinant hirudin.

Although heparin remains the sole anticoagulant used for the cardiovascular surgical procedures, the introduction of LMWH has added a new dimension to the overall management of thrombotic and cardiovascular disorders. Evidently, the LMWHs have achieved gold standard status in the management of thromboembolic disorders and now challenge other treatments, such as oral anticoagulants, for various indications. At the most recent meeting of the American Heart Association (Chicago, U.S.A., 2006), cardiologists revealed supportive data for the polytherapeutic use of LMWHs in the management of coronary syndromes, thrombotic stroke, and malignancy associated with thrombotic events. Antithrombin agents such as hirudin have also been compared with LMWHs for postsurgical prophylaxis of thromboembolism. Initial reports indicate favorable results with the use of polyethylene glycol-coupled (PEG) hirudin for treatment of coronary syndromes. In addition to the development of LMWHs, understanding the mechanisms of their antithrombotic actions and the relevance of their structural components has led to the development of synthetic analogs of heparin fragments. One remarkable approach based on the elucidation of the structure of heparin has led to the synthesis of oligosaccharides with high affinity for antithrombin III (AT III). Synthetic pentasaccharide is under evaluation in clinical trials for both thromboembolic and coronary indications. Several reports described its uses in various interventional procedures.

There is much discussion of how LMWHs mediate their effects. In addition to potentiation of AT III, several other mechanisms have been identified, including the release of tissue factor pathway inhibitor (TFPI), vascular effects, profibrinolytic effects, platelet selectin modulation, and growth factor modulation. Clinical trials in Europe have shown that subcutaneous LMWH, given once or twice daily, is at least as safe and effective as continuous intravenous heparin in the prevention of recurrent venous thromboembolism and is associated with reduced bleeding and lower mortality rates. Several recent studies have shown that home administration of LMWH is as safe and effective as hospital administration of intravenous heparin in patients with proximal venous thrombosis. Initial evidence clearly suggests that LMWH may be a useful alternative to heparin in patients with pulmonary embolism. LMWHs may also be a useful alternative to heparin for arterial indications, such as treatment of unstable angina and stroke maintenance of peripheral arterial grafts. Recognizing the usefulness of LMWHs, the pharmaceutical industry has focused its attention on their use in the management of ischemic and thrombotic stroke. The initial results of clinical trials are promising. Thus, in the near future, the use of LMWH for prevention of thrombotic or ischemic stroke will be an important goal. The success of early clinical trials also suggests that LMWH may be useful in the management of primary and secondary ischemic or thrombotic stroke.

Although LMWHs are proving to be as effective as and safer than heparin for various indications, it is important to realize that the differences in the manufacture of various LMWHs lead to differences in their pharmacological profile. Although these differences have not been clinically validated, each of the LMWHs is expected to exhibit its own therapeutic index in a given clinical setting. Thus, the interchange of LMWHs based on equivalent gravimetric or biologic potency of standardized dosages may not be feasible. Because of the newer indications and the length of therapy, some additional issues related to the optimal use of LMWHs remain to be addressed. Examples include monitoring, control of bleeding, and drug interactions. Clinical trials have been designed to obtain information related to these issues. The differential clinical efficacy of various LMWHs was evident in the trials carried out with Fragmin (FRISC and FRIC) and enoxaparin (ESSENCE) and more recently with EXTRACT and other trials.

Economic analyses of the treatment cost of heparin versus LMWH in various clinical settings show that although the cost of LMWH is marginally higher than the cost of heparin ($40–150), the expected reduction in costs for all treatment-related clinical events is much higher for LMWHs ($350–2700) than for heparin. Thus, LMWHs are an attractive alternative in an era of managed care health reform. Individual economic analysis for specific indications may provide additional information about the reduced costs, with the use of LMWHs for long-term outpatient treatment of such syndromes as unstable angina and ischemic cerebral events.

In the search for antiplatelet agents to be used as antithrombotic drugs, it was recognized that the platelet glycoprotein IIb/IIIa (GPIIb/IIIa) plays a key role in the final common pathway for platelet aggregation. Several reports have become available recently. Many synthetic GPIIb/IIIa inhibitors are currently under clinical development for various indications. In the European Prospective Investigation in Cancer trial, ReoPro (an anti-GPIIb/IIIa) has been shown to reduce thrombotic events after percutaneous coronary angioplasty (PTCA). In an EPILOG study, the combined effects of ReoPro and heparin resulted in the inhibition of restenosis. Many of the GPIIa/IIIb inhibitors, including ReoPro, have also been found to inhibit the vitronectin receptor ($\forall_1 \exists_3$ integrin), which is implicated in endothelial and smooth muscle cell migration. Thus, these agents exhibit multiple effects in addition to their antiplatelet functions. Another application of GPIIb/IIIa inhibitors is as an alternative agent to aspirin in the management of unstable angina, non-Q wave myocardial infarction, and ischemic or thrombotic stroke. The mechanism of the antiplatelet action of synthetic GPIIb/IIIa inhibitors and antibodies may be the same; however, major differences have been noted in their safety and efficacy. An emerging problem is therapeutic monitoring, which is being addressed with point-of-care systems. Thus, major clinical breakthroughs are expected with the use of these inhibitors in the management of cerebrovascular and cardiovascular disorders. The introduction of novel antiplatelet drugs has added a new dimension to the management of arterial thrombotis—in particular, thrombotic stroke. The availability of specific antagonist of adenosine diphosphate (ADP) receptor (e.g., ticlopidine) has provided a new approach for several cardiovascular and cerebrovascular indications. The second generation ADP receptor-blocking agents (e.g., clopidogrel) underwent extensive clinical trials to test their therapeutic efficacy in combined cardiovascular and cerebrovascular endpoints.

Understanding the coagulation process has led to the identification of thrombin as a key enzyme in thrombogenic processes. Several direct thrombin inhibitors have been developed over the past few years by different methods. Hirudin, the leech-derived protein, has been compared with heparin for various procedures in numerous clinical settings, including treatment and prophylaxis of venous and arterial thrombotic disorders. The use of hirudin has been reported to be associated with increased risk of bleeding, indicating that better monitoring and dose-adjustment protocols are needed as well as antidotes. So far, clinical trials comparing hirudin and heparin as adjuncts in thrombolytic therapy in myocardial infarction (TIMI 9B) and acute coronary syndromes (GUSTO IIb) have shown hirudin to be marginally (if at all) superior to heparin.

Recently, several reports comparing the effects of heparin and hirudin on various parameters have become available. A study comparing heparin and recombinant hirudin for the prophylaxis of deep venous thrombosis (DVT) provided impressive data in favor of hirudin. In a second study, LMWHs also were compared with hirudin for postsurgical prophylaxis of DVT; the results favored hirudin. Both studies emphasize an important point about the validity of well-designed clinical trials. It is important to understand that the efficacy and safety of a new drug may not be determined by trials for a single indication. Therefore, clinical trials are needed for various specific indications.

Argatroban, another smaller thrombin inhibitor, is currently under clinical development for various indications. It has been used successfully in Japan for over a decade in the treatment of thrombotic disorders. Several clinical trials in both Europe and the United States have been designed to investigate its use as an alternative to heparin in heparin-compromised patients and as a prophylactic agent to reduce late restenosis after PTCA and coronary directional atherectomy. Argatroban was successfully used for the management of anticoagulation in patients with heparin-induced thrombocytopenia and as a substitute for heparin in PTCA. Since the half-life of argatroban is rather short, it has been administered via infusion protocols. For therapeutic anticoagulation, a level of 1–2 μg/mL is indicated, whereas for interventional cardiologic procedures a level of 3–7 μg/mL is maintained.

Angiomax represents a synthetic antithrombin agent, which is shown to exhibit superior safety profile for anticoagulation in interventional procedures in comparison with heparin. Several studies have compared Angiomax with unfractionated heparin in a monotherapeutic approach and in settings with GPIIb/IIIa inhibitors. However, although the initial results show superiority in terms of efficacy and safety, the long-term outcome results have raised some questions on the mortality outcome and other complications. Like other thrombin inhibitors used parenterally, Angiomax

does not release TFPI and may compromise thrombin–thrombomodulin-mediated regulatory functions in blood vessels. Moreover, there is no antidote available for Angiomax. Therefore, heparins remain to be the anticoagulant of choice in interventional indications. Angiomax may be useful in heparin-compromised patients.

Because of their weaker anticoagulant effect in global clotting tests, direct factor Xa inhibitors were not considered the desirable anticoagulant and antithrombotic agents for developmental purposes. However, because of the favorable clinical results with pentasaccharide, strong interest in synthetic anti-factor Xa drugs has re-emerged. These agents may be useful in the prophylaxis of both arterial and venous thrombotic disorders and may offer a greater margin of safety than the existing drugs. Additional advantages of direct thrombin and factor Xa inhibitors over heparin include subcutaneous and oral bioavailability. Although their biologic half-life is usually under 30 minutes, coupling to larger agents such as dextran or albumin can prolong their half-life without affecting their pharmacologic actions. Questions about monitoring and antagonism will have to be answered before thrombin and factor Xa inhibitors can be widely explored in clinical settings. Depending on their specificity for thrombin or factor Xa, they may be used as adjuncts with other classes of drugs, such as thrombolytic agents, for treatment of acute myocardial infarction. Low-molecular-weight thrombin and factor Xa inhibitors may also be used for localized delivery, stenting, and transdermal delivery.

Because of their better bioavailabilty, a combination of thrombin and factor Xa inhibitors may be more useful in combination than as single agents. Optimal combinations for specific indications may be considered. As in the clinical development of LMWHs, thrombin and factor Xa inhibitors should be compared with heparin in terms of safety, efficacy, and cost.

Newer developments in thrombolytic therapy include recombinant tissue plasminogen activators (tPAs). Bolus-injectable Reptilase is an unglycosylated plasminogen activator consisting of the Kirngle 2 and protease domain of tPA with a three- to four-fold longer half-life than tPA. The INECT trial demonstrated that Reptilase is superior to streptokinase for management of heart failure. Different variants of wild-type (wt) tPA, recombinant staphylokinase, and RTSPA*1 (vampire bat tPA) also have undergone clinical trials. Recombinant urokinase and prourokinase are now expressed in mammalian cell lines and are undergoing active clinical development. Molecular engineering of wt recombinant tPA extended the biologic half-life for bolus dosing, whereas staphylokinase and vampire bat plasminogen activator exhibited fibrin specificity. Thrombolytic agents also have found a place in the management of acute thrombotic stroke. Optimal approaches to improve the safety/efficacy index are currently under investigation. The next few years will witness the emergence of longer-acting thrombolytics to facilitate bolus dosing and improved specificity for fibrin and other receptors to target thrombotic sites. New indications for thrombolytic therapy, such as stroke and microangiographic syndromes, will be pursued.

Restenosis after cardiac interventions remains a major challenge. An optimal therapeutic approach is still unavailable despite major scientific and financial undertakings. Even with the introduction of newer interventional cardiovascular and peripheral vascular procedures, late restenosis is commonly seen at a rate of 10% to 60%. Although the claimed efficacy of cardiovascular interventions exceeds that of medical and surgical approaches, restenosis is a major problem, resulting in angina and myocardial infarction. Several newer anticoagulant and antithrombotic drugs have been used to reduce restenosis. However, these approaches have met with limited success. Initial results with GPIIb/IIIa-targeting antibodies were encouraging. The introduction of bare metal and drug-eluting stents added a new dimension in the management of patients undergoing percutaneous coronary intervention (PCI). However, a significant number of patients treated with stents do develop thrombosis, especially those with drug-eluting stents.

With a better understanding of pathophysiology of restenosis, improved drugs can be developed. Anticoagulant drugs such as LMWHs and PEG hirudin may prove useful. Mechanical devices such as stents and localized and programmed delivery of drugs may be expected to improve outcomes. Although monotherapy may be useful in the control of abrupt closure and subchronic occlusion, its role in late restenosis may be limited. Combined pharmacologic and mechanical approaches, coupled with specialized delivery, already have provided favorable results.

The remainder of this decade will witness dramatic developments in the management of thrombotic and cardiovascular disorders. Synthetic and recombinant approaches will provide cost-effective and clinically useful drugs. LMWHs and synthetic heparin analogs are expected to have significant effects on the overall management of thrombotic and cardiovascular disorders. Factors such as managed care, regulatory issues, polytherapy, and combined pharmacologic and mechanical approaches will redirect the focus in management of DVT, thromboembolism, myocardial infarction, and thrombotic stroke. The direct thrombin agents hirudin and PEG hirudin will be of great value for surgical anticoagulation and in various acute indications. Postsurgical control of thrombotic processes may require combination therapy and LMWHs.

Conventional drugs such as heparin, oral anticoagulants, and aspirin will remain the gold standards despite their known drawbacks. They require further optimization and can be used for various indications in cost-effective manner. The newer drugs and devices, however, provide alternatives that in the next few years may lead to improved, cost-compliant treatments.

Owing to these rapid developments, several important issues related to current practices in anticoagulant therapy are recognized. Some of these issues include:

1. The replacement of unfractionated heparin by LMWHs in all indications. Although LMWHs have been used for interventional purposes, these drugs have not still gained the approval of the US FDA for this purpose. This is primarily due to the lack of clinical trial data on specific products and an understanding of the mechanisms of action. Moreover, the pharmacokinetics and pharmacodynamics of these drugs are different from that of unfractionated heparin and require further studies. LMWHs are only partially neutralized by protamine sulfate. Thus, additional data on their safety and efficacy in interventional indications are needed.

2. The potential replacement of heparins by newly developed antithrombin and anti-Xa agents. Antithrombin agents and anti-Xa agents have become the main focus for the development of oral and parenteral forms that can potentially replace heparins and oral anticoagulants. Although it is true that in heparin-compromised patients, such as those who develop heparin-induced thrombocytopenia, these agents can be used for acute anticoagulant management, there have, however, been several problematic issues related to the development of these agents. This has sensitized both the clinical and regulatory community to be cautious in recommending their unqualified use in all situations where heparins and warfarin are indicated. This is partly due to the single target effect of the two classes, which results in a relatively narrow therapeutic spectrum for these agents. Unlike heparins and oral anticoagulants, the drugs being currently developed and those undergoing trials do not have polytherapeutic effects, such as the modulation of the endothelium and interaction with endogenous proteins, growth factors, and cellular processes. Moreover, most of these agents, with the exception of the synthetic pentasaccharide, are synthetic peptidomimetics agents, with some unexplained effects on the vasculature and elevation of liver enzymes. This is particularly the case with the oral thrombin inhibitors. Thrombin inhibitors also interfere in the regulatory role of thrombin and indiscriminately inhibit the thrombin–thrombomodulin-mediated activation of protein C and thrombin activatable fibrinolysis inhibitor. In contrast, factor Xa inhibitors, being peptidomimetics, may result in the elevation of liver enzymes and produce other side effects. Currently, there is no antidote available to neutralize the effect of antithrombin and anti-Xa agents. Thus, it is unlikely that these agents will have broad indications such as the use of heparin and LMWH-s. Parenteral antithrombin agents such as argatroban, bivalirudin, and hirudins have been used in the anticoagulant management of heparin-induced thrombocytopenia. Bivalirudin has also been used in percutaneous interventions in several trials. As compared to heparin, although bleeding complications are reportedly less with the use of bivalirudin, long-term mortality outcome is less favorable. Moreover, like other thrombin inhibitors, it does not release TFPI from vascular

sites. Oral thrombin inhibitors have been developed as potential replacement for warfarin in extended antithrombotic management in such indications as atrial fibrillation, DVT, and stroke. However, the current data on the safety and efficacy are unsatisfactory. Several anti-Xa agents are also being developed for both oral and parenteral use for specific indications. The safety of these drugs is reportedly somewhat better; however, conclusive data are not available at this time. Both the anti-Xa and IIa agents may be useful in acute anticoagulant settings; however, their long-term use for extended antithrombotic management of thrombotic and cardiovascular disorders is questionable at this time.

3. The feasibility of oral anti-Xa and anti-IIa agents as potential substitutes for oral anticoagulant and heparin-related drugs. There is major interest in developing anti-Xa and-IIa agents as potential substitutes for oral anticoagulants and heparins. In this regard, synthetic agents such as argatroban and Angiomax are used currently as an anticoagulant substitute for heparin in patients with heparin-induced thrombocytopenia (HIT). These drugs are monotherapeutic, and though they may be useful in acute settings, they may not be as suitable as heparin or oral anticoagulant substitutes for long-term usage. Parenteral anti-Xa drugs have also been developed with limited amount of success. At this time, several companies are developing anti-Xa agents, mostly in the DVT and related indications with oral formulations. The usefulness of the antithrombin and anti-Xa agents in interventional cardiology has not yet been fully validated. It may be that these drugs can be used for acute settings; however, safety considerations and their inhibition of the regulatory functions of thrombin and Xa may limit their use. The claim that oral antithrombin and anti-Xa drugs will eventually replace warfarin is based on limited studies, and the clinical data are not convincing. Thus, in both the parenteral and oral formulations, the anti-Xa and -IIa drugs will be of limited value for anticoagulation in interventional cardiology and postinterventional management of patients. As heparins are polytherapeutic, it would be difficult to mimic their effect with a single target agent; thus, it is prudent to be cautious in endorsing these agents.

4. The development of synthetic heparinomimetics representing specific actions of heparins and their relative bioequivalence to heparin. The synthetic heparinomimetics represented by pentasaccharide (Arixtra) are designer heparin-derived oligosaccharides, which mimic one of the many pharmacologic actions of heparin. In interventional cardiology, their use is limited and, unless given in combination with other drugs, there effectiveness as anticoagulant may be questionable. Arixtra is a sole anti-Xa agent, which only produces this effect after interacting with antithrombin III. The therapeutic spectrum of this drug is nowhere near as broad as that of heparin and LMWHs. Arixtra has no effect on thrombin

and does not produce any anticoagulation, even at very high concentrations. This agent was developed for DVT prophylaxis and, at best, can be used for this indication. Additional derivatives of pentasaccharide are also of limited value and their use in interventional cardiovascular setting is somewhat limited. Therefore, it is reasonable to project that these heparin-derived oligosaccharides will be of limited value in interventional cardiology.

5. The development of recombinant antithrombotic agents such as activated protein C (APC), tissue factor pathway inhibitors, recombinant equivalent of serpins, and thrombomodulin, with reference to their relative applications in specific disorders. Recombinant technology offers a unique opportunity to develop anticoagulant drugs of natural origin, which are based on knowing the structure of proteins from plants and animals. One of the most widely investigated anticoagulant proteins is hirudin that is obtained from the leech, *Hirudo medicinalis*. Although initially slated for multiple indications, this agent has faced several developmental difficulties including safety issues. Moreover, like with all proteins, the development of antibodies has hampered its use in specific indications. Such may be the case with many proteins, such as the protein inhibitors of coagulation factors. Recombinant TFPI has been used in interventional cardiology; however, due to safety issues, its development has stopped. Although recombinant APC may be useful in specific hematologic indications, its use in interventional cardiology is very limited. Moreover, the cost of these proteins is rather high. Thus, the recombinant equivalent products of anticoagulant proteins will be of limited value in any interventional purposes.

6. The development of newer antiplatelet drugs such as the ADP receptor inhibitors, glycoprotein IIb/IIa receptors, phosphodiesterase inhibitors, and specific COX-1 and COX-2 inhibitors and their relevance in the management of various disorders. The relevance of on board aspirin for the therapeutic index of each of these agents also requires additional investigations. Interventional cardiology has gone through several transitions during the past 10 years for the use of antiplatelet drugs. The introduction of glycoprotein IIb/IIIa inhibitors such as the ReoPro, Integrelin, and Aggrastat were initially slated to be the standard of care and were recommended for unqualified use. Moreover, their use resulted in reducing the dosage of heparin for anticoagulation in interventional procedures. With the unexpected impact of clopidogrel on the anticoagulation management of patients undergoing PCIs, the use of GPIIb/IIIa inhibitors has undergone a re-evaluation. Currently, these drugs are only used in qualified indications with PCI. The front-loading of clopidogrel remains an open question along with the interactions of drugs with this agent. Together with the newer approaches to using LMWH, antithrombin drugs,

and possibly anti-Xa drugs, there will be complex drug interactions and safety and efficacy issues, which will require clear recommendations for the optimization of these drugs. Taking into consideration the additional effects of such drugs as statins, this polytherapeutic approach will require close monitoring.

7. The design of newer thrombolytic agents, with specific reference to their endogenous interaction and pharmacodynamic differences in terms of their relative clinical effects in stroke and myocardial infarction. The newer thrombolytic agents represent drugs with significant differences in the biochemical and pharmacologic actions. Besides dissolving the clot, these drugs also have additional effects, which are not completely understood at this time. Moreover, thrombolytic agents exhibit profound interactions with anticoagulant and antiplatelet drugs. The margin of safety in these agents is rather narrow, and although the efficacy of newer agents may be attractive, their safety consideration remains to be resolved. With the widespread use of stenting and other procedures, the use of thrombolytic drugs is reduced. Despite all of these limitations, the conventional thrombolytic agents such as the tPA and streptokinase may be useful in some indications.

8. The recent recognition of the antithrombotic actions of statins, nitric oxide donors, and other nonanticoagulant drugs, and their impact on overall therapeutic approaches. Patients who require interventional procedures are treated with multiple drugs. These drugs include statins, nitrates, calcium channel blockers, betablockers, and many other drugs. The use of anticoagulant and antiplatelet drugs is challenging from the standpoint of achieving desirable anticoagulation for the intended duration without safety compromise. At the present time, there are no guidelines or recommendations that take into account these interactions and adjust dosage for different drugs. There are pharmacokinetic and pharmacodynamic interactions. Moreover, because of the individual differences (pharmacogenomics) and population kinetic variations among patients, optimization of anticoagulation is not an easy task. Collective data from large clinical trials may be applicable, and clinical judgment on the basis of individual patient responses will be more important in achieving satisfactory results. Such interactions have not even been taken into account by some of the most recent trials on newer drugs.

9. Risks associated with drug-coated stents. The initial attempts to coat anticoagulant and antiplatelet drugs on stents have met with limited success, and results have been unsatisfactory. Because of the instant fibrosis and other occlusive lesion development, metal stents were coated with small amounts of antiproliferative (anticancer) drugs such as Paclitaxel and Sirolimus. Although these drug-coated stents have been widely used in interventional procedures, new data suggest that there is a significant increase in stent thrombosis in patients who have drug-eluting stents. The pathogenesis of the thrombotic complications associated with drug-eluted stents is not known and may be multifactorial. The CYPHER Sirolimus-eluting Coronary Stent is indicated for improving coronary luminal diameter in patients with symptomatic ischemic disease due to discrete de novo lesions of length <30 mm in native coronary arteries, with reference vessel diameter of 2.5 mm–3.5 mm. The TAXUS Express Paclitaxel-Eluting Coronary Stent System is indicated for improving the luminal diameter for the treatment of de novo lesions of <28 mm length in native coronary arteries 2.5–3.75 mm in diameter. These devices have resulted in significant reduction in the incidence of restenosis. However, because of the stent thrombosis, the US FDA has convened a panel of advisors to discuss the potential risk associated with drug-eluting stents. It is now known that cancer patients who are treated with anticancer drugs such as Sirolimus or Taxol develop therapy-associated thrombosis, requiring anticoagulant therapy. Therefore, drug-eluting stents may also produce similar effects in patients implanted with these devices. Although clopidogrel is recommended, the dosage and duration of this drug may vary with patient populations. Moreover, in complicated cases, such as patients with diabetes, acute myocardial infarction, multiple vessel decisions, or lesions involving arterial bifarcations, the left main coronary artery and long arterial segments may require individualized management. The observed thrombotic complications with drug-eluting stents are real, and clopidogrel may not be the only medication needed. In individualized risk groups, it may be that simultaneous use of oral anticoagulant drugs and/or LMWH may be warranted. The current debates on the future of drug-eluting stents and associated therapies will continue for some time to come.

Additional approaches to keep the vascular patency, structural integrity, and antithrombotic functions, especially in the coronary arteries, have also utilized stem cells and other molecular approaches. At this time, the observations based on these techniques have not provided any conclusive information. The number of drugs and devices will continue to expand for interventional procedures and postinterventional care of patients. Together with the introduction of newer devices and development of additional procedures, this entire field will continue to expand for some time. Because of these dramatic developments, additional approaches will be needed to develop newer approaches to understand the complex interplay between drugs and devices and to balance the optimized use of drugs in this field. Regardless of these remarkable developments, the basic principles behind vascular pathophysiology must be considered prior to the development of complex approaches, which may provide obscure messages and directions.

Appendix A

Pharmacokinetic comparison of various anticoagulants

Agent	COUMADIN® Warfarin	Aspirin	PLAVIX® Clopidogrel	LOVENOX® Enoxaparin	FRAGMIN® Dalteparin	INNOHEP® Tinzaparin	Heparin	ARIXTRA® Fondaparinux	ANGIOMAX® Bivalirudin	Argatroban	EXANTA™ Ximelagatran
T C_{max}	AC effect in 2 days (12); AT effect in 6 days (12); 1 hr (9.17) for C_{max}	30–40 min (9); 60.4 min (after 650 mg dose) (16)	1 hr (2.14)	3–5 hrs (3); ~3 hrs (15); 2.9 hrs for 40 mg (19)	4 hrs (4); ~3 hrs (15); 2.8 hrs for 2500 IU (19)	4–5 hrs (5); 2 hrs ~3 hrs (15)	~immediate with IV administration: 2.5 hrs for 5000 IU s.c. (15)[a]	2 hrs after 2.5 mg s.c. (6.10)	Within 5 min post 15 min IV bolus of 0.05–0.6 mg/kg and within 2 min after 0.3 mg/kg bolus inj (21)	~1 hr to steady-state after 125 mcg/kg bolus and 2.5 mcg/kg/min infusion (18)	2–3 hrs (7.8)
C_{max}	Dose-dependent; 0.65 mcg/mL for 5 mg dose (17)	5.51 mcg/mL (after 650 mg dose) (16)	3 mg/L (2.14)	0.42 IU/mL for 40 mg (15); 0.57 IU/ml for 40 mg (19)	Dose dependent; 0.49 IU/mL for 5000 IU (15); 0.22 IU/mL for 2500 IU (19)	0.18 IU/mL for 50 IU/kg (15)	0.039 IU/mL for 5000 IU s.c. (20)[a]; 0.09 IU/mL for 5000 IU s.c. (15)[a]	After 2.5 mg s.c., 0.34 mg/L (6.10)	Dose dependent; 12.3 mcg/ml after 1 mg/kg bolus and 4 hour 2.5 mg/kg/h IV infusion (11)	568 ng/ml steady-state after 125 mcg/kg bolus and 2.5 mcg/kg/min infusion (18)	0.2 μmol/L (7)
T C_{min}				12 hrs (3.15)	~12 hrs (15)	~12 hrs (15)	12 hrs (20)[a]			~2.5 hrs (18)	
Half-life[a]	For warfarin: mean of 40 hrs (1); dose-dependent, 47 hrs for 5 mg dose (17) for vitamin K dependent clotting factors: II-60 hrs. VII-4–6 hrs. IX-24 hrs, X-48–72 hrs (1)	15–20 min (9)	8 hrs (2.14)	4.5 hrs (3). 4.3 hrs for 40 mg (15); 4.4 hrs for 40 mg (19)	3–5 hrs (4). 2.4 hrs for 5000 IU (15); 2.8 hrs for 2500 IU (19)	3–4 hrs (5); 3 hrs for 50 IU/kg (15)	30–150 min: dose- and infusion time-dependent; 77 min for 5000 IU s.c. (20)[a]	17–21 hrs (6.10)	25 min (11.21)	46.2 min (18)	2–3 hrs (7.8)

(Continued)

Pharmacokinetic comparison of various anticoagulants (*Continued*)

Agent	COUMADIN® Warfarin	Aspirin	PLAVIX® Clopidogrel	LOVENOX® Enoxaparin	FRAGMIN® Dalteparin	INNOHEP® Tinzaparin	Heparin	ARIXTRA® Fondaparinux	ANGIOMAX® Bivalirudin	Argatroban	EXANTA™ Ximelagatran
Return to baseline/ duration of activity	4–5 days for INR in range 2–3 to decrease to <1.2 (22)	10 days (9)[b]	7 days (9,13)	Persistent anti-Xa activity for 12 hrs after 40 mg (3); Residual anti-Xa activity 24 hrs (19)	Residual anti-Xa activity 24 hrs (19)						
Antidote	Vitamin K_1 (1)		Platelet transfusion (2)	Protamine (3)	Protamine (4)	Protamine (5)	Protamine	None (6)	None (11)	None	None

[a]For LMWH and UFH, half-life refers to half-life of anti-Xa activity following SC injection.

[b]The platelet-inhibitory effects of aspirin last the lifetime of the platelet, due to irreversible inactivation of platelet COX-1: the average platelet lifespan is 10 days: 50% of platelets function normally 5–6 days after aspirin ingestion (9).

Abbreviations: AC, anticoagulation; AT, antithrombotic; C_{max}, maximum concentration; C_{min}, minimum concentration; T C_{max}, time to maximum concentration; T C_{min}, time to minimum concentration.

References

1 Coumadin Prescribing Information, Bristol-Myers Squibb, June 2002.

2 Plavix Prescribing Information, Bristol-Myers Squibb/Sanofi Pharmaceuticals Partnership, May 2002.

3 Lovenox Prescribing Information, Aventis Pharmaceuticals, January 2003.

4 Fragmin Prescribing Information, Pharmacia, June 2002.

5 Innohep Prescribing Information, LEO Pharmaceutical Products, January 2003.

6 Arixtra Prescribing Information, Sanofi-Synthelabo, December 2002.

7 Sarich TC, Teng R, Peters GR, et al. No influence of obesity on the pharmacokinetics and pharmacodynamics of melagatran, the active form of the oral direct thrombin inhibitor ximelagatran. Clin Pharmacokinet 2003; 42:485–492.

8 Johansson LC, Frison L, Logren U, et al. Influence of age on the pharmacokinetics and pharmacodynamics of ximelagatran, an oral direct thrombin inhibitor. Clin Pharmacokinet 2003; 42:381–392.

9 Patrono C, Coller B, Dalen JE, et al. Platelet-active drugs: the relationship among dose, effectiveness, and side effects. Chest 2001; 119:39S–63S.

10 Donat F, Duret JP, Santoni A, et al. The pharmacokinetics of fondaparinux sodium in healthy volunteers. Clin Pharmacokinet 2002; 41 Suppl 2:1–9.

11 Angiomax Prescribing Information, The Medicines Company, June 2002.

12 Hirsh J, Dalen JE, Anderson DR, et al. Oral anticoagulants: mechanism of action, clinical effectiveness, and optimal therapeutic range. Chest 2001; 119:8S–21S.

13 Weber AA, Braun M, Hohlfeld T, et al. Recovery of platelet function after discontinuation of clopidogrel treatment in healthy volunteers. Br J Pharmacol 2001; 52:333–336.

14 Caplain H, Donat F, Gaud, C, et al. Pharmacokinetics of clopidogrel. Semin Thromb Hemost 1999; 25(Suppl 2):25–28.

15 Eriksson BI, Soderberg K, Widlund L, et al. A comparative study of three low-molecular weight heparins (LMWH) and unfractionated heparin (UH) in healthy volunteers. Thromb Haemost 1995; 73:398–401.

16 Muir N, Nichols JD, Clifford JM, et al. The influence of dosage form on aspirin kinetics: implications for acute cardiovascular use. Curr Med Res Opin 1997; 13:547–553.

17 King SYP, Joslin MA, Raudibaugh K, et al. Dose-dependent pharmacokinetics of warfarin in healthy volunteers. Pharm Res 1995; 12:1874–1877.

18 Swan SK, Hursting MJ. The pharmacokinetics and pharmacodynamics of argatroban: effects of age, gender, and hepatic or renal dysfunction. Pharmacotherapy 2000; 20:318–329.

19 Collignon F, Frydman A, Caplain H, et al. Comparison of the pharmacokinetic profiles of three low molecular mass heparins-dalteparin, enoxaparin and nadroparin-administered subcutaneously in healthy volunteers (doses for prevention of thromboembolism). Thromb Haemost 1995; 73:630–640.

20 Bara L, Billaud E, Gramond G, et al. Comparative pharmacokinetics of a low molecular weight heparin (PK 10 169) and unfractionated heparin after intravenous and subcutaneous administration. Thromb Res 1985; 39:631–636.

21 Sciulli TM, Mauro VF. Pharmacology and clinical use of bivalirudin. Ann Pharmacotherapy 2002; 36:1028–1041.

22 White RH, McKittrick T, Hutchinson R, et al. Temporary discontinuation of warfarin therapy: changes in the international normalized ratio. Ann Intern Med 1995; 122:40–42.

Appendix B

Pharmacokinetic comparison of Warfarin and various antiplatelet drugs

Agent	COUMADIN® Warfarin	ASPIRIN	PLAVIX®	AZD6140	Prasugrel	AGGRASTAT® Tirofiban	INTEGRILIN® Eptifibatide	REOPRO® Abciximab
T C_{max} (Time to maximum concentration)	AC effect in 2 days (10): AT effect in 6 days (10): 1 hr (7.15) for C_{max}	30–40 min (7): 60.4 min (after 650 mg dose) (14)	1 hour (2.12)					
C_{max} (Maximum concentration)	Dose-dependent; 0.65 mcg/mL for 5 mg dose (15)	5.51 mcg/mL (after 650 mg dose) (16)	3 mg/L (2.12)					
T C_{min} (Time to minimum concentration)								
Half-life[a]	For warfarin: mean of 40 hrs (1); dose-dependent. 47 hr for 5 mg dose (15) For vitamin K dependent clotting factors: II-60 hr. VII-4–6 hr. IX-24 hr. X-48-72 hr (1)	15–20 min (7)	8 hr (2.12)					
Return to baseline/ duration of activity	4–5 days for INR in range 2–3 to decrease to <1.2 (20)	10 days (7)[b]	7 days (7.11)					
Antidote	Vitamin K_1 (1)		Platelet transfusion (2)					

(Continued)

Pharmacokinetic comparison of various anticoagulant drugs (Continued)

Agent	LOVENOX® Enoxaparin	FRAGMIN® Dalteparin	INNOHEP® Tinzaparin	HEPARIN	ARIXTRA® Fondaparinux	ANGIOMAX® Bivalirudin	ARGATROBAN
T C_{max} (Time to maximum concentration)	3–5 hr (3); ~3 hr (13); 2.9 hr for 40 mg (17)	4 hr (4); ~3 hr (15); 2.8 hr for 2500 IU (17)	4–5 hr (5); ~3 hr (13)	~immediate with IV administration; 2.5 hr for 5000 IU s.c. (13)[a]	Two hrs after 2.5 mg s.c. (6,8)	Within 5 min post 15 min IV bolus of 0.05–0.6mg/kg and within 2 min after 0.3mg/kg bolus inj (19)	~1 hr to steady-state after 125 mcg/kg bolus and 2.5 mcg/kg/min infusion (16)
C_{max} (Maximum concentration)	0.42 IU/mL for 40 mg (13); 0.57 IU/mL for 40 mg (17)	Dose dependent; 0.49 IU/mL for 5000 IU (13); 0.22 IU/mL for 2500 IU (17)	0.18 IU/mL for 50 IU/kg (13)	0.039 IU/mL for 5000 IU s.c. (18)[a]; 0.09 IU/mL for 5000 IU s.c. (13)[a]	After 2.5 mg s.c.. 0.34 mg/L (6,8)	Dose dependent; 12.3 mcg/mL after 1 mg/kg bolus and 4 hr 2.5mg/kg/hr IV infusion (9)	568 ng/mL steady-state after 125 mcg/kg bolus and 2.5 mcg/kg/min infusion (16)
T C_{min} (Time to minimum concentration)	12 hr (3,13)	~12 hr (13)	~12 hr (13)	12 hr (18)[a]			~2.5 hr (16)
Half-life[a]	4.5 hr (3). 4.3 hr for 40 mg (13); 4.4 hr for 40 mg (17)	3–5 hr (4); 2.4 hr for 5000 IU (13); 2.8 hr for 2500 IU (17)	3–4 hr (5); 3 hr for 50 IU/kg (13)	30–150 min; dose- and infusion time-dependent; 177 min for 5000 IU s.c. (18)[a]	17–21 hr (6,8)	25 min (9,19)	46.2 min (16)
Return to baseline/duration of activity	Persistent anti-Xa activity for 12 hr after 40 mg (3); Residual anti-Xa activity 24 hr (17)	Residual anti-Xa activity 24 hr (17)					
Antidote	Protamine (3)	Protamine (4)	Protamine (5)	Protamine	None (6)	None (9)	None

[a]For LMWH and UFH, half-life refers to half-life of anti-Xa activity following SC injection.

[b]The platelet-inhibitory effects of aspirin last the lifetime of the platelet, due to irreversible inactivation of platelet COX-1: the average platelet lifespan is 10 days: 50% of platelets function normally five to six days after aspirin ingestion (9).

Abbreviations: AC, anticoagulation; AT, antithrombotic; LMWH, low molecular weight heparin; UFH, unfractionated heparin.

References

1 Coumadin Prescribing Information, Bristol-Myers Squibb, June 2002.

2 Plavix Prescribing Information, Bristol-Myers Squibb/Sanofi Pharmaceuticals Partnership, May 2002.

3 Lovenox Prescribing Information, Aventis Pharmaceuticals, January 2003.

4 Fragmin Prescribing Information, Pharmacia, June 2002.

5 Innohep Prescribing Information, LEO Pharmaceutical Products, January 2003.

6 Arixtra Prescribing Information, Sanofi-Synthelabo, December 2002.

7 Patrono C, Coller B, Dalen JE, et al. Platelet-active drugs: the relationship among dose, effectiveness, and side effects. Chest 2001; 119:39S–63S.

8 Donat F, Duret JP, Santoni A, et al. The pharmacokinetics of fondaparinux sodium in healthy volunteers. Clin Pharmacokinet 2002; 41(suppl 2):1–9.

9 Angiomax Prescribing Information, The Medicines Company, June 2002.

10 Hirsh J, Dalen JE, Anderson DR, et al. Oral anticoagulants: mechanism of action, clinical effectiveness, and optimal therapeutic range. Chest 2001; 119:8S–21S.

11 Weber AA, Braun M, Hohlfeld T, et al. Recovery of platelet function after discontinuation of clopidogrel treatment in healthy volunteers. Br J Pharmacol 2001; 52:333–336.

12 Caplain H, Donat F, Gaud C, et al. Pharmacokinetics of clopidogrel. Semin Thromb Hemost 1999; 25(suppl 2):25–28.

13 Eriksson BI, Soderberg K, Widlund L, et al. A comparative study of three low-molecular weight heparins (LMWH) and unfractionated heparin (UH) in healthy volunteers. Thromb Haemost 1995; 73:398–401.

14 Muir N, Nichols JD, Clifford JM, et al. The influence of dosage form on aspirin kinetics: implications for acute cardiovascular use. Curr Med Res Opin 1997; 13:547–553.

15 King SYP, Joslin MA, Raudibaugh K, et al. Dose-dependent pharmacokinetics of warfarin in healthy volunteers. Pharm Res 1995; 12:1874–1877.

16 Swan SK, Hursting MJ. The pharmacokinetics and pharmacodynamics of argatroban: effects of age, gender, and hepatic or renal dysfunction. Pharmacotherapy 2000; 20:318–329.

17 Collignon F, Frydman A, Caplain H, et al. Comparison of the pharmacokinetic profiles of three low molecular mass heparins-dalteparin, enoxaparin and nadroparin-administered subcutaneously in healthy volunteers (doses for prevention of thromboembolism). Thromb Haemost 1995; 73:630–640.

18 Bara L, Billaud E, Gramond G, et al. Comparative pharmacokinetics of a low molecular weight heparin (PK 10 169) and unfractionated heparin after intravenous and subcutaneous administration. Thromb Res 1985; 39:631–636.

19 Sciulli TM, Mauro VF. Pharmacology and clinical use of bivalirudin. Ann Pharmacotherapy 2002; 36:1028–1041.

20 White RH, McKittrick T, Hutchinson R, et al. Temporary discontinuation of warfarin therapy: changes in the international normalized ratio. Ann Intern Med 1995; 122:40–42.

Index

T - #0543 - 071024 - C8 - 276/216/30 - PB - 9780367389024 - Gloss Lamination